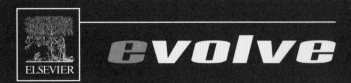

COMPREHENSIVE
NEONATAL CARE

AN INTERDISCIPLINARY APPROACH

FOURTH EDITION

COMPREHENSIVE
NEONATAL CARE

AN INTERDISCIPLINARY APPROACH

Carole Kenner, DNS, RNC, FAAN
Dean and Professor
University of Oklahoma College of Nursing
Oklahoma City, Oklahoma

Judy Wright Lott, DSN, RNC, NNP, FAAN
Dean and Professor
Louise Herrington School of Nursing
Baylor University
Dallas, Texas

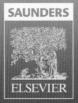

SAUNDERS

ELSEVIER

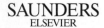

SAUNDERS
ELSEVIER

11830 Westline Industrial Drive
St. Louis, Missouri 63146

COMPREHENSIVE NEONATAL CARE:
AN INTERDISCIPLINARY APPROACH

ISBN-13: 978-1-4160-2942-7
ISBN-10: 1-4160-2942-7

Notice

Knowledge and best practice in this field are constantly changing. As new research and experience broaden our knowledge, changes in practice, treatment and drug therapy may become necessary or appropriate. Readers are advised to check the most current information provided (i) on procedures featured or (ii) by the manufacturer of each product to be administered, to verify the recommended dose or formula, the method and duration of administration, and contraindications. It is the responsibility of the practitioner, relying on his or her own experience and knowledge of the patient, to make diagnoses, to determine dosages and the best treatment for each individual patient, and to take all appropriate safety precautions. To the fullest extent of the law, neither the Publisher nor the Authors assume any liability for any injury and/or damage to persons or property arising out of or related to any use of the material contained in this book.

The Publisher

ISBN-13: 978-1-4160-2942-7
ISBN-10: 1-4160-2942-7

Acquisitions Editor: Catherine Jackson
Developmental Editor: Amanda Sunderman Politte
Publishing Services Manager: Deborah L. Vogel
Senior Project Manager: Deon Lee
Senior Designer: Jyotika Shroff
Cover Designer: Jyotika Shroff

Printed in China

Last digit is the print number: 9 8 7 6 5 4 3 2

Contributors

Leslie Altimier, MSN, RN
Manager
Neonatal ICU
Special Care Nursery
Good Samaritan Hospital
Cincinnati, Ohio

Gail A. Bagwell, MSN, RN
Clinical Nurse Specialist
Perinatal Outreach
Children's Hospital
Columbus, Ohio

Kathy Bergman, MSN, RNC, CNS
Nursing Faculty, Department of Nursing
Coordinator, Learning Resource Center
Xavier University
Cincinnati, Ohio

Susan Tucker Blackburn, PhD, RNC, FAAN
Professor
Department of Family and Child Nursing
University of Washington
Seattle, Washington

Beverly Bowers, PhD, RN, CS
Assistant Dean for Faculty Development and Professional
    Continuing Education/Assistant Professor
University of Oklahoma College of Nursing
Oklahoma City, Oklahoma

Dorothy Brooten, PhD, RN, FAAN
Professor
School of Nursing
Florida International University;
Principal
The Research A-Team, LLC
Miami, Florida

Joyce M. Butler, MSN, RNC, NNP
NNP Coordinator/Clinical Instructor
Department of Pediatrics, Division of Newborn Medicine
University of Mississippi Medical Center
Wiser Hospital for Women and Infants
Jackson, Mississippi

Waldemar A. Carlo, MD
Edwin M. Dixon Professor of Pediatrics
Director, Division of Neonatology
Director, Newborn Nurseries
University of Alabama at Birmingham
Birmingham, Alabama

Tony C. (Chris) Carnes, PhD
President and CTO
ICU Data Systems, Inc.
Gainesville, Florida

Terri A. Cavaliere, MS, RNC, NNP
Neonatal Nurse Practitioner
North Shore University Hospital
Manhasset, New York;
Clinical Assistant Professor, School of Nursing
State University of New York at Stony Brook
Stony Brook, New York

Javier Cifuentes, MD
Neored-Clinica Indisa
Providencia, Santiago;
Associate Professor, Department of Pediatrics
Catholic University of Chile
Santiago, Chile

Sergio DeMarini, MD
Director, Division of Neonatology
IRRCCS Burlo Garofolo
Trieste, Italy

Georgia R. Ditzenberger, MN, RNC, NNP
Neonatal Nurse Practitioner
Doernbecher Neonatal Care Center
Doernbecher Children's/Oregon Health Sciences University
    Hospitals
Portland, Oregon

Willa Drummond, MD, MS
CIO, CMO, and Executive VP for Medical & Regulatory
    Affairs
ICU Data Systems, Inc.
Gainesville, Florida

Susan Ellerbee, PhD, RNC, IBCLC
Associate Professor
University of Oklahoma College of Nursing
University of Oklahoma
Oklahoma City, Oklahoma

Jody A. Farrell, MSN, PNP
Nurse Coordinator
University of California, San Francisco Medical Center
The Fetal Treatment Center
San Francisco, California

Deborah L. Fike, MSN, RNC, NNP
Neonatal Nurse Practitioner
Pediatrix Medical Group of Ohio
Miami Valley Hospital
Dayton, Ohio

Rebecca Lynn Roys Gelrud, MS, RN, BC
Clinical Informatics Consultant
ICU Data Systems, Inc.
Richmond, Virginia

Lynda Harrison, PhD, RN, FAAN
Professor and Co-Deputy
School of Nursing
University of Alabama at Birmingham
Birmingham, Alabama

Kathleen Haubrich, PhD, RN
Associate Professor, Department of Nursing
Miami University—Hamilton Campus
Hamilton, Ohio

Diane Holditch-Davis, PhD, RN, FAAN
Kenan Professor and Director
Doctoral and Postdoctoral Program
School of Nursing
University of North Carolina at Chapel Hill
Chapel Hill, North Carolina

Linda MacKenna Ikuta, RN, MN, CCNS, PHN
Neonatal Clinical Nurse Specialist
Packard Children's Hospital
Stanford University Medical Center
Palo Alto, California

Jamieson Jones, MD
Attending Neonatologist
University of California, San Diego Medical Center
San Diego, California;
Kaiser Permanente
Hawaii Permanente Medical Group, Inc.
Honolulu, Hawaii

Nadine Kassity-Krich, MSA, BSN, RN
Health Care Consultant, Speaker, and Trainer
Health Care Consultant for Children's Hospital in San Diego
San Diego, California

Karen Kavanaugh, PhD, RN, FAAN
Professor
Department of Maternal Child Nursing
University of Illinois at Chicago
Chicago, Illinois

Joanne McManus Kuller, MS, RN
Neonatal Clinical Research Nurse Specialist
Children's Hospital Oakland
Oakland, California

Carolyn Houska Lund, MS, RN, FAAN
Neonatal Clinical Nurse Specialist
Children's Hospital and Research Center at Oakland
Oakland, California

Jacqueline M. McGrath, PhD, RN, NNP, FNAP
School of Nursing
Virginia Commonwealth University
Richmond, Virginia

Kristie Nix, EdD, RN
Associate Professor
University of Tulsa
Tulsa, Oklahoma

Leslie Parker, MSN, NNP, RNC
Clinical Assistant Professor
University of Florida
Gainseville, Florida

Shahirose Premji, RN(EP), PhD
Assistant Professor and Neonatal Nurse Practitioner
University of Calgary
Calgary, Alberta
Canada

Jana L. Pressler, PhD, RN
Professor and Assistant Dean for Nursing Research
University of Oklahoma College of Nursing
Oklahoma City, Oklahoma

Linda L. Rath, PhD, MSN, RN, CNNP
Assistant Professor
University of Texas School of Nursing
Galveston, Texas

Debra A. Sansoucie, EdD, RNC, NNP
Chair, Department of Parent Child Health
Director, Neonatal Nurse Practitioner Program
School of Nursing
State University of New York at Stony Brook
Stony Brook, New York

Beth Shields, PharmD
Clinical Pharmacist in Pediatrics
Department of Pharmacy
Rush University Medical Center
Chicago, Illinois

Kaye Spence, AM, RN, RM, MN, FCN
Associate Professor/Clinical Nurse Consultant
Department of Neonatology
The Children's Hospital at Westmead
Westmead NSW
Sydney, Australia

Kathleen R. Stevens, EdD, RN, MS, FAAN
Professor and Director
Academic Center for Evidence-Based Nursing
University of Texas Health Science Center at San Antonio
San Antonio, Texas

Laura Stokowski, RNC, MS
Staff Nurse
Inova Fairfax Hospital for Children
Falls Church, Virginia

Frances Strodtbeck, DNS, RNC, NNP, FAAN
Director, Graduate Program in Nursing
Professor and Coordinator
Advanced Neonatal Nursing Program
Louise Herrington School of Nursing
Baylor University
Dallas, Texas

Tanya Sudia-Robinson, PhD, RN
Director, IRB/IACUC Office
Emory University
Atlanta, Georgia

Janet Thigpen, MN, RNC, CNNP
Neonatal Nurse Practitioner
Division of Neonatology
Department of Pediatrics
Emory University School of Medicine
Atlanta, Georgia

Marlene Walden, PhD, RNC, NNP, CCNS
Baylor College of Medicine
Section of Neonatology
Texas Children's Hospital
Neonatal Nurse Practitioner Service
Houston, Texas

Sara Rich Wheeler, DNS, BC, RN, LCPC
Dean of Nursing
Lakeview College of Nursing
Danville, Illinois;
Principal
Grief, Ltd.
Covington, Indiana

Pamela Holtzclaw Williams, RN, JD
Research Staff Member
University of Oklahoma College of Nursing
Department of Case Management
Norman, Oklahoma

Contributors to the Accompanying Evolve Website

Leslie Altimier, MSN, RN
Manager
Neonatal ICU
Special Care Nursery
Good Samaritan Hospital
Cincinnati, Ohio

Christine E. Armigo, RN, BSN, PHN
Neonatal Researcher
Sonoma State University
Rohnert Park, California

Gail A. Bagwell, MSN, RN
Clinical Nurse Specialist
Perinatal Outreach
Children's Hospital
Columbus, Ohio

Susan Tucker Blackburn, PhD, RNC, FAAN
Professor
Department of Family and Child Nursing
University of Washington
Seattle, Washington

Lee Carpenter, MSN, RN
Neonatal Nurse Practitioner
Waikato Hospital in Hamilton
New Zealand

Anita Catlin, DNSc, FNP, FAAN
Ethics Consultant, Perinatal and Neonatal Ethics
Medical Advisory Board
Intersex Society of North America
Sonoma State University
Associate Professor of Nursing
Rohnert Park, California

Jody A. Farrell, MSN, PNP
Nurse Coordinator
University of California, San Francisco Medical Center
The Fetal Treatment Center
San Francisco, California

Mary M. Kaminski, RNC, MS, NNP
Clinical Instructor
The Ohio State University
Advanced Practice Nurse/NNP
Nationwide Children's Hospital
Columbus, Ohio

Nadine Kassity-Krich, MSA, BSN, RN
Health Care Consultant, Speaker, and Trainer
Health Care Consultant for Children's Hospital in San Diego
San Diego, California

Karen Kavanaugh, PhD, RN, FAAN
Professor
Department of Maternal Child Nursing
University of Illinois at Chicago
Chicago, Illinois

Valerie Kay Moniaci, MSN, RNC, NNP
Neonatal Nurse Practitioner
Pediatrix Medical Group
Dayton, Ohio;
Director, NNP Program
University of Cincinnati
Cincinnati, Ohio

Linda L. Rath, PhD, MSN, RN, CNNP
Assistant Professor
University of Texas School of Nursing
Galveston, Texas

Beth Shields, PharmD
Clinical Pharmacist in Pediatrics
Department of Pharmacy
Rush University Medical Center
Chicago, Illinois

Kaye Spence, AM, RN, RM, MN, FCN
Associate Professor/Clinical Nurse Consultant
Department of Neonatology
The Children's Hospital at Westmead
Westmead NSW
Sydney, Australia

Laura Stokowski, RNC, MS
Staff Nurse
Inova Fairfax Hospital for Children
Falls Church, Virginia

Frances Strodtbeck, DNS, RNC, NNP, FAAN
Director, Graduate Program in Nursing
Professor and Coordinator
Advanced Neonatal Nursing Program
Louise Herrington School of Nursing
Baylor University
Dallas, Texas

Heather Watson, RN(C), BA, BScN, MN
Neonatal Acute Care Nurse Practitioner
McMaster Children's Hospital—NICU
Hamilton, Ontario
Canada

Sara Rich Wheeler, DNS, BC, RN, LCPC
Dean of Nursing
Lakeview College of Nursing
Danville, Illinois;
Principal
Grief, Ltd.
Covington, Indiana

Reviewers

Geraldine Ellison, PhD, RN
Assistant Dean, Tulsa Campus
College of Nursing
University of Oklahoma–Tulsa
Tulsa, Oklahoma

Jacqueline M. McGrath, PhD, RN, NNP, FNAP
School of Nursing
Virginia Commonwealth University
Richmond, Virginia

Catherine McPherson, RN, BScN, IBCLC
Charge Nurse
Intermediate Care Nursery
Grey Nuns Community Hospital
Edmond, Alberta, Canada

Foreword

Trends associated with childbearing in the United States and other developed and developing countries continue to be a challenge to those providing care to neonates. In the United States, for example, increases in the numbers of preterm and low-birth-weight infants, the number of twin pregnancies, the number of cesarean births, and the number of births to older and to unmarried women, coupled with technologic advances, changing infectious diseases, a constantly changing health care delivery system, and changing racial and ethnic population mixes require the broadest of perspectives in providing neonatal care.

Advances in management and treatment of newborns, in knowledge of their capabilities and development, and in care of high-risk newborns, as well as the need to extend support to multicultural and multigenerational families caring for smaller and sicker newborns have challenged health care providers in many ways. First, there is the need to keep abreast of advances in knowledge regarding care of newborns and support of their families in ways that are culturally acceptable to them. Equally important is the need to keep abreast of ethical, legal, and health policy issues surrounding their care and the need for research to further improve care to this vulnerable group. A constantly changing health care delivery system requires changes in the sites of practice and shifts in where components of care can be delivered. We also constantly need evidence to support our practice. To accomplish this, textbooks for nurses caring for newborns and their families require both a cutting-edge, comprehensive approach to direct care and a thorough discussion of broader issues in areas of management and treatment. This book has both.

The authors address the breadth of issues in neonatal care, including high-risk pregnancy, fetal therapy, the need for changes in neonatal nursing education to include a competency base, evidence to support practice, care of the extremely-low-birth-weight infant, the impact of the neonatal intensive care unit (NICU) on neonatal development, use of complementary therapies, and changing sites in providing newborn and infant care. Ethics, legal issues, palliative care, and end-of-life issues are included as essentials in neonatal nursing. Whereas the breadth of content in the chapters is extensive, the text also covers major problems in depth, including respiratory, cardiovascular, metabolic, and gastrointestinal dysfunction, among many. Such breadth and depth will be an invaluable aid to health professionals providing care to neonates and their families and to educators preparing others to do so. The editors are to be applauded for contributing such an effort to the field of neonatal care.

Dorothy Brooten, PhD, RN, FAAN
Professor, Florida International University;
Principal, The Research A-Team, LLC
Miami, Florida

Preface

One of the most complex issues in health care is the care of premature infants and infants with multiple, severe congenital anomalies. Despite advanced technology and knowledge, preterm delivery continues to be a significant problem in the United States. Maternal risk factors have changed over the past decade. For example, more women with chronic illnesses such as diabetes or sickle cell anemia are giving birth to infants with consequent health problems. The rise of in vitro fertilization has resulted in increased multiple births and prematurity. Many infants in neonatal intensive care units (NICUs) have been exposed to substances or are born to mothers with other risk factors such as delayed childbearing or childhood cancers. The care of these at-risk infants requires the use of more and more complex technology. Surfactant administration, liquid ventilation, nitric oxide administration, high-frequency jet ventilators, dialysis, organ transplantation, and other extraordinary measures are becoming commonplace. However, in the midst of these high-tech interventions, developmentally supportive care interventions such as dimming lights, using visible rather than audible alarms, using more physiologically and developmentally appropriate positioning and skin-to-skin care, and cobedding multiples are emerging as important interventions, due to increasing evidence regarding the importance of maintaining a developmentally supportive NICU environment for improved long-term infant/child outcomes.

Providers of neonatal care need accurate, comprehensive information as a basis for providing care to newborns. A thorough understanding of normal physiology as well as the pathophysiology of disease processes is necessary for well-designed care practices. Knowledge about associated risk factors, genetics, critical periods of development, principles of nutrition and pharmacology, and current neonatal research findings are all essential for providing optimal care for neonates. The concepts of a family-centered approach to care are important too; parents are an integral part of the care team. Care practices need to be based on the best evidence available, rather than on tradition. A multidisciplinary approach has been replaced by an integrated approach to care. All these elements form the foundation for assessment, planning, implementation, and evaluation of effectiveness of neonatal care.

The nurse plays a vital role in the provision of integrated health care to newborns. During the last decade, the nurse's role has included added responsibilities, which are recognized at both the staff and advanced practice levels. For the purposes of this book, two definitions of advanced practice are being used. They are the National Association of Neonatal Nurses' (NANN) definitions of clinical nurse specialist and neonatal nurse practitioner (NANN, Position Statement, 1990). The Association reaffirmed these in 2000.

CLINICAL NURSE SPECIALIST

The clinical nurse specialist (CNS) is a registered nurse with a master's degree who, through study and supervised practice at the graduate level, has become an expert in the defined clinical area of nursing. The CNS provides for the diagnosis and treatment of human responses to actual or potential health problems of patients and their families within the specialized area through direct patient care and clinical consultation. In addition, the CNS may act in an educational, research, liaison, or leadership role to promote optimal nursing care for the patients served.

NEONATAL NURSE PRACTITIONER

The neonatal nurse practitioner (NNP) is a registered nurse with clinical expertise in neonatal nursing who has received formal education with supervised clinical experience in the management of sick newborns and their families. The NNP manages a caseload of neonatal patients with consultation, collaboration, and general supervision from a physician. Using extensive knowledge of pathophysiology, pharmacology, and physiology, the NNP exercises independent or intradependent (in collaboration with other health professionals) judgment in the assessment, diagnosis, and initiation of certain delegated medical processes and procedures. As an advanced practice neonatal nurse, the NNP is additionally involved in education, consultation, and research at various levels.

The American Association of Colleges of Nurses (AACN) has proposed a change in the educational preparation for advanced practice nurses. The proposal recommends that the nurse practitioner be prepared as a "doctor of nursing practice" (or DNP) level. This will likely affect the NNP role, as well as other advanced practice nurses, over the next 5 years. The role of the CNS has not been fully resolved since the last edition of this textbook. There is discussion about whether a CNS is an advanced practice role or merely a nurse role with advanced preparation. Perhaps by the next edition of this text, these issues will be resolved.

The neonatal staff nurse role requires accurate and thorough assessment skills, excellent ability to communicate with other health professionals and patients' families, and a broad understanding of physiology and pathophysiology on which to base management decisions. It requires highly developed technical skills as well as critical decision-making skills. With health care delivery changes, it also requires supervision of ancillary personnel and an informed delegation of certain patient-oriented tasks. These changes require the staff nurse to possess even better assessment skills and sound knowledge of physiology and pathophysiology than in the past because some decision making will be done in concert with other, less highly trained personnel.

PURPOSE AND CONTENT

The fourth edition of this book provides a comprehensive examination of the care of neonates from a physiologic and pathophysiologic approach appropriate for any health professional concerned with neonatal care. The format of the text has been changed to make the information more easily accessible. The clinical chapters are found in the first part of the text. This text provides a complete physiologic and embryologic foundation for each neonatal body system. Additionally, it includes medical, surgical, and psychosocial care because the integrative management approach is absolutely imperative to the well-being of the newborn and family. Appropriate diagnostic tests and their interpretation are included in each system chapter. There is extensive use of research findings in the chapters to provide evidence to support practice strategies and demonstrate the rationale for clinical decision making. Complete references for more in-depth reading are found at the end of each chapter so that the reader may pursue more specific information on a topical area. The accompanying website with weblinks contains competencies, critical thinking and study questions, case studies, and additional resources. Use of tables and illustrations to support material that is presented in the narrative portions is sure to be another help to the practicing neonatal nurse.

The thread of integrative management is interwoven throughout the text. Foundational topics such as genetics, physiologically critical periods of development, nutrition, and parenting are included, as are topics of recent interest such as iatrogenic complications, neonatal pain, use of computers or other technology in neonatal care, and neonatal AIDS. Now more than ever, neonatal care providers must examine patient outcomes and nurse outcomes to meet the demands for providing cost-effective and high-quality care. Research is critical to support both the art and the science of neonatal care. Whenever possible, the contributors remind the reader of areas in need of further study. Chapters address evidence-based practice and new trends in neonatal care, such as hospice and palliative care, management of the NICU environment, evidence-based nursing, care of the extremely-low-birth-weight infant, complementary therapies, and competency-based neonatal nursing education. Another feature is the Preemie Bill of Rights, which we felt was important as we put more emphasis on the consumer and his or her needs. Of course, for neonatal care, the consumer is the newborn/infant and family. This book is not a quick reference; it provides comprehensive in-depth discussions along with detailed physiologic principles and collaborative management strategies. It provides a sound basis for safe and effective neonatal care; however, the new format should make the information easier to find.

Each organ system is discussed in depth, including the respiratory system, its complications and new technologies, followed by assessment of and management strategies for the cardiovascular system; nutrition and the gastrointestinal system; and metabolic, endocrine, immunologic, hematopoietic, neurologic, musculoskeletal, genitourinary, integumentary, auditory, and ophthalmic systems. General areas of neonatal care—the new health care delivery environment, regionalization today, evidence-based nursing, legal/ethical issues, collaborative research, competency-based neonatal nursing education, family-centered care, bereavement, and hospice and palliative care—are included as appropriate. Bereavement and chronic sorrow are discussed along with the newer field of neonatal hospice and palliative care because a happy ending is not always possible in perinatal and neonatal nursing. Human genetics is introduced, and the impact of environmental influences on the developing fetus, as well as the nursing implications of the Human Genome Project, are discussed. This provides the transition into the aspects of perinatal care, the high-risk pregnancy, and the effects of labor on the fetus. The text then deals with more specific neonatal topics, starting with stabilization, managing the NICU environment, newborn and infant neurobehavioral development, monitoring neonatal biophysical parameters, computer technology, and assessment. This edition includes the most up-to-date information from the American Heart Association's Neonatal Resuscitation Program as well as elements of the S.T.A.B.L.E.® program used for infants undergoing transport. Diagnostic imaging and diagnostic text and laboratory values represent the section of the text that highlights the evaluative measures used by practitioners to identify the neonatal problem and its progress. This edition continues with the surgical neonate, neonatal pain, neonatal AIDS, the drug-exposed neonate, and care of the extremely-low-birth-weight infant. Because neonatal nurses are seeing more and more extremely-low-birth-weight infants, we wanted to address this population's unique care needs. The final group of chapters covers the discharge phase. Topics include principles of newborn and infant drug therapy, systematic assessment and home follow-up, neonatal behavior, assessment and management of neonatal behavior, the transition to home, and finally, home care. One topic that has been added to this edition is complementary therapies. Never before has there been so much interest in or controversy over such interventions. We address what is known and where the gaps are in this area of neonatal care. This section recognizes that many neonatal nurses now care for infants through the first year of life. It also acknowledges the need for technology in the home and some guidelines for families who feel they have set up mini-NICUs in their homes.

In this edition, each of the chapters and sections has been updated to include the newest techniques, such as the latest trends in fetal therapy; progress with the mapping of human genes; use of computers, including Internet connections opening up global neonatal care issues for examination and discussion; the latest issues in health care reform and its impact on nursing care; and the latest research findings appropriate to each of the sections.

To provide depth to these topical areas, physicians, nurses, infant developmental specialists, and other health professionals concerned with neonatal care from across the country and around the world were used as contributors in all editions. The attempt was made not only to tap the experts in the neonatal field but also to have them represent as wide a geographic area as possible. We hope that the broad geographic distribution of contributors and reviewers will help minimize the effect of regional differences in clinical practice as reflected in the text.

The accompanying Evolve website will contain additional information that can be accessed from any Internet-connected computer, making the information readily available. The website will have case studies that readers can work through to apply knowledge from the textbook. We hope that you will find the information contained in this text very useful and helpful to you in providing care to newborns and their families.

Carole Kenner, DNS, RNC, FAAN
Judy Wright Lott, DSN, RNC, NNP, FAAN

Acknowledgments

This book has been a major undertaking, one of which we are most proud. Even though this is the fourth edition, it still requires a lot of work to make sure the material is up to date and accurate. It would not have been possible without the support of many people who worked in many hidden ways. First, we would like to thank our nursing developmental editor, Amanda Politte, who provided support and helpful suggestions and whose organizational skills kept us all on target. Next, we thank Catherine Jackson from Elsevier, who encouraged us to try new avenues of learning for our readership.

We are truly grateful to our contributors, who in the midst of their very busy lives took on one more project. To those who stuck with us through a fourth edition, we are especially indebted. We also want to thank the new contributors who were willing to step in and share their expertise with us. We certainly recognize the time commitment that was made by each contributor. We believe that because of their efforts, we have been able to bring together the best and the brightest shining stars in neonatal care.

We would also like to thank our reviewers for the constructive comments that helped structure the new content of the text. We recognize that your wisdom has guided us well in restructuring parts of the book to reflect changes in neonatal care worldwide.

We also want to thank Jan Zasada, The In Bin, for her hours of correcting our manuscripts, typing, and generally getting all our "ducks lined up" for this edition. She kept us moving along every step of the way.

Finally, but certainly not least, we would both like to acknowledge the support and encouragement of our families and friends: Les Kenner and George, Bill, and Tam Lott. Their strength and positive thoughts have kept us going throughout these many months. This edition is dedicated to our mothers, who died within days of each other and who were so proud of each of the previous editions, and to the memory of Blake Lott, whose life ended much too soon.

We want to thank our readers, who have validated the need for this text. We both appreciate when we hear from those of you who are using the text around the world. Without your support, there would have been no need for a fourth edition.

Carole Kenner, DNS, RNC, FAAN
Judy Wright Lott, DSN, RNC, NNP

Contents

Chapter 39 Assessment of the Newborn and Infant, 677

Debra A. Sansoucie • Terri A. Cavaliere

Appendix Preconception and Pregnancy Risk Factors and Risk Reduction Strategies Resources, 719

Chapter **1**

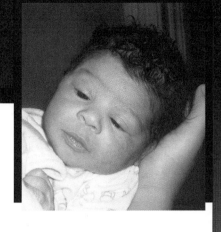

Respiratory System

Javier Cifuentes • Waldemar A. Carlo

The mechanisms that bring about normal pulmonary function are complex. The clinician must fully comprehend the physiologic processes associated with respiratory disease of the infant. Only through advanced knowledge can the clinician efficiently assess and evaluate the newborn's respiratory status. Systematic use of these assessment skills allows the clinician, as part of the collaborative team, to positively affect patient outcome.

EMBRYOLOGIC DEVELOPMENT OF THE LUNG

Pulmonary development of the embryo proceeds along a predetermined sequence throughout gestation (Greenough & Milner, 2005). Pulmonary development begins with formation of an outpouching of the embryonic foregut during the fourth week of gestation and continues on to form sufficient alveoli to maintain gas exchange in most infants by 32 to 36 weeks of gestational age. Additional alveoli continue to develop in the newborn infant and well into childhood, perhaps as late as the seventh year of life (Table 1-1). Sequential branching of the lung bud, which appears at about 4 weeks and is complete by the sixth week, marks the embryonic phase of lung development. The following 10 weeks are marked by the formation of conducting airways by branching of the aforementioned lung buds. This phase, the pseudoglandular phase, continues through week 16 and ends with completion of the conducting airways. The canalicular phase follows through week 28, when gas exchange units, known as acini, develop. Type II alveolar cells, the surfactant-producing cells, begin to form during the latter part of this phase. Mature, vascularized gas-exchange sites form during the saccular phase, which spans the 29th through 35th weeks. During this phase, the interstitial space between alveoli thins, so respiratory epithelial cells tightly contact developing capillaries. The alveolar development phase, marked by expansion of gas-exchange surface area, begins at 36 weeks and extends into the postnatal period. The alveolar wall and interstitial spaces become very thin, and the single capillary network comes into close proximity to the alveolar membrane. No firm boundaries separate these phases, and gas exchange, albeit inefficient, is possible relatively early in gestation, even before mature, vascularized gas-exchange sites form.

Lung development is a continuum that is marked by rapid structural changes. Interference at any time by premature birth or by disease introduces the possibility of inducing iatrogenic disease through intervention.

NEWBORN PULMONARY PHYSIOLOGY AND THE ONSET OF BREATHING

The fetal lung is fluid filled, underperfused, and dormant with regard to gas exchange. The fetal lung receives only approximately 10% of the cardiac output. Because the placenta is the gas-exchange organ in fetal life, a high blood flow is directed toward it rather than to the lungs. Consequently, most of the right ventricular output is shunted from the pulmonary artery across the ductus arteriosus into the aorta, bypassing the pulmonary circulation.

Within moments after the umbilical cord is clamped, the newborn undergoes an amazing transformation from a fetus floating in amniotic fluid to an air-breathing neonate. When the normal onset of breathing occurs, the ensuing chain of events converts the fetal circulation to the circulation pattern of an adult. The lung fluid is absorbed and replaced with air, thus establishing lung volume and allowing for normal neonatal pulmonary function. The process of fetal lung fluid absorption begins before birth when the rate of alveolar fluid secretion declines. Reabsorption speeds up during labor. Animal data suggest that as much as two thirds of the total clearance of lung fluid occurs during labor. This clearance probably results from the cessation of active chloride secretion into the alveolar space. Oncotic pressure favors the movement of water from the air space back into the interstitium and into the vascular space. With the onset of breathing and lung expansion, water moves rapidly from the air spaces into the interstitium and is removed from the lung by lymphatic and pulmonary blood vessels. Because a large portion of the clearance of lung fluid occurs during labor, neonates born without labor after cesarean section are at particularly high risk for delayed absorption of fetal lung fluid and thus for transient tachypnea of the newborn.

With the onset of breathing, highly negative intrathoracic pressures are generated with inspiratory efforts, filling the

TABLE 1-1	Stages of Normal Lung Growth	
Phase	**Timing**	**Major Event**
Embryonic	Weeks 4 to 6	Formation of proximal airway
Pseudoglandular	Weeks 7 to 16	Formation of conducting airways
Canalicular	Weeks 17 to 28	Formation of acini
Saccular	Weeks 29 to 35	Development of gas-exchange sites
Alveolar	Weeks 36 through postnatal life	Expansion of surface area

alveoli with air. Replacing alveolar fluid with air causes a precipitous decrease in hydrostatic pressure in the lung; therefore, pulmonary artery pressure decreases, which lowers pressure in the right atrium and increases pulmonary blood flow. These changes result in an increase in alveolar oxygen tension (PaO_2), causing constriction of the ductus arteriosus, which normally shunts right ventricular blood away from the lungs. By clamping of the cord, the large, low-resistance, placental surface area is removed from the circulation. This change in resistance causes an abrupt increase in systemic arterial pressure, reflected all the way back to the left atrium. As left atrial pressure rises, its flap valve closes the opening between the atria, known as the foramen ovale. This closure prevents blood from bypassing the lungs by eliminating the shunt across the foramen ovale from the right atrium to the left atrium. As a result of closure of fetal pathways and the decrease in pulmonary vascular resistance, systemic pressure becomes greater than pulmonary artery pressure. The infant successfully converts from the pattern of fetal circulation to neonatal circulation when blood coming from the right ventricle flows in its new path of least resistance (lower pressure) to the lungs, instead of shunting across the foramen ovale to the left atrium or across the ductus arteriosus from the pulmonary artery to the aorta.

Understanding ventilation enables the clinician to assess the infant in respiratory distress and devise strategies for management. The respiratory system is composed of the following: (1) the pumping system (the chest-wall muscles, diaphragm, and accessory muscles of respiration), which moves free gas into the lungs; (2) the bony rib cage, which provides structural support for the respiratory muscles and limits lung deflation; (3) the conducting airways, which connect gas-exchanging units with the outside but offer resistance to gas flow; (4) an elastic element, which offers some resistance to gas flow but provides pumping force for moving stale gas out of the system; (5) air-liquid interfaces, which generate surface tension that opposes lung expansion on inspiration but supports lung deflation on expiration; and (6) the abdominal muscles, which aid exhalation by active contraction.

Limitations in the respiratory system predispose the newborn to respiratory difficulty. The circular, poorly ossified rib cage, with a flat instead of angular insertion of the diaphragm, is less efficient at generating negative intrathoracic pressure to move air into the system. Small muscles and a relative paucity of type I muscle fibers hinder the strength and endurance of respiratory muscles. The newborn has a relatively low functional residual capacity (lung volume at the end of exhalation) because the comparatively floppy chest wall offers little resistance to collapse, even when a normal amount of functional surfactant is present.

An alveolar cell known as the type II pneumocyte produces pulmonary surfactant. Surfactant coats the alveoli, preventing alveolar collapse and loss of lung volume during expiration—that is, as expiration ensues and the lung deflates, the alveolar diameter becomes smaller. Surfactant coating of the alveolus reduces surface tension so that collapse is prevented and less pressure is required to re-inflate it with the next inspiration. Neonates with respiratory distress syndrome (RDS) have surfactant deficiency. In the absence of surfactant, surface tension is high, and the tendency is toward collapse of alveoli at end expiration.

Surface tension is the force that arises from the interaction among the molecules of a liquid. Molecules in the interior of the liquid bulk are attracted to each other, but molecules on the surface of the liquid are attracted to other molecules in the interior of the liquid, which results in the movement of the surface molecule toward the bulk of the liquid. This explains why a droplet of water over a surface tends to adopt a given size and not continuously expand. If we think of the alveolus as a soap bubble, the molecules of the wall of the bubble are attracted to each other, which tends to collapse the bubble. The pressures across the wall of the bubble act against the surface tension and avoid the collapse of the bubble. The relationship between the surface tension and the distending pressures and the pressure across the wall of the bubble are described by Laplace's law, as shown in the following equation:

$$P = 2\ ST/r$$

P is pressure, ST is surface tension, and r is radius of the alveolus. It is difficult to inflate a small or collapsed alveolus because it has a very small diameter. As its volume increases, the pressure needed to continue inflation becomes progressively less—that is, compliance of the alveolus and thus compliance of the lung has improved. Coating the alveoli with an agent that decreases surface tension reduces the effort required to inflate the lungs from a low volume. Pulmonary surfactant is a surface tension–reducing mixture of phospholipids and proteins found in mature alveoli. Surfactant coats the alveoli.

Compliance is the elasticity, or distensibility, of the lung. It is expressed as the change in volume caused by a change in pressure as follows:

$$C_L = V/P$$

C_L is compliance of the lung; V is volume; and P is pressure. The higher the compliance, the larger the volume delivered to the alveoli per unit of applied inspiratory pressure. Surface tension and compliance are particularly important in the preterm infant with RDS. Surface tension is a force that opposes lung expansion. Surfactant deficiency leads to increased surface tension in the alveoli. Lungs with higher surface tension are more difficult to inflate. During expiration, some alveoli collapse. This results in a decreased lung volume at the end of expiration (low functional residual capacity). Clinically, the presence of retractions and other signs of respiratory distress manifest the effects of this increased surface tension. Respiratory muscles contract to inflate the lungs against the surface tension that acts in the opposite direction. The negative pleural pressure easily deforms the floppy thoracic wall of the preterm infant. When a preterm infant with RDS is intubated, a high peak inspiratory pressure (PIP) is required to expand the thorax (i.e., tidal volume is obtained only with a high change in pressure). After surfactant is administered, chest expansion increases with the same PIP. This effect (increased compliance) is due to a decrease in surface tension (i.e., a smaller force opposing lung distention). Thus the tidal volume obtained with the same PIP is increased. Before surfactant is administered, it is very difficult to inflate the lung because compliance is low. After surfactant is administered, surface tension decreases, and it becomes easier to inflate the lung (i.e., compliance is improved).

Resistance is a term used to describe characteristics of gas flow through the airways and pulmonary tissues. Resistance can be thought of as the capacity of the lung to resist airflow. The principal component of resistance is determined by the small airways. Pressure is required to force gas through the airways (airway resistance) and to overcome the forces of the lung and chest wall, which work to deflate the respiratory system (tissue resistance). At a specific flow rate, resistance is described by the following equation:

$$R = P_1 - P_2 / \dot{V}$$

P_1 and P_2 are pressures at opposite ends of the airway, and $\dot{V}$ is the flow rate of gas (volume per unit of time). Resistance increases as airway diameter decreases. Because the infant has airways of relatively small radius, the resistance to gas flow through those airways is high. The time constant is the time necessary for airway pressure to partially equilibrate throughout the respiratory system and equals the mathematic product of compliance and resistance. In other words, the time constant is a measure of how quickly the lungs can inhale or exhale. The time constant (Kt) is directly related to both compliance (C) and resistance (R). This relationship is described by the following equation:

$$Kt = C \times R$$

An infant with RDS has decreased compliance, so the time constant of the respiratory system is relatively short. In such an infant, little time is required for pressure to equilibrate between the proximal airway and alveoli, so short inspiratory and expiratory times may be appropriate during mechanical ventilation. When compliance improves (increases), however, the time constant becomes longer. If sufficient time is not allowed for expiration, the alveoli may become overdistended, and an air leak may result.

Blood Gas Analysis and Acid-Base Balance

Oxygen diffuses across the alveolar-capillary membrane, moved by the difference in oxygen pressure between the alveoli and the blood. In the blood, oxygen dissolves in the plasma and binds to hemoglobin. Thus arterial oxygen content (CaO_2) is the sum of dissolved and hemoglobin-bound oxygen, as is shown by the following equation:

$$CaO_2 = (1.37 \times Hb \times SaO_2) (0.003 \times PaO_2)$$

CaO_2 is arterial oxygen content (ml/100 ml of blood); 1.37 is the milliliters of oxygen bound to 1 g of hemoglobin at 100% saturation; Hb is hemoglobin concentration per 100 ml of blood (g/100 ml); SaO_2 is the percentage of hemoglobin bound to oxygen (%); 0.003 is the solubility factor of oxygen in plasma (ml/mm Hg); and PaO_2 is oxygen partial pressure in arterial blood (mm Hg).

In the equation for arterial oxygen content, the first term—($1.37 \times Hb \times SaO_2$)—is the amount of oxygen bound to hemoglobin. The second term—($0.003 \times PaO_2$)—is the amount of oxygen dissolved in plasma. Most of the oxygen in the blood is carried by hemoglobin. For example, if a premature infant has a PaO_2 of 60 mm Hg, an SaO_2 of 92%, and a hemoglobin concentration of 14 g/100 ml, then CaO_2 is the sum of oxygen bound to hemoglobin ($1.37 \times 14 \times 92/100$) = 17.6 ml, plus the oxygen dissolved in plasma (0.003×60) = 0.1 ml. In this typical example, only less than 1% of oxygen in blood is dissolved in plasma; more than 99% is carried by hemoglobin. If the infant has an intraventricular hemorrhage and the hemoglobin concentration decreases to 10.5 g/dl but PaO_2 and SaO_2 remain the same, then CaO_2 ($1.37 \times 10.5 \times 92/100$) + ($0.003 \times 60$) equals 13.4 ml/100 ml of blood. Thus, without any change in PaO_2 or SaO_2, a 25% decrease in hemoglobin concentration (from 14 to 10.5 g/dl) reduces the amount of oxygen in arterial blood by 24% (from 17.6 to 13.4 ml/100 ml of blood). This is an important concept for clinicians who care for patients with respiratory disease. SaO_2 and hemoglobin should be monitored and, if low, corrected to keep an adequate level of tissue oxygenation. Besides SaO_2 and hemoglobin, cardiac output is the other major determination of oxygen delivery to the tissues.

The force that loads hemoglobin with oxygen in the lungs and unloads it in the tissues is the difference in partial pressure of oxygen. In the lungs, alveolar oxygen partial pressure is higher than capillary oxygen partial pressure so that oxygen moves to the capillaries and binds to the hemoglobin. Tissue partial pressure of oxygen is lower than that of the blood, so oxygen moves from hemoglobin to the tissues. The relationship between partial pressure of oxygen and hemoglobin is better understood with the oxyhemoglobin dissociation curve (Figure 1-1). Several factors can affect the affinity of hemoglobin for oxygen. Alkalosis, hypothermia, hypocapnia, and decreased levels of 2,3-diphosphoglycerate (2,3-DPG) increase the affinity of hemoglobin for oxygen (as shown in Figure 1-1 by a left shift of the curve). Acidosis, hyperthermia, hypercapnia, and increased 2,3-DPG have the opposite effect, decreasing the affinity of hemoglobin for oxygen, so that the hemoglobin dissociation curve shifts to the right. This characteristic of hemoglobin facilitates oxygen loading in the lung and unloading in the tissue, where the pH is lower and alveolar carbon dioxide tension ($PaCO_2$) is higher. Fetal hemoglobin, which has a higher affinity for oxygen than adult hemoglobin, is more fully oxygen-saturated at lower PaO_2 values. This is represented by a left shift on the curve of dissociation of hemoglobin.

Once loaded with oxygen, the blood should reach the tissues to transfer oxygen to the cells. Oxygen delivery to the tissue depends on cardiac output (CO) and CaO_2, as described in the following equation:

$$\text{Oxygen delivery} = CO \times CaO_2$$

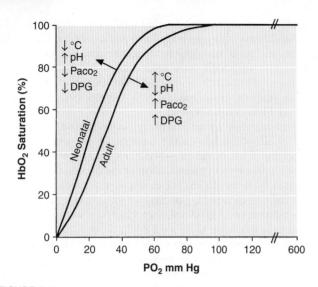

FIGURE 1-1
Oxyhemoglobin equilibrium curves of blood from term infants at birth and from adults (at pH 7.40).

In the case of the infant discussed previously, increased CO compensates for the decrease in CaO_2 that results from anemia. The key concept is that when a patient's oxygenation is assessed, more information than just PaO_2 and SaO_2 should be considered. PaO_2 and SaO_2 may be normal, but, if hemoglobin concentration is low or CO is decreased, oxygen delivery to the tissues is decreased. With this approach, the clinician should be able to better plan the interventions needed to improve oxygenation.

As in the adult, the acid-base balance in the neonate is maintained within narrow limits by complex interactions between the pulmonary system (which eliminates carbon dioxide) and the kidneys (which conserve carbon dioxide and eliminate metabolic acids). Carbon dioxide elimination, which is more efficient than oxygenation across the alveolar capillary membrane, is usually not as problematic as oxygenation. Carbon dioxide has a high solubility coefficient, so cellular diffusion is efficient and no measurable partial pressure gradient exists between venous blood and the tissues. Therefore elevated carbon dioxide tension (PCO_2) values in arterial blood samples nearly always indicate ventilatory dysfunction. Dissolved carbon dioxide moves rapidly across cell membranes of peripheral chemoreceptors, thereby making them sensitive to changes in ventilation. Increased intracellular PCO_2 elevates the cellular hydrogen ion concentration as carbon dioxide combines with water to form carbonic acid. This stimulates neural impulses to the medulla, which in turn stimulates respiration. However, excessively high PCO_2 levels can depress ventilation. Acid-base balance is controlled by homeostatic mechanisms and is expressed by the following equation:

$$pH = 6.1 \pm \log HCO_3^-/0.03 \times PCO_2$$

It can be seen from this mathematical relationship that acid-base balance depends on the interplay of bicarbonate ion (HCO_3^-) and carbon dioxide (CO_2). Serum pH is tightly regulated in the normal range. Low pH (in other words, acidosis) can contribute to vasoconstriction and can result in worsening hypoxemia caused by extrapulmonary shunt across the ductus or foramen ovale. A pH of less than 7.0 is not well tolerated and is associated with a poor survival rate in these patients.

If $PaCO_2$ rises above normal, as in hypoventilation, pH declines and the patient suffers from respiratory acidosis. The patient with a chronic respiratory acidosis may retain bicarbonate, thus self-inducing a compensatory metabolic alkalosis. A patient who is hyperventilated with a low $PaCO_2$ has respiratory alkalosis. Depressed bicarbonate ion concentration (less than approximately 20 mmol/L in plasma) is called metabolic acidosis and can be associated with any cause of anaerobic metabolism, such as poor CO from congenital heart disease—for example, hypoplastic left heart syndrome or severe aortic coarctation—or from myocardial ischemia, myocardiopathy, myocarditis, hypoxia, or septic shock. Metabolic acidosis that results from renal bicarbonate wasting commonly develops in extremely immature infants. Less common causes for prolonged and severe metabolic acidosis are the inborn errors of metabolism, including urea-cycle defects and aminoacidopathies.

The clinician should become proficient at interpreting blood gas data. With knowledge of the accepted normal values and definitions of the simple blood gas disorders and their compensatory mechanisms, the clinician can examine data in light of the disease process and interpret blood gas values in a fairly straightforward manner. Normally, the body does not overcompensate for a pH above or below the normal range. Therefore, when presented with an abnormal pH, the clinician rapidly determines whether acidosis (Figure 1-2, A) or alkalosis (Figure 1-2, B) exists. An examination of $PaCO_2$ and HCO_3^- determines whether the process is respiratory, metabolic, or mixed. The clinician should determine which derangement occurred first. For example, an acidotic, acutely ill hypoxemic infant with a high $PaCO_2$ and depressed HCO_3^- is usually hypoventilating and suffering metabolic acidosis secondary to anaerobic metabolism. The infant with a low $PaCO_2$ is hyperventilating, either spontaneously or secondary to overzealous mechanical ventilation. A concomitantly low pH and low $PaCO_2$ indicate that the infant is compensating for metabolic acidosis with hyperventilation in an effort to normalize the pH. A pure metabolic alkalosis with high pH is nearly always caused by bicarbonate administration. Infants with bronchopulmonary dysplasia usually have a compensated respiratory acidosis, with an elevated $PaCO_2$ and concomitantly elevated HCO_3^-. The pH may be in the normal range or slightly acidotic. A severely depressed pH usually indicates acute decompensation.

ASSESSMENT OF THE NEONATE WITH RESPIRATORY DISTRESS

The assessment of a neonate with respiratory distress should always begin with the compilation of a detailed perinatal history. In many cases, the history is difficult to obtain, especially when the infant has been transferred from one center to another, often with incomplete records. Even so, every effort should be made to obtain as much pertinent information as possible. The clinician is often able to gain important supplemental information from the father or visiting relatives at the bedside. A review of the maternal-perinatal history and a complete physical examination, combined with a limited laboratory and radiologic evaluation, leads to a timely diagnosis in

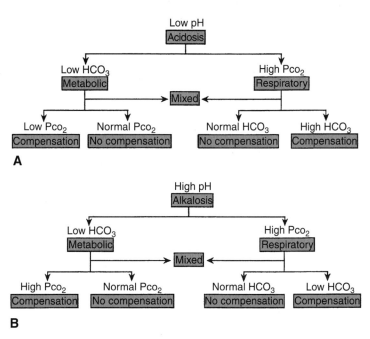

FIGURE **1-2**
Acid-base balance: diagnostic approach. **A,** Low pH. **B,** High pH.

most circumstances. Many neonatal diseases, including many with nonpulmonary origins, may manifest with signs of respiratory distress. Therefore a comprehensive differential diagnosis must be considered (Figure 1-3).

History

In most situations, data from a patient's history can direct the clinician to the correct diagnosis of neonatal respiratory distress. The prenatal record should be reviewed carefully for possible causes of the infant's difficulties. The mother's age, gravidity, parity, blood type, and Rh status should be recorded. The obstetrician's best estimate of gestational age should be documented as determined by first-trimester ultrasound or last menstrual period. Ultrasonography often provides information related to anomalies, which is useful in the anticipation of required support at birth. Historical information such as previous preterm birth is relevant as it is often associated with an increased risk of premature delivery in subsequent pregnancies. Because excessive maternal weight gain occurs with diabetes, multiple gestation, or polyhydramnios, pre-pregnancy weight and total gain should be noted. The clinician is often alerted to the possibility of gestational diabetes with abnormal glucose tolerance screening results, which will be reflected in the prenatal record.

The duration of membrane rupture, the presence of maternal fever with or without accompanying amnionitis, and the presence of meconium-stained amniotic fluid are important pieces of information that may help in the differential diagnosis of a newborn with respiratory distress. Additionally, antepartum and intrapartum administration of certain medications may affect diagnosis and management of these infants.

Administration of steroids to the mother reduces the likelihood that RDS will develop in the infant; administration of narcotics to the mother close to delivery may result in poor respiratory effort by an otherwise normal infant.

Physical Examination of the Respiratory System

One or more of the major signs of respiratory difficulty (e.g., cyanosis, tachypnea, grunting, retractions, and nasal flaring) are usually present in neonates with both pulmonary and non-pulmonary causes of respiratory distress. Observation of the distressed infant with the unaided eye and ear is the clinician's first step in the physical assessment. Cyanosis may be central, as caused by pulmonary disease and cyanotic heart disease, or peripheral, as occurs in conditions with impaired CO. Tachypnea typically manifests infants with decreased lung compliance, such as RDS, whereas patients with high airway resistance (e.g., airway obstruction) usually have deep but slow breathing. Grunting is produced by an adduction of vocal cords during expiration. Grunting holds gas in the lungs throughout expiration, which helps maintain lung volume and avoid alveolar collapse. At the end of expiration the gas is released and rapidly propelled, causing an audible grunt. Grunting is more typical of infants with decreased functional residual capacity, such as preterm infants with RDS. Chest wall retractions occur more often in very premature infants because of the highly compliant chest wall (Bates & Balistreri, 2002). When the infant is intubated, observation of the chest gives important information. Careful observation of chest wall excursions produced by the ventilator allows the clinician to adjust the magnitude of the ventilator pressure so that optimal gas exchange is achieved while risk of barotrauma is mini-

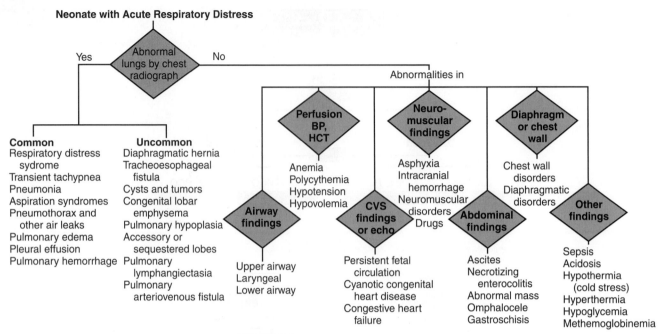

FIGURE **1-3**
Neonate with acute respiratory distress.

mized. The chest of an intubated infant should move the same or only slightly less than that of a healthy spontaneously breathing infant. The clinician should assess the appropriateness of the magnitude of the chest expansion in ventilated patients. The nurse should assess for and report changes in chest rise in an intubated infant. Abrupt decreases in the chest rise may indicate atelectasis, a plugged endotracheal tube, a pneumothorax, or ventilator failure. Slow decreases in the chest rise over the hours may indicate a deteriorating lung compliance or gas trapping. An overinflated thorax, as determined from radiographs, is a sign of gas trapping. In the intubated infant, this observation should prompt the clinician to adjust the positive end-expiratory pressure (PEEP) or expiratory time so that gas trapping and air leakage are prevented. An anguished intubated infant with cyanosis and gasping efforts may have endotracheal tube obstruction.

Careful attention should be given to the sounds that emanate from the respiratory tract, as variations in quality often aid in localization of the source of respiratory distress. Stridor is common in neonates with upper airway and laryngeal lesions. Inspiratory stridor occurs most often with upper airway and laryngeal lesions, whereas expiratory stridor suggests lower airway problems. Hoarseness is a common sign of laryngeal disorders. Forced inspiratory efforts may indicate upper airway or laryngeal involvement, whereas expiratory wheezes suggest a lower airway disease. Congenital airway disorders that may cause respiratory distress in the neonate are included in Figure 1-3.

Auscultation of the chest further aids the examiner. Because infants with RDS have low lung volumes, breath sounds are faint, usually without rales. In comparison, the infant with pneumonia may have rales indicative of alveolar filling. Auscultation allows the clinician to detect the presence of secretions in the airway and to evaluate the response to physiotherapy and suctioning. Rhonchi may be heard in neonates with airway disease, such as meconium aspiration syndrome (MAS). Unequal breath sounds may be due to a

pneumothorax or to one of the many causes of diminished ventilation to a lung lobe (e.g., atelectasis, main-stem bronchial intubation, and pleural effusion). A shift of the apex of the heart can occur with a pneumothorax, diaphragmatic hernia, unilateral pulmonary interstitial emphysema, pleural effusion, or atelectasis, which may be differentiated by transillumination of the chest. Dullness to percussion may be due to a pleural effusion or solid mass. Muffled heart tones suggest a pneumopericardium. Respiratory distress may occur in many chest wall disorders that restrict rib-cage movements. Increased oral secretions and choking with feedings are common in neonates with a tracheoesophageal fistula. Because newborns are obligate nasal breathers, those with choanal atresia typically improve with crying and have worsening respiratory distress with rest and feeding. Characteristic Potter facies and other compression deformities and contractures may be present in neonates with hypoplastic lungs secondary to oligohydramnios.

Examination of the cardiovascular system and assessment of peripheral perfusion yield many clues toward a diagnosis. Pallor and poor perfusion may indicate anemia, hypotension, or hypovolemia. Polycythemia with plethora may also cause respiratory distress. Cardiovascular signs of congestive failure (e.g., hyperactive precordium, tachycardia, and hepatomegaly), poor CO, pathologic murmurs, decreased femoral pulses, and nonsinus rhythm suggest a primary cardiac cause for the respiratory distress.

When hypotonia, muscle weakness, or areflexia accompanies respiratory distress, a neuromuscular cause should be considered (Box 1-1). In such cases, an accompanying history of less frequent fetal movement often is involved. Sometimes a history of muscular disease exists in the family. Brachial plexus injury or fracture of a clavicle may accompany phrenic nerve injury and diaphragm paralysis.

Abnormalities found on abdominal examination enlighten the examiner to other causes of respiratory difficulty.

BOX 1-1

Neuromuscular Disorders That May Cause Respiratory Distress in the Neonate

Myopathies
Myasthenia gravis
Werdnig-Hoffmann disease
Spinal cord disorder
Poliomyelitis
Others

Adapted from Battista MA, Carlo WA (1992). Differential diagnosis of acute respiratory distress in the neonate. *Tufts University School of Medicine and Floating Hospital for Children reports on neonatal respiratory diseases* 2(3):1-4, 9-11.

BOX 1-2

Causes of Late Respiratory Distress in the Neonate

Bronchopulmonary dysplasia
Pneumonia (bacterial, viral, or fungal)
Congestive heart failure
Recurrent pneumonitis or aspiration
Upper airway obstruction
Wilson-Mikity syndrome
Idiopathic pulmonary fibrosis (Hamman-Rich syndrome)
Pulmonary lymphangiectasia
Cystic fibrosis
Immature lungs

Abdominal distention that results from causes such as ascites, necrotizing enterocolitis, abdominal mass, ileus, or tracheoesophageal fistula can cause respiratory distress, whereas a scaphoid configuration of the abdomen suggests a diaphragmatic hernia.

Other nonpulmonary disorders such as sepsis, metabolic acidosis, hypothermia, hyperthermia, hypoglycemia, and methemoglobinemia may also cause respiratory distress in the neonate.

Radiographic and Laboratory Investigation

Radiographic examination is often the most useful part of the laboratory evaluation and may serve to narrow the differential diagnosis. An anteroposterior view is usually sufficient, but a lateral chest radiograph may be useful when fluid, masses, or free air is suspected. Other diagnostic imaging techniques (ultrasonography, fluoroscopy, computed tomography, or magnetic resonance imaging) may be helpful in selected patients. Bronchoscopy allows direct visualization of the upper airway. This technique, albeit invasive and technically difficult, may in selected cases be a great aid in the differential diagnosis and treatment of patients with a suspected airway lesion.

Much can be learned from a relatively small battery of laboratory tests. In the NICU setting, the clinician is often required to collect specimens for and interpret the results of physiologic testing. Considerable skill is required in sampling both venous and arterial blood from small patients who are at substantial risk for iatrogenic anemia and vascular damage. Ideally, the hospital laboratory is equipped to do most routine tests on microliter quantities of blood. The clinician must monitor total quantities of blood sampled from the infant and be alert to the development of iatrogenic anemia.

Analysis of arterial blood for pH and gas tensions is perhaps one of the most common tasks of the clinicians caring for the infant with respiratory illness. Noninvasive methods to assess gas exchange, such as transcutaneous blood gas measurements or oxygen saturation, are very useful. Because oxygen delivery to the tissues so intimately depends on circulating red blood cell volume, a hematocrit should be performed.

COMMON DISORDERS OF THE RESPIRATORY SYSTEM

A large variety of disorders may afflict neonates. The most common disorders are discussed here. Figure 1-3 lists both pulmonary and non-pulmonary disorders that cause respiratory

symptoms in the newborn infant. Several diseases may start later in the neonatal period and extend into infancy (Box 1-2). The most common is bronchopulmonary dysplasia (BPD), a chronic lung disease that affects newborns, mainly premature infants exposed to mechanical ventilation and oxygen for RDS or other respiratory problems.

Respiratory Distress Syndrome (RDS)

RDS, or hyaline membrane disease (the term *hyaline membrane disease* originated from the histological observation of alveolar space lined by an eosinophilic membrane formed by cellular debris), is the most common cause of respiratory distress in premature neonates (Bates & Balistreri, 2002). RDS occurs in about 10% of all premature infants in the United States (American Lung Association [ALA], 2006). Fifty to sixty percent of infants born before 29 weeks' gestation have RDS (ALA, 2006; Lemons et al, 2001) and account for thousands of patient days in the NICUs and millions of dollars in health care expenditures. In rare cases, RDS develops in full-term infants born to mothers with diabetes or in full-term infants who have experienced asphyxia. RDS is progressively more common the lower the infant's gestational age.

Antenatal Steroids

Acceleration of lung maturation with antenatal steroids is now the standard of care in women with preterm labor of up to 34 weeks. Antenatal corticosteroid therapy to the mothers of preterm fetuses of up to 34 weeks significantly reduces the incidence of RDS with odds ratios of around 0.5 and decreases mortality, with odds ratios of around 0.6. Subgroup analyses confirm that these benefits occur regardless of race and gender. No adverse effects have been reported with the usual single course of antenatal steroids.

Treatment

The lung is deficient in pulmonary surfactant, the surface tension–reducing agent that prevents alveolar collapse at end expiration and loss of lung volume. Treatment with surfactant is quite effective (see Chapter 2). Progressive atelectasis leads to intrapulmonary shunting, owing to perfusion of unventilated lung, and subsequent hypoxemia. The radiograph displays a characteristic ground glass, reticulogranular appearance with air bronchograms. When the lung inflation is poor, the arterial blood gas analysis usually reveals respiratory acidemia as well as hypoxemia.

Therapy is directed toward improving oxygenation as well as maintaining optimal lung volume. Continuous positive airway pressure (CPAP) or positive end-expiratory pressure (PEEP) is applied to prevent volume loss during expiration. In severe cases, mechanical ventilation via tracheal tube is required. Exogenous surfactants (artificial and natural), which are available for intratracheal instillation, improve survival and reduce some of the associated morbidity of RDS. The earlier surfactant is administered, the better the effect on gas exchange. Clinical trials indicate that prophylactic surfactant administration to extremely premature infants in the delivery room is more effective than waiting for the treatment after development of RDS (Soll & Morley, 2001). Prophylactic high-frequency ventilation for treatment of RDS has mixed results, but these new modes of ventilation should be considered as alternatives to conventional mechanical ventilation in specific circumstances, such as in infants with air leaks as interstitial emphysema or bronchopleural fistula. Infants greater than 34 weeks who have RDS and respiratory failure unresponsive to ventilatory management have responded favorably to extracorporeal membrane oxygenation (ECMO) (Thome et al, 2005).

Nursing care for infants with RDS is demanding; the most unstable infants often require a 1:1 nurse:patient ratio. The nurse must monitor the quality of respirations and observe the degree of difficulty that the infant is experiencing. Worsening retractions may signal progressive volume loss and impending respiratory failure. Arterial blood gas tensions and pH should be measured frequently, and continuous noninvasive monitoring of oxygenation may allow early identification of gas exchange problems. The risk of pneumothorax and right mainstem intubation is high, and the symmetry of breath sounds must be verified regularly. A crying infant loses airway pressure when the mouth is open and therefore must be kept calm when receiving nasal CPAP. The intubated infant must be monitored for appropriate endotracheal tube position and patency. Suctioning of the airway should be done carefully. The suction catheter should be passed only as far as the end of the endotracheal tube because overzealous suctioning can denude the tracheal epithelium (Cordero et al, 2000). Lung volume can be lost during prolonged disconnection from the ventilator. Rapid loss of lung volume can precipitate hypoxemia, so disconnection time should be minimized. Any sudden decompensation should alert the nurse to investigate for ventilator failure, pneumothorax, or tracheal tube plugging (Figure 1-4).

A common complication of RDS in the tiny premature infant is bronchopulmonary dysplasia. BPD generally refers to a chronic obstructive pulmonary disorder characterized by pulmonary fibrosis, bronchiolar metaplasia, emphysema, and interstitial edema. It is most commonly seen in survivors of extreme prematurity who were diagnosed with RDS, but extremely-low-birth-weight infants may develop BPD without history of RDS. According to the National Institute of Child Health and Human Development consensus, infants with mild BPD are those who continue to require oxygen supplementation for a total of at least 28 days, while those with moderate or severe BPD require oxygen supplementation and/or ventilatory support at 36 weeks of postmenstrual age and for more than 28 days (Jobe & Bancalari, 2001). The incidence of BPD increases as gestational age decreases. Of the infants less than or equal to 1,000 g at birth, 77% develop mild BPD, while 46% develop moderate BPD and 16% develop severe BPD (Ehrenkranz et al, 2005). Pulmonary morbidities and adverse neurodevelopmental outcomes at 18 to 22 months were more prevalent with more severe BPD. Premature infants with birth weights less than 1500 g develop moderate to severe BPD.

Air Leaks

Air leaks frequently complicate RDS and other neonatal respiratory disorders. Air leaks are characterized by air in an ectopic location (Box 1-3). Many air-leak syndromes begin with at least some degree of pulmonary interstitial emphysema, which is the result of alveolar rupture from overdistention, usually concomitant with mechanical ventilation or continuous distending airway pressure. Pulmonary interstitial emphysema occurs most commonly in preterm infants but may be seen in infants of any gestational age. Lung compliance is nonuniform, and areas of poor aeration and alveolar collapse exist. Interspersed are alveoli of normal or near-normal compliance, which become overdistended. The more normal lung units (those with better compliance) become overdistended and eventually rupture. Air is forced from the alveolus into the loose tissue of the interstitial space and dissects toward the hilum of the lung, where it may track into the mediastinum—causing a pneumomediastinum—or into the pericardium—causing a pneumopericardium. The astute clini-

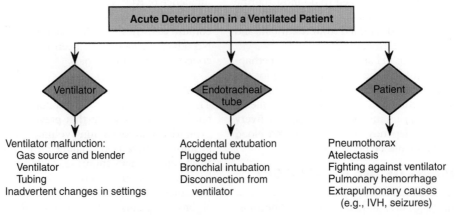

FIGURE **1-4**
Acute deterioration in a ventilated patient.

BOX 1-3

Types of Air Leaks Associated with Respiratory Distress in the Neonate

Pneumothorax
Pulmonary interstitial emphysema
Pneumomediastinum
Pneumopericardium
Pneumoperitoneum
Pulmonary venous air embolism
Subcutaneous emphysema
Pseudocyst

Adapted from Battista MA, Carlo WA (1992). Differential diagnosis of acute respiratory distress in the neonate. *Tufts University School of Medicine and Floating Hospital for Children reports on neonatal respiratory diseases* 2(3):1-4, 9-11.

TABLE 1-2 Organisms That May Cause Pneumonia in the Neonate

Bacterial	Viral	Other
Group B streptococcus	Cytomegalovirus	*Candida* (and other fungi)
Escherichia coli	Adenovirus	*Ureaplasma*
Klebsiella	Rhinovirus	*Chlamydia*
Staphylococcus aureus	Respiratory syncytial virus	Syphilis
Listeria monocytogenes	Parainfluenza	*Pneumocystis carinii*
Enterobacter	Enterovirus	Tuberculosis
Haemophilus influenzae	Rubella	
Pneumococcus		
Pseudomonas		
Bacteroides		
Others		

Adapted from Battista MA, Carlo WA (1992). Differential diagnosis of acute respiratory distress in the neonate. Tufts University School of Medicine and Floating Hospital for Children reports on neonatal respiratory diseases 2(3):1-4, 9-11.

cian may notice that an infant's chest becomes barrel-shaped with overdistention and that breath sounds become distant on the affected side. In contrast, the infant who suffers a pneumothorax usually becomes unstable, with development of cyanosis, oxygen desaturation, and carbon dioxide retention. The infant may become hypotensive and bradycardic because the high intrathoracic pressure impedes CO. A tension pneumothorax, in which the free pleural air compresses the lung, is a medical emergency, and prompt relief by thoracentesis or tube thoracostomy is indicated.

Transient Tachypnea of the Newborn

Transient tachypnea of the newborn occurs typically in infants born by cesarean section, particularly in the absence of labor. The cause of the disorder is thought to be transient pulmonary edema that results from the infant's "missed" chance during labor to absorb pulmonary alveolar fluid. The chest radiograph may show increased perihilar interstitial markings and small pleural fluid collections, especially in the minor fissure. In contrast to the infants with RDS, infants with transient tachypnea tend to have a normal or low PCO_2. Oxygenation can usually be maintained by supplementing oxygen with a hood, although some infants benefit from a short course of positive pressure support. The infant usually recovers in 24 to 48 hours.

Pneumonia

Pneumonia may be of bacterial, viral, or other infectious origin (Table 1-2). Pneumonia may be transmitted transplacentally, as has been shown with group B streptococcus, or via an ascending bacterial invasion associated with maternal amnionitis and prolonged rupture of the membranes. The usual organisms of active postamnionitis pneumonia are group B streptococcus, *Escherichia coli*, *Haemophilus influenzae*, and, less commonly, *Streptococcus viridans*, *Listeria monocytogenes*, and anaerobes.

A strong association exists between bacterial pneumonias and premature birth, which may be due to a developmental deficiency of bacteriostatic factors in the amniotic fluid. Alternatively, the infection may be a precipitating factor in preterm labor. Amnionitis can occur even in the presence of intact membranes. Blood cultures and other diagnostic tests are necessary to help direct specific antimicrobial therapy. The clinician should be attuned to the labor history. Were membranes ruptured for more than 12 to 24 hours? Did the mother have fever before delivery? Did the mother receive intrapartum antibiotics if risk factors for group B streptococcus sepsis were present? The full-term infant who exhibits tachypnea, grunting, retractions, or temperature instability should be evaluated carefully. Blood counts may be helpful, and the neutropenic infant in particular should be carefully monitored. Infection should be considered in any newborn with respiratory distress or more than transient oxygen requirements. Tracheal aspirates obtained within 8 hours of birth and that show both bacteria and white blood cells on Wright's stain are highly predictive of pneumonia.

Pending culture results, treatment is usually begun with broad-spectrum antibiotics (e.g., a penicillin) and aminoglycoside or cephalosporin. A lumbar puncture may be undertaken or may be postponed until results of blood culture are obtained. When cultures result in the identification of the organism, the study of antibiotic sensitivity allows the clinician to identify the most effective antibiotic or combination of antibiotics for the causative agent. Antibiotic treatment for up to 10 to 14 days may be necessary.

Persistent Pulmonary Hypertension of the Newborn

Persistent pulmonary hypertension of the newborn (PPHN), or persistent fetal circulation, is a term applied to the combination of pulmonary hypertension (high pressure in the pulmonary artery), subsequent right-to-left shunting through fetal channels (the foramen ovale or ductus arteriosus) away from the pulmonary vascular bed, and a structurally normal heart. The syndrome may be idiopathic or, more commonly, secondary to another disorder—such as meconium aspiration syndrome, congenital diaphragmatic hernia, RDS, asphyxia, sepsis, pneumonia, hyperviscosity of the blood, or hypoglycemia (Walsh-Sukys et al, 2000).

The neonatal pulmonary vasculature is sensitive to changes in PaO_2 and pH and, during stress, can become even hyperreactive and constrict to cause increased pressure against which the neonatal heart cannot force blood flow to the lungs. If the pulmonary artery pressure is higher than systemic pressure, blood flows through the path of least resistance, away from the lungs through the foramen ovale and the ductus arteriosus. The infant becomes progressively hypoxemic and acidemic, and the cycle perpetuates.

Collaborative management of infants with PPHN demands the greatest diligence that the health care professional can summon. Because the pulmonary vasculature is unstable, almost any event can precipitate severe hypoxemia, including routine procedures such as endotracheal tube suctioning, weighing, positioning, and diaper changes. Under these circumstances, minimal stimulation is usually practiced.

Occasionally, sedation and even muscle paralysis are necessary to prevent spontaneous episodes of hypoxemia or deterioration associated with procedures (e.g., suctioning and position changes). Alkalosis—either with bicarbonate infusion or by hyperventilation—often relaxes the pulmonary vascular bed and allows better pulmonary perfusion and thus oxygenation. The approach to therapy should be directed toward preventing hypoxemia and acidosis. The critical pH necessary for overcoming pulmonary vasoconstriction seems to be unique to the individual. High applied ventilator pressures predispose the lung to air-leak syndromes, further increasing the risk of sudden destabilization. Vasopressor therapy with dopamine and dobutamine is often used in conjunction with hyperventilation, but controlled data are not available. Presumably, they act both to improve contractility of the stressed myocardium, which improves CO, and to raise systemic arterial pressure above pulmonary artery pressure to reduce right-to-left shunting.

When conventional therapies fail, high-frequency ventilation may be attempted. Approximately 30% to 60% of patients who fail conventional mechanical ventilation respond to high-frequency ventilation. However, the exact role of high-frequency ventilation on mortality or in preventing the need for ECMO needs further evaluation. Since the early 1990s, inhalation of nitric oxide—alone and in association with high-frequency ventilation—has been shown to be an effective therapy for PPHN (The Neonatal Inhaled Nitric Oxide Study Group, 1997; Davidson et al, 1998).

When oxygenation cannot be accomplished despite the use of conventional mechanical ventilation, high-frequency ventilation, or nitric oxide, ECMO has proven to be an effective therapy (UK Collaborative ECMO Trial Group, 1996). Neonatologists disagree about the exact indications for ECMO, and some centers report impressive survival statistics without the use of ECMO (Mok et al, 1999). However, ECMO often is the only treatment that improves the outcome of some infants who fail less invasive therapies.

Meconium Aspiration Syndrome (MAS)

MAS is the most common aspiration syndrome that causes respiratory distress in neonates. The role of meconium in the pathophysiology of aspiration pneumonia has become controversial. It is unclear whether the material itself causes pneumonitis severe enough to lead to hypoxemia, acidosis, and pulmonary hypertension or whether the presence of meconium in the amniotic fluid is merely a marker for other events that may have predisposed the fetus to severe pulmonary disease.

The severely ill infant with MAS typically comes from a stressed labor and has depressed cord pH from metabolic acidosis. These infants are often postmature and exhibit classic signs of weight loss, skin peeling, and deep staining of the nails and umbilical cord.

Pharyngeal suctioning at the time of birth does not reduce MAS (Vain et al, 2004). The depressed infant with meconium-stained fluid should receive endotracheal suction at birth. If the infant has absent or depressed respirations, is hypotonic, or has a heart rate of fewer than 100 beats/min, then rapid intubation under direct laryngoscopy to allow for suctioning of the airway is recommended (International Guidelines for Neonatal Resuscitation, 2000). Endotracheal suctioning at birth is used to prevent MAS in the newly born with meconium-stained fluid but is not necessary if the infant is vigorous at birth (Wiswell et al, 2000). The American Academy of Pediatrics Neonatal Resuscitation Program suggests that if the infant is not vigorous then the trachea should be suctioned as soon as possible after delivery (Clark & Clark, 2004).

Pulmonary disease arises from chemical pneumonitis, interstitial edema, and small-airway obstruction and from concomitant persistent pulmonary hypertension. The infant may have uneven pulmonary ventilation with hyperinflation of some areas and atelectasis of others, leading to ventilation-perfusion mismatching and subsequent hypoxemia. The hypoxemia may then exacerbate pulmonary vasoconstriction, leading to deeper hypoxemia and acidosis. Infants with MAS may have evidence of lung overinflation with a barrel-chested appearance. Auscultation reveals rales and rhonchi. The radiograph shows patchy or streaky areas of atelectasis and other areas of overinflation.

As with other cases of pulmonary hypertension, nursing care of infants with MAS centers on maintenance of adequate oxygenation and acid-base balance and on the avoidance of cold stress, which contributes to acidosis. A high incidence of air leaks exists in these infants, and positive pressure ventilation is best avoided if the patient can be adequately oxygenated, even at very high-inspired oxygen concentrations. Antibiotics are often used, however, particularly in desperately ill infants, at least until a bacterial infection is ruled out, but antibiotic therapy may not be necessary. The infant is often exquisitely sensitive to environmental stimuli and should be treated in as quiet an environment as possible. Interventions should be preplanned to maximize efficiency of handling the infant. Infants with very severe respiratory failure and MAS improve with the administration of exogenous surfactant.

Although aspiration of meconium is most common, the neonate may become symptomatic as a result of the aspiration of blood, amniotic fluid, or gastrointestinal contents. The history is important in the differential diagnosis because radiographs are non-diagnostic.

Pulmonary Hemorrhage

Pulmonary hemorrhage is rarely an isolated condition and usually occurs in an otherwise sick infant. RDS, asphyxia, congenital heart disease, aspiration of gastric content or maternal blood, and disseminated intravascular coagulation and other bleeding disorders may play a role in the cause of pulmonary hemorrhage. The risk for pulmonary hemorrhage is increased by approximately 5% in infants receiving either natural or artificial surfactant. Massive bleeding may also occur as a complication of airway suction secondary to direct trauma of the respiratory epithelium.

Pulmonary hemorrhage is manifested by the presence of bloody fluid from the trachea. When massive, it may be heralded by a sudden deterioration with pallor, shock, cyanosis, or bradycardia. Attention must be given to maintenance of a patent airway because an obstructed endotracheal tube requires emergency replacement. Suctioning must be done with great care to avoid precipitation of further bleeding. Clotting factors can be consumed rapidly, and the nurse should be alert to signs of generalized bleeding.

Pleural Effusions

Pleural effusions may be caused by accumulation of fluid between the parietal pleura of the chest wall and the visceral pleura enveloping the lung. A pleural effusion may also be due to chylothorax (lymphatic fluid) or hemothorax (blood). Lymphatics drain fluid that filters into the pleural space. Fluid accumulates in the pleural space as a result of either increased filtration or decreased absorption. An increase in filtration pressure, as seen with increased venous pressure in hydrops fetalis or congestive heart failure, leads to pleural effusion. The rate of filtration into the pleural space also increases if the pleural membrane becomes more permeable to water and protein, as occurs with infection.

Pleural effusion with high glucose content in an infant who is receiving parenteral nutrition via a central venous catheter should raise the suspicion of catheter perforation into the pleural space. If the infant is also receiving lipid infusion, the fluid may appear milky and be confused with chylothorax.

Chylothorax may be congenital or acquired and is associated with obstruction or perforation of the thoracic duct. It may also be a surgical complication of repair of diaphragmatic hernia, tracheoesophageal fistula, or congenital heart defect. Congenital chylothorax may be suspected in the infant who cannot be ventilated in the delivery room. Breath sounds are difficult to hear, and chest movement with ventilation is minimal. Bilateral thoracenteses may be lifesaving. The typical pleural fluid in a chylothorax—opalescent and rich in fat—is present only if the infant has been fed.

Pleural effusions that impede respiratory function typically require drainage by thoracentesis or tube thoracostomy. It may be necessary for chest tubes placed for chylothorax and thoracic duct injury to remain in place for extended periods while the infant is given total parenteral nutrition, receiving nothing by mouth, thus minimizing thoracic duct flow.

Apnea

Apnea is the common end product of a myriad of neonatal physiologic events. Hypoxemia, infection, anemia, thermal instability, metabolic derangement, drugs, and intracranial disease can cause apnea. These causes should be ruled out before idiopathic apnea of prematurity is diagnosed.

Apnea is observed in more than half of surviving premature infants who weigh less than 1.5 kg at birth. The respiratory control mechanism and central responsiveness to carbon dioxide is progressively less mature the lower the gestational age. In contrast to adults, infants respond to hypoxemia with only a brief hyperpneic response followed by hypoventilation or apnea. In any infant who has apnea, hypoxemia should always be ruled out before the clinician embarks on any other workup or institutes therapy.

Care of the infant experiencing apneic episodes requires close observation. Obstructive apnea cannot be detected with the impedance respiratory monitor because normal or pronounced respiratory excursions of the chest wall exist. Prompt tactile stimulation for mild "spells" is often sufficient to abort the episode of apnea, obviating the need for further therapy. Infants with apneic episodes accompanied by profound bradycardia need prompt attention to their immediate needs as well as more aggressive diagnostic and therapeutic intervention.

Sensory stimulation with waterbeds or other means can sometimes be used to manage these infants, particularly those with mild apnea. Many apneic neonates respond to nasal CPAP at low pressures because the apnea may be due to airway obstruction or intermittent hypoxemia. Pressure support may also stimulate pulmonary stretch receptors, thus stimulating respiration. Nursing care that is directed toward promoting a neutral thermal environment, normoxia, optimal airway maintenance, and prevention of aspiration is essential in the care of neonates at risk for apnea.

Use of methylxanthines, such as caffeine and aminophylline, has markedly simplified the treatment of apnea in some premature infants. Xanthines appear to exert a central stimulatory effect on brainstem respiratory neurons and often markedly decrease the frequency and severity of apneic episodes. The clinician must be attuned to the toxicities of xanthines, including tachycardia, excessive diuresis, and vomiting, which may precede neurologic toxicity at inadvertently high blood drug levels. Caffeine may be associated with a lower risk of adverse effects (Schmidt et al, 2006).

CONGENITAL ANOMALIES THAT AFFECT RESPIRATORY FUNCTION

Diaphragmatic Hernia

Congenital diaphragmatic hernia (CDH) occurs at a frequency of 1 in 2500 live births and may be unsuspected until birth. Herniation of abdominal contents into the chest cavity early in gestation is accompanied by ipsilateral pulmonary hypoplasia. By mechanisms that are not well understood, there is often some degree of pulmonary hypoplasia on the contralateral side. Most infants are symptomatic at birth, with severe respiratory distress in the delivery room. The affected newborn's abdomen is usually scaphoid, and breath sounds are absent on the side of the defect (a left-sided defect occurs in 90% of cases). Bowel sounds may be heard in the chest, and heart sounds may be heard on the right side because the herniated abdominal contents push the mediastinum to the right.

As soon as the diagnosis is suspected, bag and mask ventilation should be avoided because it fills the hernia contents with gas and can compress the lungs and worsen ventilation. When CDH has been diagnosed prenatally, the infant should be intubated and mechanical ventilation should be begun immediately after birth. An orogastric tube should be placed to aid in decompression of the herniated abdominal viscera. Ventilation should be attempted with a rapid rate and low inflation pressure and tolerating hypercapnia. Symptomatic neonates often have pulmonary hypertension and progressive right-to-left shunting. Hypotension is common, and, when adequate intravascular volume is established, dopamine infusion may be helpful. Pulmonary vasodilators have been advocated by some clinicians and have met with variable success, but they should not be used unless adequate systemic blood pressure can be maintained. Although evidence of surfactant deficiency in these newborns exists, surfactant administration does not appear to improve their clinical course or outcome (Colby et al, 2004).

Survival rate is poor in infants who are symptomatic at birth, and ECMO commonly is required, often to no avail. Surgery to repair the defect is indicated. Controversy regarding the urgency of the procedure exists among pediatric surgeons, and some prefer to stabilize the patient with mechanical ventilation, vasopressors, and correction of acidosis before undertaking surgical intervention; others perform surgical repair while the patient is maintained on ECMO (see Chapter 3).

Congenital Heart Disease

Congenital heart disease commonly manifests with signs of respiratory distress. Neonates with congenital heart disease and who demonstrate right-to-left shunting and decreased pulmonary blood flow (e.g., tetralogy of Fallot, pulmonary valve atresia, and tricuspid valve atresia or stenosis) usually present with profound cyanosis unresponsive to oxygen supplementation. Neonates with congenital heart disease and who demonstrate increased pulmonary blood flow or obstruction to the left outflow tract (e.g., transposition of the great vessels, total anomalous pulmonary venous return, atrioventricular canal, hypoplastic left heart syndrome, and critical coarctation of the aorta) may transiently improve with oxygen supplementation. Neonates with non-cyanotic lesions such as patent ductus arteriosus and ventricular septal defect may present with signs of congestive heart failure (see Chapter 3).

Choanal Atresia

Choanal atresia causes upper airway obstruction in the neonate. The choanae, or nasal passages, are separated from the nasopharynx by a structure known as the bucconasal membrane, which normally perforates during gestation. Failure of this developmental event results in an obstructed airway, occurring bilaterally in 50% of cases. Most affected infants are female and half of affected infants have associated anomalies as CHARGE (coloboma, heart defects, atresia of the choanae, retardation of growth and development, genital and urinary abnormalities, and ear abnormalities and/or hearing loss) association. Because newborns are obligate nasal breathers, they have chest retractions and severe cyanosis (particularly during feeding), and paradoxically turn pink when crying. Emergency treatment consists of tracheal intubation or placement of an oral airway. Surgical correction is indicated (Park et al, 2000).

Cystic Hygroma

A variety of space-occupying lesions can impose on the airway of the newborn (Box 1-4). Most are derived from embryonic tissues. Cystic hygroma, derived from lymphatic tissue, is the most common lateral neck mass in the newborn. It is multilobular, is multicystic, and, when large, obstructs the airway. Surgery is curative, although it is sometimes technically difficult. The clinician must always be mindful of the airway and its patency. Many of these lesions are of great cosmetic concern and cause great distress in the parents. A care plan should address these parental concerns. It is sometimes helpful to facilitate contact with parents of other children with similar problems who can share similar experiences.

BOX 1-4

Thoracic Cysts and Tumors That May Cause Respiratory Distress in the Neonate

Teratoma
Cystic hygroma
- Neurogenic tumor
- Neuroblastoma
- Ganglioneuroma
- Neurofibroma
Bronchial or bronchogenic cyst
Intrapulmonary cyst
Gastrogenic cyst
Hemangioma
Angiosarcoma
Mediastinal goiter
Thymoma
Mesenchymoma
Lipoma
Cystic adenomatous malformation

Adapted from Battista MA, Carlo WA (1992). Differential diagnosis of acute respiratory distress in the neonate. *Tufts University School of Medicine and Floating Hospital for Children reports on neonatal respiratory diseases* 2(3):1-4, 9-11.

Pierre Robin Syndrome or Sequence

The major feature of Pierre Robin syndrome or sequence is micrognathia (a small mandible). The tongue is posteriorly displaced into the oropharynx, thus obstructing the airway. Sixty percent of affected patients also have a cleft palate. Obstructive respiratory distress and cyanosis are common and may be severe. In an emergency, as with all airway obstructions (obstructive apnea), tracheal intubation should be undertaken. Infants with Pierre Robin syndrome or sequence are nursed in the prone position to prevent the tongue from falling backward. Nasogastric tube feedings are usually required in the neonatal period. With good care, the infant has a good prognosis for survival; the mandible usually grows; and the problem resolves by 6 to 12 months of age.

The newer term for this condition, in many cases, is *sequence*, but syndrome can also be used because the clusters of symptoms can occur in many ways. Sequence refers to a pattern that is a result of a single problem in morphogenesis that leads to this variety of problems. Syndrome is usually used when no one determinant can be identified. For example, it may result from multifactorial inheritance, may be part of other conditions, or may be genetic (whereby one or more genes are responsible). Thus this condition is more than just an explainable, describable syndrome or a sequence of visible defects (Tewfik et al, 2006; Van den Elsen et al, 2001).

COLLABORATIVE MANAGEMENT OF INFANTS WITH RESPIRATORY DISORDERS
Supportive Care

Supportive care of the infant in respiratory distress requires attention to detail. The clinicians' primary goals are to minimize oxygen consumption and carbon dioxide production. These goals are accomplished by maintaining a neutral thermal environment. The nurse must be skilled in physical assessment to interpret signs and symptoms, such as cyanosis, gasping, tachypnea, grunting, nasal flaring, and retractions. By understanding the pathophysiology of breathing, the nurse knows that the infant with retractions has decreased lung compliance and that the cyanotic infant has poor tissue oxygenation.

Excellent communication is needed between the neonatal nurse and the rest of the neonatal team. Acutely ill neonates with respiratory disease are often unstable and their condition can deteriorate rapidly, so astute observation skills are necessary. Assessment is a continuous process, and effective communication among nurses, respiratory therapists, physicians, and support staff is necessary for proper delivery of intensive care. The nurse, who is the primary bedside caregiver, is the gatekeeper for all interactions between the patient and the environment. The nurse who is caring for an unstable patient should be the patient's advocate, whether such a role involves regulating the timing of a physical examination by the physician or venipuncture for laboratory investigation.

Technical competence is an important facet of the nurse's repertoire. The nurse is responsible for maintaining intravenous lines and tracheal tube patency, accurately measuring volumes of intravenous intake as well as urinary output, and operating advanced electronic machinery. Moreover, the nurse must also be adept at interpreting arterial blood gas and laboratory data in order to communicate these to the rest of the care team and to develop a cogent management plan. Many functions are shared to some degree with respiratory therapists. Whether nurses or respiratory therapists make ventilator changes, the nurse should become familiar with the effects of ventilator setting changes on blood gases. $PaCO_2$ is affected by changes in ventilator rate and tidal volume. Tidal volume depends on the difference between PIP and PEEP. Thus, to decrease $PaCO_2$, either rate or inspiratory pressure should be increased. PaO_2 depends on the fraction of inspired oxygen concentration (FiO_2) and mean airway pressure (MAP). MAP depends on PIP, PEEP, inspiratory to expiratory time ratio, and gas flow. To improve PaO_2, the most effective changes are to increase MAP by increasing PIP or PEEP or to increase FiO_2. Table 1-3 shows the effect of ventilator setting changes on blood gases. The nurse should also be familiar with ventilator functioning so that malfunctions can be detected promptly. The nurse should always be prepared to bag-ventilate an intubated neonate in the event that decompensation occurs while the status of the ventilatory apparatus is checked. Nurses and therapists often share such functions as airway suctioning, monitoring and recording of inspired oxygen concentration, and delivery of chest physical therapy.

The delivery of oxygen therapy should always be carefully monitored. Desired oxygenation parameters should be recorded in the nurse's notes and followed up with measurement of arterial blood gases or by noninvasive means. The acutely ill infant should have FiO_2 measured continuously and recorded frequently. The goal for oxygenation depends on the patient's diagnosis and condition. For example, in infants with PPHN, an apparently acceptable saturation may occur despite marked right-to-left shunting. In preterm infants oxygen saturation can be kept in the high 80s and low 90s, thus avoiding the risks associated with hyperoxia in preterm infants (The STOP-ROP Multicenter Study Group, 2000). Higher oxygen saturations do not improve growth or neurodevelopment (Askie et al,

TABLE 1-3	Effects of Ventilator Setting Changes on Blood Gases		
Ventilator Setting Changes		**PaCO₂**	**PaO₂**
↑ PIP		Ø	↑
↑ PEEP		↑	↑
↑ Frequency		Ø	± ↑
↑ I:E ratio		æ	↑
↑ FiO₂		æ	↑
↑ Flow		±Ø	± ↑

↑ , Increase; Ø, decrease; ±, minimal effect; æ, no consistent effect; FiO_2, fraction of O_2 in dry inspired air; PEEP, positive end-expiratory pressure; PIP, peak inspiratory pressure.
Modified from Carlo WA et al (1994). Advances in conventional mechanical ventilation. In Boynton BR et al, editors. New therapies for neonatal respiratory failure, p 144. Cambridge University Press: New York.

2003) but increase the risk for retinopathy of prematurity. Procedures such as suctioning, chest physiotherapy, and handling may lead to desaturations and may have to be minimized.

Airway suctioning is a procedure that may be associated with cardiopulmonary derangement, hypoxemia, bradycardia, and hypertension. Various techniques to perform airway suctioning exist—including preoxygenation (increase in FiO_2 before the procedure), normal saline instillation before the suctioning to improve secretion aspiration, and the use of a closed system to avoid disconnection from the ventilator. The nurse should become familiar with the techniques used in the NICU and be aware of the associated complications.

The sudden decompensation of a ventilated infant should alert the nurse to assess disconnection of the ventilator, pulmonary air leak, ventilator failure, or obstructed tracheal tube (see Figure 1-4). The very small infant who suddenly decompensates may have experienced a severe intracranial hemorrhage.

Care of the infant who is receiving CPAP can be particularly challenging. These infants should be kept calm and swaddled if necessary. Crying releases pressure through the mouth; thus lung volume is lost. Nasal CPAP can be effective, but particular attention must be given to maintaining patency of the nose, the nasal prongs, and the pharynx. The infant's nares and nasal septum should be guarded from pressure necrosis from inappropriately applied prongs. The infant who requires mechanical ventilation must be constantly assessed for airway patency. If the infant is unable to grunt against a closed glottis and maintain positive airway pressure, the condition may worsen if airway pressure is not maintained properly. Suctioning of the airway should be done only as often as necessary to remove pulmonary secretions that could occlude the airway. The suction catheter should be passed no further than the end of the tracheal tube because epithelium is easily damaged. Vibration and percussion should be used judiciously in the infant with pulmonary secretions to loosen them and allow removal via suction. There is perhaps little need to vigorously suction the intubated infant with RDS in the first days after birth because secretions are minimal and lung volume is lost with every disconnection of the ventilator circuit.

ASSESSMENT AND MONITORING

The most important aspect in monitoring patients with respiratory disease is the close and continuous observation of signs and symptoms. The color of the patient gives important clues. An infant with pink lips and oral mucosa has good oxygenation and perfusion; a cyanotic patient has poor tissue oxygenation. If the hemoglobin concentration is too low, the patient can be hypoxemic, but because the concentration of deoxyhemoglobin is low, there may be no cyanosis. An infant with tachypnea and retraction usually has decreased lung compliance. A patient with a barrel-shaped thorax, taking deep breaths, and with a normal or low respiratory rate probably has an increased airway resistance and gas trapping. Observation of the intubated patient is especially important. An anguished infant, who is cyanotic and breathing deeply, may have an obstructed endotracheal tube. An infant with RDS and increased chest expansion over time, despite no change in ventilatory pressure, is experiencing improvement in lung compliance. The same infant with later asymmetry in chest and sudden deterioration of oxygenation may have a pneumothorax. Cardiac beats, easily seen through the thoracic wall, may be caused by the presence of a symptomatic patent ductus arteriosus. A recently extubated infant, in whom increased retractions and inspiratory stridor develop, probably has upper airway obstruction. Auscultation helps in the diagnosis of increased airway resistance or the presence of secretions. It also allows the clinician to assess the response to different treatment maneuvers, such as suctioning, chest physiotherapy, and bronchodilation. Asymmetries in auscultation suggest mainstream bronchial intubation, atelectasis, pneumothorax, or pleural effusion.

Great progress has been made in noninvasive monitoring of blood gas tensions, but blood sampling is still necessary for pH determination and arterial samples are preferable. Capillary specimens are undependable, especially for PO_2. If peripheral perfusion is adequate, capillary blood approximates arterial values of pH and PCO_2. However, capillary blood PO_2 values do not reliably reflect arterial oxygenation.

Neonatal care has changed dramatically with the advent and widespread use of transcutaneous monitoring of PaO_2, $PaCO_2$, and SaO_2. The neonatal intensive care team should become familiar with the devices used in noninvasive gas monitoring. Knowing the basis for their functioning as well as how to interpret the information they provide and being aware of clinical situations in which the information provided is not reliable or needs to be complemented before any management decisions are made is essential.

Transcutaneous PO_2 ($TcPO_2$) is measured with an electrode that is applied over the skin and heated to 42° C to 44° C. The electrode measures skin PO_2, not arterial PO_2. Skin PO_2 measurement depends on skin perfusion and on oxygen diffusion across the epidermis. Warming the skin to 42° C to 44° C under the electrode increases skin perfusion so that $TcPO_2$ correlates better with arterial PO_2. For initiation of $TcPO_2$ monitoring, 10 to 15 minutes are needed to obtain a stable reading. After that, $TcPO_2$ reflects changes on FiO_2 with a 10- to 20-second delay. After 4 to 6 hours, the method becomes unreliable because of changes in skin secondary to hyperthermia, so the electrode position should be changed. In premature infants with more labile skin, the electrode placement should be changed even more frequently to avoid skin burns. The nurse should be aware of situations that make $TcPO_2$ lose its reliability. Overestimation of oxygenation occurs when an air bubble or leak between the electrode and the skin occurs or when the calibration is improper. Underestimation occurs with skin hypoperfusion, in older infants (increased thickness of the skin), with insufficient heating of the electrodes, or with improper calibration.

$TcPO_2$ monitoring has been largely supplanted by continuous pulse oximetry. Arterial oxygen saturation is computed from absorption of emitted low-intensity red or infrared light. The probe is attached to a finger or toe in large infants or to a hand or foot in small premature infants. Pulse oximetry offers the following advantages over transcutaneous oxygen monitoring: (1) avoidance of heating the skin and the risk of burns; (2) elimination of a delay period for transducer equilibration; (3) accurate measurement regardless of presence of edema or patient age; (4) in vitro calibration not required; and (5) frequent position changes not required. However, the nurse should be aware that SaO_2 higher than 97% may be associated with PaO_2 higher than 100 mm Hg. This is important in premature infants who are at risk for retinopathy of prematurity. SaO_2 between 85% and 95% probably is associated with a safe range of PaO_2. With SaO_2 over 95% to 97%—and especially when it is 100%—the clinician cannot predict a patient's PaO_2. When the saturation is 100%, the PaO_2 can be approximately 100 mm Hg or much higher (see Figure 1-1). This situation is particularly important in infants with PPHN because the decision whether to wean ventilator settings depends on PaO_2. In these patients, the simultaneous use of $TcPO_2$ and pulse oximetry is a useful alternative.

A common problem of pulse oximetry is the presence of motion artifact, an altered signal caused by movement of the part of the body where the sensor is applied. Because the pulse waveform is not detected, this movement is recognized by the loss of correlation between the oximeter pulse rate and the electrical monitor heart rate. With new technology the motion artifacts have been minimized (Malviya et al, 2000). Peripheral pulse oximetry may not detect pulse signals in patients with hypotension and poor perfusion. $TcPO_2$ may also give false readings in this situation. The clinician should be aware that pressure of the probe over the skin can produce skin pressure necrosis. This consideration is particularly important in the premature infant. Phototherapy may interfere with accuracy of SaO_2 monitoring, but this problem can be avoided by covering the sensor with an opaque material (e.g., a diaper).

$TcPO_2$ monitoring and pulse oximetry are useful in several clinical situations. They may be used in neonates with mild respiratory distress, such as transient tachypnea, to assess the oxygen requirement and to allow weaning without placement of an arterial catheter. In infants receiving mechanical ventilation, $TcPO_2$ or pulse oximetry helps to assess the effects of ventilator setting changes, thus reducing the need for arterial blood sampling. Continuous oxygenation monitoring reduces the risk of hyperoxemia or hypoxemia during interventions such as airway suctioning, position change, lumbar puncture, or venous cannulation. This monitoring is particularly helpful in the care of infants who do not tolerate excessive stimulation, such as those with PPHN. $TcPO_2$ and pulse-oximetry monitoring are also useful in caring for patients with PPHN because simultaneous monitoring of preductal (head, right arm, right upper chest) and postductal (left arm, abdomen, legs) $TcPO_2$ or SaO_2 allows assessment of the magnitude of ductal shunting or the response to therapies such as vasodilation or alkalinization.

Transcutaneously measured PCO_2 is accomplished with a glass electrode that is pH-sensitive. Transcutaneous PCO_2 response is slower than that of $TcPO_2$, and the value measured must be corrected for skin production of carbon dioxide. Thus transcutaneously measured values are approximately 1.3 to 1.4 times higher than arterial PCO_2 values. Most modern monitors display an electronically corrected value to $TcPO_2$. This modality is especially useful for monitoring chronically ventilated patients without indwelling catheters. Blood gas values during arterial puncture or vigorous crying during the procedure are often affected by breath holding and shunting and thus may be misleading.

ENVIRONMENTAL CONSIDERATIONS

Maintenance of the therapeutic environment is an important nursing function. Much attention has been given recently to the effects of sensory stimulation on the infant with respiratory distress. The sick newborn often has unstable pulmonary vasculature and may be particularly prone to hypoxic vasoconstriction. This phenomenon may be triggered in some individuals by excess stimulation, such as loud noise, handling, or venipuncture. It has been shown that the agitated neonate has more difficulty with oxygenation and that a quiet, minimally stimulating environment allows for more stable oxygena-tion (Als, 1998). The nurse should develop a care plan that allows the baby long periods of undisturbed rest by clustering interventions into short periods whenever possible. Positioning the infant in the flexed or fetal position or "nesting" may help in calming some infants.

FAMILY CARE

Neonates with respiratory distress frequently require multiple instrumentation. They may have endotracheal tubes, umbilical catheters, oximeter probes, chest leads, and other paraphernalia attached or applied to the skin. All of these interventions can give parents an unnatural feeling or increased separation from the infant. The nurse should explain the equipment surrounding the bedside as well as the function of invasive catheters, monitoring leads, and tracheal tubes. Terminology appropriate to the parents' level of understanding should be used. Even the most astute parents may be bewildered, and repetition is necessary. Staff should maintain consistent terminology so that the parents do not become confused between "respirators" and "ventilators." Whenever possible, the use of frightening or inaccurate terms should be avoided. Imagine the fear engendered by the phrase, "We paralyzed your baby last night."

Parents should be involved in developing and implementing the plan of care as much as possible. The mother who plans to breastfeed can be assisted in pumping her breasts and

Case Study

IDENTIFICATION OF THE PROBLEM

A term infant was admitted to the NICU. The infant developed respiratory distress soon after birth. Birth weight was 4000 g. Since birth, the infant had an increasing oxygen requirement and because of a recent desaturation episode, he is now receiving 100% oxygen on a ventilator. The ventilatory settings are peak inspiratory pressure of 25 cm H_2O, positive end-expiratory pressure of 5 cm H_2O, ventilator rate 60 per minute, and inspiratory time 0.4 seconds.

ASSESSMENT: HISTORY AND PHYSICAL EXAMINATION

The infant was born by emergency C-section because of late desaturations and thick meconium-stained fluid. No signs of infection were observed. The infant was not vigorous at birth and was intubated and received endotracheal suction. No meconium was aspirated from the endotracheal tube. Blow-by oxygen was given and the infant responded well, initially weaning to 40% oxygen. However, after transfer to the NICU, he had increasing oxygen requirements.

The physical examination is now pertinent for excellent chest rise, equal breath sounds, central cyanosis with oxygen saturations in the mid-80s, good color and perfusion, and normal tone and reflexes.

DIFFERENTIAL DIAGNOSIS

Many conditions may be considered the differential diagnosis in this patient.

1. **Persistent pulmonary hypertension of the neonate.** This is a likely possibility given the severity and persistence of the very abnormal alveolar to arterial oxygen gradient ($AaDO_2$). Pulmonary hypertension may be associated with meconium aspiration syndrome. It is important to consider that right-to-left shunting can occur associated with disorders such as myocardial dysfunction, sepsis, metabolic abnormalities, and others.

2. **Meconium aspiration syndrome.** Meconium aspiration syndrome with intrapulmonary (ventilation-perfusion mismatch) or extrapulmonary shunting (atrial or ductal shunting with pulmonary hypertension) may lead to desaturation despite high oxygen supplementation.

3. **Pneumothorax.** Infants with meconium aspiration syndrome are at high risk for pneumothorax. A pneumothorax can cause severe desaturation.

4. **Gas trapping.** Because this infant has a large tidal volume for the given pressure gradient (positive inspiratory pressure [PIP] minus positive end-expiratory pressure [PEEP]) and thus high compliance, a long-time constant of the respiratory system leading to gas

Continued

Case Study—cont'd

trapping at a borderline high ventilator rate should be considered.

5. **Other causes.** There are other less frequent causes in the differential diagnosis.

DIAGNOSTIC TESTS

The chest radiograph was obtained, repeat blood gases were followed, and pre- and postductal pulse oximetry and transcutaneous measurements of gases were monitored continuously. In addition, a CBC and blood culture were obtained. Four extremity blood pressures and an echocardiogram were obtained.

WORKING DIAGNOSIS

The chest radiograph showed bilateral gas trapping. The CBC and the blood cultures were negative. The echocar-

diogram was consistent with persistent pulmonary hypertension.

DEVELOPMENT OF MANAGEMENT PLAN

The infant was given surfactant and initial improvement was seen. However, during the next 24 hours there were episodes of repeated intracardiac and ductal shunting, which lead to the initiation of nitric oxide.

IMPLEMENTATION AND EVALUATION OF EFFECTIVENESS

Nitric oxide resulted in a marked reduction of the shunting episodes. The infant was gradually weaned off FiO_2 and subsequently weaned off nitric oxide before extubation. He was entirely weaned off the ventilator and FiO_2 over the subsequent 3 days.

---

freezing the milk, even if enteral feedings are delayed for some time. This pumping may be the only thing that she alone can do for her baby.

Often lost in the bustle of critical care is the need for privacy. The perceptive nurse senses this need and backs away from the bedside when appropriate, allowing the parent some time with the infant.

SUMMARY

Most infants admitted to the NICU present with breathing difficulty. Nursing care of these infants requires a broad knowledge of newborn physiology and practical skills in the application of therapies that are directed toward solving the many problems that sick infants can have. The nurse often must anticipate these problems. While managing the nursing care for several patients, the neonatal nurse must also care for the sickest of infants. Parents and family of all infants in the NICU require special attention not only to achieve an understanding of the complex issues surrounding the infant's illness but also to calm fears and guilt that are often experienced. The rewards of being part of the accomplishments in the NICU may be overlooked as they are usually slowly achieved. But, when they are recognized, the victories surpass the greatest of expectations.

REFERENCES

Als H (1998). Developmental care in the newborn intensive care unit. *Current opinion in pediatrics* 10:138-142.

American Lung Association (ALA) (2006). Lung disease data at a glance: Respiratory distress syndrome (RDS). Available at: http://www.lungusa.org/site/pp.asp?c=dvLUK9O0E&b=327819. Accessed May 28, 2006.

Askie LM et al (2003). Oxygen-saturation targets and outcomes in extremely preterm infants. *New England journal of medicine* 349:959-967.

Bates MD, Balistreri WF (2002). The neonatal gastrointestinal tract: part one: development of the human digestive system. In Fanaroff AA, Martin RJ, editors. *Neonatal-perinatal medicine: diseases of the fetus and infant*, ed 7. St Louis: Mosby.

Clark DA, Clark MB (2004). Meconium aspiration syndrome. eMedicine from WebMD. Available at: http://www.emedicine.com/PED/topic768.htm. Accessed May 27, 2006.

Colby CE et al (2004). Surfactant replacement therapy on ECMO does not improve outcome in neonates with congenital diaphragmatic hernia. *Journal of pediatric surgery* 39:1632-1637.

Cordero L et al (2000). Comparison of a closed (trach care MAC) with an open endotracheal suction system in small premature infants. *Journal of perinatology* 20:151-156.

Davidson D et al (1998). Inhaled nitric oxide for the early treatment of persistent pulmonary hypertension of the term newborn: a randomized, double-masked, placebo-controlled, dose-response multicenter study. *Pediatrics* 101:325-334.

Ehrenkranz RA et al (2005). Validation of the National Institutes of Health consensus definition of bronchopulmonary dysplasia. *Pediatrics* 116:1353-1360.

Greenough A, Miner AD (2005). Pulmonary disease of the newborn. In Rennie JM, editor. *Roberton's textbook of neonatology*, 4th ed. London, England: Churchill Livingstone.

International Guidelines for Neonatal Resuscitation (2000). An excerpt from the Guidelines 2000 for Cardiopulmonary Resuscitation and Emergency Cardiovascular Care: International Consensus on Science. *Pediatrics* 106(3):E29. Available at: http://www.pediatrics.org/cgi/–content/—full/106/3/e29.

Jobe AH, Bancalari E (2001). Bronchopulmonary dysplasia. *American journal of respiratory critical care medicine* 163:1723-1729.

Lemons JA et al (2001). Very low birth weight outcomes of the National Institute of Child Health and Human Development Neonatal Research Network, January 1995 through December 1996. *Pediatrics* 107:E1.

Malviya S et al (2000). False alarms and sensitivity of conventional pulse oximetry versus the Masimo SET technology in the pediatric postanesthesia care unit. *Anesthesia & analgesia* 90(6):1336-1340.

Mok Q et al (1999). Persistent pulmonary hypertension of the term neonate: a strategy for management. *European journal of pediatrics* 158:825-827.

Park AH et al (2000). Endoscopic versus traditional approaches to choanal atresia. *Otolaryngology clinics of North America* 33:77-90.

Schmidt B et al (2006). Caffeine therapy for apnea of prematurity. *New England journal of medicine* 354(20):2179-2180.

Soll RF, Morley CJ (2001). Prophylactic versus selective use of surfactant for preventing morbidity and mortality in preterm infants. *Cochrane database of systematic reviews* 2:CD000510.

The Neonatal Inhaled Nitric Oxide Study Group (1997). Inhaled nitric oxide in full-term and nearly full-term infants with hypoxic respiratory failure. *New England journal of medicine* 336(9):597-604.

The STOP-ROP Multicenter Study Group (2000). Supplemental therapeutic oxygen for prethreshold retinopathy of prematurity (STOP-ROP): a randomized, controlled trial. I: Primary outcomes. *Pediatrics* 105:295-310.

Tewfik TL et al (2006). Pierre Robin syndrome. eMedicine from WebMD. Available at: http://www.emedicine.com/ent/topic150.htm. Accessed May 27, 2006.

Thome UH et al (2005). Ventilation strategies and outcome in randomised trials of high frequency ventilation. *Archives of disease in childhood: fetal and neonatal edition* 90:F466-473.

UK Collaborative ECMO Trial Group (1996). UK collaborative randomised trial of neonatal extracorporeal membrane oxygenation. *Lancet* 348(9020):75-82.

Vain NE et al (2004). Oropharyngeal and nasopharyngeal suctioning of meconium-stained neonates before delivery of their shoulders: multicentre, randomised controlled trial. *Lancet* 364:597-602.

Van den Elsen AP et al (2001). Diagnosis and treatment of the Pierre Robin sequence: results of a retrospective clinical study and review of the literature. *European journal of pediatrics* 160:47-53.

Walsh-Sukys MC et al (2000). Persistent pulmonary hypertension of the newborn in the era before nitric oxide: practice variation and outcomes. *Pediatrics* 105:14-20.

Wiswell TE et al (2000). Delivery room management of the apparently vigorous meconium-stained neonate: results of the multicenter, international collaborative trial. *Pediatrics* 105:1-7.

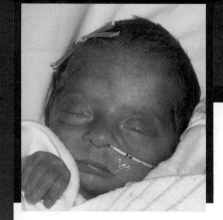

Chapter 2

Emerging Technologies for the Management of Respiratory Disorders

Waldemar A. Carlo

This chapter focuses on innovative technologies and newer strategies for the management of intractable hypoxemia and respiratory failure in the newborn. These include exogenous surfactant administration, conventional and high-frequency ventilation, inhaled nitric oxide, extracorporeal membrane oxygenation, and liquid ventilation. Discussion of these technologies and strategies requires understanding of the pathophysiology of neonatal hypoxemia as well as the standard treatments for hypoxemia in the newborn. Neonatal cardiorespiratory physiology and the physiology of transition are discussed in depth later in this book and will only briefly be covered in this chapter.

NEONATAL HYPOXEMIA

In the neonate, the transition from complete dependence on the maternal-placental unit for oxygenation to complete respiratory self-reliance must occur rapidly and requires a cascade of immediate responses (Table 2-1). The central nervous system responds to changes in oxygen and carbon dioxide tensions by generating the necessary efferent signals to establish a regular respiratory pattern. The chest wall and its respiratory muscles must have sufficient stiffness and strength to respond to the signals received from the central nervous system. The pulmonary blood flow must be adequate for the delivery of oxygen from the alveolus to the body, and shunting through the ductus arteriosus and foramen ovale must be minimal. Adequate cardiac output is needed to deliver oxygen to the tissues, and the affinity of hemoglobin for oxygen must allow oxygen release to the tissues. All of the above responses need to occur within minutes of birth, and, unsurprisingly, a large proportion of the problems in the neonatal intensive care unit (NICU) relate to tissue oxygenation.

For numerous reasons outlined in the following sections, preterm newborns are at particular risk for hypoxemia during extrauterine transition. The respiratory control center of the preterm infant often lacks sufficient maturity to sustain regular respiration, as manifested by the frequent occurrence of periodic breathing and apnea. The chest wall may be highly compliant, which leads to inefficient breathing and causes inward or expiratory movement of the rib cage (retractions) during inspiration. The highly compliant chest wall is often confronted with a stiff lung (low compliance) because of surfactant deficiency. This problem causes increased work for the respiratory muscles. The preterm ductus arteriosus also may remain patent and shunt blood away from the systemic organs. Furthermore, the preterm newborn's blood hemoglobin concentration is lower than that of the full-term newborn, thereby limiting oxygen-carrying capacity. Finally, there are limits to how much the preterm infant can increase cardiac output to respond to increased oxygen demand or other deficits in oxygen delivery.

Term newborns have different problems that may interfere with the ability to establish adequate tissue oxygenation at birth. Aspiration of meconium, infectious pneumonia, retained fetal lung fluid, and air-leak syndromes are some examples of respiratory disorders that can cause intrapulmonary shunting, hypoxemia, and increase work of breathing. Hypoxemia, whether caused by a known respiratory disorder or idiopathic in nature, can result in pulmonary arterioles that remain constricted rather than dilate normally. Constricted pulmonary arterioles elevate pulmonary vascular resistance and lead to a vicious cycle of right-to-left (pulmonary-to-systemic) shunting, maintenance of pulmonary vasoconstriction, and protracted neonatal hypoxemia. This condition is called persistent pulmonary hypertension of the newborn (PPHN).

Two additional threats to normal tissue oxygenation at birth are anemia and polycythemia. A variety of events may lead to neonatal anemia—including abruptio placenta, placenta previa, fetal-maternal hemorrhage, trauma to the cord or fetal placental vessels, and timing of cord clamping. Anemia results in a diminished oxygen-carrying capacity and thus an increased risk for inadequate tissue oxygenation. Polycythemia may be caused by intrauterine events such as chronic hypoxia and twin-to-twin transfusion or extrauterine events such as delayed cord clamping. Paradoxically, polycythemia increases blood oxygen-carrying capacity but may decrease tissue oxygen delivery by causing poor tissue blood flow from hyperviscosity.

CONVENTIONAL MANAGEMENT OF NEONATAL HYPOXEMIA

The perinatal caregiver's first line of defense for the prevention or treatment of hypoxemia is an increased inspired oxygen

TABLE 2-1	The Neonatal Respiratory System
Components	**Functions**
Central and peripheral nervous system	Control of breathing
Chest wall (ribs and respiratory muscles)	Pump
Pulmonary circulation	Oxygen uptake from alveoli
Hemoglobin	Oxygen transport
Systemic cardiac output	Oxygen delivery
Mitochondria	Oxygen-dependent energy production

concentration. Although fetal hypoxemia does not respond dramatically to an increase of maternal inspired oxygen concentrations, providing oxygen by mask or nasal cannula to mothers whose fetuses show signs of hypoxia is an accepted mode of therapy in most obstetrical units. Administration of oxygen dramatically increases maternal arterial oxygen tension (PaO_2) but increases fetal PaO_2 by only a few millimeters of mercury. However, because fetal PaO_2 is on the steep portion of the oxygen-hemoglobin dissociation curve, small changes in fetal PaO_2 are associated with relatively large increases in fetal blood-oxygen content.

After birth, the response to an increased inspired oxygen concentration in the hypoxic newborn depends on the cause of the hypoxemia. When hypoxemia is caused by hypoventilation, PaO_2 increases in an approximately one-to-one relationship with alveolar oxygen tension. Thus the PaO_2 increases by approximately 60 mm Hg in the hypoventilating newborn who is placed in 30% oxygen. On the other hand, when hypoxemia is caused by an intrapulmonary or extrapulmonary right-to-left shunt (pulmonary-to-systemic shunt), the neonatal PaO_2 increases minimally in response to an increased inspired oxygen concentration. For example, a newborn with a 50% right-to-left shunt (i.e., 50% of right ventricular output does not pass through the lungs) has a PaO_2 of approximately 50 to 55 mm Hg in room air. Placing the newborn in a head hood that contains 100% oxygen may raise the PaO_2 to only 60 to 65 mm Hg. In infants with right-to-left shunts who are placed on oxygen, blood oxygen content may increase significantly because of the position and shape of the oxygen-hemoglobin dissociation curve, although little is gained in terms of PaO_2. Although increasing the inspired oxygen concentration in the hypoxemic newborn may be essential to prevent permanent cell injury or cell death, this benefit must be weighed against the risk for chronic lung disease due to the toxic effects of pulmonary oxygen.

Another technique used in the newborn at risk for hypoxemia is the maintenance of an adequate oxygen-carrying capacity by intermittent blood transfusion. Although few scientific studies have been published, it is empirically accepted that prevention and treatment of anemia in the newborn with cardiorespiratory disease are important aspects of management. For example, transfusion of infants with bronchopulmonary dysplasia results in decreased use of oxygen. Some studies support the administration of human erythropoietin combined with iron supplementation to reduce the risk of repeated blood transfusions. In one study using this treatment, patients received significantly fewer transfusions (1.0 vs 2.9) than did controls (Carnielli et al, 1998). However, this treatment may not be cost-effective because donor blood is usually split into quad packs, and therefore a small but significant reduction in number of transfusions would not reduce exposure to different blood donors.

Decreasing oxygen demand and thus minimizing the newborn's metabolic rate can reduce the risk for cell injury secondary to tissue hypoxia. Depending on the specific thermal environment, the neonatal energy (and oxygen) expenditure necessary to keep warm may be great or small. This relationship has been recognized for more than 40 years and has led to studies designed to define the thermal environment in which energy expended to keep warm is minimal (known as a neutral thermal environment). Attempts to create a near-neutral thermal environment have shown improved survival of sick premature newborns, presumably by favorably affecting the balance between oxygen demand and oxygen supply.

Another critical factor that affects the delivery of oxygen to the tissues is the adequacy of organ blood flow. Organ blood flow may be globally decreased because of decreased cardiac output, thus increasing the risk for tissue hypoxia. Methods commonly employed for maintenance of adequate cardiac output include volume expansion of the hypovolemic newborn and inotropic drugs to stimulate the poorly contractile myocardium. Clinical evaluation often is used to estimate cardiac output, including determination of the rate of capillary refill; determination of the presence or absence of acrocyanosis, skin mottling, or relative coolness of the extremities; and determination of pulse strength and blood pressure. Laboratory aids, including serial hematocrit determinations to diagnose acute blood loss and echocardiography to evaluate cardiac contractility, are at times helpful. Bedside evaluation of neonatal cardiac output is difficult, remains an inexact science, and has little benefit over the long term. Therefore, it will not be addressed in this text. Determination of the distribution of organ blood flow is also almost impossible. Even when cardiac output is normal or nearly normal, some organs suffer hypoxic insults because of low blood flow. If, for example, necrotizing enterocolitis results in part from decreased intestinal blood flow and thus decreased intestinal oxygenation, it would be useful to be able to estimate that flow. Similarly, decreased urine output may indicate decreased renal blood flow; however, waiting for changes in blood and urine chemistries (e.g., elevated creatinine) may mean that an irreversible renal hypoxic injury already has occurred. Rapid determination of the distribution of neonatal organ blood flow awaits the development of new methods.

A discussion of strategies now available in NICUs for the management of hypoxemia would not be complete without at least mentioning the widespread use of techniques for measuring or estimating blood-oxygen tension or blood-oxygen saturation. The direct measurement of PaO_2 and oxygen saturation in small samples of blood (0.1 to 0.2 ml) has been available for several years. Although they are not in widespread use, indwelling vascular catheters for the continuous measurement of blood PaO_2 or oxygen saturation are available. Perhaps the most significant technologic development for aiding the management of potentially hypoxic sick newborns has been noninvasive methods of measuring transcutaneous PaO_2 and transcutaneous oxygen saturation nearly continuously to provide fairly reliable estimations of blood-oxygen levels.

TREATMENT OF NEONATAL LUNG DISEASE WITH EXOGENOUS SURFACTANT

It has generally been accepted for more than 30 years that respiratory distress syndrome (RDS), or hyaline membrane disease, is associated with an abnormal gas-liquid interface in the lung. Normal airways contain a surface-active substance, now called surfactant that reduces airway and alveolar surface tension and therefore increases lung compliance. In the late 1950s, studies determined that the liquid found in the airways of premature infants and of infants whose mothers had diabetes and who died with RDS had a diminished ability to decrease surface tension in vitro (Avery & Mead, 1959; Pattle, 1958). Thus the hypothesis that decreased lung compliance in infants with RDS was due to lack of surfactant was developed.

RDS is characterized by diffuse pulmonary microatelectasis. Atelectasis causes tachypnea, low tidal-volume breathing, and increased work of breathing. Clinically, infants with RDS have retractions as a consequence of decreased lung compliance, expiratory grunting to prevent further atelectasis, and hypoxemia secondary to intrapulmonary shunting. RDS is therefore defined as the immediate onset after birth of tachypnea, retractions, grunting, and cyanosis in a premature infant or in an infant of a mother with diabetes. The chest radiograph in these patients usually confirms the presence of diffuse microatelectasis with uniform increased opacity of the alveolar portions of the lung and widespread air bronchograms. The arterial carbon dioxide tension ($PaCO_2$) may be either increased or normal, thus reflecting the infant's ability to compensate for decreased lung compliance. When the infant breathes room air, the PaO_2 is always decreased because of intrapulmonary shunting. The arterial hydrogen ion concentration (pH) reflects the presence or absence of an elevated $PaCO_2$ and the adequacy of tissue oxygenation. Infants with RDS often have both a metabolic and a respiratory acidosis.

Surfactant Biochemistry and Physiology

Surfactant is generally defined as the noncellular liquid found in the more distal airways and alveoli of normal lungs. Although surfactant contains a mixture of various phospholipids, proteins, and neutral lipids, the extent to which each of these components contributes to the surface tension decreasing properties of surfactant is not certain.

Surfactant is produced and secreted by cuboid type II pneumocytes that line the distal airways. Phospholipids and surfactant-specific proteins are packaged within intracellular lamellar bodies. These are secreted by exocytosis into the liquid lining layer of the airway. Within the hypophase of this liquid interface between the pneumocytes and lung gas, surfactant forms a regular microscopic latticework called tubular myelin. It is thought that surfactant exerts its surface tension decreasing activity by the movement of certain surfactant components from the hypophase to the gas-liquid interface. Surface tension is decreased by molecular interactions as the gas-liquid interface is compressed during expiration. An intrapulmonary conservation of surfactant, in which "used surfactant" is reabsorbed by the type II pneumocyte, is repackaged, and is resecreted, probably exists.

Surfactant Therapy

Surfactant therapy has been one of the major advances in the care of preterm infants (Table 2-2). Prophylactic and rescue administration of synthetic and natural surfactants have reduced important adverse outcomes, including mortality (Shah et al, 1999; Soll, 1998a, 1998b, 1999, 2000; Soll & Morley, 2001; Soll & Blanco, 2001; Yost & Soll, 1999). Specifically, neonatal mortality [relative risk (RR), confidence interval (CI), and number needed to treat (NNT)] is decreased with prophylactic (vs rescue) administration of both synthetic (23% to 17%; RR 0.70; CI 0.58, 0.85; NNT 15) and natural surfactant (12% to 7%; RR 0.61; CI 0.48, 0.77; NNT 24) (Shah et al, 1999; Soll, 1998a, 1998b). Prophylactic administration of surfactants decreases the risk for pneumothorax and pulmonary interstitial emphysema. The lack of reduction in bronchopulmonary dysplasia (BPD) rates following surfactant replacement is probably due in part to the increased survival (Cifuentes, 1996).

Trials have been conducted to determine if early (vs delayed) rescue therapy with surfactant improves important outcomes. Early (less than 2 hours) vs delayed rescue surfactant (Yost & Soll, 1999) resulted in decreased risk for neonatal mortality (22% to 20%; RR 0.87; 0.77, 0.99; NNT 36). Early rescue administration reduced both pneumothorax (14% to 12%, RR 0.70; CI 0.59, 0.82; NNT 50) and pulmonary interstitial emphysema (15% to 10%; RR 0.63; CI 0.43, 0.93; NNT 19). An alternative to early administration in many infants is to treat infants with surfactant before ventilation is needed. Temporary endotracheal intubation for surfactant administration when infants are requiring only continuous positive airway pressure (CPAP) reduces the subsequent need for mechanical ventilation and may reduce mortality and/or BPD (Verder et al, 1994, 1999).

Trials of natural and synthetic surfactants report superiority of the natural surfactants. Natural (vs synthetic) surfactants (Hudak et al, 1996; Soll & Blanco, 2001) resulted in decreased rates of pneumothoraces (12% to 7%; RR 0.63; CI 0.53, 0.75; NNT 22) and mortality (18% to 16%; RR 0.86; CI 0.76, 0.98; NNT 37).

Initial protocols of surfactant administration used single-dose therapies. However, when compared to a strategy of single dose of surfactant, a policy of administration of multiple doses of surfactant when indicated according to the protocol resulted in decreased pneumothorax risk (18% to 9%; RR 0.63; CI 0.30, 0.88; NNT 11) and a trend for less mortality.

Thus, a review of all the current evidence supports the use of prophylactic or early use of natural surfactants as early as when infants are requiring CPAP. More than one dose of surfactant should be administered, if indicated, to optimize the benefits of this therapy.

TABLE **2-2**	Exogenous Surfactants
Name	**Source**
Calf lung surfactant extract	Bovine
Human	Amniotic fluid
Curosurf	Porcine
Survanta	Bovine
Infasurf	Bovine
Exosurf	Artificial

Collaborative Care: Surfactant Therapy

Nurses in particular play an important role in caring for infants who receive surfactant replacement therapy in the NICU. The care of the infants before, during, and after surfactant administration is unique to this treatment modality. It is important for nurses to have a working knowledge of the specific care needs of infants treated with surfactant.

Before administration of surfactant, several factors should be considered. Accurate weights of the infants must be determined to ensure the proper doses of surfactant to be given. Confirmation of proper placement of the infants' endotracheal tubes by chest radiographs must be documented. These infants should have continuous cardiac and respiratory monitoring. Cardiac monitoring may include electrocardiograms as well as arterial catheters. Respiratory monitoring may include transcutaneous measurement of PO_2 or PCO_2 and pulse oximetry. Nurses or physicians may also suggest increases in ventilator settings before dosing for infants who do not tolerate handling or who become hypoxic quickly. Endotracheal suctioning is another essential part of the care prior to the administration of surfactant. These infants should be suctioned approximately 15 minutes before surfactant dosing to rid the infants of secretions that may inhibit the administration of the surfactant.

The care of infants during surfactant dosing is also unique to this treatment modality. Of utmost importance during dosing is the ongoing assessment and monitoring of the infants. Because dosing with surfactant may impair ventilation transiently, nurses and physicians must be alert for signs that indicate the need to slow or stop the dosing momentarily to allow the infants to recover. Some signs that ventilation may be impaired include bradycardia, duskiness, and decrease in transcutaneous PO_2 or oxygen saturation. Optimal positioning of infants during surfactant administration is another critical facet of care. Infants receive some surfactants, such as Survanta (Columbus, OH: Ross Labs), in four aliquots, each in a different body position.

The infants are positioned head down, head turned to the right; head down, head turned to the left; head up, head turned to the right; and head up, head turned to the left. The infants are held in each position for 30 seconds after the dose is administered into the endotracheal tube. Administration of Exosurf requires only turning the head from midline to the right, then midline to the left.

Lastly, nurses have specific responsibilities after surfactant is administered to infants. Immediately after dosing, the nurse should assess the infant's skin color, respirations, oxygen saturation, and transcutaneous monitoring. Arterial blood gas should be sampled, and the ventilator should be weaned appropriately. Surfactant produces changes in pulmonary compliance that generally requires rapid weaning of ventilator settings, but some infants may also experience respiratory distress immediately after dosing. Endotracheal suctioning is delayed after dosing of surfactant for at least 1 to 2 hours to prevent removal of the instilled surfactant. Other side effects of this effective therapy are sudden changes in cerebral blood flow, which makes intraventricular hemorrhage a real possibility, and changes in retinal blood flow, which increases chances for retinopathy of prematurity.

CONVENTIONAL VENTILATORY SUPPORT AND RESPIRATORY CONSIDERATIONS

This chapter focuses on the ventilator technologies and strategies. Both continuous positive airway pressure (CPAP) and conventional mechanical ventilation (CMV) continue to be the mainstay of the care of infants with respiratory failure.

Continuous Positive Airway Pressure

Continuous positive airway pressure can be defined as the use of positive pressure continuously throughout the respiratory cycle. The use of CPAP requires that the infant be breathing spontaneously without the full support of a ventilator. Three devices are commonly used to administer CPAP (nasal prongs, endotracheal tubes, and nasopharyngeal tubes), each with its own advantages and disadvantages. Nasal prongs are noninvasive but may not always transmit optimal pressure to the airway because they are easily dislodged and may cause damage to the nasal septum with prolonged use. Endotracheal tubes give optimal transmission of pressure and can be converted easily to mechanical ventilation but can cause pharyngeal grooves or subglottic stenosis with prolonged use. Nasopharyngeal CPAP is more stable than prongs but can result in nasopharyngeal irritation and plugging with secretions.

Physiologic effects of CPAP are increased transpulmonary pressure with a resultant increase in functional residual capacity, stabilization of collapsed alveoli, and improvement in ventilation-perfusion matching. These improvements lead to better oxygenation and ventilation. In preterm infants with relatively floppy airways, CPAP can provide increased pressure to the posterior pharynx and prevent airway collapse during inspiration and prevent obstructive apnea (Hansen, 1998). Although CPAP is relatively safe, some complications are associated with its use. Excessive levels of CPAP can raise intrathoracic pressure and compress the right atrium and vena cava, thus compromising venous return. Excessive CPAP may also overdistend alveoli and result in air leaks.

Conventional Mechanical Ventilation

The two types of conventional ventilators commonly used in neonatal intensive care units are pressure or volume ventilators. Pressure ventilators are used more frequently than volume ventilators. These ventilators are constant-flow, time-cycled, and pressure-limited devices. This means there is a constant flow of gas through the endotracheal tube, breaths are given at fixed intervals, and a preset peak inspiratory pressure (PIP) is maintained through the duration of the inspiration. In a pressure-limited ventilator an increase in ventilation (decrease in pO_2) can be achieved by increasing ventilator rate or increasing tidal volume. Oxygenation improvement is achieved by increasing the mean airway pressure (increasing PIP, increasing Ti, increasing PEEP, increasing flow, and increasing rate) or by increasing the FiO_2. An increase in ventilation (decrease in pCO_2) can be achieved by increasing ventilator rate or increasing tidal volume. If compliance changes in a compression ventilator, no change in pressure is delivered. The disadvantages are decreases in tidal volume if the compliance decreases or overdistention if compliance improves.

Volume ventilators deliver the same tidal volume with each breath, regardless of the pressure needed to achieve the preset volume. In a volume-limited ventilator, an increase in ventilation is achieved by increasing the ventilator rate or increasing delivered tidal volume. An increase in oxygenation will occur if the FiO_2, PEEP, or tidal volume is increased. The disadvantage to the volume ventilator is that a fixed volume will be delivered regardless of changes in compliance and can lead to the use of very high PIPs.

The newer conventional ventilators can use a variety of different operating modes. In this chapter, intermittent mandatory ventilation (IMV), synchronous IMV, and assist control will be briefly discussed. IMV provides a continuous flow of oxygen/air mixture through the ventilatory circuit; however, the neonate can breathe spontaneously. The term *mandatory* refers to the number of mandatory breaths per minute that are set by the caregiver. The settings allow PIP, rates, inspiratory time, and flow to be adjusted to individual ventilation. This very simply means giving intermittent breaths at a fixed rate. If the infant is breathing faster than the preset rate, then the ventilator does not support those breaths. The disadvantage with this mode is that infants may exhale during the ventilator's inspiratory cycle and thus "fight" against the ventilator. SIMV is similar to IMV except that the ventilator senses the infant's spontaneous respirations and mechanically delivered breaths are synchronized to those efforts. If the infant is breathing faster than the set SIMV rate, those breaths are not supported, which is similar to the IMV mode. SIMV is more flexible than IMV and can be used for primary ventilatory support and weaning. However, in some cases SIMV may fail as a weaning mode because at low set rates the infant must exert a considerable work of breathing. Assist/control ventilation (A/C) is also known as patient-triggered ventilation (PTV). This therapy uses the spontaneous respiratory efforts of the infant to "trigger" a mechanical breath by the ventilator. In PTV a sensor is used to detect a variety of stimuli such as airflow, airway pressure, chest wall movement, and esophageal pressure. When the machine detects an inspiration, it delivers a breath with a preset PIP, inspiratory time, and airflow. PTV is therefore similar to SIMV and has the theoretical advantage of supporting all breaths by the ventilator, even those above the set rate. A disadvantage of PTV is that very immature infants have weak respiratory effort that does not trigger this machine (Carlo & Ambalavanan, 1999). Backup respiratory rates may be used to reduce this problem.

There is emerging consensus that ventilator support, by itself, may inflict lung injury (Artigas et al, 1998; Clark et al, 2001). A strategy to minimize ventilator-associated lung injury is the use of CPAP instead of endotracheal intubation. Several retrospective studies suggest that the decreased need for ventilator support with the use of CPAP may allow lung inflation to be maintained but may prevent volutrauma due to overdistention and/or atelectasis. However, preliminary summaries of three large multicenter randomized controlled trials including a total of 495 preterm infants do not report benefits of early CPAP (Finer et al, 2005; Sandri et al, 2004; Thomson, 2002). Further research on the use of early CPAP is ongoing. Interestingly, nasal intermittent mandatory ventilation (vs nasal CPAP) reduces extubation failure in small trials (18% to 7%; RR 0.39; CI 0.16, 0.97; NNT 9) and this could be an alternative to prevent intubation (Greenough et al, 2000).

The strategy most evaluated with conventional mechanical ventilation is the use of high rates and presumably small tidal volumes as $PaCO_2$ levels were kept in comparable ranges. Meta-analyses of the randomized controlled trials of high (>60 per min) vs low (usually 30 to 40 per min) rates (and presumed low vs high tidal volumes, respectively) revealed that the high ventilatory rate strategy led to fewer air leaks (28% to 19%; RR 0.69; CI 051, 093; NNT 11) and a trend for increased survival.

If mechanical ventilation is needed, a ventilatory approach of small tidal volumes and permissive hypercapnia can be employed (Carlo et al, 2002; Hargett, 1995; Mariani et al, 1999). Permissive hypercapnia is a strategy for the management of patients receiving ventilatory support in which priority is given to the prevention or limitation of lung injury secondary to the ventilator by tolerating relatively high levels of $PaCO_2$ rather than maintenance of normal blood gases (Acute Respiratory Distress Syndrome Network, 2000; Carlo et al, 2002; Mariani et al, 1999). A multicenter trial of infants <1000 g reported that permissive hypercapnia (target $PaCO_2$ >50 mm Hg) during the first 10 days led to a trend for reduced BPD or death at 36 weeks (68% vs 63%). Furthermore, the strategy of permissive hypercapnia reduced severity of BPD as evidenced by a decreased need of ventilator support at 36 weeks from 16% to 1% (P <0.005). In summary, a gentle ventilator strategy of small tidal volumes, higher rates, and permissive hypercapnia may reduce BPD in very preterm infants, but further research is needed.

Hyperoxia may also contribute to lung injury in preterm infants. Thus, permissive hypoxemia is another strategy that may reduce BPD. Trials to target different levels of oxygen saturations performed for treatment of retinopathy of prematurity (STOP-ROP Pediatrics, 2000) or BPD (Askie et al, 2003) revealed that the groups with lower saturation targets (89% to 94% and 91% to 94%, respectively) had less need for oxygen supplementation and fewer BPD/BPD exacerbations. Further trials of permissive hyperoxemia are needed before this strategy can be recommended. Technological advances, including improvement in flow delivery systems, triggering of inspiration, breath termination criteria, guaranteed tidal volume delivery, stability of PEEP, air-leak compensation, prevention of pressure overshoot, and on-line pulmonary function monitoring have resulted in better ventilators. Patient-initiated mechanical ventilation, patient-triggered ventilation, and synchronized intermittent mandatory ventilation are being used increasingly in neonates.

HIGH-FREQUENCY VENTILATION

In contrast to high-frequency ventilation (HFV), CMV uses ventilator rates and tidal volumes that correspond to the spontaneous ventilation patterns of newborns. High mean and peak airway pressures may be required during CMV to adequately ventilate noncompliant lungs. Exposure to high inflating pressures may lead to lung and airway injury, including pulmonary interstitial emphysema, pneumothoraces, bronchopleural fistulas, and bronchopulmonary dysplasia. HFV attempts to avoid these complications by delivering low tidal volumes at high frequencies. HFV may be used as a "rescue" technique to prevent further damage in infants who have developed complications secondary to CMV. HFV allows severely ill infants to be adequately ventilated at lower volumes than with CMV while improving gas exchange. HFV may be used perioperatively and postoperatively to reduce movement of the airway and thoracic cavity. HFV may be beneficial to infants who have preexisting pneumothoraces or bronchopleural fistulas. There is no generally accepted ventilator rate, which defines the term *high frequency*. Accepted definitions generally include ventilator rates at 2 to 4 times the natural breathing frequency and ventilation with tidal volumes smaller than anatomic dead space. Gas transport during high frequency cannot be explained by conventional concepts of ventilation and lung mechanics.

TABLE 2-3	Classification of High-Frequency Neonatal Ventilators		
Type		**Maximal Rate (breaths/min)**	**Expiration**
Pressure-limited, time-cycled		150	Passive
Jet		250 to 300	Passive
Oscillator		1800	Active

Three types of HFV are approved for use in the United States: the high-frequency oscillatory ventilator (HFOV), the high-frequency jet ventilator (HFJV), and the high-frequency flow interrupter (HFFI) (Table 2-3). The HFOV has a diaphragm or piston that oscillates a flow of gas, thus creating both positive and negative pressure changes. Mean airway pressure is generated by gas flow through a filter, which acts as a resistor. The respiratory therapist or clinician can adjust the mean airway pressure, frequency, and amplitude. The mean airway pressure affects lung inflation and can be increased by increasing MAP oxygenation. The piston amplitude affects ventilation, and increases in ventilation occur when amplitude is increased. The HFOV is the only HFV in which inspiration and exhalation are active.

HFJV delivers tidal volumes that may be less than or greater than anatomic dead space at frequencies of 60 to 600 breaths per minute. HFJV operates similarly to constant-flow time-cycled ventilation with passive expiration. With an HFJV, a high-pressure gas source is connected to a small airway cannula with use of a high-frequency flow interrupter valve. This valve opens and closes rapidly, thus propelling the pressurized gas into the airway. HFJV requires a specific endotracheal tube with a lumen for the jet gas flow and a lumen for the fresh gas flow. The fresh gas flow allows entrainment of gases and addition of PEEP. There is a port, near the jet gas flow lumen, for the instillation of nebulized saline to prevent tracheal erosion. A conventional ventilator may be used with a jet ventilator to provide "background" ventilation or sighs at a low rate. Background ventilation may decrease the risk for microatelectasis that may occur with long-term HFJV. The operator can adjust the PIP of the jet and the CMV as well as the PEEP and frequency. To increase the pO₂, the operator adjusts PEEP and FiO₂. Elimination of carbon dioxide is dependent mostly on the PIP-to-PEEP pressure difference.

The HFFIs have both conventional and high-frequency options. A high-pressure source of gas is delivered into a standard ventilator circuit, and this flow of gas is interrupted by a valve mechanism that is operated by a microprocessor. The operator can adjust the PIP, PEEP, and frequency. The conventional ventilator is often used to give intermittent "sigh" breaths. Oxygenation depends primarily on the PEEP that is delivered by the conventional ventilator, whereas ventilation depends primarily on the difference between the PIP and the PEEP.

HFOV and high-frequency flow interruption have been evaluated in 12 randomized controlled trials including more than 3000 stable preterm infants. Even though there is some heterogeneity in results between the trials, meta-analysis reveals no clear evidence that high-frequency oscillatory ventilation is superior to conventional as the initial mode of ventilatory support (Thome et al, 2005). There are trends for reduction in mortality and BPD (Thome & Carlo, 2003; Henderson-Smart et al, 2003) despite a significant increase in air leaks with HFOV (OR 1.23; CI 1.04-1.46; NNT 30). Also, there are trends for an increase in grade 3 to 4 intraventricular hemorrhage and periventricular leukomalacia but the results are inconsistent (Thome & Carlo, 2003). Long-term outcome studies do not show an advantage of high-frequency ventilation over conventional ventilation. HFJV in stable preterm infants resulted in less BPD at 36 weeks' (33% to 20%; RR 0.59, 0.35, 0.99; NNT 8) but the data are limited (Bhuta & Henderson-Smart, 2002).

HFV has also been used as a rescue mode in several randomized controlled trials. A trial in infants with severe RDS observed a reduction in air leaks and development and progression of air leaks in infants randomized to HFOV (HiFO Study Group, 1993). However, there was no improvement in other major outcome measures. HFJV in preterm infants with pulmonary interstitial emphysema led to a more frequent and faster resolution of emphysema but no reduction in mortality or other adverse outcomes (Keszler et al, 1991).

Few data from large, multicenter, randomized trials that examine the use of HFV for lung diseases other than RDS exist. It is generally accepted that HFV is useful in the management of newborns with severe pulmonary interstitial emphysema because airway pressures may be significantly reduced and thus theoretically decrease the risk for further air leak, other pressure-related airway injury, and decreased cardiac output.

Complications Associated with High-Frequency Ventilation

HFV can provide adequate ventilation to infants, but its use is associated with the possibility of complications. The gases that are used during HFV need to be heated to avoid the delivery of cold gas into the airway. Cold air can lead to hypothermia and necrotizing tracheobronchitis (NTB). NTB is a lesion of the airway that is caused by epithelial erosion and loss of cells in the airway; it is commonly found near the distal end of the endotracheal tube. It leads to formation of granulation tissue that can cause impaired gas exchange, airway obstruction, or atelectasis. With high ventilatory frequencies, the inspiratory and expiratory times are decreased, which may increase the risk for gas trapping in the lungs. Gas trapping occurs less often during HFOV because it is the only form of HFV in which expiration is active. With some high-frequency ventilators, such as the jet-and-flow interrupter, expiration occurs by passive recoil of the distended respiratory system (lung and chest).

Nursing Care—High-Frequency Ventilation

Caring for infants who receive HFV presents many challenges to NICU nurses. Nurses must adopt new skills and alter those used in caring for infants who are conventionally ventilated. Specific care needs unique to infants who receive HFV include physical assessment, airway management, positioning, and comfort (Tables 2-4 and 2-5).

One of the most challenging yet critical aspects of caring for these infants is the physical assessment. Recognizing subtle changes in the physical exam is critical because these changes may signify changes in the infant's condition. Of extreme

TABLE 2-4	Nursing Responsibilities and Interventions for Oscillated Infants Before High-Frequency Ventilation
Responsibility	**Intervention**
Obtain and record baseline physiologic data	Record temperature, heart rate, respiratory rate, systolic and diastolic blood pressures, transcutaneous PO_2, and PCO_2
Obtain and record baseline biochemical data	Draw blood samples for arterial gases
Maintain current ventilation	Record ventilator parameters: rate, PIP, PEEP, MAP, inspiratory:expiratory ratio, FiO_2
Assemble and prepare equipment	Ensure that infant is attached to monitoring devices for heart rate, intra-arterial blood pressure, transcutaneous oxygen and carbon dioxide
	Check alarms on all monitors
	Assist with arterial line insertion

From Inwood MS (1991). High-frequency oscillation. In Nugent J, editor. Acute respiratory care of the neonate. Petaluma, CA: NICU Ink.

TABLE 2-5	Nursing Responsibilities and Interventions for Oscillated Infants During Oscillation
Responsibility	**Intervention**
Monitor and document physiologic parameters	Record hourly temperature, heart rate, spontaneous respirations, systolic and diastolic blood pressure
	Measure and record accurate intake and output of fluids every 8 hours
Monitor and document biochemical parameters	Draw arterial blood gas samples as ordered
Maintain patent airway	Monitor for continuous vibration of chest
	Assess transcutaneous PO_2 and PCO_2 hourly
	Perform endotracheal suctioning every 2 hours and prn
	Record amount, color, and consistency of secretions
	Assess bilateral air entry while hand bagging at sigh pressures, before and after suctioning
	Ensure adequate humidification of gas flow
Prevent pneumothorax	Maintain ordered MAP
	Observe for decreased vibrations of the chest
	Assess infant for signs of respiratory difficulty: increased spontaneous respirations, increased chest retraction, diminished air entry, increased FiO_2 requirements, increased transcutaneous PCO_2 readings
	Obtain chest radiograph as required and ensure that oscillator is stopped during filming
Provide pulmonary support	Monitor and record MAP, amplitude, frequency, and FiO_2 hourly
	Perform a sustained inflation after endotracheal suctioning and disconnection at ordered pressure and duration
	Record infant's response to sigh
Provide physical care	Reposition infant from side to side or from prone to supine every 2 hours
Provide emotional support to family	Provide accurate, consistent information
	Promote bonding by encouraging nurse specialist or social worker for assistance with coping skills
	Encourage parents to attend parents' support group

From Inwood MS (1991). High-frequency oscillation. In Nugent J, editor. Acute respiratory care of the neonate. Petaluma, CA: NICU Ink.
MAP, Mean airway pressure.

importance is the assessment of chest wall vibration, which is an indicator of tidal volume. Even small changes in the vibrations may indicate a change in the neonate's condition. Decreased chest vibration may indicate pneumothorax, endotracheal secretions, and mechanical malfunction. The noise of the ventilator and the constant vibration of the infants make auscultation of breath sounds, heart tones, and bowel sounds difficult. If oscillating ventilators are used, this evaluation is best done when the infants are momentarily removed from the ventilator (for routine circuit changes) or when the ventilator is in standby (interruption of oscillation

but not from ventilator mean airway pressure). Disconnection from HFV is discouraged because of possible alveolar collapse and loss of lung volume. Therefore, when necessary, disconnection from HFV should be limited to short periods. If the infant is receiving HFOV, it is also important to auscultate breath sounds to assess the symmetry of oscillatory intensity while he or she is being oscillated.

The second specific area of care unique to infants who receive HFV is airway management. Suctioning of these infants requires two people—one person to suction and another to either manually ventilate or return the infants to

HFV. Remember that disconnection from HFV may lead to alveolar collapse, so the infants may need to be manually ventilated or the mean airway pressure increased after suctioning. It is generally accepted practice to suction infants while they are disconnected from HFOV and HFJV. Positioning and comfort of infants who are receiving HFV are also important facets of care. Because of the physical restraints of the delivery devices and the importance of disconnecting the infant from the ventilator for only short durations, positioning and repositioning become challenging. Two caregivers should be used for repositioning—one to turn the infant and stabilize the endotracheal tube and another to reposition the circuit and ventilator. Although water mattresses are not recommended, sheepskins, lamb's wool, and egg-crate mattresses may be used to provide comfort and prevent skin breakdown. However, there is rising concern that infants may inhale fibers from sheepskin, so it may not be used in some units.

Sedatives, paralytics, and analgesics may be necessary to facilitate comfort for infants while they are receiving HFV. Interventions such as bundling and soothing music may decrease the need for pharmacologic agents. Whereas some believe that the noise and the constant vibration may be disturbing to the infants, others believe them to have a calming effect.

INHALED NITRIC OXIDE

In the past 20 years, it has become apparent that vascular endothelium has an important role in the regulation of blood vessel smooth muscle tone as well as in other important physiologic functions. Relaxation of vascular smooth muscle in response to acetylcholine requires an intact endothelium. Nitric oxide (NO) is thought to be the molecule released from the endothelium that is responsible for vascular smooth muscle relaxation. These findings were the catalyst for additional investigations of the biologic effects of NO.

NO has an unpaired electron and therefore rapidly combines with other free radicals. The biologic half-life of the molecule is estimated to be 110 to 130 msec. In vivo, biologic activity of NO is limited because it is rapidly inactivated within the vessel lumen. Inactivation occurs because NO has a high affinity for hemoglobin and avidly binds to the iron of heme proteins to form a biologically inactive compound, nitrosyl-hemoglobin. Nitrosyl-hemoglobin is then oxidized to form methemoglobin and nitrate.

The NO molecule is synthesized from the amino acid L-arginine in a reaction that is catalyzed by a group of enzymes called the nitric oxide synthases (NOS). The by-product of this reaction is L-citrulline: L-arginine + molecular O_2 → NO + L-citrulline.

Three major types or isoforms of NOS exist. The first isoform is the endothelial or constitutive type, which is located in vascular endothelial cell wall, endocardium, myocardium, and platelets. Neuronal NOS is the isoform located in both the peripheral and central nervous systems. The third isoform, inducible NOS, is not present under normal physiologic conditions but is produced in response to various inflammatory stimuli. Excitation of the inducible NOS causes production of much greater quantities of NO than activation of other isoforms. Activation of inducible NOS during sepsis plays a major part in producing vasodilation and consequent hypotension.

The biologic actions of NO are mediated through the guanylate cyclase–cyclic guanosine monophosphate (cGMP)

system. After formation from L-arginine in the endothelial cell, NO readily diffuses into the cytosol of smooth muscle because it is a small, lipophilic molecule. Once inside the smooth muscle cell, NO binds soluble guanylate cyclase, which in turn catalyzes the formation of cGMP from guanosine triphosphate. Increases in cGMP lead to activation of cGMP-dependent protein kinase, which triggers a reduction in intracellular calcium concentration through extrusion and sequestration. The decreased calcium concentration causes smooth muscle relaxation.

NO is a biologic mediator of a variety of physiologic responses in numerous systems in the body. In the healthy state, the arterial circulation is partially dilated by basal production of NO in the endothelium. At birth, production of endogenous NO in response to rhythmic distention of the lung, shear stress, and acetylcholine release plays a major role in mediating a decrease in pulmonary vascular resistance. In addition to being an important determinant of basal tone in small arteries and arterioles, NO inhibits platelet aggregation and adherence and may alter vascular permeability. In the nervous system, NO may have a role in memory formation, pain perception, and electrocortical activation, but more research is needed to support this hypothesis. In the gastrointestinal and genitourinary tracts, NO participates in control of signals that regulate smooth muscle relaxation. NO is produced in large quantities in response to various immunologic stimuli. It may also have a role in nonspecific immunity because it is generated when macrophages are activated.

A particularly frustrating problem for caregivers in the NICU is the treatment of acute hypoxic respiratory failure due to pulmonary arterial vasoconstriction. Successful adaptation for extrauterine life depends on the ability of the fetus to make a transition from fetal to postnatal circulation. A variety of factors, probably related to adverse intrauterine events, may alter the ability of the newborn to decrease pulmonary vascular resistance at birth and make this adaptation. When pulmonary vascular resistance remains elevated postnatally, blood is shunted right to left across the ductus arteriosus and foramen ovale and away from the lungs, thus causing hypoxemia. This condition, PPHN, is seen either in isolation or in conjunction with various diseases such as meconium aspiration syndrome, severe birth asphyxia, sepsis, congenital diaphragmatic hernia, and RDS. In the past, pharmacologic interventions—such as tolazoline, an alpha-adrenergic blocker with histamine-like properties—have been used to decrease pulmonary vascular resistance. However, the effects of these drugs are unpredictable and inconsistent, and because they are not selective for the pulmonary bed, nearly 50% of patients develop systemic hypotension. Sodium nitroprusside is another drug that causes vasodilation through activation or release of NO, but it is not selective for the pulmonary arterial bed and decreases systemic vascular resistance as well. Other intravenous vasodilators, such as prostaglandin I2 and adenosine triphosphate–magnesium chloride, may selectively decrease pulmonary vascular resistance. The ideal agent for the treatment of pulmonary hypertension would be one that causes pulmonary vasodilation without decreasing systemic vascular resistance.

The early 1990s saw the development of theories that inhaled NO would diffuse from the alveolar space across the epithelium to directly mediate vascular smooth muscle relaxation. Ultimately, NO would diffuse into the lumen of the pulmonary blood vessels and be inactivated on binding hemoglobin, thus avoiding effects on the systemic circulation. Theoretically, inhaled NO could increase systemic oxygenation by two mechanisms: by global pulmonary arterial vasodilation with increased pulmonary blood flow and cardiac output or by improved matching of ventilation and perfusion in the lung.

Concern grew, however, with potential toxic effects that might be associated with the use of inhaled NO. One potential problem is the formation of excess amounts of methemoglobin, thus causing the clinical condition known as methemoglobinemia. This serious condition is associated with hypoxemia because of the inability of methemoglobin to carry oxygen. The body's defense mechanism against the formation of methemoglobin is the enzyme methemoglobin reductase, which readily converts methemoglobin back to hemoglobin. If the rate of accumulation of methemoglobin is slow, this enzyme will limit increases in methemoglobin. To date, significant methemoglobin levels have not been noted in trials in which low concentrations of inhaled NO have been used in neonates.

Another possible problem is the production of nitrogen dioxide and higher oxides of nitrogen such as peroxynitrite when NO is used with high concentrations of oxygen. Nitrogen dioxide and peroxynitrite in high concentrations can directly damage the lung. Using low concentrations of NO and limiting the time of mixing of NO and oxygen minimizes the formation of these toxic molecules.

Large multicenter, double-masked, randomized, placebo-controlled studies have determined that inhaled nitrous oxide (INO) can decrease the need for ECMO in infants with PPHN. The NINOS study enrolled 235 patients under the age of 2 weeks with PPHN and compared responses to either 20 ppm of INO or placebo gas, which was 100% oxygen. The primary hypothesis was that INO would result in a reduction in the risk of death or need for ECMO by 120 days from 50% in controls to 30% in infants who received INO (Finer, 2000). This study encouraged the use of all other aggressive modalities in the treatment of PPHN and was terminated early by an External Data Safety Monitoring Committee when treated infants were shown to have a statistically significant lower risk of death or need for ECMO. Another well-conducted multicenter trial matched control and treatment infants for diagnoses, blood gases, oxygen indices, and ventilator settings (Roberts et al, 1992). The trial was stopped early at interim analysis when it demonstrated a significant increase in systemic oxygenation when INO-treated infants were compared to controls. A third multicenter randomized trial compared high-frequency oscillatory ventilation (HFOV) to INO in term and near-term infants with hypoxic respiratory failure (Kinsella & Abman, 1995). This study showed an equivalent response to either modality. In this study, if infants failed to respond to either treatment used alone ($n = 125$), they would then receive treatment with both. Thirty-two percent of infants who failed with a single modality improved with a combination of both treatments, which led the investigators to speculate that INO works better with maximized lung recruitment. A recent, large randomized study had similar results to the NINOS trial despite the use of lower doses of nitric oxide (Clark et al, 2000). A total of 248 infants with hypoxemic respiratory failure were randomly assigned to be controls or to receive treatment with 24 hours of INO at 20 ppm followed by another 96 hours of INO at 5 ppm. The two groups were then compared with regard to ECMO requirements. Sixty-four percent of controls vs 38% of treated infants ($P = 0.001$) required ECMO. Mortality was not different in the two groups, but treated infants showed a lower incidence of bronchopulmonary dysplasia. INO significantly improves oxygenation and lowers the oxygenation index 30 to 60 minutes after treatment. A significant overall reduction in the combined incidence of need for ECMO and death in infants treated with INO also occurs. Extensive data on long-term outcome of infants treated with INO are not yet available. Some existing data on neurodevelopmental follow-up after the NINOS trial have been gathered (Finer & Barrington, 2001). Of the 173 infants seen at follow-up, no differences exist between control and INO-treated infants with respect to incidence of cerebral palsy, mental or psychomotor development index scores, or hearing loss. The currently published trials of inhaled nitric oxide for preterm infants present heterogeneous results (Barrington & Finer, 2006; Field et al, 2005; Schreiber et al, 2003; Van Meurs et al, 2005) and do not support the routine use of inhaled nitric oxide in this subpopulation. Further clinical trials are ongoing.

NO gas is supplied in aluminum tanks that contain high concentrations of gaseous NO in equilibrium with inert nitrogen. This gas is added to the inspiratory limb of the ventilator circuit by flowmeters and blenders. Use of high flow rates limits NO mixing time with oxygen and decreases the formation of nitrogen dioxide. Scavenging equipment at the expiratory limb of the ventilator eliminates potentially toxic exhaust gases. In-line monitoring of NO and a chemoluminescence analyzer performs nitrogen dioxide tests to determine levels. Samples of gas in the ventilator circuit are aspirated, and the concentrations of these two molecules are determined. Blood is periodically monitored for methemoglobin levels when patients receive INO.

INO holds promise as a selective pulmonary vasodilator that may soon be added to the clinician's armamentarium. Several small pilot studies suggest that INO may be effective in decreasing pulmonary vascular resistance and improving oxygenation without reducing systemic blood pressure or cardiac output. Extreme care must be taken to monitor blood levels of methemoglobin and the formation of higher oxides of nitrogen when NO is used. Until larger controlled trials are completed, the benefit-to-risk ratio of INO as a possible treatment for neonatal pulmonary hypertension remains unknown.

Collaborative Care: Nitric Oxide

Multicenter trials have shown that INO decreases the chance that some critically ill infants will need ECMO. Future studies are currently underway to determine the most effective and safe doses of INO in the management of term and preterm infants with respiratory dysfunction. Over the next several years the use of this treatment modality will slowly increase, and the nursing care of these infants as we know it today will change. Like liquid ventilation, NO therapy will bring with it many new challenges to NICU nurses and physicians.

TREATMENT OF NEONATAL HYPOXEMIA WITH EXTRACORPOREAL MEMBRANE OXYGENATION (ECMO)

ECMO is a complex and expensive therapy for infants with severe respiratory failure. Because this therapy has limited applicability to most NICU nurses, it will be discussed only briefly. The first heart-lung machines, designed to serve the function of cardiopulmonary bypass during pediatric cardiac surgery, were developed in the 1950s. Blood was removed from the patient and pumped through an oxygenator before return to the systemic circulation. At the end of the surgical procedure, the patient was disconnected from the machine, and pulmonary and systemic flows were restored with the patient's own heart as the pump. In the mid-1970s, the first attempts at prolonged cardiopulmonary bypass in infants with potentially reversible hypoxemia were made. The differences between these efforts and those employed during cardiac surgery were that the duration of bypass was measured in days rather than hours and that the underlying disease that led to hypoxemia was potentially reversible lung disease rather than primary cardiac disease.

In the past 20 years, prolonged cardiopulmonary bypass, also known as extracorporeal membrane oxygenation (ECMO) or extracorporeal life support, has been used in thousands of newborn infants with hypoxemia that appears to be intractable to aggressive nonsurgical management. A few controlled clinical trials of ECMO have shown its effectiveness (UK Collaborative Trial Group, 1996). Despite its efficacy in improving oxygen delivery in sick newborns and markedly increasing survival, there is concern for morbidity associated with its use.

ECMO is widely used in the United States as well as in several other industrialized nations. Neonatal ECMO is used in the management of intractable hypoxemia in near-term newborns with meconium aspiration syndrome, RDS, pneumonia/sepsis, and congenital diaphragmatic hernia. Contraindications to the use of ECMO exist. The most important contraindication is prematurity. Early reports of ECMO use in premature infants revealed alarmingly high rates of intracranial hemorrhage. Whether intracranial hemorrhage in these patients is related to the systemic anticoagulation required with ECMO or to the abnormal cerebrovascular pressures and flows associated with ECMO is unknown. Other contraindications to ECMO include preexisting intracranial hemorrhage and hypoxemia that is not potentially reversible, such as that seen in patients with cyanotic congenital heart disease.

The follow-up study of the 4-year-old children enrolled in a trial of ECMO revealed that ECMO resulted in a decrease in death/disability (37% vs 59%, RR 0.55; CI 0.47–0.86) with a number needed to treat of only 4 to 5 (Bennett et al, 2001). This study provides strong evidence for the efficacy and safety of ECMO.

ECMO is an expensive and labor-intensive procedure. Two caretakers are required 24 hours per day—one to provide nursing care directly to the patient and one to monitor the functional integrity of the circuit and its various components because a variety of technical malfunctions can occur. During ECMO the circuit must be heparinized, and the most frequently reported ECMO complication is hemorrhage secondary to this. Table 2-6 lists other common complications of ECMO.

Although it is used widely, ECMO is likely to be replaced by less invasive and less risky preventive and therapeutic procedures. However, at this time, referral to an ECMO center is a logical approach when infants with severe hypoxic respiratory failure do not respond to surfactants, conventional or high-frequency ventilation, or inhaled nitric oxide therapy.

LIQUID VENTILATION

The skills, technologies, and resources for managing respiratory compromise in neonates have continued to improve. Despite these advancements, prematurity and respiratory distress are still associated with significant morbidity and mortality. Modern therapies can cause lung injury that eventually may lead to a chronic lung disease. To decrease lung injury, efforts have concentrated on decreasing inspired oxygen concentration and decreasing inspiratory pressure. To decrease inspiratory pressure, surface tension in the alveoli must be uniformly decreased. This surface tension arises because of the air-liquid interface at the lining of the alveolar membrane. Surfactant therapy is used to decrease surface tension but is not always successful in improving acute respiratory distress or preventing chronic lung disease. Liquid ventilation has been studied as a therapy that could reduce surface tension in the alveoli. Because this therapy is still considered experimental, it will only briefly be discussed.

As early as the 1920s, it was demonstrated that oxygenated saline could be used to inflate the lung and improve ventilation. However, saline proved to be inadequate because of its low gas-carrying ability and its high viscosity. In 1966, it was first demonstrated that perfluorochemical liquids could support the respiration of animals. Perfluorochemical liquids are inert, have high solubility for respiratory gases, and minimize surface tension. They appear to be absorbed only minimally through the mature epithelium. Limited clinical experience and extensive work in animals suggest that these compounds are relatively nontoxic, even when given intravenously.

A liquid gel surfactant that acts to decrease surface tension, enhance alveolar stability, and protect the respiratory epithelium lines the alveolus. The surface-tension forces within the alveolus are the result of the air-fluid interface and are dramatically increased by the absence of surfactant. Surfactant production and function are usually deficient in preterm infants. This deficiency results in noncompliant alveoli that tend to collapse spontaneously. Because surfactant deficiency tends to be nonhomogeneous, alveolar surface tension varies from one portion of the lung to another. Respiratory function in preterm infants is characterized by stiff lungs, increased work of breathing, uneven ventilation, and ventilation-perfusion mismatch. One way to decrease alveolar surface tension is to eliminate the air-liquid interface in the alveolus by filling it with liquid. Elimination of the air-liquid interface can improve alveolar compliance, reverse ventilation-perfusion abnormalities, and—if the liquid contains oxygen—increase oxygen uptake (Shaffer et al, 1999).

Tidal Liquid Ventilation

Efforts were initially made to entirely replace gas breathing with liquid respiration. In tidal liquid ventilation (TLV), a liquid is used to transport dissolved oxygen and carbon dioxide; inhaled liquid brings dissolved oxygen to the lungs, and exhaled liquid carries off carbon dioxide. During TLV, both functional residual capacity and tidal volume are replaced by perfluorocarbon liquid. Technically, TLV is difficult. Clinically, provisions need to be made to mechanically deliver and withdraw liquid from the lung. Equipment is needed for eliminating carbon dioxide from the liquid and for equilibrating it with oxygen. TLV requires new equipment and procedures. Moreover, the high viscosity of the perfluorocarbon

TABLE **2-6**	Complications of Extracorporeal Membrane Oxygenation
Complication	**Rationale and Treatment**

PHYSIOLOGIC

Electrolyte/glucose/ fluid imbalance	Sodium requirements decrease to 1 to 2 mEq/kg/day; potassium requirements increase to 4 mEq/kg/day secondary to action of aldosterone
	Calcium replacement may be required if citrate is a component of prime blood anticoagulant
	Hyperglycemia may occur if citrate-phosphate-dextrose anticoagulated blood is used; reduce dextrose concentration of maintenance and heparin infusions
	Maintain total fluid intake of 100 to 150 ml/kg/day
	Fluid intake should balance output; furosemide may be required if positive fluid balance occurs
Central nervous system deterioration: cerebral edema, intracranial hemorrhage, seizures	This significant complication of ECMO can be related to pre-ECMO hypoxia, acidosis, hypercapnia, or vessel ligation
	Drug of choice for seizures is phenobarbital
	Serial electroencephalograms and cranial ultrasound examinations may be required
Generalized edema	Extracellular space is enlarged by distribution of crystalloid solution from the prime fluid and action of aldosterone and antidiuretic hormone
	Furosemide or hemofiltration may be indicated if edema causes brain or lung dysfunction
Renal failure	Acute tubular necrosis results from pre-ECMO hypotension and hypoxia
	Monitor output and indicators of renal failure: blood urea nitrogen, creatinine
	Increase renal perfusion by increasing pump flow and use of dopamine (5 mcg/kg/min)
	Hemodialysis may be added to the circuit if necessary
Bleeding/thrombocytopenia	Most frequent cause of death
	Large foreign surface of ECMO circuit lowers platelet function and count
	Most common in infants requiring surgery or chest tubes
	Minimize with good control of ACT (180 to 200 seconds) and judicious use of platelets and frozen plasma
	All surgical procedures must be done with electrocautery
Decreased venous return/hypovolemia	Infant must have adequate circulating volume to obtain adequate flow rates
	Manifested by collapsing silicone bladder triggering bladder box alarm and decrease in extracorporeal flow rate, arterial pressure, and arterial pulse amplitude
	Blood sampling, wound drainage, or peripheral dilatation may account for hypovolemia
	Check for pneumothorax, partial venous catheter occlusion, or malposition, which may decrease venous drainage and return
	Replace volume with packed cells, fresh frozen plasma
	Treat pneumothorax with chest tube placement
	Raise level of bed to enhance gravity drainage of venous blood
Hypervolemia	Caused by overinfusion of blood products, which causes a larger percentage of blood to flow through malfunctioning lungs
	Can also be caused by renal ischemia and excretion of renin/angiotensin
	Manifested by widening pulse amplitude and decreasing systemic oxygenation at an extracorporeal flow rate
	Treat overinfusion by removing blood from the circuit; renal hypertension may dictate use of captopril or labetalol
Patent ductus arteriosus	Left-to-right shunting may occur, thus causing increased blood flow to the lungs and necessitating high pump flows without expected increase in PaO_2
	Ligation may be indicated because weaning will not be successful

MECHANICAL

Tubing rupture, air in oxygenator	Increase ventilator to pre-ECMO parameters; take patient off bypass (repair circuit, aspirate air, replace malfunctioning oxygenator); be prepared to resuscitate infant
Power failure	Always plug pump into hospital's emergency power supply; hand crank until emergency power is available
Decannulation	Apply firm pressure; come off bypass; increase ventilator parameters; repair vessel; replace blood volume; be prepared to resuscitate infant

From Askin DF, editor (1997). Acute respiratory care of the neonate, ed 2. Santa Rosa, CA: NICU Ink. Adapted from Nugent J (1986). Extracorporeal membrane oxygenation in the neonate. Neonatal network 4(5):33.
ACT, *Activated coagulation time;* ECMO, *extracorporeal membrane oxygenation.*

liquid limits the number of breaths that can be delivered per minute.

Partial Liquid Ventilation (PLV)

PLV, also known as perfluorocarbon-associated gas exchange (PAGE), is a hybrid method that attempts to overcome some of the limitations of TLV while retaining the advantages of liquid ventilation. During PLV, functional residual capacity is replaced by liquid, but tidal ventilation is conventional, using oxygen-enriched gas and standard ventilator equipment. The lung is filled with perfluorocarbon liquid to a volume equivalent to the normal pulmonary functional residual capacity. This volume of liquid is left in the lung, and gas ventilation is resumed with use of conventional gas ventilators. On inspiration, oxygen is pushed down the airway into the liquid-filled alveoli, where it forms bubbles and where oxygen and carbon dioxide are exchanged in the liquid from bubbles to the alveoli. This process oxygenates the alveolar perfluorocarbon reservoir and purges it of carbon dioxide. On exhalation, the gas is expelled from the lung. Breaths can be delivered at a frequency appropriate for the size and needs of the patient because the viscosity of the liquid does not limit respiratory rate. PLV has been shown to be effective in surfactant-deficient premature lambs. PLV improved oxygenation and carbon dioxide elimination as well as lung compliance. It has also been shown to work in two models of ARDS, oleic acid lung injury, and saline lavage. A small, nonrandomized study treated 13 preterm infants who failed conventional management of severe respiratory distress with PLV (Leach et al, 1996). In this study when PaO_2 and compliance improved, the oxygen index decreased significantly within 1 hour of treatment. Six term infants with respiratory failure and no improvement after ECMO were treated with PLV in another study (Greenspan et al, 1997). The study concluded that PLV appeared to be safe, improved lung function, and recruited lung volume. However, this therapy remains experimental as randomized trials have not been performed in neonates.

Collaborative Care: Liquid Ventilation

The care of infants with respiratory compromise may be greatly affected if future advances prove liquid ventilation to be safe and effective. Because of the complexity of the delivery systems, a specialized team, similar to an ECMO team, would be required to care for these infants. These specialists will need to be trained in fluid pharmacologic mechanics and liquid breathing techniques.

PHARMACOLOGIC THERAPIES FOR VENTILATED INFANTS

Several pharmacologic options are available to the clinician for the treatment of RDS and prevention of its complications. Selected treatments are reviewed in this section.

A large multicenter randomized controlled trial and other smaller trials have shown benefits of vitamin A administration in preterm infants. Vitamin A supplementation given largely to infants less than 1 kg resulted in a decrease in death and/or BPD at 36 weeks (66% to 60%; RR 0.87; CI 0.83, 0.99; NNT 17) and trends for less nosocomial sepsis and retinopathy of prematurity (Tyson et al, 1999; Darlow & Graham, 2002). Nonetheless, vitamin A supplementation is only used in the minority of the infants less than 1 kg currently in the United States (Ambalavanan et al, 2003).

Systemic corticosteroids have been used to treat infants with RDS, to selectively treat infants who continue to require respiratory support, and to treat those who develop BPD. Mortality and/or BPD at 36 weeks decreases (from 72% to 45%; RR 0.63; CI 0.51, 0.78; NNT 4) with moderately-early (7 to 14 days) administration of corticosteroids. Early (<96 hours) and delayed (>3 weeks) administration of systemic steroids has also been assessed with meta-analyses and the results are qualitatively similar. However, there are short-term adverse effects including hyperglycemia, hypertension, gastrointestinal bleeding, gastrointestinal perforation, hypertrophic obstructive cardiomyopathy, poor weight gain, poor growth of the head, and a trend toward a higher incidence of periventricular leukomalacia (American Academy of Pediatrics/Canadian Paediatric Society, 2002). Furthermore, data including an increased incidence of neurodevelopmental delay and cerebral palsy in infants randomized to systemic corticosteroids raise serious concerns about adverse long-term outcomes. Thus, routine use of systemic corticosteroids is not recommended for the prevention or treatment of BPD by the Consensus Group of the American Academy of Pediatrics and the Canadian Paediatric Society. Administration of inhaled steroids to ventilated preterm infants during the first 2 weeks after birth reduced the need for systemic steroids (45% to 35%; RR 0.78; CI 0.62, 0.99; NNT 10) and tended to decrease death and/or BPD at 36 weeks without an increase in adverse effects (Shah et al, 1999).

Inhaled nitric oxide has been evaluated in preterm infants following the observation of its effectiveness in term and near-term infants with hypoxemic respiratory failure. Despite optimistic results from a large randomized controlled trial (Schreiber et al, 2003), trials in preterm infants report heterogeneous effects on bronchopulmonary dysplasia, mortality, and other important outcomes (Barrington & Finer, 2001; Schreiber et al, 2003; Van Meurs et al, 2005). The most current data do not support the routine administration of inhaled nitric oxide in preterm infants with hypoxemic respiratory failure, but this is an area of much research.

Prevention of extubation failure has been attempted using various pharmacologic approaches. Methylxanthines appear to have a large effect on reducing extubation failure (51% to 25%; RR 0.47; CI 0.32, 0.70; NNT 4). Similarly, systemic steroids before extubation reduces need for reintubation (10% to 1%; RR 0.18; CI 0.04, 0.97; NNT 11). In contrast, racemic epinephrine post extubation does not improve pulmonary function or extubation failure (Davies & Davis, 2001).

Other medications that have been evaluated include diuretics, bronchodilators, and antioxidants. Administration of furosemide to ventilated preterm infants improved pulmonary function (various measures with heterogeneity of results) but did not result in important or long-term benefits (Brion et al, 2003). Bronchodilators have been used to treat preterm infants with evolving or established BPD. Improvement in pulmonary mechanics (both resistance and compliance) has been reported without effect on long-term or important outcomes. Vitamin E or superoxide dismutase therapy did not reduce BPD.

SUMMARY

Hypoxemia continues to contribute significantly to both morbidity and mortality in NICUs. As our understanding of the pathophysiology of neonatal hypoxemia improves, new approaches to prevention and treatment are suggested. The

Case Study

IDENTIFICATION OF THE PROBLEM

A female infant was born after an elective repeat cesarean section. The amniotic fluid was clear. The infant developed respiratory distress in the first hours after birth while in the newborn nursery. She was placed on a radiant warmer for observation, and pulse oximetry revealed a saturation of 90% while breathing room air.

ASSESSMENT: HISTORY AND PHYSICAL EXAMINATION

The infant was born after elective repeat cesarean section, but decreased beat-to-beat variability of the fetal heart rate had been noted for the first time during routine monitoring just before the cesarean section. The pregnancy had been uncomplicated. Amniotic fluid was clear. Apgar scores were 7 and 8 at 1 and 5 minutes, respectively. There was no history of infection or other complications during pregnancy. At half an hour after birth, the infant was taken from the mother to the normal newborn nursery for routine care. During the subsequent hours she was noted to have occasional grunting and retractions.

DIFFERENTIAL DIAGNOSIS

The differential diagnosis for a term infant with mild respiratory distress in the first hours after birth by cesarean section include transient tachypnea of the newborn, hypothermia, hypoglycemia, and other less common conditions.

DIAGNOSTIC TESTS

The initial arterial blood gas values were as follows: pH 7.35, PCO_2 48, PO_2 43, bicarbonate 27. The blood sugar was 29 mg/dL. The infant was given 100% oxygen, and oxygen saturations remained around 90%. A chest radiograph, blood culture and CBC, and serial blood gases were obtained. Because of persistent low saturations, the infant was intubated.

WORKING DIAGNOSIS

The preductal and postductal oxygen saturations persisted around 90% despite 100% oxygen and endotracheal intubation. The chest radiograph showed clear lungs with decreased perfusion. The blood pressures were normal. The CBC and white blood cell count were normal.

DEVELOPMENT OF MANAGEMENT PLAN

Nitric oxide was initiated because of a suspicion of pulmonary hypertension. Because of persistent low saturations, congenital cyanotic heart disease was also suspected. An echocardiogram was obtained to assist in the diagnosis. A prostaglandin E drip was initiated while the echocardiogram was obtained. The echocardiogram confirmed the diagnosis of interrupted aortic arch. No evidence of pulmonary hypertension was seen, but moderate-to-severe obstruction to left cardiac output was observed. The nitric oxide was discontinued. The infant was continued on prostaglandin E_1 until surgical repair was performed. The serum calcium level was 7.5 mg/dl.

IMPLEMENTATION AND EVALUATION OF EFFECTIVENESS

The infant was continued on a prostaglandin E_1 intravenous infusion. Because of the association of interrupted aortic arch and other outcome obstruction lesions with DiGeorge syndrome, the DiGeorge probe was obtained, which confirmed this diagnosis. The infant had intractable hypocalcemia treated with high doses of calcium. In addition, she had a decreased T cell count. Surgical repair of the interrupted aortic arch was successful.

---

development of new therapeutic techniques—such as surfactant replacement, ECMO, HFV, NO, and liquid ventilation—holds the promise of improved neonatal outcome. There is a paucity of data regarding long-term outcome with some of these newer therapies and whether they hold significant benefits over older conventional methods. The evaluation and discovery of newer and safer methods to prevent and treat neonatal hypoxemia requires the collaborative efforts of basic scientific research and ongoing large, multicenter, randomized clinical trials.

REFERENCES

Acute Respiratory Distress Syndrome Network (2000). Ventilation with lower tidal volumes as compared with traditional tidal volumes for acute lung injury and the acute respiratory distress syndrome. *New England journal of medicine* 342:1301-1308.

Ambalavanan N et al (2003). Vitamin A supplementation in extremely low birth weight (ELBW) infants: prevalence and factors inhibiting its widespread use. *Pediatric research* 371A:2108.

American Academy of Pediatrics/Canadian Paediatric Society (2002). Postnatal corticosteroids to treat or prevent chronic lung disease in preterm infants. *Pediatrics* 109:330-340.

Anonymous (2000). Supplemental therapeutic oxygen for pre-threshold retinopathy of prematurity (STOP-ROP), Randomized, Controlled Trial. I: Primary outcomes. *Pediatrics* 105:295-310.

Artigas A et al (1998). The American-European Consensus Conference on RDS, Part 2. Ventilation, pharmacologic, supportive therapy, study design strategies, and issues related to recovery and remodeling. *American journal of respiratory critical care medicine* 157:1332-1347.

Askie LM et al (2003). Oxygen-saturation targets and outcomes in extremely preterm infants. *New England journal of medicine* 349:959-967.

Avery ME, Mead J (1959). Surface properties in relation to atelectasis and hyaline membrane disease. *American journal of diseases of children* 97:517-523.

Barrington KJ, Finer NN (2001). Inhaled nitric oxide for respiratory failure in preterm infants. Neonatal Collaborative Review Group. *NICHD Cochrane neonatal reviews*. Available at: http://156.40.88.3/cochrane/barrington/barring1.htm.

Barrington KJ, Finer NN (2006). Inhaled nitric oxide for respiratory failure in preterm infants. *Cochrane database of systematic reviews*, 2001(4):CD000509.

Bennett CC et al (2001). UK collaborative randomised trial of neonatal extracorporeal membrane oxygenation: follow-up to age 4 years. *Lancet* 357(9262):1094-1096.

Bhuta T, Henderson-Smart DJ (2002). Elective high frequency jet ventilation versus conventional ventilation for respiratory distress syndrome in preterm infants. *NICHD Cochrane neonatal reviews*. Available at: www.cochrane.org/reviews/en/ab000104.html.

Brion LP et al (2003). Diuretics acting on the distal renal tubule for preterm infants with (or developing) chronic lung disease. Neonatal Collaborative Review Group. *NICHD Cochrane neonatal reviews.* http://156.40.88.3/cochrane/brion5/brion.htm.

Carlo WA, Ambalavanan N (1999). Conventional mechanical ventilation: traditional and new strategies. *Pediatrics in review* 20:e117-e126.

Carlo WA et al (2002). Minimal ventilation to prevent bronchopulmonary dysplasia in extremely-low birth-weight infants. *Journal of pediatrics* 141:370-374.

Carnielli VP et al (1998). Iron supplementation enhances response to high doses of recombinant human erythropoietin in preterm infants. *Archives of disease in childhood: fetal and neonatal edition* 79(1):F4448.

Cifuentes J (1996). Does surfactant administration reduce the incidence of bronchopulmonary dysplasia (BPD)? *Pediatric research* 39:1192.

Clark RH et al (2000). Low-dose nitric oxide therapy for persistent pulmonary hypertension of the newborn. Clinical inhaled nitric oxide research group. *New England journal of medicine* 342(7):469-474.

Clark RH et al (2001). Lung injury in neonates: causes, strategies for prevention, and long-term consequences. *Journal of pediatrics* 139:478-486.

Darlow BA, Graham PJ (2002). Vitamin A supplementation for preventing morbidity and mortality in very low birth weight infants. Neonatal Collaborative Review Group. *NICHD Cochrane neonatal reviews.* http://156.40.88.3/cochrane/Darlow/Darlow.htm.

Davies MW, Davis PG (2001). Nebulized racemic epinephrine for extubation of newborn infants. Neonatal Collaborative Review Group. *NICHD Cochrane neonatal reviews.* Available at: http://156.40.88.3/cochrane/Davies/Davies.htm.

Field D et al (2005). Neonatal ventilation with inhaled nitric oxide versus ventilatory support without inhaled nitric oxide for preterm infants with severe respiratory failure: the INNOVO multicentre randomised controlled trial (ISRCTN 17821339). *Pediatrics* 115(4):926-936.

Finer NN (2000). Inhaled nitric oxide in term and near-term infants: neurodevelopmental follow-up of the neonatal inhaled nitric oxide study group (NINOS). *Journal of pediatrics* 136(5):611-617.

Finer NN, Barrington KJ (2001). Nitric oxide for respiratory failure in infants born at or near term. *Cochrane database of systematic reviews,* Issue 2.

Finer et al (2005). NICHD Neonatal Network. Delivery room continuous positive airway pressure/positive end-expiratory pressure in extremely low birth weight infants: a feasibility trial. *Pediatrics* 115:197-198.

Greenough A et al (2000). Synchronized mechanical ventilation for respiratory support in newborn infants. *Cochrane database of systematic reviews,* Issue 4.

Greenspan JS et al (1997). Pulmonary sequelae in infants treated with extracorporeal membrane oxygenation. *Pediatric pulmonology* 23(1):31-38.

Hansen TN (1998). *Contemporary diagnosis and management of neonatal respiratory disease,* ed 2. Newton, PA: Handbooks in Health Care.

Hargett KD (1995). Mechanical ventilation of the neonate. In Barnhart SL, Czervinske MP, editors. *Perinatal and pediatric respiratory care.* Philadelphia: Saunders.

Henderson-Smart DJ et al (2003). Elective high frequency oscillatory ventilation versus conventional ventilation for acute pulmonary dysfunction in premature infants. *Cochrane database of systematic reviews* 2003(3):CD000104.

HiFO Study Group (1993). Randomized study of high-frequency oscillatory ventilation in infants with severe respiratory distress syndrome. *Journal of pediatrics* 122:609-619.

Hudak ML et al (1996). A multicenter randomized, masked comparison trial of natural versus synthetic surfactant for the treatment of respiratory distress syndrome. *Journal of pediatrics* 128(3):396-406.

Keszler M et al (1991). Multicenter controlled trial comparing high-frequency jet ventilation and conventional mechanical ventilation in newborn infants with pulmonary interstitial emphysema. *Journal of pediatrics* 119:85-93.

Kinsella JP, Abman SH (1995). Recent developments in the pathophysiology and treatment of persistent pulmonary hypertension of the newborn. *Journal of pediatrics* 126(6):853-863.

Leach CL et al (1996). Partial liquid ventilation with perflubron in premature infants with severe respiratory distress syndrome. The liquivent study group. *New England journal of medicine* 335(11):761-767.

Mariani G, Cifuentes J, Carlo WA (1999). Randomized trial of permissive hypercapnia in preterm infants. *Pediatrics* 104:1082-1088.

Pattle RE (1958). Properties, function and origin of alveolar lining layer. *Proceedings of the Royal Society of London* B148:217-240.

Roberts JD et al (1992). Inhaled nitric oxide in persistent pulmonary hypertension of the newborn. *Lancet* 340(8823):818-819.

Sandri F et al (2004). Prophylactic nasal continuous positive airway pressure in newborns 28-31 weeks gestation: multicenter randomized controlled trial. *Archives of disease in childhood: fetal and neonatal edition* 89:F394-F398.

Schreiber MD et al (2003). Inhaled nitric oxide in preterm infants with respiratory distress syndrome. *New England journal of medicine* 349(22):2099-2107.

Shaffer TH et al (1999). Liquid ventilation: current status. *Pediatrics in review* 20e:134-142.

Shah V et al (1999). Early administration of inhaled corticosteroids for preventing chronic lung disease in ventilated very low birth weight preterm neonates. Neonatal Collaborative Review Group. *NICHD Cochrane neonatal reviews.* Available at: http://156.40.88.3/cochrane/shah2/shah.htm.

Soll RF (1998a). Synthetic surfactant treatment for preterm infants with respiratory distress syndrome. Neonatal Collaborative Review Group. *NICHD Cochrane neonatal reviews.* Available at: http://156.40.88.3/cochrane/SOLL8/SOLL.htm.

Soll RF (1998b). Prophylactic synthetic surfactant in preterm infants. Neonatal Collaborative Review Group. *NICHD Cochrane neonatal reviews.* Available at: http://156.40.88.3/cochrane/SOLL5/SOLL.htm.

Soll RF (1999). Multiple versus single dose natural surfactant extract for severe neonatal respiratory distress syndrome. Neonatal Collaborative Review Group. *NICHD Cochrane neonatal reviews.* Available at: http://156.40.88.3/cochrane/SOLL/SOLL.htm.

Soll RF (2000). Natural surfactant extract versus synthetic surfactant for neonatal respiratory distress syndrome. *Cochrane database of systematic reviews,* Issue 4.

Soll RF, Blanco F (2001). Natural surfactant extract versus synthetic surfactant for neonatal respiratory distress syndrome. Neonatal Collaborative Review Group. *NICHD Cochrane neonatal reviews.* Available at: http://156.40.88.3/cochrane/SOLL2/SOLL.htm.

Soll RF, Morley CJ (2001). Prophylactic versus selective use of surfactant in preventing morbidity and mortality in preterm infants. Neonatal Collaborative Review Group. *NICHD Cochrane neonatal reviews.* Available at: http://156.40.88.3/cochrane/SOLL4/SOLL.htm.

The STOP-ROP Multicenter Study Group (2000). Supplemental therapeutic oxygen for prethreshold retinopathy of prematurity (STOP-ROP): a randomized, controlled trial. I: Primary outcomes. *Pediatrics* 105:295-310.

Thome UH, Carlo WA (2003). High-frequency ventilation: when is it beneficial? *Neonatal respiratory diseases* 13:1-11.

Thome UH et al (2005). Ventilation strategies and outcome in randomized trials of high frequency ventilation. *Archives of disease in childhood: fetal and neonatal edition* 90(6):F466-F473.

Thomson MA on behalf of the IFDAS study group (2002). Early nasal continuous positive airways pressure (nCPAP) with prophylactic surfactant for neonates at risk of RDS. The IFDAS multi-centre randomized trial. *Pediatric research* 379A:2204.

Tyson JE et al (1999). Vitamin A supplementation for extremely-low-birth-weight infants. NICHD Neonatal Research Network. *New England journal of medicine* 340:1962-1968.

UK Collaborative Trial Group (1996). UK collaborative randomized trial of neonatal extracorporeal membrane oxygenation. *Lancet* 348:75-82.

Van Meurs KP et al (2005). Inhaled nitric oxide for premature infants with severe respiratory failure. *New England journal of medicine* 353(1):13-22.

Verder H et al (1994). Surfactant therapy and nasal continuous positive airway pressure for newborns with respiratory distress syndrome. Danish-Swedish Multicenter Study Group. *New England journal of medicine* 331:1051-1055.

Verder H et al (1999). Nasal continuous positive airway pressure and early surfactant therapy for respiratory distress syndrome in newborns of less than 30 weeks' gestation. *Pediatrics* 103:E25.

Yost CC, Soll RF (1999). Early versus delayed selective surfactant treatment for neonatal respiratory distress syndrome. Neonatal Collaborative Review Group. *NICHD Cochrane neonatal reviews.* Available at: http://156.40.88.3/cochrane/YOST/YOST.htm.

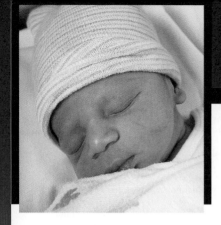

Chapter 3

Cardiovascular System

Judy Wright Lott

This chapter presents the physiology of normal cardiac function, including fetal circulatory patterns and the changes that occur during transition to extrauterine life. The most common congenital heart defects (CHDs) and cardiac complications are described. Information about incidence, hemodynamics, manifestations, diagnosis, and medical and surgical management is included. Because some CHDs are not identified during the neonatal period, information about presentation of some defects in older infants is also included. The chapter concludes with a discussion about the support of the family of an infant with a CHD. A case study is used to illustrate the complex care infants and families of infants with cardiac disorders require. Additional case studies and supplemental material can be accessed on the website.

CARDIOVASCULAR ADAPTATION

Fetal Circulation

Knowledge of the normal route of fetal blood flow is essential for understanding the circulatory changes that occur in the newborn at delivery. The pattern of fetal circulation is illustrated in Figure 3-1. Fetal circulation involves four unique anatomic features.

In fetal life, the placenta serves as the exchange organ for oxygen and carbon dioxide and for nutrients and wastes. The ductus venosus is a shunt that permits the majority of blood from the placenta to bypass the liver and enter the inferior vena cava. The foramen ovale, an opening in the septum between the atria, permits a portion of the blood to flow from the right atrium directly to the left atrium and reduce the flow of blood through the pulmonary system. The patent ductus arteriosus (PDA), a tubular communication between the pulmonary artery and the descending aorta, that allows blood to flow from the right ventricle through the pulmonary artery to the descending aorta, further decreases the amount of blood circulation through the fetal lungs (Friedman, 2001; Keane et al, 2006; Lott, 2002; Park et al, 2002).

Oxygen diffuses into the fetal circulation from the maternal uterine arteries in the placenta. From the placenta, the oxygenated blood flows through the umbilical vein to the fetus. The fetal circulation divides at the liver, with about half of the blood entering the liver and the remainder bypassing the liver through the *ductus venosus*. Blood from the ductus venosus enters the inferior vena cava. In the inferior vena cava blood of lower oxygen content coming from the gastrointestinal tract, legs, and liver mixes with the blood of higher oxygen content coming from other parts of the body. The mixed blood then enters the right atrium (Friedman, 2001; Lott, 2002; Park et al, 2002).

From this point, the blood from the right atrium flows directly to the left atrium through the *foramen ovale*. From the left atrium, the blood goes to the left ventricle, and then it travels to the head and neck through the ascending aorta. This circulatory pattern ensures that the fetal brain constantly receives well-oxygenated blood (Friedman, 2001; Lott, 2002; Park et al, 2002).

The blood returns from the head and neck through the superior vena cava to the right atrium. This blood then flows into the right ventricle. From the right ventricle, the blood enters the pulmonary arteries. Only a small portion of this blood enters the pulmonary circuit to perfuse the lungs; the majority of the blood is shunted through the ductus arteriosus into the aorta to supply oxygen and nutrients to the trunk and lower extremities (Friedman, 2001; Lott, 2002; Park et al, 2002).

Most of the blood flow from the lower extremities rejoins the fetal circulation through the internal iliac arteries via the umbilical cord to the placenta, where it is reoxygenated and recirculated. A small amount of the blood from the lower extremities passes back into the ascending vena cava, mixed with fresh blood from the umbilical vein, and recirculated without reoxygenation. Thus, fetal circulation can be described as two parallel circuits rather than as the serial circuit present in extrauterine life (Friedman, 2001; Lott, 2002; Park et al, 2002).

Extrauterine Circulation

The cardiac and pulmonary systems undergo drastic changes at birth; these changes usually occur functionally immediately at onset of respirations. The most significant change is that the primary oxygenation organ becomes the lungs rather than the placenta. Immediate circulatory changes in the newborn occur as a result of the clamping of the umbilical cord and subsequent removal of the placenta. With the first breath and occlusion of the umbilical cord, the newborn's systemic resistance is elevated, causing a decrease in the amount of blood flow through the ductus arteriosus. Cord occlusion causes a prompt increase in blood pressure and a corresponding stimulation of the aortic baroreceptors and the sympathetic nervous system. The onset of respirations and consequent lung expansion causes a decrease in pulmonary vascular resistance because of the direct effect of oxygen and carbon dioxide on the blood vessels. Pulmonary vascular resistance decreases as arterial oxygen increases and arterial carbon dioxide decreases (Lott, 2002; Park et al, 2002).

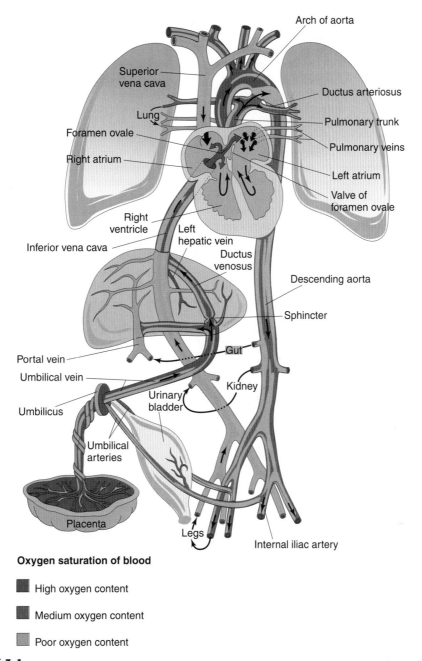

Arch of aorta

Superior vena cava

Ductus arteriosus

Lung

Pulmonary trunk

Foramen ovale

Pulmonary veins

Right atrium

Left atrium

Valve of foramen ovale

Right ventricle

Left hepatic vein

Inferior vena cava

Ductus venosus

Descending aorta

Sphincter

Portal vein

Gut

Umbilical vein

Kidney

Umbilicus

Urinary bladder

Umbilical arteries

Placenta

Legs

Internal iliac artery

Oxygen saturation of blood

■ High oxygen content

■ Medium oxygen content

■ Poor oxygen content

FIGURE **3-1**
Fetal circulation. From Moore KL, Persaud TVN (2003). *The developing human: clinically oriented embryology,* ed 7. Philadelphia: Saunders.

Most of the right ventricular output flows through the lungs and increases the pulmonary venous return to the left atrium. The increased amount of blood in the lungs and the heart causes pressure in the left atrium of the heart. The increased pressure in the left atrium, combined with the increased systemic vascular resistance, functionally closes the foramen ovale.

The ductus arteriosus normally closes within 15 to 24 hours after birth in response to increased arterial oxygen content caused by pulmonary respiratory effort of the newborn and the effects of sympathomimetic amines and prostaglandins. The ductus arteriosus is anatomically obliterated by constriction by 3 to 4 weeks of age. Clamping of the umbilical cord causes the cessation of blood flow through the ductus venosus; it is anatomically obliterated by approximately 1 to 2 weeks after

birth. After birth, the umbilical vein and arteries no longer transport blood and are obliterated.

Functional closure refers to the cessation of flow through the structure caused by changes in pressure. *Anatomic closure* refers to obliteration of the structure by constriction or growth of tissue.

Because anatomic closure of the fetal pathways lags behind functional closure, the shunts may open and close intermittently before anatomic closure, resulting in transient functional murmurs.

Pulmonary artery pressure remains high for several hours after birth. As the pulmonary vascular resistance diminishes, the direction of blood flow through the ductus arteriosus reverses. Initially bi-directional, the flow becomes entirely left to right; it is functionally insignificant by approximately 15 hours after birth. Intermittent or functional murmurs do not cause any cardiovascular compromise for the newborn and are not clinically significant. Conditions that cause transient opening of fetal shunts, allowing unoxygenated blood to shunt from the right side of the heart to the left, thereby bypassing the pulmonary circuit, produce transient cyanosis. Any murmur or cyanosis in the newborn should be carefully evaluated and monitored to detect cardiovascular abnormalities (Friedman, 2001; Lott, 2002; Park et al, 2002). Hypoxemia can cause a constricted ductus arteriosus to reopen and may reestablish increased pulmonary vascular resistance, leading to persistent pulmonary hypertension of the newborn (PPHN). The ductus arteriosus responds to hypoxemia by opening, whereas the pulmonary arterioles respond by constricting (Lott, 2002; Park et al, 2002).

NORMAL CARDIAC FUNCTION

The normal anatomy of the heart is shown in Figure 3-2.

Cardiac Valves

Blood flow through the heart is directed through two sets of one-way valves. The *semilunar valves* consist of the *pulmonary valve* and the *aortic valve*. The pulmonary valve connects the right ventricle and the pulmonary artery. The aortic valve connects the left ventricle and the aorta. The *atrioventricular valves* (AV) consist of the *tricuspid valve* and the *mitral valve*. The tricuspid valve connects the right atrium and the right ventricle. The mitral valve connects the left atrium and the left ventricle (Lott, 2002).

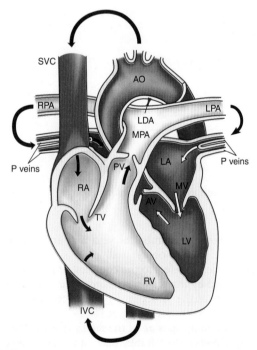

FIGURE **3-2**
Normal cardiac anatomy and circulation. *AO*, Aorta; *AV*, aortic valve; *IVC*, inferior vena cava; *LA*, left atrium; *LDA*, ligamentum ductus arteriosus; *LPA*, left pulmonary artery; *LV*, left ventricle; *MPA*, main pulmonary artery; *MV*, mitral valve; *PV*, pulmonary valve; *P veins*, pulmonary veins; *RA*, right atrium; *RPA*, right pulmonary artery; *RV*, right ventricle; *SVC*, superior vena cava; *TV*, tricuspid valve.

Cardiac Cycle

Normal cardiac function involves two stages: *systole* and *diastole*. During systole, contraction of the ventricle causes the pressure inside the ventricle to increase to approximately 70 mm Hg in newborns (approximately 120 mm Hg in adults). When sufficient pressure is generated, the aortic and pulmonary valves open and blood is ejected from the ventricles. As the blood flows from the ventricles, the pressure decreases, causing the aortic and pulmonary valves to close.

During diastole, the mitral and tricuspid valves open and 70% of the blood in the atria flows into the ventricles. A small portion of the blood flows back into the aorta and enters the coronary arteries for perfusion of the heart. At the end of diastole, a small atrial contraction occurs (4 to 6 mm Hg on the right side; 7 to 8 mm Hg on the left side), and the mitral and tricuspid valves close. Metabolism of the heart is decreased during diastole. The average newborn's cardiac cycle is approximately 0.4 second, with 0.2 second for diastole and 0.2 second for systole (based on a heart rate of approximately 150 beats per minute) (Opie, 2001).

Cardiac Output

Cardiac output is the amount of blood pumped by the left ventricle in 1 minute. Cardiac output is equal to the stroke volume times the heart rate (CO × SV × HR). The stroke volume is the volume of blood pumped per beat from each ventricle. The greater the stroke volume, the greater the volume of blood is in the systemic circulation. An increase in cardiac output increases systole and decreases diastole. Cardiac output is influenced by changes in heart rate, pulmonary vascular resistance, and systemic resistance to flow.

Cardiac output is influenced by the amount of blood returned to the heart, as explained by the Frank-Starling law, which states that within physiologic limits, the heart pumps all the blood that enters it without allowing excessive accumulation of blood in the veins. Venous return is determined by the passive movement of blood through the veins, the thoracic pump, and the venous muscle pump. Normally, when increased volume enters the heart, contractility is increased as a response to stimulation of stretch receptors in the heart muscle. The newborn's heart has fewer fibers and is unable to stretch sufficiently to accommodate increased volume; therefore, increased heart rate is the only effective mechanism by which the newborn can respond to increased volume (Colucci & Braunwald, 2001; Lott, 2002; Opie, 2001).

Cardiac failure occurs when the volume exceeds the ability of the heart to pump. Local factors that affect venous return to the heart include hypoxia, acidosis, hypercarbia, hyperthermia, increased metabolic demand, and increased metabolites (potassium, adenosine triphosphate, and lactic acid).

Other factors that influence cardiac output include vascular pressure and resistance. Pressure and resistance are inversely related: if pressure in the arterial bed is increased, resistance is decreased and flow is improved. The size (radius) of vessels influences resistance: the greater the radius of a vessel, the lower the resistance. Vessels obstructed by thromboses or constriction have greater resistance to vascular flow (Colucci & Braunwald, 2001; Lott, 2002; Opie, 2001).

Autonomic Cardiac Control

Cardiovascular function is modulated by the autonomic nervous system. Baroreceptors and chemoreceptors in the aorta and carotid sinus provide feedback to the autonomic nervous system. Feedback from these receptors stimulates the parasympathetic or sympathetic nervous system.

The parasympathetic nervous system is less powerful than the sympathetic system. Stimulation of the parasympathetic and sympathetic nervous systems results in vagal nerve stimulation and a decrease in heart rate. Most parasympathetic and sympathetic nervous system effects are on the atria, but decreased ventricular contractility may also occur. Right vagal stimulation affects the sinoatrial (SA) node, and left vagal stimulation affects the AV node. Acetylcholine is the active neurotransmitter for the parasympathetic and sympathetic nervous systems (Colucci & Braunwald, 2001; Lott, 2002; Opie, 2001).

Stimulation of the sympathetic nervous system through the ganglionic chain releases norepinephrine and epinephrine, which act on the SA node, the AV node, the atria, and the ventricles. Maximal stimulation of the sympathetic nervous system can increase heart rate to 250 to 300 beats per minute. Contractility can be improved by approximately 100%. Alpha- and beta-adrenergic receptors are stimulated. Alpha receptors cause increased contractility (inotropic) and increased rate (chronotropic); beta$_2$-receptors cause vasodilation, bronchodilatation, and smooth muscle relaxation (Kaplan, 2001).

Term newborns have a decreased number of receptors but are capable of normal cardiovascular system function. The preterm newborn is not able to smoothly maintain autonomic function, and energy expenditure is increased. Hence, the cardiovascular signs such as color changes and bradycardia may occur as a result of an excessive demand for autonomic nervous system function.

CARDIAC ASSESSMENT

Early recognition of signs and symptoms of congenital heart disease leads to earlier diagnosis and treatment and may improve outcome (Goh, 2000). Thus careful newborn assessment is a crucial component of newborn care. Cardiac assessment includes history taking, physical assessment, and interpretation of diagnostic tests. Review of the maternal, fetal, and neonatal history is helpful in cardiac evaluation of the newborn. Associated with CHDs are (1) maternal infections, especially viral and protozoal infections early in pregnancy, (2) maternal use of tobacco, alcohol, or drugs, and (3) maternal diseases. Table 3-1 lists heart defects commonly associated with maternal history. Birth weight may also aid in the identification of a CHD. Macrosomia is associated with maternal diabetes and transposition of the great arteries (TGA), whereas infants of mothers with viral diseases are frequently small for gestational age (Little, 2001; Park et al, 2002).

Methods of Assessment

Assessment for evidence of a cardiovascular disorder begins with a careful history and is followed by a thorough physical examination. Family history of hereditary disease, congenital heart disease, or rheumatic fever is significant. Certain hereditary diseases have a CHD as part of the expression (Table 3-2). The overall incidence of CHDs is approximately 1%, or 8 per 1000 live births, excluding persistent patent ductus arteriosus (PDA) in preterm newborns. If the mother had a CHD, however, the incidence increases in the offspring to approximately 3% to 4% (Park et al, 2002; Pyeritz, 2001).

TABLE 3-1	Maternal Condition and Associated Congenital Heart Defects
Condition	**Defect**
MATERNAL DISEASE	
Diabetes mellitus	Cardiomyopathy, TGA, VSD, PDA
Lupus erythematosus	Congenital heart block
Collagen disease	Congenital heart block
Congenital heart defect	Increased risk for congenital heart defect (3%–4%)
VIRAL DISEASE	
Rubella	
First trimester	PDA, pulmonary artery branch stenosis
Later	Various cardiac and other defects
Cytomegalovirus	Various cardiac and other defects
Herpesvirus	Various cardiac and other defects
Coxsackievirus B	Cardiomyopathy
DRUGS	
Amphetamines	VSD, PDA, ASD, TGA
Phenytoin	PS, AS, COA, PDA
Trimethadione	TGA, TOF, HLHS
Progesterone/estrogen	VSD, TOF, TGA
Alcohol	VSD, PDA, ASD, TOF

Data from Hazinski MF (1984). Cardiovascular disorders. In Hazinski MF, editor. Nursing care of the critically ill child (pp 63–252). St Louis: Mosby; and Park MK (1988). Pediatric cardiology for practitioners. St Louis: Mosby.
AS, *Aortic stenosis;* ASD, *atrial septal defect;* COA, *coarctation of the aorta;* HLHS, *hypoplastic left heart syndrome;* PDA, *patent ductus arteriosus;* PS, *pulmonary stenosis;* TGA, *transposition of the great arteries;* TOF, *tetralogy of Fallot;* VSD, *ventricular septal defect.*

A neonatal history of cyanosis, tachypnea without pulmonary disease, sweating, poor feeding, edema, or, in older infants, failure to gain weight is suggestive of congenital heart disease. Careful evaluation of the maternal, fetal, and neonatal history, in conjunction with a thorough physical assessment identifies infants for whom further diagnostic testing is indicated.

Physical examination of the newborn with a suspected cardiovascular dysfunction includes inspection, palpation, and auscultation (Park et al, 2002; Perloff & Braunwald, 2004).

Inspection

Valuable information about the cardiovascular system of the newborn can be obtained by observation of the infant's general appearance before examination. The following states of the newborn should be observed: sleeping or awake, alert or lethargic, anxious or relaxed. Respiratory effort, including signs of respiratory distress such as nasal flaring, expiratory grunting, stridor, retractions, or paradoxical respirations, should be observed. Tachypnea and tachycardia are early signs of left ventricular failure. Severe left ventricular failure also causes dyspnea and retractions (Park et al, 2002; Perloff & Braunwald, 2004).

The color of the neonate should be observed. Cyanosis refers to the bluish color of the skin, mucous membranes, and nail beds that occurs when at least 5 g/100 ml of deoxygenated

TABLE **3-2**	Congenital Heart Defects Associated with Specific Genetic or Chromosomal Abnormalities
Disease or Syndrome	**Defect**
Trisomy 13, 18	PDA, VSD
Trisomy 21	ECD, VSD, PDA
Turner syndrome	COA
Marfan syndrome	AS, MVS, aortic aneurysms, TAPVR
Williams syndrome (elfin facies)	AS, PPAS
DiGeorge syndrome	Interrupted aortic arch
Neurofibromatosis	PVS

Data from Park MK (1988). Pediatric cardiology for practitioners. St Louis: Mosby.
AS, *Aortic stenosis;* COA, *coarctation of the aorta;* ECD, *endocardial cushion defect;* MVS, *mitral valve stenosis;* PDA, *patent ductus arteriosus;* PPAS, *peripheral pulmonic arterial stenosis;* PVS, *pulmonic valvular stenosis;* TAPVR, *total anomalous pulmonary venous return;* VSD, *ventricular septal defect.*

hemoglobin is present in the circulation. If cyanosis is present, note whether it is peripheral or central cyanosis and whether it improves with crying, does not change, or becomes worse with crying. Cyanosis can result from pulmonary, hematologic, central nervous system, or metabolic diseases, as well as from cardiac defects. Pulmonary and cardiac defects are the two most common causes of central cyanosis in the newborn.

Pallor may indicate vasoconstriction resulting from congestive heart failure (CHF) or circulatory shock caused by severe anemia. Prolonged physiologic jaundice may occur in infants with CHF or congenital hypothyroidism, which is associated with PDA and pulmonary stenosis (PS). A ruddy or plethoric appearance is often seen in polycythemia. These infants may appear cyanotic without significant arterial desaturation.

The presence of sweating is very suggestive of a CHD in the newborn. The cause of sweating is sympathetic overactivity as a compensatory mechanism for decreased cardiac output. Precordial activity is a reliable parameter of cardiac dysfunction. Precordial bulging is suggestive of chronic cardiac enlargement. Precordial activity without bulging may be associated with acute onset of cardiac dysfunction. Pectus excavatum may cause a pulmonary systolic ejection murmur or a large cardiac silhouette on an anteroposterior chest radiograph because of the decreased anteroposterior chest diameter. Pectus excavatum does not cause cardiac dysfunction (Park et al, 2002).

Palpation

Palpation includes the palpation of the precordium and peripheral pulses. Palpation of the precordium detects hyperactivity, thrill, and the point of maximal impulse (PMI). Irregularities or inequalities of rate or volume can be detected by counting the peripheral pulse rate. Evaluation of the carotid, brachial, femoral, and pedal pulses detects differences between sides and upper and lower extremities. If pulses are unequal, four extremity blood pressures should be measured. Weak leg pulses with strong arm pulses suggest coarctation of the aorta (COA). Supravalvular aortic stenosis or coarctation

proximal to or near the origin of the left subclavian artery may be present if the right brachial pulse is stronger than the left (Park et al, 2002).

Heart defects that lead to "aortic runoff," such as PDA, aortic insufficiency, large arteriovenous fistula, or persistent truncus arteriosus, cause bounding pulses. However, preterm newborns frequently have a bounding pulse because of relatively decreased subcutaneous tissue. Also, preterm infants frequently have PDA secondary to their prematurity. Cardiac failure or circulatory shock causes weak or thready pulses (Park et al, 2002).

The hyperactive precordium indicates a heart defect with increased volume, such as CHDs with large left to right shunts (e.g., PDA, ventricular septal defect [VSD]) or heart disease with valvular regurgitation (e.g., aortic regurgitation or mitral regurgitation). The location of the PMI depends on whether the right or left ventricle is dominant. With right ventricular dominance, the PMI is at the lower left sternal border (LLSB). Left ventricular dominance places the PMI at the apex. A diffuse, slow-rising PMI is called a *heave*. Heaves are associated with volume overload. A sharp, fast-rising PMI is called a *tap* and is associated with pressure overload. The normal newborn has a right ventricular dominance (Park et al, 2002).

The apical impulse of the newborn is normally felt in the fourth intercostal space to the left of the midclavicular line. Displacement of the apical impulse downward or laterally may indicate cardiac enlargement (Park et al, 2002).

The presence and location of a thrill provide important diagnostic information. The palms of the hands, rather than the fingertips, should be used to feel for a thrill, except in the suprasternal notch and carotid arteries. The examiner should palpate for the presence of thrills in the upper left, upper right, and lower left sternal border, in the suprasternal notch, and over the carotid arteries. A thrill in the upper left sternal border is derived from the pulmonary valve or pulmonary artery. Thrills in the lower left sternal border suggest pulmonary stenosis, pulmonary artery atresia, or, occasionally, PDA. A thrill felt in the upper right sternal border signifies aortic origin, usually aortic stenosis or, less frequently, PS, PDA, or COA. A thrill over the carotid arteries along with a thrill in the suprasternal notch suggests COA or aortic stenosis (AS), or other defects of the aorta or aortic valve (Park et al, 2002).

Palpation of the abdomen is performed to determine the size, consistency, and location of the liver and spleen. Increased liver size is a frequent finding with CHF (Park et al, 2002).

Auscultation

Careful auscultation by a skilled evaluator is an essential component of any cardiovascular assessment. Auscultation includes heart rate and regularity, heart sounds, systolic and diastolic sounds, and heart murmurs. The skillful evaluation of cardiac sounds requires systematic auscultation and much practice.

Identification of Heart Sounds. Individual heart sounds should be identified and evaluated before evaluation of cardiac murmurs is attempted. The four individual heart sounds are S_1, S_2, S_3, and S_4. However, S_3 and S_4 are rarely heard in the newborn. S_1 is the sound resulting from closure of the mitral and tricuspid valves following atrial systole and is best heard at the apex or lower left sternal border. S_1 is the beginning of ventricular systole. Splitting of S_1 is infrequently heard in newborns. Wide splitting of S_1 is heard in right bundle branch block or Ebstein's anomaly (Park et al, 2002).

S_2 is the sound created by closure of the aortic and pulmonary valves, which marks the end of systole and the beginning of ventricular diastole. S_2 is best heard in the upper left sternal border or pulmonic area. Evaluation of the splitting of S_2 is important diagnostically. The timing of the closure of the aortic and pulmonary valves is determined by the volume of blood ejected from the aorta and pulmonary artery and the resistance against which the ventricles must pump. In the immediate newborn period, there may be no appreciable splitting of S_2. Because the right and left ventricles pump similar quantities of blood and the pulmonary pressure is close to the aortic pressure, these valves close almost simultaneously. Thus, S_2 is heard as a single sound. As the pulmonary vascular resistance decreases, the pulmonary resistance decreases and becomes lower than the aortic pressure, causing a splitting of S_2 as the valve leaflets on the left side of the heart (aortic valve) close before those on the right (pulmonary valve). By 72 hours of life, S_2 should be split. The absence of a split S_2 or the presence of a widely split S_2 usually indicates an abnormality. A fixed, widely split S_2 occurs in conditions that prolong right ventricular ejection time or shorten left ventricular ejection time. It occurs in (1) atrial septal defect (ASD) and partial anomalous pulmonary venous return (PAPVR) (amount of blood ejected by right ventricle is increased, resulting in volume overload), (2) pulmonary stenosis (stenosis delays right ventricular ejection time, resulting in pressure overload), (3) right bundle branch block (delayed electrical activation of right ventricle), (4) mitral regurgitation (decreased forward output, decreased left ventricular ejection time), and (5) idiopathic dilated main pulmonary artery (increased capacity of main pulmonary artery produces less recoil to close the valves, delaying closure) (Park et al, 2002).

A narrowly split S_2 may be caused by early closure of the pulmonary valve (pulmonary hypertension) or a delay in aortic closure. A single S_2 is significant because it could represent the presence of only one semilunar valve (e.g., aortic or pulmonary atresia and truncus arteriosus). A single S_2 may also occur with a critical pulmonary stenosis, transposition of the great arteries, or tetralogy of Fallot (TOF), in which the pulmonary closure is not audible. Severe aortic stenosis may also cause a single S_2 because aortic closure is delayed. Severe pulmonary hypertension may cause early closure of the pulmonary valve, thus causing a single S_2.

The relative intensity of the aortic and pulmonary components of S_2 must be assessed. In the pulmonary area (upper left sternal border), the aortic component is usually louder than the pulmonary component. Increased intensity of the pulmonary component, compared with the aortic component, occurs with pulmonary hypertension. Conditions that cause decreased diastolic pressure of the pulmonary artery (e.g., critical pulmonary stenosis, TOF, tricuspid atresia) may cause decreased intensity of the pulmonary component. Evaluation of intensity is difficult, requiring frequent practice listening to heart sounds (Park et al, 2002).

As discussed, S_3 and S_4 are rarely heard in the neonatal period; their presence denotes pathologic origin. Likewise, a gallop rhythm, the result of a loud S_3 and S_4, and tachycardia are abnormal. After evaluation of individual heart sounds, the systolic and diastolic sounds are evaluated. The ejection sound, or click, occurs after S_1 and may sound like splitting of S_1. The ejection click is best heard at the upper left or right sternal border or base. The pulmonary click can best be heard at the second or third left intercostal space and is louder with expiration. The aortic click, best heard at the second right intercostal space, does not change in intensity with change in respiration. Ejection clicks are associated with pulmonary or aortic stenosis or with the dilated great arteries seen in systemic or pulmonary hypertension, idiopathic dilation of the main pulmonary artery, TOF, or truncus arteriosus (Park et al, 2002).

CARDIAC MURMURS

Cardiac murmurs should be evaluated for intensity (grades 1 to 6), timing (systolic or diastolic), location, transmission, and quality (musical, vibratory, or blowing).

The grade scale for murmurs is as follows:

Grade 1: barely audible
Grade 2: soft but easily audible
Grade 3: moderately loud; no thrill
Grade 4: loud; thrill present
Grade 5: loud; audible with stethoscope barely on chest
Grade 6: loud; audible with stethoscope near chest

The murmur grade is recorded as 1/6, 2/6, and so on. Again, practice in auscultation improves the listener's evaluation skills. The intensity of the murmur is affected by cardiac output; anything that increases cardiac output (e.g., anemia, fever, exercise) increases the intensity of the murmur (Park et al, 2002; Perloff & Braunwald, 2004).

The next step in evaluating a murmur is its classification in relation to S_1 and S_2. The three types of murmurs are systolic, diastolic, and continuous.

Systolic Murmurs

Most heart murmurs are systolic, occurring between S_1 and S_2. Systolic murmurs are either ejection or regurgitation murmurs. Ejection murmurs occur after S_1 and end before S_2. Ejection murmurs are caused by flow of blood through stenotic or deformed semilunar valves or increased flow through normal semilunar valves. Systolic ejection murmurs are best heard at the second left or right intercostal space. Regurgitant systolic murmurs begin with S_1, with no interval between S_1 and the beginning of the murmur. Regurgitation murmurs generally continue throughout systole (pansystolic or holosystolic). Regurgitation systolic murmurs are caused by flow of blood from a chamber at a higher pressure throughout systole than the receiving chamber. Regurgitation systolic murmurs are associated with only three conditions: (1) VSD, (2) mitral regurgitation, and (3) tricuspid regurgitation (Park et al, 2002).

Location

The location of the maximal intensity of the murmur is helpful in evaluation of the cardiac murmur. Figure 3-3 shows the locations at which various systolic murmurs can be heard.

Related to the location is the transmission of the murmur. Knowledge of transmission can assist in determining the origin of the murmur. A systolic ejection murmur that transmits well to the neck is usually aortic in origin, whereas one that transmits to the back is usually pulmonary in origin. An apical systolic murmur that transmits well to the left axilla and lower back is characteristic of mitral regurgitation, but one that transmits to the upper right sternal border and neck is likely to be aortic in nature (Park et al, 2002).

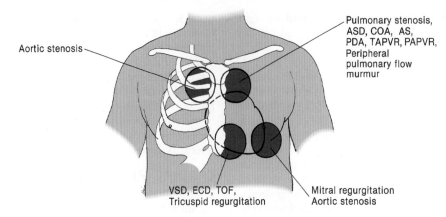

FIGURE **3-3**
Location of systolic murmurs. *AS*, Aortic stenosis; *ASD*, atrial septal defect; *COA*, coarctation of the aorta; *ECD*, endocardial cushion defect; *PAPVR*, partial anomalous pulmonary venous return; *PDA*, patent ductus arteriosus; *TAPVR*, total anomalous pulmonary venous return; *TOF*, tetralogy of Fallot; *VSD*, ventricular septal defect.

Quality

Murmurs are described as musical, vibratory, or blowing (Park et al, 2002). VSDs or mitral regurgitation murmurs have a high-pitched, blowing quality. Aortic stenosis and pulmonary valve stenosis murmurs have a rough, grating quality. Establishing the quality of the murmur is subjective, and expertise is gained only after extensive practice.

Diastolic Murmurs

Diastolic murmurs occur between S_1 and S_2. Diastolic murmurs are classified according to their timing in relation to heart sounds as early diastolic, mid-diastolic, or presystolic.

Early diastolic (protodiastolic) murmurs occur early in diastole, right after S_2, caused by incompetence of the aortic or pulmonary valve. Aortic regurgitation murmurs are high-pitched and are best heard with the diaphragm of the stethoscope at the third left intercostal space. Aortic regurgitation murmurs radiate to the apex. Bounding pulses are present with significant regurgitation. Aortic regurgitation murmurs occur with bicuspid aortic valve, subaortic stenosis, and subarterial infundibular VSD. Pulmonary regurgitation murmurs are medium pitched unless pulmonary hypertension is present, in which case they are high pitched. Diastolic regurgitation murmurs are heard best at the second left intercostal space, radiating along the left sternal border. Pulmonary regurgitation murmurs occur with postoperative TOF, pulmonary hypertension, postoperative pulmonary valvotomy for pulmonary stenosis, or other deformity of the pulmonary valve (Park et al, 2002; Perloff & Braunwald, 2004).

Mid-diastolic murmurs result from abnormal ventricular filling. These murmurs are low pitched and can best be heard with the bell of the stethoscope placed lightly on the chest wall. The murmur results from turbulent flow caused by stenosis of the tricuspid or mitral valve. Mitral mid-diastolic murmurs are best heard at the apex and are referred to as *apical rumbles*. Mitral mid-diastolic murmurs are associated with mitral stenosis or large VSDs with a large left to right shunt or PDA, producing relative mitral stenosis because of increased flow across the normal-sized mitral valve. Tricuspid mid-diastolic murmurs can best be heard along the lower left sternal border and are associated with ASD, total or partial anomalous pulmonary venous return, endocardial cushion defects, or abnormal stenosis of the tricuspid valve. Presystolic or late diastolic murmurs result from flow through AV valves during ventricular diastole as a result of active atrial contraction ejecting blood into the ventricle. These are low-frequency murmurs found with true mitral or tricuspid valve stenosis (Park et al, 2002; Perloff & Braunwald, 2004).

Continuous Murmurs

Continuous murmurs begin in systole and continue throughout S_2 into all or part of diastole. Continuous murmurs are caused by (1) aorticopulmonary or AV connection (e.g., PDA, AV fistula, or persistent truncus arteriosus), (2) disturbances of flow in veins (e.g., venous hum), and (3) disturbances of flow in arteries (e.g., COA or pulmonary artery stenosis) (Park et al, 2002).

PDA is the most commonly heard continuous murmur in the newborn. The PDA murmur is described as a machinery murmur, louder during systole, peaking at S_2, and decreased in diastole. PDA murmurs are loudest in the left infraclavicular area or the upper left sternal border (Park et al, 2002; Perloff & Braunwald, 2004).

Other Murmurs

Functional or innocent cardiac murmurs are common in children and can occur in newborns. Innocent murmurs occur in the absence of abnormal cardiac structures. Functional murmurs are asymptomatic. The presence of any unusual or abnormal finding warrants consultation. Findings such as cyanosis, enlarged heart size on examination or enlarged cardiac silhouette on radiograph, abnormal electrocardiogram (ECG), diastolic murmur, grade 3/6 systolic murmur or a less intense murmur with a thrill, weak or bounding pulses, or other abnormal heart sounds have pathologic origins and must be investigated (Park et al, 2002).

The pulmonary flow murmur is commonly found in low-birth-weight infants. Infants with a pulmonary flow murmur have relative hypoplastic right and left pulmonary arteries at birth, which are a result of the small amount of blood flow during fetal life. The increased flow after birth creates turbulence in the small vessels, which is transmitted along the smaller branches of the pulmonary arteries. This murmur is best heard at the upper left sternal border. The pulmonary flow murmur has a grade of 1/6 to 2/6 intensity, but is transmitted to the right and left chest, both axillae, and back. No other significant cardiac findings are seen. It usually disappears by 3 to 6 months after birth. Persistence beyond this period should lead to further evaluation for anatomic pulmonary artery stenosis (Park et al, 2002).

CONGENITAL HEART DEFECTS
Etiology
Cardiac development occurs during the first 7 weeks of gestation. Major structural defects can be caused by interference with the maternal-placental-fetal unit during this critical period. Causes of CHDs are classified as chromosomal (10% to 12%), genetic (1% to 2%), maternal or environmental (1% to 2%), or multifactorial (85%) (Wernovsky & Gruber, 2005). Table 3-2 lists congenital heart defects associated with specific genetic or chromosomal disorders.

Many chromosomal abnormalities are associated with structural heart defects. From 30% to 50% of infants with trisomy 21 (Down syndrome) have a structural heart defect. In one study of 243 children with trisomy 21, 44% had associated congenital heart defects. The most common CHDs with trisomy 21 are endocardial cushion defects (ECD); the most common ECD was an ASD and VSD (Freeman et al, 1998). Specific genetic abnormalities account for only a small percentage of CHDs. Marfan syndrome is associated with defects of the aorta, such as aortic insufficiency or an aortic aneurysm (Ardinger, 1997; Park et al, 2002; Pyeritz, 2001).

Maternal or environmental factors include maternal illness and drug ingestion. Maternal rubella during the first 7 weeks of pregnancy carries a 50% risk of congenital rubella syndrome (CRS) with major defects of multiple organ systems. Heart defects seen with CRS include PDA and pulmonary artery branch stenosis. Other viral diseases, such as cytomegalovirus, or protozoal diseases, such as toxoplasmosis, are also associated with CHDs. The diagnosis of a CHD calls for a careful maternal history to identify viral-like illnesses that may have been unrecognized or unreported at the time of occurrence and careful examination to rule out the presence of other congenital defects (Ardinger, 1997; Park et al, 2002; Pyeritz, 2001).

Maternal drug use may also cause cardiac malformations. Fifty percent of newborns with fetal alcohol syndrome (FAS) have a CHD. Only a few drugs are proven teratogens (e.g., thalidomide); however, *no* drugs are known to be completely safe. The threat of environmental hazards to fetal development has only recently been recognized.

Metabolic disease of the mother increases the risk for CHDs. Infants of diabetic mothers have a 10% risk of having a CHD. TGA, VSD, or generalized hypertrophic cardiomyopathy are the most common types of defects found in infants of diabetic mothers (Ardinger, 1997; Park et al, 2002).

Most CHDs are considered to be of multifactorial origin; these defects are probably the result of an interaction effect of the other causes. Research into genetic causes of cardiac defects may identify specific genetic causes for some heart defects that are currently thought to have multifactorial origin. Infants with other congenital defects often have associated CHDs. Multiple defects affect the development of structures that

are forming at the time of the interference with normal development.

Incidence
Estimates of incidence of CHD vary from 4.05 to 10.2 per 1000 live births. The overall incidence of CHD is slightly less than 1%, or 8 per 1000 live births, excluding PDA in the preterm newborn (Nouri, 1997; Park et al, 2002). Congenital heart defects are the single largest factor for infant mortality due to all birth defects, with hypoplastic left heart syndrome being the largest specific cause of congenital heart defect (Kochanek & Smith, 2004). Recent reviews of the incidence of congenital heart defects have demonstrated an overall prevalence of congenital heart defects. It is surmised that some of the increase can be attributed to better diagnosis and reporting; however, changes in the distribution of risk factors may account for actual increases. The prevalence of VSDs, TOF, atrioventricular septal defects, and pulmonary stenosis increased from 1968 through 1997. The prevalence of TGA decreased during that same time period (Botto et al, 2001). Because the overall incidence of CHD is approximately 1% of all live births and because the incidence of individual defects is less than 1%, the incidence of individual defects is usually given as a percent of total CHDs. The incidence of a specific defect within the overall incidence of CHDs is included in the discussion of that defect. Identification of cardiovascular abnormalities and prompt institution of appropriate therapy is extremely important in the care of newborns, as approximately 95% of congenital heart defects can be partially or fully corrected (Cooley, 1997).

Some CHDs are not detected in the neonatal period; others are identified, but are initially managed medically. Thus, the following discussion of CHDs extends beyond the neonatal period. Table 3-3 is an overview of the diagnosis of CHDs.

The discussion of defects is based on the common pathophysiologic features. CHDs can be classified in numerous ways. The simplest classification is based on whether the defect produces cyanosis, a method described by Taussig in 1947. Cyanosis is the bluish discoloration of the skin that occurs when approximately 5 g/100 ml of desaturated hemoglobin is present in the circulating volume (Taussig, 1947). Thus, the appearance of cyanosis depends on the hemoglobin concentration. An infant with low hemoglobin may be hypoxic but may not appear cyanotic; thus, low hemoglobin cannot be the sole criterion for determining pathologic origin. Cyanosis in the extremities, or acrocyanosis, is frequently seen in newborns because of reduced blood flow through the small capillaries. Oxygen is extracted from the hemoglobin in the capillaries, giving the skin a blue appearance. This blue appearance is a normal phenomenon in the newborn. Differentiation of central cyanosis from peripheral or acrocyanosis is essential.

The presence or absence of cyanosis depends on whether deoxygenated blood is oxygenated by going through the lungs. Thus CHDs that allow the blood to go through the lungs and then shunt from the left side of the heart and back to the right side of the heart are generally acyanotic. Defects that shunt deoxygenated blood directly to the left side of the heart, bypassing the lungs, are cyanotic heart defects. Some defects have mixed anatomic or functional features and do not fit into this schema, or overlap exists between the classifications. For this discussion, the following categories will be used: (1) defects with communication between the systemic and pulmonary circulations (i.e., those with a left to right shunt or

TABLE **3-3**	Diagnosis of Congenital Heart Defects				
Defect	**Chest Radiograph**	**ECG**	**Echocardiogram**	**Catheterization**	**Lab Tests**
PDA	Increased pulmonary vascularity; cardiac enlargement; left aortic arch	Left atrial and ventricular enlargement; abnormal QRS axis for age	LA:AO ratio >1.3 (term), 1.0 (preterm); increased left atrium and ventricle (2-D)	Increased O$_2$ saturation in pulmonary artery; increased right ventricular and pulmonary artery pressure (with pulmonary hypertension)	NA
ASD	Mild heart enlargement; prominent main pulmonary artery; increased pulmonary vascularity	Right axis deviation; deviation; incomplete right bundle branch block; right ventricular hypertrophy	Dilated right ventricle; paradoxical movement of ventricular septum	Increased O$_2$ in right atrium; normal right side atrium; normal right side pressure; 10%: PAPVR	NA
AS	Normal heart size; slight prominence of left ventricle and aorta	Normal or mild left ventricular hypertrophy; inverted T waves	Prominent septal thickening; abnormal mitral valve motions	Anatomic and physiologic alterations in cardiac function	NA
VSD	Enlarged heart; increased pulmonary markings	Left and right ventricular hypertrophy	Large left atrium (M-mode); presence or absence of other defects (2-D)	Increased O$_2$ in right ventricle; increased systolic pressure in right ventricle and pulmonary artery	NA
ECD	Cardiomegaly; increased pulmonary vascularity	Left axis deviation; prolonged P-R interval; right and left atrial enlargement; right ventricular hypertrophy; incomplete right bundle branch block	Ventricular dilation; abnormal mitral and tricuspid valves	Increased O$_2$ in right atrium; increased right ventricular and/or pulmonary artery pressure; with angiography, a "gooseneck" deformity of ventricular outflow area	NA
TOF	Normal heart size; boot-shaped contour; decreased pulmonary markings; prominent aorta; right aortic arch in 1 of 3 cases	Right axis deviation; right ventricular hypertrophy	Large VSD, aortic dextroposition, and PS; size of main, right, and left pulmonary arteries (2-D)	Demonstrates anatomy of right ventricular outflow region; microcytic anemia	Increased Hgb and HCT clotting time
PS	Normal heart size; normal pulmonary vascularity; enlarged pulmonary artery; right ventricle filling (lateral)	Right axis deviation; right atrial enlargement; right ventricular hypertrophy	Decreased valve eaflet motion; small changes in right ventricular wall thickness	Elevated right ventricular pressure; normal or slightly lowered pulmonary artery pressure	NA
TA	Cardiomegaly; absence of main pulmonary artery segment; large aorta; increased pulmonary vascularity	Right and/or left ventricular hypertrophy	Absence of two semilunar valves	Left to right shunt at level of ventricle; pressure equal in ventricles, truncus, and pulmonary arteries	Increased Hgb and HCT
TGA	Enlarged heart with narrow base; enlarged ventricles; increased pulmonary vascularity	Right axis deviation; right ventricular hypertrophy	Abnormal origin of great vessels	Increased right ventricular pressure; catheter can enter aorta from right ventricle; pulmonary artery can be entered only through PDA or ASD	Increased Hgb and HCT; polycythemia

TABLE 3-3	Diagnosis of Congenital Heart Defects—cont'd				
Defect	Chest Radiograph	ECG	Echocardiogram	Catheterization	Lab Tests
COA	Cardiomegaly; postcoarctation dilation (by age 5 years); notching of ribs from collateral vessels	Left ventricular hypertrophy; inverted T waves in left precordial leads; right ventricular hypertrophy (severe)	Visualization of narrowed aorta and location of associated defects; allows evaluation of aortic valve movement, structure, and function and left ventricular size and function	Performed to determine exact location and evaluation	NA
HLHS	Cardiomegaly; increased pulmonary vascularity; interstitial emphysema	Prominent right ventricular forces; decreased left ventricular forces	Small left ventricle	Performed for evaluation for surgical intervention or if echocardiogram is inconclusive	NA
TAPVR	Cardiac enlargement; large pulmonary artery; increased pulmonary flow	Right ventricular hypertrophy; right axis deviation; right atrial hypertrophy (after 1 month)	Presence of right atrial enlargement; patent foramen ovale; inability to demonstrate continuity between the pulmonary veins and left atrium (2-D)	Higher O_2 saturation in right atrium; angiography reveals opacification of pulmonary arterial circulation, pulmonary venous circulation, and abnormal circulation	NA

AS, Aortic stenosis; ASD, atrial septal defect; COA, coarctation of the aorta; ECG, electrocardiogram; HCT, hematocrit; Hgb, hemoglobin; HLHS, hypoplastic left heart syndrome; LA:AO, left atrium to aortic root; Lab, laboratory; NA, not applicable; PAPVR, partial anomalous pulmonary venous return; PDA, patent ductus arteriosus; PS, pulmonary stenosis; TA, truncus arteriosus; TAPVR, total anomalous pulmonary venous return; TGA, transposition of the great arteries; TOF, tetralogy of Fallot; VSD, ventricular septal defect.

acyanotic defects); (2) defects that have obstructions of the vascular system or valvular systems, with or without right to left shunt; and (3) defects with abnormalities in the origin of the pulmonary arteries or veins.

Defects Involving Communication Between the Systemic and Pulmonary Circulations with Left to Right Shunt (Acyanotic Defects)

Typically, these defects do not produce cyanosis because sufficient oxygenated blood is in the circulation. The left to right shunts produce increased pulmonary blood flow and increased workload on the heart. The acyanotic heart defects discussed here are patent ductus arteriosus (PDA), ventricular septal defect (VSD), atrial septal defect (ASD), endocardial cushion defect (ECD), aortic stenosis (AS), tetralogy of Fallot (TOF), pulmonary atresia, pulmonary stenosis (PS), and persistent truncus arteriosus (PTA).

Patent Ductus Arteriosus

The ductus arteriosus is a wide muscular connection between the pulmonary artery and the aorta. The ductus arteriosus originates from the left pulmonary artery and enters the aorta below the subclavian artery; it allows oxygenated blood from the placenta to bypass the lungs and enter the circulation. The ductus arteriosus closes functionally by about 15 hours after birth. During the first 24 hours after birth, some shunting of blood may occur, but the ductal opening must be greater than 2 mm for shunting to be significant.

Closure of the ductus arteriosus occurs in response to increased arterial oxygen concentration after the initiation of pulmonary function. Other factors that contribute to closure of the ductus arteriosus include a decrease in prostaglandin E (PGE) and an increase in acetylcholine and bradykinin (Park et al, 2002). The persistence of the ductus arteriosus beyond 24 hours after birth is considered a PDA in the term newborn. PDA in the preterm newborn presents a different clinical problem and is discussed separately from PDA in the term newborn (Park et al, 2002).

Patent Ductus Arteriosus in the Term Newborn

Incidence. PDA accounts for approximately 5% to 10% of all CHDs, excluding those in preterm newborns. The incidence is higher in females (about 3:1) (Park et al, 2002).

Hemodynamics. In extrauterine life, the flow of blood through the ductus arteriosus is reversed. The PDA allows blood to flow from left to right, thereby reentering the pulmonary circuit and increasing pulmonary blood flow. The amount of blood flow through the PDA and the effects of the ductal flow depend on the difference between systemic and pulmonary vascular resistance and the diameter and length of the ductus. High pulmonary blood flow causes increased pulmonary vascular resistance, pulmonary hypertension, and right ventricular hypertrophy. Figure 3-4 depicts the hemodynamics of PDA.

Manifestations. A small PDA may be asymptomatic. A large PDA with significant shunting may cause signs of CHF with tachypnea, dyspnea, and hoarse cry. Frequent lower respi-

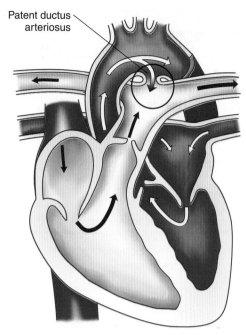

Patent ductus arteriosus

FIGURE 3-4
Patent ductus arteriosus is a communication between the pulmonary artery and the aorta.

ratory tract infections, coughing, and poor weight gain are common in older infants with PDA.

Diagnosis. The diagnosis of PDA is based on history and physical examination findings, radiograph, and echocardiogram. Characteristic findings on physical examination include bounding peripheral pulses, widened pulse pressure (>25), and a hyperactive precordium. A systolic thrill may be felt at the upper left sternal border. A grade 1/6 to 4/6 continuous "machinery" murmur is audible at the upper left sternal border or left infraclavicular area. The murmur is heard throughout the entire cardiac cycle because of the pressure gradient between the aorta and the pulmonary artery in both systole and diastole. In severe PDA with a large shunt, the S_2 may be accentuated because of pulmonary hypertension (Park et al, 2002).

A small PDA may not be distinguishable on a chest radiograph. With more severe shunting, cardiomegaly and increased pulmonary vascularity may be seen. An ECG may show left atrial and ventricular enlargement and an abnormal QRS axis for age. The definitive diagnosis is made by echocardiogram. With two-dimensional echocardiogram, PDA can be directly visualized. A ductus is considered to be hemodynamically significant if the left atrium to aortic root ratio (LA:AO) is greater than 1:3 in term newborns or greater than 1:0 in preterm newborns (Park et al, 2002).

Management. Medical management includes prophylactic antibiotics against bacterial endocarditis. No exercise restrictions are needed in the absence of pulmonary hypertension. Definitive treatment is surgical ligation through a posterolateral thoracotomy. Corrective surgery is performed in patients between 1 and 2 years of age, unless CHF, recurrent pneumonia, or pulmonary hypertension is a factor. The mortality rate is less than 1% (excluding preterm newborns). The prognosis is excellent, and complications are rare (Park et al, 2002).

Patent Ductus Arteriosus in the Preterm Newborn

Patent ductus arteriosus is a common complicating factor in the care of preterm newborns. As the newborn recovers from respiratory distress, pulmonary vascular resistance decreases as oxygenation improves. The ductus arteriosus in the preterm newborn is not as responsive to increased oxygen content as it is in term newborns and does not close. Decreased pulmonary vascular resistance causes blood to shunt from left to right and reenter the pulmonary circuit, leading to increased pulmonary venous congestion, which decreases lung compliance and stiff lungs. Consequences of large shunts include symptoms of CHF, inability to wean from ventilatory support, or an increased oxygen requirement.

Clinical findings indicative of PDA include bounding peripheral pulses, hyperactive precordium, widened pulse pressures (greater than 25), and a continuous murmur, best heard at the upper left and middle sternal border. Radiographic findings include increased pulmonary vascularity and cardiomegaly. PDA can be directly visualized by two-dimensional echocardiogram and Doppler flow studies (Park et al, 2002).

Management of PDA depends on the severity of the symptoms. Conservative management consists of fluid restriction and diuretic therapy. Use of cardiac glycosides is controversial in the preterm newborn. The preterm newborn's myocardium has a higher amount of connective tissue and water, which may decrease the distensibility of the left ventricle; thus, digitalis would have no effect. Digitalis toxicity may occur because of poor elimination of the drug. If digitalis is used, the dose should be decreased and monitored carefully (Park et al, 2002).

Indomethacin, a prostaglandin synthetase inhibitor, may be used to close the ductus arteriosus. PGE_2 is produced in the walls of the ductus arteriosus to prevent closure during fetal life. Indomethacin inhibits the production of PGE_2 and promotes ductal closure. Smaller babies may require a higher dose to obtain effective plasma levels. Indomethacin works best if used in newborns younger than 13 days of life; it is not effective later than 4 to 6 weeks after birth. Indomethacin dosage is 0.2 mg/kg intravenously every 12 hours for three doses. Indomethacin is highly nephrotoxic, so the blood urea nitrogen (BUN) and creatinine levels must be monitored.

Contraindications to using indomethacin include renal failure, low platelet count, bleeding disorders, necrotizing enterocolitis, and hyperbilirubinemia (Park et al, 2002). Ibuprofen has been suggested as an alternative to indomethacin for closure of the ductus arteriosus in preterm infants; however, further study is necessary to show that ibuprofen is as effective or is safer than indomethacin (Chotigeat et al, 2003; Leonhardt & Seyberth, 2003; Su et al, 2003). Surgical ligation is reserved for cases in which indomethacin fails or is contraindicated. The mortality rate for ligation is slightly less than 2%. The mortality rate is highest in the more preterm, sicker infants, especially if pulmonary hypertension has developed (Park et al, 2002).

Ventricular Septal Defect

A VSD is a defect or opening in the ventricular septum caused by imperfect ventricular division during early fetal development. The defect can occur anywhere in the muscular or membranous ventricular septum. The size of the defect and the degree of pulmonary vascular resistance are more important in determining the severity than the location. With a small defect, there is a large resistance to the left to right shunt at the defect and the shunt is

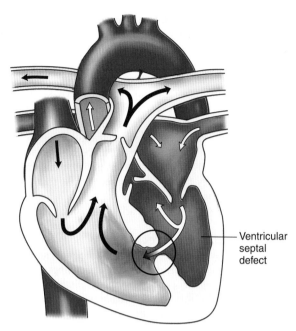

FIGURE **3-5**
Ventricular septal defect is a communication between the right and left ventricles.

not dependent on the pulmonary vascular resistance. With a large VSD, there is little resistance at the defect and the amount of left to right shunt is dependent on the level of pulmonary vascular resistance (Park et al, 2002; Turner et al, 1999).

Incidence. VSD is the most common CHD. It accounts for approximately 20% to 25% of all CHDs. Figure 3-5 shows a VSD.

Hemodynamics. The hemodynamic consequences of a VSD depend on its size: small, moderate, or large.

Small Ventricular Septal Defect. Small VSDs produce minimal shunting and may not be symptomatic. Chest radiograph and ECG are generally normal. A loud, harsh pansystolic heart murmur may be best heard in the third and fourth left intercostal space at the sternal border (Park et al, 2002; Turner et al, 1999).

Moderate Ventricular Septal Defect. With moderate-sized VSDs, the blood is shunted from the left to the right ventricle because of higher pressure in the left ventricle and higher systemic vascular resistance. The shunt of blood occurs during systole, when the right ventricle contracts, so that the blood enters the pulmonary artery rather than remaining in the right ventricle. This prevents the development of right ventricular hypertrophy.

Large Ventricular Septal Defect. With large VSDs, blood is shunted from the left to the right ventricle. The larger the VSD, the greater the volume of blood shunted, and the higher the pressure in the right ventricle and pulmonary artery. If pulmonary artery pressure is significantly increased, thickening of the walls of the pulmonary arterioles may develop and the increased resistance may decrease the left to right shunt. Pulmonary vascular disease can lead to right to left shunting and cyanosis.

Manifestations. Manifestations of VSD depend on the degree of shunting. Small VSDs may produce no hemodynamic compromise and be asymptomatic. Larger defects are associated with decreased exertional tolerance, recurrent pul-

monary infections, poor growth, and symptoms of CHF. With severe VSD, pulmonary hypertension and cyanosis may be seen.

Diagnosis. In VSD, a systolic thrill may be palpated at the lower left sternal border. A precordial bulge may be seen with very large VSDs. A grade 2/6 to 5/6 regurgitant systolic murmur is heard at the lower left sternal border. An apical diastolic rumble also may be heard, and the pulmonary heart sound may be loud.

Radiography can be of use in detecting intermediate to large VSDs (Danford et al, 2000). Radiographs show cardiomegaly involving the left atrium, left ventricle, and possibly the right ventricle, as well as increased pulmonary vascularity. An ECG may reveal left ventricular hypertrophy. Right ventricular hypertrophy may also be present in severe cases. An echocardiogram (M-mode) shows a large left atrium. A two-dimensional echocardiogram shows other defects and the size and location of the VSD (Park et al, 2002).

Physical examination of infants with a large VSD not detected in the neonatal period may reveal inadequate weight gain, cyanosis, and clubbing of the digits.

Managements. Treatment of the VSD depends on the severity of the defect and the symptoms produced. The VSD can close spontaneously, so defects that cause no compromise may be observed to allow time for spontaneous closure. Small VSDs generally spontaneously close by approximately 6 years of age. Muscular VSDs have a higher spontaneous closure rate than do perimembranous VSDs (29% vs 69%) (Turner et al, 1999).

Initial management of the hemodynamically significant VSD includes monitoring for signs of CHF and prompt initiation of therapy. Congestive heart failure in the older infant is treated with diuretics and digitalis. In the absence of pulmonary hypertension, there is no need to restrict activities. Prophylaxis against bacterial endocarditis is indicated.

Surgical management involves direct closure of the VSD. Cardiopulmonary bypass is required for the surgical correction. The timing of the surgery depends on the severity of the circulatory and pulmonary compromise. Infants with significant left to right shunting with evidence of severe compromise require surgery. Signs of CHF that do not respond to conservative medical management or increasing pulmonary vascular resistance are indications for surgical correction. Asymptomatic children with a moderate VSD usually have surgical correction between 2 and 4 years of age. Thomson et al (2000) reported using a cardiac catheter across a muscular VSD to aid closure, a technique that allowed improved visualization of the defect from the right side of the heart and minimized the size of the surgical incision of the left ventricle. The mortality rate for VSD correction is approximately 5%. The mortality rate is higher among smaller infants, those with other defects, and those with multiple VSDs.

Atrial Septal Defect

An ASD is a defect or opening in the atrial septum that develops as a result of improper septal formation early in fetal cardiac development.

There are three types of ASDs (Park et al, 2002):
1. Ostium secundum, commonly associated with mitral valve
2. Ostium primum, an endocardial cushion defect associated with anomalies of one or both AV valves

3. Sinus venosus, often associated with partial anomalous pulmonary venous connection

Incidence. ASDs account for 5% to 10% of all CHDs.

Hemodynamics. An ASD usually does not produce symptoms until pulmonary vascular resistance begins to decrease and right ventricular end-diastolic and right atrial pressures decline. All types of ASDs produce some blood flow alterations. With an ASD, blood shunts from left to right across the defect because the right ventricle, which is more compliant than the left, offers less resistance to filling. Any factors that decrease right ventricular distensibility or obstruct flow into the right ventricle (e.g., pulmonary stenosis or tricuspid stenosis) can reduce or reverse the shunt direction (Massin et al, 1998). The left to right shunt increases right ventricular volume, but pulmonary vascular resistance decreases, so pulmonary artery pressure is almost normal. The large pulmonary blood flow gradually leads to increased pulmonary artery pressures. Figure 3-6 shows an ASD.

Manifestations. Newborns with ASDs are usually asymptomatic, although a grade 2/6 to 3/6 systolic ejection murmur may be found, which can best be heard at the upper left sternal border. S_2 may be widely split and fixed. With a large ASD, a mid-diastolic rumble caused by the relative tricuspid stenosis may be audible at the lower left sternal border (Park et al, 2002). On chest radiograph, the heart is enlarged, with a prominent main pulmonary artery segment and increased pulmonary vascularity. Electrocardiogram enhances detection of ASD, showing right axis deviation and mild right ventricular hypertrophy. Incomplete right bundle branch block may be seen (Danford et al, 2000; Park et al, 2002).

An echocardiogram by M-mode shows increased right ventricular dimension and paradoxical movement of the ventricular septum. Diagnosis can be made by two-dimensional echocardiogram, which shows the location and size of the defect. Children with ASDs are usually thin and may be easily fatigued. By late infancy, a precordial bulge caused by enlargement of the right side of the heart may be seen.

Management. Untreated ASD can lead to CHF, pulmonary hypertension, and atrial dysrhythmias in adults.

Spontaneous closure of ASDs occurs in the first 5 years of age in up to 40% of children (Park et al, 2002). Medical management of ASD consists of prevention or treatment of CHF. There is no need to limit activity. Surgical correction is accomplished by a simple patch or with direct closure during open-heart surgery using cardiopulmonary bypass. Timing of surgery depends on the severity of the defect. The presence of a significant left to right shunt is an indication for surgical correction. Surgery is performed when the patient is between 2 and 5 years of age. The surgery is not performed in infants unless CHF that is unresponsive to medical management is a factor. The mortality rate of the surgery is less than 1%. The highest risk is for small infants with CHF or increased pulmonary vascular resistance (Park et al, 2002).

Endocardial Cushion Defects

Endocardial cushion defects result from inappropriate fusion of the endocardial cushions during fetal development. Endocardial cushion defects produce abnormalities of the atrial septum (ostium primum), ventricular septum, and AV valves. Endocardial cushion defects take many forms and are characterized by downward displacement of the AV valves as a result of deficiency in ventricular septal tissue and an elongation of the left ventricular outflow tract. The term *complete AV canal* describes the large opening in the center of the heart between the atria and the ventricles. The following defects can occur in the AV canal: (1) an ostium primum ASD, (2) a VSD in the inlet portion of the ventricular septum, (3) a cleft in the anterior mitral valve leaflet, and (4) a cleft in the septal leaflet of the tricuspid valve, which results in common anterior and posterior cusps of the AV valve (Park et al, 2002). Figure 3-7 shows the anatomy of an endocardial cushion defect.

Incidence. Endocardial cushion defects account for 2% of all CHDs; 30% of ECDs appear in infants with Down syndrome. Of infants with ECDs, 10% also have PDA, and 10% have TOF (Park et al, 2002).

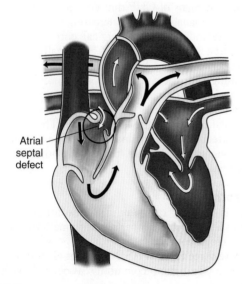

Atrial septal defect

FIGURE 3-6
Atrial septal defect is a communication between the right and left atria.

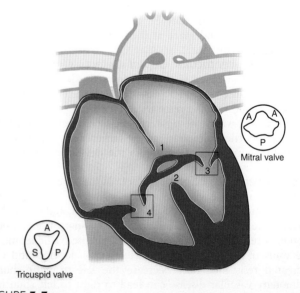

Mitral valve

Tricuspid valve

FIGURE 3-7
Endocardial cushion defect. *1,* Ostium primum atrial septal defect; *2,* a ventricular septal defect in the inlet portion of ventricular septum; *3,* cleft in anterior mitral valve leaflet; *4,* cleft in septal leaflet of the tricuspid valve, resulting in common anterior and posterior cusps of the atrioventricular valve. *A,* Anterior; *S,* septal; *P,* posterior.

Hemodynamics. The hemodynamic consequences of endocardial cushion defects depend on the type and severity. There may be interatrial and interventricular shunts, left ventricle to right atrium shunts, or AV valve regurgitation.

Manifestations. The manifestations of ECDs result from the increased pulmonary blood flow caused by the abnormal connection between both ventricles and the atria and by absent or malformed AV valves. The newborn may have respiratory distress, signs of CHF, tachycardia, and a cardiac murmur. The mitral regurgitation may be heard as a grade 3/6 to 4/6 holosystolic regurgitant murmur audible at the lower left sternal border, which transmits to the left back and may be audible at the apex. A mid-diastolic rumble is also heard at the lower left sternal border or at the apex caused by the relative stenosis of tricuspid and mitral valves. S_1 is accentuated, and S_2 is narrowly split. The sound of the pulmonary closure is increased in intensity (Kwiatkowska et al, 2000; Park et al, 2002).

A chest radiograph reveals generalized cardiomegaly with increased pulmonary vascularity and a prominent main pulmonary artery segment. An ECG shows left axis deviation with a prolonged P-R interval, right and left atrial enlargement, right ventricular hypertrophy, and incomplete right bundle branch block. An infant with an endocardial cushion defect may demonstrate signs of CHF, recurrent respiratory infections, and failure to thrive. Physical examination reveals a poorly nourished infant with signs of respiratory distress and tachycardia (McElhinney et al, 2000; Kwiatkowska et al, 2000; Park et al, 2002).

Management. Initial medical management is aimed at preventing or treating CHF with diuretics and digitalis. Prophylaxis against bacterial endocarditis is required before and after surgical correction. Definitive management consists of surgical closure of the ASD and VSD, with reconstruction of the AV valves under cardiopulmonary bypass, deep hypothermia, or both. In some cases, pulmonary artery banding may be performed as a palliative procedure if significant mitral regurgitation is not a factor. This procedure carries a slightly higher mortality risk than when primary surgical repair is performed.

Surgery is indicated with CHF that is unresponsive to medical therapy, recurrent pneumonia, failure to thrive, or a large shunt with development of pulmonary hypertension and increasing pulmonary vascular resistance. The repair is performed in patients aged approximately 6 months to 2 years of age. The mortality rate has declined in recent years to approximately 5% to 10%. The mortality rate for patients who undergo pulmonary banding is approximately 15%. Factors that increase the risks of this procedure include (1) very young age, (2) severe AV valve incompetence, (3) hypoplastic left ventricle, and (4) severe symptoms before surgery (Park et al, 2002).

Aortic Stenosis

Aortic stenosis is one of a group of defects that produce obstruction to ventricular outflow. Aortic stenosis may be valvular, subvalvular, or supravalvular. Valvular stenosis is the most common, and supravalvular is the least common (Park et al, 2002).

In valvular stenosis, a bicuspid valve is usually present. Subvalvular stenosis can involve either a simple diaphragm or a long tunnel-like ventricular outflow tract. Idiopathic hypertrophic subaortic stenosis is a form of subvalvular stenosis that manifests as a cardiomyopathy. Supravalvular stenosis is associated with Williams syndrome, or elfin facies, characterized by mental retardation, short palpebral fissures, and thick lips (Park et al, 2002).

Incidence. Aortic stenosis accounts for 5% of all CHDs. It is four times more common in males.

Hemodynamics. Aortic stenosis causes increased pressure load on the left ventricle, leading to left ventricular hypertrophy. The resistance to blood flow through the stenosis gradually causes a pressure gradient between the ventricle and the aorta. Eventually, coronary blood flow decreases. Aortic stenosis is illustrated in Figure 3-8.

Manifestations. Symptoms depend on the severity of the defect. Mild aortic stenosis may not cause symptoms. More severe defects can cause activity intolerance, chest pain, or syncope. With severe defects, CHF develops.

Diagnosis. Physical examination reveals normal development without cyanosis. A narrow pulse pressure and a higher systolic pressure may be found in the right arm with severe supravalvular aortic stenosis. A systolic murmur of approximately grade 2/6 to 4/6 may occur that is best heard at the second right or left intercostal space with transmission to the neck. With valvular aortic stenosis, an ejection click may be heard. Severe aortic stenosis may produce paradoxical splitting of S_2. Aortic insufficiency may cause a high-pitched, early diastolic decrescendo murmur if there is bicuspid aortic valve or subvalvular stenosis (Park et al, 2002).

Chest radiographs may be normal or may show a dilated ascending aorta or, in the case of valvular stenosis, a prominent aortic "knob" caused by post-stenotic dilation (Park et al, 2002). Cardiomegaly is present if CHF or severe aortic regurgitation is a factor. An ECG may be normal or may show mild left ventricular hypertrophy and inverted T waves. An echocardiogram shows prominent thickening of the septum and abnormal mitral valve motions. A two-dimensional echocardiogram shows the anatomy of the aortic valve (bicuspid, tricuspid, or unicuspid) and that of subvalvular and supravalvular aortic stenosis.

Cardiac catheterization may be performed. Its purpose is to identify the exact anatomy and to analyze pressure gradients.

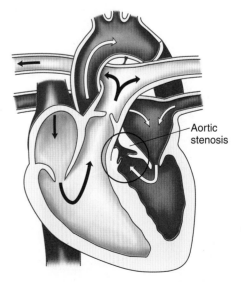

FIGURE **3-8**
Aortic stenosis is a narrowing or thickening of the aortic valvular region.

Management. Management is aimed at preventing or treating the CHF with fluid restriction, diuretics, and digitalis. In children with moderate to severe aortic stenosis, activity is restricted to prevent increased demand on the heart. Balloon valvuloplasty is sometimes performed at the time of cardiac catheterization to improve circulation. In critical aortic stenosis, maintenance of the patency of the ductus arteriosus with PGE_1 is necessary to prevent hypoxia.

The type of surgical correction depends on the exact location and severity of the defect. The procedure may consist of aortic valve commissurotomy or valve replacement with a prosthetic valve or a graft. The placement of prosthetic valves is usually deferred until adult-sized prosthetic valves can be inserted. The timing of the surgery depends on the severity of the defect. Infants with critical aortic stenosis with CHF must have corrective surgery. Surgery is performed on children when a peak systolic pressure gradient greater than 80 mm Hg or symptoms of chest pain are present.

The mortality risk for infants and small children is 15% to 20%. As in all cases, the sicker, smaller infants have the highest mortality rate. The mortality rate in older children is approximately 1% to 2% (Park et al, 2002).

Tetralogy of Fallot

TOF was first described in 1888. Tetralogy of Fallot is caused by lack of development of the subpulmonary conus during fetal life. TOF consists of a large VSD, pulmonary stenosis or other right ventricular outflow tract obstruction, overriding aorta, and hypertrophied right ventricle. The right ventricle may not be hypertrophied initially. Pulmonary valve atresia is seen in the most severe form of TOF.

Incidence. TOF accounts for 10% of all CHDs. Because repair is generally not carried out in the first year of life, TOF is the most common cyanotic heart defect beyond infancy.

Hemodynamics. In TOF, the VSD causes equalization of pressure in the ventricles. Unsaturated blood flows through the VSD into the aorta because of the obstruction to blood flow from the right ventricle into the pulmonary artery. TOF is shown in Figure 3-9.

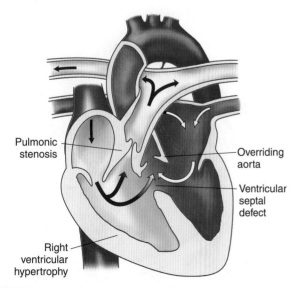

FIGURE **3-9**
Tetralogy of Fallot consists of pulmonary stenosis, ventricular septal defect, overriding aorta, and hypertrophy of the right ventricle.

Pulmonic stenosis

Overriding aorta

Ventricular septal defect

Right ventricular hypertrophy

Manifestations. Cyanosis, hypoxia, and dyspnea are the cardinal signs of TOF. Newborns may have just a loud murmur or they may be cyanotic. Severe decompensation or "tet" spells are common in infants or children but can also occur in neonates. Children instinctively assume a squatting position, which traps venous blood in the legs and decreases systemic venous return to the heart. Chronic arterial desaturation stimulates erythropoiesis, causing polycythemia. Increased viscosity of the blood caused by the increased red blood cells and microcytic anemia may lead to cerebrovascular accident (stroke). Brain abscesses may also occur as a result of bacteremia and compromised cerebral flow in the microcirculation. The chronic hypoxemia and polycythemia cause (1) an increased risk of hemorrhagic diathesis because decreased platelet survival time and reduced platelet aggregation cause thrombocytopenia and (2) impaired synthesis of vitamin K–dependent clotting factors.

Diagnosis. Neonates with TOF exhibit varying degrees of cyanosis, depending on the severity of the obstruction of blood flow through the right ventricular outflow tract. A long, loud, grade 3/6 to 5/6 systolic ejection murmur is heard at the middle and upper left sternal border. A ventricular tap may also be audible along the lower left sternal border and a systolic thrill at the lower and middle left sternal border. A PDA murmur may also be heard in severe TOF (Park et al, 2002).

A chest radiograph demonstrates decreased or normal heart size with decreased pulmonary vascularity. The contour of the heart may be a typical boot shape caused by the concave main pulmonary artery segment with upturned apex. Right atrial enlargement and a right aortic arch may also be found.

Echocardiography shows a large VSD and overriding aorta. The anatomy of the right ventricular outflow tract and pulmonary valve can be identified by two-dimensional echocardiogram.

In addition to the manifestations present in the neonate, clubbing of the fingers may be present in the infant or child with TOF.

Management. The definitive therapy for TOF is surgical repair under cardiopulmonary bypass. The surgical correction can sometimes be delayed with careful medical management. Neonates with only mild cyanosis improve when the pulmonary vascular resistance decreases. Medical management is aimed at prevention or treatment of hypoxemia, polycythemia, infection, and microcytic hypochromic anemia. Careful follow-up is essential to detect signs of clinical deterioration. Parents need adequate education and support for home management (Dipchand et al, 1999; Park et al, 2002).

Dehydration must be avoided to prevent increased risk of cerebral infarcts caused by hemoconcentration. Polycythemia develops as a compensatory mechanism to increase the oxygen-carrying capacity of the blood. In the presence of decreased volume, however, the increased viscosity of the blood may further impede cerebral circulation.

Parents must be taught how to recognize the early signs and symptoms of decompensation. They must also be taught to recognize and treat hypercyanotic or tet spells (Table 3-4). Tet spells are precipitated by events that lower the systemic vascular resistance, producing a large right to left ventricular shunt. Increased activity, crying, nursing, or defecation may trigger a hypoxemic episode. The right to left shunt causes a decreased PO_2, increased PCO_2, and decreased pH, which stimulates the respiratory center, causing increased rate and

TABLE 3-4	Recognition and Treatment of Hypercyanotic (Tet) Spells
Manifestations	

Irritability, crying
Hyperpnea
Cyanosis
Diaphoresis
Loss of consciousness
Seizures
Decreased murmur
Metabolic acidosis

Treatment	**Rationale**
Knee–chest or squatting position	Traps blood in lower extremities to decrease systemic venous return; increases pulmonary blood flow
Oxygen administration	Improves arterial oxygen saturation
Morphine sulfate (0.1 to 0.2 mg/kg/dose)	Suppresses respiratory center to decrease hyperpnea
Bicarbonate	Corrects acidosis and eliminates stimulation of respiratory center
Propranolol (Inderal) (0.15 to 0.25 mg/kg/dose) to stabilize the infant's condition	May decrease spasm of right ventricular outflow tract or may act peripherally

depth of respirations (hyperpnea). The hyperpnea causes increased systemic venous return by increasing the efficiency of the thoracic pump. The right ventricular outflow tract obstruction prevents the increased blood flow from entering the pulmonary artery, so the increased flow is shunted through the aorta, which further decreases the arterial PO_2. Severe, uninterrupted hypercyanotic spells lead to loss of consciousness, hypoxemia, seizures, and death.

Surgical treatment is indicated in the presence of hypercyanotic (tet) spells that result in increased hypoxemia, metabolic acidosis, inadequate systemic perfusion, increased cyanosis, or polycythemia. Systemic perfusion can be evaluated by observing peripheral pulse intensity, urine output, capillary filling time, blood pressure, or peripheral vasoconstriction.

Surgical management can be either palliative or corrective. Palliative procedures are undertaken to improve pulmonary blood flow by creating a pathway between the systemic and pulmonary circulation. In addition, these procedures allow time for the right and left pulmonary arteries to grow. Palliative procedures are indicated for newborns with TOF and pulmonary atresia, severely cyanotic infants younger than 6 months of age, infants with medically unmanageable tet spells, or children with a hypoplastic pulmonary artery, in whom corrective surgery is difficult (Park et al, 2002). Common cardiac surgical procedures are listed in Table 3-5.

Surgical correction is performed under cardiopulmonary bypass after the infant is 6 months old. Surgery may be delayed until 2 to 4 years of age in asymptomatic children or in children who undergo palliative procedures. The defect is repaired by patch closure of the VSD and resection and widening of the right ventricular outflow tract. Postoperative care of the newborn requires careful assessment and monitoring so that complications can be prevented or quickly identified and treated (Russo & Russo, 2005). Complications of cardiac surgery are listed in Box 3-1 and Table 3-6. The mortality rate for TOF varies with the severity of the circulatory compromise caused by the defect. The postoperative mortality

rate is 5% to 10% in the first 2 years for uncomplicated TOF. More severe cases have a higher mortality rate, exhibit residual pulmonary outflow tract obstruction, and may require further surgery. Because myocardial damage may occur from the restriction of the right ventricular blood flow during the surgery, cardiac support is needed to ensure adequate myocardial perfusion. Extracorporeal membrane oxygenation (ECMO) is being used by some centers to support the cardiovascular perfusion. ECMO is also being attempted after surgical procedures for TGA and total anomalous pulmonary venous return (TAPVR), but infants with TOF make up the largest group of patients who benefit from its use. Many of these infants experience pulmonary hypertension because of the cardiac problem or the surgical correction. With ECMO, management of cases can focus on decreasing pulmonary vascular resistance and diminishing right to left shunting during the immediate postoperative period.

Pulmonary Atresia

Pulmonary atresia results in the absence of communication between the right ventricle and the pulmonary artery. The atresia can be at the level of the main pulmonary artery or the pulmonary valve. Atresia of the pulmonary valve, with a diaphragm-like membrane, is the most common type. The right ventricle is usually hypoplastic, with thick ventricular walls. Less frequently, the right ventricle is of normal size with tricuspid regurgitation. The presence of a PDA, ASD, or patent foramen ovale to allow mixing of blood is crucial for survival.

Incidence. Pulmonary atresia accounts for less than 1% of all CHDs (Park et al, 2002).

Hemodynamics. Pulmonary atresia with ASD results in a small, hypoplastic right heart. The absence of a right ventricular outflow tract results in high right ventricular end-diastolic pressures. Tricuspid insufficiency occurs and right atrial pressures increase, causing systemic venous blood to shunt from the right to the left atrium through the patent foramen ovale or ASD. Mixed venous blood flows into the left ventricle and aorta.

TABLE **3-5**	Common Cardiac Surgical Procedures		
Procedure	**Type**	**Defect**	**Description**
Blalock-Hanlon	Palliative	TGA	Surgical creation of an ASD: rarely used; still useful for complex TGA or mitral atresia and single ventricle
Blalock-Taussig	Palliative	TOF, PA, PS, VSD	Anastomosis of the subclavian artery and pulmonary artery to improve pulmonary blood flow
Brock	Corrective	PVA	Blind pulmonary valvotomy incision of PV
Fontan	Corrective	HLHS (stage 2), tricuspid atresia, tricuspid stenosis	Bypass of the right ventricle by connection of the right atrium to pulmonary artery
Gore-Tex shunt	Palliative	TOF	Interposition of Gore-Tex between subclavian artery and ipsilateral pulmonary artery
Jatene	Corrective	TGA	Switching of transposed great arteries to their anatomically correct position
Mustard	Corrective	TGA	Use of a pericardial or synthetic baffle in the atria so that venous blood is shunted across the right atrium to the left ventricle and into the pulmonary artery; systemic blood is shunted across the left atrium to the right ventricle, which delivers blood to the aorta
Norwood	Palliative	HLHS (stage 1)	1. The main pulmonary artery is divided, and the proximal stump is anastomosed to the descending aorta; distal main pulmonary artery is closed 2. Right-sided Gore-Tex shunt is performed to increase pulmonary blood flow 3. The atrial septum is excised to allow interatrial mixing
Potts	Palliative	TOF	Surgical creation of a window between descending aorta and left pulmonary artery; difficult to take down; rarely used
Pulmonary artery banding	Palliative	VSD, single ventricle	Placement of a band around the pulmonary artery to decrease the blood flow to the lungs
Rashkind	Corrective	PA, TGA	Atrial septostomy created at cardiac catheterization by passing a balloon-tipped catheter through the patent foramen ovale, inflating the balloon, and snapping it back through the patent foramen
Rastelli	Corrective	TGA, TOF, PA, TA	Commonly applied to all valved conduits from the right ventricle to the pulmonary artery
Senning	Corrective	TGA	Creation of an intra-atrial baffle, using atrial tissue, to shunt blood from the vena cava to the left ventricle and from the pulmonary veins to the right ventricle
Waterston	Palliative	TOF	Creation of a window between the ascending aorta and the pulmonary artery, improving oxygenation of systemic blood; rarely used because of the distortion or obstruction of pulmonary artery

ASD, Atrial septal defect; HLHS, hypoplastic left heart syndrome; PA, pulmonary artery; PS, pulmonary stenosis; PV, pulmonary valve; PVA, pulmonic valve atresia; TA, truncus arteriosus; TGA, transposition of the great arteries; TOF, tetralogy of Fallot; VSD, ventricular septal defect.

The PDA produces the only pulmonary blood flow. Closure of the PDA causes severe cyanosis, hypoxemia, and acidosis.

In the presence of a VSD, right ventricular size is usually adequate. Systemic venous blood shunts from the right ventricle through the VSD to the left ventricle and enters the aorta. The PDA still provides the only pulmonary blood flow. Pulmonary atresia is shown in Figure 3-10.

Manifestations. Pulmonary atresia usually is seen with cyanosis at birth. Tachypnea is present, but there is no obvious respiratory distress. S_2 is single and a soft systolic PDA murmur can be heard in the upper left sternal border. Tricuspid insufficiency may produce a harsh systolic murmur along the lower right and left sternal border (Park et al, 2002).

The heart may be normal size or enlarged on the chest radiograph. The main pulmonary artery segment is concave and similar to the radiographic appearance of tricuspid atresia. Pulmonary vascular markings are decreased and continue to decrease as the PDA closes.

An ECG may reveal a normal QRS axis, left ventricular hypertrophy (type I), or, less frequently, right ventricular hypertrophy (type II). Right atrial hypertrophy is seen in approximately 70% of cases (Park et al, 2002). A two-dimensional echocardiogram reveals the atretic pulmonary valve and the hypoplastic right ventricular cavity and tricuspid valve. The location and size of the atrial communication are estimated by echocardiography.

BOX 3-1

Complications of Cardiac Surgery

Low Cardiac Output
Hypovolemia
Hemorrhage
Diuresis
Inadequate fluid volume
Tamponade
Mediastinal bleeding
Inadequate mediastinal drainage
Decreased cardiac contractility
Hypervolemia
Electrolyte imbalance
Cardiac dysfunction
Increased systemic vascular resistance
Increased pulmonary vascular resistance
Arrhythmias
Hypothermia

Congestive Heart Failure
Uncorrected congenital heart defect (CHD) (after palliative
    procedure)
Corrected CHD, causing alterations in ventricular preload,
    contractility, and afterload
Hypervolemia
Electrolyte imbalance
Arrhythmias

Respiratory Distress
Atelectasis
Pneumothorax
Hemothorax
Pleural effusion
Chylothorax

Congestive heart failure
Low cardiac output
Pulmonary hypertension
Inadequate ventilatory support
Ineffective pleural drainage
Hypoventilation caused by pain

Renal Dysfunction or Failure
Poor systemic and renal perfusion
Intravascular hemolysis
Thromboembolus
Nephrotoxic drugs

Electrolyte Imbalance
Effects of cardiopulmonary bypass
Diuretics
Stress response
Fluid administration
Blood administration
Renal failure

Neurologic Abnormalities
Hypoxia
Acidosis
Poor systemic perfusion
Thromboembolism
Electrolyte imbalance

Infection
Surgery
Prosthetic material
Invasive monitoring or procedures
Inadequate nutrition

TABLE 3-6 Complications of Cardiac Surgery: Postoperative Syndromes

Syndrome	Cause	Symptoms	Management
Postcoarctectomy syndrome	Results from changes in pressure and flow	Severe intermittent abdominal pain, fever, and leukocytosis; abdominal distention, melena, and ascites with gangrenous bowel; rebound systemic hypertension	Monitor blood pressure; prevent hypertension; delay postoperative feeding
Postpericardiotomy syndrome	Immunologic syndrome in response to blood in the pericardial sac	Fever, chest pain, pericardial and pleural effusions, hepatomegaly, leukocytosis, left shift, increased erythrocyte sedimentation rate, persistent ST and T wave changes on electrocardiogram. Rare in children younger than 2 years of age	Rest, aspirin for pain, corticosteroids in severe cases, pericardiocentesis if tamponade develops, diuretics
Postperfusion syndrome	Cytomegalovirus	Onset 3 to 6 weeks after surgery; fever, splenomegaly, atypical lymphocytosis	Supportive care; self-limiting disease process
Hemolytic anemia syndrome	Trauma of red blood cells or autoimmune action	Onset 1 to 2 weeks postoperatively; fever, jaundice, hepatomegaly, reticulocytosis	Iron supplementation or blood transfusions, correction of turbulent flow

Management. Immediate management of pulmonary atresia is administration of prostaglandin to maintain ductal patency. PGE_1 (Prostin) is given as a continuous intravenous infusion. The initial dose is started at 0.1 mcg/kg/min. When the desired effect is achieved, the dose is incrementally decreased to a maintenance dose of 0.01 mcg/kg/min. Careful attention to the site of the infusion is important.

A balloon atrial septostomy is performed at cardiac catheterization to promote better mixing of systemic and

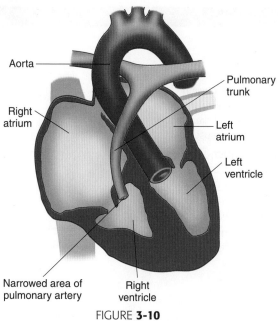

FIGURE **3-10**
Pulmonary atresia.

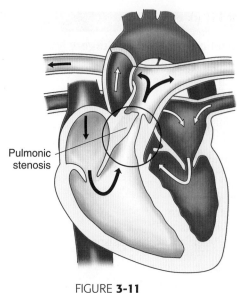

FIGURE **3-11**
Pulmonary stenosis.

pulmonary venous blood in the atria. As soon as the newborn's condition has been stabilized, surgical correction is performed. Initially, a systemic-pulmonary artery shunt using Gore-Tex between the left subclavian artery and the left pulmonary artery (Blalock-Taussig procedure) is performed. If pulmonary valve atresia is present, a closed heart pulmonary valvotomy (Brock's procedure) may be performed. The mortality rate for these procedures is 10% to 25%.

If the initial systemic-pulmonary shunt is not effective, a second shunt is attempted in another location. Right ventricular outflow tract reconstruction can be attempted if the right ventricle size is adequate. This procedure has a mortality rate of 25%. The Fontan procedure is attempted in the presence of a hypoplastic right ventricle in late childhood. The mortality rate for this procedure can be as high as 40%.

The prognosis for pulmonary atresia depends on the size of the pulmonary outflow tract established through surgery and the degree of fibrosis of the right ventricle. If there is severe fibrosis and significant outflow tract obstruction, there is an increased risk of development of dysrhythmias and right ventricular dysfunction (Park et al, 2002).

Pulmonary Stenosis

Pulmonary stenosis is caused by abnormal formation of the pulmonary valve leaflets during fetal cardiac development. Pulmonary stenosis can be valvular, subvalvular (infundibular), or supravalvular. Valvular pulmonary stenosis is the most common, accounting for 90% of cases. Pulmonary stenosis is frequently seen in Noonan syndrome. It is one of the four defects found in TOF. Isolated infundibular pulmonary stenosis is uncommon.

Incidence. Pulmonary stenosis makes up 5% to 8% of all CHDs. It is often associated with other defects.

Hemodynamics. Pulmonary stenosis results in obstruction to blood flow from the right ventricle to the pulmonary artery. The right ventricle hypertrophies in response to the increased pressure caused by the obstruction to outflow. Pulmonary blood flow volume is normal in the absence of

intracardiac shunting. Pulmonary stenosis is shown in Figure 3-11.

Manifestations. Pulmonary stenosis may be asymptomatic if it is mild. Moderate pulmonary stenosis may cause easy tiring. Severe or critical pulmonary stenosis causes CHF.

Diagnosis. The findings of pulmonary stenosis depend on the severity of the defect. A pulmonary systolic ejection click can be heard at the upper left sternal border. S$_2$ may be widely split, and the pulmonary component may be soft and delayed. A systolic ejection murmur (grade 2/6 to 5/6) is audible at the upper left sternal border and transmits across the back. The severity of the pulmonary stenosis is directly related to the loudness and duration of the murmur. A systolic thrill can sometimes be felt at the upper left sternal border. Hepatosplenomegaly may be present along with CHF.

The ECG is normal in mild pulmonary stenosis. There may be right axis deviation and right ventricular hypertrophy with moderate stenosis. Right atrial hypertrophy and right ventricular strain occur with severe pulmonary stenosis.

Radiographically, the heart size is normal, with a prominent main pulmonary artery segment. In mild to moderate pulmonary stenosis, pulmonary markings are normal. The critical type of pulmonary stenosis causes decreased pulmonary markings. CHF results in increased heart size. An echocardiogram demonstrates decreased motion of the pulmonary valve leaflets and poststenotic dilation of the main pulmonary artery segment (Danford et al, 1999; Park et al, 2002).

Management. Management of pulmonary stenosis is determined by the severity of the obstruction to flow. The mild type generally requires no therapy except antimicrobial prophylaxis against subacute infective endocarditis (SAIE). Moderate pulmonary stenosis is treated through balloon valvuloplasty during cardiac catheterization. Surgical correction is performed in children when the right ventricular pressure measures 80 to 100 mm Hg and balloon valvuloplasty is not successful or when the pulmonary stenosis is infundibular in origin. Infants with critical pulmonary stenosis and CHF require PGE$_1$ infusion to maintain ductal patency until surgery is performed (Park et al, 2002). Careful fluid and electrolyte management requires balancing the need for fluids against the prevention of further expansion of the extracellular fluid volume and consequent strain on the heart's ability to pump (Burlet et al, 1999).

The overall prognosis for pulmonary stenosis is excellent. The mortality rate is less than 1% in older infants. The mortality rate is higher in newborns with critical pulmonary stenosis and CHF (Park et al, 2002).

Persistent Truncus Arteriosus (PTA)

The truncus arteriosus is a large vessel located in front of the developing fetal heart. The truncus arteriosus gives rise to the coronary and pulmonary arteries and the aorta. The persistence of the truncus arteriosus results from inadequate division of the common great vessel into a separate aorta and pulmonary artery during fetal cardiac development. A single, large great vessel arises from the ventricles and gives rise to the systemic, pulmonary, and coronary circulations. Inadequate closure of the conal ventricular septum results in a VSD. Four types of this defect have been described; see Table 3-7 for the classifications (Park et al, 2002).

Incidence. Persistent truncus arteriosus accounts for less than 1% of all CHDs.

Hemodynamics. Desaturated blood from the right ventricle and oxygenated blood from the left ventricle are received in the truncus arteriosus. The pressures of both ventricles are equal. The truncus arteriosus supplies blood to the systemic and pulmonary circuits. The amount of flow depends on the resistance of the two circulations. Pulmonary vascular resistance is high at birth, so pulmonary and systemic flow is relatively equal initially. Pulmonary resistance gradually decreases, causing increased pulmonary blood flow. CHF may develop as a result of increased pulmonary blood flow. If the defect is not corrected, pulmonary vascular disease develops in response to high pressure and increased pulmonary blood flow, subsequently decreasing pulmonary blood flow. These changes, although compensatory initially, complicate the hemodynamics after surgical correction. The volume overload is compounded by incompetent truncal valves, which allow regurgitation of blood into the ventricles. Truncus arteriosus is illustrated in Figure 3-12.

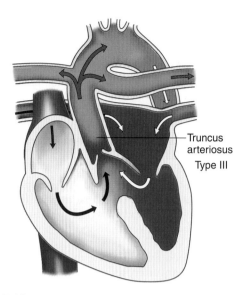

FIGURE **3-12**
Persistent truncus arteriosus is a single arterial vessel that gives rise to the coronary arteries, pulmonary arteries, and aorta.

Manifestations. The presence of cyanosis depends on the amount of pulmonary blood flow. Signs of CHF may be the first indication of persistent truncus arteriosus. On auscultation, there may be a systolic click at the apex and upper left sternal border. The VSD may produce a harsh, grade 2/6 to 4/6 systolic murmur heard along the lower sternal border. Increased pulmonary blood flow may produce an atrial rumble. Truncal valve insufficiency produces a high-pitched, early diastolic decrescendo murmur. There may be bounding arterial pulses and a widened pulse pressure. S_2 is single. If truncus arteriosus is not detected in the newborn period, symptoms of poor feeding, failure to thrive, frequent respiratory infections, and signs of CHF appear.

Diagnosis. On a chest radiograph, the heart size is increased and pulmonary blood flow may be increased. In 50% of cases a right aortic arch is present (Park et al, 2002). An ECG reveals a normal QRS axis and ventricular hypertrophy. Echocardiography demonstrates the presence of the truncus arteriosus overriding a VSD and the absence of the pulmonary valve (Park et al, 2002).

Management. Medical management consists primarily of treatment of CHF and prophylaxis with antimicrobials. Pulmonary artery banding, instituted as a palliative measure, may be performed in small infants with increased pulmonary blood flow and CHF unresponsive to medical management. The mortality rate for this group of infants is close to 30% (Park et al, 2002).

The definitive surgical correction is Rastelli's procedure. (See Table 3-5 for a description of common cardiac surgical procedures.) Surgery is performed in infants because there is a high mortality rate for uncorrected truncus arteriosus. The mortality rate associated with surgery is also high, ranging from 20% to 60%. Repeated surgery may be required to enlarge the conduit as growth occurs (Park et al, 2002).

Defects with Abnormalities in the Origin of the Pulmonary Arteries or Veins

These defects arise from a defect in the bending and rotation of the heart as it grows and elongates during fetal development.

TABLE **3-7**		Four Major Types of Truncus Arteriosus
Type	**Incidence (%)**	**Description**
I	60	Main pulmonary artery arises from truncus and divides into left and right pulmonary artery; results in increased pulmonary blood flow
II	20	Pulmonary artery arises from posterior portion of truncus arteriosus; pulmonary blood flow is normal
III	10	Pulmonary artery arises from sides of truncus arteriosus; pulmonary blood flow is normal
IV	10	Bronchial arteries arise from descending aorta to supply lungs; pulmonary blood flow is decreased

The result is abnormal alignment of the heart vessels and resulting cyanosis.

Transposition Defects

Transposition defects include a group of malformations that have in common an abnormal anatomical relationship between the cardiac chambers and the great arteries.

Complete Transposition of the Great Arteries or Vessels (TGA or TGV)

TGA is the result of inappropriate septation and migration of the truncus arteriosus during fetal cardiac development. TGA may be dextrotransposition of the great arteries (D-TGA) or levotransposition of the great arteries (L-TGA). In D-TGA, the aorta arises from the right ventricle and the pulmonary artery arises from the left ventricle. The aorta receives unoxygenated systemic venous blood and returns it to the systemic arterial circuit. The pulmonary artery receives oxygenated pulmonary venous blood and returns it to the pulmonary circulation.

In L-TGA, the great vessels are transposed, with the aorta arising from the right ventricle and the pulmonary artery arising from the left ventricle. The aorta is to the left and anterior to the pulmonary artery. This type of transposition is called *corrected* because, functionally, the hemodynamics are normal. The oxygenated blood comes into the left atrium, enters the right ventricle, and goes through the aorta to the systemic circulation. However, frequently there are other associated cardiac defects (Park et al, 2002).

Incidence. TGA accounts for 5% of all CHDs. It is more common in males (3:1). D-TGA is the most common cyanotic heart defect in newborns.

Hemodynamics. Hemodynamically, two separate parallel circulations result from complete D-TGA. Oxygenated blood from the lungs is returned to the left atrium, enters the left ventricle, and goes through the pulmonary artery to the lungs again. Desaturated blood from the systemic circulation enters the right atrium, goes to the right ventricle, enters the aorta, and is directed back into the systemic circulation. The end result is that the heart and brain and other vital tissues are perfused with desaturated blood. This defect is incompatible with life. A communication between the two circulations must exist to allow mixing of the oxygenated and desaturated blood. This communication can be at the ductal, atrial, or ventricular level. The best mixing occurs with a large VSD. Figure 3-13 shows TGA (Park et al, 2002).

Manifestations. Marked cyanosis is the prominent sign of TGA. The degree of cyanosis varies with the amount of communication between the two circulations. Signs of CHF are present. S_2 is loud and single. If a VSD is present, a loud, harsh systolic murmur of variable intensity can be heard. Hypoglycemia, hypocalcemia, and metabolic acidosis are frequently present.

Diagnosis. On radiographic study of TGA, the heart is enlarged and has a narrow base because the aorta is over the pulmonary artery. The heart is described as egg shaped (Park et al, 2002). Pulmonary blood flow is increased. An ECG shows right axis deviation of the QRS and right ventricular hypertrophy. Echocardiography reveals the abnormal origin of the great arteries from the ventricles. Associated defects can also be visualized by echocardiography.

Management. TGA is a cardiac emergency. Immediate medical management includes correction of acidosis,

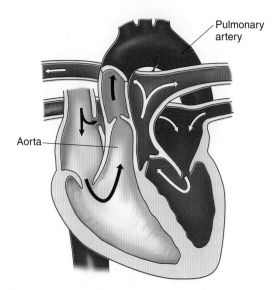

FIGURE **3-13**
Transposition of the great arteries or vessels is a condition in which the aorta arises from the right ventricle and the pulmonary artery arises from the left ventricle. The result is two distinct circulatory (parallel) pathways.

hypoglycemia, and hypocalcemia; administration of oxygen and infusion of PGE_1; and treatment of CHF. A cardiac catheterization is performed and a balloon atrial septostomy is carried out to promote mixing of oxygenated and desaturated blood in the atria. If the septostomy and PGE_1 infusion do not sufficiently improve oxygenation, surgical excision of the posterior aspect of the atrial septum (Blalock-Hanlon procedure) is performed without cardiopulmonary bypass as a palliative measure. This procedure has a 10% to 25% mortality rate (Park et al, 2002).

Definitive surgical correction involves switching the right- and left-sided structures at the ventricular level (Rastelli's procedure), the artery level (Jatene's procedure), or the atrial level (Senning's or Mustard's procedure).

See Table 3-5 for a description of these procedures.

The prognosis for TGA without surgical intervention is poor; 90% of patients die within the first year of life. The surgical procedures have high mortality rates and a high rate of postoperative complications (e.g., dysrhythmias, obstruction to systemic or pulmonary venous return, and right ventricular dysfunction). Jatene's procedure is newer but seems to minimize many complications associated with the intra-atrial repair operations. Long-term results of this procedure must be evaluated. The type and timing of surgical correction depend on the condition of the patient and the anatomic defect, so each case must be decided individually. A typical management approach is presented in the flow diagram in Figure 3-14.

Defects That Have Obstructions of the Vascular or Valvular Systems, With or Without Right to Left Shunt

These are congenital heart defects resulting from a defect of either the vascular or the valvular system with a consequent obstruction of blood flow with a right to left shunt with either reduced or increased pulmonary blood flow. The defects described in this section include coarctation of the aorta (COA), hypoplastic left heart syndrome (HLHS), and total anomalous pulmonary venous return (TAPVR).

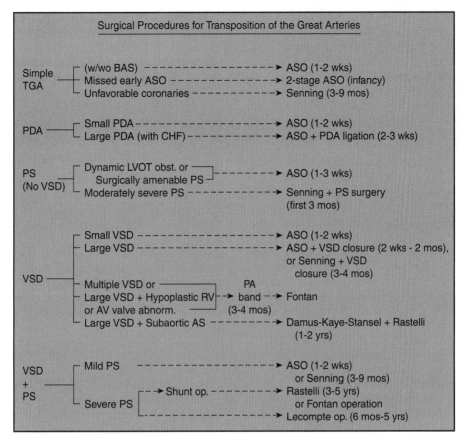

Surgical Procedures for Transposition of the Great Arteries

Simple TGA
- (w/wo BAS) ----------------→ ASO (1-2 wks)
- Missed early ASO -----------→ 2-stage ASO (infancy)
- Unfavorable coronaries -------→ Senning (3-9 mos)

PDA
- Small PDA ------------------→ ASO (1-2 wks)
- Large PDA (with CHF) --------→ ASO + PDA ligation (2-3 wks)

PS (No VSD)
- Dynamic LVOT obst. or Surgically amenable PS -------→ ASO (1-3 wks)
- Moderately severe PS --------→ Senning + PS surgery (first 3 mos)

VSD
- Small VSD ------------------→ ASO (1-2 wks)
- Large VSD ------------------→ ASO + VSD closure (2 wks - 2 mos), or Senning + VSD closure (3-4 mos)
- Multiple VSD or Large VSD + Hypoplastic RV or AV valve abnorm. → PA band (3-4 mos) → Fontan
- Large VSD + Subaortic AS ----→ Damus-Kaye-Stansel + Rastelli (1-2 yrs)

VSD + PS
- Mild PS --------------------→ ASO (1-2 wks) or Senning (3-9 mos)
- Severe PS → Shunt op. -------→ Rastelli (3-5 yrs) or Fontan operation ----→ Lecompte op. (6 mos-5 yrs)

FIGURE 3-14

Management of transposition of the great arteries: flow diagram. "Senning" on the diagram represents an intra-atrial repair, either Senning's operation or Mustard's operation. From Park MK (1996). *Pediatric cardiology for practitioners*, ed 3. St Louis: Mosby.

Coarctation of the Aorta

COA is a narrowing or constriction of the aorta in the aortic arch segment. The most common location is below the origin of the left subclavian artery. Coarctation may occur as a single lesion due to improper development of the aorta or may occur because of constriction of the ductus arteriosus. The severity of the circulatory compromise depends on the location of the constriction and the degree of constriction. Coarctation proximal to the ductus arteriosus (preductal COA) has associated defects in 40% of cases. Associated defects include VSD, TGA, and PDA. Collateral circulation is poorly developed with preductal COA. Postductal COA is usually not associated with other defects, and collateral circulation is more effective. Infants with postductal COA may not be symptomatic. More than half of infants with COA have a bicuspid aortic valve (Park et al, 2002).

Incidence. COA accounts for 8% of all CHDs. Coarctation occurs twice as often in males. It is found in 30% of infants with Turner syndrome (Park et al, 2002).

Hemodynamics. Coarctation causes obstruction to flow, which leads to varying pressure across the aortic segment. The portion of aorta proximal to the constriction has an elevated pressure, which leads to increased left ventricular pressure. The increased left ventricular pressure results in left ventricular hypertrophy and dilation. Collateral circulation develops from the proximal to distal arteries, bypassing the constricted segment of the aorta. This is a compensatory mechanism to increase flow to the lower extremities and abdomen, producing lower pulses in the lower extremities. COA is shown in Figure 3-15 (Park et al, 2002).

Manifestations. The severity and time of appearance of symptoms of coarctation depend on the location and degree

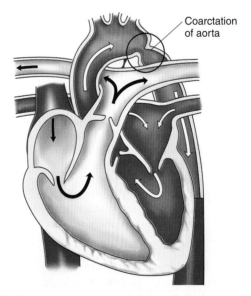

Coarctation of aorta

FIGURE 3-15

Coarctation of the aorta is a narrowing or constriction of the aorta near the ductus arteriosus.

of constriction, as well as the presence of associated cardiac defects. Symptoms of coarctation include signs of CHF and absent, weak, or delayed pulses in the lower extremities with bounding pulses in the upper extremities. In the presence of CHF, however, all pulses may be weak. With severe COA, S_2 is loud and single. A systolic thrill may be felt in the suprasternal notch. An ejection click may be audible at the apex if there is a bicuspid aortic valve or if systemic hypertension is present. A systolic ejection murmur of grade 2/6 to 3/6 can be heard at the upper right and middle or lower left sternal border, and at the left interscapular area in the infant's back; however, no murmur is heard in more than half of infants with COA. Correction of CHF may produce the murmur (Park et al, 2002).

Diagnosis. Diagnosis of COA is based on the history, physical findings, radiographs, ECGs, and echocardiographic data. In asymptomatic infants and children, radiographs may show a normal or slightly enlarged heart. Dilation of the ascending aorta may be evident. The "E" sign on barium swallow is characteristic, but is usually not evident until at least 4 months of age. The "E" appearance is due to the large proximal aortic segment or prominent subclavian artery above and the poststenotic dilation of the descending aorta below the constricted segment (Park et al, 2002). In symptomatic infants and children, radiographs show cardiomegaly and increased pulmonary venous congestion.

The ECGs of asymptomatic children may show left axis deviation of the QRS and left ventricular hypertrophy. In symptomatic children, the ECG reveals normal or right axis deviation of the QRS. Right ventricular hypertrophy or right bundle branch block is present in infants, whereas left ventricular hypertrophy is present in older children (Park et al, 2002). A two-dimensional echocardiogram demonstrates the location and degree of the constriction and the presence of associated defects.

Management. Surgical correction of COA is the definitive treatment. Surgery is performed in patients 3 to 5 years of age if signs and symptoms can be medically controlled. Earlier surgery is indicated if medical management is not successful.

Medical management is aimed at providing adequate oxygenation, preventing or treating CHF, and preventing SAIE. PGE_1 may be needed to maintain ductal patency if the constricted segment is at the level of the ductus arteriosus (Park et al, 2002).

Surgical intervention of COA involves the excision of the constricted segment of the aorta with end-to-end anastomosis, patch graft, bypass tube graft, or Dacron graft (Park et al, 2002). Alternatively, a subclavian flap aortoplasty may be performed. Surgery is indicated in the presence of CHF with or without circulatory shock. In the presence of a large VSD, pulmonary artery banding may be performed at surgery to reduce pulmonary blood flow in an attempt to prevent pulmonary hypertension. The pulmonary artery banding is removed and the VSD is repaired at 6 months to 2 years of age. The mortality rate for surgical corrections is less than 5%. Postoperative complications include renal failure and recoarctation.

Hypoplastic Left Heart Syndrome

HLHS consists of a group of cardiac defects, including a small aorta, aortic and mitral valve stenosis or atresia, and a small left atrium and ventricle. The great vessels are usually normally related (Norwood et al, 1983).

Incidence. HLHS accounts for 1% to 2% of all CHDs, but it accounts for 7% to 8% of heart defects producing symptoms in the first year of life; it is the leading cause of death from CHDs in the first month of life. HLHS is not associated with abnormalities in other organ systems.

Hemodynamics. Left ventricular output is greatly reduced or eliminated because of the valvular obstruction and the small size of the left ventricle. Left atrial and pulmonary venous pressures are elevated, and pulmonary edema and pulmonary hypertension are seen. With a PDA, blood shunts from the pulmonary artery into the aorta. The PDA provides the only cardiac output, because there is little or no flow across the aortic valve. Retrograde flow through the aortic arch supplies the head, upper extremities, and coronary arteries.

Although circulation is abnormal in utero, the high pulmonary vascular resistance and the low systemic vascular resistance make survival possible. The right ventricle maintains normal perfusion pressure in the descending aorta by a right to left ductal shunt. At birth, the onset of pulmonary ventilation causes the pulmonary vascular resistance to decrease. The systemic vascular resistance increases because the placenta is eliminated. Closure of the ductus arteriosus further decreases systemic cardiac output and aortic pressure, leading to metabolic acidosis and circulatory shock. Increased pulmonary blood flow causes increased left atrial pressure and pulmonary edema (Park et al, 2002). Figure 3-16 shows HLHS.

Manifestations. Progressive cyanosis, pallor, and mottling are presenting symptoms of HLHS. Tachycardia, tachypnea, dyspnea, and pulmonary rales are present. The S_2 is loud and single. Poor peripheral pulses and vasoconstriction of the extremities are noted on examination. A cardiac murmur may be absent, or a grade 1/6 to 3/6 nonspecific systolic murmur may be heard (Park et al, 2002).

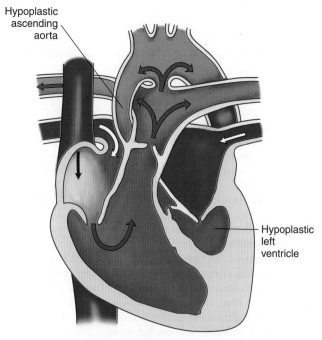

Hypoplastic ascending aorta

Hypoplastic left ventricle

FIGURE **3-16**
Hypoplastic left heart syndrome.

Diagnosis. On radiographic study of HLHS, there is mild to moderate heart enlargement and pulmonary venous congestion or pulmonary edema. Metabolic acidosis found on arterial blood gas study is a result of decreased cardiac output. Right ventricular hypertrophy is the characteristic finding on ECG. Echocardiography is usually diagnostic. Findings demonstrate the components of the small left-sided heart structures and the dilated or hypertrophied right-sided heart structures. Findings include a small left ventricle, small ascending aorta and aortic root, absent or abnormal mitral valve, and enlarged right ventricle. An abnormal left ventricle to right ventricle end-diastolic ratio is present (Park et al, 2002).

Management. Medical management of HLHS is aimed at prevention of hypoxemia and correction of metabolic acidosis. PGE_1 is administered through continuous infusion to maintain ductal patency. Balloon atrial septostomy may be performed to decompress the left atrium.

Surgical correction of the HLHS is experimental and has a high mortality rate. However, this defect was once considered 100% fatal. Surgical correction is performed in stages. The first stage, the modified procedure, is performed in the neonatal period to maintain pulmonary blood flow and create interatrial mixing of blood. The second stage, a modified Fontan procedure, is performed in patients at 6 months to 2 years of age. This procedure closes the Gore-Tex shunt, closes the atrial communication, and forms a direct anastomosis of the right atrium and pulmonary artery. See Table 3-5 for a description of these procedures (Park et al, 2002).

The mortality rate for HLHS remains high. The first-stage surgical repair has a mortality rate of nearly 75%. For the survivors, there is a 50% mortality rate with the second-stage operation (Park et al, 2002). Nursing care is critical after the first-stage repair. Nursing care must focus on assessment of homeostasis and pulmonary blood flow during the immediate postoperative period. Attention to nutritional status is important for the long-term recovery. Postoperative care requires close monitoring of vital signs, chest tube output, platelet counts, liver function tests, guaiac tests, and pulmonary and circulatory status.

Dopamine at 5 to 10 mcg/kg/min may be used to decrease pulmonary vasoconstriction. Dobutamine or isoproterenol are avoided because they dilate the pulmonary arterioles, making the situation worse. Fentanyl may be used to balance pulmonary vascular resistance. Diuretics or peritoneal dialysis may be necessary to maintain a fluid balance. High-frequency ventilation is sometimes used to support pulmonary function when acidosis and stiffening lungs is present. ECMO has also been used in these infants.

Initially, nutritional support is provided through total parenteral nutrition (TPN). Monitoring of daily weights, of urine for ketones, glucose, and protein, and of serum levels of electrolytes and trace minerals is necessary to adjust the parenteral fluids. Enteral feedings may be started in the first 2 weeks postoperatively if the infant is stable and when the greatest danger of necrotizing enterocolitis is past.

Pericardial effusion may occur several days or weeks after the Fontan procedure; alterations in tissue perfusion and changes in systemic blood flow return may be present if pericardial effusion occurs. Cardiac transplantation, although experimental, may provide improved prognosis for infants with HLHS. It is essential that parents be informed of all available treatments, including risks and prognosis if surgical intervention is an option.

Total Anomalous Pulmonary Venous Return (TAPVR)

With TAPVR, the pulmonary veins drain into the right atrium (rather than the left atrium) directly or through connection with the systemic veins. There is no direct connection between the pulmonary veins and the left atrium. Four types of TAPVR have been identified (Park et al, 2002).

Incidence. TAPVR accounts for 1% of all CHDs. There is a 1:1 male to female ratio of occurrence.

Hemodynamics. If there is an ASD or patent foramen ovale in TAPVR, a portion of the mixed blood from the right atrium can cross into the left atrium, into the left ventricle, and on into the systemic circulation. The direction of the blood flow and the amount that crosses the atrial communication into the left atrium or that enters the left ventricle are determined by the compliance of the ventricles.

Two clinical hemodynamic states exist with TAPVR. If pulmonary blood flow is unobstructed, this flow is greatly increased. The result is highly saturated blood in the right atrium and mild cyanosis. If obstruction to pulmonary blood flow does exist, the volume of flow is decreased and cyanosis is severe. Pulmonary edema is often caused by elevated pulmonary venous pressure. Obstruction to pulmonary blood flow is a common occurrence when the TAPVR is below the diaphragm (Park et al, 2002). TAPVR is shown in Figure 3-17.

Manifestations. The manifestations of TAPVR depend on the presence of pulmonary venous obstruction (PVO). TAPVR without PVO includes a history of mild cyanosis, frequent pulmonary infections, poor growth, and CHF. TAPVR with PVO involves severe cyanosis and respiratory distress in the neonatal period, with progressive growth failure. Feeding is associated with increased cyanosis caused by the compression of the common pulmonary vein by the filled

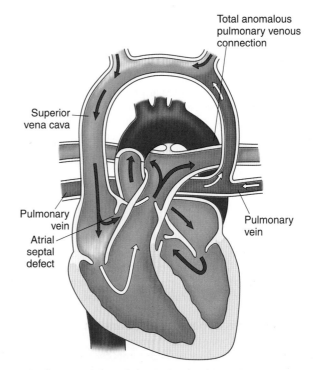

FIGURE **3-17**
Total anomalous pulmonary venous return is a condition in which all the pulmonary veins empty into the right atrium.

esophagus (Park et al, 2002). Signs and symptoms of CHF are also present.

Diagnosis. TAPVR without PVO produces a precordial bulge with hyperactive right ventricular impulse. The PMI is at the xiphoid process or lower left sternal border. S_2 is widely split and fixed; the pulmonic sound may be pronounced. A grade 2/6 to 3/6 systolic ejection murmur can be heard at the upper left sternal border, and a mid-diastolic rumble is always audible at the lower left sternal border. The rhythm is a quadruple or quintuple gallop (Park et al, 2002).

TAPVR with PVO may produce minimal cardiac findings. S_2 is loud and single and there is a gallop rhythm. There may be a faint systolic ejection murmur at the upper left sternal border. Pulmonary rales may be audible.

Radiographic findings of TAPVR without PVO include mild to moderate cardiomegaly and increased pulmonary markings. The characteristic "snowman" sign occurs because of the anatomic appearance of the left superior vena cava, the left innominate vein, and the right superior vena cava. This sign is seldom visible before the patient is 4 months of age. With TAPVR with PVO, the heart size is normal on radiographs and there are signs of pulmonary edema (Park et al, 2002).

On an ECG, TAPVR without PVO has right axis deviation of the QRS and sometimes right atrial hypertrophy. TAPVR with PVO has right axis deviation for age and right ventricular hypertrophy in the form of tall R waves in the right precordial leads.

Echocardiography of TAPVR without PVO reveals the pulmonary veins draining into a common chamber posterior to the left atrium. The ASD and small left atrium and left ventricle are visualized. A dilated coronary sinus protruding into the left atrium or a dilated innominate vein and superior vena cava can be visualized, if present. Two-dimensional echocardiography of TAPVR with PVO shows the small left atrium and left ventricle. Anomalous pulmonary venous return below the diaphragm can be directly visualized. Doppler echocardiography can be used to detect the venous flow pattern (Park et al, 2002).

Management. Management of TAPVR is surgical, and surgery is emergent when PVO is below the diaphragm. Medical management is aimed at preventing or treating CHF and preventing hypoxemia. Diuretics may be required to manage pulmonary edema. Balloon atrial septostomy at cardiac catheterization is performed to enlarge the interatrial communication and promote better mixing of blood. Surgery may be delayed when response to medical management is good, but it is usually performed when the patients are infants (Park et al, 2002).

The surgical procedure depends on the site of the anomalous drainage. Cardiopulmonary bypass is required. Surgery involves the anastomosis of the pulmonary veins to the left atrium, closure of the ASD, and division of the anomalous connection. The surgical mortality rate is high, 10% to 25%, but it is lower than with medical management alone. The highest mortality rate is with the infracardiac type (Russo & Russo, 2005).

Emerging Postoperative Treatments. As discussed, morbidity and mortality rates remain high after surgery in many of the cardiac defects. Treatments that are aimed at decreasing pulmonary vascular resistance, decreasing persistent pulmonary hypertension, and improving cardiac output are being tried at many centers. These include ECMO, especially in infants with TOF, and high-frequency jet ventilation in infants who have undergone stage 1 repair of the Norwood procedure for stage 1 HLHS. Newer therapies that are under study include nitric oxide (NO) administration and ultrafiltration.

Inhaled NO is a pulmonary dilator and directly affects pulmonary and systemic vascular resistance. Its use is being researched in infants who have undergone procedures that require cardiac bypass, such as bidirectional Glenn or Fontan procedures.

Ultrafiltration is an experimental procedure undertaken after open-heart surgery. This process is similar to peritoneal dialysis in that it removes water and solutes to increase the hematocrit and blood pressure and to decrease cardiac workload and pulmonary vascular resistance. The action is probably due to a change in the pressure gradient between the blood and the dialyzing solution. The result is restoration or maintenance of blood volume, which reduces the need for transfusions. The better perfusion lessens the edema. As contractility of the heart improves, cardiac workload decreases, possibly because cardiodepressant proteins that are present after cardiac surgery are removed. The exact action of this procedure is being researched. It does appear to be a potential treatment for the capillary leak syndrome that is prevalent after cardiac surgery (Park et al, 2002).

Congenital Arrhythmias

Cardiac arrhythmias in infants generally arise from primary cardiac lesions, usually from abnormal conduction pathways. Alternatively, cardiac arrhythmias can develop following corrective cardiac surgery. It is not clear whether the arrhythmia is caused by the surgical procedure or by the initial heart defect. Other factors that contribute to the development of arrhythmias include electrolyte imbalances, neurologic conditions, or infections. Generally in infants, rhythm disturbances are not the primary manifestation of a cardiac problem; instead congestive heart failure or cyanosis is present before dysrhythmias occur (Sacchetti et al, 1999). However, there are some conditions that appear with rhythm disturbances in the newborn period. The most commonly occurring include congenital complete heart block (CCHB) and supraventricular tachycardia (SVT). These two dysrhythmias will be discussed.

Congenital Complete Heart Block

The AV node and the bundle of His arise as separate structures that join together. Congenital heart block is a result of a discontinuity between the atrial musculature and the AV node or the bundle of His and the AV node. For the majority of cases, the exact cause of the discontinuity is unknown and the remainder of the heart anatomy is normal. Certain antibodies passed from mothers with systemic lupus erythematosus (SLE) are associated with congenital heart block. Congenital heart block can be a manifestation of congenital heart defects, including congenitally corrected transposition of the great arteries.

CCHB can be diagnosed by detection of consistent fetal bradycardia (heart rate of 40 to 80 beats/min) by auscultation, fetal echocardiography, or electronic monitoring. A newborn with a ventricular rate less than 50 beats/min and an atrial rate greater than 150 beats/min is at significant risk. If the newborn has an associated heart defect, the risk for mortality is higher.

Treatment. Asymptomatic infants do not require treatment. If the infant is in congestive heart failure, digitalization is generally the first line of treatment. Insertion of a pacemaker is necessary for infants in congestive heart failure that does not respond to digitalization. Children with pacemakers implanted need close follow-up because of complications or adverse effects of the pacemakers (Bevilacqua & Hordof, 1998).

Supraventricular Tachycardia

Supraventricular tachycardia (SVT) can arise in utero or in the neonatal period. The most common arrhythmias that produce signs are paroxysmal SVT with or without ventricular preexcitation, atrial flutter, and junctional tachycardia. If the SVT occurs in utero, it can lead to heart failure and hydrops fetalis. SVT in the fetus is treated through maternal administration of digitalis. If digitalization is not successful, propranolol, quinidine, felcainide, or amiodarone are used. The fetus is delivered if there is evidence of fetal lung maturity.

In most cases of SVT, no cause is found. Long-acting thyroid stimulators and immune gamma-2-globulin from hyperthyroid mothers, hypoglycemia, and Ebstein's anomaly of the tricuspid valve can be the cause in other cases. Of infants with SVT, 10% to 50% have Wolfe-Parkinson-White (WPW) syndrome in which the atrial impulse activates the whole or some part of the ventricle or the ventricular impulse activates the whole or some part of the atrium earlier than would be expected if the impulse traveled via the normal pathway. WPW is characterized by a normal QRS, regular rhythm, ventricular rates of 150 to 200 beats/min, sudden onset, and sudden termination (Rubart & Zipes, 2005).

Symptoms produced by the SVT after birth are subtle and often are undetected until signs of congestive heart failure have been present for 24 to 36 hours. Treatment with digitalis or adenosine, cardioversion, transesophageal atrial pacing, or elicitation of a diving reflex by covering the face with a cold washcloth for 4 to 5 seconds generally is successful in establishing normal sinus rhythm. After conversion, digitalis is continued for 9 to 12 months. Therapy is discontinued abruptly, without weaning dosages.

Recurrence is more likely in patients with WPW and is treated with the foregoing drugs, alone or in combination. Recurrence decreases between 2 and 10 years of age. Prognosis for SVT is good (Rubart & Zipes, 2005).

Congestive Heart Failure (CHF)

CHF is a condition in which the blood supply to the body is insufficient to meet the metabolic requirements of the organs. CHF is a manifestation of an underlying disease or defect, rather than a disease itself. Before development of CHF, compensatory mechanisms are activated to maintain adequate cardiac output (Park et al, 2002; Wernovsky & Gruber, 2005). Normal mechanisms for regulation of cardiac output are listed in Box 3-2. CHF is classified according to the cause. Box 3-3 shows common causes of CHF in newborns.

Increased fluid volume may be caused by fluid overload or fluid retention. In the normally functioning myocardium, fluid retention does not cause CHF; however, fluid retention complicates CHF from other causes. In neonates, the most common cause of increased volume is CHD or altered hemodynamics, as in PDA.

CHF caused by obstruction to outflow occurs when the normal myocardium pumps against increased resistance. This

---

BOX 3-2

Regulation of Cardiac Output

Sympathetic Nervous System
* Activated by
Vasomotor center through peripheral sympathetic fibers
Secretion of norepinephrine from the adrenal medulla ("fight or flight" response)
* Characterized by tachycardia, increased contractility, peripheral vasoconstriction, pupil dilation

Parasympathetic Nervous System
* Activated by vagal fibers
Atria: stimulation causes decreased heart rate
Ventricles: stimulation causes decreased contractility

Baroreceptor Reflexes
* Located in walls of carotid sinuses and in aortic arch
* Pressure receptors stimulated by blood pressure
* Stimulation causes inhibition of the sympathetic portion of the vasomotor center and stimulation of the parasympathetic (vagal) center; decreased arterial blood pressure

---

BOX 3-3

Causes of Congestive Heart Failure in the Newborn

Causes of Congestive Heart Failure
Increased volume
Obstruction to flow
Ineffective myocardial function
Arrhythmias
Excessive demand for cardiac output

Congenital Heart Defects
Hypoplastic left heart syndrome
Interrupted aortic arch
Coarctation of the aorta
Total anomalous pulmonary venous return with obstruction
Arteriovenous malformation (cranial or hepatic)
Transposition of the great arteries
Patent ductus arteriosus (in preterm infants)

Acquired Heart Defects
Myocardial dysfunction
Anemia
Polycythemia or hyperviscosity
Tachyarrhythmias
Myocarditis

---

increased resistance may be caused by structural defects, such as valvular stenosis or COA, or by pulmonary disease or pulmonary hypertension. CHF caused by pulmonary disease is called *cor pulmonale*. Severe systemic hypertension can also cause increased resistance.

CHF in the neonate usually results from abnormal stresses placed on the heart rather than from an ineffective myocardium. However, electrolyte imbalances, acidosis, and myocardial ischemia affect the ability of the heart to function effectively. Conditions such as rheumatic fever, infectious myocarditis,

Kawasaki disease, and anomalous origin of the left coronary artery reduce the effectiveness of the heart.

Dysrhythmias that may produce CHF include complete AV block or sustained primary tachycardia. AV block results in a severe bradycardia that prohibits adequate circulation of blood. Tachycardia causes insufficient time for ventricular filling, decreasing cardiac output.

Severe anemia can cause CHF because of excessive demand for cardiac output. Because the oxygen-carrying capacity of the blood is diminished, the heart must pump more blood per minute to meet the tissue oxygenation requirements. If the heart cannot meet the excessive demand, CHF develops (Park et al, 2002).

Compensatory mechanisms function to meet the body's increased demand for cardiac output. These mechanisms are regulated by the sympathetic nervous system and mechanical factors. The compensatory mechanisms can sustain adequate cardiac output for only a short period of time. If the underlying condition is not corrected, CHF develops.

Sympathetic Nervous System Compensatory Mechanisms.
Decreased blood pressure stimulates vascular stretch receptors and baroreceptors in the aorta and carotid arteries, which trigger the sympathetic nervous system. Decreased systemic blood pressure inactivates baroreceptors, causing (1) increased sympathetic stimulation, (2) increased heart rate, (3) increased cardiac contractility, and (4) increased arterial blood pressure. Catecholamine release and beta-receptor stimulation increase the rate and force of myocardial contraction. Catecholamines also increase venous tone, so that blood is returned to the heart more effectively. Circulation to the skin, kidneys, extremities, and splanchnic bed is decreased, allowing better circulation to the brain, heart, and lungs. Decreased renal blood flow stimulates the release of renin, angiotensin, and aldosterone. This release causes retention of sodium and fluid, resulting in increased circulating volume. The increased volume puts additional work on the heart.

Mechanical Compensatory Mechanisms.
The heart muscle thickens to increase myocardial pressure. The hypertrophy is effective in the early stages, but as soon as the muscle mass increases, compliance decreases. This change in compliance requires greater filling pressure for adequate cardiac output. The hypertrophied heart eventually becomes ischemic because it does not receive adequate circulation to meet its metabolic needs. Ventricular dilation occurs as myocardial fibers stretch to accommodate heart volume. Initially, this increases the force of the contraction, but it, too, fails after a point.

Effects of Congestive Heart Failure.
When the right ventricle is unable to pump blood into the pulmonary artery, less blood is oxygenated by the lungs, there is increased pressure in the right atrium and systemic venous circulation, and edema occurs in the extremities and viscera. When the left ventricle is unable to pump blood into the systemic circulation, there is increased pressure in the left atrium and pulmonary veins. The lungs become congested with blood, causing elevated pulmonary pressures and pulmonary edema.

The end effects of CHF include decreased cardiac output, decreased renal perfusion, systemic venous engorgement, and pulmonary venous engorgement, and their consequent effects. Decreased cardiac output stimulates the sympathetic nervous system, causing tachycardia, increased contractility, increased vasomotor tone, peripheral vasoconstriction, and diaphoresis.

Decreased renal perfusion stimulates the renin-angiotensin-aldosterone mechanism, causing sodium and water retention. Systemic venous engorgement leads to hepatomegaly, jugular venous distention, periorbital and facial edema, and, occasionally, ascites and dependent edema. Pulmonary venous engorgement results in tachypnea, decreased tidal volume, decreased lung compliance, increased airway resistance, early closure of the small airways with air trapping, increased work of breathing, and increased respiratory effort, grunting, and rales. Stimulation of the j-receptors in the lung causes the infant to become apprehensive and irritable.

Diagnosis. The diagnosis of CHF is based on clinical signs and symptoms, laboratory data, and chest radiography. In contrast to infants with cyanotic heart disease, infants with CHF usually have significant respiratory distress with tachypnea, grunting, and retractions. They exhibit peripheral pallor, appearing to be ashen or gray in color. The precordium is active, and loud murmurs can usually be heard throughout systole and diastole. Pulses are usually full, but there may be a difference between the upper and the lower extremities. Hepatomegaly is common. The infants are irritable.

In addition to demonstrating hypoxemia, arterial blood gas may reveal a metabolic acidosis resulting from the decreased systemic blood flow. If acidosis is severe, concurrent respiratory acidosis may be seen because of the pulmonary edema caused by left-sided heart failure. Pulmonary ventilation-perfusion mismatch may cause hypoxemia. Hypocalcemia is often present in infants with CHF because they have an inappropriate response to stress. In addition, infants with DiGeorge syndrome may have hypocalcemia because of absent parathyroids. Aortic arch abnormalities (e.g., interrupted aortic arch, hypoplastic left heart, and COA) are commonly associated with DiGeorge syndrome (Park et al, 2002).

Hypoglycemia may be present in infants with severe CHF. The myocardium is dependent on glucose; decreased glucose levels diminish the ability of the heart to compensate for CHF. On chest radiographs, the heart is enlarged and there is increased pulmonary congestion. An ECG generally is not diagnostic unless the CHF is caused by an arrhythmia. There may be nonspecific changes in the T waves, changes in the ST segment, and an increase in the height of the P wave.

Electrolyte imbalances usually include relative hyponatremia, which is due to the increase in free water. Hypochloremia and increased bicarbonate may result from respiratory acidemia and the use of loop diuretics. Hyperkalemia results from the release of intracellular cations, which is related to poor tissue perfusion. Elevated lactic acid levels are also indicative of tissue hypoxia. Atrial natriuretic factor (ANF), a peptide hormone, may be important in the regulation of volume and blood pressure. ANF is released from the atria when they are distended. ANF release causes natriuresis, diuresis, and vasodilation. ANF acts with other volume regulators, such as renin, aldosterone, and vasopressin. An increased ANF level may be found when there is increased pulmonary blood flow, increased left atrial pressure, or pulmonary hypertension.

Children with corrected or uncorrected congenital heart defects frequently have abnormal homeostasis, suggesting a chronic compensated disseminated intravascular coagulopathy, with reduced synthesis of clotting factors or deranged platelet aggregation that can lead to bleeding problems (Goel et al, 2000).

Treatment. The goal of management of CHF is to improve cardiac function while identifying and correcting the underlying cause. General measures that decrease the demand on the heart are helpful; however, pharmacologic intervention is the most efficacious therapy.

General Measures. General measures to manage CHF include the administration of oxygen to improve ventilation and perfusion at the alveolar level. Ventilation with positive end-expiratory pressure at 6 to 10 cm H_2O may relieve the effects of CHF by reducing pulmonary edema.

Fluid restriction may decrease the circulating volume. Careful monitoring of serum electrolytes, intake and output, and weight is essential. It is imperative that *all* fluid be counted in the total daily fluid volume. Infants with CHF do not usually feed well and may require caloric supplementation with hyperalimentation or gavage feedings (Park et al, 2002).

Infants with CHF are irritable and agitated, which further complicates their status. Sedation with continuous infusions of morphine sulfate or fentanyl may improve the infant's comfort and oxygenation. Other measures that reduce cardiac demand include maintenance of a normal hematocrit, maintenance of the thermoneutral environment, and minimal stimulation. Cautious use of sedation may reduce anxiety and agitation, increasing comfort and decreasing the demand for oxygen (Verklan & Walden, 2004).

Pharmacologic Interventions. Table 3-8 lists the medications most commonly used in the management of cardiac conditions. The mainstay of management of CHF beyond the neonatal period is digitalis (digoxin). Digoxin slows conduction through the AV node, prolongs the refractory period, and slows the heart rate through vagal effects on the SA node.

The use of digoxin in preterm or term neonates is controversial. The preterm newborn is at risk for digitalis toxicity because of the narrow range between therapeutic and toxic drug levels. The preterm infant requires a lower maintenance dose because of limited renal excretion of the drug (Table 3-9). If digoxin is used, the neonate must be carefully monitored for signs and symptoms of digitalis toxicity. Lead II ECGs should be obtained before each dose for the first 3 days; the dose should be withheld if the P-R interval is greater than 0.16 second or if an arrhythmia is found. Digoxin levels should be monitored and should be less than 2.0 ng/ml (Park et al, 2002). Blood samples for digoxin levels should be drawn after the drug has achieved equilibrium in the body, approximately 6 to 8 hours after administration.

Other inotropic agents can be used to improve cardiac output. Dopamine, a norepinephrine precursor, has direct and indirect beta-adrenergic effects that are dose dependent. At low doses (2 to 5 mcg/kg/min), there is increased renal blood flow with minimal effect on heart rate, blood pressure, or contractility. Medium doses (5 to 10 mcg/kg/min) increase renal blood flow, heart rate, blood pressure, and contractility. Pulmonary artery pressure may be increased; peripheral resistance is not affected. High doses (10 to 20 mcg/kg/min) cause alpha effects, resulting in peripheral vasoconstriction, increased cardiac rate, and increased contractility (Park et al, 2002).

Dobutamine is a synthetic catecholamine that acts on beta- and alpha-adrenergic receptors. Dobutamine (2 to 10 mcg/min) has decreased effects on the heart rate and rhythm and causes less peripheral vasoconstriction.

Isoproterenol (Isuprel), a synthetic epinephrine-like substance, has beta$_1$- and beta$_2$-adrenergic effects. The usefulness of Isuprel in the neonate is limited because it produces increased heart rate, arrhythmias, and decreased systemic vascular resistance, which may worsen the hypotension (Park et al, 2002).

Diuretics. Diuretics are useful in the treatment of CHF to decrease sodium and water retention. The primary goal is to increase renal perfusion (with inotropic agents or vasodilators) and to increase sodium delivery to distal diluting sites of the renal tubules. Diuretic agents increase the renal excretion of sodium and other anions by inhibition of tubular reabsorption of sodium (Park et al, 2002).

Furosemide (Lasix), a loop diuretic, blocks sodium and chloride reabsorption in the ascending limb of the loop of Henle. Loop diuretics interfere with the formation of free water and free water reabsorption by preventing the transport of sodium, potassium, and chloride into the medullary interstitium. Loop diuretics cause increased excretion of potassium by delivering increased quantities of sodium to sites in the distal nephron, where potassium can be excreted. Furosemide also increases excretion of calcium, but does not affect the ability of the kidney to regulate acid-base balance.

An aldosterone antagonist such as spironolactone (Aldactone, Chicago, IL: Searle LLC) may be useful because it is a potassium-sparing diuretic. Spironolactone works by binding to the cytoplasmic receptor sites and blocking aldosterone action, thus impairing the reabsorption of sodium and the secretion of potassium and hydrogen ion. Spironolactone has no effect on free water production and absorption. Thiazide diuretics (chlorothiazide and hydrochlorothiazide) inhibit sodium and chloride reabsorption along the distal tubules. They are not as effective as the loop diuretics and are infrequently used (Park et al, 2002).

Complications of Diuretic Therapy. Diuretic therapy can provide severe electrolyte imbalances if not monitored carefully. The complications of diuretic therapy include (1) volume contraction, (2) hyponatremia, (3) metabolic alkalemia or acidemia, and (4) hypokalemia or hyperkalemia. Administration of water and electrolytes is needed to maintain fluid and electrolyte balance when diuretics are given. The adequacy of the volume can be determined by monitoring serum electrolytes, BUN, creatinine, urinary output, weight, specific gravity, and skin turgor.

The increased renal losses of sodium can lead to hyponatremia, unless adequate amounts of sodium are provided. Release of antidiuretic hormone may also increase because of changes in the osmoreceptors or inhibition of antidiuretic hormone action. This can best be managed by decreasing the amount of total water and improving the cardiac output, thus increasing renal perfusion.

Metabolic alkalosis can result from administration of loop diuretics that interfere with sodium- and potassium-dependent chloride reabsorption. Hypochloremia results in a greater aldosterone production and an increase in bicarbonate concentration. Hypokalemia is a frequent complication of loop diuretic therapy. An increased ratio of intracellular to extracellular potassium results in the clinical signs and symptoms of hypokalemia. Hypokalemia increases the risk for digoxin toxicity. In contrast, hyperkalemia may result when the cardiac output is low and tissue perfusion is severely compromised. Other complications of diuretic therapy include increased calcium excretion, hyperuricemia, and glucose intolerance.

TABLE 3-8	Drugs Used in the Management of Congenital Heart Defects			
Drug (Brand Name)	**Dosage**	**Action**	**Onset**	**Comments**
DIURETICS				
Furosemide (Lasix)	1 mg/kg/dose given intravenously (IV) 1 to 3 mg/kg/dose	Loop diuretic; inhibits sodium and chloride reabsorption in proximal tubule	15 to 30 min 30 to 60 min	Associated with increased patent ductus arteriosus; calcium loss
Spironolactone (Aldactone)	1.5 to 3.0 mg/kg/day given orally (PO)	Competitive antagonist of aldosterone	3 to 5 days	Potassium sparing
Chlorothiazide	20 to 40 mg/kg/day PO	Inhibits sodium and chloride reabsorption along the distal tubules	1 to 2 hours	
INOTROPIC AGENTS				
Dopamine	Low: 2 to 5 mcg/kg/min Moderate: 5 to 10 mcg/kg/min High: 10 to 20 mcg/kg/min	Increased renal blood flow; beta-adrenergic effects Increased renal blood flow; heart rate, BP, and contractility Peripheral vasoconstriction, increased heart rate, and contractility		Monitor electrocardiogram, blood pressure (BP)
Dobutamine	2 to 10 mcg/kg/min	Increased renal blood flow; increased contractility	Rapid	Decreased systemic vascular resistance; increased pulmonary wedge pressure
Isoproterenol	0.05 to 0.5 mg/kg/min	Increased venous return to heart and decreased pulmonary vascular resistance		Tachycardia, dysrhythmias, decreased renal perfusion
VASODILATORS				
Sodium nitroprusside (Nipride)	0.5 to 6 mcg/kg/min	Directly relaxes smooth muscles in arteriolar and venous walls; increases cardiac output if the decrease is caused by myocardial dysfunction	Seconds	Monitor BP and thiocyanate levels; light sensitive; monitor heart rate
PROSTAGLANDINS				
PGE_1	0.05 to 0.1 mg/kg/min	Produces vasodilation and smooth muscle relaxation of ductus arteriosus and pulmonary and systemic circulations; increased arterial saturation by 25% to 100%	Rapid	Monitor BP; vasopressors may be required; apnea, flush, fever, seizure-like activity; decreased heart rate
PROSTAGLANDIN SYNTHETASE INHIBITOR				
Indomethacin	0.2 mg/kg IV every 24 hours (first dose) 0.1 mg/kg IV (second and third doses) *Infant age over 48 hours but less than 14 days:* 0.3 mg/kg IV and 3 doses every 24 hours *Infant age over 14 days but less than 6 weeks:* 0.2 to 0.3 mg/kg every 12 hours	Promotes ductal closure by inhibition of PGE_2 in the walls of the ductus	12 to 24 hours	Monitor renal function, bilirubin, electrolytes, glucose, platelets, bleeding

TABLE **3-9**	Digoxin Prescription Information
Total Digitalizing Dose (TDD)	**Maintenance Dose**
PRETERM	
0.025 to 0.05 mg/kg	0.008 to 0.012 mg/kg/day
TERM	
0.04 to 0.08 mg/kg	0.01 to 0.02 mg/kg/day ($\frac{1}{8}$ TDD)

To digitalize:
1. Give $\frac{1}{2}$ the TDD.
2. Six to 8 hours later, give $\frac{1}{4}$ the TDD.
3. Six to 8 hours later, get a rhythm strip; if normal, give $\frac{1}{4}$ the TDD.
4. Give maintenance dose ($\frac{1}{8}$ the TDD) 12 hours after last digitalizing dose and then every 12 hours.

Slow digitalization, with decreased risk of toxicity, can be achieved by starting with the maintenance dose.

Vasodilators may be used in severe CHF to reduce the right and left ventricular preload and afterload to improve cardiac function. Vasodilators cause arterial and venous dilation, resulting in decreased systemic and pulmonary vascular resistance. Sodium nitroprusside (Nipride, Nutley, NJ: Roche Pharmaceuticals) is a smooth muscle relaxant that decreases ventricular afterload by decreasing pulmonary and systemic vascular resistance and decreases venous return and ventricular preload. This leads to decreased ventricular end-diastolic volume, increased ejection fraction, increased heart rate and cardiac index, and decreased pulmonary and systemic resistance. Sodium nitroprusside is sensitive to light and must be stored in dark containers. Side effects are cyanide toxicity and decreased platelet function (Park et al, 2002). The prognosis for CHF depends on the severity of the underlying condition and on the degree of CHF.

Subacute Bacterial Infective Endocarditis (SBIE)

SBIE can be a complication of CHD. Two factors are important in the development of SBIE: (1) structural abnormalities that create turbulent flow or pressure gradients and (2) bacteremia. All cardiac defects that produce turbulent flow or have a significant pressure gradient predispose the patient to bacterial invasion of the cardiac endothelium. The turbulent flow damages the endothelial lining and platelet-fibrin thrombus formation. Prevention of bacterial SBIE requires scrupulous daily oral care as well as prophylactic antimicrobials for dental procedures (Park et al, 2002). All CHDs, except secundum-type ASDs, predispose the patient to SBIE. VSDs, TOF, and aortic stenosis are the CHDs most commonly associated with SBIE (Park et al, 2002).

Vegetation of SBIE usually occurs on the low-pressure side of the defect, where endothelial damage is established by the jet effect of the defect. More than 90% of SBIE cases are caused by *Streptococcus viridans*, *Streptococcus faecalis* (enterococcus), and *Staphylococcus aureus*. Other organisms include *Haemophilus influenzae*, *Pseudomonas*, *Escherichia coli*, *Proteus*, *Aerobacter*, and *Listeria*. *Candida* may infect infants who have been on long-term antimicrobial or steroid therapy.

Prevention. Procedures for which SBIE prophylaxis is indicated include (1) all dental procedures, (2) tonsillectomy or adenoidectomy, (3) surgical procedures involving the respiratory mucosa, (4) bronchoscopy, (5) incision and drainage of infected tissue, and (6) gastrointestinal or genitourinary procedures.

For complete prescribing and dosing information, refer to the Committee on Rheumatic Fever and Infective Endocarditis of the Council on Cardiovascular Diseases in the Young. The recommendations for children are listed in Box 3-4.

Family Support

Families of infants who are critically ill or who have congenital defects generally experience confusion, guilt, anger, and fear. The family must cope with short- and long-term consequences of the congenital heart defect. Severity of the defect, availability of treatment, and prognosis influence the amount and kind of support required. Parents may be overwhelmed by the knowledge of their infant's heart defect, regardless of the severity. With treatment now available, over 95% of congenital heart defects can be partially or fully corrected through a combination of medical and surgical management (Cooley, 1997). However, residual defects or cardiovascular sequelae after surgical correction are common (Meberg et al, 2000). Parents need to be able to discuss quality-of-life issues with health care professionals in order to ensure that parents can make informed decisions about possible treatment options (Moyen et al, 1997). All options must be explained and described objectively. The impact of the cardiac defect on other systems must also be included when giving parents information, as the parents may not be aware of the associated complications, such as respiratory problems, that often accompany cardiac defects (Lubica, 1996). Although often overlooked, neurological prognosis is a key factor in determining the overall quality of life of a child with a congenital heart defect. Pediatric neurologists can be integrated into the health care team to assist parents in assessing the neurological prognosis of their child as well as to begin early intervention programs to facilitate the best outcome (Shevell, 1999). Parents need frequent contact with members of the health care team. Caretakers should speak with the parents routinely, not just when there are major changes in the infant's condition.

Although the majority of congenital heart defects do not have an identifiable genetic pattern, genetic counseling should be offered to all parents with a newborn with a congenital heart defect. Parents will want answers to questions about the cause of the defect, the likelihood of a recurrence in future pregnancies, and if there may be associated defects (Ardinger, 1997; Welch & Brown, 2000). However, recent work on the Human Genome Project and other advances in the study of genetics offer promise of determination of specific genetic causes of heart defects (Belmont, 1998). These advances may offer improved specific information to fully answer parents' questions. In addition, future innovation may greatly improve the ability to diagnose congenital heart defects prenatally (DeVore, 1998), thus increasing the opportunity for fetal surgery for correction of some defects, improved immediate management at birth, or, in some cases, termination of the pregnancy. The majority of congenital heart defects can be identified through targeted transvaginal or transabdominal ultrasound; however, they evolve in utero at different stages, and thus a single sonogram may not be sufficient to detect all CHDs (Yagel et al, 1997). Health care professionals

BOX **3-4**

Antimicrobial Prophylaxis to Prevent Subacute Infective Endocarditis in Children with Cardiac Defects

I. Dental procedures and oral respiratory tract surgery
   A. Standard regimen
      1. Amoxicillin 50 mg/kg 1 hour before procedure, followed by 25 mg/kg 6 hours after procedure.
   B. Alternative regimens
      1. Allergic to penicillin or amoxicillin: erythromycin ethylsuccinate or erythromycin stearate 20 mg/kg orally 2 hours before procedure, followed by erythromycin 10 mg/kg 6 hours after initial dose.
      2. Children unable to take oral medications: ampicillin 50 mg/kg given intravenously (IV) or intramuscularly (IM) 30 minutes before procedure, followed by ampicillin 25 mg/kg IV or IM 6 hours after initial dose.
      3. Allergic to penicillin and/or amoxicillin and unable to take oral medications: clindamycin 10 mg/kg IV 30 minutes before procedure, followed by clindamycin 5 mg/kg IV 6 hours after initial dose.
      4. High-risk children not candidates for standard regimen: ampicillin 50 mg/kg IV or IM plus gentamicin 2.0 mg/kg IV or IM 30 minutes before procedure, followed by amoxicillin 25 mg/kg orally 6 hours after initial dose or a repeat of the ampicillin plus gentamicin regimen.
      5. High-risk children allergic to ampicillin, amoxicillin, or penicillin: vancomycin 20 mg/kg IV over 1 hour, starting 1 hour before procedure. No repeat dose necessary.
II. Gastrointestinal or genitourinary procedure
   A. Standard regimen
      1. Ampicillin 50 mg/kg plus gentamicin 2.0 mg/kg IV or IM 30 minutes before procedure, followed by amoxicillin 25 mg/kg 6 hours after initial dose; or repeat ampicillin plus gentamicin regimen 8 hours after initial dose.
   B. Alternative regimens
      1. Ampicillin/amoxicillin/penicillin-allergic children: vancomycin 20 mg/kg IV over 1 hour plus gentamicin 2.0 mg/kg IV or IM 1 hour before procedure; repeat the vancomycin plus gentamicin regimen 8 hours after initial dose.
      2. Low-risk patient alternative regimen: amoxicillin 50 mg/kg orally 1 hour before procedure, followed by amoxicillin 25 mg/kg 6 hours after initial dose.

Data from Dajani AS et al (1997). *Prevention of bacterial endocarditis. Recommendations by the American Heart Association.* Dallas, TX: American Heart Association.

must be keenly aware of all options to ensure that parents receive the most up-to-date information on which to base decisions.

Family members should be given an accurate description of the defect; diagrams and models illustrating the defect should be used. Parents need frequent reassurance and repetition of information. Parents of infants who do not require immediate surgery but who will eventually require surgical correction must be educated about all aspects of the infant's care, including signs and symptoms of deterioration, medication administration, activity limitations, and normal development. Because growth failure with a cardiac defect is common, efforts to maximize nutrition are important; extra support is needed if the mother planned to breastfeed her baby (Lambert & Watters, 1998; Varan et al, 1999). Careful follow-up is important to prevent complications.

Identification of support persons for the family is extremely valuable. Parents may be encouraged to talk to other parents of newborns with the same or similar defects. Many neonatal intensive care units have active support groups consisting of parents of patients. Care should be taken in selection of supporters. Parents with a term newborn with a CHD may not be able to relate to parents of a preterm neonate. Other family members or friends should not be overlooked; they can become valuable support persons if they are provided appropriate guidance and education. The needs of siblings should also be assessed. Siblings need support, education, and guidance appropriate for their age and comprehension of the situation. Parents may not recognize their needs because of the overwhelming situation. Health care providers can facilitate the parent-child relationship during the initial period and throughout the course of management.

Financial resources should be addressed because preoperative, operative, and postoperative care is expensive. Many parents need assistance in obtaining aid to which they are entitled. Even the most knowledgeable of parents may not be aware of resources available to them. If experimental surgery is contemplated, parents may need assistance in speaking with private insurance companies regarding coverage. Referrals to appropriate local, state, federal, or private organizations that pertain to the CHD should be made for the parents. These include the Department of Family and Children Services, the March of Dimes, and Children's Medical Services. The family may qualify for the Special Supplemental Nutrition Program for Women, Infants, and Children.

Discharge planning must be comprehensive for the neonate who will receive medical management for a CHD before corrective surgery. A thorough assessment of the home should be obtained before discharge. Contact with the primary care provider who will perform the routine management of the infant is imperative. Initial contact by telephone should be followed up with a copy of the complete medical record and discharge summary. If the infant requires any special equipment for home care, the equipment should be obtained before discharge so that the parents can be taught how to use it. Also, practical details such as whether there are enough electrical outlets in the infant's room must be determined. Notification of local emergency medical services, power companies, and other relevant companies should be completed before discharge.

Case Study

IDENTIFICATION OF THE PROBLEM

The NICU in a large women's and children's hospital received a call for assistance on the adjacent mother and baby unit to evaluate an infant for cyanosis. Nurse Johnson responded to the call and discovered that Baby Johanna was pale, cyanotic, and tachypneic. Nurse Johnson positioned the baby for optimal oxygenation and supplied oxygen via blow-by. Baby Johanna responded to the blow-by oxygen with improved color and tone. Nurse Johnson told the mother that she would take the baby to the NICU for further evaluation and would update her as soon as possible. In the NICU, the baby's pediatrician was called and the birth history was obtained from the medical record, supplied by the mother and baby unit personnel. Baby Johanna was put in an Oxyhood, and vital signs were obtained. The baby was now pink, heart rate was 164 beats/min, respiratory rate was 76 breaths/min, and the mean blood pressure was 58 mm Hg.

ASSESSMENT: HISTORY AND PHYSICAL EXAMINATION

Johanna was born to a gravida 1, para 0 (now 1), 24-year-old mother with uncomplicated pregnancy and delivery. Her birth weight was 3.3 kg, and her Apgar scores were 8/9 (–1 color, –1 tone; –1 color). Johanna showed no distress, and the pediatrician's examination at 3 hours after birth was within normal limits, with some slight acrocyanosis of the hands and feet present. Johanna had been in the mother and baby unit, and the mother was nursing. At this feeding, the mother had offered the baby a bottle following nursing. She called the floor nurse because the baby seemed to turn blue during the feeding.

On auscultation, a soft ejection-type murmur was noted at the left upper sternal border. Right radial arterial blood gas showed a partially compensated metabolic acidosis on 70% FiO_2 per hood. The pulse oximeter registered an oxygen saturation of 58% on arms and legs. A hyperoxia test using 100% FiO_2 showed no improvement in arterial oxygenation. The cardiac murmur had increased and was determined to be systolic in origin and probably tricuspid regurgitation. Chest radiograph showed a normal heart size and decreased pulmonary markings.

DIFFERENTIAL DIAGNOSIS

The presence of a cardiac murmur in a cyanotic newborn without apparent respiratory distress is characteristic of a significant cardiac defect. Cyanosis commonly occurs in defects that result in decreased oxygenated blood flow through the heart. Because the infant is cyanotic, the defect could be a ductal-dependent cardiac defect. A continuous infusion of prostaglandin E_1 (PGE_1) was started after the chest radiograph was obtained to maintain ductal patency.

DIAGNOSTIC TESTS

A stat echocardiogram was ordered to determine whether a cardiac defect was present.

WORKING DIAGNOSIS

Echocardiography revealed the presence of pulmonary atresia with intact intraventricular septum and reverse flow into the pulmonary system through the patent ductus arteriosus.

DEVELOPMENT OF MANAGEMENT PLAN

Immediate management of any ductal-dependent cardiac defect, such as pulmonary atresia, is administration of prostaglandin E_1 to maintain the patency of the ductus arteriosus. PGE_1 must be administered as a continuous infusion. A balloon atrial septostomy is performed through cardiac catheterization to provide adequate mixing of systemic and pulmonary venous blood at the atrial level. Surgical correction is performed as soon as the newborn is stable; the most common procedure is the Blalock-Taussig operation.

IMPLEMENTATION AND EVALUATION OF EFFECTIVENESS

Johanna had a balloon atrial septostomy, which improved blood flow, and she underwent a Blalock-Taussig operation at 4 days of life. The procedure was successful, and Johanna went home with her parents at 17 days of age.

SUMMARY

The most common congenital heart defects were described based on the effects on cardiovascular circulation. The most common dysrhythmic disorders seen in the newborn were discussed. The diagnosis and management of the most frequent complications of congenital heart defects, congestive heart failure, and subacute bacterial infective endocarditis was included. Parental support of families with newborns and children with congenital heart defects was discussed.

REFERENCES

Ardinger RH (1997). Genetic counseling in congenital heart disease. *Pediatric annals* 26(2):99-104.

Belmont JW (1998). Recent progress in the molecular genetics of congenital heart defects. *Clinical genetics* 54(1):11-19.

Bevilacqua L, Hordof A (1998). Cardiac pacing in children. *Current opinion in cardiology* 13(1):48-55.

Botto LD et al (2001). Racial and temporal variations in the prevalence of heart defects. *Pediatrics* 107(3):1-8.

Burlet A et al (1999). Renal function in cyanotic congenital heart disease. *Nephron* 81(3):296-300.

Chotigeat U et al (2003). A comparison of oral ibuprofen and intravenous indomethacin for closure of patent ductus arteriosus in preterm infants. *Journal of the medical association of Thailand* 86(Suppl 3):S563-S569.

Colucci WS, Braunwald E (2001). Pathophysiology of heart failure. In Braunwald E, editor. *Heart disease: a textbook of cardiovascular medicine* (pp 503-533). Philadelphia: Saunders.

Cooley DA (1997). Early development of congenital heart surgery: open heart procedures. *The annals of thoracic surgery* 64(5):1544-1548.

Danford DA et al (1999). Pulmonary stenosis: defect-specific diagnostic accuracy of heart murmurs in children. *Journal of pediatrics* 134(1):76-81.

Danford DA et al (2000). Effects of electrocardiography and chest radiography on the accuracy of preliminary diagnosis of common congenital cardiac defects. *Pediatric cardiology* 21(4):334-340.

DeVore GR (1998). Influence of prenatal diagnosis on congenital heart defects. *Annals of the New York Academy of Sciences* 847:46-52.

Dipchand AI et al (1999). Tetralogy of Fallot with non-confluent pulmonary arteries and aortopulmonary septal defect. *Cardiology in the young* 9(1):75-77.

Freeman SB et al (1998). Population-based study of congenital heart defects in Down syndrome. *American journal of medical genetics* 80(3):213-217.

Friedman WF (2001). Congenital heart disease in infancy and childhood. In Braunwald E et al, editors. *Heart disease: a textbook of cardiovascular medicine*. Philadelphia: Saunders.

Goel M et al (2000). Haemostatic changes in children with cyanotic and acyanotic congenital heart disease. *Indian heart journal* 52(5):559-563.

Goh TH (2000). Common congenital heart defects: the value of early detection. *Australian family physician* 29(5):429-435.

Kaplan NM (2001). Systemic hypertension therapy. In Braunwald E, editor. *Heart disease: a textbook of cardiovascular medicine* (pp 972-994). Philadelphia: Saunders.

Keane JF et al (2006). *Nadas' pediatric cardiology*, ed 2. Philadelphia: Saunders.

Kochanek KD, Smith BL (2004). *Deaths: preliminary data for 2002*. National vital statistics reports, vol 52, no 13. Hyattsville, MD: National Center for Health Statistics.

Kwiatkowska J et al (2000). Atrioventricular septal defect: clinical and diagnostic problems in children hospitalized in 1993-1998. *Medical science monitor: international medical journal of experimental and clinical research* 6(6):1148-1154.

Lambert JM, Watters NE (1998). Breastfeeding the infant/child with a cardiac defect: an informal survey. *Journal of human lactation* 14(3):205-206.

Leonhardt A, Seyberth HW (2003). Do we need another NSAID instead of indomethacin for treatment of ductus arteriosus in preterm infants? *Acta paediatrica* 92(9):996-999.

Little WC (2001). Assessment of normal and abnormal cardiac function. In Braunwald E, editor. *Heart disease: a textbook of cardiovascular medicine* (pp 479-502). Philadelphia: Saunders.

Lott JW (2002). Fetal development: environmental influences and critical periods. In Kenner CA, Lott JW, editors. *Comprehensive neonatal care: a physiologic perspective*, ed 3(pp 151-172). Philadelphia: Saunders.

Lubica H (1996). Pathologic lung function in children and adolescents with congenital heart defects. *Pediatric cardiology* 17(5):314-315.

Massin MM et al (1998). Heart rate behavior in children with atrial septal defect. *Cardiology* 90(4):269-270.

McElhinney DB et al (2000). Aortopulmonary window associated with complete atrioventricular septal defect. *Journal of thoracic and cardiovascular surgery* 119(6):1284-1285.

Meberg A et al (2000). Outcome of congenital heart defects—a population-based study. *Acta paediatrica* 89(11):1344-1351.

Moyen LK et al (1997). Quality of life in children with congenital heart defects. *Acta paediatrica* 86(9):975-980.

Norwood WI et al (1983). Physiologic repair of aortic atresia—hypoplastic left heart syndrome. *New England journal of medicine* 308(1):3-26.

Nouri S (1997). Congenital heart defects: cyanotic and acyanotic. *Pediatric annals* 26(2):95-98.

Opie LH (2001). Mechanisms of cardiac contraction and relaxation. In Braunwald E, editor. *Heart disease: a textbook of cardiovascular medicine* (pp 443-478). Philadelphia: Saunders.

Park MK et al (2002). *Pediatric cardiology for practitioners*, ed 4. St Louis: Mosby.

Perloff JK, Braunwald E (2004). Physical examination of the heart and circulation. In Braunwald E et al, editors. *Braunwald's heart disease: a textbook of cardiovascular medicine*, ed 7 (pp 15-52). Philadelphia: Saunders.

Pyeritz RE (2001). Genetics and cardiovascular disease. In Braunwald E, editor. *Heart disease: a textbook of cardiovascular medicine* (pp 443-478). Philadelphia: Saunders.

Rubart M, Zipes DP (2005). Mechanisms of sudden cardiac death. *Journal of clinical investigation* 115(9):2305-2315.

Russo P, Russo JG (2005). Congenital heart defects in newborns and infants: cardiothoracic repair. In Spitzer R, editor. *Intensive care of the fetus & neonate*, ed 2 (pp 939-953). Philadelphia: Elsevier.

Sacchetti A et al (1999). Primary cardiac arrhythmias in children. *Pediatric emergency care* 15(2):95-98.

Shevell MI (1999). The role of the pediatric neurologist in the management of children with congenital heart defects: a commentary. *Seminars in pediatric neurology* 6(1):64-66.

Su PH et al (2003). Comparison of ibuprofen and indomethacin therapy for patent ductus arteriosus in preterm infants. *Pediatrics international* 45(6):665-670.

Taussig WB (1947). *Cyanosis in congenital malformations of the heart*. New York: Oxford University Press.

Thomson JD et al (2000). Cardiac catheter guided surgical closure of an apical ventricular septal defect. *Annals of thoracic surgery* 70(4):1402-1404.

Turner SW et al (1999). The natural history of ventricular septal defects. *Archives of disease in childhood* 81(5):413-416.

Varan B et al (1999). Malnutrition and growth failure in cyanotic and acyanotic congenital heart disease with and without pulmonary hypertension. *Archives of disease in childhood* 81(1):49-52.

Verklan MT, Walden M (2004). *Core curriculum for neonatal intensive care nursing*. St Louis: Elsevier.

Welch KK, Brown SA (2000). The role of genetic counseling in the management of prenatally detected congenital heart defects. *Seminars in perinatology* 24(5):373-379.

Wernovsky G, Gruber PJ (2005). Common congenital heart disease: presentation, management, and outcomes. In Taeusch WH et al, editors. *Avery's diseases of the newborn*, ed 8 (pp 827-871). Philadelphia: Elsevier.

Yagel S et al (1997). Congenital heart defects: natural course and in utero development. *Circulation* 96(2):550-555.

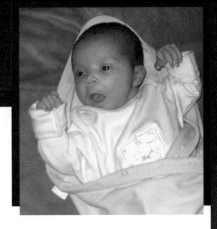

Chapter 4

Integumentary System

Carolyn Houska Lund • Joanne McManus Kuller

Skin phenomena, along with other examination findings, are used to assess maturity, duration of pregnancy, and neonatal vitality. The skin of a preterm infant makes up 13% of the body weight, compared with 3% in adults. This large organ provides a barrier against infection, protects internal organs, contributes to temperature regulation and prevention of insensible water loss, stores fats, excretes electrolytes and water, and provides tactile sensory input. The sensations of touch, pressure, temperature, pain, and itch are received by millions of microscopic dermal nerve endings. The skin is instrumental in early establishment of the mother-infant relationship, in that the quality of touch and stimulation that an infant receives is responsible for the infant's later responses to other people and to the environment. Thus, the skin fulfills a task of vital importance, particularly in the area of maternal-child nursing.

Care practices that affect the fragile, underdeveloped skin of the premature infant present major concerns as well as dilemmas for care providers. Life support and monitoring equipment must be securely attached and frequently removed or replaced; this practice can cause trauma to the skin. Necessary invasive procedures, such as vascular access, blood sampling, and chest tube insertion, invade the skin's barrier. Trauma to skin can result in the diversion of an excessive proportion of caloric intake to tissue repair. Other effects of trauma to premature skin include the energy demands of electrolyte imbalances and increased evaporative heat loss through damaged or immature skin and the risk of toxicity when substances are applied to the skin surface.

Trauma to the skin creates portals for bacteria and fungus in an already immune-compromised host. Even common resident skin flora—such as coagulase-negative staphylococci and *Candida* species—become serious pathogens in neonates; they often enter the system through mucocutaneous inoculation. Thus, significant morbidity and mortality can be attributed to practices that cause either trauma to skin or alterations in normal skin function.

Iatrogenically caused skin problems—including burns and caustic lesions from isopropyl alcohol and erythema and skin craters from transcutaneous oxygen monitoring—have been reported. Increased skin permeability and percutaneous toxicity from drugs and chemicals have also been documented in neonates.

This chapter covers the development and structure of skin, the normal physiologic variations in newborn skin, and dermatologic diseases. This information is then incorporated into the management of the neonatal skin.

SKIN STRUCTURE AND FUNCTION

Skin consists of three anatomically distinct layers: the epidermis, the dermis, and the subcutaneous tissue. The principal functional compartment of the epidermis is the stratum corneum epidermidis, the horny outer layer of the epidermis, primarily composed of closely packed dead cells that are being continually brushed off by clothing and washing. These exfoliated cells form part of the vernix caseosa, the cheese-like substance that covers and protects fetal skin. The bottom, living basal layer constantly replaces these cells. It takes approximately 26 days for cells from this layer to migrate up to the stratum corneum. Approximately 20% of an adult's protein requirement is needed for this purpose. Keratin-forming cells—which cornify the outer layer of the epidermis—and melanocytes are contained in the lower levels of the epidermis. Melanocytes begin producing melanin, or pigment, before birth and distribute it to the epidermal cells. Active pigmentary activity can be observed before birth in the epidermis of infants of dark-skinned races, but little evidence of such activity exists in white fetuses (Moore & Persaud, 2003).

The dermis lies directly under the epidermis and is 2 to 4 mm thick at birth. It is a closely woven layer of collagen, which is a fibrous protein, and elastin fibers. This fibrous complex provides mechanical strength as well as elasticity and allows the skin to withstand frictional stress while extending easily over joints. At term, the dermis is thick and well organized but is thinner and has a higher water content compared to the adult dermis (Loomis & Birge, 2001). Many nerves and a rich supply of blood vessels are contained there. They nourish the skin cells and act as carriers of the sensations of heat, touch, pressure, and pain from the skin to the brain.

Hair originates from deep in the dermis. Down-growths, called epidermal ridges, which extend into the developing dermis, result from a proliferation of cells in the basal layer. These ridges are permanently established by 17 weeks' gestation and produce ridges and grooves on the surface of the palms—including the fingers—and on the soles of the feet—including the toes.

Determined genetically, this type of pattern constitutes the basis for the use of fingerprints in criminal investigations and medical genetics. Dermatoglyphics is the study of the pattern of these epidermal ridges. The presence of abnormal chromosome complements affects the development of the ridge patterns. For example, infants with Down syndrome exhibit distinctive hand and feet patterns that are of diagnostic value (Moore & Persaud, 2003).

65

The major component of the subcutaneous layer is fatty connective tissue. The subcutaneous fat functions as a heat insulator, a shock absorber, and a calorie reserve area. Fat accumulation occurs predominantly in the last trimester. Sebaceous glands are found in both the dermis and the subcutaneous layer. Well-developed and potentially functional at birth, these glands have only minimal function until puberty. Sweat glands are also found in the dermis and the subcutaneous layer and are affected directly by external environmental temperature. In premature infants, sweat gland maturation occurs between 21 and 33 days of age. In term infants, this maturation occurs at about 5 days of age. Poor sweat production in the premature infant is caused by sweat gland immaturity. However, adult function is not achieved until the second or third year of life.

Term infant skin is soft, wrinkled, velvety, and covered with vernix caseosa. Transformation of the fetal circulation is evident soon after the cord is cut, as the skin develops the intense red coloration characteristic of the newborn. This color may remain for hours. A blue, blotchy appearance may occur if the infant is exposed to a cool environment.

The insulating layer of vernix is usually lost during the first few days of life through traditional newborn skin care. This results in a loss of insulation for the stratum corneum, which then peels off, thus resulting in skin with a grayish-white or yellowish hue. Visible desquamation of newborn skin comes to an end after about 7 days. Vernix may provide bactericidal protection and may contribute to the development of epidermal barrier function, heat flux, and surface electrical activities (Hoath & Pickins 2003; Hoath et al, 2001).

In comparison with the skin of the term infant, the premature infant's skin is more transparent, gelatinous, and unwrinkled. Lanugo, which has been lost in the full-term infant, may be present in varying degrees and is one criterion used to estimate gestational age. Additionally, subcutaneous edema may be present and is clinical evidence of a cutaneous excess of water and sodium. This edema decreases within the first few days of life, and the skin then lies loosely over the infant's entire body. The immaturity of the infant's skin is linked to the premature newborn's difficulty maintaining body temperature. A poorly developed fat supply and a large body surface area in relation to body weight add to temperature instability.

The skin of the full-term infant has a well-developed epidermis; the stratum corneum is structured to perform efficiently to control transepidermal water loss (TEWL) and prevent absorption of toxic substances, similar to the function of the adult epidermis. The stratum corneum, the nonliving layer of the epidermis, contains 10 to 20 layers in adults and term infants. The stratum corneum of term newborns has been shown to have lower TEWL and stratum corneum hydration (SCH) than adults, with the lowest levels seen on the first day of life. This suggests that the barrier is relatively impermeable to water to protect from maceration in utero and that a gradual drying process occurs over the first few days of life. In addition, the TEWL in different areas—such as the forehead, palms, and soles—is lower in newborns, whereas levels are higher on the forearm region (Yosipovitch et al, 2000).

The premature infant has been shown to have a less well-developed stratum corneum; at less than 30 weeks' gestation there may be only two to three layers of stratum corneum (Figure 4-1). This immaturity results in the premature infant's decreased capacity to resist particles, viruses, parasites, and bacteria in the external environment, thus leaving the infant readily susceptible to infection and irritation of the skin.

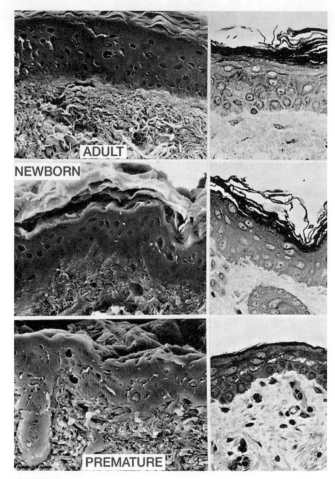

FIGURE **4-1**
Photomicrograph of stratum corneum in an adult, in a full-term newborn, and in a premature infant of 28 weeks' gestation. From Holbrook KA (1982). A histological comparison of infant and adult skin. In Maibach HI, Boisits EK, editors. *Neonatal skin: structure and function*. New York: Marcel Dekker. Reprinted with permission.

Transferring from the intrauterine aquatic environment to the external atmospheric environment stimulates and accelerates maturation of skin function. Harpin and Rutter (1983) reported that by 10 days' postnatal age or with increasing gestational age, the integrity of the premature infant's skin improves and approaches that of the term infant or adult. However, other authors cite a slower process in premature infants less than 27 weeks' gestation with rates of TEWL nearly double adult levels even at 28 days of life (Agren et al, 1998). In infants of 23 to 25 weeks' gestation, skin barrier function has been shown to reach mature levels at a much slower rate, with mature levels seen at 30 to 32 weeks' postconceptional age (Kalia et al, 1998). Embryologic skin development is described in Box 4-1.

Developmental Variations

Several factors are responsible for the functional differences between premature and term infants' skin. These differences subside with increasing gestational and postnatal age (Table 4-1).

Thickness of the Stratum Corneum and Permeability

The stratum corneum layer provides the barrier properties of the skin. This barrier is composed of keratinocytes coated by intercellular lipids. The stratum corneum begins to develop in

TABLE 4-1	Structural Differences Between Infant and Adult Skin		
	Premature	**Full-Term**	**Adult**
Epidermis	Thinner cells compressed Fewer desmosomes Fewer layers of stratum corneum Melanin production low	Stratum corneum appears as adherent cell layers Melanin production low	Good resistance to penetration
Dermoepidermal junction	Fewer hemidesmosomes Less cohesion between layers		
Dermis	Fewer elastin fibers Thinner than in the adult	Fewer elastin fibers Thinner than in the adult	Full complement of elastin fibers
Eccrine glands	May be more typical of fetus than adult Ducts patent Secretory cells undifferentiated	Equivalent in structure to adult Denser distribution Vellus hair characteristic	Distribution less dense than in infant Both vellus and terminal hairs
Hair	Lanugo hair may be present Hair growth synchronous	Hair growth synchronous Large and active but diminishing rapidly in both size and activity for several weeks after birth	Hair growth dyssynchronous
Sebaceous glands	Large and active	Vascular system not fully organized until 3 months Cutaneous nerve network not fully developed; may continue to develop until puberty Most nerves are small in diameter, unmyelinated, sensory, and autonomic Meissner's touch receptors not fully formed	Large and active
Nerve and vascular system	Not fully organized Most nerves are small in diameter, unmyelinated, sensory, and autonomic Unmyelinated nerves are typically fetal in structure Meissner's touch receptors not fully formed	Good resistance to penetration Higher penetrability of fat-soluble substances Greater absorption because of higher skin surface: body weight ratio	Adult pattern
Permeability	Highly permeable Higher penetrability of fat-soluble substances Greater absorption because of higher skin surface: body weight ratio	Reduced sweating capability, especially for first 2 to 5 days	Good resistance to penetration
Eccrine sweating	Reduced sweating capability, especially for first 13 to 24 days	Melanin production low; will sunburn readily	Full sweating capability
Photosensitivity	Melanin production low; will sunburn readily	Reduced ability to ward off infection	Sensitivity to sun depends on skin type
Related conditions	Reduced ability to ward off infection because of deficient immune system Low reactivity to allergens	Low reactivity to allergens	Readily sensitized to allergens

From Shalita A (1981). Principles of infant skin care. Skillman, NJ: Johnson & Johnson Baby Products.

the fetus after 21 weeks' estimated gestational age (EGA). The stratum corneum in infants of 28 weeks' gestation consists of only a few cell layers and is markedly thinner than that of term infants (see Figure 4-1). These findings correlate with the immaturity of barrier function of the stratum corneum; this immaturity is characterized by increased permeability and increased TEWL. By 32 to 34 weeks' EGA, the stratum corneum has developed sufficiently to offer some protection. The full-term infant has a fully functional stratum corneum.

After birth, rapid postnatal maturation occurs with thickening of the epidermis and development of the stratum corneum. As noted previously, the stratum corneum of premature infants is thought to rapidly mature and reach adult barrier function within approximately 2 weeks after birth. A slower process in premature infants less than 27 weeks' gestation is noted; rates of TEWL are nearly double adult levels, even at 28 days of life. In infants of 23 to 25 weeks' gestation, skin barrier function reaches mature levels much more slowly (Agren et al, 1998), as long as 8 weeks after birth in a 23-week gestation infant (Kalia et al, 1998).

The undeveloped stratum corneum of the premature infant's skin also produces increased transepidermal water loss and evaporative heat loss and contributes to the difficulty the premature newborn experiences in maintaining fluid balance and body temperature. Neonatal skin is 40% to 60% thinner than adult skin, and the body surface/weight ratio is nearly five

BOX **4-1**

Embryologic Development of Skin

The skin consists of two morphologically different layers, derived from two different germ layers. The epithelial structures (epidermis, pilosebaceous-apocrine unit, eccrine unit, and nails) are ectodermal derivatives. The ectoderm also gives rise to the hair, the teeth, and the sense organs of smell, taste, hearing, vision, and touch—everything involved with events that occur outside the organism. Mesenchymal structures (collagen, reticular, and elastic fibers; blood vessels; muscles; and fat) originate from the mesoderm. These developments are outlined in Table 4-2.

The epidermis, which develops from the surface ectoderm, consists of one layer of undifferentiated cells in a 3-week-old embryo. By 4 weeks' gestational age, it has an inner germinative layer of cuboidal cells with dark, compact nuclei and an outer layer of slightly flatter cells covered by microvilli. About the middle of the second month of gestation, some of the cells begin to be crowded to the surface and form a thin, protective layer of flattened cells known as the periderm. The cells of this layer continually undergo keratinization and desquamation and are replaced by cells arising from the basal layer. The periderm is often called the epitrichial ("upon the hair") layer of the epidermis because the hairs that later grow up from the deeper layers are said not to penetrate this thin surface layer but to push it up on their growing tips, thus causing it to be cast off if it has not already disappeared. These exfoliated cells form part of the vernix caseosa.

During the later part of the second month, the epithelium tends to become thicker. This occurs (at first) by a staggering of the nuclei and the beginning of cell rearrangement, which leads rapidly to the formation of an intermediate layer between the flattened cells of the epitrichial layer and the basal layer adjacent to the underlying dermis. The cells of this intermediate layer tend to become enlarged and show a high degree of vacuolation. The basal layer of the epidermis is later called the stratum germinativum (Moore & Persaud, 2003).

At the end of the second month of gestation, the cutaneous nerves, which are detectable in embryonic dermis about the fifth week of gestation, appear to be functional, although the skin is primitive by comparison with that of an adult.

At about 10 weeks' gestation, fingernail development begins at the tips of the digits. A thickened area of epithelium on the dorsum of each digit is the first sign of nail formation. Our nails are adaptations of the epidermis, homologous to the claws and hoofs of lower mammals, and are formed by a modified process of keratinization. Development of the fingernails is begun and completed (30 to 34 weeks) before that of the toenails (35 to 38 weeks).

By about 11 weeks' gestation, collagen and elastic connective-tissue fibers begin to develop in the dermis. The epidermal-dermal junction, which has been smooth up to this time, now becomes wavy as epidermal thickenings grow down into the dermis of the palm and the soles of the feet. Dermal papillae develop in these dermal projections. Capillary loops develop in some dermal papillae, and Meissner's corpuscles, which are the sensory nerve endings of touch, form in others (Moore & Persaud, 2003). These epidermal ridges produce ridges and grooves in a genetically determined pattern and are the basis for fingerprinting and footprinting. The development of these ridges can be distinctly affected by the presence of abnormal chromosome complements (e.g., as occurs in Down syndrome). These ridges are permanently established by about 17 weeks' gestation.

During the third to fourth month of gestation, the stratum germinativum differentiates from the rest of the epithelium. These cells are termed the germinative layer because they undergo the repeated cell divisions that are responsible for the growth of the epidermis.

During the fourth month of gestation, the epithelium starts to become many cells thick, and keratin begins to accumulate in the cells above the stratum germinativum layer. Daughter cells from the basal layer are crowded upward and undergo progressive changes in each layer and finalize in cornification. The thin stratum granulosum epidermidis, which contains keratohyaline granules, is the layer directly above the stratum germinativum. The next higher layer is the thin and clear stratum lucidum epidermidis, the content of which is a fluid—eleidin—that replaces the granules. Above that is the keratinized multilayered stratum corneum epidermidis (Moore & Persaud, 2003). As the keratin accumulates in these cells, they become more and more sluggish and finally die, so that the surface layer of the epidermis is made up of tough, scale-like, dead cells that form a relatively impermeable membrane.

In areas such as the soles of the feet and the palms of the hands, where the skin is subjected to more than ordinary wear, the keratinization of the outer layer is much heavier than in the general body surface. Of interest, however, is that the greater thickness of palmar and plantar epidermis becomes evident in the embryo long before it is possible for these areas to have been subjected to any more wear than other parts of the skin. When the aforementioned layers are all completely differentiated, the structure of fetal epidermis resembles that of adult epidermis.

During the early fetal period, neural crest cells migrate into the dermis and differentiate into melanoblasts. At about 17 to 20 weeks of gestation, these melanoblasts differentiate into melanocytes, migrate to the epidermal-dermal border, and begin to produce melanin. Fetal melanocytes in white races contain little or no pigment, whereas in dark-skinned races, they produce melanin granules. The skin of black newborns is only a little darker than that of white newborns. The skin at the bases of the fingernails and toenails is often noticeably darker, however.

The skin of black infants continues to darken after birth, as increased melanin production occurs in response to light. When melanocytes remain behind in the dermis, they appear bluish through the overlying cutaneous tissue and are called mongolian spots. Some believe that it is not the number of melanocytes present that is important but, rather their activity level. The hormone secreted by the pituitary gland that controls the clumping or dispersion of the melanin granules is melanocyte-stimulating hormone.

BOX **4-1**

Embryologic Development of Skin—cont'd

Around 20 weeks of gestation, the eyebrows, upper lip, and chin hair are first recognizable. On the general body surface, the hair makes its appearance about a month later. These fine hairs are called lanugo. As stated earlier, the emergence of this hair breaks off the periderm, and the periderm becomes one component of the vernix caseosa. The other components of vernix are sebum from the sebaceous glands, fetal hair, and desquamated cells from the amnion (Moore & Persaud, 2003). Vernix protects the epidermis against a macerating influence that would be exerted by the amniotic fluid and acts as a lubricant to prevent chafing injuries from the amnion as the growing fetus becomes progressively confined in its fluid-filled sac.

Between 21 and 24 weeks' gestation, the fetus's skin is wrinkled, translucent, and pinkish-red because blood in the capillaries has become visible. Head and lanugo hair are well developed in a 26- to 29-week fetus. At this same time, eccrine sweat glands are anatomically developed and are found over the entire body. Their function, however, is somewhat immature in the perinatal period.

Brown adipose tissue cells begin to differentiate in the 7th month of gestation, and the accumulation of subcutaneous fat begins to smooth out the many skin wrinkles. Between the 30th and 34th week of gestation, the skin is pink and smooth, and the lanugo is beginning to shed. The fingernails reach the fingertips, but the distal part of the nail is still thin and soft (Moore & Persaud, 2003). During the last trimester of pregnancy, subcutaneous fat accumulates, and the fetus acquires a plump appearance. The composition of amniotic fluid tested at this time reflects skin function. The number of anucleated cells and keratinized lipid-containing skin flakes increases.

TABLE **4-2**	Embryonic and Fetal Development of Skin*
Weeks of Gestation	**Development**
3	Epidermis, which develops from surface ectoderm, consists of one layer of cells.
5	Cutaneous nerves are detectable in embryonic dermis.
6 to 7	Periderm, a thin, protective layer of flattened cells, is formed.
11	Collagen and elastic fibers are developing in the dermis.
	Epidermal ridges (fingerprints) are forming.
	Nails begin to develop at the tips of the digits.
13 to 16	Scalp hair patterning is determined.
17 to 20	Melanocytes migrate to the epidermal-dermal junction and begin to produce melanin.
	Skin is covered with vernix caseosa and lanugo.
	Keratin is accumulating in the epidermis.
21 to 25	Skin is wrinkled, translucent, and pink to red because blood in the capillaries has become visible.
26 to 29	Subcutaneous fat begins to be deposited and starts to smooth out the many wrinkles in the skin.
	Eccrine sweat glands are anatomically developed and found over the entire body; their function, however, is somewhat immature in the perinatal period.
30 to 34	Skin is pink and smooth.
	Fingernails reach fingertips.
	Lanugo begins to shed.
35 to 38	Fetuses are usually plump.
	Skin is usually white or bluish-pink.
	Toenails reach toe tips.

Data from Ackerman A (1985). Structure and function of the skin. In Moschella S, Hurley H, editors. Dermatology, vol 2, ed 2. Philadelphia: Saunders.

*Embryonic period: undoubtedly the most important period of human development because the beginnings of all major external and internal structures develop. Fetal period (9th week to birth): primarily concerned with growth and differentiation of tissue and organs that started to develop during the embryonic period.

times greater, making the newborn at risk for toxicity from topically applied substances (Mancini, 2004; Siegfried, 2001). The skin of a premature infant is remarkably permeable; permeability correlates inversely with gestational age. Sekkat et al (2004) have developed an in vitro model to examine the biophysical characteristics of TEWL in premature infants. This model will help clinicians understand how procedures coupled with gestational age can affect skin integrity, permeability, and TEWL.

Toxicity due to topically applied substances secondary to the increased permeability of both preterm and term infants' skin has been reported in numerous cases (Siegfried, 2001). All topical solutions during the first 2 to 3 weeks of life should be carefully evaluated as to potential benefits, risks, and effectiveness.

Dermal Instability

Collagen in the dermis increases with gestational age as the tendency toward water fixation and edema decreases. The other component of the dermis, the elastin fibers, is formed mostly after birth and may not become fully mature until 3 years of age. Protection from pressure and ischemic injury includes routine turning and repositioning on surfaces such as gelled pads or water mattresses (Lund, 1999).

Diminished Cohesion

Another variation in the premature infant's skin structure and function is the diminished cohesion between the dermis and the epidermis. The junction of the epidermis and the dermis, which is normally connected by numerous fibrils, has fewer and more widely spaced fibrils in the premature infant than in term infants or adults (Figure 4-2). These fibrils become stronger with increasing gestational and postnatal age. Because the premature infant in the neonatal intensive care unit (NICU) is usually covered with some type of adhesive to secure intravenous lines, cardiorespiratory electrodes, endotracheal tubes, and umbilical artery catheters, the premature infant is at higher risk for blistering and stripping of the epidermis when adhesives are removed. The cohesion between many of the currently used adhesives and the stratum corneum may be stronger than the bond between the dermis and the epidermis.

Skin pH

Another developmental variation of infant skin resides in the functional capacity of the skin to form a surface pH of less than 5.0, which is the acid mantle. A skin surface pH of less than 5 is ordinarily seen in both children and adults.

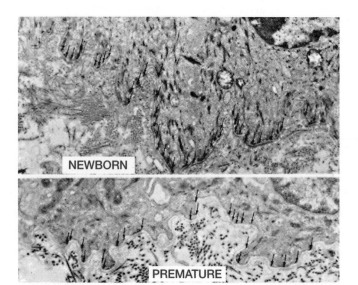

FIGURE 4-2
Arrows indicate anchoring fibrils at dermoepidermal junction in a full-term and a premature infant. From Holbrook KA (1982). A histological comparison of infant and adult skin. In Maibach HI, Boisits EK, editors. *Neonatal skin: structure and function.* New York: Marcel Dekker. Reprinted with permission.

In the large number of term newborns studied, the skin was found to have a mean pH of 6.34 immediately after birth. Within 4 days, the pH decreased to a mean of 4.95, and between 7 and 30 days it further decreased to 4.7. In a later study of 127 low-birth-weight infants, these authors documented that the mean pH decreased from 6.7 (day 1) to 5.04 (day 9). However, a different technique for measuring pH was used than in the previous study; thus the absolute values for pH may not be comparable. They concluded that acidification of the skin is independent of gestational age (Fox et al, 1998).

An acidic skin surface is credited with having bactericidal qualities against some pathogens and serves in the defense against microorganisms. Microbial colonization also begins immediately after birth. An increased skin pH, from acidic to neutral, can increase the total numbers of bacteria and TEWL and shift the species present.

Melanin Production

One of the primary functions of melanin is to screen the skin from the sun's harmful rays by absorbing their radiant energy. Although melanin production—and therefore pigmentation—are lower during the neonatal period than later in life, certain areas—such as the linea alba, the areola, and the scrotum—are often deeply pigmented as a result of high circulating levels of maternal and placental hormones. Melanin production in premature infants is even less than in term infants, thus placing them at greater risk for damage from sunlight and ultraviolet light (Williams, 2001).

ASSESSMENT AND PHYSIOLOGIC VARIATIONS

Acrocyanosis, or peripheral cyanosis involving the hands, feet, and circumoral area, is a common finding in the newborn. It occurs because of sluggish blood flow in the feet and hands that results from limited development of the peripheral capillary circulation. Acrocyanosis usually resolves within the first few days of life but may reappear with cold stress.

Pallor is most commonly a sign of anemia, hypoxia, or poor peripheral perfusion that results from hypotension or infection. Meconium staining is caused by the passage of meconium in utero and usually requires at least 6 hours of meconium contact to stain the skin.

Jaundice, which occurs in 50% to 70% of newborns, is a yellowing of the skin and develops because of the presence of indirect bilirubin in the blood. Bilirubin is normally processed by the liver and is eliminated in the urine and feces. In newborns, the body cannot eliminate bilirubin as fast as it is produced.

For visible staining of the skin and sclera, a bilirubin level of at least 5 mg/100 ml is required. The head-to-toe progression of jaundice over the body gives a crude estimate of the level of bilirubin.

Linea nigra is a line of increased pigmentation from the umbilicus to the genitals. This area of benign pigmentation may become less noticeable as the infant's skin darkens. Mongolian spots are collections of melanocytes located in the dermis that are most frequently seen at birth. They are slate blue, gray, or black, shaped as irregular, bruise-like spots that are seen primarily over the sacrum and the buttocks but may extend over the back and shoulders. Most commonly seen in newborns with darkly pigmented skin, they are found in 96% of African American, 86% of Asian, and 13% of Caucasian infants (Lucky, 2001). Although they look like bruises, they are harmless and resolve over several years.

Lanugo is the fine downy hair that is most commonly seen over the back, shoulders, and facial areas of a premature newborn. It is shed at the seventh to eighth month of gestation and is one criterion used to estimate gestational age.

Milia are common papules that occur primarily on the face but may also occur in other locations. They are seen as small, white, pinhead-sized bumps that are scattered over the chin, cheeks, noses, and forehead of 25% to 40% of full-term babies (Margileth, 2005). They spontaneously resolve within the first month of life. Mothers should be instructed not to squeeze or prick these pimple-like spots. Milia can develop on the foreskin of infant boys; these are called epidermal inclusion cysts. When they occur on the palate, they are called Epstein's pearls.

Miliaria is a general term for describing obstructions of the eccrine duct. The cause is retention of sweat as a result of edema of the stratum corneum; this edema blocks eccrine pores, thus resulting in four types of miliaria: rubra (prickly heat), crystallina, pustulosa, and profunda.

Miliaria pustulosa and miliaria profunda are rarely seen in temperate climates. Miliaria rubra is commonly observed in infants exposed to excessive environmental temperatures with humidity. It appears as pink or white pimples with a little redness around them. They resolve when the infant is moved to cooler temperatures. Miliaria crystallina presents as clear, 1- to 2-mm superficial water blisters without inflammation (Margileth, 2005). The distribution and grouping of vesicles that contain no eosinophils help to differentiate them from erythema toxicum neonatorum.

Harlequin color change is a dramatic but benign phenomenon in which the color on the dependent half of an infant in a side-lying position turns deep red while the upper half is pale. The color reverses when the infant is turned. Attributed to a temporary imbalance in the autonomic regulatory mechanism of the cutaneous vessels, this phenomenon is more common in low-birth-weight infants—whether well or sick.

Vernix caseosa is a grayish-white cheesy substance that is protective to the fetal skin while the fetus is in utero and helps the infant slide through the birth canal. The vernix covering diminishes as the fetus reaches term and is one determinant of gestational age.

Cutis marmorata, or mottling, is a normal physiologic vascular response to cool air. This generalized mottling reflects the infant's vasomotor instability. The marbling disappears with rewarming and is uncommon after several months of age. Mottling is often prominent in infants with Cornelia de Lange syndrome and Down syndrome.

Erythema toxicum neonatorum, the most common rash of newborns, usually occurs within 5 days of birth and affects approximately half of term infants, although it is almost never seen in premature infants or those weighing less than 2500 g. It appears as small, firm, white or pale yellow pustules with an erythematous margin. Lesions may first appear on the face and spread to the trunk and extremities, but may appear anywhere on the body, except the soles and palms (Lucky, 2001). A smear and Wright's stain of the pustules reveal numerous infiltrates of eosinophils that are devoid of bacteria. The differential diagnosis includes transient neonatal pustular melanosis, candidiasis, staphylococcal pyoderma, and miliaria. No treatment is necessary.

Neonatal and infantile acne are two distinct conditions distinguished by the time of onset and clinical features. Neonatal acne involves inflammatory, erythematous papules and pustules located primarily on the cheeks, often scattered over the face and extending into the scalp. Recently, a hypothesis that neonatal acne may be an inflammatory response to *Malassezia* species of fungus has been proposed (Niamba et al, 1998; Rapelanoro et al, 1996). Other experts suggest that neonatal acne is related to sebum excretion rate while the infantile form is related to high androgen levels, but both have genetic influences (Herane & Ando, 2003). Infantile acne is considered to result in hyperplasia of sebaceous activity. It is found primarily on the face. Neonatal acne generally resolves without treatment. Infantile acne may be more persistent and even cause scarring. Infantile acne may benefit from treatment with topical benzyl alcohol peroxide or erythromycin (Lucky, 2001). Some success has been reported with oral isotretinoin (Torrelo et al, 2005).

Transient neonatal pustular melanosis is a lesion that is similar to miliaria but is present at birth, usually causing the infant to be unnecessarily isolated. It occurs most commonly on the face, the palms of the hands, and the soles of the feet. It is most commonly seen in black infants. The differential diagnosis includes erythema toxicum neonatorum, staphylococcal impetigo, neonatal candidiasis, miliaria crystallina or rubra, and acropustulosis of infancy. If the lesions are ruptured, smeared on a slide, and stained, the contents are found to be amorphous debris. The lesion is neither infectious nor contagious. It is self-limiting and requires no treatment.

Sucking blisters that contain sterile, serous fluid may be seen on the thumb, index finger, or lip. Presumably, they are the result of vigorous sucking in utero and resolve without treatment.

Pigmentary Lesions

Hyperpigmented lesions may be present at birth or during the first weeks of life. Some pigmentary problems are benign, such as mongolian spots, whereas others can be signs of a systemic or genetic disorder. Some of the more common are included in this section.

Café au lait spots are irregularly shaped, oval lesions. Their color resembles coffee to which milk has been added. They should be noted on the newborn's initial physical examination, and if they are larger than 4 to 6 cm or if more than six are present, a diagnosis of neurofibromatosis should be considered (Landau & Krafchik, 1999).

Hyperpigmentation that presents in a diffuse pattern is unusual in the newborn. When present, it may be caused by congenital Addison's disease, hepatic or biliary atresia, metabolic disease (Hartnup disease, porphyria), nutritional disorders (pellagra, sprue), hereditary disorders (lentiginosis, melanism), or unknown causes (the bronze discoloration seen in Niemann-Pick disease). Hyperpigmentation of the labial folds with clitoral hypertrophy may result from the transplacental passage of androgens (Margileth, 2005).

Hypopigmentation that presents as a diffuse or localized loss of pigment in the neonate may stem from metabolic (phenylketonuria), endocrine (Addison's disease), genetic (vitiligo, piebaldism, tuberous sclerosis, albinism), traumatic, or postinflammatory causes (Margileth, 2005).

Partial albinism (piebaldism) is an autosomal dominant disorder that is present at birth and is easily detected in the dark-skinned infant. Off-white macules are seen on the scalp, widow's peak, and forehead and extend to the base of the nose, trunk, and extremities. Differential diagnoses are Klein-Waardenburg syndrome, vitiligo, nevus anemicus, Addison's disease, and white macules of tuberous sclerosis. When illuminated with a Wood light, the amelanotic areas of piebaldism exhibit a brilliant whiteness (Margileth, 2005). Albinism refers to a group of genetic disorders involving abnormal melanin synthesis. It may occur in any race, with the incidence approximately 1 in 20,000, with a slightly higher rate in African Americans (Sethi et al, 1996). An autosomal recessive gene usually causes it, but rare cases of autosomal dominant inheritance have occurred (Margileth, 2005).

White leaf macules are the earliest cutaneous manifestations of tuberous sclerosis, an autosomal dominant neurocutaneous syndrome. They vary in size and shape but most often resemble a mountain ash leaflet. They may be difficult to see in a newborn infant and may be more readily observed by examination with a Wood lamp, which heightens the contrast between the macule and normal skin. Normal infants occasionally have a single lesion, but the presence of one or more of these macules in an infant with neurologic problems strongly suggests the diagnosis of tuberous sclerosis. Skin biopsy is nondiagnostic. A careful family history, physical examination, and, when appropriate, additional diagnostic studies are indicated in infants with these lesions.

Lesions Related to the Birth Process

Caput succedaneum is a diffuse, generalized edema of the scalp that is caused by local pressure and trauma during labor. The borders are not well defined, and the swelling crosses suture lines. Cephalhematoma is a subperiosteal hemorrhage caused by the trauma of labor and delivery. The margins of the suture lines are clearly demarcated, and the swelling never crosses suture lines. Sclerema neonatorum may have the same cause and adipose tissue abnormality in the subcutaneous tissues as those noted in fat necrosis. However, sclerema more commonly affects the premature or debilitated infant. It is a diffuse hardening of the subcutaneous tissue that results in cold, nonpitting skin. Low environmental temperature alone can produce this injury. The extremities may be involved at first, but generalized involvement occurs within 3 to 4 days. Infants with this disorder are usually critically ill, but if they survive, the sclerematous changes rarely last beyond 2 weeks. Treatment is based on therapy for the underlying systemic disease, restoration of body temperature, and adequate nutrition.

Forceps marks are identified by their rounded contours and position. The bruised area should be checked for underlying tissue and nerve damage. Scalp lacerations can occur in many ways. A laceration can be caused by the placement of an internal monitoring lead or by the artificial rupture of membranes. A circular red or ecchymotic area may be caused by the use of a vacuum extractor. Any abraded area may serve as a portal of entry for infection; therefore a scalp laceration should be carefully and continuously assessed for the presence of infection. Lacerations can also occur to other body surfaces from scalpel injuries during cesarean birth; an incidence of 1.9% was noted in a series of 896 cesarean section deliveries (Smith et al, 1997).

Subcutaneous fat necrosis is an uncommon disorder that occurs primarily in full-term infants. It has been associated with birth trauma, shock, asphyxia, hypothermia, seizures, preeclampsia, meconium aspiration, and intrapartum medications. One or several indurated, violet or red plaques or sharply defined subcutaneous nodules on the buttocks, thighs, trunk, face, or arms may appear (Cohen, 2001). Most areas of subcutaneous fat necrosis gradually reabsorb over weeks to months if left alone. Residual atrophy or scarring is unusual.

Internal fetal monitoring sites are at risk for infection, owing to the introduction of the maternal vaginal flora directly into the subcutaneous tissue of the fetus. Scalp abscesses caused by implantation of a fetal electrode are generally benign, self-limited occurrences. Rare instances of major complications have been reported, however—including significant areas of cellulitis, osteomyelitis, and sepsis.

DERMATOLOGIC DISEASES

Diseases of the skin in newborns often present patterns that are different from the presentation of the same disease in adults. Therefore a careful physical examination of the skin is necessary for an accurate dermatologic diagnosis to be made. All lesions should be described and their location and pattern noted.

Lesions can be classified as either primary or secondary. Primary lesions are described as the initial or principal lesion that is identified when the disease begins. Primary lesions are classified as macule, patch, papule, plaque, nodule, tumor, vesicle, bulla, wheal, pustule, or abscess. Secondary lesions are brought about by the modification of a primary lesion. The secondary lesion may be called a crust, scale, erosion, ulcer, fissure, lichenification, atrophy, or scar.

Terminology

Ecchymoses appear as black and blue bruises of varying sizes anywhere over the body. Primarily seen over the presenting part in a difficult vertex delivery or a vaginal breech delivery, ecchymosis is most frequently due to trauma associated with labor and delivery. It occurs more commonly in the fragile premature infant. This bruising, however, can be indicative of serious infection or bleeding disorders.

Petechiae are pinpoint hemorrhagic areas, less than 1 mm in diameter, scattered over the upper trunk and face as a result of pressure during the descent and rotation of birth. Their incidence is increased when the umbilical cord has been around the neck or when the cervix clamps down after delivery of the head. They usually fade within 24 to 48 hours. If they continue to develop or are unusually numerous, a complete workup for infection or bleeding disorders should be performed.

Intracutaneous hemorrhage may be caused by thrombocytopenia, inherited disorders of coagulation, transient deficiency of vitamin K, disseminated intravascular coagulation, and trauma.

Disseminated intravascular coagulation should be suspected in an acutely ill infant who has an intracutaneous hemorrhage. Thrombocytopenia and disorders of coagulation generally occur in infants who seem well otherwise. Thrombocytopenia should be suspected when the infant presents with general cutaneous petechiae. It frequently accompanies neonatal infections and is most commonly associated with the TORCH diseases (toxoplasmosis, rubella, cytomegalovirus, and herpes simplex).

Ecchymoses and petechiae are purple discolorations caused by hemorrhage into the superficial skin layers. They do not disappear with blanching because the blood is contained in the tissues. Macules are nonpalpable, nonraised lesions less than 1 cm in diameter that are identified only by color change. They are seen in measles, rubella, scarlet fever, roseola, typhoid fever, and drug reactions.

Papules are superficial elevated solid lesions less than 1 cm in diameter. They are firm and not fluid-filled. They may follow the macular stage in many eruptive diseases. Vesicles are skin elevations that contain serous fluid (blisters). They are commonly seen with herpes simplex, insect bites, and poison ivy.

Pustules are localized accumulations of pus in or just beneath the epidermis. They are often centered around appendageal structures (e.g., hair follicles) and are usually caused by bacterial infections or skin abscesses. When a pustule breaks, the degree of crusting is more marked than occurs with the rupture of a vesicle.

Nodules are deep solid lesions larger than 1 cm in diameter. Nodules are similar to papules but are larger. Because of their size, they are more likely to have a dermal component than are papules.

Developmental Vascular Abnormalities

The following two major groups of vascular birthmarks are seen:
1. Vascular malformations composed of dysplastic vessels
2. Vascular tumors that demonstrate cellular hyperplasia

Vascular malformations have various subcategories determined by the anomalous vessels involved—including capillary, venous, arteriovenous, or lymphatic. Hemangiomas or vascular nevi are the most common cutaneous congenital malformations seen during early infancy. They may be either involuting or noninvoluting vascular lesions, as well as flat (telangiectatic) or raised (hemangiomatous). The common involuting types include salmon patch, spider nevi (telangiectases), and strawberry and cavernous hemangiomas. Noninvoluting lesions, which are seen less commonly in newborns, are the port-wine stain and, rarely, the pyogenic granuloma (Enjolras & Garzon, 2001).

Pigmented Nevus

Pigmented nevi are benign tumors of the skin that contain nevus cells. Nevus cells can produce melanin and are closely related to melanocytes. In contrast to melanocytes, they tend to lie in groups or nests. Congenital pigmented nevi are different from pigmented nevi that arise later in that they are usually larger and more extensive. As the infant grows, the area becomes thicker and darker (Margileth, 2005).

Flat, junctional nevi are seen in about 1% of newborns. They are brown or black, and their size varies from one to several centimeters. When they are present at birth, they may be associated with neurofibromatosis, tuberous sclerosis, or bathing trunk nevi. Therapy is rarely needed, but lesions larger than 3 cm should be removed.

Giant Hairy Nevus

A giant hairy nevus is characterized by a pigmented, hairy, and softly infiltrated area. The color varies from pale brown to black. When the nevi are large, they tend to have a dermatomic distribution, and their location and size give them their name (e.g., bathing trunk nevus, vest nevus, shoulder stole nevus) (Figure 4-3). On histologic examination of a biopsy specimen, the nevus cells are seen penetrating deeply into the dermis and subcutaneous tissue.

When a giant nevus is situated on the head or neck, it may be associated with mental retardation, epilepsy, or hydrocephalus. Spina bifida or meningocele may occur when this nevus is present over the spine (Margileth, 2005). Other abnormalities that are sometimes associated with a giant

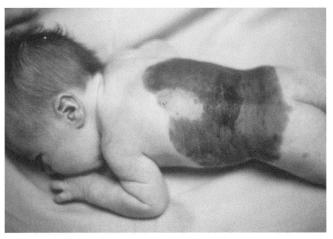

FIGURE **4-3**
The giant pigmented hairy nevus of this infant involves the thorax, abdomen, and back and is commonly called a "bathing trunk" nevus. It is raised with fleshy elements and has a somewhat leathery texture. From Clark D, Thompson J (1986). Dermatology of the newborn. Parts 1 and 2. In *Pathology of the neonate slide series* (vol 3, no 4). Philadelphia: Wyeth-Ayerst Laboratories. Copyright © Wyeth; used with permission.

pigmented nevus are clubfoot, hypertrophy or hypotrophy of the affected limb, and von Recklinghausen's disease (neurofibromatosis). Besides being a cosmetic problem, the giant nevus is associated with a higher incidence of malignancy. Malignant melanomas develop in as many as 15% of these patients. Management involves surgical excision of the entire lesion at or near puberty to prevent the development of skin cancer in the lesion. Plastic surgical reconstruction may be needed if the excision is extensive.

Hemangiomas

Hemangioma of infancy is an angiomatous disorder characterized by the proliferation of capillary endothelium and multilamination of the basement membrane and accumulation of mast cells, fibroblasts, and macrophages. Hemangiomas appear on 1% to 3% of infants at birth and develop on another 10%, usually within the first 3 to 4 weeks of life. The incidence is 22% in preterm babies who weigh less than 1000 g and 15% in infants with birth weights of 1000 to 1500 g. When examined microscopically, hemangiomas are one of two kinds: capillary or cavernous. They most often appear in the skin as a single tumor, but multiple cutaneous lesions also occur, often with involvement of other organ systems.

The natural history of the hemangioma is characterized by their appearance during the first few weeks of life, rapid postnatal growth for 8 to 18 months (proliferative phase), which is followed by very slow but inevitable regression for the next 5 to 8 years (involutive phase). Hemangiomas completely resolve in more than 50% of children by 5 years of age and in more than 70% by 7 years of age, and continued improvement occurs in the remaining children until 10 to 12 years of age. The rate of regression does not seem to be related to the sex or age of the infant or to the site, size, or appearance of the hemangioma or the duration of the proliferative phase.

Strawberry hemangiomas consist of a dilated mass of capillaries in the dermal and subdermal layers that protrude above the skin surface. They are bright red, soft, compressible tumors

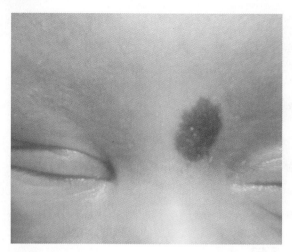

FIGURE **4-4**
This photograph shows the early hemangioma in a 28-weeks'-gestation premature infant. Approximately 5 weeks after birth the first area of discoloration appeared. The irregular surface with sharp demarcation is typical of strawberry hemangioma, which eventually enlarges to twice the size it appears in this photograph before involution. From Clark D, Thompson J (1986). Dermatology of the newborn. Parts 1 and 2. In *Pathology of the neonate slide series* (vol 3, no 4). Philadelphia: Wyeth-Ayerst Laboratories. Copyright © Wyeth; used with permission.

that can appear anywhere on the body (Figure 4-4). These marks require no treatment, and no permanent scars occur if the marks are left alone. However, when these lesions interfere with vital functions such as vision, feeding, and respiration, intervention is required.

Cavernous hemangiomas are more deeply situated in the skin than are strawberry hemangiomas. They are bluish-red and feel spongy when touched. Most hemangiomas are small, harmless birthmarks that involute to leave either normal or slightly blemished skin. However, even a small hemangioma can obstruct the airway or impair vision. A large hemangioma in the liver or an extensive cutaneous hemangioma can divert a considerable volume of blood through its extensive labyrinth of capillaries and produce high-output heart failure. The increased capillary endothelial surface that characterizes a giant hemangioma can also trap platelets and may cause thrombocytopenic coagulopathy (Kasabach-Merritt syndrome).

A few hemangiomas grow to an alarming size or proliferate simultaneously in several organs and cause life-endangering conditions, such as soft-tissue destruction, deformation or obstruction of vital structures, serious bleeding, congestive heart failure, and sepsis. Large lesions can expand the skin, and even after they regress, they can result in excess slack skin, pigment changes, and a fibro-fatty residuum.

Visceral hemangiomas may arise in many organs, most commonly in the liver and larynx, with or without cutaneous involvement; a singe lesion or multiple hemangiomas may occur. Flow through extensive hemangiomas increases the total blood volume, causes hemodeviation, and disturbs the hemodynamic equilibrium. The hyperdynamic cardiovascular state of the hemangiomas decreases or shunts blood away from other tissues, thus resulting in hypoperfusion of other tissues. This hypoperfusion may cause brain hypoxia and acidosis and predispose to seizures, as seen in some cases. Close

surveillance of the cardiovascular system is necessary to determine the proper time to begin digitalization.

Management. Management of both strawberry and cavernous hemangiomas consists of a detailed history; close scrutiny of the lesion or lesions, including three-dimensional measurements; and evaluation of the growth pattern of the hemangioma. As involution progresses, the color gradually changes from grayish-pink to white or pink, and the tension of the lesion decreases. Ulcerated hemangiomas should be treated with topical antibiotics to prevent infection.

While the cutaneous lesions are being monitored, the infant's clinical course and physical development must be closely observed for poor growth, altered cry, stridor, dyspnea, cyanosis, feeding difficulties, or swallowing impairment. If any abnormal sign or symptoms appear—such as tachycardia, heart murmur, hepatomegaly, or bruit heard over the liver—the infant should be examined for evidence of heart failure. Ultrasonography, echocardiography, and computed tomography may be needed.

In general, management consists of planned neglect, which is essential in avoiding disfiguring scars. Complications of therapy may be significant, but residual scarring after complete involution is uncommon. Hemangiomas located in exposed areas often cause great parental anxiety, which increases as the hemangioma grows. This anxiety often puts pressure on the physician to do something. However, the hemangioma should be left to regress spontaneously, and preconceived notions about birthmarks should be discussed with the family.

Treatment of hemangiomas may be needed. The following indications for treatment have been proposed: life-threatening or function-threatening hemangiomas, including those that cause impairment of vision, respiratory compromise, or congestive heart failure; hemangiomas occurring in certain anatomic locations such as the nose, lip, glabellar areas, and ear and that may cause permanent deformity or scars; large facial hemangiomas, especially those with a large dermal component; and ulcerated hemangiomas (Enjolras & Garzon, 2001).

Alarming hemangiomas is a term used to categorize lesions that impair vital functions or cause life-threatening complications. A vascular mark was present at birth in 68% of these infants. Visceral hemangiomas are associated with cervicocephalic hemangiomas or with small hemangiomas scattered over the body. About a third of these life-threatening hemangiomas respond to treatment with corticosteroids, but for the others, no safe and effective treatment exists. The mortality rate can be as high as 54% for life-threatening visceral or hepatic hemangiomas and may be up to 30% to 40% with platelet-consumptive coagulopathy, despite the administration of steroids.

High-dose corticosteroid therapy is the primary means of controlling hemangiomas pharmacologically. These agents inhibit the activators of fibrinolysis in vessel walls, decrease plasminogen activator content of endothelium, and increase sensitivity to vasoactive amines, thus causing constriction of arterioles. When steroids fail, less conventional modalities, such as embolization, operative excision, and radiotherapy, are used.

Subcutaneous interferon alpha-2a (2 million units per square meter of body surface area) has been used with life-threatening or vision-threatening hemangiomas that failed to respond to corticosteroid therapy. Their mechanisms of action include inhibition of motility and proliferation of endothelial cells and interference with new capillary vessel formation, thereby preventing platelet trapping. These daily injections seemed to reduce the local and systemic complications and appeared to shorten the length of time to involution in some infants. Sustained therapy for 9 to 14 months appeared to be desirable because earlier withdrawal was followed by regrowth of the lesion that was halted and reversed by reintroduction of the drug. Interferon alpha therapy was not found to have toxic effects.

Tranexamic acid has been used in the treatment of giant hemangiomas. It is a fibrinolytic inhibitor that exerts its effect through inhibition of plasminogen activator and plasmin and through inhibition of tumor vessel proliferation. One of the infants had a measurable response in the size of the hemangioma and the extent of the coagulopathy. The other two had progression of their lesions. It appears that tranexamic acid is an additional agent for treatment of giant hemangiomas, but its efficacy is limited. Further study of this treatment is needed to determine which patients may respond best. Surgical therapy involves either laser removal, or surgical excision is also a treatment option. Excision is usually done once the hemangioma has involuted, so as to remove residual tissue and redundant skin. Early excision is generally not recommended.

Port-Wine Stain

Port-wine stain is a capillary angioma consisting of dilated and congested capillaries lying directly beneath the epidermis. It appears in approximately 3 of 1000 newborns. This birthmark appears pink at birth but gradually darkens to purple. Most commonly found on the face and neck, it is a permanent developmental defect. Although a port-wine stain is primarily a cosmetic problem, it is occasionally an indicator of a multisystem disorder, such as Sturge-Weber syndrome or Klippel-Trenaunay-Weber syndrome. The presence of convulsions, mental retardation, hemiplegia, or intracortical calcification suggests the presence of Sturge-Weber syndrome. An ophthalmologic examination is extremely important in these infants. Gradual thickening and nodule formation can occur with port-wine stain and thus support the need for early treatment in infancy and childhood. Recent advances in laser therapy techniques are shown to be more effective in previously resistant lesions. Although the timing of intervention is somewhat controversial, many dermatologists now advise laser treatment as early as possible in infancy to decrease the stigma associated with this lesion and to prevent skin thickening (Enjolras & Garzon, 2001).

Blistering Diseases
Epidermolysis Bullosa

Epidermolysis bullosa (EB) is a group of rare congenital blistering disorders, all of which are inherited. They are considered mechanobullous diseases, meaning that trauma to or friction on the skin induces blister formation. EB is caused by defects in the complex meshwork of proteins in the epidermis, dermis, and dermoepidermal junction that allow the skin to adhere in the presence of frictional stress. The underlying defect appears to be a lack of cellular glue in squamous epithelium, which is responsible for the maintenance of cellular integrity. Diagnostic studies should include a skin biopsy for light and electron microscopy.

EB is classified by the clinical extent and ultrastructural level of blistering, by inheritance pattern, and by specific molecular defect (Fine et al, 1999, 2000; Marinkovich, 1999). Although some subtypes of EB are severe in the neonatal period and milder later, others can be fatal in the first weeks as a result of severe generalized blistering and complications that arise from this. EB can be nonscarring or scarring. Inheritance may be either autosomal dominant or autosomal recessive.

Epidermolysis bullosa simplex is the mildest form of EB. Most cases are autosomal dominant. The lesions occur at the basal layer of epidermis and do not lead to scarring and hyperkeratosis. Usually present at birth, the vesicles and bullae appear over the joints and the bony protuberances and at sites subjected to repeated trauma. The differential diagnosis may be aided by the absence of milia, which are commonly seen in the dystrophic types of epidermolysis bullosa. Little or no scarring is seen with EB simplex.

Junctional epidermolysis bullosa is the least common type of EB with autosomal recessive inheritance. In junctional EB, severe generalized blistering is present at birth, with subsequent extensive denudation. Marked mucosal blistering occurs, and erosions of the larynx, respiratory, gastrointestinal, and urinary tract may also be present. It may be fatal in a few days to a few months because of fluid loss or sepsis. Histopathologically, a separation occurs between the plasma membrane of the basal cells and the basal lamina. In junctional EB, healing is poor, and scarring is extensive.

Dystrophic EB results in blistering that occurs below the dermoepidermal junction and has either dominant or recessive inheritance. In the recessive form, blistering is severe, begins at birth, and can lead to marked scarring and joint contractures.

The dominant form of dystrophic EB is milder, with moderately severe blisters seen on the distal extremities and bony protuberances (Figure 4-5). Some scar formation occurs, and the nails may be mildly dystrophic. Atrophy may occur with healing. The external skin layer can be easily rubbed off by slight friction or injury. Milia, due to a functional disorder of the sweat glands, are found on the rims of the ears, the dorsa of

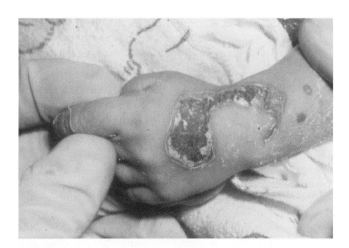

FIGURE **4-5**
This photograph of epidermolysis bullosa shows the scaling, broken bullae with underlying erythroderma. From Clark D, Thompson J (1986). Dermatology of the newborn. Parts 1 and 2. In *Pathology of the neonate slide series* (vol 3, no 4). Philadelphia: Wyeth-Ayerst Laboratories. Copyright © Wyeth; used with permission.

the hands, and the extensor surfaces of the arms and legs. The oral, anal, and esophageal mucosa are frequently involved. Complications include infections and hemolytic, nutritional, orthopedic, gastrointestinal, and psychiatric sequelae. These vary according to the severity of the disease.

Management. EB can be a great challenge in the newborn period, particularly with the more severe forms. Nursing care centers around three main issues: (1) skin breakdown; (2) prevention of infection; and (3) dysphagia. Many of the techniques used to protect the skin of very premature infants are useful with EB patients. Avoiding the use of tape and preventing traumatic injuries is important. Clean, soft dressings may be helpful over bony pressure points. Wound care involves providing a moist healing environment by covering open lesions with a thick coating of petrolatum-based emollients combined with topical antibiotic ointments and covering with nonstick dressings.

Many dermatologists will rotate topical antibiotics every few months to prevent resistance, and may use wound cultures to guide selection of agents. Nonstick dressings include petrolatum gauze, Exu-dry or silicone-based products such as Mepitel (Direct Medical Inc., Houston, TX). After this layer, the wound is further protected by wrapping with nonadhesive cotton gauze; some practitioners prefer cotton mesh, and others use Coban (3M, Indianapolis, IN), a wrap that adheres to itself without adhesives. When blisters are tense and fluid filled, they should be "unroofed" to prevent extension. This procedure is done with sharp, clean scissors, leaving the blister roof in place. Dressings are changed daily and removed gently; some prefer to remove dressings during immersion bathing (Frieden & Howard, 2001).

From birth to 6 months of age, the environment is easy to control through the use of sheepskin, loose-fitting clothes, and mittens for the infant's hands and feet. Cloth diapers softened with fabric softener are preferred over rougher, disposable diapers. Any person handling the infant should avoid wearing jewelry. Protection of the infant becomes more difficult once the infant is mobile.

The infant should always wear long pants, and foam rubber pads sewn into the knees help avoid trauma during crawling. Contractures may form quickly as scarring begins to occur. The pathologic increase in elastic skin fiber adds to this process. Gentle range-of-motion exercises lessen contracture formation.

Dysphagia can occur from facial and pharyngeal scarring, which is secondary to erosions on the buccal mucosa, tongue, palate, esophagus, and pharynx. Feedings should be performed slowly and carefully to avoid aspiration and to maintain adequate nutrition. The metabolic needs of these infants are high because of the continuous sloughing of epithelium, which results in large protein, fluid, and electrolyte losses. Adding additional puncture holes to a nipple may help prevent oral mucosal trauma. If oral ulcerations occur, several weeks of hyperalimentation and high-dose steroid therapy are instituted. Gavage feedings are discouraged because of the possibility of trauma. It is essential that the family receive genetic counseling regarding the inheritance pattern associated with epidermolysis bullosa; a negative family history does not exclude its occurrence.

Infections of the Skin

Normal skin flora includes 13 species of coagulase-negative staphylococci (CONS) (Darmstadt & Dinulos, 2001). CONS colonize the skin of newborns within 2 to 4 days after birth. Skin infections and skin manifestations of systemic infection can be of bacterial, viral, or fungal origin. In this section, the various skin infections from each type of microorganism are discussed, along with implications for nursing care.

Bacterial

Staphylococcus aureus. Infections resulting from *Staphylococcus aureus* are seen in newborns and can result in two types of skin lesions. Nonbullous impetigo is a superficial infection localized to the epidermis and is characterized by erythematous, honey-colored crusted plaques. Bullous impetigo of the newborn involves blisters that originate in the subcorneal portion of the epidermis and are filled with clear or straw-colored fluid. Bullous impetigo often presents during the first 2 weeks of life. Few or many blisters may be dispersed widely over all areas of the body and may rupture easily, thus leaving denuded areas of skin. *S. aureus* is most commonly cultured, but other bacteria, such as group A streptococci and beta-hemolytic streptococci, are sometimes seen.

Management. Medical and nursing management is focused on treatment of the affected infant and on prevention of the spread of infection to other infants, because this condition is highly contagious. Systemic antibiotics are administered parenterally initially and may be followed by oral treatment once the infection begins to subside. Antibiotics include oxacillin, nafcillin, or methicillin; vancomycin is used if the culture indicated methicillin-resistant *S. aureus*. Topical antibiotics are not indicated for treatment of bullous impetigo (Darmstadt & Dinulos, 2001). Fluid and electrolyte monitoring is necessary if the denuded areas cover a large surface or if the infant is of low birth weight. Isolation of the affected infant is necessary to prevent the spread of the infection throughout the nursery.

Scalded Skin Syndrome. *S. aureus* can also result in a severe bullous eruption called scalded skin syndrome. Initially, the infant's skin is bright red and resembles a scald. This finding is followed by the formation of large flaccid blisters that quickly progress to large sheets of shed skin (Figure 4-6). The entire epidermis is often shed during the course of this disease. The mechanism for this severe injury involves the production of an endotoxin, called exfoliatin, that causes the skin manifestations. Usually, the skin lesions do not culture positive for the responsible organism; thus culturing the nasopharynx, blood, conjunctiva, and normal skin is recommended to recover the organism for appropriate sensitivity assessment (Drolet & Esterly, 2002).

Management. Medical and nursing management also involves administration of the appropriate antibiotic regimen and supportive measures in terms of fluid and electrolytic replacement, prevention of secondary infection through the damaged epidermis, and comfort. Applying local antibiotic solutions or ointments is not recommended; cleansing open skin areas with gentle irrigation using half normal saline promotes healing and prevents secondary infection. The infant may be more comfortable in an incubator rather than in a radiant warmer because the incubator is a convective heat source that does not have a direct cutaneous effect, whereas the radiant heat source heats directly through the skin. In addition, the radiant heat source may further increase the degree of insensible water loss through the damaged epidermis. Usually, a flaking process is observed on the skin during the

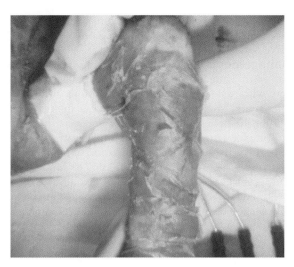

FIGURE **4-6**
The peeling, scaling skin of this premature infant had an acute onset at approximately 2 weeks of age. This is the scalded skin syndrome that results from *Staphylococcus aureus*. From Clark D, Thompson J (1986). Dermatology of the newborn. Parts 1 and 2. In *Pathology of the neonate slide series* (vol 3, no 4). Philadelphia: Wyeth-Ayerst Laboratories. Copyright © Wyeth; used with permission.

healing process. Emollients may be helpful in treating dry skin at this point.

Listeria monocytogenes. Another bacterial skin disease is listeriosis, caused by *L. monocytogenes*. This organism, which can cause severe systemic disease, can also result in a disseminated miliary granulomatosis in neonates (Drolet & Esterly, 2002). In some cases, miliary abscesses can occur; occasionally, more generalized erythema or petechiae may be present. Systemic listeriosis is a severe infection that causes blood hemolysis and a high mortality rate. Prompt recognition and treatment with intravenous penicillin or ampicillin are indicated for the best prognosis. No direct skin therapy has been described as being necessary in this disease.

Syphilis. Congenital syphilis is another bacterial infection that has skin manifestations. If the infant with congenital syphilis is not treated after birth, a maculopapular or bullous skin eruption develops between 2 and 6 weeks of age (Margileth, 2005). Sometimes the bullous lesions may be observed at birth on the palms or the soles, thus signifying the presence of more severe disease. Fluid contained in the blisters contains spirochetes.

The lesions most commonly seen in congenital syphilis are copper-colored and maculopapular and are located on the soles and palms. In addition, open lesions may be present around the mouth, anus, or genitals, and a highly contagious nasal discharge is occasionally seen. If the syphilis remains untreated, the lesions regress in 1 to 3 months, leaving areas on the skin with either hyperpigmentation or hypopigmentation.

Management. Medical and nursing management for the infant with congenital syphilis involves prompt, consistent administration of penicillin—usually a 10-day course. Titers are obtained over the next year at 3-month intervals, and a negative serologic finding is expected at 1 year. Care of the skin lesions is primarily directed toward preventing the spread of infection during the active phase of the illness, especially when bullous lesions or open areas are apparent. No direct topical therapies have been advocated in the literature.

Viral
Viral infections can display a broad range of cutaneous manifestations in the neonate and can occur in utero, perinatally, or postnatally. Skin manifestations can be a direct result of skin infection or be a consequence of viral infection in other tissues. Viral infections that have skin symptoms include several of the herpes conditions, cytomegalovirus, and rubella. Toxoplasmosis, which has cutaneous manifestations and is caused by a parasite, is also discussed in this section.

Herpes Simplex. Herpes simplex virus types 1 and 2 are serious pathogens in newborns. The majority of newborns acquire infections from infectious vaginal secretions at the time of delivery. Infections range from systemic, disseminated infections to CNS infection and infection involving the skin, eye, or mouth. Vesicles that occur on the skin with this disease vary; a few faint scars may be present, or actual vesicle formations may be present with either one large swelling or discrete groups of vesicles. Vesicles may recede and then recur over months.

Management. Medical and nursing management is centered primarily on early recognition and treatment with the antiviral medication acyclovir. The prognosis of systemic herpes simplex is extremely poor if encephalitis develops, with a high risk of either death or severe mental retardation. An important consideration in the care of infants with known or suspected herpes simplex infection is isolation from other patients to prevent transmission.

Varicella. Another viral infection with manifestation in the skin is varicella. Varicella infection is rare, but when it occurs in the first 10 days of life, it is generally thought to have been acquired in utero. The vesicular eruptions are the same as those in chickenpox acquired at any age. A mortality rate of 20% is associated with varicella infection in newborns, and certainly this infection poses a significant risk for the immunocompromised infants in premature and intensive care nurseries. No systemic medication or topical treatment is required for these lesions. Occasionally scarring can occur. Strict isolation is absolutely necessary to protect other infants from exposure because this virus is airborne. Passive immunization of infants exposed to the affected infant may also be necessary.

Toxoplasmosis. Toxoplasmosis, which is caused by an intracellular parasite (*Toxoplasma gondii*), can be transmitted transplacentally and can result in systemic infection. Some infants may have a generalized maculopapular rash as well as hepatosplenomegaly, jaundice, fever, and anemia. The rash may progress to desquamation and hypopigmentation in very severe cases. Direct topical therapy is not reported to be necessary or efficacious; systemic therapy may be considered.

Cytomegalovirus and Rubella. Both cytomegalovirus and rubella have symptoms that are manifested in the skin. Petechial lesions can occur with both infections. These are the result of thrombocytopenia and usually disappear in 2 to 6 weeks. In severe rubella infection, and very rarely in cytomegalovirus, bluish-red papules that are 2 to 8 mm in diameter can occur on the head, trunk, and extremities (Figure 4-7). This so-called blueberry muffin syndrome is the result of erythropoiesis in the dermis and usually subsides in 2 to 3 weeks. Neither of these lesions requires topical therapy (for a complete discussion of infections, see Chapter 9).

Fungal
Candida albicans infection is the primary fungal infection with cutaneous manifestations, although other species—such as

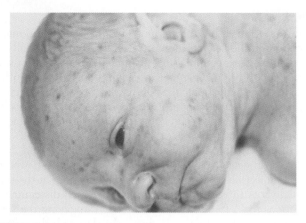

FIGURE **4-7**
This is an example of the "blueberry muffin" syndrome, seen in an infant with congenital cytomegalovirus infection. The infant has multiple petechiae and purpura from thrombocytopenia in this systemic infection. From Clark D, Thompson J (1986). Dermatology of the newborn. Parts 1 and 2. In *Pathology of the neonate slide series* (vol 3, no 4). Philadelphia: Wyeth-Ayerst Laboratories. Copyright © Wyeth; used with permission.

C. parapsilosis, C. tropicalis, C. lusitaniae, C. glabrata, and *Malassezia furfur*—can also potentially colonize the skin of term and preterm newborns, particularly those who are hospitalized in an intensive care nursery. Manifestations of infection with *Candida* species can range from diaper dermatitis or other localized skin or mucous membrane eruptions to disseminated candidiasis, thus resulting in significant morbidity and mortality. *Candida* is not normally found in the skin flora of the newborn. The gastrointestinal system is the primary reservoir, but the skin may also be colonized during passage through a colonized vaginal canal. The incidence of *Candida* colonization is also increased with the frequent use of broad-spectrum antibiotics that alter normal skin flora in infants after delivery.

Infants with systemic candidiasis may demonstrate cutaneous involvement. This cutaneous pattern may be a diffuse burn-like dermatitis that affects large areas on the lower back, buttocks, chest, and abdomen. In a few infants, the axilla and groin are affected. Scaling followed the erythematous macular patches, and severe cases desquamation develops in a manner similar to that seen in staphylococcal scalded skin syndrome. These infants do not always have the satellite papules and pustules normally seen with *Candida* diaper dermatitis. The onset of the generalized rash often occurs within the first 3 days of life, but it can appear later.

A monilial diaper rash was the other dermatologic condition exhibited by some infants. This rash consisted of a red, scaling dermatitis in the groin, and the rash spread to other body parts. Erosive crusting lesions in a cohort of extremely premature infants as an invasive fungal dermatitis, leading also to systemic disease, was reported (Rowen et al, 1995). Although the lesions were primarily due to *Candida albicans* or other *Candida* species, other fungal species were also seen and included *Aspergillus, Trichosporum beigelii,* and *Curvularia.* Cutaneous fungal infections with *Aspergillus* have been reported by others as well (Woodruff & Herbert, 2002). Skin biopsies performed on patients with this condition revealed fungal invasion that extended beyond the epidermis into the dermis. The onset is several days after birth, and associated factors included maternal colonization with vaginal birth, steroid administration, hyperglycemia, and skin trauma from adhesive removal.

Management. Medical and nursing management of infants with systemic or local *Candida* infection involves therapy with systemic antifungal medications and antifungal ointments and creams. Cutaneous *Candida* in the extremely premature infant less than a week of age requires aggressive monitoring for systemic infection and may warrant parenteral antifungal agents to prevent dissemination of the fungal infection. Yeast is sometimes difficult to culture; techniques include obtaining urine to look for hyphae or budding yeast, blood cultures, and skin scrapings prepared with potassium hydroxide (KOH) obtained from the margins of the affected areas since this is the area of active growth, and examined for pseudohyphae (Cunningham & Wagner, 2001). Nursing observation in low-birth-weight infants for evidence of the diffuse burn-like dermatitis or a spreading monilial diaper rash is essential and may expedite the initiation of parenteral antifungal therapy with amphotericin B for systemic candidiasis.

Scaling Disorders

A scaly appearance in the skin of a newborn can have a range of causes, from relatively benign to long-term and potentially life-threatening. In this section, scaly skin due to postmaturity, essential fatty acid deficiency, congenital ichthyosis, and eczema is discussed, and areas of nursing management are determined.

Postmaturity

Many term infants born between 40 and 42 weeks' gestation experience a period of shedding, or desquamation that is considered to be a normal physiologic process. Postmature infants born after 42 weeks' gestation may also have this appearance, but other characteristics are different. The postmature infant may have a lean appearance, with little subcutaneous fat; the weight is low in relationship to length. The skin resembles parchment paper and may literally peel off in sheets. Fingernails may be stained with meconium and may be long. Long hair may also be present.

Skin care is not the major problem, nor is it the focus of medical or nursing management. Eventually, the skin underneath the peeling layers predominates; even during the period of desquamation, the skin functions well as a barrier because these infants have all the layers of stratum corneum of a term infant or adult. Aside from bathing with a mild soap initially, moisturizing with a petrolatum-based ointment may be used. More careful attention is paid to the more compelling problems associated with postmaturity, such as hypoglycemia and meconium aspiration.

Essential Fatty Acid Deficiency

In some newborns who are unable to receive an adequate diet because of other illnesses or surgical condition, scaly dry skin may signify the development of essential fatty acid deficiency syndrome. Infants may be more prone to the development of this syndrome, especially if they are premature or postmature because of the decreased fat stores available. It may also occur in infants with severe fat malabsorption, such as those with cystic fibrosis.

The skin appearance in essential fatty acid deficiency includes a superficial scaling and, in some cases, desquamation.

Later presentation may involve oozing and irritation in the neck, groin, or perianal region.

This syndrome is sometimes confused with other conditions that cause scaling or other skin disruptions, including ichthyosis, acrodermatitis enteropathica, and candidal infection. Laboratory findings that confirm this diagnosis are decreased serum essential fatty acid levels, possibly in conjunction with thrombocytopenia and impaired platelet aggregation, because essential fatty acids are necessary to ensure platelet function.

Management. Medical and nursing management consists of replacement of essential fatty acids through the administration of intravenous lipid solutions or diet. Human breast milk and most infant formulas contain more than adequate amounts of essential fatty acids. However, if the gastrointestinal system is not functioning well in the digestion and absorption of nutrients, intravenous therapy is required.

Once skin symptoms are present, administration of intravenous lipid solution can reverse the process in 1 to 2 weeks. Dietary replacement takes longer and is effective only in the presence of healthy gastrointestinal function.

Prevention of essential fatty acid deficiency is possible and should be the goal. The development of essential fatty acid deficiency can be prevented by early administration of intravenous lipid solutions in the first weeks of life in a dose as low as 0.5 g/kg per day.

Ichthyosis

The most serious cause of scaly skin in the newborn is ichthyosis dermatosis. Four major types of ichthyosis exist: (1) X-linked ichthyosis; (2) lamellar ichthyosis; (3) bullous congenital ichthyosiform erythroderma, which is present at birth; and (4) ichthyosis vulgaris, which usually appears after the third month of life. Terms commonly used to describe infants with ichthyosis may include harlequin fetus and collodion baby, but these terms do not define which form of ichthyosis is present.

In the X-linked type of ichthyosis, males are affected. Some female heterozygotes may exhibit mild scaling of the arms and lower extremities. Affected male newborns have large yellow or brown plaques that cover the whole body, except the palms, soles, and midface and over joints. At birth, some affected males may appear scaly, whereas others are often called collodion babies.

Lamellar ichthyosis, formerly called nonbullous congenital ichthyosiform erythroderma, is an autosomal recessive disorder. Initially, affected newborns may have a bright red appearance that rapidly progresses to desquamation; rarely is a collodion-baby appearance present at birth. Later, scales develop that are yellow to brown and that may eventually become thick, horny plates. Although the prognosis is usually good, infants who are severely affected—the so-called harlequin fetuses—may die of sepsis or require extensive plastic surgery (Figure 4-8).

In bullous congenital ichthyosiform erythroderma, autosomal dominance is the mode of heredity; thus several family members may be affected. Large bullae are initially seen, as are erythema and dry scaly skin; the blistering that recurs throughout childhood differentiates this form from the lamellar type. Extensive denuded areas of the skin can present a problem in the newborn as the blisters burst because secondary infections with *Streptococcus* or *Staphylococcus* can occur and are life-threatening.

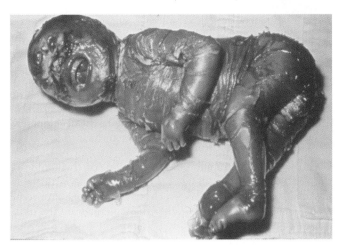

FIGURE **4-8**
This harlequin infant is an example of the most severely affected ichthyotic infant. The skin is hard and thick, with deep crevices. The lack of elasticity of the skin results in fleshy deformities of joints and limbs. From Clark D, Thompson J (1986). Dermatology of the newborn. Parts 1 and 2. In *Pathology of the neonate slide series* (vol 3, no 4). Philadelphia: Wyeth-Ayerst Laboratories. Copyright © Wyeth; used with permission.

Management. Medical and nursing management of all forms of ichthyosis involves the continual use of topical therapies and prescription bathing techniques and the prevention of infection. Bathing is performed with a water-dispersible bath oil, and soaps that are excessively drying or irritating should be avoided. Collodion babies should be placed in a high-humidity incubator to increase hydration. Emollients that preserve moisturization, such as Aquaphor ointment (Beiersdorf, Inc., Wilton, CT), should be applied several times daily.

Infants with severe skin involvement from ichthyosis may require protective isolation if they receive care in an intensive care nursery because of the higher risk of contact with nosocomial infections. Incubators provide a barrier to infection. Use of sterile linen and sterile gloves and other measures are needed if larger areas of denuded skin are present.

Comfort is another key nursing concern in the care of the infant who is significantly affected with ichthyosis. Fussy, irritable agitation may be seen and is related to pruritus or inflammation. Some form of analgesia may help, although the topical therapies prescribed have the most direct effect. Some authors describe the use of diphenhydramine (Benadryl, Pfizer, Morris Plains, NJ) if severe pruritus exists, but this would be hard to determine in a neonate, who lacks verbal or fine motor skills to communicate this symptom. A trial of this medication with careful observation might be helpful in the case of a frantic or irritable infant when other measures (e.g., topical treatment, pacifiers, feeding) are unsuccessful.

Working with the parents of an infant with ichthyosis has many facets. The appearance of the infant, especially if he or she is severely affected, could be shocking and traumatic to the parents and could require careful interventions. As with parents of infants with other congenital abnormalities, a period of shock, denial, and grief occurs over the loss of a perfect baby. In addition, the genetic nature of this disorder and the implications for future children must be comprehended. Parents of these infants need genetic counseling, support, and education as they come to terms with this disease.

Eczema

Eczema, which is a skin disorder that causes several degrees of skin irritation and has multiple causes, is rarely seen in the newborn period. It is more commonly seen after 2 months of age and involves an eruption that proceeds to the development of microvesicles and oozing, which later turns into scaling of the epidermis. The scaling is due to an attempt of the skin layer to regenerate rapidly. Lichenification, or thickening of the skin, which occurs in adult skin with eczema, is not seen in infants. Primary irritants—such as saliva, feces, and some soaps or skin preparations—rather than allergies are the usual causes of eczema in infants. It is important to have a good history of all products that have been applied to the skin to sort out the causes. If external agents have been ruled out, other diagnoses are considered, such as seborrheic dermatitis and Leiner's disease, which involves a total exfoliation of the entire body.

Management. Medical and nursing treatment of eczema involves prevention by avoiding the primary irritant source, if it has been identified, or protection, as in the use of zinc oxide paste to the perianal area to prevent contact with feces. For more generalized eruptions, short-term therapy with topical steroids may be used. Bathing should be carried out in tepid water with water-dispersible oil; use of irritating or drying soaps should be avoided. If large areas of skin are involved, thermoregulation may be a concern, especially in dry climates. Humidification may be desirable in some climates, especially during the summer months. Air conditioning may also be necessary during the summer months. Discomfort is a significant concern because infants with eczema may experience considerable pruritus. Topical therapy is generally the first consideration, followed by the judicious use of diphenhydramine in severe cases.

SKIN CARE PRACTICES

The most basic aspects of skin care for newborns include daily bath; moisturizing with emollients; skin preparation with disinfectant solutions; and use of adhesives for life-support devices, monitoring of vital signs, and oxygenation, if the newborns are hospitalized. During all these practices, the skin of the newborn has the potential for trauma or alterations in normal barrier function and pH. The literature is reviewed to determine what is currently known about these and other common nursing practices and the impact on the skin of newborns.

Bathing

The purpose of bathing newborns includes providing overall hygiene, aesthetics, and protection of health care workers by removing blood and body fluids. However, bathing is not an innocuous procedure and during the immediate postbirth period can result in hypothermia, increased oxygen consumption, and respiratory distress. The first bath should be delayed until the infant's temperature has been stabilized in the normal range for 1 to 4 hours (Penny-MacGillivray, 1996; Varda & Behnke, 2000) Bathing has also been shown to destabilize vital signs and temperature in premature infants.

Bathing with antiseptic soaps and cleansers is still practiced in some nurseries. Studies have shown that although hexa-

chlorophene reduced the number of *Staphylococcus aureus* strains, toxicity was reported, especially in premature infants and was associated with absorption through the skin; thus it should not be used (American Academy of Pediatrics, 1997). Both povidone-iodine and chlorhexidine are sometimes used for the initial bath in newborn nurseries, although the effect on bacterial colonization is transient. Chlorhexidine has proven effective in reducing colonization for up to 4 hours but can also be absorbed. Although toxicity from chlorhexidine has not been identified, many nurseries do not use chlorhexidine for routine bathing because of the potential risk. No guidelines from the Centers for Disease Control or the American Academy of Pediatrics recommend that antimicrobial cleansers be used for the newborn's first or subsequent baths (American Academy of Pediatrics, 1997).

Products used in bathing include soaps made with lye and animal fats that are alkaline (pH >7.0) and cleansing bars and liquids made with synthetic detergents that are formulated to a more neutral pH of 5.5 to 7.0. All soaps and cleansers are at least mildly irritating and drying to skin surfaces. Study of bathing with soap, cleansing liquid, or cleansing bar in infants ages 2 weeks to 16 months showed alterations in fat content, hydration, and skin surface pH—most significantly with alkaline soap (Gfatter et al, 1997). In addition, the degree to which the skin is irritated also depends on the length of contact and the frequency of bathing.

Selecting cleansers that have a neutral pH and minimal dyes and perfumes to reduce risk of future sensitization to these products and bathing only 2 to 3 times per week is the best course to follow. Reducing the frequency of bathing even to 4-day intervals did not increase colonization with pathogens or result in infections in a study of healthy premature infants (Franck et al, 2000). For extremely premature infants, skin surfaces should be cleaned with warm water for the first week, with soft materials such as cotton balls or cloth. A rinsing technique is best during cleansing because rubbing is irritating to immature skin and potentially is uncomfortable. If areas of skin breakdown are evident, use warm sterile water.

Immersion bathing may be beneficial, when clinically possible, from a developmental perspective (Anderson et al, 1995). Immersion bathing places the infant's entire body, except the head and neck, into warm water (100.4° F), deep enough to cover the shoulders. Stable premature infants (after umbilical catheters are removed) and term infants with umbilical clamp in place can safely be bathed in this way (AWHONN/NANN Guideline, 2001). A recent study of immersion versus sponge bathing in 102 newborns for their first and subsequent baths showed that the immersion-bathed infants had significantly less temperature drop, appeared more content, and their mothers reported more pleasure with the bath; there was no difference in cord healing scores with either immersion or sponge bathing (Bryanton, 2004). Bathing is also an excellent time to educate parents about how to physically care for their babies and may also integrate information about their children's neurobehavioral status and social characteristics (Karl, 1999).

Emollients

The skin surface of term newborns is drier than that of adults but becomes gradually better hydrated as the eccrine sweat glands mature during the first year of life. Maintaining the hydration of the stratum corneum is necessary for an intact skin surface and normal barrier function. Skin that is dry, scaly, or cracking not only is uncomfortable but also can be a portal of entry for microorganisms. Products used to counteract dryness are called moisturizers, emollients, or lubricants. Common emollients include mineral oils, petrolatum, and lanolin and its derivatives. Emollients are divided into oil-in-water or water-in-oil emulsions (Hoath & Narendran, 2000).

Emollient use to prevent dermatitis and improve skin integrity in premature infants has been studied recently. Premature infants of 29 to 36 weeks' gestation treated daily with Eucerin cream (Beiersdorf, Inc., Wilton, CT) had less visible dermatitis but no differences in direct measurements of TEWL with an evaporimeter.

In a later study, premature infants of both younger gestation and postnatal age were treated with Aquaphor ointment (Beiersdorf, Inc., Wilton, CT), a water-miscible oil-in-water preparation that contains neither dyes nor perfumes. In this study, both TEWL and visual scale dermatitis improved. No increase in skin surface temperatures or thermal burns was seen, even when the emollient was applied to infants under radiant heaters or phototherapy lights. In addition, cutaneous cultures revealed no increase in bacterial or fungal colonization on skin treated with emollients, and fewer treated infants had positive blood or cerebrospinal fluid cultures compared with controls (Nopper et al, 1996).

A large, randomized controlled trial of 1191 infants with birth weights of 501 to 1000 g was conducted to determine whether a twice-daily application of Aquaphor ointment would reduce combined outcome measures of mortality and sepsis. Although skin integrity appeared improved with routine emollient use, no effect on the outcomes of sepsis plus mortality was seen. Of note, an increase in coagulase-negative *Staphylococcus epidermidis* bloodstream infections was seen in infants with birth weights <750 g although the mechanism and relationship to emollient use are not clearly understood (Edwards et al, 2004). Although a small case-control study had previously associated petrolatum-based emollients to a higher incidence of fungal infections (Campbell et al, 2000), this was not seen in this larger, randomized, controlled trial. The effects of emollients on TEWL or fluid balance were not studied in this trial (Edwards et al, 2004).

The benefits of emollient use must be carefully weighed against the risk of infection. In general, emollients can be safely used to treat skin with excessive drying, skin cracking, and fissures. They may also be beneficial in reducing TEWL and evaporative heat loss, although other methods, such as using a high-humidity environment or transparent adhesive dressings, are also available for this purpose (AWHONN/NANN Guideline, 2001). Avoiding products with perfumes or dyes is prudent because these can be absorbed and are potential contact irritants. Small tubes or jars for single-patient use are recommended to prevent contamination with microorganisms.

Disinfectants

Disinfection of the skin before invasive procedures such as venipuncture and placement of umbilical catheters and chest tubes is common practice in neonatal intensive care nurseries. Anecdotal reports of skin injury include blistering, burns, and sloughing from both isopropyl alcohol and povidone-iodine use in premature infants. High iodine levels, iodine goiter, and hypothyroidism associated with povidone-iodine use in pre-

mature infants have also been reported. Several prospective studies of routine povidone-iodine use in intensive care nurseries (Linder et al, 1997; Parravicini et al, 1996) and one study of presurgical skin preparation of infants under 3 months of age found alterations in iodine levels and potential thyroid effects from povidone-iodine exposure due to absorption through the skin. Although one study did not find thyroid effects from iodine absorption in neonates (Gordon et al, 1995), the study period (10 days) may be too short a period of time to see the effect.

Efficacy of the solutions is another important aspect of skin disinfection. During skin preparation before blood culture sampling in children and adults, lower rates of microbial colonization were seen with povidone-iodine compared to isopropyl alcohol. A larger study of blood culture sampling in adults found fewer contaminated cultures with chlorhexidine compared to povidone-iodine (Mimoz et al, 1999). Two studies in premature infants compared skin and peripheral intravenous catheter colonization with bacteria after skin preparation with either chlorhexidine or povidone-iodine. Malathi et al (1993) found that the rate of colonization was no different between disinfectants but that the technique of application was important; the authors recommended longer periods of cleansing (>30 seconds) or two consecutive cleansings for maximum reductions of colonization. Garland et al (1995) reported that chlorhexidine reduced the rate of catheter colonization in premature infants: 4.3% with chlorhexidine, in comparison to 9.3% with povidone-iodine. A comparison of isopropyl alcohol, povidone-iodine, and 2% chlorhexidine aqueous solution for disinfection of 668 central venous catheters in adults during insertion and routine dressing changes showed chlorhexidine to be significantly more effective in reducing catheter related infections (Maki et al, 1991).

Skin disinfectants used for newborns include both chlorhexidine gluconate or povidone-iodine solutions and, less frequently, 70% isopropyl alcohol. Chlorhexidine gluconate is available as a 2% aqueous solution in 4-ounce bottles that must be poured onto sterile gauze for application, and as a tincture of 2% chlorhexidine in isopropyl alcohol (Chloraprep™, Medi-Flex, Inc., Leawood, KS) in single-use packaging of foam sponges or small "sepp" style applicators. This product has been approved for infants >2 months of age, although many nurseries use Chloraprep tincture because it is more convenient and single-use packaging is optimal in terms of infection control practices. However, the combination of two disinfectants (CHG and isopropyl alcohol) has the potential for damaging or irritating skin, particularly in premature infants less than 30 weeks' gestation because of their immature stratum corneum.

Chlorhexidine should not be used as preoperative skin disinfection on the face or head, because misuse has been reported to result in injury if it remains in contact with either the eye or ear during surgical procedures. However, careful use before scalp intravenous or central-line insertion is acceptable, providing that splashing or using excessive amounts of chlorhexidine is avoided. Chlorhexidine is applied in two consecutive wipings or for a 30-second scrubbing period and is removed with sterile water or saline when the procedure is completed.

Povidone-iodine is available in a 10% aqueous solution in a variety of single-use applications. It is also applied in two consecutive wipings or for a 30-second scrubbing period and then allowed to dry for at least 30 seconds before the procedure, and completely removed with sterile water or saline to prevent any further absorption.

Disinfection with isopropyl alcohol is questionable in the neonatal intensive care nursery because it is less efficacious than either povidone-iodine or chlorhexidine and can be irritating and drying to skin surfaces. All disinfectants can cause skin injury, and isopropyl is one of the most irritating (Harpin & Rutter, 1982); using two disinfectants together likely increases this risk (Figure 4-9). There is a need for future studies of disinfectants that may have fewer side effects and comparable efficacy in neonates, such as ethanol products currently used for hand hygiene.

Use of disinfectants for umbilical cord care is debatable. The use of antibiotic ointments and antiseptics can prolong the time to cord separation and seems to have no beneficial effect on the frequency of infection (Zupan & Gardner, 2000). A study of 1811 newborns randomized to receive either routine isopropyl alcohol with each diaper change or natural drying found no umbilical infections in either group, and time to cord separation was reduced from 9.8 days in the alcohol-treated group to 8.16 days in the natural drying group (Dore et al, 1998). Another study randomized 766 newborns to receive either triple dye applied to the umbilical cord immediately after delivery followed by twice daily applications of isopropyl alcohol, or "dry care" without any treatment. Infants in the dry care group were more likely to be colonized with bacteria than the treatment group, and one infant in the dry care group

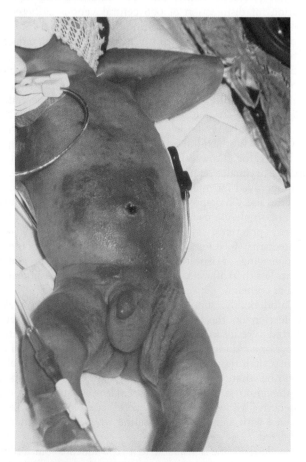

FIGURE **4-9**
Skin injury resulting from skin disinfectant.

developed omphalitis on the third day of life. The days to cord separation were not reported (Janssen et al, 2003). The development of omphalitis is not necessarily related to cord disinfection, as it also occurs in infants who have received topical disinfectants. However, vigilant attention to the signs and symptoms is necessary by health professionals, and parents need guidance about how to manage the umbilical cord and when to consult their health care provider (AWHONN/ NANN Guideline, 2001).

Adhesives

One of the most common practices in the neonatal intensive care nursery is the application and removal of adhesives that secure endotracheal tubes, IV devices, and monitoring probes and electrodes. A research utilization project that involved 2820 premature and term newborns found that adhesives were the primary cause of skin breakdown among NICU patients (Lund et al, 2001a).

Changes in TEWL and skin-barrier function are seen in adults after 10 consecutive removals of adhesive tape and after one removal of adhesive tape in a premature infant. Types of damage from adhesive removal include epidermal stripping, tearing, maceration, tension blisters, chemical irritation, sensitization, and folliculitis (Hoath & Narendran, 2000).

Solvents are sometimes used to prevent discomfort and skin disruption from adhesive removal. They contain hydrocarbon derivatives or petroleum distillates that have potential or proven toxicities. Toxicity is a major concern, especially in premature infants with their underdeveloped stratum corneum, increased skin permeability, larger surface area to body weight, and immature hepatic and renal function. A case report of toxic epidermal necrosis in a premature infant resulted from the use of a solvent. Mineral oil or petrolatum products may be helpful in removing adhesives but cannot be used if the site must be used again for reapplication of adhesives, such as with the retaping of an endotracheal tube.

Skin-bonding agents promote adherence. Unfortunately, they may create a stronger bond between adhesive and epidermis than the fragile cohesion of the epidermis to the dermis; when they are removed, epidermal stripping may result. Plastic polymers have been studied and are reported to reduce skin trauma. An alcohol-free skin protectant is available that is less irritating to skin surfaces in adults than comparable products that contain alcohol. This product has been approved for infants over 30 days of age to treat mild diaper dermatitis and to prevent skin injury from adhesive removal (3M Health Care, 2000). Although a single study from England reports positive effects when using this skin protectant to tape intravenous lines in newborns (Irving, 2001), it has not yet been approved for use in premature infants or term newborns in the United States.

Skin barriers such as karaya rings and pectin products have been used to protect the peristomal skin in adult ostomy patients. A comparison of regular adhesive electrodes and karaya electrodes found less skin disruption, as measured by TEWL, from the karaya electrodes in premature infants. However, some premature infants developed skin irritation from the karaya electrodes, and they are no longer available. Pectin barriers (Hollihesive, Hollister, Libertyville, IL; Duoderm, Conbatec, Gillman, NJ; Comfeel, Coloplast North America, Marietta, GA) have been used beneath adhesives in premature infants and are reported as leaving less visible skin trauma when removed (Dollison & Beckstrand, 1995). Following these reports, a controlled trial of pectin barrier (Hollihesive), plastic tape (Transpore, 3M), and hydrophilic gelled adhesive was done and found significant skin disruption, as measured by TEWL and visual inspection, occurred after removal of both the pectin barrier and plastic tape. Because the adhesives were left in place 24 hours before removal in this study, a time effect of peak adhesive aggressiveness may have been reached. It is interesting to note that significant changes were identified after a single adhesive removal in all three weight groups that were studied (<1000 g, 1001 to 1500 g, >1501 g), thus indicating that even larger premature infants are at risk for skin injury from tape removal.

Prevention of skin trauma from adhesive removal includes minimizing tape use when possible by using smaller pieces, backing the adhesive with cotton, and delaying tape removal until adherence is reduced. Pectin barriers and hydrocolloid adhesives may prove helpful because they mold and adhere well to body contours and often attach better in moist conditions. As with tape, removal of pectin barriers and hydrocolloid should be delayed, if possible, until the adherence lessens. Soft gauze wraps to secure probes and the use of hydrogel ECG electrodes and hydrogel tapes are helpful. Adhesives should be removed with warm water and cotton balls slowly and carefully, and removal by gently pulling the adhesive parallel to the skin surface while holding the skin gently may facilitate removal with fewer traumas (Lund & Tucker, 2003). Mineral oil or an emollient may facilitate adhesive removal if reapplication of adhesives at the site of removal is not necessary.

Transepidermal Water Loss

Because of the poorly keratinized stratum corneum, which provides minimal resistance to the diffusion of water, the preterm infant is subjected to transepidermal water loss (TEWL) and heat loss via evaporation that results in low body temperatures during the first few days after birth. Characteristic skin factors that predispose infants to water loss include larger surface area in relation to body weight, thinner epidermis, increased water content, increased permeability, and increased blood supply that is closer to the skin surface.

TEWL is directly correlated to gestational age and degree of maturation of the epidermal stratum corneum. Mature keratin, which is a major component of the tough, nonliving outer layer of the epidermis, is relatively water impermeable. Because keratin formation is directly related to gestational age, the extremely premature infant is at increased risk for increased evaporative losses. Water easily diffuses across the permeable skin barrier and evaporates. TEWL is influenced by many factors: ambient humidity, gestational age at birth, postnatal age, ambient temperature, weight, activity, and body temperature. Term infants have been shown to have lower TEWL levels compared to adults, with the exception of the antecubital region (Yosipovitch et al, 2000). Infants who are small-for-gestational-age have a lower TEWL in the first day after birth than that of infants of the same gestational age whose weight is appropriate for gestational age.

The highest TEWL levels are seen in extremely premature infants. Water losses of 130 to 160 ml/kg/day have been measured in infants of 23 to 25 weeks' gestation (Agren et al, 1998). Mature barrier function—at one time thought to advance rapidly over a 2-week period in premature infants less than 30 weeks' gestation—has been shown to take longer in extremely premature infants of 23 to 24 weeks' gestation and occurs when the infant reaches approximately 30 to 31 weeks' postconceptional age (Kalia et al, 1998).

Several techniques that have been shown to reduce evaporative heat and TEWL in very-low-birth-weight infants include the use of double-walled incubators, increased ambient humidity, transparent adhesive dressings, and coating the skin with petrolatum-based emollients.

For the past two decades it has been known that insensible water loss is greater under radiant warmers than in incubators without shields. The addition of the heat shield reduced insensible water loss in the incubator but not under the radiant warmer. A plastic blanket under a radiant warmer reduces oxygen consumption, insensible water loss, and radiant-warmer demands. In 1995, Kjartansson et al measured the rate of evaporation from the skin of 12 full-term and 16 preterm infants (gestational age of 25 to 34 weeks), both during incubator care and in care under a radiant warmer. They concluded that the evaporative water loss from the skin depends on the ambient water vapor pressure, irrespective of whether the infant is nursed under a radiant warmer or in an incubator. The higher rate of evaporation during care under a radiant warmer is due to the lower ambient water vapor pressure and not to any direct effect of the nonionizing radiation on the skin. The immediate "microclimate" of the infant needs to be assessed with consideration given to the effect of any heating device being used. This assessment should consider the temperature and relative humidity (RH). A RH below 40% is drying to the skin and leads to excessive TEWL in the extremely premature infant.

Plastic wraps and transparent adhesive dressings have also been shown to reduce TEWL and evaporative heat loss. Immediately after delivery, infants <28 weeks' gestation wrapped with occlusive polyethylene bags covering their torso and extremities had significantly better temperatures than infants who received drying and radiant heat in the delivery room due to significantly reduced evaporative heat and water loss; the wrapping was removed upon admission to the NICU. Mortality also significantly decreased in the infants who were wrapped (Vohra et al, 1999).

Transparent adhesive dressings such as Tegaderm (3M Health Care, St. Paul), OpSite (Smith-Nephew, Inc., Largo, FL), or Bioocclusive (3M) applied to large areas of skin surfaces reduce TEWL. Mancini et al (1994) studied the effect of a nonadhesive semipermeable dressing on the epidermal barrier of 15 premature infants by measuring TEWL on control and on treated skin. Treated skin showed a significantly decreased TEWL on the treated site; TEWL was measured after temporary dressing removal on days 1, 2, 4, and 7. Increased cellular proliferation was documented; this phenomenon is associated with improved epidermal barrier function. High humidity (>70% RH) added to the incubator has been shown to effectively reduce evaporative heat loss and TEWL; using incubators that actively heat and evaporate water separately from circulating heat prevents contamination with microorganisms (Figure 4-10) (Drucker & Marshall, 1995; Marshall, 1997). Application of petrolatum-based emollients, such as Aquaphor ointment (Beiersdorf, Inc., Wilton, CT), every 6 to 12 hours also reduces TEWL and can be used on infants on radiant warmers or under phototherapy without temperature increases or burns (Nopper et al, 1996). Although each of

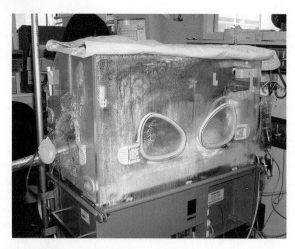

FIGURE **4-10**
Incubator with >70% relative humidity; humidity is generated by heating system that is separate from circulating convective heat to prevent contamination with microorganisms.

three techniques has been shown to be effective, none have been compared; thus it is not clear which is most effective with the fewest side effects. However, addressing the important area of reducing excessive heat loss and TEWL is necessary in the care of the small premature with lung disease to maintain adequate hydration without excessive fluid intake. The goal of maintaining hydration and normal serum sodium levels on an intake of less than 150 ml/kg/day is optimal and achievable using one of these preventive strategies.

MANAGEMENT OF SKIN CARE PROBLEMS

The stratum corneum can be traumatized by a variety of insults, including epidermal stripping from removal of adhesives; burns from transcutaneous oxygen electrodes; pressure sores; infection; nutritional inadequacies, such as zinc and essential fatty acid deficiency; extravasation of intravenous fluids; and diaper dermatitis. The goal of all skin care for neonates should be the maintenance of skin integrity; however, even with meticulous care, skin breakdown can occur.

Skin Assessment

A thorough examination of all skin surfaces on a daily basis will reveal the state of skin integrity in critically ill or extremely premature infants in the NICU. Early signs of skin abrasions or small excoriations may call for either diagnostic or treatment procedures. A skin-assessment tool such as the Neonatal Skin Condition Score (NSCS) (Box 4-2, Figure 4-11), used in the AWHONN/NANN research-based practice project may be beneficial when assessing skin conditions (Lund et al, 2001a, 2000b). The NSCS was found to have both inter- and intrarater reliability, and validity was confirmed by the relationship of the skin scores with birth weight, number of observations over time, and prevalence of infection (Lund & Osborne, 2004). Identifying risk factors for skin injury in individual patients may include gestational age <32 weeks, use of paralytic medications and vasopressors, multiple tubes and lines, numerous monitors and probes, surgical wounds, ostomies, and technologies that limit patient movement such as high-frequency ventilation and extracorporeal membrane oxygenation (ECMO).

From the Association of Women's Health, Obstetric, and Neonatal Nurses (AWHONN) and the National Association of Neonatal Nurses, Skin Care Utilization Project. Copyright 2001, AWHONN.

Skin Excoriations

When a skin excoriation is noted, the first step is to identify the cause of the injury before determining a treatment strategy. In cases in which no trauma has been known to occur, ruling out infectious causes—such as staphylococcal scalded skin syndrome and cutaneous candidiasis—is especially important because these conditions may require culturing and either systemic or topical treatment.

Ointments are sometimes used because of their antibacterial or antifungal properties and also because covering the wound with a semiocclusive layer promotes healing by facilitating the migration of epithelial cells across the surface. Petrolatum-based emollients and ointments are used to cover wounds and provide a semiocclusive layer that facilitates the migrations of epithelial cells across the surface and may actually become part of the stratum corneum layer during the healing process. Antibacterial ointments such as Polysporin, Bacitracin, or Bactroban are useful to treat gram-positive colonized surfaces, but can actually promote the growth of gram-negative organisms (Smack et al, 1996). Many dermatologists recommend against the use of Neosporin because of the potential for developing later sensitization to this ointment, although sensitization to Bacitracin is being reported with increasing frequency (Marks et al, 1995). If fungal infection is suspected, Nystatin ointment is used and can also be applied to surrounding intact skin to prevent extension of the infection. In general, ointments are preferable to creams in this application because of better adherence and healing properties.

Transparent adhesive dressings are made from a polyurethane film, backed with an adhesive that is impermeable to water and bacteria, but allows airflow. There must be a rim of intact skin around the wound to attach the dressing. Uses include wound care, dressings for IV devices—including central venous lines and percutaneous silicone catheters—and prevention of friction injuries to areas such as the knees or sacrum. When used for wound care, a transparent adhesive dressing promotes "moist healing" that allows the rapid migration of epithelial cells across the site. These dressings

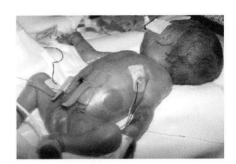

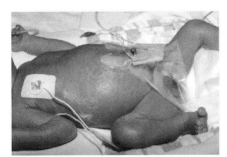

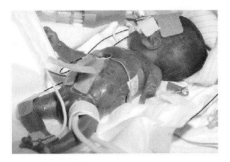

Dryness: 1 = normal, no
                   sign of dry skin
Erythema: 2 = visible
                   erythema <50%
                   body surface
Breakdown: 3 = extensive

Dryness: 2 = dry skin,
                   visible scaling
Erythema: 1 = no evidence of
                   erythema
Breakdown: 1 = none
                   evident

Dryness: 2 = dry skin,
                   visible scaling
Erythema: 3 = visible erythema
                   >50% body surface
Breakdown: 3 = extensive

FIGURE **4-11**
Examples of skin assessments in three infants using the Neonatal Skin Condition Score (NSCS).

should only be used on "clean wounds" (uninfected) because bacteria and fungus can proliferate under the dressing. When placed over a clean wound, a serous or milky exudate often forms and is composed of leukocytes that actually aid in the prevention of infection. The dressings can be left in place for days at a time or until they become loose. Removing and reattaching the dressings on a daily basis is not recommended because the adhesive can injure the intact skin around the wound and further impede healing.

Some of the skin excoriations seen in the patient in the NICU cannot be easily covered with transparent adhesive dressings if no rim of intact skin exists around the site or if it is located in close proximity to other skin that cannot be separated or folds over the excoriation, such as the neck folds and the groin. Treatment of excoriations includes irrigating with sterile normal or half-normal saline every 4 to 6 hours and then leaving the area exposed to air. This simple, basic procedure is effective in keeping the excoriation clean, and it promotes healing with little risk of sensitization or infection. Other types of dressings used in wound management include hydrogel dressings (Vigilon, C Bard Inc., Covington, GA) and hydrocolloid and pectin dressings (Duoderm, Conbatec, Gillman, NJ), both of which promote moist healing. Hydrogel dressings can be used after irrigation of the wound and in conjunction with either antibacterial or antifungal ointment if the wound is infected. These dressings must be changed every 8 to 12 hours because they can dry out. No adhesive can attach these dressings. It is best to avoid placing hydrogel dressings on intact skin surfaces because they can macerate the skin and actually reduce barrier function. Hydrocolloid dressings are used over uninfected wounds and can be left in place for 5 to 7 days while healing takes place (Lund, 1999). Surgical wounds that open or dehisce are infrequent but require expert wound management. Nutrition is often a part of the process in getting these wounds to heal, as is the prevention of infection. Often the surgeon or enterostomal therapist will design the appropriate wound management program for these situations.

Nutritional Deficiencies

Zinc is an essential trace element—essential because it is crucial for growth and development and a trace element because it is present in humans in quantities equal to or less than the quantities in which iron is present. Zinc is a cofactor in the reaction of more than 15 enzymes in many areas of metabolism. It is essential for lymphocyte transformation and is important for the metabolism of proteins, nucleic acids, and mucopolysaccharides of the skin and subcutaneous tissues. It is also an essential part of the enzyme structure of alkaline phosphatase (Prasad, 1995). In addition, zinc is required for normal taste, smell, and wound healing.

Zinc deficiency can result from inadequate intake, malabsorption, excessive loss, or a combination of factors (Coelho et al, 2006; Stevens & Lubitz, 1998). Absorption and excretion of zinc occur primarily through the gastrointestinal tract. Deficiencies are related to abnormal losses of zinc in stool or urine, poor stores, or increased demands, as occur during rapid growth phases or stress. Total body zinc doubles between 32 and 40 weeks' gestation, with two thirds of the maternal-fetal transport occurring during the last 10 weeks of gestation. Premature infants are at special risk for developing a zinc deficiency. Because they have trouble absorbing zinc and have not received adequate stores before birth, they may be in negative zinc balance for several weeks after birth. Other infants at risk for zinc deficiency include those with gastrointestinal pathology, chronic diarrhea, short-gut or short-bowel syndrome with jejunoileal bypass, necrotizing enterocolitis, or an ileostomy.

The clinical manifestations of zinc deficiency include lethargy, growth retardation, skin lesions, alopecia, and diarrhea; the striking sign of zinc deficiency, however, is some form of skin lesions. Common sites of involvement are the groin and perianal area, the neck folds, and the face, particularly the angles of the mouth and the cheeks. Lesions have also been noted at sites of trauma, such as endotracheal and cardiac monitor tape sites. The skin lesions are reddened, scaly, and moist. The skin eruption of zinc deficiency strongly resembles acrodermatitis enteropathica, a rare autosomal recessive disorder of zinc malabsorption and deficiency, in its morphologic features and distribution.

Zinc deficiency can result from inadequate intake of zinc. The routine supplementation of trace minerals in parenteral nutrition solutions has eliminated much of the zinc deficiency seen in the past. It is still seen in some premature infants who are exclusively breastfed. For infants receiving total parenteral nutrition, zinc supplementation is 250 mcg/kg/day for term infants under 3 months of age and 400 mcg/kg/day for premature infants (Zenk, 1999). Oral supplementation with zinc sulfate ranges from 1 to 3 mg/kg/day. Recovery from zinc deficiency is dramatic once adequate zinc supplementation has begun. In general, skin conditions caused by nutritional deficiencies are often confused with infections and other irritants but do not respond until the deficiency state itself is treated.

Intravenous Extravasations

The extravasation of intravenous fluids and medications can result in skin injury and, in some cases, deep-tissue injury to muscle and nerves (Figure 4-12). The most serious extravasation injuries are iatrogenic complications that can lead to pain, prolonged hospitalization, and increased morbidity, such as infection. Extravasation injuries can also result in increased hospital costs and the potential for legal action. Despite vigilant nursing assessment, intravenous extravasations do occur in about 11% of patients in the NICU. Tissue sloughing occurs in as many as 43.6% of these infants. Therefore nursing actions such as the monitoring of intravenous sites and other preventive strategies as well as immediate interventions that can reduce the extent of tissue injury are important considerations for all nurseries that care for newborns with intravenous devices for fluid administration and medications. Some of the risk factors for tissue injury from intravenous extravasations in NICU patients are listed in Box 4-3.

Another risk factor is compromised perfusion to the skin, as evidenced by the poor capillary refill exhibited by the most critically ill neonates or by the obstructed venous circulations seen with taping methods that constrict the extremities in which the intravenous device is placed.

Prevention of skin injury after infiltration is the first important consideration. Strategies include ensuring that the insertion site is clearly visible by using transparent adhesive dressing or clear tape to secure the device and observing the site with appropriate documentation every hour. In addition, the tape should be carefully placed on the extremity to avoid obstruction of venous return. Tape placed loosely over a bony promi-

---

BOX 4-3

Risks for Tissue Injury from Intravenous Extravasations

Some of the factors known to increase the risk of tissue injury include:
- The length of exposure after extravasation occurs, especially when the patients are unable to verbalize the discomfort of pain or pressure.
- The nature of the drug or solution; hypertonic solutions with high concentrations of calcium, potassium, glucose, or amino acids and medications such as nafcillin have been identified as high-risk for causing injury.
- The mechanical compression caused by electronic infusion pumps.

---

nence, such as the knee or elbow, permits extravasated fluids and medications to disperse over a larger surface area and thus reduce the risk of injury, compared with extravasation that is limited to a small surface area. Avoiding extremities with poor perfusion in favor of better-perfused scalp veins (except, of course, those on the forehead) may also be prudent; in some cases, the wiser choice may be the placement of central venous lines for access. Nursery policies that limit the glucose (<12.5%), amino acid (<2%), and calcium (10%) concentrations are also strategies to reduce the risk of tissue injury from the extravasation of intravenous fluids and medications.

Once an intravenous extravasation has been identified, immediate measures to reduce injury are instituted. The device should be carefully removed, and the extremity should be elevated (if it is an arm or leg). Treatment with heat or moisture is not recommended because the delicate tissue could be further injured by a burn or the effects of maceration. If tissue damage is visible, the use of a topical antimicrobial ointment and petrolatum-impregnated gauze to facilitate healing is instituted. In the most severe cases of deep-tissue necrosis after extravasation injury, a surgical or plastic surgery consultation is necessary, and skin grafts may be needed (Figure 4-13). In all cases of tissue injury, the open wound should be considered to be a potential portal for infection, and topical or systemic treatment may be required.

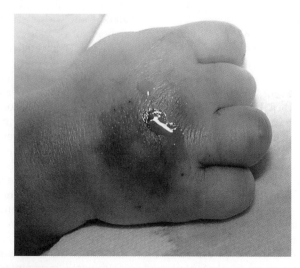

FIGURE 4-12
IV extravasation injury with swelling, discoloration, and leaking of fluid.

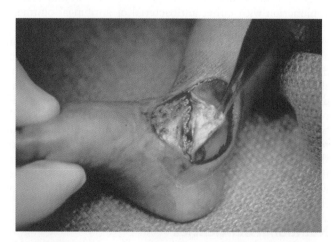

FIGURE 4-13
This IV extravasation injury will require plastic surgery.

Hyaluronidase is an enzyme that facilitates diffusion of the extravasated fluids by temporarily dissolving the normal interstitial barriers, reducing tissue damage (Banta & Noerr, 1992; Raszka et al, 1990; Laurie et al, 1984). It is currently available as Vitrase (Ista Pharmaceuticals, Inc., Irvine, CA) or Amphadase (Amphastar Pharmaceuticals, Inc., Rancho Cucamonga, CA), although this formulation contains thimerosal as a preservative, whereas Vitrase does not. An alternative to intervention with hyaluronidase includes making multiple puncture holes over the area of greatest swelling and squeezing or allowing the fluid to leak out of the tissue to release the infiltrated fluid and potentially prevent skin injury (Chandavasu et al, 1986).

Diaper Dermatitis

A common skin disruption that occurs in neonates and infants is diaper dermatitis (diaper rash). This term encompasses a range of processes that affect the perineum, groin, thighs, buttocks, and anal area of infants who are incontinent and wear some covering to collect urine and feces. Diaper dermatitis can be caused by many different mechanisms, but the condition of the skin has a direct role in the progression of skin injury.

The pathogenesis of diaper dermatitis is partly related to the degree of wetness of the skin. Skin that is moist and macerated becomes more permeable and susceptible to injury because wetness increases friction. In addition, moisture-laden skin is more likely to contain microorganisms than dry skin is.

Another component in the process of skin injury from diaper dermatitis is the effect of an alkaline pH. The normal skin pH is acidic—ranging between 4.0 and 5.5—but can become alkaline when it is exposed to urine, which generally has a higher pH. It is the resulting increased pH of the skin—not the effect of ammonia in urine, as previously thought—that increases its vulnerability to injury and penetration by microorganisms. Another problem associated with increased pH of the skin is that it stimulates fecal enzyme activity. Specifically, both protease and lipase, which are found in stool, can injure the skin, which is made up of protein and fat components. These enzymes can cause significant injury to the epidermis fairly quickly and are responsible for the contact irritant diaper dermatitis that is commonly seen.

Once the epidermis has been impaired or becomes a less efficient barrier because of one of the aforementioned mechanisms, invasion by bacteria or fungus can occur. Thus a contact irritant diaper dermatitis can turn into a staphylococcal or fungal rash if this progression occurs. S. aureus can be found in large numbers on the skin surface, especially if it is inflamed or impaired, and can result in secondary infection. The classic presentation for S. aureus is pustule formation at the site of hair follicles, although the overall incidence of S. aureus complicated diaper dermatitis is quite low.

Fungal rashes, primarily those caused by C. albicans, may have different mechanisms of invasion. Many researchers have identified C. albicans as a secondary invader of skin that has been injured by other mechanisms, whereas others suggest that C. albicans is a primary causative factor in diaper dermatitis. This theory is based on the ability of C. albicans to penetrate the stratum corneum, especially in a warm and moist environment, such as that found under an occlusive diaper. The resulting intense inflammation is significant and appears as brightly erythematous, sharply marginated dermatitis that involves the

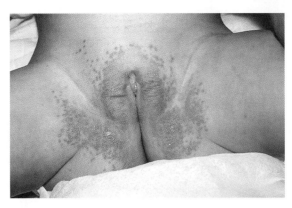

FIGURE **4-14**
Candida diaper dermatitis involving labia and inguinal folds with characteristic satellite lesions.

inguinal folds as well as the buttocks, thighs, abdomen, and genitalia, characteristically with satellite lesions that may extend the rash over the trunk (Figure 4-14). The gastrointestinal tract is often the reservoir for C. albicans, and it can frequently be recovered in stool. Thus oral therapy may be indicated, especially if evidence of oral infection, such as thrush, is apparent.

Some diaper dermatitis can be the result of a primary dermatologic condition, such as psoriasis, eczema, and seborrheic dermatitis. Significant family history of these skin conditions may identify infants who are especially vulnerable to developing severe reactions to inflammation in the diaper area.

Management

Prevention is the first goal of intervention and is paramount in breaking the cycle of diaper dermatitis. Frequent diaper changes result in skin that is drier with a more normal pH and thus maintain the functional barrier of the skin. Strategies to keep the skin dry also include the use of highly absorbent gelled diapers that act to "wick" moisture away from the skin. Use of talcum powders has been discouraged because of the risk of inhalation of silicone particles into the respiratory tract.

Once diaper dermatitis occurs—and it is not completely avoidable in most infants—protection of injured skin during healing is the primary goal. Use of a generous layer of protective skin barriers that contain zinc oxide prevents further trauma and allows impaired skin to heal (Figure 4-15). Opening the skin to light and air is not effective if the fecal contents are allowed to have direct contact with already injured areas. Because protective skin barriers tend to adhere well to the skin, it is neither necessary nor desirable to completely remove them during diaper changes before more cream is applied. It is best to generously apply more cream to the site to protect the area from further injury.

Multiple products are used in the care of diaper dermatitis—including topical emollients, diaper rash balms, and wipes—but product selection is often affected by myth and tradition, rather than science. A damp diaper covered with a plastic coating enhances the risk of irritation and percutaneous absorption. The risk of absorption is even greater in newborns and premature infants because of their large surface area to body weight ratio and immature skin. The various compounds and numerous chemicals used have been described extensively (Siegfried & Shah, 1999; Siegfried, 2001), with concerns raised

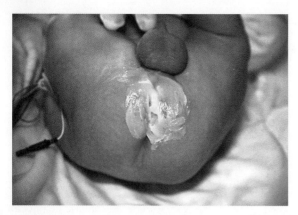

FIGURE **4-15**
Use of thick layer of a skin barrier such as zinc oxide or pectin paste will prevent reinjury of skin damage in diaper dermatitis.

From the Association of Women's Health, Obstetric, and Neonatal Nurses (AWHONN) and the National Association of Neonatal Nurses Skin Care Utilization Project. Copyright 2001, AWHONN.

> ### BOX **4-4**
>
> ## Elements of the AWHONN/NANN Evidence-Based Practice Guideline: Neonatal Skin Care
>
> 1. Newborn skin assessment
> 2. Bathing, including first bath, routine, and immersion bathing
> 3. Cord care
> 4. Circumcision care
> 5. Disinfectants
> 6. Diaper dermatitis
> 7. Adhesives
> 8. Transepidermal water loss (TEWL)
> 9. Skin breakdown
> 10. IV infiltration
> 11. Skin nutrition

about potential toxicity, irritancy, and later sensitization. Simple, inexpensive products such as zinc oxide ointment are recommended over more complex compounds.

Treatment of diaper dermatitis that is solely due to invasion with *C. albicans* requires the use of antifungal creams or ointments. Some of the antifungal preparations include nystatin, miconazole, and clotrimazole. If the diaper dermatitis involves both fungus and a contact irritant component, alternating applications of the topical creams or ointments is effective.

Severe diaper dermatitis with deep excoriations can be seen in infants with severe malabsorption syndrome secondary to intestinal resection or mucosal injury. Other infants at risk for severe diaper dermatitis include those with symptomatic opiate withdrawal, spina bifida, and exstrophy of the bladder with loss of anal sphincter tone. In these cases, the stool is extremely caustic and contains a higher level of enzyme activity, a lower pH as the result of rapid transit through the intestine, and significant amounts of undigested carbohydrates. Stool frequency is often greatly increased. In cases of loss of sphincter tone, fecal material constantly dribbles to the perianal area.

Although skin disruption frequently becomes the focus of nursing interventions, this symptom may be a significant indication of more serious physiologic concerns. These infants' stools should be carefully monitored by documentation of number, volume, pH, and carbohydrate testing. The infants must be observed for the dehydration caused by extensive water losses in diarrhea. Once dietary manipulations and hydration have stabilized the general physiologic status, a program of skin protection is imperative because some level of chronic diarrhea may be ongoing for many weeks or months. Products such as pectin-based powders or pectin-containing pastes without alcohol may be better barriers to the caustic, constant fecal irritation if traditional zinc oxide creams do not work adequately. If yeast is present, antifungal creams may be applied in conjunction with protective barriers.

EVIDENCE-BASED SKIN CARE GUIDELINE

Many intensive care and newborn nurseries have written protocols for various aspects of neonatal skin care. Recently, two national nursing organizations, the Association of Women's Health, Obstetrics and Neonatal Nurses (AWHONN) and the National Association of Neonatal Nurses (NANN), collaborated in the development of a comprehensive evidence-based neonatal skin care guideline. An extensive review of the scientific basis for neonatal skin care was undertaken by a team including advanced practice nurses and a pediatric dermatologist (Lund et al, 1999), and a neonatal skin guideline was written to address 11 aspects of skin care (Box 4-4). Following this report, 50 nurseries agreed to participate in a research-based practice project to implement and evaluate this guideline for their patients. The project involved identifying coordinators at each site who were willing to collect baseline information about the skin condition of infants in their units, implement the practice guideline in their respective units, and then collect skin condition information again once the guideline had been introduced. Issues of safety and feasibility were important, as was the evaluation of the impact of evidence-based practice on skin condition.

More than 11,000 skin observations using the Neonatal Skin Condition Score (NSCS) were performed on 2820 newborns of varying gestational ages and weights. An improvement in skin condition was observed after implementation of the guideline, as evidenced by overall lower scores on the NSCS during the observation period. Initial scores were similar in both the preguideline and postguideline groups but improved more rapidly after the guideline had been implemented. The results were more dramatic in the low-birth-weight infants, but improvement was seen in the "well-baby" sample as well. Reduction in the frequency of bathing and fewer baths given with cleansers were noted, thus showing compliance with the guideline. An increase in the use of emollients was also documented.

Positive blood cultures did not increase after the guideline had been implemented (Lund et al, 2001a). AWHONN and NANN both offer the neonatal skin care evidence-based clinical practice guideline as well as educational materials for both members and nonmembers (AWHONN/NANN Guideline 2001).

SUMMARY

Neonatal skin management is a complex problem that requires a collaborative approach. Some research has been conducted in this area, but a lot remains to be done regarding the use of routine NICU equipment and its impact on neonatal skin, the use of skin barriers for protection, and the effect of a consistent approach to skin care on the integrity of neonatal skin. This chapter has outlined the development and structure of the skin. It has addressed differences in the skin based on gestational age variations. Normal physiologic as well as common dermatologic abnormalities have been presented. Evidence-based neonatal skin care is recommended and has proven to be feasible and safe and to result in improvement in skin condition for newborns.

Case Study

IDENTIFICATION OF THE PROBLEM

This extremely premature infant was admitted to the NICU 3 days ago with RDS; birthweight 650 g, gestational age 24 0/7 weeks. He has an endotracheal tube and is receiving assisted ventilation; catheters are inserted in both the umbilical artery and vein for blood sampling, blood pressure monitoring, and administration of IV fluids. An area of skin breakdown is noted on the abdomen where a temperature probe had been placed and removed on the first day of life. By day 3 the area is erythematous and oozing a yellow-tinged fluid. Surrounding areas are also quite red.

ASSESSMENT: HISTORY AND PHYSICAL EXAMINATION

The infant, a baby boy, was born via vaginal delivery to a 30-year-old G1P1 mother. The pregnancy was complicated by preterm labor starting at 20 weeks, and a cervical circlage was performed. A month later the mother was again hospitalized with PROM and preterm labor. This time the efforts to stop labor were unsuccessful, and the infant was delivered vaginally 48 hours after a single course of betamethasone was administered.

The infant's Apgars were 4 and 7. Birthweight was 650 g, and gestational age was 24 0/7 weeks. The infant was intubated in the delivery room due to poor respiratory effort, and an initial dose of surfactant was administered. The infant was placed immediately into a polyurethane bag for reduction of evaporative heat and fluid loss in the delivery. Upon arrival in the NICU, the infant was placed on a combination radiant warmer/incubator table for insertion of umbilical catheters. After catheters were placed and position confirmed with a radiograph, the top of the heating device was lowered and converted to a convectively heated incubator with relative humidity set at 80%.

The infant's skin was very moist and fragile in appearance. After placement of the umbilical catheters, the periumbilical skin was cleansed with sterile water to remove the skin disinfectant; however, the skin was noted to be more erythematous than prior to insertion. A temperature probe was attached to the abdomen with a hydrogel electrode, which promptly slid off as a result of the high humidity in the environment. An adhesive-backed foil probe cover was used to secure the catheter.

DIFFERENTIAL DIAGNOSIS

The chief differential diagnoses for an extremely premature infant with skin breakdown includes trauma from adhesive removal, chemical burn from disinfectant used for periumbilical skin preparation, and infection. Although the original problem may be trauma, the wound can also be infected by microorganisms on the skin surface.

DIAGNOSTIC TESTS

A skin culture with Gram stain and KOH prep is obtained from the area of breakdown. A CBC is obtained, as well as a blood culture. Although a catheter urine culture is requested, this is not obtained due to the extremely small size of the infant's penis and urethra; a "clean" bag specimen is collected instead.

WORKING DIAGNOSIS

The Gram stain and KOH prep show budding yeast within 24 hours. The skin culture later shows a heavy growth of *Candida albicans*. The blood and urine show no growth of microorganisms after 72 hours. The CBC shows the WBC remain unchanged from the first sample sent on the day of admission, but the platelet count has dropped from 100,000 to 60,000.

DEVELOPMENT OF MANAGEMENT PLAN

After the Gram stain and KOH prep report, the area of breakdown appeared more extensive and the skin over the abdomen erythematous. The excoriated skin was gently debrided using a 30 ml syringe with warmed, one half normal saline gently squirted through a 20-gauge Teflon catheter. Antifungal ointment, rather than cream or powder, was selected for topical treatment because of the potential healing benefits of ointments. The humidity level of the incubator was empirically decreased to 60%.

Because of the proximity of the excoriation to the umbilical catheters, a decision was made to place a percutaneous central line and peripheral arterial line so that the umbilical catheters could be discontinued.

IMPLEMENTATION AND EVALUATION OF EFFECTIVENESS

After receiving the preliminary culture report and noting the drop in platelet count, it was determined that further evaluation for systemic illness would be necessary. A subsequent platelet count was 45,000, and this, coupled with the need for dopamine infusion for hypotension, prompted the medical decision to initiate systemic antifungal treatment. Amphotericin B infusion was begun, and a platelet transfusion was also administered.

Continued

Case Study—cont'd

After a second platelet transfusion, the platelet count had stabilized at 90,000 by the fifth day of treatment with Amphotericin B. Careful monitoring for hypokalemia and renal and hepatic function as potential toxicity from Amphotericin therapy was carried out.

Despite having no growth of *Candida albicans* from blood or urine samples, fungal infections in extremely premature infants can initially be cutaneous infections. If not treated early, this can quickly progress to disseminated *Candida* infections involving the blood, urinary tract, cerebrospinal fluid, or other organs.

Factors associated with cutaneous fungal infections in the first week of life are instrumentation procedures, such as circlage placement, and PROM. The infant can thus be colonized from maternal fungal or bacterial flora. Additional risk factors are skin breakdown from trauma or irritation, and glucosuria. Several authors recommend early, aggressive management of cutaneous manifestations of fungal infection to prevent further dissemination and systemic complications.

REFERENCES

3M Health Care (2000). *3M Cavilon No Sting Skin Barrier Film* (brochure). St Paul, MN: Author.

Agren J et al (1998). Transepidermal water loss in infants born at 24 and 25 weeks of gestation. *Acta paediatrica* 87:1185-1190.

American Academy of Pediatrics (1997). *Red book: report of the committee on infectious diseases*, ed 24. Elk Grove Village, IL: Author.

Anderson GC et al (1995). Axillary temperature in transitional newborn infants before and after tub bath. *Applied nursing research* 8:123-128.

Association of Women's Health, Obstetric, and Neonatal Nurses (AWHONN) and National Association of Neonatal Nurses (NANN) (2001). *Evidence-based clinical practice guideline: neonatal skin care*. Washington, DC: AWHONN.

Banta C, Noerr B (1992). Hyaluronidase. *Neonatal network* 11:103-105.

Bryanton J et al (2004). Tub bathing versus traditional sponge bathing for the newborn. *Journal of obstetric, gynecologic, and neonatal nursing* 33:704-712.

Campbell J et al (2000). Systemic candidiasis in extremely low birth weight infants receiving topical petrolatum ointment for care: a case control study. *Pediatrics* 1055:1041-1045.

Chandavasu O et al (1986). A new method for the prevention of skin sloughs and necrosis secondary to intravenous infiltration. *American journal of perinatology* 3:4-5.

Coelho S et al (2006). Transient zinc deficiency in a breast fed, premature infant. *European journal of dermatology* 16(2):193-195.

Cohen BA (2001). Disorders of the subcutaneous tissue. In Eichenfield LA et al, editors. *Textbook of neonatal dermatology*. Philadelphia: Saunders.

Cunningham BB, Wagner AM (2001). Diagnostic and therapeutic procedures. In Eichenfield LA et al, editors. *Textbook of neonatal dermatology*. Philadelphia: Saunders.

Darmstadt GL, Dinulos JG (2001). Bacterial infections. In Eichenfield LA et al, editors. *Textbook of neonatal dermatology*. Philadelphia: Saunders.

Dollison E, Beckstrand J (1995). Adhesive tape vs. pectin-based barrier use in preterm infants. *Neonatal network* 14:35-39.

Dore S et al (1998). Alcohol versus natural drying for newborn cord care. *Journal of obstetrics, gynecology, and neonatal nursing* 27:621-627.

Drolet BA, Esterly NB (2002). The skin. In Fanaroff AA, Martin RJ, editors. *Neonatal-perinatal medicine: diseases of the fetus and infant*, ed 7. St Louis: Mosby.

Drucker D, Marshall N (1995). Humidification without risk of infection in the Draeger incubator 8000. *Neonatal intensive care* 8:44-46.

Edwards W et al (2004). The effect of prophylactic ointment therapy on nosocomial sepsis rates and skin integrity in infants of birthweights 501–1000 grams. *Pediatrics* 113:1195-1203.

Enjolras O, Garzon MC (2001). Vascular stains, malformations, and tumors. In Eichenfield LA et al, editors. *Textbook of neonatal dermatology*. Philadelphia: Saunders.

Fine JD et al (1999). *Epidermolysis bullosa: clinical, epidemiologic, and laboratory advances and the findings of the National Epidermolysis Bullosa Registry*. Baltimore: Johns Hopkins University Press.

Fine JD et al (2000). Revised classification system for inherited epidermolysis bullosa: report of the Second International Consensus Meeting on diagnosis and classification of epidermolysis bullosa. *Journal of the American Academy of Dermatology* 42:700-702.

Fox C et al (1998). The timing of skin acidification in very low birth weight infants. *Journal of perinatology* 18:272-275.

Franck L et al (2000). Effect of less frequent bathing of preterm infants on skin flora and pathogen colonization. *Journal of obstetrics, gynecology, and neonatal nursing* 29:584-589.

Frieden IJ, Howard R (2001). Vesicles, pustules, bullae, erosions, and ulcerations. In Eichenfield LA et al, editors. *Textbook of neonatal dermatology*. Philadelphia: Saunders.

Garland J et al (1995). Comparison of 10% povidone-iodine and 0.5% chlorhexidine gluconate for the prevention of peripheral intravenous catheter colonization in neonates: a prospective trial. *Pediatric infectious disease journal* 14:510-516.

Gfatter R et al (1997). Effects of soap and detergents on skin surface pH, stratum corneum hydration and fat content in infants. *Dermatology* 195:258-262.

Gordon C et al (1995). Topical iodine and neonatal hypothyroidism. *Archives of pediatric and adolescent medicine* 149:1336-1339.

Harpin V, Rutter N (1982). Percutaneous alcohol absorption and skin necrosis in a preterm infant. *Archives of disease in childhood* 57:477-479.

Harpin VA, Rutter N (1983). Barrier properties of the newborn infant's skin. *Journal of pediatrics* 102(3):419-425.

Herane MI, Ando I (2003). Acne in infancy and acne genetics. *Dermatology* 206(1):24-28.

Hoath S, Narendran V (2000). Adhesives and emollients in the preterm infant. *Seminars in neonatology* 5:112-119.

Hoath S, Pickins WL (2003). The biology and role of vernix. In Hoath S, Maibach H, editors. *Neonatal skin: structure and function*, ed 2. New York: Marcel Dekker.

Hoath S et al (2001). The biology and role of vernix. *Newborn and infant nursing reviews* 1:53-58.

Irving V (2001). Reducing the risk of epidermal stripping in the neonatal population: an evaluation of an alcohol free barrier film. *Journal of neonatal nursing* 7:5-8.

Janssen PA et al (2003). To dye or not to dye: a randomized, clinical trial of a triple dye/alcohol regime versus dry cord care. *Pediatrics* 111:15-20.

Kalia YN et al (1998). Development of the skin barrier function in premature infants. *Journal of investigative dermatology* 111:320-326.

Karl D (1999). The interactive newborn bath: using infant behavior to connect parents and newborns. *American journal of maternal/child nursing* 24:280-286.

Kjartansson S et al (1995). Water loss from the skin of term and preterm infants nursed under a radiant heater. *Pediatric research* 37(2):233-238.

Landau M, Krafchik B (1999). The diagnostic values of café au lait macules. *Journal of the American Academy of Dermatology* 40:877-890.

Laurie S et al (1984). Intravenous extravasation injuries: the effectiveness of hyaluronidase in their treatment. *Annals of plastic surgery* 13:191-194.

Linder N et al (1997). Topical iodine-containing antiseptics and subclinical hypothyroidism in preterm infants. *Journal of pediatrics* 131:434-439.

Loomis CA, Birge MB (2001). Fetal skin development. In Eichenfield LA et al, editors. *Textbook of neonatal dermatology*. Philadelphia: Saunders.

Lucky AW (2001). Transient benign cutaneous lesions in the newborn. In Eichenfield LA et al, editors. *Textbook of neonatal dermatology.* Philadelphia: Saunders.

Lund C (1999). Prevention and management of infant skin breakdown. *Nursing clinics of North America* 34:907-920.

Lund C, Osborne JW (2004). Validity and reliability of the neonatal skin condition score. *Journal of obstetrics, gynecology, and neonatal nursing* 33:320-327.

Lund C, Tucker J (2003). Skin adhesion. In Hoath S, Maibach H, editors. *Neonatal skin: structure and function,* ed 2. New York: Marcel Dekker.

Lund C et al (1999). Neonatal skin care: the scientific basis for practice. *Journal of obstetrics, gynecology, and neonatal nursing* 28:241-254.

Lund C et al (2001a). Neonatal skin care: clinical outcomes of the AWHONN/NANN evidence-based clinical practice guideline. *Journal of obstetrics, gynecology, and neonatal nursing* 30:41-51.

Lund C et al (2001b). Neonatal skin care: evaluation of the AWHONN/NANN research-based practice project on knowledge and skin care practices. *Journal of obstetrics, gynecology, and neonatal nursing* 30:30-40.

Maki D et al (1991). Prospective randomized trial povidone-iodine, alcohol, and chlorhexidine for prevention of infection associated with central venous and arterial catheters. *Lancet* 338:339-343.

Malathi I et al (1993). Skin disinfection in preterm infants. *Archives of disease in children* 69:312-316.

Mancini AJ (2004). Skin. *Pediatrics* 113:114-119.

Mancini A et al (1994). Semipermeable dressings improve epidermal barrier function in premature infants. *Pediatric research* 36:306-314.

Margileth AM (2005). Dermatologic conditions. In Avery G et al, editors. *Neonatology: pathophysiology and management of the newborn,* ed 6. Philadelphia: Lippincott.

Marinkovich MP (1999). Update on inherited bullous dermatoses. *Dermatology clinics* 17(3):473-485.

Marks J et al (1995). North American Contact Dermatitis Group standard tray patch test results. *American journal of contact dermatitis* 6:160-165.

Marshall A (1997). Humidifying the environment for the premature neonate: maintenance of a thermoneutral environment. *Journal of neonatal nursing* 3:32-36.

Mimoz O et al (1999). Chlorhexidine compared with povidone-iodine as skin preparation before blood culture. *Annals of internal medicine* 131:834-837.

Moore KL, Persaud TVN (2003). *The developing human: clinically oriented embryology,* ed 7. Philadelphia: Saunders.

Niamba P et al (1998). Is common neonatal cephalic pustulosis (neonatal acne) triggered by *Malassezia furfur?* *Archives of dermatology* 134(8):995-998.

Nopper A et al (1996). Topical ointment therapy benefits premature infants. *Journal of pediatrics* 128:660-669.

Parravicini E et al (1996). Iodine, thyroid function, and very low birth weight infants. *Pediatrics* 98:730-734.

Penny-MacGillivray T (1996). A newborn's first bath: when? *Journal of obstetrics, gynecology, and neonatal nursing* 25:481-487.

Prasad AS (1995). Zinc: an overview. *Nutrition* 11:93-99.

Rapelanoro R et al (1996). Neonatal *Malassezia furfur* pustulosis. *Archives of dermatology* 132:190-193.

Raszka W et al (1990). The use of hyaluronidase in the treatment of intravenous extravasation injuries. *Journal of perinatology* 10:146-149.

Rowen JL et al (1995). Invasive fungal dermatitis in the <1000 gram neonate. *Pediatrics* 95:682-687.

Sethi R et al (1996). Oculocutaneous albinism. *Cutis* 57:397-400.

Sekkat N et al (2004). Development of an in vitro model for premature neonatal skin: biophysical characterization using transepidermal water loss. *Journal of pharmacological sciences* 93(12):2936-2940.

Siegfried EG (2001). Neonatal skin care and toxicology. In Eichenfield LA et al, editors. *Textbook of neonatal dermatology.* Philadelphia: Saunders.

Siegfried EC, Shah PY (1999). Skin care practices in the neonatal nursery: a clinical survey. *Journal of perinatology* 19:31-39.

Smack DP et al (1996). Infection and allergy incidence in ambulatory surgery patients using white petrolatum vs. bacitracin ointment: a randomized controlled trial. *Journal of the American Medical Association* 276:972-977.

Smith JF et al (1997). Fetal laceration injury at cesarean delivery. *Obstetrics and gynecology* 90:344-346.

Stevens J, Lubitz L (1998). Symptomatic zinc deficiency in breastfed term and premature infants. *Journal of paediatric child health* 34:97-100.

Torrelo A et al (2005). Severe acne infantum successfully treated with isotretinoin. *Pediatric dermatology* 22(4):357-359.

Varda K, Behnke R (2000). The effect of timing of initial bath on newborn's temperature. *Journal of obstetrics, gynecology, and neonatal nursing* 29:27-32.

Vohra S et al (1999). Effect of polyethylene occlusive skin wrapping on heat loss in very low birth weight infants at delivery: a randomized trial. *Journal of pediatrics* 134:547-551.

Williams ML (2001). Skin of the premature infant. In Eichenfield LA et al, editors. *Textbook of neonatal dermatology.* Philadelphia: Saunders.

Woodruff CA, Herbert AA (2002). Neonatal primary cutaneous aspergillosis: case reports and review of the literature. *Journal of pediatric dermatology* 19:439-444.

Yosipovitch G et al (2000). Skin barrier properties in different body areas in neonates. *Pediatrics* 106:105-108.

Zenk K (1999). *Neonatal medications and nutrition: a comprehensive guide.* Santa Rosa, CA: NICU Ink.

Zupan J, Gardner P (2000). Topical umbilical cord care at birth. *The Cochrane database of systematic reviews* 3:34-82.

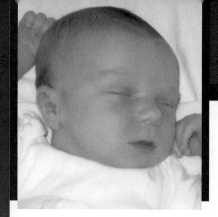

Chapter 5

Gastrointestinal System

Janet Thigpen

The intake and digestion of foodstuffs and the elimination of waste products are critical to long-term survival. Although many complex metabolic processes are involved, the ability to maintain adequate nutrition ultimately requires that the gastrointestinal (GI) tract be patent and structurally intact. With only a few exceptions, the vast majority of conditions that cause GI dysfunction are the result of congenital anatomic malformations. The discovery and management of GI dysfunction requires knowledge of both embryogenesis and normal anatomy. Although some anomalies involve external defects and are immediately apparent, most causes of dysfunction may initially cause few symptoms unless allowed to progress to the point at which serious pathophysiologic changes present a major threat to life. The input and support of a variety of nursing, medical, and other specialists are required for optimal outcomes—that is, the infant's physiologic well-being and the parents' psychosocial stability. The emotional needs of parents and their work through the process of grief over the loss of the expected "perfect" child cannot be underestimated. Visible defects, especially those involving the face, appear to be particularly difficult for parents to accept. Frequently GI malformations are associated with other congenital anomalies and prematurity, and the need for transport to a distant center where corrective surgery can be accomplished places additional demands on parental coping.

The GI tract is the site of the many complex transport and enzymatic mechanisms required for the biologic absorption and digestion of nutrients. The successful intake and assimilation of these nutrients, however, rests on the capability of the gut to act as a conduit for ingestion, digestion, and elimination. Congenital malformations, particularly those involving anatomic or functional obstruction, clearly hinder this process. Even when structurally intact, the supporting gastric and intestinal musculature of the newborn is relatively deficient, making peristaltic movements more infrequent and irregular when compared with those of adults, thus increasing the tendency toward distention. Transport of materials through the tract is further diminished in premature infants who may have poor sucking and swallowing abilities, small gastric capacity, and incompetent cardioesophageal sphincter. Debilitated, hypotonic infants may similarly exhibit poor sucking and swallowing and decreased motility. In addition, the bowel seems particularly susceptible to ischemic conditions in which blood flow is preferentially directed away from the GI tract (as well as the kidneys and peripheral vascular bed) toward the brain and heart.

Untoward effects of drugs commonly used in the nursery may further compromise intestinal function or integrity. Morphine, for example, in addition to its desired analgesic effect, also slows gastric emptying and reduces propulsive peristalsis. Conversely, the antibiotic erythromycin has been shown to accelerate gastric emptying. Ulceration of the GI tract with possible bleeding and perforation are reported side effects of tolazoline, dexamethasone, and indomethacin (Zenk et al, 2003). Mydriatics administered for ophthalmologic examination in the preterm infant decrease duodenal activity and gastric emptying (James, 2002). Xanthines may cause or exacerbate gastroesophageal reflux (Jadcherla, 2002). The major purposes of this chapter are to discuss the normal anatomic structure of the GI tract and to describe common causes of neonatal dysfunction and their implications for care.

PHYSIOLOGY OF THE GASTROINTESTINAL TRACT

The major function of the GI tract is to transfer food and water from the external to the internal environment, where they can be digested, absorbed, and distributed to the cells of the body by the circulatory system. While these processes are occurring, contractions of the smooth muscle lining the walls of the intestine move the contents through the lumen, releasing any material not digested and absorbed during transit back into the external environment. This released material is composed of very few "waste products." Although some end products, such as the breakdown products of hemoglobin, are contained in the stool, most metabolic end products are actually eliminated from the body by the kidneys and lungs.

Structure

The GI tract consists of a tube of variable diameter with the same general structure throughout most of its length. Moving from the outside inward toward the lumen, six concentric layers in the wall of the intestine can be identified (Figure 5-1). The first, outermost layer is composed of connective tissue. In the esophagus, where the connective layer is continuous with the deep fascia, it is called the adventitia; in all other portions of the gut, the connective-tissue layer is covered with peritoneal epithelial cells and is called the serosa. The next two layers are both made up of smooth muscle—but with each exhibiting a different orientation of its muscle fibers. The outer layer of muscle has its fibers running longitudinally along the gut; the fibers in the inner muscle layer circle the gut. The fourth layer, the submucosa, is composed primarily of connective tissue as well as a few exocrine gland cells, blood vessels, and lymphatics. The fifth layer is again composed of smooth muscle but is of mixed orientation with both longitudinal and circular fibers. The last layer, which actually lines the lumen of the gut, is known as the mucosa and contains most of the exocrine

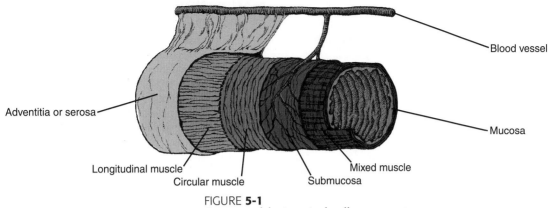

FIGURE **5-1**
Anatomy of the intestinal wall.

gland cells as well as epithelial cells. The mucosal surface is highly convoluted in the small intestine, with many ridges and valleys giving it a larger surface area for absorption. Elsewhere, the mucosa has a smoother surface. In addition to these six structural layers, two major nerve plexuses are found in the gut wall; they regulate the contraction of the smooth muscles. The myenteric plexus lies between the longitudinal and circular layers of muscle and is largely motor in function. The submucosal plexus, as its name implies, is located in the submucosa and is mainly sensory. Synaptic connections between the two nerve networks allow one plexus to stimulate activity in the other and vice versa, leading to activity that is conducted both up and down the length of the gut.

Circulation

Blood flow and oxygen delivery to the newborn intestine is double that during fetal life. After birth, the intestine is a site for intense metabolic activity. Blood flow increases significantly from days 1 to 3, and then plateaus until day 12, and declines progressively until day 30. The change in flow is mediated by nitric oxide (NO), a vasodilator, and myogenic response and endothelin (ET-1), which provide vasoconstriction. Infants have altered capacity to respond to systemic circulatory problems such as decreased arterial pressure and hypoxemia. Introduction of feedings causes vasodilation and increased oxygen delivery (postprandial hyperemic response) from capillary to cell to meet increased demand for digestion (Reber et al, 2002).

Motility

Once food enters the esophagus, it is moved along by peristaltic waves initiated by impulses from autonomic nerves—more specifically, the enteric nervous system (ENS)—and coordinated by the swallowing center in the medulla. The ENS is regulated by a series of genes that influence receptor sites, transcription, and translation of neuronal signals (Bates, 2002; Bates & Balistreri, 2002). As the wave of contractions begins, the gastroesophageal sphincter temporarily relaxes to allow the bolus to enter the stomach. Although this sphincter is anatomically indistinct from the remainder of the esophagus, it normally remains tonically contracted so that the contents of the stomach, which are under relatively higher internal pressure in relation to that experienced in the esophagus, do not reflux.

When the stomach is filled with food, peristaltic waves spread across the stomach toward the small intestine. The con-

tractions are no longer mediated by the medulla but rather by the nerve plexuses and the effect of smooth muscle stretching. Because the muscle layers are thicker in the distal portion of the stomach (antrum) in comparison with the relatively thin layer surrounding the upper portion of the stomach (fundus), the contractions are most powerful and intense in the antrum. These strong antral contractions fulfill two functions. First, they are the primary force acting to break up the gastric contents and mix them with enzymes to form a semifluid mixture called chyme. Second, they force the chyme past the pyloric sphincter into the duodenum. Normally the rate of gastric emptying is controlled by the chemical composition and amount of chyme, but when the stomach is distended or subjected to increased caloric density or high loads of carbohydrate, fat, or acid, the gastric motility may actually decrease so that more time can be devoted to digestion and absorption in the small intestine. In general, formula empties more slowly than breast milk. Right lateral positioning increases gastric emptying, but is associated with increased occurrence of GER as compared to left lateral positioning (Omari et al, 2004).

The contractions that sweep strongly over the stomach become more oscillatory in nature in the small intestine, promoting the digestive and absorptive processes that occur there. Assisting in the process are pancreatic secretions and bile secreted by the liver into the duodenum just below the stomach. Although contractions become progressively slower in the small intestine as chyme passes from the duodenum to the jejunum to the ileum, the muscular activity is sufficient to move the contents slowly downward toward the colon. Distention and luminal injury may bring muscular activity to a halt.

Interruption of normal peristaltic activity results in overgrowth of anaerobic bacteria in the small intestines and malabsorption of nutrients. The coordination of peristalsis may not be developed fully until late in the third trimester, around 34 to 35 weeks (Neu & Bernstein, 2002).

The colon functions primarily as a storage area. Consequently, its structure differs from that of the small intestine in several major ways. Because only a minuscule amount (approximately 4%) of the total intestinal contents is absorbed here, no digestive enzymes are secreted, the lumen is no longer convoluted, and it lacks villi. In addition, the longitudinal smooth-muscle layer is incomplete. The contractions of the remaining circular smooth muscle layer therefore produce only segmental, not propulsive, movement. Consequently, when the luminal contents enter the colon through the ileocecal sphincter, they are merely concentrated (through the reabsorption of water) until distention of the rectum initiates the defecation reflex and the fecal matter is expelled.

Immunity

The neonatal gut is in constant exposure to bacteria and antigens. Complex host defenses, both immune and nonimmune, are present in the newborn and serve to enhance the neonate's immune response.

Motility, as discussed earlier, is important to decrease time for colonization in the lumen of the gut. The release of gastric acid and pancreatico-biliary secretions inhibits bacterial growth and activates proteolysis, altering antigen structure. Unfed infants have decreased release of these secretions, which may impair the host defense. The mucus lining of the gut provides a protective physical barrier to larger molecules.

Epithelial cells, goblet cells, the M cells, and subepithelial cells provide innate immune defense by retarding cellular penetration or large macromolecules and delivering foreign molecules and microorganisms to lymphoid tissue. T cells, B cells, and macrophages are present in the fetal intestine by 20 weeks' gestation, but antigenic stimulation of lymphoid tissue is not demonstrated until 46 weeks (Neu & Bernstein, 2002; Berseth, 2005a; Burrin & Stoll, 2002).

Cytokines are soluble proteins that are important in stimulating chemotaxis of neutrophils, promotion of IgA expression, and epithelial cell proliferation after mucosal injury. Several nutrients (immunonutrients) may play a role in the immune defenses of the neonate. Some of the most studied include glutamine, arginine, short-chain fatty acids, long-chain fatty acids, nucleotides, probiotics, and prebiotics. Glutamine helps in maintaining epithelial cell integrity, cell growth, and mounting inflammatory response. Probiotics are live microbes that improve intestinal microbial balance. Prebiotics are nondigestible food ingredients that enhance growth of nonpathogenic organisms. Manipulation of the microenvironment of the newborn intestine may provide a way for improving outcomes (Berseth, 2005a; Burrin & Stoll, 2002; Neu & Bernstein 2002).

MATURATION OF GASTROINTESTINAL FUNCTION

Anatomic structures of the gastrointestinal tract are well formed by the second trimester. Functional maturation of these structures occurs later (Berseth, 2005a) (Table 5-1). Many GI functions are still immature in the term infant at birth.

The gross anatomy of the supporting musculature and the functional development of GI motility have not been as well studied as has the development of the secretory and absorptive capabilities of the bowel. In general it appears that these supporting structures are relatively thinner in the newborn, especially in the premature newborn, than in the adult. The muscular layers of the stomach are somewhat deficient, with the longitudinal muscle layer being especially thin over the greater curvature. Similarly, the musculature of the intestine is also relatively thin, constituting approximately 50% of the bowel wall in the newborn, as compared with approximately 60% in the adult.

The presence of lanugo and squamous cells in meconium in the newborn bowel indicates that at least some movement of materials from swallowed amniotic fluid occurs. Under normal circumstances, however, little propulsive peristaltic muscle activity appears to occur until late in gestation, and even at term such activity is somewhat irregular and slowed in comparison with that occurring in the adult. Measurable duodenal contractions have been demonstrated by indwelling intraluminal manometry to be present in the infant born as early as the 26th week of gestation, although they occur infrequently (mean of 1.9 contractions per minute) and are relatively weak (mean of 6.3 mm Hg at peak pressure). Between 29 and 32 weeks of gestation, motility spontaneously and significantly improves, with contractions occurring at an average rate of 6.5 per minute and with an average force of 17.1 mm Hg. Neither postnatal age nor type of enteral feed given (breast milk vs formula) nor mode of feeding (instillation by orogastric vs transpyloric tube) appears to affect the timing of this narrow maturational window.

Evidence does point to a somewhat enhanced maturation in infants who receive early enteral feedings with volumes as small as 10 to 20 ml/kg/day for 4 to 7 days (Schanler, 2005).

TABLE 5-1	Anatomic and Functional Maturation of the Gastrointestinal Tract				
Postconceptional Age (weeks)					
15	**20**	**25**	**30**	**35**	**40**
Mouth	Salivary glands	Swallow	Lingual lipase	*Sucking*	
Esophagus	Muscle layers present	Striated epithelium present	*Poor lower esophageal sphincter tone*		
Stomach	Gastric glands present	G cells appear	*Gastric secretions present*	*Slow gastric emptying*	*
Pancreas	Exocrine and endocrine tissue differentiate	Zymogen present	*Reduced trypsin lipase*	*	
Liver	Lobules form	*Bile secreted*	*Fatty acids absorbed*		*
Intestine	Crypt and villus form	*Glucose transport present*	*Dipeptidase, sucrase, and maltase active*	*Lactose active*	
Colon		Crypts and villi recede		*Meconium passed*	

From Berseth CL (2005). *Developmental anatomy and physiology of the gastrointestinal tract. In Taeusch HW et al, editors.* Avery's diseases of the newborn, *ed 8. Philadelphia: Saunders. Reprinted with permission.*
Full functional maturation postnatally.
Italics indicate functional maturation.

Use of diluted formula for these early feedings is, however, controversial because the onset, strength, and duration of motor activity appear to be inversely related to the concentration of formula. Manometric studies, in fact, indicate that the routine use of diluted formula (even one-third strength) may not provide an optimal stimulus for gut motility (Koenig et al, 1995). Antenatal corticosteroid treatment to initiate production of pulmonary surfactant does appear to promote gut maturation, but maturation appears to be delayed in infants affected with significant central nervous system insult or abnormality such as asphyxia and hydrocephalus. After 32 weeks' gestation, duodenal function steadily improves and by term reaches a contraction frequency of approximately 10 per minute. Thus the duodenal contraction rate at term approaches but is less than that found in fasting adults of roughly 11 per minute. Furthermore, the number of contractions that occur in a burst or rapid sequence is often fewer than that measured in adults.

The motor mechanism of the colon also appears to be affected by maturation and illness. Although virtually all healthy, full-term newborns (99.8%) pass meconium within 48 hours of delivery, the first passage of stool is frequently delayed in premature infants. Over 90% of infants with birth weight less than 2500 g, 80% of infants weighing less than 1500 g at birth, and 43% of infants with birth weight less than 1000 g have passed their first stool by the end of 48 hours. Low-birth-weight infants who are ill, especially those with severe respiratory distress syndrome, in whom enteral feedings are consequently delayed, may experience further delay. Data for such infants with birth weights less than 1500 g reveal a mean time of passage of the first stool at 91 hours for those receiving early feedings vs an average of 168 hours for those receiving delayed feedings. Thus even in the absence of congenital GI problems, very-low-birth-weight infants might not be expected to pass their first stool until as late as 7 to 12 days of age.

Bacterial Colonization

As the gut matures postnatally, bacteria are introduced to the GI tract through feedings and invasive procedures. The once-sterile gut rapidly changes, depending on whether the infant is being fed and what feeding is received. *Lactobacillus* is passed to the infant through breast milk and assists with lactose reduction. Secretory IgA and bactericidal enzymes are also passed on to breastfed infants, thus affecting the bacterial growth in the gut. Aerobic organisms appear within a few hours and anaerobic organisms by 24 hours. The organisms are important in metabolizing bile acids, nonabsorbed proteins, lipids, and carbohydrates (Berseth, 2005a). The colonization is disrupted by the introduction of medications, especially antibiotics that change the normal flora. Profound intestinal dysfunction can occur when the gut flora is altered.

Delayed Transit

Even when structurally intact, the relatively deficient supporting musculature and immature motor mechanisms of the newborn, particularly the premature newborn, at best allow only irregular peristaltic activity that occurs in somewhat disorganized patterns. This infrequent and irregular activity increases the tendency toward distention in the ill or premature infant, thus increasing the likelihood of delayed transit and stooling. Complete and thorough assessment of the GI tract therefore becomes essential to distinguish the expected physiologic deficiencies of the newborn from pathologic causes of dysfunction.

ASSESSMENT OF THE GASTROINTESTINAL TRACT

History

Assessment of the newborn infant ideally begins during the prenatal period. Although newly born, each infant has a history dating to the time of conception. Consequently, historical antecedents to birth may serve as an indicator of increased likelihood of dysfunction of a specific organ system such as the GI tract. Although most cases of isolated abdominal and GI defects occur sporadically, some (such as cleft lip or palate, or both, and pyloric stenosis) may exhibit familial recurrence patterns, thus suggesting at least some degree of genetic influence mediated by environmental factors. Therefore any initial history taking should include a screen to identify parents who have had a previous child with related genetic or congenital anomaly or other positive family history. Major syndromes that have frequently associated GI anomalies are listed in Table 5-2.

Although a certain degree of risk may be established through genetic screening, the best evidence of fetal GI anomalies is obtained through prenatal ultrasonography. The fetal abdomen can be identified as early as 10 weeks from the last menstrual period, and the stomach can be visualized at 13 weeks' gestation. The transient herniation of the intestine into the umbilical cord has even been documented by ultrasonography. However, because embryogenesis is still underway at this time, first-trimester diagnosis of defects, particularly small ones, is exceptionally difficult. It is generally not until the second and third trimesters, when the GI structures are established, that reliable visualization becomes possible. Scanning at that point would include a survey of the abdominal wall and insertion of the umbilical cord, visualization of the fluid-filled stomach, and a search for bowel dilation or abnormal echolucencies that resemble cysts and that might indicate collection of fluid within the bowel owing to obstruction. Prenatal echogenic bowel has been associated with cystic fibrosis, chromosomal abnormalities, congenital infections, uteroplacental insufficiency, meconium peritonitis, and various causes of intestinal obstruction (Cass & Wesson, 2002). Abnormal facial features such as clefting may even be identified if fetal position allows and if examination is targeted for that area. The presence of polyhydramnios may provide an additional clue to defects high in the GI tract. Normally, in utero the fetus swallows, absorbs, and metabolizes amniotic fluid. Polyhydramnios results when the fetus is unable to swallow effectively because of a GI obstruction.

Postnatally, three cardinal signs point to the possibility of GI obstruction, whether structural or functional: (1) persistent vomiting, especially if it is bile stained; (2) abdominal distention; and (3) failure to pass meconium within the first 48 hours of birth in the term infant.

Vomiting, as differentiated from reflux, indicates an attempt by an irritated or overdistended bowel to rid itself of its contents. Although vomiting may be initiated by distention or irritative stimuli at any point along the length of the gut, the stomach and duodenum appear to be the most sensitive to these stimuli. Consequently, vomiting is most often considered an indicator of defects high in the GI tract. The presence of

TABLE 5-2	Major Syndromes Associated with Gastrointestinal Dysfunction
Syndrome	**Gastrointestinal Component**
Apert's syndrome	Narrow palate with or without cleft palate or bifid uvula
	Pyloric stenosis
	Ectopic anus
Beckwith-Wiedemann syndrome	Omphalocele
Fetal hydantoin syndrome	Cleft lip and palate
	Pyloric stenosis
	Duodenal atresia
	Anal atresia
Meckel-Gruber syndrome	Cleft palate with or without cleft lip
	Bile duct proliferation fibrosis, cysts
	Omphalocele
	Malrotation
	Imperforate anus
Sirenomelia (mermaid syndrome)	Imperforate anus
	Esophageal atresia with tracheoesophageal fistula
Trisomy 13	Cleft lip with or without cleft palate
	Omphalocele
	Incomplete rotation of colon
Trisomy 18	Cleft lip with or without cleft palate
	Pyloric stenosis
	Biliary atresia
	Omphalocele
	Incomplete rotation of colon
	Imperforate anus
Trisomy 21	Short palate
	Tracheoesophageal fistula
	Duodenal atresia
VATER association	Imperforate anus with or without fistula
	Esophageal atresia with tracheoesophageal fistula

Data from Jones KL (1988). Smith's recognizable patterns of human malformation: genetic, embryologic and clinical aspects, ed 4. Philadelphia: Saunders.

bile further indicates that the point of obstruction is distal to the ampulla of Vater, where bile is emptied from the common bile duct into the duodenum. Conversely, nonbilious vomiting would be noted if obstruction were proximal to the ampulla. Because the mechanism for vomiting requires expulsion of the offending contents up through the esophagus, a patent esophagus is required for true vomiting to occur.

Abdominal distention occurs when large amounts of swallowed air and fluid collect in the bowel and, because of obstruction, cannot pass through the gut. The situation is compounded as digestive fluids and electrolytes continue to be secreted and proteins are lost from the circulation into the lumen of bowel that becomes progressively edematous as the result of distention. Because the stomach is shielded by the rib cage, such distention is generally observed when obstruction occurs in the lower small intestine or colon.

Most normal full-term infants pass their first stool by 48 hours of age. Failure to pass meconium within the first 2 days of life therefore generally indicates obstruction of the large intestine, unless such delay can be attributed to the case of an oversedated, debilitated, or premature infant.

Physical Assessment

A systematic approach to assessment of the newborn GI tract includes inspection, auscultation, and palpation. Percussion,

although useful in the examination of adults, is unreliable and difficult to perform in the infant because the internal abdominal organs are so small and close together. Consequently, the examiner tends to rely on radiography and other diagnostic procedures instead of percussion.

Inspection

Because many of the GI defects are grossly apparent even to the untrained eye, inspection is a fundamental part of assessment. The mouth is observed for its position, shape, size, and symmetry, and the lips, palate, and uvula are evaluated for clefts. Although complete separation of the lip extending up into the nasal area is obvious, close attention must also be paid for any niche in the lip that might easily be overlooked. Abundant oral secretions or saliva provides an early clue to esophageal atresia, particularly when a history of polyhydramnios has been reported.

The abdomen is next inspected for contour, symmetry, and integrity. Distention of the abdomen, which is normally slightly rounded, serves as a hallmark of obstruction. Although the decreased muscle tone in a premature infant may allow visualization of peristalsis, such movement is not normally observed, and when noted in the presence of vomiting or distention, it again suggests the possibility of obstruction. The character of the umbilical cord and site of insertion are checked. Although most cases of omphalocele are obvious, an abnormal thickness to the stump or cord itself should raise suspicion of a single herniated loop of intestine. Any such enlargement must be differentiated from a Wharton's jelly cyst or umbilical hernia through the lax rectus muscles. The anus is examined for position, and the perineal area is inspected for fistulas. The muscle tone of the anal sphincter can be determined by stroking the anal area with a gloved finger and observing for the contraction "wink" that normally occurs around the anal opening. If clinically indicated, the examiner can assess for anal patency by digital examination using the gloved little finger. Insertion of a rectal thermometer presents the risk of perforating the rectum and should not be performed for assessment purposes.

Auscultation

Although initially absent, bowel sounds generally become audible within the first 15 to 30 minutes of life, as the bowel fills with swallowed air and peristaltic activity is activated by the parasympathetic nervous system. Normally these sounds should be of a metallic tinkling quality and occur approximately two to five times per minute. Sounds may be hyperactive, absent, or even normal in the case of neonatal obstruction. The presence and intensity of bowel sounds must be interpreted in relation to other pertinent historical and clinical findings. Hyperdynamic sounds in a recently fed infant with a benign history and otherwise insignificant examination should be considered normal. Marked concern should be raised if hyperdynamic sounds are found in an infant with concurrent findings of distention and vomiting. More often than not, however, the abdomen is misleadingly silent.

Palpation

Abdominal palpation is performed with the infant in a supine position and is best carried out when the infant is quiet and preferably during the first 24 hours of life, when the abdominal musculature is lax. Holding the infant's knees and hips in a flexed position also helps to relax the abdominal musculature. The liver, spleen, and kidneys should be felt with a warm hand using slow, gentle pressure, using the pads of the fingers. Care to perform abdominal palpation in as gentle a manner as possible cannot be overemphasized. The multiple maneuvers involved are often distressing to the newborn, and the pressure applied even during a routine examination may result in significant, although transient, elevations in both systolic and diastolic blood pressures.

The liver is found by placing the index finger just above and to the right of the groin and slowly advancing upward until the edge of the liver can be felt to slip beneath the pad of the finger. Normally the organ is firm (but not hard) with a sharp edge that extends 1 to 2 cm below the right costal margin and can be followed across the abdomen into the left upper quadrant. The spleen is found on the left side in a similar manner, but generally only the tip of the organ is felt at the left costal margin—or it may be entirely unpalpable. The kidneys are located in the flank areas above the level of the umbilicus and are normally 4.5 to 5 cm in length in the term infant. Palpation may be performed bimanually (with one hand supporting and stabilizing the flanks posteriorly while the thumb or a finger of the free hand is moved anteriorly over the same area), or a single hand may be used (with the fingers of

the hand supporting the flank posteriorly while the free thumb of the same hand explores the flank anteriorly). Although the overlying liver may obscure the upper position of the right kidney, the entire left kidney should be felt easily. The remainder of the abdominal examination consists of a gentle search for pathologic masses. Although most masses found are of renal origin, it may be possible to detect stool-filled bowel, particularly in the case of meconium ileus.

Related Findings

Prenatal ultrasonography and direct postnatal visualization of external defects are diagnostic of GI anomalies. In the absence of these obvious signs, a history of maternal polyhydramnios, vomiting, distention, and failure to pass stool are most indicative of GI dysfunction. Other relatively subtle—and oftentimes nonspecific—signs may also be noted.

Respiratory difficulty may arise as the result of an inability to handle the abundant oral secretions commonly found in esophageal atresia or may develop as a result of aspiration of gastric contents by way of an associated tracheoesophageal fistula. Abdominal distention may impede diaphragmatic excursions and therefore decrease ventilation. Frank airway obstruction may even occur in the case of cleft palate, if the negative inspiratory pressure pulls the tongue into the hypopharynx.

Jaundice may occur if the removal of bilirubin is hampered. In the case of biliary atresia, the conjugated bilirubin, which is a normal component of bile, is unable to pass into the duodenum for excretion in the stool. In cases of intestinal atresias, meconium ileus, and Hirschsprung's disease, the enterohepatic circulation becomes exaggerated as stasis of the luminal contents promotes intestinal reabsorption of the bilirubin that is present.

Systemic hypertension may be an additional—although rarely noted—subtle sign. This increase in blood pressure may be appreciated in situations in which masses or distention significantly increases intra-abdominal pressure.

Risk Factors

Maternal, neonatal, and other risk factors associated with GI dysfunction may be found in Table 5-3. These factors are discussed in the sections outlining the management of specific problems.

Genetic Consultation

Once the family history has been obtained, it may be clear that a genetic history is important. Some GI disorders are related to chromosomal and single-gene defects, or as part of multisystem syndromes (see Table 5-2). Omphalocele, duodenal atresia, and stenosis have a high association with trisomy disorders. At least 95% of cases of meconium ileus occur in infants with cystic fibrosis (Merenstein & Gardner, 2006). Because cystic fibrosis is inherited as an autosomal recessive disease, a family history of the disease may or may not exist. There is a familiar association with pyloric stenosis. Five percent of infants of affected men have pyloric stenosis, and approximately 20% of infants of affected women are also affected by the disease. Genetic consultation is suggested for infants with these disorders to provide additional counseling to parents on the risk of recurrence. Chromosomal studies should be performed if additional physical findings associated with GI anomaly are found.

TABLE **5-3**	Risk Factors Associated with Gastrointestinal Dysfunction	
Risk Factor	**Gastrointestinal Dysfunction**
MATERNAL	
Cigarette smoking	Cleft lip with or without cleft palate
Diabetes	Small left colon syndrome
Hypovitaminosis	Cleft lip with or without cleft palate
Influenza with fever	Cleft lip with or without cleft palate
Ionizing radiation exposure	Biliary atresia
Polyhydramnios	Esophageal atresia with or without TE fistula, duodenal atresia, meconium ileus
Stress and anxiety	Pyloric stenosis
MEDICATIONS	
Doxylamine succinate–pyridoxine hydrochloride	Pyloric stenosis
Benzodiazepines	Cleft lip with or without cleft palate
Cortisone	Cleft lip with or without cleft palate
Phenytoin	Cleft lip with or without cleft palate
Magnesium sulfate	Meconium plug syndrome
Opiates	Cleft lip with or without cleft palate
Penicillin	Cleft lip with or without cleft palate
Salicylates	Cleft lip with or without cleft palate
POSITIVE FAMILY HISTORY	
"Apple peel" type of jejunoileal atresia	Similar anomaly
Cleft lip with or without cleft palate	Similar anomaly
Cystic fibrosis	Meconium ileus
Hirschsprung's disease	Similar anomaly
NEONATAL	
Apnea	Necrotizing enterocolitis
Aseptic environment	Necrotizing enterocolitis
Asphyxia or ischemic episodes	Biliary atresia, necrotizing enterocolitis
Cyanotic spells	Necrotizing enterocolitis
Exchange transfusion	Necrotizing enterocolitis
Feeding practices	Pyloric stenosis, necrotizing enterocolitis
Hyperbilirubinemia	Duodenal atresia, jejunoileal atresia
Polycythemia	Necrotizing enterocolitis
Respiratory distress	Necrotizing enterocolitis
Vascular catheterization	Necrotizing enterocolitis
INFECTIONS	
Cytomegalovirus	Biliary atresia
Gastroenteritis	Intussusception
Hepatitis A and B	Biliary atresia
Reovirus type 3	Biliary atresia
Respiratory infection	Intussusception
Rubella	Biliary atresia
Viral infection	Pyloric stenosis
MEDICATIONS	
Hyperosmolar medications	Necrotizing enterocolitis
Indomethacin	Isolated bowel perforation, ulcer
Xanthines	Gastroesophageal reflux
OTHER	
Abdominal wall defect	Gastroesophageal reflux, malrotation
Congenital deafness	Hirschsprung's disease

TABLE 5-3	Risk Factors Associated with Gastrointestinal Dysfunction—cont'd
Risk Factor	**Gastrointestinal Dysfunction**
OTHER	
Congenital heart disease	Esophageal atresia with or without TE fistula, duodenal atresia, biliary atresia, omphalocele, anorectal atresia, malrotation
Diaphragmatic hernia	Malrotation, gastroesophageal reflux
Genitourinary anomalies	Esophageal atresia with or without TE fistula, duodenal atresia, biliary atresia, omphalocele, Hirschsprung's disease, malrotation, anorectal atresia
Imperforate anus	Esophageal atresia with or without TE fistula, duodenal atresia
Intestinal atresia or obstruction	Gastroesophageal reflux, esophageal atresia with or without TE fistula, biliary atresia, omphalocele gastroschisis, malrotation
Malrotation	Duodenal atresia, jejunoileal atresia
Meckel's diverticulum	Malrotation, intussusception
Meconium ileus	Jejunoileal atresia
Neurologic abnormalities	Hirschsprung's disease, meconium plug syndrome, gastroesophageal reflux
Ocular neurocristopathies	Hirschsprung's disease
Pancreatic defects	Meconium ileus
Tracheoesophageal anomalies	Duodenal atresia, anorectal atresia, gastroesophageal reflux
Vertebral malformations	Esophageal atresia with or without TE fistula

Diagnostic Procedures
Radiologic Examination
Air in the GI tract serves as a naturally occurring contrast medium that makes radiologic evaluation of the abdomen a useful tool in the diagnosis of obstruction. At birth, the gut is fluid-filled, but as the infant swallows air after delivery, the radiolucent gas may be followed radiographically as it passes through the bowel. Within the first 30 minutes of life, air should be present in the stomach. By 3 to 4 hours, gas should be seen in the small bowel. After 6 to 8 hours, the entire gut including the colon and rectum should be filled with air. This normal progression of gas through the GI tract cannot occur if obstruction is present. Since no air is able to pass beyond the point of obstruction, the portion of the intestine distal to the obstruction is generally airless. Nevertheless, air continues to be swallowed so that the part of the alimentary tract that lies above the obstruction can become quite distended and is demonstrated on radiography by often-dramatic radiolucent (black) bubbles. Flat and upright radiographic studies of the chest and abdomen may suffice for identifying esophageal or intestinal atresias. Cross-table lateral radiographs may be helpful by identifying air in the rectum of infants suspected of having intestinal obstruction. A left lateral decubitus film may determine the presence of free air in the intestinal wall or the peritoneal cavity.

Upper gastrointestinal series is often used to diagnose GER, pyloric stenosis, and malrotation. Contrast material, such as barium or Gastrograffin, is swallowed or administered by nasogastric tube and observed by fluoroscopy as it passes through the digestive tract. Gastrograffin, meglumine diatrizoate, is preferred if perforation is suspected because it is a water-soluble solution (Kee, 2001). The procedure may last 30 minutes to 4 hours, depending on the rate of small intestine motility. The patient need not be placed on a nothing-by-mouth status before the examination and may continue feedings after the examination.

Barium or Gastrograffin enema is used for examination of the large intestine after contrast solution is instilled through the rectum. It may be diagnostic in cases of malrotation, suspected Hirschsprung's disease, meconium ileus, and meconium plug syndrome. The procedure should be performed prior to any planned upper GI examination because contrast material from the upper GI tract may take several days to clear. No special preparation is made other than placing the infant on a nothing by mouth status 4 to 6 hours before the study. Gentle saline enemas may be helpful in clearing barium and trapped air after the contrast procedure. If barium is allowed to harden and form concretions that can become impacted, more aggressive procedures may be required for evacuation.

Ultrasonography
Ultrasonography may be diagnostic in cases of pyloric stenosis, enteric duplication, or biliary atresia if the intrahepatic or proximal extrahepatic tracts are dilated. Conducting gel is placed on the abdomen, and the transducer is placed against the gel on the abdomen. The computer transforms reflected sound waves from tissues into scans, graphs, or audible sound (Kee, 2001).

Gastric Aspirate
A gastric aspirate may be obtained to measure the pH of the gastric contents. A premeasured feeding tube is passed into the stomach. At least 1 ml of gastric contents is gently aspirated into a syringe, and the feeding tube is withdrawn. The syringe is capped, labeled, and sent for testing.

Apt Test
The Apt test may be used to determine the origin of blood in vomitus or stool by differentiating neonatal GI blood loss from swallowed maternal blood. Bloody aspirate or bloody stool is centrifuged in 5 ml water. One part 0.25% sodium hydroxide is added to five parts supernatant. The fluid remains pink in the

presence of fetal blood but turns brown in the presence of maternal blood.

Stool Culture

A stool culture may differentiate between an intestinal lining insult and an infection as the cause of bloody diarrhea. A stool sample is taken from a diaper, placed in a specimen container, labeled, and sent for testing.

Stool Hematest

A stool Hematest is a rapid and convenient method for detection of fecal occult blood—a possible indication of GI disease. The test is based on the oxidation of guaiac by hydrogen peroxide, thus resulting in a blue compound. A thin smear of stool is placed on guaiac paper. Developer is applied over the smear. Results are read in 60 seconds. Any blue colorization on or at the edge of the smear indicates a positive occult blood result. Fecal samples need not be tested if hematuria or obvious rectal bleeding is present. Drugs that influence positive results include iron preparations, indomethacin, potassium preparations, salicylates, and steroids. Large amounts of ascorbic acid may cause a false-negative result (Kee, 2001).

Stool-Reducing Substances

Carbohydrate intolerance is detected by the presence of reducing substances in the stool. A stool sample is placed in a specimen container and sent for testing. If the stool is watery, the liquid portion of stool, which can be collected in a diaper, is aspirated into a syringe. A 1:2 ratio of stool to water is obtained. Fifteen drops of this supernatant are placed in a clean test tube, and a Clinitest (test for urinary glucose) tablet is added. After 15 seconds, the test tube is shaken gently, and the color of the liquid is compared with the color chart provided with the Clinitest tablets. More than 0.5% glucose in the stool indicates an abnormal amount of sugar.

pH Probe Test

The 24-hour pH probe test is considered the gold standard for the diagnosis of GER. A thin, flexible, pH-sensitive electrode is placed into the distal esophagus. The study is scored by determining the amount of time the esophagus is exposed to an acid pH level, which is usually less than 4 minutes. Scoring for abnormal results is based on frequency of reflux, number of episodes greater than 4 minutes' duration, time of longest episode, and the percentage of time in reflux. A dual sensor may be used, which places an electrode in the distal esophagus and another in the pharyngeal area of the esophagus.

The use of formula feedings may obscure episodes of reflux by buffering the gastric acid. Many clinicians use acid feeding, such as apple juice, to better estimate the true amount of gastric reflux in the esophagus. Interpretation of the data is complex due to confounding factors such as position, activity, frequency and composition of feeding, and medication. Nursing responsibilities include recording the time of feedings and describing the activity level of the infant throughout the test.

Scintigraphy

Gastroesophageal scintigraphy, by feeding radionucleotide-tagged formula to the infant, may be used to measure gastric emptying, aspiration with swallowing, and reflux with aspiration. A technetium radioisotope is used because it has relatively low radiation and is easily added to formula.

Endoscopy

Flexible endoscopy with biopsy of the distal esophagus is used to diagnose esophagitis. Biopsy findings suggestive of esophagitis include basal cell hyperplasia, increased stromal papillary length, and demonstration of intraepithelial eosinophils.

Fecal Fat

A fecal fat test may be helpful to screen for malabsorption. Fecal fat content of >6 g/24 hr is predictive of malabsorption syndrome. A very small stool sample can cause false test results.

COLLABORATIVE MANAGEMENT
General Principles

Early recognition accompanied by medical or surgical intervention for infants with GI obstructions or alterations is necessary to decrease the likelihood of a poor outcome. The general considerations that guide nursing care in alterations of the GI system include GI decompression, fluid and electrolyte balance, thermoregulation, positioning, prevention of infection, nutrition, and pain management.

Gastric Decompression

Gastric decompression is extremely important to prevent aspiration, respiratory compromise, or gastric perforation. If the intestinal obstruction is not relieved, abdominal distention may become severe and the upward pressure on the diaphragm may compromise respirations. Connection of an orogastric tube to low intermittent suction minimizes the risk of aspiration and prevents distention from swallowed air. Tube patency is essential if gastric decompression is to be maintained. A 10 French soft vinyl, double-lumen gastric sump tube provides sufficient decompression for most infants. Irrigating the tube every 2 to 4 hours with 2 ml air helps ensure that the tube remains open and functioning.

Fluid and Electrolytes

Large amounts of extracellular fluid pass into and out of the GI tract as part of the normal digestive process. In intestinal obstruction, the fluids that are normally reabsorbed by the intestine become trapped. Additionally, infants with obstruction often experience "third-spacing," with a shift of fluid from the vascular into the interstitial compartment. This third-spacing is also referred to as capillary leak syndrome. If severe, this loss of intravascular volume can result in relative hypovolemia and hypoperfusion with all their attendant risks. Furthermore, vomiting, diarrhea, and gastric suction can cause excessive volume depletion and electrolyte abnormalities, especially losses of sodium, potassium, and chloride.

The goal of collaborative management is to maintain fluid and electrolyte balance. Maintenance fluids are usually run at 60 to 80 ml/kg for the first 24 hours of life and are increased by 10 ml/kg/day or as needed to 120 to 160 ml/kg/day (Zenk et al, 2003). A rate should be maintained at which urine output is at least 1 to 2 ml/kg/hr and maintains a specific gravity of 1.005 to 1.012. Sodium is provided at a rate of 2 to 3 mEq/kg/day and potassium at 2 mEq/kg/day, as serum electrolytes indicate.

For the infant who is receiving gastric suction, the amount of gastric loss is determined by measuring drainage every 4 to 8 hours. The total volume of gastric output should be replaced every 4 to 8 hours with one half normal saline with 10 to 20 mEq KCl/L. The replacement fluids are given in addition to maintenance fluids. Fluid-volume deficit and electrolyte imbalances may occur if replacement therapy is inadequate. The adequacy for fluid replacement is assessed by changes in vital signs, amount of urinary output, urine specific gravity, levels of electrolytes and blood urea nitrogen, and hematocrit values.

Metabolic alkalosis may occur with pyloric stenosis or high jejunal obstruction because of loss of acidic gastric juice. In obstructions in the distal segment of the small intestine, larger quantities of alkaline fluids than acidic fluids may be lost, thus resulting in metabolic acidosis. If the obstruction is below the proximal colon, acid-base balance may be maintained because most of the GI fluids are absorbed before reaching the obstruction. Respiratory acidosis may develop in patients with abdominal distention because of carbon dioxide retention from hypoventilation. Correction of acid-base imbalances would be made in the instance of a pH less than 7.35 or greater than 7.45 or for a base excess below −4 or above +4 (Merenstein & Gardner, 2006).

Thermoregulation

Thermoregulation is vital in the care of all newborns and becomes more critical for the stressed neonate. Cold stress dramatically increases oxygen requirements and predisposes the infant to hypoglycemia, hypoxia, and metabolic acidosis. An appropriate heat source and monitoring must be ensured for any infant with GI dysfunction. Gastroschisis and omphalocele in particular cause profound heat loss from exposed bowel. Preoperative nursing intervention includes provision of an external heat source and head covering, hourly monitoring of temperature, and, in the case of exposed bowel, use of warm saline soaks over the defect, with bowel bag or plastic wrap from the feet to the axillae.

Positioning

Head-up positioning accomplishes two management goals in the infant with GI dysfunction. In suspected GER, a 30-degree prone position or left lateral position has been shown to be the most effective position to decrease reflux. For the infant with tracheal esophageal fistula, elevating the head of the bed 30 to 40 degrees helps to avoid reflux of gastric contents into the trachea via a distal fistula. In the case of an isolated esophageal atresia, a flat or head-down position may assist gravity drainage from an overflowing esophageal pouch.

Prevention of Infection

Newborn infants are uniquely at risk for infections acquired prenatally, intrapartally, and postnatally. Infants who require specialized care as the result of medical or surgical problems have an increased susceptibility for infection. Broad-spectrum antibiotics are administered immediately in presumed neonatal infections. Many institutions administer antibiotics preoperatively to prevent infection.

Pain Management

Infants with gastrointestinal disorders are at high risk for pain pre- and postoperatively. It is important to constantly monitor the infant's physiologic and behavioral cues to pain as well as to factor in the infant's risk for pain (Walden, 2001). Both nonpharmacologic and pharmacologic therapies are used in pain management. Containment and positioning strategies are utilized as well as a quiet and low-lighted environment. Opioids, particularly morphine and fentanyl, are the most commonly used agents for analgesia. Postoperatively it may be useful to implement analgesia every 2 to 4 hours around the clock in anticipation of expected pain. Pain levels must be assessed and reassessed at regular intervals. Pain scores, intervention, and responses are critical to evaluate for effective relief.

Nutrition

Meeting the caloric and metabolic needs postoperatively in the infant with GI dysfunction is challenging. Enteral feeding is delayed owing to surgery of the alimentary tract. Hyperalimentation is indicated to supply these needs. Peripherally inserted central catheters or surgically placed central catheters are needed in order to manage the nutritional needs of most infants with gastrointestinal disorders. When the infant is ready to begin enteral feedings, clear liquids are begun and may progress to elemental feedings such as Pregestimil (protein hydrolysate formula). Bowel loss or severity of the defect influences the infant's tolerance to feedings. Initial feedings are small, frequent, or continuous-drip; are supplemented with intravenous hyperalimentation; and are gradually advanced. Advancement of feeding should be stopped if signs of intolerance, such as diarrhea, vomiting, abdominal distention, or presence of reducing substances in stool, appear (Zenk et al, 2003).

General Preoperative Management

In an infant already afflicted by GI dysfunction, surgery presents an additional stress that the baby is often ill-equipped to tolerate. The principles of preoperative management revolve around the prevention or minimization of identified stressors by replacing all fluid losses, decompressing the distended bowel, and supporting failing organ systems by means of assisted ventilation, radiant heating, parenteral nutrition, pain management, and other interventions as needed. Appropriate fluid and electrolyte balance is challenging due to third-space losses in the infant with bowel obstruction or necrotizing enterocolitis. The third-space fluid losses are isotonic and have an electrolyte composition like that of serum. Fluid losses from the GI tract due to vomiting or nasogastric suction additionally contribute to negative fluid balance and electrolyte depletion. Nasogastric fluid losses need to be replaced at full volume using one-half normal saline with potassium chloride at 10 to 20 mEq/L. Careful monitoring of the clinical status, which includes the heart rate, blood pressure, perfusion, capillary refill, and urine output, helps guide the rate of fluid replacement. Laboratory monitoring for potential derangements is essential.

Antibiotics should be started early in the neonate with bowel dysfunction, until the etiology is clear. Antibiotic regimens usually include combining a penicillin and an aminoglycoside, such as ampicillin and gentamicin. Clindamycin may be added to cover anaerobic infection.

General Postoperative Management

Hydration, maintenance of electrolyte balance, gastric decompression, fluid loss replacement, and pain management are continued postoperatively, along with respiratory and other therapy that the individual case warrants. Most patients will have extraneous tubes or devices such as gastrostomy tubes, chest tubes, or drains as well as incision sites. Meticulous care is needed to maintain skin integrity. Skin must be kept dry as much as possible. When tape or adhesive has been placed directly on the skin, gentle and careful removal is mandatory. Pectin-based skin barriers can be used to protect the skin from tape. If enteral feedings are expected to be delayed beyond 3 to 5 days, total parenteral nutrition should be instituted to prevent excessive catabolism. Feedings are generally started when bowel sounds are present, stools are being passed normally, and the gastric drainage clears and lessens in amount.

Ostomy Care

Infants with ostomies require special management. The primary diagnoses leading to fecal diversion in infants are necrotizing enterocolitis, imperforate anus, and Hirschsprung's disease. A colostomy/ileostomy/jejunostomy is formed surgically by opening part of the bowel to the outside of the abdomen for the evacuation of feces. It may be temporary or permanent, depending on the indication for surgery. The opening is called a stoma, which is made from the innermost lining of the intestine. Stomas are insensate (no sensory nerves) and incontinent (no sphincter control) and usually shrink for the first 6 to 8 weeks after surgery. If there is more than one stoma, the proximal stoma is the functioning one and the distal stoma(s) are called mucous fistula(s). If two stomas are close together, they may both be pouched together. If not, the distal stomas can be covered with dry gauze.

The primary goal in ostomy care is to keep stool off of the skin. Pouching of the stomas is necessary when drainage begins, usually 1 to 2 days postoperatively. The area around the stoma is washed with warm water, rinsed well, and dried. Soap is not used because it may irritate the skin. The skin and stomas are observed for swelling, change in color, or bleeding. A pattern is drawn for the pectin-based skin-barrier wafer and pouch, to be used for further pouch changes. The opening of the pouch is cut out so it fits up close to the stoma with no peristomal skin exposed to stool. If the hole is cut too large, stool will leak out and irritate skin or cause the wafer to lose its seal. If the pattern size is too small, the pouch's wafer will sit on the wet stoma, and the pouch will not stick. The hole in the wafer should not be more than $1/8$ inch larger than the stoma and the hole in the pouch should be about $1/4$ inch larger than the hole in the wafer. The wafer is applied to the skin and the pouch is applied to the top of the wafer. The bottom of the pouch is folded and tied with a rubber band.

The length of time that the pouch stays on depends on how active the baby is, how liquid the stool is, and how "budded" the stoma is. Usually an infant pouch will stay on 2 to 4 days. To improve the pouch's seal, the peristomal skin needs to be dry before applying the pouch and the pouch held in place for 5 minutes after applying. The bag is emptied as needed, usually when it is a third to half full. If it gets too full, it may break the seal of the wafer and cause the pouch to come off.

Complications

Complications are inherent in postoperative surgical patients and may include infection, respiratory distress, fluid and electrolyte imbalances, third spacing of fluids, oliguria, pain management issues, skin breakdown around surgical sites and tubes, and intestinal obstruction related to adhesions, strictures, or volvulus.

The short-bowel syndrome is an unfortunate complication of many neonatal surgeries that involve extensive resection of the GI tract. The loss of considerable absorptive surface results in a complex malabsorptive problem with episodic diarrhea, steatorrhea, and dehydration, which, if allowed to progress, may cause metabolic derangements and ultimately poor growth and development.

Peritonitis, chemical or bacterial, is a concerning complication of infants with gastrointestinal disorders, with a mortality rate of 33% to 80%. Meconium peritonitis can result from intestinal perforation related to meconium ileus, intussusception, volvulus, incarcerated internal hernia, imperforate anus, and meconium plugs (Berseth, 2005b). Infectious peritonitis is usually caused by mixed anaerobic and aerobic organisms associated with necrotizing enterocolitis, appendicitis, biliary tract disease, rupture of visceral abscess, or infection of indwelling foreign objects. *Candida* is also associated with approximately 10% of cases of peritonitis, seen primarily in extremely premature infants, extended use of umbilical arterial catheters, prolonged intubation, or prolonged use of antibiotics (Berseth, 2005b). Treatment includes surgical drainage and administration of antibiotics or antifungal agents.

CONSIDERATION OF ETHICAL ISSUES

Congenital malformations often have associated organ defects. When another defect or organ system dysfunction represents a major threat to life, decisions regarding the timing of surgical intervention must be made. For example, repair of a serious heart lesion may necessarily precede repair of esophageal atresia, but the resection of necrotic bowel must precede both conditions. Such scheduling decisions are made difficult when it is recognized that some conditions may be improved only at the expense of others. Even when surgical correction of GI dysfunction can be achieved successfully, in the face of multiple malformations (which may not be equally amenable to operative treatment or may result in early demise), the appropriateness of intervention must be reevaluated. Each affected newborn deserves individual consideration. The wishes of the parents and the opinion of each member of the management team must be considered.

MANAGEMENT OF PROBLEMS WITH INGESTION

Cleft Lip and Palate

Anatomy

Generally defined, cleft lip is the term that signifies a congenital fissure in the upper lip, whereas cleft palate indicates a congenital fissure in either the soft palate alone or in both the hard and soft palates. The two conditions may occur in isolation or together. Isolated cleft lip may be either unilateral or bilateral and may range in severity from a slight notch in the lip to a complete cleft into the nostril. Isolated cleft palate may also be unilateral or bilateral and may be as mild as a submucous cleft characterized by a notch at the posterior edge of the hard palate, an imperfect muscle union across the palate, a thin mucosal surface, and a bifid uvula. In this mild form, the diagnosis may never be made. Combined clefts of the lip and palate are the most severe form of the defect, particularly if they are bilateral.

Pathophysiology

Although cleft lip and cleft palate are often associated, these defects are embryologically distinct disorders. Cleft lip occurs when the maxillary process fails to merge with the medial nasal elevation on one or both sides. Cleft palate occurs when the lateral palatine processes fail to meet and fuse with each other, the primary palate, or the nasal septum. When both cleft lip and cleft palate occur together, studies indicate that the failure of the secondary palate to close may be a developmental consequence of the abnormalities in the primary palate associated with the cleft lip, rather than an intrinsic defect in the secondary palate. It is possible, therefore, that isolated cleft lip and cleft lip with an associated cleft palate represent varying degrees of the same embryologic defect.

Rates of cleft lip with or without an associated cleft palate have been reported to be 1/500 to 1/2500 in different populations, depending on geographic location, ethnic group, and socioeconomic conditions (Spritz, 2001). The defects appear in both syndromic and non-syndromic forms. Rates are higher in males than in females and in Asians than in whites. Isolated cleft palate has a lower incidence rate, occurring more frequently in females, and has no clear racial variation. Approximately 70% of infants with unilateral cleft lip and 85% of infants with a bilateral cleft lip will also have a cleft palate (Merritt, 2005a). These defects are usually isolated, but 10% of infants with cleft lip and cleft palate will have an associated syndrome. When a parent has cleft lip/palate, there is a 3% to 5% risk of having an affected child. Recurrence rate for parents with one affected child rises to 40% for another affected child (Merritt, 2005a). No single gene has been identified to explain clefts, but many genes are associated in specific ethnic groups. Mutations of 1q24, 2p, 3p20, 3q, 4q32, 10p15, 17q, 18q, and 21q have been found in cases of cleft lip and/or palate (Merritt, 2005a). MSX1 mutations are found in 2% of cases of clefting and would warrant genetic counseling in families with dental anomalies associated with clefting phenotypes (Jezewski et al, 2003). Although rates of recurrence risks indicate that genetic factors are often involved, environmental factors also appear to contribute in some way, indicating a multifactorial mode of inheritance.

Maternal medication during the first trimester—especially benzodiazepines, phenytoin, opiates, penicillin, salicylates, cortisone, and high doses of vitamin A—has been associated with clefting. Occurrence of fever and influenza during the first trimester has also been demonstrated as a possible factor; however, it is questionable as to whether the viral agent or the therapeutic drugs are the causative factors. Threatened abortion in the first and second trimesters and premature delivery of neonates with clefts has also been reported, but it is uncertain whether this indicates an unfavorable intrauterine environment or simply a symptom of an already malformed fetus (e.g., Pierre Robin syndrome or sequence). An association between clefting and variables such as maternal smoking, maternal alcohol use, maternal diabetes, hypovitaminosis, and hypervitaminosis—especially of vitamin A—has also been supported. The role of folic acid in preventing orofacial clefts remains controversial (Spritz, 2001). Maternal age does not appear to be a factor, although there may be a small but nonsignificant increase in the incidence of clefting with increasing paternal age (Ryckman & Balistreri, 2002; Spilson et al, 2001).

Clearly, cleft lip or cleft palate—or both—can have multiple causes and, consequently, may represent a malformation, a disruption, or a deformation. When the defect is the result of an inherently abnormal developmental process, as in the case of genetic derangement, it is appropriately called a malformation. An example is pits within the lower lip that lead to a cleft associated with Van der Woude's syndrome, autosomal dominant condition. Holoprosencephaly is associated with a median cleft lip. Smith-Lemli-Opitz syndrome is another condition that has deviations along the palatal ridges and can result in a cleft palate. When the developmental process is originally normal but goes awry because of extrinsic factors, as in the case of teratogenic exposure, it is called a disruption. Last, when mechanical forces interfere with normal development, as in the case of Pierre Robin syndrome or sequence—in which mandibular hypoplasia causes the tongue to be posteriorly displaced, thus interfering with the fusion of the lateral palatine shelves—the result is called a deformation.

Treatment

The management of an individual born with a cleft defect is beyond the capabilities of any one professional. Effective care requires the services of a team of individuals: pediatrician, plastic surgeon, audiologist, speech pathologist, dental specialist, geneticist, social worker, and nursing personnel at various levels.

Emotional preparation of the parents is frequently the most immediate and demanding nursing problem encountered. The birth of a defective child comes as both a shock and a disappointment to the parents. Information and reassurance are desperately needed at this critical time. Nurses can also provide a role model to influence the parents' attitude toward the child positively and to provide guidance and support as the family copes with the reactions of others. "About Face USA" (www.aboutfaceUSA.org) is an organization that provides information, emotional support, and educational programs to patients and families experiencing facial differences.

Understanding of the etiology of the defect is assisted through the familial history, antenatal exposure to potential teratogens, chromosomal analysis and thorough systematic physical exam (Merritt, 2005b).

Surgical repair is a priority—not only to achieve closure of the defect but also to minimize maxillary growth retardation, to limit dental deformity, and to allow normal speech development. If the infant is healthy and no complications are expected, a cleft lip can be repaired at about 3 months of age. Repair of an associated cleft palate is generally postponed until a later time to allow medial movement of the palatal shelves, which appears to be initiated by lip closure. Depending on the involvement, palate closure may occur as a two-step process, with the hard palate being corrected at 14 to 16 months of age, followed by soft palate repair by 18 months of age. The timing of repair is controversial and some surgeons perform the correction in the neonatal period. If additional repair of the lip or nose is required for aesthetic purposes, it is postponed until sufficient structural growth has been achieved, generally after 12 years of age.

Feeding is another important aspect in the care of an infant with cleft lip or palate and is one that requires a great deal of patience and attention to technique. In the presence of cleft lip, the infant may have difficulty not only in holding the nipple in the mouth but also in creating the vacuum necessary for adequate sucking. The bottle should be held securely and the cheeks grasped so that the cleft is pushed closed. Even then, large amounts of air may be swallowed; therefore frequent burping should be performed. The infant with cleft palate should be held in an upright or semiupright position to avoid choking, and the flow of milk should be directed to the side of the mouth. Use of a "preemie" nipple or a special cleft palate nipple and squeeze bottle may also be helpful. Frequent, small feedings help in preventing fatigue and frustration. Squeeze bottles appear to be easier to use than rigid bottles, but there is no evidence in the difference of growth outcomes of infants fed either way (Glenny et al, 2005). Breastfeeding is certainly possible, although considerable creativity may be required. A pillow placed between the infant's back and the mother's arm can maintain the infant in an upright position. Because the clefted areas easily become encrusted with milk and are therefore prone to excoriation and infection, a small amount of sterile water should be offered after each feeding. Some craniofacial centers fit infants with cleft palate with a prosthetic device to occlude the cleft. This device is made of hard or soft plastic and molded to fit the infant's mouth. It is thought to help in feeding and speech development until repair is possible. The device is removed and rinsed with water after each feeding (Merritt, 2005b).

The major condition that requires differential diagnosis is Van der Woude's syndrome, which is inherited as an autosomal dominant trait. This syndrome ranges in appearance from a single, barely visible lower lip depression to frank pits or fistulas usually occurring in pairs on the vermilion of the lower lips, with clefting of the lip with or without palate involvement (Merritt, 2005a).

Although an excellent prognosis for survival can be expected, an individual born with a cleft defect is faced with more than just a cosmetic problem. Language and speech tend to be retarded in affected individuals. This retardation is further compounded by a higher incidence of hearing impairment. Olfactory defects have also been demonstrated in males with cleft palate; however, females appear to be affected less frequently. Dental problems, such as malocclusion, irregularity of the teeth, and increased frequency of caries, may also be encountered in affected individuals. Although the majority of cases of cleft lip or palate or both are not associated with any recognizable syndrome, there are more than 300 syndromes that include cleft lip or palate, or both, as a feature (Merritt, 2005a). Obviously, the prognosis in such cases varies with the associated anomalies involved.

Esophageal Atresia/Tracheoesophageal Fistula

Anatomy

Esophageal atresia (EA) is defined as a complete interruption in the continuity of the esophagus. Tracheoesophageal fistula (TEF) is a congenital fistulous connection of the proximal and/or distal esophagus and the airway. They can exist as separate congenital anomalies, but most patients will have both EA and TEF.

Pathophysiology

Esophageal atresia and tracheoesophageal (TE) fistula occur when the trachea fails to differentiate and separate from the esophagus. The atresia appears most likely to be the result of either a spontaneous posterior deviation of the esophago-tracheal septum or some mechanical force that pushes the dorsal wall of the foregut in an anterior direction. A fistula occurs when the lateral ridges of the septum fail to close completely in their normal zipper-like fashion so that a com-

munication is left between the foregut and the primitive respiratory tree.

The infant with esophageal atresia may appear well at birth, but oral secretions and saliva collect in the upper esophageal pouch and appear in the mouth and around the lips because effective swallowing is not possible. The body does not produce greater amounts of secretions; they simply cannot be handled properly and thus become more visible. Respiratory difficulty may be encountered if the secretions and mucus fill the esophageal pouch and overflow into the upper airway or find their way into the trachea through a proximal fistula. Any attempts at feeding are generally accompanied by coughing, choking, and cyanosis. If a distal fistula is present, crying may force air into the stomach, where it collects and causes progressive distention. This gastric distention may impede diaphragmatic excursions, thus leading to worsening respiratory status or a reflux of gastric contents back up through the fistula into the trachea. If there is no distal fistula, the abdomen is more likely to appear scaphoid owing to the lack of swallowed air. True vomiting is not possible (except in the case of an isolated TE fistula) because the esophagus and stomach are not connected. This triad of "excessive" secretions, reflux, and respiratory distress, particularly in association with a maternal history of polyhydramnios, indicates esophageal atresia until proved otherwise (Ryckman & Balistreri, 2002). The clinical presentation may vary slightly, depending on the specific type of anomaly found (Figure 5-2). There are five major pathologic types of esophageal atresia with or without TE fistula; however, approximately 100 subtypes have been described.

Esophageal atresia with or without TE fistula occurs approximately once in every 2400 to 4500 live births (Cass & Wesson, 2002; Kovesi & Rubin, 2004). Isolated TEF occurs 5% in the absence of EA. Symptoms include coughing, cyanosis, and choking with feedings, and recurring pneumonia. Although rare cases of familial occurrence have been reported, most cases represent an accident of embryology. A history of maternal polyhydramnios is reported in 14% to 90% of cases of esophageal atresia. The higher rates are found with an isolated esophageal atresia; the lower rates are found when a fistula allows passage of swallowed amniotic fluid around the obstruction. Associated malformations are present in 30% to 70% of infants. Congenital heart disease is reported most frequently (25% to 40%), with ventricular and atrial septal defects being the most common lesions. Other associated anomalies include vertebral malformations (13%), atresias of the small intestine (5%), imperforate anus (10% to 20%), and genitourinary anomalies (10% to 24%). Congenital lung anomalies such as pulmonary and lobar agenesis, horseshoe lung, and pulmonary hypoplasia have been reported in infants with EA/TEF (Kovesi & Rubin, 2004). Approximately 25% present as part of the VATER association. This acronym represents a complex of V, vertebral and ventricular septal defects; A, anal atresia; TE, tracheoesophageal fistula with E, esophageal atresia; and R, radial and renal anomalies (Spoon, 2003). Some experts describe the same cluster of symptoms but use the VACTERL association. The C stands for congenital heart defects, and the L is for limb deformities. Overall, 20% to 30% of these infants are premature or small for gestational age, but in the case of isolated esophageal atresia, the incidence of prematurity approaches 50%. EA/TEF has also been associated in patients with DiGeorge syndrome, Down syndrome, Pierre-Robin syndrome and CHARGE association.

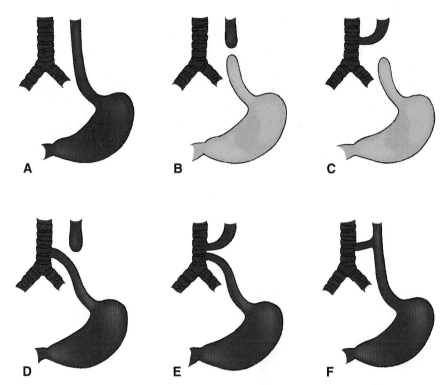

FIGURE **5-2**
Esophageal atresia and transesophageal (TE) fistula. Shading represents areas of lucency typically found on radiographs. Percentages reflect relative occurrence. **A**, Normal. **B**, Isolated esophageal atresia (8%), characterized by excessive salivation. **C**, Esophageal atresia with proximal TE fistula (1%), characterized by respiratory distress, especially with feeding. **D**, Esophageal atresia with distal TE fistula (86%), characterized by excessive salivation, respiratory distress, and reflux. **E**, Esophageal atresia with both proximal and distal TE fistulas (1%), characterized by respiratory distress, especially with feeding, and reflux. **F**, Isolated (H-type) TE fistula (4%), characterized by respiratory distress, especially with feeding, and reflux. Data from Cassani VL (1984). Tracheoesophageal anomalies. *Neonatal network* 3(2):20-27; Desjardins JG (1987). Esophageal atresia. In Stern L, Vert P, editors. *Neonatal medicine*. New York: Masson Publishing; and Sunshine P et al (1983). The gastrointestinal system. In Fanaroff AA, Martin RJ, editors. *Behrman's neonatal-perinatal medicine: diseases of the fetus and infant*, ed 3. St Louis: Mosby.

Treatment

Diagnosis of esophageal atresia is confirmed by attempting to pass a radiopaque catheter from the nares through the esophagus into the stomach. If the esophagus is atretic, the catheter cannot be advanced further than a depth of approximately 9 to 12 cm before meeting resistance, and any contents that are aspirated are alkaline rather than acidic. A chest radiograph shows the tube ending or coiling in the upper esophageal pouch (Figure 5-3). Air in the bowel indicates the presence of a distal TE fistula. If the abdomen is airless, no such fistula is present. Contrast studies are generally contraindicated owing to the danger of aspiration but may become necessary in the diagnosis of an isolated or H-type TE fistula. In these cases, which are more difficult to diagnose, bronchoscopy or endoscopy may be required to allow direct visualization of the fistulous site.

Surgical correction involves esophageal anastomosis (esophagoesophagostomy) and obliteration of any fistula that is present. The procedure may be done thoracically or laparoscopically. The exact technique varies with the type of defect present, but if a great distance separates the two ends of the esophagus, the repair is made more difficult and must often be staged. In this case, the ends may be brought into closer approximation either preoperatively by stretching the upper esophageal pouch daily with a bougie to produce progressive

elongation or intraoperatively by performing multiple circular myotomies so that the upper esophageal segment can be lengthened in a telescoping fashion. Alternatively, a combination of the two methods may be used. If these procedures are not effective or if the gap is particularly large, a segment of the small or large intestine or an inverted tube of gastric tissue may be used for esophageal replacement. Such a dramatic procedure is generally delayed until 1 year of age. If the gap makes primary repair impossible, the upper esophageal pouch can be brought to the surface as a cervical esophagostomy ("spit fistula") to allow the drainage of saliva, with gastrostomy performed for feeding. In these protracted cases, sham feeding may be attempted, wherein orally fed milk is collected with saliva in the ostomy bag attached to the esophagostomy stoma and refed through the gastrostomy tube into the stomach.

Generally, repair is performed through an incision at the base of the neck, but if the lesion is exceptionally low within the chest, a thoracic approach may be used, thus necessitating chest tube placement. A gastrostomy may also be performed to allow feeding during healing.

Preoperative care is focused primarily on the reduction of symptoms. To prevent overflow of secretions, a sump catheter (Replogle tube) is placed in the upper esophageal pouch and

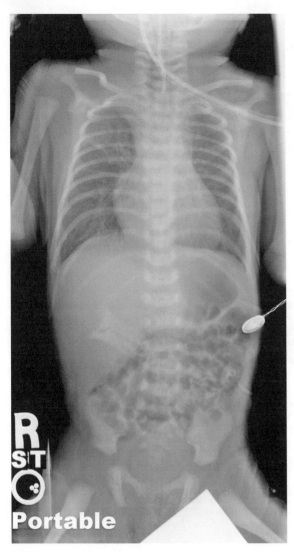

FIGURE **5-3**
Esophageal atresia with TE fistula. Catheter is seen with the tip in the distal end of the proximal esophageal pouch. Air is seen in the stomach and bowel indicating a distal tracheoesophageal fistula. Courtesy Radiology Department of Children's Healthcare of Atlanta.

connected to low continuous suction. The tube lumen becomes easily occluded by tenacious secretions and should therefore be changed daily. Periodic catheter irrigations are usually required to maintain patency. If the secretions are particularly thick, humidified air may assist in liquefying them for easier removal. Elevating the head 30 to 40 degrees helps avoid reflux of gastric secretions into the trachea via a distal fistula. Comfort measures to prevent crying reduce the amount of air swallowed through the fistula, thus limiting gastric distention and further reducing the risk of reflux. If no TE fistula is present, a flat or head-down position may be preferable to avoid gravity drainage of saliva from an overflowing esophageal pouch. Intravenous fluids are used for hydration. Electrolytes are monitored closely. Supplemental oxygen and intubation may be needed if respiratory distress occurs. However, use of positive-pressure ventilation increases the propensity for gastric distention and may even necessitate preoperative gastrostomy for decompression.

Postoperatively, vital signs are monitored closely, and frequent assessment is made to look for potential leaking at the anastomotic site. If a chest tube has been placed, such leakage presents as persistent or increased drainage. The endotracheal tube is generally left in place for at least 24 hours to allow full recovery from anesthesia and relaxants. For suctioning of the airway, the catheter should be well marked and inserted to a predetermined depth above the site to avoid disruption or trauma. The quantity and appearance of secretions and any respiratory difficulties are reported. Feeding by gastrostomy may be started within 48 hours, with oral feedings generally withheld for 5 to 10 days to ensure healing. Gastroesophageal reflux is a common complication because of the upward pull on the lower esophageal pouch and stomach and generally poor peristalsis, occurring in 40% to 70% of infants, and should be managed as described in the next section. Postoperative complications that are frequently seen arising over time include anastomotic leak (17%), stricture of the anastomosis (40% to 50%), recurrence of the fistula (5% to 12%), and abnormal esophageal peristalsis (75% to 100%) (Kovesi & Rubin, 2004; Berseth & Poenaru, 2005a).

With early diagnosis and efforts to prevent aspiration pneumonia, most full-term infants do well, with a survival rate of 97%. However, mortality dramatically increases in the presence of prematurity or associated major anomalies, particularly cardiac disease. When birth weight is less than 1500 g or when major cardiac disease is present, survival is approximately 85%. Morbidity and mortality rates depend very much on coexisting conditions such as syndromes or associations. In premature infants with coexisting conditions, mortality is about 50% (Kovesi & Rubin, 2004; Ryckman & Balistreri, 2002). Support and communication are the cornerstones of parental care throughout hospitalization.

Gastroesophageal Reflux
Anatomy
Gastroesophageal reflux (GER) is the effortless retrograde passage of acidic gastric contents from the stomach into the esophagus. The term *chalasia* refers to an abnormal relaxation of the gastroesophageal junction. Infants are at greater risk for GER because of altered esophageal motility and peristalsis; lower esophageal sphincter (LES) position and immaturity; limited gastric volume and delayed gastric emptying; and impaired intestinal motility.

The distal esophagus possesses a physiologic sphincter, which is approximately 0.5 cm long in the infant, called the esophageal vestibule. In adults, the upper portion of the esophagus lies in the thorax, the middle section at the diaphragm, and the lower segment in the abdomen. This segment of terminal esophagus has a higher pressure than that of the stomach below or the esophagus above and helps prevent retrograde flow of gastric contents into the esophagus. LES tone normally increases in response to abdominal pressure, thus protecting against reflux. In infants, this protective mechanism is less effective because the LES is primarily above the diaphragm and subjected to intrathoracic pressure. An immature LES in the preterm infant may not allow effective pressure to be generated and may cause inappropriate relaxation of the muscle. LES pressure remains low for the first 2 weeks of life and increases markedly between 2 and 4 weeks. Adult LES pressures are achieved usually between 12 and 15 months of life. By 18 to 24 months, the esophagus has grown such that the LES is below the diaphragm. Any condition delaying or altering the maturation of this valve may cause reflux of stomach contents in the infant.

Pathophysiology

GER may be asymptomatic; present with nonspecific symptoms such as inconsolability, irritability, sleep disturbance, food refusal, and failure to thrive; or present with more obvious symptoms of postprandial regurgitation or vomiting. It has also been implicated in the pathogenesis of apnea, hoarse cry, stridor, reactive airway disease, recurrent bronchopulmonary infections, bronchopulmonary dysplasia (BPD), chronic lung disease, and ventilator dependence. Persistent vomiting due to GER often leads to failure to thrive. Such infants tend to be pale, thin, hypoactive, listless, and underweight and may be misdiagnosed with a nutritional deficiency. The most commonly recognized pulmonary symptom associated with GER is recurrent aspiration pneumonia, characterized by fever, cough, poor appetite, and typical findings on radiography.

Apneic spells, most commonly seen in the early weeks of life, may be caused by reflux. Gastroesophageal reflux is capable of causing laryngospasm, with cardiac slowing or arrest. Acid in the esophagus can lead to apnea or bronchospasm with wheezing or stridor. Worsening of chronic lung disease or BPD has also been associated with GER. Near sudden infant death syndrome (SIDS) episodes have been linked with GER, although the associated is unclear. Well-documented recurrent apneic spells have been completely eliminated in many cases after antireflux surgery. Asthma or asthma-like symptoms related to reflux are rare during the first year of life but have been seen occasionally in infants. Esophagitis is generally not seen in the early months of life. Infants who suffer from esophagitis caused by GER are usually fussy, irritable, and colicky. Frank bleeding is rare but may be present with anemia and guaiac-positive stools.

Healthy premature infants often demonstrate behavior that in symptomatic older infants is associated with acid reflux but in the preterm infant is not reflux. Reflux specific behavior such as irritability, crying, or grimacing that is established in older term infants may be inappropriate as diagnostic criteria for GER in preterm infants and may lead to unnecessary use of antireflux medications.

Premature infants are at risk for weak junction with the LES not maturing normally and have a 63% risk of GER. Approximately 50% of healthy infants at the age of 2 months may have symptomatic reflux. Regurgitation peaks at 3 months of age and usually resolves by 6 to 12 months of age (Khalaf et al, 2001). Symptomatic GER has been reported in 3% to 10% of very-low-birth-weight infants (VLBW) (<1500 g).

Infants with high bowel obstructions have delayed maturation of the valve mechanism and are at risk for chalasia resulting from structural weakness. Most infants with congenital diaphragmatic hernia experience reflux after repair—most likely caused by deviation of the esophagus to the affected side, malposition of the stomach, increased intra-abdominal pressure, gastric dysmotility, or a combination of these factors. Additionally, infants who have undergone operative repair of tracheoesophageal fistula or esophageal atresia have extremely high incidence of GER, as do infants with congenital abdominal wall defects. A high percentage of infants with neurologic damage exhibit GER, possibly due to reduced swallowing frequency and weaker esophageal sphincter control. Some medications such as diazepam, calcium-channel blockers, theophylline, caffeine, and anticholinergics may worsen GER (Khalaf et al, 2001; Jadcherla, 2002).

Treatment

Most infants can be safely treated medically for 3 months before it may be judged that conservative therapy has failed. Seventy-five percent recover when treated medically; 10% to 15% require prolonged medical management; and 10% to 15% require surgery. When symptoms are controlled by medical means, reflux ceases by 15 months of age and therapy can be discontinued. Surgical long-term results are good, with reported 95% total clinical cures assessed at check-ups after 10 years or more. Adverse side effects, including mild gas bloating, slow eating, and inability to burp or vomit, are seen in approximately one third of surgically treated patients.

Careful history and clinical evaluation are needed to rule out a host of diseases that present with emesis. Differential diagnosis includes ruling out other causes of vomiting, such as distal outlet obstruction as in pyloric stenosis or antral web; volvulus; intussusception; meconium ileus/plug; Hirschsprung's disease; sepsis; abnormalities of amino acid metabolism such as urea cycle defects, galactosemia, or congenital adrenal hyperplasia; increased intracranial pressure; necrotizing enterocolitis; gastroenteritis; formula intolerance; pancreatitis; cholecystitis; pyelonephritis; hydronephrosis; rumination; and drug toxicity.

A barium swallow is a poor test for diagnosing GER, but is useful for confirming normal esophageal, gastric, and intestinal anatomy. The 24-hour pH probe test is considered the gold standard for the diagnosis of GER. The study is scored by determining the amount of time the esophagus is exposed to an acid pH level. Scoring for abnormal results is based on frequency of reflux, number of episodes greater than 4 minutes in duration, time of longest episode, and percentage of time in reflux. Interpretation of the data is complex because of confounding factors such as position, activity, frequency and composition of feeding, and medication. Nursing responsibilities include recording the time of feedings and describing the activity level of the infant throughout the test. Technetium scintigraphy may be used to measure gastric emptying, aspiration with swallowing, and reflux with aspiration. A technetium radioisotope is used because it has relatively low radiation and is easily added to formula. Flexible endoscopy with biopsy of the distal esophagus is used to diagnose esophagitis. Laryngoscopy and bronchoscopy can be helpful in assessing vocal cord erosion or inflammation or finding milk-laden macrophages (Berseth, 2005b).

A multidisciplinary approach in the assessment of the infant with GER and its related problems is important in the diagnostic process. The history, physical examination, and test results of upper GE series or pH probe testing confirm or deny the diagnosis. A clinical distinction must be made as to whether the GER is physiologic or pathologic based on the infant's ability to thrive well. In the face of pathologic GER, nursing and medical collaboration is necessary to assess the effectiveness of conservative treatment modalities. These methods include positioning, thickening of feedings, monitoring for apnea, pharmacologic management, and parental support.

A 30-degree prone or left lateral position after feedings is better than the upright and supine positions, when the infant is both awake and asleep. Contrary to popular thinking, infants placed in infant seats have 50% more reflux episodes that last twice as long as those that occur in the prone position. Slouching increases pressure on the stomach and the risk of reflux. When infants are positioned in infant seats or car seats, their trunks must be supported to minimize abdominal compression. Kangaroo care has been anecdotally reported to offer benefit by holding the infant in a prone elevated position. Positioning the infant at a 45- to 60-degree angle during feedings has been shown to reduce reflux.

Thickened feedings with 1 tablespoon of rice cereal added to 1 to 2 ounces of formula may reduce vomiting and crying and increase sleep time after feedings for some infants. Thickened feedings have not been shown to reduce reflux during concurrent pH probe studies unless the infants were also in an elevated prone position. For some infants, thickened feedings increase the length of reflux episodes, thus causing increased coughing and pulmonary complications.

Apneic episodes and recurrent aspiration pneumonia have been associated with GER. Infants suspected of and documented as having clinically significant reflux should therefore undergo continuous respiratory monitoring. This monitoring is particularly important when xanthines are used to treat the apnea. Although xanthines are used to improve respiratory function and reduce apnea, they also increase gastric acid secretion and decrease lower esophageal sphincter pressure, which may further increase GER (Zenk et al, 2003).

Histamine-2 antagonists (cimetidine, famotidine, or ranitidine) are used to reduce acidity and associated esophageal pain and damage from acid reflux. Omeprazole, pantoprazole, lansoprazole, and rabeprazole are proton pump antagonists, blocking acid production. They have been used in infants with severe esophagitis who do not respond to other agents. Antacids such as aluminum hydroxide and magnesium hydroxide are rarely used due to side effects of constipation and diarrhea (Bell, 2003). The pharmacologic mainstay of treatment for GER is the prokinetic drug metoclopramide, a dopamine receptor antagonist, which decreases gastric emptying time and enhances LES pressure. It has a narrow therapeutic range with onset of 30 to 34 minutes. Extrapyramidal side effects sometimes include restlessness, lethargy, and abnormal posturing. Less commonly seen side effects include nausea, vomiting, diarrhea. Bethanecol and erythromycin are prokinetic drugs used rarely to treat GER in the infant because of cardiac and gastrointestinal side effects (Hammer, 2005; James, 2002). Cisapride, a prokinetic agent that enhances gastric motility, was widely used in the 1980s and 1990s to manage GER in infants. Concern about its use in preterm infants due to prolonged QT intervals prompted warning from the Food and Drug Administration and the subsequent discontinuance of use.

If medical management fails to control life-threatening complications, surgical intervention is indicated. Although many procedures have been devised, the Nissen fundoplication is most widely used in the neonate. In this procedure, the proximal stomach is wrapped around the distal esophagus, creating a junction that is effective in preventing reflux. Laparoscopic techniques have been successful in even the smallest of infants. Complication rates are comparable and there appears to be less pain, less gastric ileus, and shorter hospital stay (Cass & Wesson, 2002). Infants may have a temporary gastrostomy placed to vent swallowed air and decrease bloating. The tube is usually removed after 3 to 6 weeks. Rate of revision of the fundoplication has been reported to be as high as 24%; the highest failure occurs in infants with

associated anomalies such as TEF, lung abnormalities, congenital diaphragmatic hernia (CDH), and neurologic disorders. Parental support is essential in nursing management of the infant with GER. The nurse can help parents to identify feeding, positioning, and soothing techniques. Parents need to learn the etiology of GER and its usual course as well as interventions, including medication administration. Parents can also be referred to local support groups or PAGER (Pediatric and Adolescent Gastroesophageal Reflux) at http://www.reflux.org/, for additional information and support.

Pyloric Stenosis
Anatomy
Although many cases of pyloric stenosis may be acquired postnatally, this disorder is properly referred to as congenital hypertrophic pyloric stenosis. The pathologic picture consists of marked hypertrophy of the pylorus with spasm of the muscular coat, creating a tumor-like nodule resulting in a partial gastric outlet obstruction.

Pathophysiology
The infant typically appears healthy for the first 2 weeks of life and then begins vomiting (nonbilious), which worsens to frequent projectile vomiting. The infant may be anxious, irritable, and excessively hungry; have decreased frequency of stool; and lose weight. Vomiting may cause dehydration, metabolic alkalosis, hypochloremia, and hypokalemia. The level of indirect bilirubin is significantly elevated in 5% of affected infants but resolves when stenosis is corrected.

The cause is poorly understood but probably has a genetic basis with a polygenic mode of inheritance, modified by gender. The prevalence rate typically ranges from 1 to 3 per 1000, with higher rates in whites than in blacks. More males, specifically first-born males, have the disease than do females, and approximately 5% of affected infants are born to women who themselves have the disease (Merenstein & Gardner, 2006).

Associated factors include maternal stress and anxiety, feeding practices, and antenatal exposure to doxylamine succinate–pyridoxine hydrochloride (Bendectin). Seasonal factors, such as infection, have also been reported.

Treatment
Medical and nursing assessment and management of the infant are critical throughout the process of management. Diagnosis of pyloric stenosis may be made by palpation of the hypertrophied pylorus, an olive-like mass in the deep right upper quadrant of the abdomen. Most surgeons are not comfortable with palpatory findings alone and request confirmatory ultrasound before surgical intervention (Berseth & Poenaru, 2005a).

There is no effective medical treatment. The repair is by pyloromyotomy. A simple incision is made in the hypertrophied longitudinal and circular muscles of the pylorus, thus releasing the obstruction. Laparoscopic pyloromyotomy, introduced in 1991, is an alternative, leaving essentially no scar, and may reduce postoperative pain and the duration of gastric ileus (Cass & Wesson, 2002; Hall et al, 2004).

Preoperatively, fluid and electrolyte management is paramount. A nasogastric tube connected to low intermittent suction is maintained to prevent distention and vomiting and to decrease the risk of aspiration. Thermoregulation is maintained to prevent exacerbation of symptoms.

Postoperatively, intravenous hydration and electrolyte balance must be maintained. Nasogastric suction is continued for 4 to 24 hours. The tube may be removed when the infant is fully awake and bowel sounds are present. Assessment of the suture line is made for signs of infection or skin breakdown. Feedings are begun 4 to 24 hours after surgery when the baby is fully awake.

Once it is diagnosed and surgically treated, the prognosis is excellent, with complete relief of symptoms. The mortality rate is less than 1%, provided that the infant has not become too dehydrated and malnourished.

MANAGEMENT OF PROBLEMS WITH DIGESTION

Biliary Atresia

Anatomy

Biliary atresia is the complete obstruction of bile flow due to fibrosis of the extrahepatic ducts. Infants appear normal at birth and pass stools with appropriate pigmentation. Clinical signs are subtle, with jaundice persisting after the first week of life. The direct bilirubin level slowly increases and results in a greenish bronze appearance of the skin. Gradually stools become clay-colored to pale to yellowish tan, and the urine becomes dark as the result of bile excretion.

Over a 2- to 3-month period, the liver becomes cirrhotic. Portal hypertension is a major complication. The reverse blood flow results in enlargement of esophageal, umbilical, and rectal veins, which is manifested as splenomegaly, hemorrhoids, enlarged abdominal veins, ascites, and blood in the stools. Additional complications include decreased clotting ability, anemia, and ineffective metabolism of nutrients. End-stage liver disease may lead to rupture of veins in the esophagus and stomach or hepatic coma with eventual death from liver failure.

Case Study

IDENTIFICATION OF THE PROBLEM

Baby B was a male infant born to a 34-year-old, G3, P2002 mother, by primary cesarean section for nonreassuring fetal heart tones. Amniocentesis had revealed a prenatal diagnosis of trisomy 21. He did well after delivery with Apgar scores of 7 at 1 minute and 9 at 5 minutes of life. He was taken to the term nursery where he developed feeding intolerance and bilious emesis. Abdominal radiograph revealed a large gastric bubble, a smaller duodenal bubble, and no distal bowel gas. He was made NPO and given IV fluid of D10W started at 80 ml/kg/day. Blood cultures were drawn and ampicillin and gentamicin were administered. An orogastric tube was placed to low intermittent suction.

ASSESSMENT: HISTORY AND PHYSICAL EXAMINATION

This mother had a history of being group B streptococcus (GBS) positive, serology negative, and had polyhydramnios and hypertension. She received a partial course of antibiotics prior to the baby's delivery. Rupture of membranes was at delivery with clear amniotic fluid. The baby was preterm with gestational age assessed by physical exam of 36 weeks, and he weighed 1800 g. The facies were consistent with trisomy 21 and the head appeared disproportionately large. He was acyanotic, well perfused, breath sounds clear bilaterally, no heart murmur was noted. The abdomen was soft and flat. There was slight hypotonia.

DIFFERENTIAL DIAGNOSIS

Bilious emesis is a hallmark for high gastrointestinal obstruction. The classic radiographic finding of "double bubble" reflects the localization of swallowed air in stomach and duodenum, with the rest of the bowel being airless. If air is present elsewhere, other anomalies causing partial obstruction must be ruled out (duodenal stenosis, duodenal web, annular pancreas, or malrotation with volvulus).

DIAGNOSTIC TESTS

Radiographic findings of "double bubble" were noted, and the abdomen was gasless beyond the duodenum. An upper GI study may be helpful if there is incomplete obstruction by identifying duodenal stenosis, duodenal web, annular pancreas, or associated malrotation.

Loss of gastric secretions through suction can cause dramatic shifts in fluid and electrolyte balance. Electrolytes must be monitored closely and replacement fluids altered as needed. Blood cultures and CBC with differential in the face of abdominal distention are needed to rule out septic ileus. Blood cultures must be drawn prior to administration of antibiotics. Because of a high association of Down syndrome and cardiac defects, an echocardiogram was done that showed a structurally normal heart with patent foramen ovale.

WORKING DIAGNOSIS

Prenatal chromosome results revealed trisomy 21, and the physical examination was consistent with Down syndrome. The infant plotted in the 9th percentile of weight for gestational age of 36 weeks. The radiographic findings showed "double bubble." There was risk of sepsis due to intestinal obstruction and a GBS positive maternal history. The working diagnoses were trisomy 21, preterm, small for gestational age (SGA), duodenal atresia, and suspected sepsis.

DEVELOPMENT OF MANAGEMENT PLAN

Initial management after identification of the problem was to stabilize the infant with IV fluids, to decompress the stomach to prevent vomiting and aspiration of stomach contents or perforation due to overdistention, and to treat with antibiotics until sepsis is ruled out as cause of bilious vomiting. Baby B was transferred to a tertiary center for pediatric surgery intervention and genetic consultation.

Continued

Case Study—cont'd

IMPLEMENTATION AND EVALUATION OF EFFECTIVENESS

Excision of the atretic site was performed on day 2 of life. Post-operative care included continued decompression of the stomach with low intermittent suction. Morphine was given prn for pain control. Antibiotics were continued 48 hours post-operatively. Initial blood cultures were negative. The baby was ventilated for 24 hours post-op and was extubated to room air. Parenteral nutrition was provided. Electrolytes were carefully monitored due to loss of gastric fluid. Replacement fluid of one-half normal saline with 2 mEq KCl/100 ml was given ml/ml q8h equaling the volume of gastric aspirate. Oral feedings were begun 10 days after surgery. Some nasogastric feeds were required because of poor PO feeding and a speech therapy consult obtained. Coordination improved and he was able to advance to all PO feeds by 8 days post-op. He was discharged home on full enteral feeding and given appointments for Pediatric Surgery 2 weeks after discharge and Genetics in 2 months. Referral was made for early intervention.

Pathophysiology

Biliary atresia is the most common form of ductal cholestasis and occurs in approximately 1 in every 10,000 births, with a female predominance. The cause remains unclear. Some clinicians theorize that the obstruction is due to injured bile ducts leading to atresia; others describe the disease as an inflammatory process, whereas still others propose an intrauterine insult from environmental factors or failure of ducts to recanalize. Pathologically, the obstruction of the common bile duct prevents bile from entering the duodenum. Consequently, digestion and absorption of fat are impaired, thus leading to deficiencies in fat-soluble vitamins and vitamin K, which affect bleeding tendencies. Owing to the obstruction, bile accumulates in the ducts and gallbladder and causes distention of these structures. The atresia appears to progress to the intrahepatic ducts, leading to biliary cirrhosis and ultimately death if the bile flow is not established.

Associated congenital defects, found in 15% of reported cases, include congenital heart disease, polysplenic syndrome, small bowel atresia, bronchobiliary atresia, and trisomies 17 and 18. Teratogenic factors include ionizing radiation, drugs, ischemic episode, and viruses such as reovirus type 3, cytomegalovirus, rubella, and hepatitis A and B.

Treatment

Medical, surgical, and nursing staff must strive diligently in the diagnostic workup and ultimate treatment. Consultation and follow-up care by a gastroenterologist provides guidance for feeding and drug therapy modalities. Parents of these infants can profit from ongoing support from social services, chaplains, or support counseling sources.

Surgical intervention involves a hepatic portoenterostomy, called the Kasai procedure, which consists of dissection and resection of the extrahepatic bile duct. The porta hepatis, where the ducts normally occur, is cut, and a loop of bowel is brought up to permit bile drainage from the liver surface to the GI tract. If the Kasai procedure is unsuccessful, the only alternative for treatment is transplantation.

Nurses take an active role in the complex task of diagnosis and treatment of the infant with biliary atresia. Because of the portal hypertension and bleeding tendencies, careful monitoring of vital signs and blood pressure is important. Efficient collection of multiple blood samples is required for tests, including bilirubin, aspartate transaminase (AST), alanine transaminase (ALT), alkaline phosphatase, albumin, protein, and cholesterol determinations; prothrombin time; complete blood count; reticulocyte count; Coombs' test; measurement of platelets and red blood cell morphologic features, thyroxine, thyroid-stimulating hormone, and glucose determinations; cultures; and TORCH titers. Urine is collected for urinalysis, culture, and metabolic screens. Radiography, ultrasonography, liver biopsy, and hepatobiliary scan (using hydroxyiminodiacetic acid) or HIDA scan may be performed. The last is used to determine adequacy of the liver function (Karpen, 2002).

Meeting nutritional requirements is difficult because the infant needs one and one-half to two times the normal caloric requirements owing to affected metabolism, yet ascites and pressure on the stomach make it difficult for the child to eat. Formulas must contain medium-chain triglycerides for easier absorption. Supplementation with fat-soluble vitamins is required because of impaired absorption. Parenteral nutrition is often given to provide adequate calories. Phenobarbital, Actigall, and cholestyramine may be an ongoing therapy to stimulate bile flow. Vitamin K may be given for coagulopathy.

The whole family requires comprehensive psychosocial support. Family and work life are disrupted by lengthy, repeated hospitalizations. The emotional and physical toll is high because of complex care demands, and dealing with the suffering of the child places further stress on the parents. Social support systems need to be explored to assist families in dealing with the long-term health crisis of an infant with biliary atresia.

Multiple causes of cholestasis in the infant exist. All causes must be considered in the presence of conjugated hyperbilirubinemia, other causes excluded, and proper therapy instituted. The differential diagnosis includes neonatal hepatitis, choledochal cyst, errors of metabolism, trisomies 18 and 21, α_1-antitrypsin deficiency, neonatal hypopituitarism, cystic fibrosis, TORCH infectious agents, bacterial sepsis, drug-induced cholestasis, and cholestasis associated with parenteral nutrition.

Survival in untreated cases of biliary atresia is less than 2 years. Approximately 23% of patients with a Kasai portoenterostomy will survive more than 20 years without liver transplantation (Lykavieris et al, 2005). One third of the patients drain bile but develop complications of cirrhosis and require liver transplantation before the age of 10. The remaining third of patients have bile flow that is inadequate after the Kasai procedure and develop fibrosis and cirrhosis. Only 18% of infants with biliary atresia who have corrective surgery avoid liver transplant. The overall survival rate after the Kasai procedure and transplantation is >90% (Kobayashi & Stringer, 2003). Sequential surgical treatment of Kasai portoenterostomy in infancy followed by selective liver transplantation for children with progressive hepatic deterioration yield improved overall survival. Limited donor availability and increased complications after liver transplantation in infants less than 1 year of age militate against the use of primary liver transplantation without prior Kasai procedure in infants with biliary atresia (Ryckman & Balistreri, 2002).

Predictors of poor outcome after portoenterostomy include operative age greater than 2 months of age, presence of cirrhosis at first biopsy, total nonpatency of extrahepatic ducts, absence of bile ducts at transected liver hilus, and subsequent development of varices or ascites.

Duodenal Atresia
Anatomy
Thirty percent of all atresias occur in the duodenum (Berseth & Poenaru, 2005a). Although atresias may be located at any point along the duodenum, most obstructions (80% to 90%) are situated below the ampulla of Vater. Consequently, bilious vomiting is a common presenting sign. Failure to pass meconium is noted in approximately 70% of patients. Both the onset of vomiting and the ability to pass stool are related to the site of obstruction. Proximal duodenal obstructions tend to present with vomiting within a few hours of birth, although stool may be passed normally. Distal obstructions tend to present with a later onset of vomiting and failure to pass stool. Abdominal distention is generally not noted, but when present is confined to the upper abdomen, thus giving the lower abdomen an almost scaphoid appearance in contrast.

Pathophysiology
Duodenal atresia occurs as the result of incomplete recanalization of the lumen. The mechanism by which recanalization is prevented is not known but most likely occurs when the proliferative villi adhere abnormally to one another. The result is the formation of a transverse diaphragm of tissue that completely obstructs the lumen. Almost half of all duodenal or postampullary obstructions are due to duodenal atresia (Ryckman, 2002). Overall occurrence is approximately 1 in every 6,000 to 10,000 live births. Over one quarter of these cases are related to Trisomy 21 or Down syndrome (Ryckman, 2002). Most infants with duodenal atresia have related anomalies such as Down syndrome, cardiac malformations, malrotation, esophageal atresia, small bowel lesions, and anorectal lesions (Berseth & Poenaru, 2005a).

Polyhydramnios has been identified as a significant risk factor that occurs in one quarter to one half of women who deliver affected infants. Associated anomalies, present in 60% to 70% of patients, are numerous and include trisomy 21, malrotation, TE anomalies, imperforate anus, congenital heart disease, VATER or VACTERL association, and renal anomalies. An annular pancreas—resulting from the failure of the two pancreatic buds to fuse normally, allowing the deformed pancreas to encircle the duodenum—is found in approximately 20% of patients. Nearly half of all infants are premature

or of low birth weight and 40% acquire hyperbilirubinemia (Bates & Balistreri, 2002; Ryckman, 2002).

Treatment
The significance of polyhydramnios has been noted previously, but in its absence a large amount of gastric aspirate may be obtained on routine delivery room screening. Normally, only small amounts of aspirate are expected (4 to 7 ml), but if more than 10 to 15 ml is obtained, atresia should be suspected (Bloom, 2002).

Radiographic examination provides confirmation of duodenal atresia with the classic finding of a "double bubble" (Figure 5-4). These bubbles reflect the localization of swallowed air in the stomach and in the distended portion of the duodenum lying above the obstruction; the remainder of the bowel is totally airless. If gas is present elsewhere, other anomalies causing partial obstruction must be presumed. An upper GI series may be helpful in identifying incomplete obstructions such as duodenal stenosis, duodenal web, or annular pancreas or in ruling out associated malrotation.

Surgical treatment involves excision of the atretic site (unless the area so closely approximates the pancreatic and bile ducts that injury to these structures is risked) and side-to-side anastomosis of the free ends. The level of the obstruction determines whether a duodenoduodenostomy or a duodenojejunostomy is carried out. Tapering of a distended duodenum may be done to reduce future duodenal dysmotility. A gastrostomy may also be performed for decompression to avoid trauma to the anastomotic site. A combined nursing and medical approach facilitates both preoperative stabilization and postoperative recuperation.

Preoperative care is directed toward hydration and gastric decompression. Intermittent gastric suction by use of a sump tube reduces the risk of aspiration or perforation due to

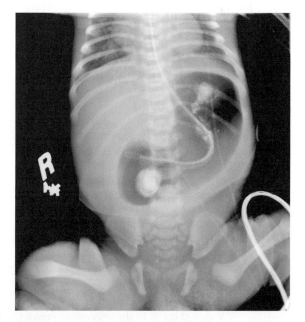

FIGURE **5-4**
Duodenal atresia with the hallmark radiographic finding of abdominal "double bubble" as seen when air fills the stomach and the duodenum and can progress no further. Courtesy Radiology Department of Children's Healthcare of Atlanta.

overdistention. Vital signs, fluid intake and output, urine specific gravity, and serum electrolytes must be closely monitored, and fluids, electrolytes, and crystalloid must be provided as needed. Antibiotics may be instituted for preoperative prophylaxis or when perforation or sepsis is suspected.

Continued decompression and nutrition are the major postoperative concerns. Total parenteral nutrition is given initially. Oral feedings are generally begun at 10 to 14 days with an oral electrolyte solution and advanced to low-osmolality formulas such as Nutramigen or Pregestimil (protein hydrolysate formulas) before moving to regular formula. Often enteral feedings will be given as jejunal ones so that it is introduced distal to the surgical site (Ryckman, 2002).

Late complications such as peptic ulcers, adhesions, and need for revision of correction have been reported in 12% of patients (Escobar et al, 2004). A 65% to 84% survival rate is reported, with deaths attributed to associated cardiac or renal anomalies or to infectious or respiratory complications.

Jejunal/Ileal Atresia
Anatomy

Fifty percent of all atresias occur in the jejunum or ileum where there is complete obstruction of the intestinal lumen. Signs and symptoms generally present at 1 or 2 days of age and are virtually the same for all types of jejunoileal atresia

(Figure 5-5). Presentation includes bilious vomiting, failure to pass stool, and generalized abdominal distention.

Pathophysiology

Atresias of the jejunum and ileum are thought to result from mesenteric vascular compromise with necrosis and eventual resorption of the involved area. The presence of bile, meconium, epithelial cells, and lanugo distal to the atresia indicates that this ischemic injury occurs relatively late in utero, possibly as late as 3 to 6 months' gestation (Ryckman, 2002). The occurrence rate is 1 in 20,000 live births, with an apparently equal distribution of atresias between the jejunum and the ileum. There is no linkage to gender and the development of this form of atresia (Berseth & Poenaru, 2005a).

Owing to the surface area available for absorption proximal to the obstruction, maternal polyhydramnios does not generally present as a risk factor, as it does in the higher atresias of the esophagus and duodenum. Polyhydramnios is reported in only one third of those with jejunal atresia; ileal atresias rarely present with polyhydramnios. Because this group of defects arises after embryogenesis is complete, associated anomalies are rare. When they do occur, they are primarily restricted to the GI tract, with malrotation and meconium ileus being most common. Between 25% and 30% of patients experience hyperbilirubinemia, and 25% to 38% are born

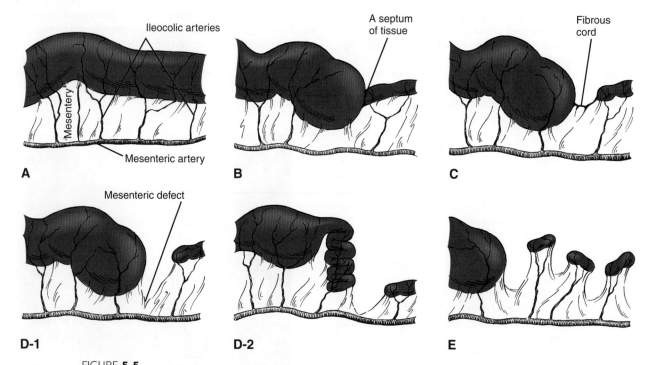

FIGURE **5-5**
Jejunoileal obstruction. Percentages reflect relative occurrence. **A,** Normal anatomy. **B,** Type I or diaphragmatic form (20%): single atresia in which the integrity of the bowel wall is preserved, but its lumen is obstructed by a septum of tissue; the mesentery is intact. **C,** Type II or cord anomaly (30% to 35%): single but discontinuous atresia with opposing ends connected by a long, fibrous cord; the mesentery is intact. **D-1,** Type IIIa or mesenteric defect (35% to 45%): single but discontinuous atresia with a V-shaped defect in the intervening mesentery. **D-2,** Type IIIb or "apple peel" (<1%): single but discontinuous atresia with a V-shaped defect in the intervening mesentery; the intestine coils around a single ileocolic artery, which is its sole source of circulation. **E,** Type IV or multiple atresias (5% to 10%): multiple discontinuous atresias with intervening V-shaped mesenteric defects, giving it the appearance of sausage links. Data from Gryboski J, Walker WA (1983). *Gastrointestinal problems in the infant*. Philadelphia: Saunders; and Touloukian RJ (1978). Intestinal atresia. *Clinics in perinatology* 5(1):3-18.

prematurely. Of the different types of jejunoileal atresia that have been identified (Figure 5-5), only the "apple peel" or "Christmas tree" type is typically familial, thus indicating that this one form alone may involve some autosomal recessive or multifactorial type of inheritance.

Although it is the most rare form of jejunoileal atresia, it carries the highest mortality rate (54%) and higher rates of prematurity and malrotation in comparison with the more conventional types.

Treatment

Abdominal radiographs show multiple bubbles that reflect dilation and collection of swallowed air proximal to the obstruction (Figure 5-6). Intraperitoneal calcifications are present in 10% of patients, which indicates antenatal intestinal perforation with resultant meconium peritonitis. The peritonitis in this case is due to chemical irritation (there is no infection because the bowel and meconium are sterile before birth), thus causing fibrosis, granuloma formation, and ultimately calcifications. The perforated site usually heals spontaneously before delivery and leaves no evidence of what occurred other than the residual calcifications. The airless, unused distal portion of the gut is generally contracted and of a much smaller caliber than normal. Visualization of this distal "microcolon" by barium or meglumine diatrizoate (Gastrograffin) enema may be necessary to rule out malrotation and meconium ileus (Bates & Balistreri, 2002).

Surgical management begins with resection of the dilated proximal gut and atretic, bulbous ending and a search for multiple distal atresias. Primary closure by end-to-end or side-to-end anastomosis generally follows, but preliminary tapering of the distended distal segment may be required; as a third alternative, an end-to-oblique closure may be performed. If there is considerable discrepancy (more than 2:1) between the dilated proximal portion and the distal microcolon, an ostomy (either double-barrel or single) is created. Once surgical correction is

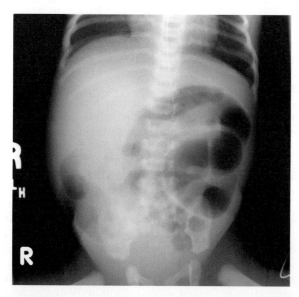

FIGURE **5-6**
Bowel distention in neonate with ileal atresia. Multiple bubbles reflect dilation and collection of swallowed air proximal to the obstruction. Courtesy Radiology Department of Children's Healthcare of Atlanta.

complete, collaboration with the nutritional support team and enterostomal therapist is essential.

The principles of preoperative care involve bowel decompression and intravenous hydration with the correction of any electrolyte imbalance that may occur as the result of vomiting or third-spacing-capillary leak syndrome. Antibiotics may be given prophylactically, or therapeutically in the case of peritonitis. Recovery of bowel peristalsis and enzymatic integrity may be delayed, thus necessitating parenteral nutrition. When started, initial feedings are of a clear electrolyte solution and progress serially to elemental formulas such as Nutramigen or Pregestimil (protein hydrolysate formulas) until standard formula can be tolerated. The nurses should assess diligently for evidence of short-bowel syndrome, commonly seen with atresias that are multiple or of the "apple peel" variety, which necessitate excision of an extensive length of bowel.

With the availability of parenteral alimentation, survival rates have risen to as high as 84% to 96%. Deaths are generally the result of prematurity, postoperative short-bowel syndrome, or infectious complications.

Omphalocele
Anatomy

Omphalocele is generally an immediately apparent anomaly and ranges between 2 and 15 cm in size. However, the small defects that involve perhaps a single loop of intestine may be easily overlooked unless the physical examination is carried out in an unhurried fashion and the umbilical ring is clearly absent on palpation. The larger defects generally contain the intestine and possibly the liver, spleen, stomach, bladder, ovaries and tubes, or testicles. These two extremes most likely reflect the difference in the time at which normal embryogenesis is interrupted. If the interruption is early, around the 3- to 4-week window when infolding is in its last stages, the defect is large. If the interruption occurs later, at about 9 to 10 weeks when migration is generally completed, the defect is smaller. However, in both cases, the intestine—and possibly other abdominal organs—herniate into the umbilical cord. A thin, transparent membrane composed of peritoneum and amnion covers the viscera, and the visible bowel has a normal appearance (Figure 5-7). The abdominal cavity is often relatively small and underdeveloped, having never held the growing intestine.

Pathophysiology

Omphalocele results from the failure of the intestines to return from the umbilical cord into the abdominal cavity. Because some defects can be sufficiently large that they also contain the liver and other organs that do not normally participate in the migratory process, it has been further proposed that their passage can be accommodated only when there is incomplete folding of the embryonic disk so that the future abdominal wall cannot close completely, thus resulting in an unusually large umbilical ring.

Omphalocele occurs in roughly 1 of every 3000 to 6000 live births, with a male predominance. Mothers tend to be younger (93% <29 years old) (Hwang & Kousseff, 2004). Multiple and often life-threatening syndromes and anomalies occur with an unusually high frequency (30% to 70%) and include trisomy 13, trisomy 18, Beckwith-Wiedemann syndrome, pentalogy syndrome, congenital heart defects, diaphragmatic and upper midline defects, malrotation, intestinal atresia, and genitourinary anomalies. Additionally, 30% to 33% of affected infants

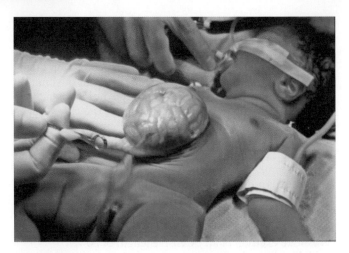

FIGURE **5-7**
Omphalocele with membranous covering prior to reduction. Courtesy Richard R. Ricketts, MD. Department of Pediatric Surgery, Emory University School of Medicine.

are premature, and approximately 19% are small for gestational age (Hwang & Kousseff, 2004). Of the infants with a central omphalocele, about one quarter will have cardiac anomalies, especially Cantrell pentalogy (cleft sternum, anterior midline diaphragmatic defects, a pericardial defect, congenital cardiac abnormalities which may include ectopia cordis, and an upper abdominal omphalocele) (Ryckman, 2002). Lower omphaloceles are associated in some cases with Beckwith-Wiedemann syndrome (omphalocele, macroglossia, macrosomia, and hypoglycemia) (Ryckman, 2002).

Treatment

Prenatal diagnosis has become so sophisticated that most incidences of abdominal wall defects are known well in advance of delivery. This knowledge allows preparation of the family and of the fetus. Ideally, maternal transport to a tertiary center saves the emergency situation of transporting an infant with such a defect. With the improved diagnostics, karyotyping can also be done to determine whether life-threatening chromosomal conditions exist, with the abdominal problem only being one part of the condition. Omphalocele is often used as an indicator for cesarean section, yet studies have shown no significant difference in morbidity and mortality according to delivery mode (Heider et al, 2004).

If surgery is contraindicated because of coexisting chromosomal or other syndromes, the defect may be treated medically by repeatedly painting the sac with silver nitrate solution, silver sulfadiazine mercurochrome, thimerosal (Merthiolate), polymer substances, or alcohol (Ryckman, 2002). These topical agents promote eschar formation and epithelialization with complete coverage by skin within 6 to 8 weeks. Should the patient survive, a later repair of the muscle wall becomes necessary. Biologic dressings have also been used to provide temporary protection. In some cases porcine and human skin grafts are also used.

The definitive surgical treatment is return of the viscera into the abdominal cavity and closure of the defect. This can be done via skin-flap closure or staged reduction. The procedure employed varies with the size of the defect. Primary closure is preferred, but larger defects (>5 cm) may require a staged repair with a polymeric silicone (Silastic) pouch or

chimney (silo) used to suspend the viscera above the patient. Reduction maneuvers are carried out daily to return the suspended organs into the relatively small abdominal cavity. A forceful return and closure under pressure would risk compression of the inferior vena cava, with reduced filling of the heart and decreased cardiac output and impedance of the diaphragmatic excursions, thus resulting in respiratory compromise. A gastrostomy to provide decompression and an appendectomy to avoid atypically presenting appendicitis in later life may be carried out with both primary and staged procedures, depending on the preferences of the surgical team. If a staged repair is performed, complete return of the organs into the abdominal cavity is generally achieved over a period of 7 to 10 days. At that time, the infant is returned to surgery for final closure of the abdominal wall.

These children often require aggressive postoperative respiratory management followed by prolonged total parenteral nutrition. Early psychosocial support of parents must be provided to promote their involvement in what is commonly an extended hospital stay. Genetic counseling may also be warranted.

The cornerstones of preoperative management include protection of the eviscerated organs, decompression of the gut, and hydration (Berseth & Poenaru, 2005b). Thermoregulation is a particular concern because massive evaporative and radiant heat losses may occur through the exposed defect. Care directed in these four areas may overlap, but all are necessary. The first step is to loosely apply sterile, warmed, saline-soaked gauze in a turban style around the defect, wrapping the ends around the body. Great care must be taken to prevent tight application, which might create pressure; two fingers should fit easily between the trunk and the encircling gauze. Some clinicians suggest that an outer, dry sterile dressing also be applied. The dressing is then covered with plastic wrap. As an alternative, sterile bowel bags may be used. Both wrapping and bag techniques provide protection to the defect from trauma and infection and help limit the loss of fluids and body heat. Clearly, sterile gloves must be worn during the necessary manipulation of the bowel. If the defect is small, the infant may be positioned on the back, but if the defect is large, it may be best to place the infant on the side. In the side-lying position, a small blanket or diaper may be slipped between the covered viscera and the bed surface so that no traction is placed on the bowel, which might cause physical injury to the gut or impede circulation. A gastric tube should be passed and set to low intermittent suction for decompression. Appropriate comfort measures to reduce or prevent crying with concomitant air swallowing should also be employed. Intravenous fluids should be started immediately to counteract direct fluid losses from exposure and the loss of fluids from the circulation caused by inflammation and third-spacing. Poor venous return from the lower extremities is also a concern owing to the ever-present potential for vena cava compression. Hydration status, fluid intake and output, and vital signs should be monitored closely for any evidence of hypovolemia, such as tachycardia, thready pulses, hypotension, poor perfusion, and decreased output of urine with increased specific gravity. Umbilical catheterization for venous access is contraindicated because of the nature and site of the defect. Prophylactic antibiotic administration should also be started.

Postoperative support varies slightly according to the repair procedure used, but both methods should generally include measures of hydration, decompression, and a search for evidence of increased intraabdominal pressure. Third-spacing, or capillary leak syndrome, may continue to be a problem and may actually be exacerbated by the trauma of surgical manipulation of the bowel. Assessment for signs of hypovolemia should be documented. Serum electrolytes, albumin, and total serum protein values should also be followed, with fluid and other replacements made as necessary. Decompression by gastric tube or gastrostomy is generally required for a considerable time until peristaltic activity returns. Ileus and cholestasis are common following repair, so enteral feedings may be considerably delayed, and parenteral alimentation is provided during the interval. When feedings are begun, an elemental formula may be used initially. Respiratory support with increased pressures may be required to achieve adequate ventilation if diaphragmatic movements are hampered. Inspection of the lower extremities and palpation of pedal pulses are helpful in assessing for impaired circulation. Elevating the extremities may promote venous return to the heart. In addition to these measures, if a staged repair is undertaken, particular attention must be paid to the infant's tolerance of daily reduction attempts. Furthermore, the silo provides an open port for bacterial invasion. Povidone-iodine or silver sulfadiazine (Silvadene) ointment may be applied with dressing changes, and most certainly antibiotic therapy is continued postoperatively.

Although a membrane generally covers omphaloceles, intrauterine rupture of that membrane occurs in 11% to 23% of patients. As a consequence of prolonged exposure to the amniotic fluid, the bowel becomes matted and edematous in appearance and difficult to differentiate from gastroschisis. Closer examination may reveal the sac remnants, but if none is noted, one need only look to the base of the cord. In gastroschisis, the umbilical cord is intact, inserted normally at the abdominal wall, and separated from the defect by a small amount of skin.

The overall mortality rate is reported as 5% to 50% depending on the size of the defect, associated chromosomal and other anomalies, early detection, and coincidental prematurity or low birth weight (Ryckman, 2002). Malrotation with the resultant danger of volvulus, ischemia, and necrosis is common. Antenatal membrane rupture may also add the dimension of potential sepsis.

Gastroschisis
Anatomy
Gastroschisis is a full-thickness defect in the abdominal wall through which the uncovered intestines protrude (Figure 5-8). Although it is often confused with a ruptured omphalocele, in gastroschisis the umbilical cord is inserted normally. The defect is next to rather than in the umbilical cord, and there is no protective sac, nor remnants thereof.

The liver and other solid organs generally remain in the abdominal cavity, although evisceration is possible. The defect is usually small (2 to 5 cm) and located to the right of the umbilicus, from which it is separated by a narrow margin of skin. The bowel is uncovered and, as a consequence of chemical peritonitis caused by long exposure to the amniotic fluid, appears as an edematous and matted mass with no identifiable loops. The abdominal cavity is small and underdeveloped.

Pathophysiology
Gastroschisis is generally thought to arise as the result of incomplete lateral infolding of the embryonic disk. As a result

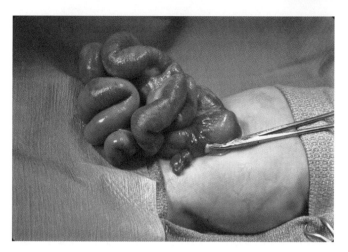

FIGURE **5-8**
Preoperative gastroschisis. Forceps attached to umbilicus. Courtesy Richard R. Ricketts, MD. Department of Pediatric Surgery, Emory University School of Medicine.

of this primary failure, the abdominal wall is incompletely formed, allowing herniation of the gut. Three other accepted theories have also been offered. The first suggests that the umbilical coelom (cavity) fails to form, so normal herniation of the midgut into the cord cannot occur. Consequently, during its rapid growth phase the intestine ruptures through the embryonic body wall. Another view considers that a vascular accident occurring in utero leads to occlusion of the omphalomesenteric artery. With its circulation removed, the base of the cord becomes necrotic, leaving an opening through which the intestine can eviscerate. The last theory proposes that gastroschisis may simply be a variant of omphalocele, with early intrauterine rupture of its membranous covering. The membrane remnants are subsequently reabsorbed, and the umbilical cord is reformed around the offset umbilical vessels. For the last two theories, the gap between the evisceration and cord base is presumably filled in by skin.

Prematurity (58%) and low birth weight (92%) are extremely common. Malrotation is found in all affected infants, and a few may exhibit intestinal atresia, but anomalies of systems other than the GI tract are infrequent and relatively minor. The overall incidence of gastroschisis has been steadily rising over the past several decades with incidence of approximately 1 per 5000 live births. Males are affected 1.5 times more often than females (King & Askin, 2003). It appears to be more common in mothers less than 20 years of age and rarely occurs in women over 30 years old. Nutritional alterations are noted in some mothers who give birth to an infant with gastroschisis. These changes are β-carotene, total glutathione, and high nitrosamine intakes (Ryckman, 2002).

Treatment
Cesarean section is often chosen for delivery to avoid injury to exposed bowel. Several studies have shown no difference in mortality or morbidity for infants born vaginally or by cesarean section. Some clinicians have proposed premature delivery when there is evidence of bowel compromise. Routine preterm delivery of infants with gastroschisis is not recommended because of inherent risk factors of prematurity and the

reversibility of most intestinal damage (King & Askin, 2003; Salihu et al, 2004).

A primary closure is the preferred surgical technique; however, the majority of defects are closed by staged repair using a fabricated spring-loaded silo that can be inserted at the bedside (Figure 5-9). This gradual approach to closure has shown fewer ventilation days, decreased time to full feeds, and shorter hospital days (Cass & Wesson, 2002; Schlatter, 2003). Although gastroschisis is a smaller defect than omphalocele, the distortion of the viscera with typical thickening and edema of the bowel make primary closure more difficult. Often the defect must be surgically enlarged to allow thorough inspection of the entire length of the GI tract and to avoid restricting the passage of the eviscerated intestine back into the abdominal cavity. All display some degree of malrotation, predisposing them to both intestinal atresias and infarction. Bowel resection and anastomosis are often necessary; however, primary anastomosis is contraindicated in the face of peritonitis or inflammation. In such situations, an enterostomy is performed away from the defect, with anastomosis delayed until final closure of the abdominal wall. The visceral mass is returned to the abdominal cavity as a whole. Because of the potential for bowel injury and blood loss, no attempt is made to unravel the adherent loops of bowel.

Preoperative nutritional and respiratory support is essential. Consultation with social services is helpful in providing parental support and establishing healthy parent-child relationships. The care of patients with gastroschisis is much like that for omphalocele. The intestines should be covered to protect them from injury and to reduce the loss of fluids and heat. Preoperative care is rounded out by use of gastric decompression, fluid resuscitation, and antibiotic prophylaxis.

Following surgery, the major concerns are venous stasis, respiratory compromise, infection, and nutrition. Edema and cyanosis of the lower extremities and evidence of decreased cardiac output should be reported immediately. Intensive respiratory support is provided, and oxygenation and ventilation are monitored closely. Infection is prevented by careful aseptic dressing changes, daily applications of bacteriostatic solutions or ointments, and systemic administration of antibiotics. Total parenteral nutrition is generally continued for several weeks until intestinal function returns. Feedings are usually begun with elemental formula, eventually progressing to standard formula, with diligent assessment for evidence of intestinal obstruction during the process.

A less than 8% mortality rate is reported for gastroschisis, with all deaths directly related to the defect. Early deaths are largely attributable to a combination of shock, sepsis (associated with perforation or contamination of the exposed bowel), and hypothermia. Profound hypothermia (temperature lower than 35° C [95° F]) is reported to occur in 67% of affected infants. Late deaths come as a result of sepsis, respiratory failure, and the inability of the bowel to sustain nutrition.

Malrotation with Volvulus
Anatomy
Malrotation is an anomaly of intestinal rotation and fixation where the base of the mesentery becomes short, placing all small bowel at risk of volvulus and ischemia. Of all the affected infants, only about half will present with symptoms in the first week of life. In those who do, the symptoms are generally intermittent or recurrent, indicating that most of these obstructions are partial rather than complete. Most infants demonstrate progressive bilious vomiting. When a previously well infant presents with sudden bilious vomiting, a malrotation with volvulus should be the clinician's first thought. In the case of volvulus, the abdomen may become distended, and the stools may be bloody. Bleeding occurs when twisting is severe enough to interfere with venous return from the bowel, thus causing the vessels to become engorged and leak blood into the gut.

Pathophysiology
The abnormality most likely arises between the 8th and 10th week of gestation as the intestine rotates around the axis of the superior mesenteric artery during its entry into and movement from the umbilical cord. Once returned to the abdominal cavity, the intestinal mesentery lies along and eventually adheres to the posterior abdominal wall, thus fixing the intestine in place. The normal 270-degree counterclockwise rotation can be interrupted or deviated at any time, and consequently a variety of rotation and fixation anomalies are possible (Figure 5-10).

The major danger with malrotation is that the intestinal loops may become kinked, knotted, or otherwise obstructed. This knotting and twisting of the bowel is called a volvulus. The resultant occlusion of the intestinal tract or its blood

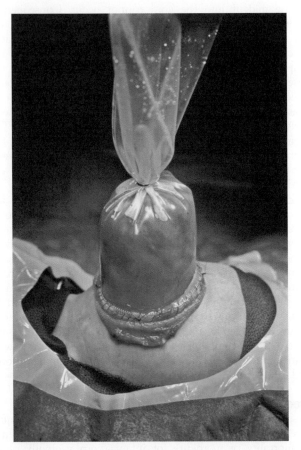

FIGURE **5-9**
Gastroschisis in polyurethane silo. Intestines are slowly reduced into the abdomen over several days. Courtesy Richard R. Ricketts, MD. Department of Pediatric Surgery, Emory University School of Medicine.

supply can lead to widespread ischemia and necrosis. Nearly two thirds of all cases of malrotation are complicated by volvulus, with the incidence varying with age at the onset of symptoms, but 80% occurring in the neonatal period (Berseth & Poenaru, 2005a). Eighty-five percent of patients less than 1 month of age have volvulus, compared with 43% of older children.

Intestinal rotational anomalies occur in approximately 1 in 6000 live births. The anomaly does appear to predominate in males with no specific cause identified.

Because of the nature of these defects, almost all cases of omphalocele, gastroschisis, and diaphragmatic hernia entail some component of malrotation. The frequency is in fact so high that many clinicians do not consider malrotation an anomaly associated with these conditions but rather an expected component of them. Associated anomalies such as intestinal atresias, annular pancreas, Meckel's diverticulum, and urinary tract malformation as well as congenital heart disease are found in patients with malrotation.

Treatment
On plain radiograph, the stomach and upper small intestine are generally distended with air and may mimic the characteristic "double-bubble" of duodenal atresia. However, the

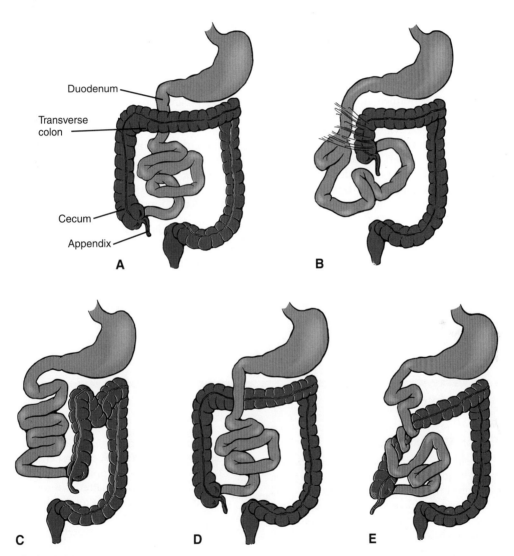

FIGURE **5-10**
Anomalies of rotation and fixation. **A,** Normal anatomy: cecum lies in right lower quadrant; transverse colon overlies duodenum. **B,** Incomplete rotation (Ladd bands): cecum lies just below and anterior to the duodenum, where it becomes fixed to the posterior wall by abnormal peritoneal bands; the bands cross over, compress, and obstruct the duodenum. **C,** Nonrotation ("left-sided colon"): entire small intestine lies in the right side of the abdominal cavity, whereas all of the large intestine lies on the left; volvulus may occur, but the condition is more frequently asymptomatic. **D,** Reverse (clockwise) rotation: duodenum overlies and may obstruct the transverse colon. **E,** Nonfixation ("midgut volvulus"): mesentery fails to adhere to the posterior abdominal wall so that the small intestine hangs loosely from the superior mesenteric artery and is free to twist around it or on itself to create a volvulus, typically involving the duodenum. Data from Chang JHT (1980). Neonatal surgical emergencies: Part IV—malrotation of the intestine. *Perinatalogy/neonatology* 4(1):50-52; Moore KL Persuad TVN (1993). *Before we are born: Basic embryology and birth defects,* ed 4. Philadelphia: Saunders; and Sadler TW (1985). *Langman's medical embryology,* ed 5. Baltimore: Williams & Wilkins.

presence of small amounts of gas in the distal positions of the gut is more reflective of a partial obstruction by malrotation than of an atresia in the jejunum or ileum. A contrast enema can be given to locate the position of the cecum under fluoroscopy. If a misplaced colon is seen, the diagnosis of malrotation is confirmed. However, some malrotations (notably reverse rotation) may not be demonstrated. An upper GI series is diagnostic in all cases and allows the exact position of the duodenum to be seen. When volvulus is present, the contrast column is noted to end with a peculiar "beaking" effect that is caused by the twisting of the bowel into a sharp point.

The goals for surgical management are the release of obstruction and counterclockwise rotational reduction of the bowel. The volvulus is relieved by counterclockwise rotation, and the viability of the bowel is determined with necrotic sections removed. When necrosis is not expected, successful laparoscopic surgery for repair has been reported (Cass & Wesson, 2002). If the necrosis is extensive, rather than perform massive bowel resection, the abdomen may be closed. A return "second look" surgery is performed in 24 to 48 hours, at which time it becomes mandatory to remove any unrecovered, infarcted bowel. If the bowel appears viable, the Ladd bands (if present) are divided, and the entrapped duodenum is freed. The entire length of the bowel is then inspected for patency and associated defects and returned to the abdominal cavity; the small intestine is placed on the right and the colon on the left side of the abdominal cavity. Suture fixation of the replaced bowel generally is not necessary. Appendectomy and gastrostomy may be performed as well.

The major postoperative complication is short-bowel syndrome, which results from the excision of major portions of the gut. The complex malabsorption problems and prolonged hospitalization with total parenteral nutrition call for consultation and close collaboration with members of the nutritional support team and social services. Wound problems and prolonged ileus may also be noted.

The principles of preoperative stabilization include gastric decompression and correction of fluid and electrolyte deficits. The presence of volvulus places the infant at particular risk for both hypovolemia and metabolic acidosis. Hypovolemia occurs as a result of fluid accumulation in the bowel wall, which effectively reduces the circulating blood volume. Clinically, as the infant worsens, the abdomen becomes distended, erythematous, and tender, and blood is passed into the stool. The heart rate quickens in an attempt to maintain cardiac output, and the infant's color may become ashen. This state constitutes a true surgical emergency.

The same principles of decompression and fluid and electrolyte resuscitation apply postoperatively. Total parenteral nutrition is instituted and continued, often for months in the case of short-bowel syndrome, until the intestine has had an opportunity to recover and grow. When feedings are begun, elemental or dilute formula is given initially; the volume and then the concentration are gradually increased until a normal amount of full-strength formula can be tolerated. This feeding progression is often a tedious process fraught with many setbacks that are frustrating to both the nurse and the parents.

When the condition is uncomplicated by infarction or associated anomalies, the survival rate is excellent and may be as high as 99%. However, in the presence of necrosis, survival falls to 35%. An increased risk of dying is also noted with younger age (<3 months) at the time of surgery.

MANAGEMENT OF PROBLEMS WITH ELIMINATION

Hirschsprung's Disease

Anatomy

Hirschsprung's disease (also known as congenital megacolon or aganglionic megacolon) is an abnormality of the colon marked by the congenital absence of ganglion cells (aganglionosis).

Case Study

IDENTIFICATION OF THE PROBLEM

Baby C is an 18-day-old male infant who presented to an ER with listlessness and abdominal distention. Two days prior, his mother had brought him to the hospital because he was irritable and lethargic and feeding poorly. He was evaluated and sent home. On the current visit he was admitted with a diagnosis of failure to thrive. The birth weight had been 3220 g and present weight was 2980 g. When an IV could not be started, an orogastric tube was placed and Pedialyte given. He was then transferred to a tertiary care center.

ASSESSMENT: HISTORY AND PHYSICAL EXAMINATION

Prenatal history was unremarkable. Baby C was born by NSVD to a 28-year-old, G4, P3003 mother and had Apgar scores of 8 at 1 minute and 9 at 5 minutes of life. He was discharged from his birth hospital at 4 days of age after being watched for failure to stool. A contrast enema on day 2 showed movable stool in the colon and no anatomical problems and he was discharged to home after passing two stools.

Evaluation for this admission included checking electrolytes which were normal. The CBC was shifted with 10 segs and 24 bands; C-reactive protein (CRP) was 11.7. Blood cultures were drawn and ampicillin, gentamicin, and clindamycin were started. The abdomen was grossly distended and tender to touch. A peripheral IV was inserted and parenteral nutrition started. Abdominal radiographs revealed extremely gaseous, distended bowel with no air in the rectum. Baby C was active and irritable, well perfused and slightly pale. Breath sounds were clear bilaterally; no murmur was present. The anus was patent and normally placed.

Case Study—cont'd

DIFFERENTIAL DIAGNOSIS

Hirschsprung's disease presents similarly to jejunoileal atresia, meconium ileus, meconium plug syndrome, and small left colon syndrome. A contrast enema can be helpful in diagnosing the disease by determining the caliber of the colon. Microcolon is typically seen with jejunoileal atresia and meconium ileus. Normal or enlarged colon is seen with Hirschsprung's disease, meconium plug, and small left colon syndrome. Retention of contrast material 24 hours after exam is suggestive of Hirschsprung's disease. Final diagnosis can be made by rectal biopsy through the anus with histologic examination of the specimen. Absence of ganglionic cells in the submucosa confirms the diagnosis of Hirschsprung's disease.

DIAGNOSTIC TESTS

An abdominal radiograph is needed to evaluate the abdominal distention. Because of the lack of air in the rectum, a contrast enema was performed. After finding a transitional zone in the colon, a rectal biopsy was performed. To rule out sepsis, blood cultures and CBC with differential were drawn prior to starting antibiotics.

WORKING DIAGNOSIS

The abdominal radiograph showed no air in the rectum. Contrast enema was consistent with Hirschsprung's disease with a transitional zone at the level of the mid to distal descending colon. The rectal biopsy revealed absence of ganglionic cells. The working diagnoses for this baby were term infant with Hirschsprung's disease, colitis due to tender abdomen, and clinical sepsis due to elevated CRP, shifted CBC, and lethargy.

DEVELOPMENT OF MANAGEMENT PLAN

Initial management was directed toward abdominal decompression, maintenance of fluid and electrolyte balance, nutrition, and treatment of sepsis. Gastric suction was placed to low intermittent suction. Normal saline enemas were continued until corrective surgery. The baby remained NPO with IVF at 120 to 150 ml/kg/day. Antibiotics were continued. Electrolytes and CBC were checked daily. After diagnostic examinations were completed, there was discussion that a colon endorectal pull-through was probable, but a colostomy might be needed as sequential histologic examination made during surgery showed higher involvement.

IMPLEMENTATION AND EVALUATION OF EFFECTIVENESS

A laparoscopic subtotal protocolectomy–right colon endorectal pull-through was successfully performed. He was ventilated 3 days postoperatively and extubated to room air. Ampicillin, gentamicin, and clindamycin were discontinued postoperatively and he was treated with flagyl and rocephin for 5 days. Pain was controlled with morphine and Ativan prn. Parenteral nutrition was provided at 135 ml/kg/day with 3 g/kg/day protein and intralipids at 3 g/kg/day. Enteral feeds were begun on the fifth postoperative day and advanced slowly with full feeds reached in 4 days. He was discharged to home in room air, on full feedings, and no medications. Follow-up was with his pediatrician in 1 week and pediatric surgeon in 2 weeks after discharge.

The signs and symptoms of Hirschsprung's disease in the newborn are primarily those of intestinal obstruction, including bilious vomiting, distention, and failure to pass meconium. The rectum is empty of stool unless the aganglionic segment is very short, in which case rectal examination with the gloved little finger may cause explosive release of gas and evacuation of meconium. If the disease goes undiagnosed, fecal stagnation may lead to increased intraluminal pressures, reduced colonic blood flow, and bacterial overgrowth with resultant enterocolitis. This severe bowel irritation and inflammation may cause "overflow" diarrhea, with complicating dehydration, hypoproteinemia, electrolyte imbalance, and sometimes perforation and shock.

Pathophysiology

Failure of the neural crest cells to migrate in their usual craniocaudal fashion results in aberrant bowel innervation and interrupted neuromuscular conduction of the messages that promote peristalsis of the anal sphincter. This local failure of relaxation results in functional intestinal obstruction. Fecal matter accumulates in the normally innervated proximal bowel, producing dilation (megacolon) and hypertrophy of the muscular wall as normal peristaltic activity works against the obstruction. The distal, aganglionic segment is unused and may appear narrowed in relation to the proximal dilation, but it is in fact of normal caliber. Between the ganglionic proximal section and the distal aganglionic section is a "transition zone" of tapered bowel (Ryckman, 2002).

The rectum is always involved, and most cases (85%) involve the sigmoid colon as well. Rarely, aganglionosis may also be found in the upper portion of the colon or throughout the entire intestine (Cass & Wesson, 2002). Atypical forms of Hirschsprung's disease, in which areas of normal innervation are found between aganglionic areas, have also been described, but the presence of such "skip areas" is extremely rare.

The cause of the interrupted migration of ganglion cells is not known, but anoxia is often cited. The theory is that local anoxemia, because of an interference with the source of oxygen to the site, may lead to ischemia, atrophy, and regression of the cells. There is increasing evidence that Hirschsprung's disease is linked to genetic defect in neural crest stem cell function. RET mutations have been found in 30% to 50% of patients with familial Hirschsprung's disease, and 20% EDNRB mutations (Berseth, 2005a; Iwashita et al, 2003; Puri & Shinkai, 2004).

The incidence of Hirschsprung's disease is 1 in 5000 live births and accounts for 20% to 25% of neonatal intestinal obstruction. There is a 4:1 male to female predominance. Associated anomalies are relatively infrequent but include trisomy 21, Waardenburg's syndrome, Smith-Lemli-Opitz syndrome, central hypoventilation syndrome, and asymptomatic urologic anomalies. The ganglionic plexuses of the bowel are derived from the same craniocervical neural crest as are the oral, facial, and cranial ganglia. Consequently, a limited number of infants may also exhibit congenital deafness and ocular neurocristopathies, most commonly in association with Waardenburg's syndrome. Approximately 5% have associated neurologic abnormalities ranging from developmental delay to mental retardation or cerebral palsy.

Treatment

Hirschsprung's disease may be clinically indistinguishable from jejunoileal atresia, meconium ileus, meconium plug syndrome, and small left colon syndrome. Plain radiographic examination offers little or no help in differentiation. All conditions show large gas-filled loops of bowel consistent with intestinal obstruction. The rectum may or may not contain air, but when air is present, it generally is of a reduced amount consistent with partial or functional obstruction.

Barium contrast studies may be indicated to determine the caliber of the distal colon. Microcolon is typically found with jejunoileal atresia and meconium ileus, but if the colon is of normal size or somewhat enlarged, the obstruction may be the result of Hirschsprung's disease, meconium plug syndrome, or small left colon syndrome. In about 60% of studies barium enema demonstrates the "pigtail" or "funnel" sign characteristic of Hirschsprung's disease. This sign is simply a demonstration of the tapering transition zone lying between the dilated, innervated proximal segment and the normal-caliber, aganglionic distal bowel. When the sign is present, usually in infants older than 2 months of age, it highly suggests Hirschsprung's disease, but it may also be found in small left colon syndrome. The margins of the distal colon generally have a sawtooth appearance in Hirschsprung's disease, whereas smooth margins are typically described with small left colon syndrome. Retention of contrast material or barium noted by follow-up film 24 hours later is suggestive of Hirschsprung's disease but may also be noted in its absence.

Anorectal manometry has been used as an alternative diagnostic tool. The test is performed to determine the ability of the internal sphincter to relax. Findings should not be considered conclusive but only suggestive in neonates (Ryckman, 2002). Further tests must be done to confirm the diagnosis.

Definitive diagnosis is made only by suction or punch rectal biopsy through the anus and histologic examination of the specimen obtained. No anesthesia is required, but sedation and pain management are used. The procedure can easily be performed in the nursery. If ganglionic bowel is obtained, either meconium plug syndrome or small left colon syndrome is possible. The absence of ganglionic cells in the submucosal plexus firmly establishes the diagnosis of Hirschsprung's disease. Should questions regarding diagnosis persist, a full-thickness operative biopsy under general anesthesia may be performed to collect deeper nerve plexuses, but this is rarely needed.

Although older children with mild symptoms of Hirschsprung's disease may be managed medically with a daily colonic lavage of normal saline to evacuate the bowel, such conservative therapy is inappropriate in the neonatal period owing to the risk of fatal enterocolitis with perforation, peritonitis, and septicemia.

The surgical goal is to bring normal bowel down to the anus. In the past this was done in a two- to three-stage pull-through with a preliminary stoma. There has been a gradual transition to primary repair with endorectal pull-through. Laparoscopic approach has been established as the standard surgical approach in many centers (Cass & Wesson, 2002). This technique is less invasive, but relies heavily on accurate biopsy location of normal ganglionic cells. In a two-stage procedure, a temporary colostomy is placed proximal to the aganglionic segment, to decompress the bowel and divert the fecal contents. The definitive repair is carried out between 6 and 12 months of age and involves resection of the affected, aganglionic bowel and anastomosis of the normal bowel to the anus. The enterostomal therapist is clearly an important member of the patient care team.

The surgical procedure may be one of several—the Swenson procedure: abdominoperineal sphincter-saving proctectomy and end-to-end anastomosis in the rectal area; the Duhamel procedure: oblique end-to-side anastomosis between the proximal ganglionic colon and the anterior aganglionic anorectal wall, thus forming a new rectum, with the posterior portion pulled through the intestine and making a sleeve of good tissue; and the Soave procedure: an endorectal mucosal dissection in the area of the rectum where the muscular tissue is preserved and a sleeve of good, innervated tissue is pulled through to create a viable bowel surface (Ryckman, 2002).

No matter what the surgical procedure, the initial nursing care is directed toward abdominal decompression, return of fluid and electrolyte balance, and the treatment of sepsis. A gastric tube is set to low intermittent suction, and all drainage is measured. Fluids with appropriate electrolytes for the maintenance and replacement of gastric losses should be provided. Actions to combat the fluid shifts that are common following contrast studies with hyperosmolar media may also be necessary. Prophylactic antibiotic therapy is initiated because of the high risk of enterocolitis. If enterocolitis is present, aggressive therapy with fluids, blood, or plasma may be required. The infant should be monitored closely after rectal biopsy. Bleeding can usually be controlled with digital pressure.

A preoperative colonic lavage or enema may be given to evacuate and prepare the bowel for surgery. Only isotonic solutions such as normal saline should be used to avoid water intoxication and resultant hyponatremia. Following colostomy, the infant must be assessed frequently for respiratory compromise, abdominal distention, hemorrhage, wound dehiscence, and infection. The stomal perfusion and appearance should also be noted and appropriate skin care provided. Intravenous fluids and/or parenteral nutrition is continued until oral feedings can be started.

As the infant becomes ready for discharge, the focus of care shifts to readying the parents for home management of the colostomy. Family teaching should include skin care, normal stomal appearance and stool output, and the construction and application of appliances.

The mortality rate for Hirschsprung's disease is generally less than 5% but may be as high as 15% to 20% in the neonatal period, when diagnosis is often delayed and enterocolitis develops. Good surgical results can be expected in the vast majority of patients (90%), but diarrhea, constipation with distention, and intermittent colitis may occur as the result of residual aganglionosis, postoperative stricture formation, overactivity of the sphincter, or motility disorders. Delayed toilet training is frequently reported, with the actual rate varying in direct proportion to the length of the aganglionic segment.

Small Left Colon

Anatomy

Neonatal small left colon syndrome is a condition of functional immaturity of the large bowel in which the left colon is uniformly narrowed from the anus to the splenic flexure. The proximal colon above the flexure is dilated and distended with meconium. A cone-shaped transition zone lies between the dilated and narrowed distal segments.

Presenting signs and symptoms are those associated with low intestinal obstruction. These manifestations include bile-stained vomitus, abdominal distention, and failure to pass meconium spontaneously. Rectal examination may be followed by the passage of very small amounts of meconium in approximately a third of patients.

Pathophysiology

The cause of small left colon syndrome is unclear, but is generally thought to involve the myenteric plexuses that innervate the GI tract in a cephalocaudal direction between 5 and 12 weeks' gestation. Once the plexuses are in position, their maturation and function are largely determined by gestational age. The impression that this condition results from intramural immaturity is supported by histologic findings of increased numbers of small, immature neuronal elements in contrast to the larger, multipolar ganglion cells that normally predominate at term. The neuronal plexuses are present but immature; morphologically they resemble the structure expected at approximately 32 weeks' gestation. The syndrome might therefore be best described as a disease of decreased intestinal motility.

Approximately 40% of those with small left colon syndrome are the infants of mothers with diabetes. Fifty percent of asymptomatic infants of mothers with diabetes have shown a demonstrable narrowed colonic configuration in the absence of frank symptoms. Variable degrees of hypoglycemia, hypocalcemia, and hyperbilirubinemia have also been reported, but these findings may simply reflect the predisposition for hyperinsulinemia and polycythemia in the general population of infants of mothers with diabetes.

Treatment

On clinical presentation and with plain radiographic studies, this condition is indistinguishable from Hirschsprung's disease and meconium plug syndrome. Multiple gas-filled loops of bowel are seen proximally, with decreased air noted distally.

Barium enema shows the uniformly small left colon with a zone of transition at the splenic flexure. Although a zone of transition may also be noted with Hirschsprung's disease, the margins of the distal colon generally appear smooth with small left colon syndrome rather than jagged or serrated as described in Hirschsprung's disease. Perhaps more distinguishing from Hirschsprung's disease is the incidental finding that following contrast studies, the majority (71%) of infants with small left colon syndrome promptly evacuate the barium and begin passing stools spontaneously. As a consequence, the signs and symptoms of low intestinal obstruction disappear. The meconium rarely (5%) contains a significant rubbery plug.

Rectal biopsy for the presence of ganglion cells, although they may appear atypically immature in small left colon syndrome, may ultimately be required to differentiate this syndrome from Hirschsprung's disease. If the possibility of meconium plug persists, a follow-up contrast examination should be performed. Despite the passage of meconium, the transition zone persists in infants suffering from small left colon syndrome.

Management is generally conservative. The diagnostic barium enema is generally curative. Only in the rare case of significant intermittent obstruction or cecal perforation is a colostomy required. If the diagnosis of small left colon syndrome is made in the face of a negative maternal history, the suggestion of maternal diabetes may be made to the obstetric team.

As with all intestinal obstructions, initial management involves decompression, intravenous fluids for hydration, and the treatment of electrolyte imbalance. Symptoms generally resolve following barium enema, and oral feeding may be instituted gradually. The nurse must be diligent in looking for evidence of persistent or recurrent obstruction and report abnormal findings accordingly. Although the initial presentation may be dramatic, many cases are apparently asymptomatic and go undiagnosed. In either case, the condition spontaneously resolves within the neonatal period with no subsequent stooling problems encountered. Late intermittent obstruction with or without cecal perforation is reported rarely.

Meconium Ileus

Anatomy

Meconium ileus is an obstruction of the distal ileum due to an accumulation of abnormally thick, tarry meconium.

Meconium ileus generally presents first with progressive abdominal distention (within 12 to 24 hours of birth), followed by bilious vomiting and failure to pass meconium. On physical examination the meconium mass may be palpated as a movable, doughy or putty-like ball; smaller pellet-like concretions of inspissated meconium may be felt distally. Rectal examination should produce no meconium, but normal sphincter tone should be felt.

Pathophysiology

The condition is a result of pancreatic insufficiency. Pancreatic hydrolytic enzymes are normally responsible for the metabolism of fat and protein. Consequently, if these enzymes are absent, the meconium has an unusually high protein content and abnormal mucous glycoprotein, which makes it more viscid than usual. The resultant thick, tenacious material literally becomes impacted within the ileal lumen, thus producing a functional obstruction.

Virtually all children (90%) with meconium ileus have cystic fibrosis, although only a small proportion (10% to 15%) of infants with cystic fibrosis present with meconium ileus. Rarely (5%) meconium ileus occurs in the absence of cystic fibrosis, but pancreatic duct stenosis or partial pancreatic aplasia generally can be demonstrated. The cause of these isolated findings is not known. Additional findings associated with meconium ileus include maternal polyhydramnios (5% to 10%) and prematurity (10% to 33%).

Treatment

Plain abdominal films show distended loops proximal to the point of obstruction, but unlike the uniformly lucent areas seen in jejunoileal atresia, the dilated areas typical of meconium ileus are of varying sizes and have a "soap-bubble" or "ground-glass" appearance. This appearance reflects the mixture of trapped air and meconium. Calcifications that are the result of antenatal intestinal perforation and consequent meconium peritonitis may also be noted. Barium enema demonstrates a distally unused microcolon, thus differentiating this condition from Hirschsprung's disease. The smaller pellet-like masses of meconium may also be noted in the distal segment. A history of cystic fibrosis in siblings virtually ensures the diagnosis of meconium ileus. An immunoreactive trypsin test using a dry blood spot provides a screen for cystic fibrosis, with confirmation by sweat test and DNA analysis for cystic fibrosis mutations.

In the case of uncomplicated meconium ileus, the bowel can generally be evacuated using a hyperosmolar contrast enema such as meglumine diatrizoate. Because of the hyperosmolarity, of the contrast, fluid is drawn from the interstitial and intravascular spaces into the intestinal lumen, softening the impacted meconium and allowing it to pull away from the intestinal wall. The mass can then be evacuated by normal peristalsis.

If repeated enemas are not productive, or if meconium ileus is complicated by bowel ischemia, sepsis, or hypovolemic shock, the obstructing meconium may be surgically removed. A temporary ileostomy may be established. Such an ileostomy is irrigated daily with dilute acetylcysteine until any residual meconium is softened and evacuated. Chest physiotherapy, acetylcysteine sodium aerosols (Mucomyst, New York: Bristol-Myers, Squibb), and extra humidity may be helpful in preventing postoperative pulmonary complications (such as atelectasis and pneumonia), to which infants with cystic fibrosis are particularly prone.

All infants with meconium ileus need to be evaluated for cystic fibrosis. Genetic counseling should be provided to parents of affected children, with appropriate referral to a geneticist or genetic counselor. A social worker or other mental health professional may help parents explore their feelings concerning their child's prognosis and their future reproductive plans. Extensive parent teaching of pulmonary toilet and enzyme supplementation is needed. Respiratory therapy personnel and the nutritional support team should consequently be included in parent teaching. Many larger communities have special follow-up clinics for cystic fibrosis patients that may be used to ensure continuity and coordination of care after discharge.

Immediate stabilization of the child with meconium ileus requires decompression with gastric suction and the correction of fluid and electrolyte imbalances. Hydration is particularly important in patients being treated medically with hyperosmolar enemas. Fluids drawn into the intestinal lumen to allow softening and evacuation of the meconium are by default removed from the effective circulation, thus placing the infant at risk for severe hypovolemia and vascular collapse. The extracted fluids should be replaced accordingly. Generally 4 ml of one-half normal saline solution is given for every 1 ml of retained enema. Fluids and suction are continued until the meconium is evacuated and the clinical manifestations of obstruction resolve. When intestinal function is deemed adequate, elemental formula feedings may be started, together with a pancreatic enzyme.

If the obstruction is not relieved, decompression, fluids, and electrolytes are continued until surgical treatment can be carried out. Postoperatively, ostomy care becomes a part of

nursing management, along with assistance in providing pulmonary toilet. The infant's respiratory status should be monitored closely. If adhesions secondary to meconium peritonitis or surgical manipulation are noted or if the meconium is incompletely removed, signs of obstruction may recur. These signs of persistent or recurrent obstruction must be reported immediately to allow early intervention and reoperation as needed. Feedings are delayed until the obstruction is relieved, the ileostomy is functioning, and bowel activity has returned. Many of these infants feed quite poorly, however, and total parenteral nutrition may be required for an extended period of time.

Cystic fibrosis is a condition of delayed mortality, with a mean survival of 22 years. At this age, death comes as a result of obstructive pulmonary disease and infection. The intervening period is marked by poor growth and chronic respiratory and GI dysfunction. The infant mortality rate in cystic fibrosis is 13%, with these early deaths attributed to malabsorption and malnutrition.

Meconium Plug
Anatomy
Meconium plug syndrome is a condition in which intestinal obstruction (generally of the lower colon and rectum) occurs as the result of unusually thick meconium in the absence of demonstrable enzymatic deficiency.

The signs are those of low intestinal obstruction with failure to stool, followed by abdominal distention and bilious vomiting. Hyperactive bowel sounds are often noted on auscultation, and normal sphincter tone is generally felt on rectal examination. The meconium plug and flatus are often passed after digital examination (Bates & Balistreri, 2002).

Pathophysiology
The syndrome is most likely the result of abnormal gut motility associated with immaturity or hypotonia; ganglion deficiency is not found. The plug is formed primarily from mucus and secretions and therefore appears yellowish white and is gelatinous in consistency, lacking the usual flow properties of normal meconium.

Premature infants are especially prone to meconium plug syndrome; however, the condition may also be found in hypotonic infants with central nervous system damage, and some infants of mothers with diabetes are also affected. In the latter case, meconium plug syndrome is considered to be a variant of small left colon syndrome. Treatment of the mother with magnesium sulfate is an additional risk factor that has been noted by some clinicians (Bates & Balistreri, 2002). Meconium plugs are found in about 1 of every 100 newborns, but only a quarter of these infants are unable to evacuate the plug spontaneously and thus experience intestinal obstruction.

Treatment
Plain radiographs indicate a low intestinal obstruction with multiple distended loops of proximal bowel, thus bringing to mind a number of possible conditions, including jejunoileal atresia, meconium ileus, Hirschsprung's disease, small left colon syndrome, or meconium plug syndrome. On barium enema examination, the colon is generally described as being of normal caliber with no evidence of microcolon, thus eliminating the diagnosis of jejunoileal atresia or meconium ileus. The presence of normal ganglion cells on rectal biopsy

removes Hirschsprung's disease from the differential diagnosis. In the absence of a history of maternal diabetes, meconium plug syndrome becomes the most logical cause for the symptoms presented (Bates & Balistreri, 2002).

Small enemas of warm saline, meglumine diatrizoate, or acetylcysteine are usually all that are needed to dislodge the obstructing meconium plug if it has not already been expelled following rectal examination. Normal stooling patterns should follow. Surgical intervention is rarely needed (Bates & Balistreri, 2002).

Decompression, hydration, and electrolyte balance are the immediate concerns. Once the plug is evacuated, symptoms have resolved, and normal intestinal function has returned, feedings can be started. Once the meconium plug is expelled, complete recovery should follow.

Anorectal Agenesis
Anatomy
Anorectal agenesis (imperforate anus) refers to a group of congenital malformations that involve the anus or rectum or the junction between the two structures. If the urorectal septum deviates during its growth, the cloaca is abnormally or incompletely partitioned, thus resulting in rectal stenosis or atresia. Rectourethral and rectovaginal fistulas frequently occur in association with these defects. If the anal membrane fails to rupture, the result is a membranous anal atresia.

A whole spectrum of defects is possible, but they are generally classified into four major types (Figure 5-11). Presenting signs and symptoms vary slightly with the particular type of defect present. For the majority (those with type III agenesis), the anus is clearly imperforate. Owing to the high incidence of fistulas, meconium may be passed in the urine (in males), or its presence may be noted at the vaginal outlet (in females). With anal stenosis (type I), the anus and rectal vaults are patent but narrowed so that the pasty stools of the newborn may be passed. The stenosis is generally suspected by the microscopic appearance of the anus and is confirmed on rectal examination. With the remaining two types, the anus may appear misleadingly normal on first inspection. In the membranous type (type II), the anal membrane may become

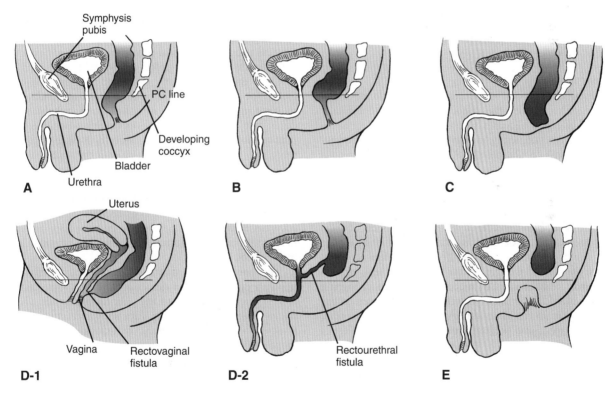

FIGURE **5-11**
Anorectal agenesis. Shading represents areas of lucency typically found on radiograph. Percentages reflect relative occurrence. **A,** Normal anatomy. **B,** Type I or anal stenosis (5% to 6%): anus or lower rectum is narrowed but patent. **C,** Type II or anal membrane (5% to 7%): anal opening covered by a membranous diaphragm. **D,** Type III or anal agenesis (85%): anus is clearly imperforate; fistulas are present in three quarters of cases. **D-1,** Type IIIA or low agenesis: bowel ends as a blind pouch below the pubococcygeal (PC) line; most common in females. **D-2,** Type IIIB or high agenesis: bowel ends as a blind pouch above the pubococcygeal line; most common in males. **E,** Type IV or anal atresia (3%): rectum and anus are present as blind pouches but are separated by a variable distance. Data from Avery ME, Taeusch HW (1984). *Schaffer's diseases of the newborn,* ed 5. Philadelphia: Saunders; Chang JHT (1980). Neonatal surgical emergencies: Part V—Intestinal obstruction. *Perinatology/neonatology* 4(2):34; deVries PA, Cox KL (1985). Surgery of anorectal anomalies. *Surgical clinics of North America* 65(5):1139-1169; Gryboski J, Walker WA (1983). *Gastrointestinal problems in the infant,* ed 2. Philadephia: Saunders; Moore KL, Persuad TVN (1993). *Before we are born: basic embryology and birth defects,* ed 4. Philadelphia: Saunders; and Sadler TW (1985). *Langman's medical embryology,* ed 5. Baltimore: Williams & Wilkins.

visible within 24 to 48 hours as meconium bulges from beneath the thin epithelial covering, but by then the signs of low intestinal obstruction (distention, bilious vomiting, and failure to pass stool) are also becoming apparent. The atretic type (type IV), which is fortunately rare, generally first presents with the full-blown manifestations of obstruction.

Pathophysiology

The cause of deviated or arrested anorectal development is not known. Anorectal agenesis occurs in 1 of every 5000 live births with a slight male predominance. Greater than 50% of all affected infants have an associated anomaly (Berseth & Poenaru, 2005a). Considering its common origin from the cloaca, it is not surprising that genitourinary tract abnormalities are found most frequently (25% to 50%); approximately 4% of affected infants have the lethal defects of bilateral renal agenesis or dysplasia. Cryptorchidism is noted in 3% to 19% of affected males. Congenital heart disease and esophageal atresia are also reported occasionally, and when the latter is found, the VATER and VACTERL associations should be considered. Approximately half of affected patients have spinal dysraphism, ranging from occult spina bifida (2.2%) to myelomeningocele (2% to 4.4%)—including scoliosis (13.3 %), hemivertebra (6.7%), extra segments (8.9%), tethered cord (4% to 13.3%), and fibrolipoma of the cord (8.9% to 38%) (Ryckman, 2002).

Treatment

The treatment of anorectal anomalies varies with the nature of the defect. The higher the lesion, the more technically complicated its repair becomes. Reconstruction techniques are usually done laparoscopically, minimizing trauma to surrounding tissue (Sydorak & Albanese, 2002). Careful perineal examination is generally diagnostic. In the presence of a fistula, the urine may also be examined for meconium epithelial cells.

An inverted lateral radiograph (upside-down Wangensteen-Rice technique) or cross-table prone film may demonstrate air collected in the blind-ending upper rectal pouch, but is generally unreliable for determining the level of obstruction, owing to the considerable time required for swallowed air to reach this portion of the gut. Even when sufficient time is given, air may be prevented by meconium from reaching the end of the pouch. If a fistula is present, air may be seen in the bladder or vagina on the plain film. An abdominal ultrasound, cardiac echography, and skeletal films are needed to rule out associated defects.

The treatment of anal stenosis (type I defect) consists of repeated dilation using Hegar dilators. If the infant is otherwise stable, and the anus is sufficiently enlarged, the patient is discharged with daily digital dilation (using the little finger) to be performed by the parents. Membranous defects (type II) require minimal surgical therapy. The membrane is simply punctured with a hemostat or excised using a scalpel. Repeated dilation is performed as needed.

Low agenesis (translevator, type III lesion) is corrected by perineal anoplasty. After locating the position of the superficial external sphincter using a nerve stimulator, the rectal pouch is brought down through the sphincter to the opening on the anal skin. The fistulous connection, if present, is removed. Gentle irrigations help facilitate stooling and keep the anastomotic site clean until daily dilations can be started, generally between 10 and 14 days postoperatively.

High agenesis (intermediate or high supralevator, type III lesions) and atresia (supralevator, type IV lesions) generally are treated in two phases. The first step is immediate placement of a colostomy for decompression and diversion of fecal contents. If present, the urethrorectal fistula is generally closed or excised to avoid "spill-over" fecal contamination with resultant urinary tract infection. The definitive repair is generally delayed 3 to 12 months to allow growth and pelvic enlargement. At that time, an abdominal-perineal pull-through procedure is performed in which the rectal pouch is literally pulled through the levator sling and anchored to the skin. The colostomy is left intact until healing is complete.

Nonemergent cases (typically stenosis) usually require little in the way of stabilization other than replacement and correction of fluid and electrolyte imbalance. If a fistula is present, these infants are at risk for the development of hyperchloremic acidosis owing to the absorption of urine from the colon. Gastric suction for decompression is instituted prophylactically (in the case of agenesis when the defect is obvious on inspection) or therapeutically (when membranous and atretic types begin to display symptoms of obstruction).

Postoperatively, wound care and monitoring for postoperative complications are added to the regimen. If anoplasty is performed, the site should be inspected (as allowed by the surgical team) for mucosal prolapse, which may occur if there is inadequate sphincter preservation. Mineral oil may be used to clean meconium gently from the anal area. A colostomy placed for higher defects should receive the standard care and monitoring. The surgeon initially carries out dilatory procedures, but when digital dilation becomes possible, the nurse may assume this task, making sure to provide bedside parent teaching. Throughout recuperation, the urine (or vaginal outlet) should be closely observed for the presence of meconium, which would indicate a recurrent fistula. If such a fistula is suspected, electrolyte and acid-base status should also be monitored for hyperchloremic acidosis. Otherwise, feeding may begin when the colostomy or anoplasty is sufficiently healed and intestinal function resumes. Stool-softening agents may be required.

The outcome for infants with anorectal anomalies largely depends on the type of defect and on the level of the upper rectal pouch in relation to the puborectal muscle, which is the main muscle of sphincter function and continence. This muscle is a central component of the levator ani muscle, which spans the pelvis much like a sling to support the lower end of the rectum. On radiography, the position of this muscle can be estimated by drawing an imaginary line between the symphysis pubis and the developing coccyx (see Figure 5-11). Based on the relation of the pouch to this pubococcygeal line, anorectal anomalies can be classified into three groups that indicate low-, high-, or intermediate-level defect. In low (translevator) types, the rectum descends through and is surrounded by the puborectalis and levator ani muscles so that the sensorimotor mechanisms are generally intact. With high (supralevator) defects, the rectal pouch ends above the puborectalis and levator ani muscles so that the neurologic and muscular mechanisms of continence may be impaired. In intermediate types (supralevator), the rectum again ends above the puborectalis, but the pouch is cradled in the muscular hammock formed by the levator ani so that neuromuscular function is variable and repair more complicated.

The overall mortality rate is approximately 20%, with death largely a reflection of the nature of the defect and the presence of associated anomalies.

For survivors, the main criterion for outcome is fecal continence. When anorectal anomalies are reviewed as a whole, 74% of patients can be expected to have good results, with normal anal function and control of defecation; 14% have fair results, with only occasional soiling on straining; and 12% have poor results, being nearly or completely incontinent or requiring permanent colostomy.

Intussusception
Anatomy
Intussusception is an acquired obstruction in which a part of the intestine prolapses into the lumen of an adjoining distal intestinal segment (Figure 5-12). This luminal prolapse may occur at any site in the GI tract, but typically there are four varieties: (1) enteric intussusception, in which the small intestine prolapses into itself; (2) colic intussusception, in which the large intestine prolapses into itself; (3) ileocecal intussusception, in which the ileocecal valve is inverted and pushed into the cecum, pulling a segment of ileum with it; and (4) ileocolic intussusception, in which the ileocecal valve remains in place but the ileum prolapses through it into the colon. Rarely, a retrograde intussusception may occur in which a distal intestinal segment prolapses upward into a proximal part. In the neonate, the majority of cases (80%) are of the enteric (most often involving the terminal ileum) or ileocecal type.

Regardless of the site, the intussusception gives rise to two problems. First, it causes a simple mechanical obstruction as the result of the blockage of the distal intestinal lumen by the prolapsed proximal segment. Second, as the intestinal walls are telescoped into one another, the mucosal blood vessels become compressed, congested, and prone to ischemia or infarction. Thus the symptoms of intussusception typically include vomiting, colicky pain, and bloody stools or red "currant jelly" stools.

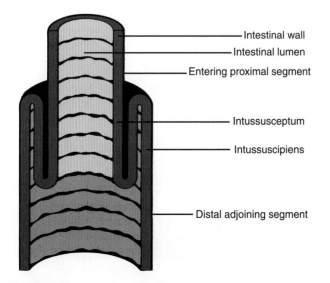

FIGURE **5-12**
Schematic representation of intussusception. The proximal intestinal segment has prolapsed into the lumen of an adjacent distal intestinal segment.

Pathophysiology
Intussusception is an acquired condition and therefore not easily explained by any one causative factor. A small proportion of cases (2% to 12%) appear to have a "lead point," a demonstrable anatomic lesion or defect that may have been the cause of intussusception. Such lead points may include Meckel's diverticula, duplication defects, polyps, hematomas, and lymphomas. The viscid stool common in cystic fibrosis may even be a potential cause. In most situations, the cause is not known (idiopathic intussusception); however, there is often a history of preceding upper respiratory infection or gastroenteritis. Nearly half of all patients demonstrate infection with adenovirus on stool culture. The role played by infection in the phenomenon of intussusception has not yet been determined. The inflammatory response of the intestine to infection may possibly cause an abnormal hyperplasia of lymphoid tissue. The hyperplastic site might then serve as a lead point for intussusception.

Intussusception is extremely rare in the newborn period and even more unusual in preterm infants with an overall incidence rate of less than 0.3% (Nock & Wilson-Costello, 2002). The usual age for intussusception is between 3 and 24 months, with males predominating.

Treatment
Plain radiographs may not be helpful in the diagnosis, with 20% to 30% showing only a general picture of intestinal obstruction with dilated proximal loops and an airless distal bowel. On ultrasonography, the affected area often appears as a "doughnut sign" on cross-section. Definitive diagnosis is by barium enema, with the contrast media outlining the gut and ending proximally in a characteristic "coiled spring" pattern. Intussusception is so rare that little medical research has been undertaken to determine the best approach for treatment. In older children and adults, an attempt is first made to reduce the intussusception by using the hydrostatic pressure produced by a barium enema. Barium is injected into the rectum and allowed to flow distally until the "coiled-spring" pattern appears. A balloon-tipped catheter is then inserted into the rectum. The balloon is inflated with air, and gentle traction is applied until the balloon is pulled back against the muscular sling of the levatores, thus preventing any outflow of barium. The administration of barium is restarted, which causes the intraluminal pressure to rise slowly as more and more contrast medium is added without an avenue for escape. The pressure is maintained until the intussusception is pushed distally and freed. If the intussusception is fully reduced, the barium is seen suddenly to flow freely into the proximal bowel, and the clinical status of the patient should immediately improve. Unfortunately, in infants, full reduction is generally not accomplished, and surgical reduction is required.

Surgical intervention involves a manual reduction of the intussusception using a "milking" motion on the proximal bowel. The pressure and squeezing are continued until the loop is freed; traction and pulling should never be applied. The bowel is carefully inspected; any necrotic tissue is removed; and lead points are resected.

The major concerns before reduction are sepsis and shock. In light of the strong association with adenovirus and the frequent history of gastroenteritis or respiratory infection, sepsis should be expected. Antibiotic therapy is initiated pending culture results. Fluid lost into the wall of the trapped intestine or blood lost from congested vessels into the lumen of the intestine, or a combination of both, predisposes to shock and should be appropriately managed with fluid resuscitation and volume expansion. Decompression by gastric suction is also recommended.

Postoperative care is fairly routine. Fluids, electrolytes, and decompression are provided as needed. The recurrence risk is 2% to 20% and is more common following hydrostatic reduction (8% to 13%) than after surgical reduction (0% to 4%). Consequently, even though the intussusception has presumably been resolved, the nurse must be alert for the return of associated signs and symptoms.

The prognosis for intussusception in newborns is not good, basically because they present with so few of the signs that classically appear in infants and older children. Consequently, intussusception is rarely considered in the differential diagnosis of intestinal obstruction. When diagnosed, the mortality rate is approximately 41%.

Necrotizing Enterocolitis
Anatomy
Necrotizing enterocolitis (NEC) is an acquired disorder characterized by necrosis of the mucosal and submucosal layers of the GI tract. Any portion of the bowel can be affected, but the ileocecal area predominates, with the antimesenteric side most typically being involved. Symptoms generally present on an overall average (mean) at 12 days of age, with the most common age at onset (mode) of 3 days. Cases have been reported to occur in infants as old as 90 days. Early signs are highly variable but generally include nonspecific signs of GI compromise (abdominal distention, gastric residuals, vomiting that may or may not be bilious, and bloody stools) or nonspecific signs of infection (lethargy, temperature instability, apnea, and bradycardia), or both. Laboratory findings include abnormal blood gases caused by apnea and acidosis, abnormal blood counts resulting from sepsis, thrombocytopenia resulting from consumption by the necrotic process and infection, and reducing substances in the stool caused by carbohydrate malabsorption. As the disease progresses, hypovolemia occurs as the result of the third-spacing of fluids in the interstitial compartments of the damaged intestine; blood pressure falls; urinary output decreases; and the poorly perfused, often septic infant appears gray, pale, or mottled. Peritonitis is evident by erythema, edema, and tenderness of the abdominal wall. If clotting factors continue to be consumed, disseminated intravascular coagulation may occur.

Pathophysiology
NEC is the most common GI disorder seen in the intensive care nursery and affects approximately 5% of all admissions (10% in infants weighing less than 1500 g), although wide differences are reported from center to center (from a low of 1% to a high of 8%). Any condition or situation that leads to ischemia and bacterial overgrowth in the presence of formula feedings can logically be considered a risk factor. However, prematurity is probably the greatest risk factor of all. Although cases in term infants are noted, NEC is almost exclusively a disease of the prematurely born. Of all infants affected, 62% to 94% are premature, with the highest rates in those with lowest birth weight and gestational age. No consistent associations between NEC and sex, race, socioeconomic status, or season of the year have been found. It is not clear if NEC is caused by infectious agents, but the occurrence of NEC is epidemic with outbreaks occurring usually during times of nursery crowding (Berseth & Poenaru, 2005c).

Pathologically the affected intestine appears irregularly dilated with patchy areas of discoloration ranging from pale to dark purple. The pale color indicates areas of ischemic necrosis where the tissues have been deprived of their blood supply; the purple color indicates areas of hemorrhagic necrosis where blood has leaked into the tissues from capillary hemorrhage. Gas-containing cysts (pneumatosis) may be seen in the wall of the intestine as the result of gas dissecting beneath the serosa or submucosa (Figure 5-13). If perforation has occurred, it is usually found in the ileocecal area. On microscopic examination, the mucosa appears edematous, and the necrotic areas may extend beyond the mucosa and submucosa into the muscular layers. Microthrombi may also be noted in the tiny arterioles and venules of the mesentery, but frank thrombosis of the larger arteries or veins rarely occurs.

The etiology and pathogenesis of NEC have been the focus of extensive debate and research for the past 30 years. Many theories have been offered concerning the factors that cause the disease and their method of introduction to the neonate, but few absolute answers have been found. At present the sum of knowledge indicates that three major pathologic mechanisms occur in combination that lead to the development of NEC. These three mechanisms involve selective ischemia of the bowel, establishment of bacterial flora, and the effect of feeding.

The selective bowel ischemia is really an asphyxial defense mechanism that serves to protect the brain and heart from hypoxia by shunting blood away from the mesenteric, renal, and peripheral vascular bed. This redistribution of blood flow is similar to the "diving reflex" typical of aquatic birds and mammals. Unfortunately, in human infants this relative circulatory insufficiency to the bowel may result in intestinal ischemia. Asphyxiated infants and those suffering respiratory distress syndrome, apneic episodes, or cyanosis are most commonly affected. Although these conditions undoubtedly affect intestinal perfusion, such compromise may be intermittent in

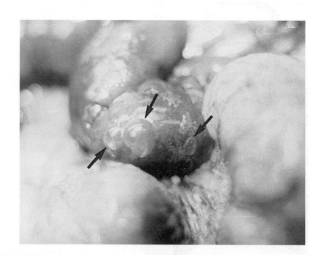

FIGURE **5-13**
Gross operative findings in necrotizing enterocolitis. The gas-filled intramural cysts (*arrows*) are typical of pneumatosis intestinalis. Courtesy Drs. David A. Clark and Jeffery E. Thompson and Wyeth-Ayerst Laboratories, Philadelphia, PA. Copyright © Wyeth.

nature and of insufficient magnitude alone to induce necrosis without some additional factor. Any condition or procedure that holds potential for causing hemodynamic change may also be at fault. Polycythemia, umbilical artery catheterization, exchange transfusion, patent ductus arteriosus, indomethacin administration, and cyanotic heart disease, as well as maternal cocaine abuse, have been implicated in bowel ischemia (Berseth & Poenaru, 2005c).

Colonization of the intestine with bacteria that normally reside within its lumen is a postnatal process. In utero the intestines are sterile, but during the process of delivery and subsequent contact with the surrounding environment, the gut becomes seeded with a wide variety of aerobic and anaerobic bacteria, which then multiply and spread with enteral feedings. In healthy newborn infants, the intestinal flora is established by about 10 days of age; however, in premature and sick infants, the colonization may be delayed, with fewer species of bacteria than are normally present. Attempts at controlling infectious disease within the special care nursery and skill at employing aseptic technique may in large part be responsible. Nevertheless, the result is a newborn with a GI tract that is both structurally and immunologically immature and susceptible to injury from bacterial toxins—that is, the passage of bacteria or bacterial products (such as endotoxins) across the mucosal wall. This decreased immunity and lack of resistance may explain the fact that most of the bacteria cultured from affected infants are of species that are otherwise considered a part of the normal intestinal flora. The organisms that are typically isolated include *Escherichia coli* and *Enterobacter*, *Klebsiella*, and *Clostridium* species. These enteric bacilli do not usually invade normal tissue but are opportunistic pathogens.

Based on these observations, work is underway to develop a means of prophylaxis. Although the administration of oral antibiotics to modify intestinal flora has provided mixed results, oral administration of an immunoglobulin preparation (IgA or IgG, or both) appears promising (Berseth & Poenaru, 2005c). Other preventive strategies being explored include administration of glucocorticoids to accelerate maturation of the GI system, enhancement of platelet activating factor acetyl hydrolase activity, the use of platelet-activating factor receptor antagonists, and administration of immunonutrients such as glutamine, arginine, long-chain polyunsaturated fatty acids, and probiotics (Berseth & Poenaru, 2005c; Lin et al, 2004; Neu & Bernstein, 2002).

Formula feedings have also been cited as an important factor in making the gut susceptible to NEC. In fact, virtually all infants in whom the disease develops (98%) have previously been fed either formula or dextrose solution. It is believed that such intake may simply provide a substance on which bacteria can feed and flourish. In comparison, infants who receive fresh breast milk are 60% less often affected with NEC, presumably being protected by the secretory immunoglobulin (IgA) and anti-inflammatory components it provides (Horton, 2005; Schanler, 2005).

Hyperosmolar loads of formula or medications may present additional risk factors. In response to the osmotic gradient and in a futile attempt to reduce the osmolarity, intestinal secretions are increased and fluid moves into the lumen of the GI tract. As a result of this fluid shift, blood volume is decreased; GI blood flow is reduced; and the intestinal mucosa becomes relatively ischemic, thus increasing the risk of NEC. Furthermore, in vitro studies have demonstrated that the tissue

fluid content of the bowel wall itself is also decreased as fluid moves into the lumen. This dehydration of the epithelium causes both morphologic and functional alterations in the mucosal lining of the intestine. The height and width of the villi decrease; the intercellular spaces close; and, as a result, the overall absorptive capacity of the bowel is decreased. Malabsorption with varying degrees of stasis and ileus in turn allows the development of abnormal flora, which further increases the risk of NEC. The complex mechanism of vascular and cellular changes that occur in response to hyperosmolar loads is believed to be responsible for the increased incidence of NEC historically reported for low-birth-weight infants who receive hyperosmolar feedings and certain oral medications. Even when diluted in formula, a medication such as phenobarbital elixir can increase the osmolality of a feeding by more than twofold. In many cases it may be preferable to give the intravenous preparation of the drug by the oral route to avoid such hypertonic feedings.

Injured by ischemia, the mucosal cells lining the gut stop secreting protective enzymes. Digestive enzymes that are present will autodigest the unprotected luminal cells. Enteric bacteria proliferate in the substrate-rich but immunologically deficient environment and invade the intestinal wall, where they release toxins and produce hydrogen gas. The gas is formed as a result of the catalytic activity of bacterial enzymes acting on formula as a substrate. The gas initially dissects beneath the serosal and submucosal layers of the intestine (pneumatosis intestinalis), but if this gas ruptures into the mesenteric vascular bed, it can be distributed through the systemic vessels into the venous system of the liver (portal venous gas). The bacterial toxins together with ischemia result in necrosis. If the full thickness of the intestinal wall is damaged, perforation can result, releasing free air into the peritoneal cavity (pneumoperitoneum) and producing a true surgical emergency.

Treatment

Aggressive medical management may be successful in approximately half of all affected neonates (Ricketts, 1994). Such management is based on three traditional principles: (1) bowel rest, (2) prevention of progressive injury, and (3) normalization of systemic responses. Enteral nutrition is discontinued; the stomach is decompressed by low intermittent suction through a large-bore orogastric tube; and fluids and electrolytes are closely monitored and adjusted. Antibiotic therapy, early intubation and ventilation, management of acid-base derangements, and efforts to support blood pressure and blood flow to the gut are undertaken both to prevent continuing injury and to correct systemic responses. Serial abdominal films are made at 6- to 8-hour intervals during acute illness to monitor progression of the disease and to detect perforation.

Because of the high incidence of NEC in the intensive care nursery, a premature infant who experiences any of the early signs of obstruction (vomiting, distention, increased gastric aspirates), one who demonstrates increased episodes of apnea and bradycardia, or one who passes bloody stools should be regarded with a high index of suspicion. Should two or more of the early signs appear together, one should presume NEC until other diagnostic studies can be performed. Feedings are immediately stopped and venous access obtained. A gastric tube is set to intermittent suction for decompression. Vigorous hydration and total parenteral nutrition is initiated as soon as possible. Antibiotic coverage usually includes ampicillin or a cephalosporin and an aminoglycoside. In the event of perforation, anaerobic coverage is added. Circulatory status must be evaluated frequently by monitoring perfusion, vital signs—including blood pressure—and urinary output. Stools are routinely checked for blood. Hematologic studies are performed to look for anemia, thrombocytopenia, and disordered coagulation. Blood, platelets, and fresh frozen plasma are given as needed. Oxygenation and acid-base status are also monitored, with respiratory support provided accordingly. Careful, gentle reexamination of the abdomen should be carried out every 6 to 8 hours for the first 48 to 72 hours to evaluate for progression of the disease and presence of free air.

Radiographic findings change as the disease progresses. Radiographs taken early in the course of the disease generally exhibit little more than fixed, dilated bowel loops with thickened walls, all due to local edema. The invasion of gasforming bacteria into the intestinal wall produces the diagnostic picture of pneumatosis intestinalis (Figure 5-14). This intraluminal air, found in 85% of affected infants, generally appears as tiny, lucent bubbles that may come so close together in some places that they coalesce to form curvilinear or crescent-shaped streaks. If extensive disease is

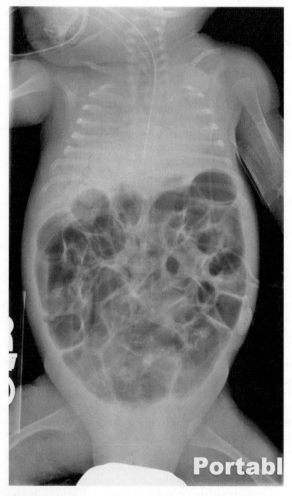

FIGURE 5-14
Extensive pneumatosis intestinalis and necrotizing enterocolitis in a premature infant. Courtesy Radiology Department at Children's Healthcare of Atlanta.

present, air may enter the venous system and outline the hepatic veins. Portal venous gas, found in 15% to 30% of patients, is also diagnostic of NEC. Ultimately, perforation may occur, thus presenting the characteristic appearance of pneumoperitoneum with a layer of free air lying immediately inferior to the abdominal wall. This free air is best seen by a lateral view, but on anteroposterior view it may be noted by the characteristic "football sign" due to air outlining the falciform ligament (Horton, 2005).

Surgical intervention is required in approximately one-fourth to one-half of infants with NEC. Criteria for surgery are somewhat controversial and vary from institution to institution. Expedient laparotomy is ideally performed after the advent of intestinal gangrene but prior to perforation. Absolute indications are pneumoperitoneum or confirmation of intestinal gangrene by positive paracentesis. Nonspecific but supportive findings include clinical deterioration in spite of vigorous clinical management (metabolic acidosis, ventilatory failure, thrombocytopenia, leukopenia or leukocytosis with shift to the left, oliguria, portal venous air, erythema of the abdominal wall, or persistently dilated and fixed bowel loop (Kosloske, 1994; Ricketts, 1994).

The principles of surgical management include careful examination of the bowel with resection of all grossly necrotic intestine or perforated sites. If the viability of extensive portions of the gut is in question, resection is deferred, with a follow-up second-look operation carried out in 24 to 48 hours. Otherwise the bowel ends are brought to the surface to create an ostomy. In the smallest and sickest infants, peritoneal drains are placed as a temporary measure to relieve symptoms of abdominal compartment syndrome and sepsis. Many of the extremely small neonates do not require further surgery (Cass & Wesson, 2002; Ricketts, 1994).

Extensive respiratory therapy may be required throughout hospitalization, especially when marked abdominal distention may interfere with ventilation. Long-term parenteral nutrition can be anticipated, thus making collaboration with the nutritional support team essential.

Ventilatory and circulatory support are maintained in the postoperative period, and antibiotic therapy is continued for 10 to 14 days past resolution of pneumatosis. Ostomy care is performed as previously described. When stabilized GI function has resumed (generally in 7 to 14 days), feedings are cautiously and slowly begun with small amounts of dilute elemental formula. The amount and concentration of feedings are advanced as tolerated, but these attempts are frequently frustrated by malabsorption associated with short-bowel syndrome or the development of strictures. Recurrent distention, residuals, vomiting, intractable constipation, or bloody stools may be noted with partial or complete obstruction due to such strictures.

Mortality rates have dramatically decreased over time with improved medical-surgical care and the use of total parenteral nutrition, falling from a rate of 24% to 65% in the 1960s and 1970s to a rate of 9% to 28% in the 2000s. Within groups, mortality varies with treatment. Lower rates occur in those who are managed medically as opposed to those requiring surgical intervention. Persistent acidosis, severe pneumatosis, and the presence of portal venous air are poor prognostic indicators (Kosloske, 1994; Berseth & Poenaru, 2005c).

Of those who survive, approximately 10% to 30% experience strictures (mostly colonic) as the result of structural changes in nonperforated, healed ischemic sites. Surgical resection of the stricture is required. Somewhat fewer patients suffer from short-bowel syndrome (9% to 23%). Recurrent NEC has been reported in 5% of patients, with an average onset of symptoms approximately 4 to 5 weeks after the original episode. Neither the type or timing of enteral feedings nor the anatomic site or method of management of the initial episode appears to be an influencing factor. Those affected tend to be recovering premature infants (63%), although recurrence is also seen in mature infants with major congenital anomalies (31%), primarily cyanotic congenital heart disease. The mortality rate is similar to that seen with primary NEC (Berseth & Poenaru, 2005c; Ricketts, 1994).

OTHER GASTROINTESTINAL DISORDERS

The majority of gastrointestinal disorders are categorized as problems of ingestion, digestion, or elimination. Additional disorders that overlap or do not fit these categories are presented, including short-bowel or short-gut syndrome, spontaneous bowel and gastric perforation, peptic ulcer, umbilical hernia, and lactobezoars.

Short-Bowel Syndrome

Anatomy

The short-bowel (short-gut) syndrome is an unfortunate complication of many neonatal surgeries that involve extensive resection of the GI tract. The loss of considerable absorptive surface results in a complex malabsorptive problem with episodic diarrhea, steatorrhea, and dehydration, which, if allowed to progress, may cause metabolic derangements and ultimately poor growth and development. In the presence of short-bowel syndrome, a 1- to 2-year hospitalization may not be unusual. The duration of initial hospitalization and length of dependence on parenteral nutrition are both inversely related to the length of bowel that remains.

The median length of newborn small intestine is 200 to 300 cm (Hwang & Schulman, 2002). Infants with as little as 15 cm and an intact ileocecal valve have survived. The ileocecal valve delays transit time and allows for increased digestion and absorption. Additionally it acts as a barrier to prevent overgrowth of colonic bacteria in the small intestine. If the ileocecal valve is removed, 30 to 45 cm of bowel is probably needed for survival (Berseth & Poenaru, 2005c).

Pathophysiology

The short-bowel syndrome is a complication of surgeries involving extensive resection of the GI tract, such as necrotizing enterocolitis, gastroschisis, megacystic microcolon, intestinal atresia, Hirschsprung's disease, and volvulus. Congenital short bowel is extremely rare, but has been reported in about 30 patients (Hwang & Shulman, 2002). Overall incidence of short-bowel syndrome is 21 per 1000 NICU admissions and 24.5 per 100,000 live births. Incidence is higher is preterm infants (Wales et al, 2004).

Most infants eventually experience progressive small bowel adaptation, and the surgically shortened intestine grows; the mucosal wall hypertrophies; and the villi become hyperplastic so that the absorptive area is increased. Blood flow to the residual intestine and the proportion of the villus that is enzymatically active are both initially increased but gradually decline as the surface area and length continue to increase with time (Neu & Bernstein, 2002). However, completely

normal absorption may never be achieved in cases of extensive resection in which less than 75 cm of the bowel remains, especially if the ileocecal valve is removed.

Infants with short-bowel syndrome postoperatively often fail to tolerate even small amounts of enteral nutrition and exhibit diarrhea and malabsorption. Months to years of hospitalization may not be unusual (DiBaise et al, 2004). The duration of initial hospitalization and length of dependence on parenteral nutrition are both inversely related to the length of remaining bowel. Most infants eventually experience progressive small-bowel adaptation, and the surgically shortened intestine grows; the mucosal wall hypertrophies; and the villi become hyperplastic so that the absorptive area is increased. Blood flow to the residual intestine and the proportion of the villus that is enzymatically active are both initially increased but gradually decline as the surface area and length continue to increase with time (Hwang & Shulman, 2002).

Treatment

Treatment of short-bowel syndrome is difficult because of the length of time it takes for intestinal adaptation to take place. Parenteral nutrition is initiated soon after surgery and continued throughout the period of refeeding. Elemental formula is required usually by continuous infusion and is very gradually increased. Refeeding ostomy drainage into the distal bowel has been shown to improve weight gain and decrease parenteral nutrition usage (Gardner et al, 2003). Medications such as loperamide, diphenoxylate, phenothiazines, ocreotide, and dietary fiber have been used in individual patients to help control diarrhea. Cholestyramine may be used to help bind bile acid and thereby decrease diarrhea. Trimethoprim-sulfamethoxazole and metronidazole are used in the treatment of bacterial overgrowth. Gastroenterology consultation is essential for guidance in feeding practices, medication therapies, vitamin supplementation, and referral for transplantation if needed.

Infants who show no adaptive response after months of feeding attempts may have radical surgery to slow intestinal transit (e.g., intestinal valves, reversed segment, colon interposition, intestinal pacing, intestinal lengthening, tapering enteroplasty, or neomucosa). Small-bowel transplantation presents a lifesaving option for these patients. Results of intestinal transplantation continue to improve, with survival rates of 55% to 78% (Cass & Wesson, 2002; Hwang & Schulman, 2002; Kelly, 2002). Higher survival rates may be achieved with improved operative technique and postoperative management as well as better patient selection and timing of transplant.

Nursing care of the infant with short-bowel syndrome includes collaborative management with team members to monitor fluid, electrolyte, acid-base balance, and nutritional status. Prevention of skin breakdown due to diarrhea and infection are critical. Parents must be involved in their infants' care, and every effort must be made to stimulate normal growth and development.

Infant survival after massive bowel resection is related to the maturity of the infant at the time of resection, length of the remaining intestine, presence of distal small intestine, presence of the ileocecal valve, presence of an intact colon, intactness of pancreatic and liver function, and absence of other complicating congenital anomalies. Patients with short-bowel syndrome with chronic dependence on TPN usually have poor quality of life and numerous readmissions for abdominal surgeries, central venous catheter-related infections, dislodgement of central line catheters and/or feeding tubes, wound infections and dehiscence, developmental delay, and TPN-associated liver failure.

Spontaneous Bowel or Gastric Perforations
Anatomy

Spontaneous bowel or gastric perforations result in free air into the peritoneum. The infant is usually several days old at the time symptoms appear. The third or fourth day is the most common time. There is marked abdominal distention that is tender to the touch and respiratory distress that worsens as the distention increases. There may or may not be vomiting. If the perforation has progressed, hypovolemic shock is possible. This condition is considered a neonatal surgical emergency.

Pathophysiology

Spontaneous bowel or gastric perforations can be caused by a variety of factors. NEC and ischemia of the bowel are two of the more common problems. Iatrogenic trauma that is secondary to an invasive procedure such as gastric intubation or hyperinflation of the stomach is another potential causative factor. Spontaneous bowel or gastric perforations can also be secondary to mechanical ventilation or distal bowel obstruction that leads to ischemia (Berseth & Poenaru, 2005a; Ryckman, 2002). Steroid therapy, especially long-term therapy, has been linked to such perforations (Ryckman, 2002).

Prematurity and perinatal stress have some association with spontaneous perforations. Isolated intestinal perforation is seen in very-low-birth-weight infants, usually before feedings have been initiated, associated with patent ductus arteriosus and indomethacin therapy. Although indomethacin has been minimally associated with isolated bowel perforation, the incidence markedly increases when coupled with stress doses of glucocorticoids (Clyman, 2005). They do not have pneumatosis intestinalis, but develop distended abdomen with blue-gray discoloration from the perforation. These infants usually have better outcomes than infants with perforation caused by NEC (Neu & Bernstein, 2002).

Treatment

Radiographic studies will confirm perforations with the presence of free air. The initial treatment is abdominal decompression by paracentesis. Fluid resuscitation, insertion of a nasogastric tube for decompression, and broad-spectrum antibiotic administration are required. Surgery is performed to remove any torn tissue and to close the perforation.

Postoperative care centers on maintenance of fluids and electrolytes, blood volume, gastric suction, and broad-spectrum antibiotics (Ryckman, 2002). The prognosis is directly related to how quickly the situation is recognized, the age of the infant (maturity), and the severity of the perforation. Early recognition and treatment are associated with high survival rates (Berseth & Poenaru, 2005a).

Peptic Ulcer
Anatomy

Ulceration may occur in the gastric or duodenal mucosa. Ulcers are rare in newborn and are usually related to underlying systemic disorders.

Pathophysiology

The cause of ulcers in newborns is probably multifactorial including genetic, dietary, and environmental factors; the amount of hydrochloric acid; and local tissue resistance. Drugs such as indomethacin or conditions such as acidosis and shock may precipitate mucosal destruction and ulcer formation (Berseth & Poenaru, 2005a).

Treatment

Bloody emesis may be acute with considerable blood loss, or there may be gradual bleeding seen as "coffee ground" emesis or occult blood in the stools. Fibroscopic endoscopy is effective in diagnosing gastric ulcers.

The treatment is aimed at prompt replacement of blood loss. A normal saline lavage is used to evacuate bloody residue. Antacids and/or histamine H2 receptor antagonists are administered for up to 6 to 8 weeks. Sucralfate has been effective when used for a short term after gastric bleeding (Zenk et al, 2003). Feedings can be resumed after 24 hours if there is no further bleeding (Berseth & Poenaru, 2005a).

Umbilical Hernia
Anatomy

Umbilical hernias are outpouching of intestines through the umbilical ring. The defect size ranges from 1 to 4 cm in diameter (Berseth & Poenaru, 2005b).

Pathophysiology

Umbilical hernias occur because of failure of closure of the umbilical ring. The hernia contains a loop of bowel that is easily reduced. The occurrence rate is 30% in African American infants and 4% in white infants. It is more common in low-birth-weight infants and infants with Down syndrome. There is a familial association. Approximately 80% of hernias spontaneously close by 3 to 4 years of age.

Treatment

In the absence of clinical symptoms, no treatment is necessary. Surgical closure is indicated in large defects in children more than 4 years of age or when there are signs of incarceration.

Lactobezoars
Anatomy

Lactobezoars are an adverse effect of high-caloric feedings. They are firm balls of fat that form in the infant's intestinal tract about 3 to 12 days after enteral feedings have started (Ryckman, 2002). The most common symptoms are those associated with an intestinal obstruction; they include abdominal distention, vomiting, diarrhea, and increasing gastric aspirates (Ryckman, 2002). The infant may or may not have guaiac-positive stools, depending on how long the bezoar has been present and the amount of pressure it is exerting on the intestinal wall.

Pathophysiology

Prematurity, low birth weight, and the introduction of high-calorie, highly dense formulas are the most common risk factors. Infants who have received antacids have also been known to form these bezoars (Ryckman, 2002). They may be secondary to delayed gastric emptying, but in most cases there is no known etiology.

Treatment

The diagnosis can be made either by palpation of a firm ball or mass usually in the upper left quadrant or by radiographic studies (Ryckman, 2002). Contrast studies following injection of a small amount of air into the gastric area can also help with the diagnostic evaluation, as the mass will appear on a radiograph.

The treatment is aimed at relief of the intestinal obstruction. Gastric decompression may or may not be needed to relieve the distention. Gastric perforation, although rare, is always a possibility, and evaluation of the infant for this complication is wise. Ryckman (2002) advocates prevention as the best treatment by delaying the introduction of highly caloric feedings until 2 to 3 weeks of age. The prognosis is good and in most cases with minimal complications.

SUPPORT OF FAMILY WITH AN INFANT WITH A GASTROINTESTINAL SYSTEM DISORDER

The birth of an infant with a congenital anomaly or the birth of an infant who is acutely ill elicits feelings of loss, guilt, and confusion for parents. Nurses and other health professionals must expect grief reactions and help the family cope with the crisis. Strategies to help parents cope include support for early contact between parents and infant and explanation with factual information of the infant's condition and plan of care. The lines of communication must be kept open to reinforce information that the family has not been able to process and to assist the family in responding to their grief. Understanding of the disease process is essential for parents to deal later with the prognosis and ongoing health care needs.

SUMMARY

The gastrointestinal system is vital to human growth and development and ultimately long-term survival. The vast majority of conditions that cause GI dysfunction in the infant are the result of congenital anatomic malformations. Additionally, any condition or situation that leads to ischemia and bacterial overgrowth places an infant at risk of necrotizing enterocolitis and resultant long-term sequelae. The input and support of a variety of nursing, medical, and other specialists are required for optimal outcomes of the infant's physiologic well-being and the parents' psychosocial stability. The major purposes of this chapter are to present the embryologic development of the GI tract and resultant anatomic structure and to describe common causes of neonatal dysfunction with implications for care.

Case Study

IDENTIFICATION OF THE PROBLEM

Baby Girl A was born at 40 weeks' gestation, weighing 3040 g, to a 28-year-old mother, G2,P1001, with history of polyhydramnios this pregnancy. She was born by normal spontaneous vaginal delivery without complications. Apgar scores were 8 at 1 minute and 9 at 5 minutes of life. At 1 hour of life she was put to mother's breast. Excessive secretions and drooling were noted prior to coughing, choking, and cyanosis requiring suctioning and blow-by oxygen. Baby A was taken to NICU. Chest radiograph revealed slight infiltrates with good lung expansion.

ASSESSMENT: HISTORY AND PHYSICAL EXAMINATION

The maternal history was unremarkable except for polyhydramnios. Physical examination was normal except for a slight heart murmur. Excessive secretions continued. A suction catheter was used to clear oral secretions. Deep suction was attempted, but resistance to the catheter was noted shortly postpharyngeal.

DIFFERENTIAL DIAGNOSIS

An esophagus ending in a short pouch is most likely esophageal atresia. Additional workup is needed to differentiate associated tracheoesophageal fistula or other associated anomalies (30% to 70% incidence). Imperforate anus and limb anomalies were ruled out on physical examination. Related diagnoses still to be ruled out include tracheoesophageal atresia, heart defects, vertebral anomalies, intestinal atresias, and renal anomalies.

DIAGNOSTIC TESTS

A chest radiograph was done with a feeding tube inserted until resistance was met. The radiograph on the baby was consistent with esophageal atresia with tracheoesophageal fistula (EA/TEF) with a blind esophageal pouch approximately three vertebral body spaces from the distal esophagus with accompanying air in the stomach and throughout the intestine to the rectum. Hemivertebrae were present in the lumbar region. Contrast studies are generally contraindicated because of danger of aspiration, but may be necessary to diagnose an isolated or H-type tracheoesophageal fistula. Additional tests were required to rule out associated cardiac, vertebral, renal, and lower gastrointestinal disorders. An echocardiogram showed isolated ventricular septal defect (VSD). Spinal ultrasound and renal ultrasounds were normal. Anal opening and positioning was normal. Extremities were normal in appearance and movement.

WORKING DIAGNOSIS

Because of findings from the chest and abdominal radiographs and the echocardiogram, the working diagnoses for this baby included esophageal atresia with tracheoesophageal fistula, ventricular septal defect, and hemivertebrae.

Continued

Case Study—cont'd

DEVELOPMENT OF MANAGEMENT PLAN

Prevention of aspiration and providing adequate nutrition are the primary goals in initial management of an infant with esophageal atresia. A sump catheter was placed in the esophageal pouch to low continuous suction. Patency of this tube is paramount and irrigation of the tube may be needed every 2 to 4 hours. If primary repair is not possible within the first week of life, as in this case, a gastrostomy tube is needed to provide enteral nutrition and relieve the stomach of distending pressure. The tracheoesophageal fistula was to be repaired at this time to prevent stomach contents from refluxing through the fistula to the lungs. Parenteral nutrition would be given until enteral feeds can be started. Supplemental oxygen or ventilation may be needed if respiratory complications occur. Cardiology evaluated the baby in light of the VSD prior to decision for repair of EA/TEF, assessing no contraindication with proceeding with TEF repair and gastrostomy. Furosemide 1 mg/kg/day was given every 12 hours for treatment of VSD.

IMPLEMENTATION AND EVALUATION OF EFFECTIVENESS

Repair of the TEF and placement of the gastrostomy tube were done on day 1 of life. A chest tube was placed to water seal drainage. The baby remained on the ventilator 24 hours post-operatively. A sump catheter remained in place to the esophageal pouch to low continuous suction. Morphine was given for pain control. Gastrostomy feedings were started on day 2 after surgery and advanced to full feeds in 3 days. At 2 weeks of life, esophageal dilatations were initiated using a 10 Fr catheter every 4 hours. Acetaminophen was given prn for discomfort. At 1 month of life, fluoroscopic examination instilling contrast material in the stomach and a radiopaque catheter in the esophageal pouch showed a gap equal to one vertebral body space. Surgery for repair of the esophageal atresia was done the next day. Feedings were resumed on postoperative day 2 via the gastrostomy tube. One week later an upper GI revealed no leak at the site of esophageal anastomosis. Oral feeds were begun and advanced to full oral feeds in 5 days. The gastrostomy tube was clamped off, but maintained after discharge to assess if oral feedings could be maintained long-term. The mother was taught care of the gastrostomy tube and administration of furosemide. The baby was discharged home with follow-up with Cardiology in 1 month and Pediatric Surgery in 2 weeks following discharge.

REFERENCES

Bates MD (2002). Development of the enteric nervous system. In Berseth CL, editor. *Clinics in perinatology: recent advances in neonatal gastroenterology* (pp 97-114). Philadelphia: Saunders.

Bates MD, Balistreri WF (2002). The neonatal gastrointestinal tract: part one: development of the human digestive system. In Fanaroff AA, Martin RJ, editors. *Neonatal-perinatal medicine: diseases of the fetus and infant,* ed 7. St Louis: Mosby.

Bell SG (2003). Gastroesophageal reflux and histamine2 antagonists. *Neonatal network* 22(2):53-57.

Berseth CL (2005a). Developmental anatomy and physiology of the gastrointestinal tract. In Taeusch HW et al, editors. *Avery's diseases of the newborn,* ed 8 (pp 1071-1085). Philadelphia: Saunders.

Berseth CL (2005b). Physiologic and inflammatory abnormalities of the gastrointestinal tract. In Taeusch HW et al, editors. *Avery's diseases of the newborn,* ed 8 (pp 1103-1112). Philadelphia: Saunders.

Berseth CL, Poenaru D (2005a). Structural anomalies of the gastrointestinal tract. In Taeusch HW et al, editors. *Avery's diseases of the newborn,* ed 8 (pp 1086-1102). Philadelphia: Saunders.

Berseth CL, Poenaru D (2005b). Abdominal wall problems. In Taeusch HW et al, editors. *Avery's diseases of the newborn,* ed 8 (pp 1113-1122). Philadelphia: Saunders.

Berseth CL, Poenaru D (2005c). Necrotizing enterocolitis and short bowel syndrome. In Taeusch HW et al, editors. *Avery's diseases of the newborn,* ed 8 (pp 1123-1133). Philadelphia: Saunders.

Bloom RS (2002). Delivery room resuscitation of newborn. In Fanaroff AA, Martin RJ, editors. *Neonatal-perinatal medicine: diseases of the fetus and infant,* ed 7. St Louis: Mosby.

Burrin DG, Stoll B (2002). Key nutrients and growth factors for the neonatal gastrointestinal tract. In Berseth CL, editor. *Clinics in perinatology: recent advances in neonatal gastroenterology* (pp 65-96). Philadelphia: Saunders.

Cass DL, Wesson DE (2002). Advances in fetal and neonatal surgery for gastrointestinal anomalies and disease. In Berseth CL, editor. *Clinics in perinatology: recent advances in neonatal gastroenterology* (pp 1-22). Philadelphia: Saunders.

Clyman RI (2005). Patent ductus arteriosus in the preterm infant. In Taeusch HW et al, editors. *Avery's diseases of the newborn,* ed 8 (pp 816-826). Philadelphia: Saunders.

DiBaise JK et al (2004). Intestinal rehabilitation and the short bowel syndrome. Part 2. *American journal of gastroenterology* 99(9):1823-1832.

Escobar MA et al (2004). Duodenal atresia and stenosis: long-term follow-up over 30 years. *Journal of pediatric surgery* 39(6):867-871.

Gardner VA et al (2003). A case study utilizing an enteral refeeding technique in a premature infant with short bowel syndrome. *Advances in neonatal care* 3(6):258-271.

Glenny AM et al (2005). Feeding interventions for growth and development in infants with cleft lip, cleft palate, or cleft lip and palate. *The Cochrane database of systematic reviews,* vol 1. Available from: http://gateway.ut.ovid.come/gwl/ovidweb.cgi. Accessed April 23, 2005.

Hall N et al (2004). Meta-analysis of laparoscopic versus open pyloromyotomy. *Annals of surgery* 240(5):774-778.

Hammer D (2005). Gastroesophageal reflux and prokinetic agents. *Neonatal network* 24(2):51-58.

Heider AL et al (2004). Omphalocele: clinical outcomes in cases with normal karyotypes. *American journal of obstetrics and gynecology* 190(1):135-141.

Horton KK (2005). Pathophysiology and current management of necrotizing enterocolitis. *Neonatal network* 24(1):37-46.

Hwang P, Kousseff BG (2004). Omphalocele and gastroschisis: an 18 year review study. *Genetics in medicine* 6(4):232-236.

Hwang ST, Shulman RJ (2002). Update on management and treatment of short gut. In Berseth CL, editor. *Clinics in perinatology: recent advances in neonatal gastroenterology* (pp 181-194). Philadelphia: Saunders.

Iwashita T et al (2003). Hirschsprung disease is linked to defects in neural crest stem cell function. *Science* 301(5635):972-976.

Jadcherla SR (2002). Gastroesophageal reflux in the neonate. In Berseth CL, editor. *Clinics in perinatology: recent advances in neonatal gastroenterology* (pp 135-158). Philadelphia: Saunders.

James LP (2002). Pharmacology for the gastrointestinal tract. In Berseth CL, editor. *Clinics in perinatology: recent advances in neonatal gastroenterology* (pp 115-134). Philadelphia: Saunders.

Jezewski PA et al (2003). Complete sequencing shows a role for MSX1 in non-syndromic cleft lip and palate. *Journal of medical genetics* 40(6):399-407.

Karpen SJ (2002). Update on the etiologies and management of neonatal cholestasis. In Berseth CL, editor. *Clinics in perinatology: recent advances in neonatal gastroenterology* (pp 159-180). Philadelphia: Saunders.

Kee JL (2001). *Laboratory and diagnostic tests with nursing implications*, ed 4. Upper Saddle River, NJ: Prentice-Hall.

Kelly D (2002). Transplantation—new beginnings and new horizons. *Journal of pediatric gastroenterology and nutrition* 34(suppl 1):551-553.

Khalaf MN et al (2001). Clinical correlations in infants in the neonatal intensive care unit with varying severity of gastroesophageal reflux. *Journal of pediatrics and gastroenterology and nutrition* 32(1):45-49.

King J, Askin DF (2003). Gastroschisis: etiology, diagnosis, delivery options, and care. *Neonatal network* 22(4):7-12.

Kobayashi H, Stringer MD (2003). Biliary atresia. *Seminars in neonatology* 8(5):383-391.

Koenig WJ et al (1995). Manometrics for preterm and term infants: a new tool for old questions. *Pediatrics* 95(2):203-206.

Kosloske AM (1994). Indications for operation in necrotizing enterocolitis revisited. *Journal of pediatric surgery* 29(5):663-666.

Kovesi T, Rubin S (2004). Long-term complications of congenital esophageal atresia and/or tracheoesophageal fistula. *Chest* 126(3):915-925.

Lin H et al (2004). Oral probiotics reduce the incidence and severity of necrotizing enterocolitis in very low birth weight infants. *Pediatrics* 115(1):1-4.

Lykavieris P et al (2005). Outcome in adulthood of biliary atresia: a study of 63 patients who survived for over 20 years with their native liver. *Hepatology* 41(2):366-371.

Merenstein GB, Gardner SL (2006). *Handbook of neonatal intensive care*, ed 6. St Louis: Mosby.

Merritt L (2005a). Part 1: Understanding the embryology and genetics of cleft lip and palate. *Advances in neonatal care* 5(2):64-71.

Merritt L (2005b). Part 2: Physical assessment of the infant with cleft lip and/or palate. *Advances in neonatal care* 5(3):125-134.

Neu J, Bernstein H (2002). Update on host defense and immunonutrients. In Berseth CL, editor. *Clinics in perinatology: recent advances in neonatal gastroenterology* (pp 41-64). Philadelphia: Saunders.

Nock ML, Wilson-Costello D (2002). Intussusception in a premature neonate. *Clinical pediatrics* 41(9):721-724.

Omari TI et al (2004). Paradoxical impact of body positioning on gastroesophageal reflux and gastric emptying in the premature neonate. *Journal of pediatrics* 145(2):194-200.

Puri P, Shinkai T (2004). Pathogenesis of Hirschsprung's disease and its variants: recent progress. *Seminars in pediatric surgery* 13(1):18-24.

Reber KM et al (2002). Newborn intestinal circulation: physiology and pathophysiology. In Berseth CL, editor. *Clinics in perinatology: recent advances in neonatal gastroenterology* (pp 23-40). Philadelphia: Saunders.

Ricketts RR (1994). Surgical treatment of necrotizing enterocolitis and the short bowel syndrome. *Clinics in perinatology* 21(2):365-387.

Ryckman FC (2002). The neonatal gastrointestinal tract: Part IV: selected anomalies and intestinal obstructions. In Fanaroff AA, Martin RJ, editors. *Neonatal-perinatal medicine: diseases of the fetus and infant*, ed 7. St Louis: Mosby.

Ryckman FC, Balistreri WF (2002). The neonatal gastrointestinal tract: part two: upper gastrointestinal disorders. In Fanaroff AA, Martin RJ, editors. *Neonatal-perinatal medicine: diseases of the fetus and infant*, ed 7. St Louis: Mosby.

Salihu JM et al (2004). Mode of delivery and neonatal survival of infants with isolated gastroschisis. *Obstetrics and gynecology* 104(4):678-683.

Schanler RJ (2005). Enteral nutrition for the high-risk neonate. In Taeusch HW et al, editors. *Avery's diseases of the newborn*, ed 8 (pp 1043-1060). Philadelphia: Saunders.

Schlatter M (2003). Preformed silos in the management of gastroschisis: new progress with an old idea. *Current opinion in pediatrics* 15(3):239-242.

Spilson SV et al (2001). Association between maternal diabetes mellitus and newborn oral cleft. *Annals of plastic surgery* 47(5):477-481.

Spoon JM (2003). VATER association. *Neonatal network* 22(3):71-75.

Spritz R (2001). The genetics and epigenetics of orofacial cleft. *Current opinion in pediatrics* 13(6):556-560.

Sydorak RM, Albanese CT (2002). Laparoscopic repair of high imperforate anus. *Seminars in pediatric surgery* 11(4):217-225.

Walden M (2001). *Pain assessment and management: guideline for practice*. Glenview, IL: National Association of Neonatal Nurses.

Wales PW et al (2004). Neonatal short bowel syndrome; population-based estimates of incidence and mortality rates. *Journal of pediatric surgery* 39(5):690-695.

Zenk KE et al (2003). *Neonatal medications and nutrition, comprehensive guide*, ed 3. Santa Rosa, CA: NICU Ink.

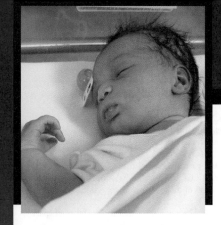

Chapter 6

Metabolic System

Laura Stokowski

Metabolic disorders, or inborn errors of metabolism (IEMs), encompass a group of disorders in which gene mutations cause clinically significant blocks in metabolic pathways. Most IEMs are inherited in an autosomal recessive fashion; a few are X-linked. The major categories are disorders of amino acid metabolism, organic acidemias, fatty acid oxidation disorders, congenital lactic acidoses, disorders of carbohydrate metabolism, lysosomal disorders, peroxisomal disorders, cholesterol biosynthetic disorders, and disorders of metal metabolism. Into these categories fall hundreds of individual disorders of metabolism, many of which have their onset in the neonatal period. The inherited metabolic disorders manifesting in the early neonatal period will be the focus of this chapter.

GENERAL PRINCIPLES: THE NEONATE WITH A METABOLIC DISORDER
Pathophysiology of IEMs
The primary gene defect causing an inborn error of metabolism results in an accumulation of precursors before a blocked step in a metabolic pathway or a deficiency of a metabolic product. In disorders involving the intermediary metabolism of small molecules (such as maple syrup urine disease), the accumulated molecules give rise to an "intoxication syndrome" because of the profoundly toxic nature of these substances and their effect on the CNS. Disorders involving energy metabolism (such as pyruvate dehydrogenase deficiency) lead to a failure of energy production or utilization with a broad range of symptoms and physiologic consequences. Other disorders, such as lysosomal storage diseases, involve complex molecules, and the symptoms that arise from these disorders are permanent, progressive, and independent of intercurrent events (Saudubray et al, 2002).

Clinical Manifestations of IEMs
The vast majority of neonates who are eventually diagnosed with IEMs appear essentially normal at birth and have no history of antepartum or intrapartum complications. The placenta and maternal circulation protect the fetus from damaging effects of toxins. Birth is followed by a symptom-free interval of variable duration. Some metabolic disorders are unmasked by the ingestion of formula, milk, or fructose. Others are unrelated to feeding or may be brought on by fasting, infection, or stress.

Common presentations include feeding problems (poor intake, vomiting), progressive neurologic symptoms, multisystem involvement (liver, kidneys, GI system), or nonspecific symptoms such as respiratory distress. The presentation may be consistent with neonatal sepsis, because the neonate has a limited repertoire of responses to severe illness (Saudubray et al, 2002). The infant often deteriorates rapidly and does not respond to symptomatic therapy. Metabolic acidosis with an increased anion gap, significant hyperammonemia, unexplained hepatic dysfunction, or ketonuria should always raise suspicion of an inborn error of metabolism (Leonard, 2005a). Although a minority of IEMs are associated with dysmorphism, the possibility of an inborn error of metabolism should not be discounted in the neonate with congenital malformations or unusual features.

A complete family history should be obtained to determine if other individuals in the family have had similar symptoms or the same disorder, or if there is a history of unexplained infant death, SIDS, mental retardation, or consanguinity (Leonard, 2005a).

Diagnosis of IEMs
The initial laboratory investigation of a suspected inborn error of metabolism includes a broad range of tests of both blood and urine (Box 6-1). Screening tests do not provide a diagnosis; at best they will confirm that there is a high likelihood that the infant does have a metabolic disorder and suggest a specific category of disease (e.g. organic acidemia, fatty acid oxidation disorder). Interpretation of results can be tricky. Conditions of sampling can profoundly affect results. Blood and urine samples must be obtained prior to the initiation of therapy, and whenever possible, both should be collected when the infant is symptomatic. Extra blood and urine samples should be obtained and frozen for later testing. Secondary metabolic derangements can interfere with test interpretation, and biochemical abnormalities might be present only during acute episodes. Laboratory abnormalities can be transient; a result within the reference range does not necessarily rule out a metabolic disorder. Studies may need to be repeated at specific times. Clinicians might be falsely reassured by screening tests that are inadequate to exclude certain conditions. Therefore, consultation with a metabolic specialist is recommended. Furthermore, a clinical history and as much information as possible about the infant's symptoms and the suspected diagnosis should be provided to the referral laboratory to improve the accuracy of testing and interpretation of results (Garganta & Smith, 2005; Kenner & Moran, 2005).

Postmortem Diagnosis
If a neonate with a possible metabolic disorder dies suddenly, it is of great importance to continue to try to establish the proper diagnosis for purposes of genetic counseling and future ante-

---

BOX 6-1

General Screening Tests for Inborn Errors of Metabolism

Blood Tests	Urine Tests
Glucose	Glucose
Complete blood count (CBC) with differential	Ketones
Blood gases	pH
Electrolytes (and anion gap*)	Reducing substances
Liver function tests	Ferric chloride reaction
Blood urea nitrogen (BUN) and creatinine	Dinitrophenylhydrazine reaction
Total and direct bilirubin	Amino acids
Prothrombin time (PT) and partial thromboplastin time (PTT)	Organic acids
Uric acid	Odor
Ammonia	Orotic acid (if blood NH_4
Lactate	elevated)
Pyruvate	
Amino acids	
Free fatty acids	
Ketones ($_3$OH-butyrate, acetoacetate)	
Creatinine phosphokinase (CPK)	
Newborn metabolic screen/blood acylcarnitine analysis	
Cerebrospinal fluid (CSF) glycine (to rule out nonketotic hyperglycinemia)	

*Anion gap is (sodium – [chloride + bicarbonate]). Normal is less than 15 mEq/L.

---

natal diagnosis (Olpin, 2004). In addition to standard blood and urine samples, a sample of cerebrospinal fluid (CSF) should be obtained if possible, and whole blood and bile should be collected on filter paper. The routine state newborn screening card should be completed and sent. If the family declines a full autopsy, tissue biopsies should be obtained. Tissue samples of value are skin, liver, kidney, and muscle (Garganta & Smith, 2005).

Neonatal Screening

The development of tandem mass spectrometry (MS/MS) has greatly improved the presymptomatic detection of a large number of inborn errors of metabolism. With MS/MS, it is possible to measure 30 or 40 different metabolites in less than 2 or 3 minutes, using a single dried blood spot (McCandless, 2004). Tandem mass spectrometry works by applying a charge to the compounds in solution, sending them through an electromagnetic field, and sorting them out and weighing them according to their mass-to-charge ratio. Expanded newborn screening using MS/MS is mandated in some states as part of the routine newborn screening program. It is also available to parents who wish to purchase it from a number of private laboratories at a nominal cost. Currently, MS/MS screens only for disorders of intermediary metabolism, including amino acid disorders, organic acid disorders, and fatty acid oxidation disorders (Banta-Wright & Steiner, 2004). A normal neonatal screen, even an expanded newborn screen by MS/MS, does not rule out an inborn error of metabolism in a suspicious clinical setting (Kenner & Moran, 2005; McCandless, 2004).

Collaborative Management of IEMs. As soon as it becomes apparent that the infant has some type of metabolic disorder, it is important to consult a metabolic specialist/geneticist. In addition to general supportive measures as indicated by the infant's symptoms, both general and specific treatments should be initiated. Oral feedings and amino acid solutions (all protein sources) are withheld and 10% glucose solution with electrolytes is administered temporarily until the precise diagnosis is ascertained. A glucose infusion rate of at least 5 mg/kg/min (and higher if tolerated) is administered because many metabolic disorders are exacerbated by tissue catabolism. Intralipids are withheld until disorders of fatty acid oxidation have been ruled out. Acute hypoglycemia, metabolic acidosis, dehydration, hypovolemia, and electrolyte imbalances are corrected as part of the overall supportive management of a metabolic disorder. Many disorders with rapid neonatal or prenatal onset are lethal and all that can be offered are palliative and symptomatic care.

UREA CYCLE DISORDERS

Urea cycle disorders (UCDs) are caused by inherited defects in genes encoding enzymes or membrane transporters involved in ureagenesis (Summar & Tuchman, 2001). All are transmitted as autosomal recessive traits except ornithine transcarbamylase (OTC) deficiency, which is X-linked, and the most common of the primary defects. The prevalence of UCDs is believed to be approximately 1:10,000 live births (Burton, 2000).

Pathophysiology of UCDs

The hepatic urea cycle is the mechanism used by the body to detoxify and eliminate ammonia generated from nitrogen waste. Five enzymatic reactions make up the urea cycle, leading to the incorporation of ammonia into urea and enabling its excretion in the urine (Figure 6-1). The first two steps, the carbamyl phosphate synthetase (CPS) and OTC reactions, take place in the mitochondria and lead to the synthesis of citrulline. In a subsequent cytosolic reaction citrulline is converted to argininosuccinate, which is hydrolyzed to

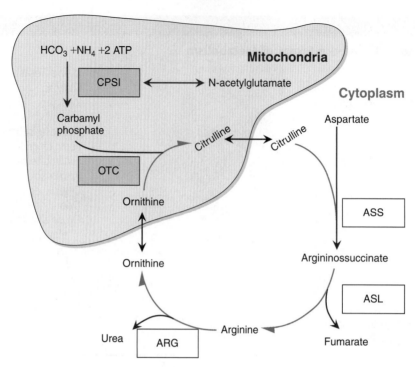

FIGURE **6-1**
The urea cycle and alternative pathways of nitrogen excretion. Nitrogen is converted to ammonia (NH_4) and transported to the liver where it is processed via the urea cycle, composed of five enzymes in the direct pathway: (1) carbamyl phosphate synthase I *(CPSI)*; (2) ornithine transcarbamylase *(OTC)*; (3) argininosuccinic acid synthetase *(ASS)*; (4) argininosuccinic acid lyase *(ASL)*; (5) arginase *(ARG)*. From GeneReviews: Genetic Disease Online Reviews, University of Washington, Seattle, WA.

arginine and fumarate. Arginine is then hydrolyzed to urea and ornithine is regenerated.

A block of the urea cycle can result from a deficiency of any one of the first five enzymes in the urea cycle pathway: carbamyl phosphate synthetase I (CPS deficiency), ornithine transcarbamylase (OTC deficiency), argininosuccinic acid synthetase (citrullinemia), argininosuccinic acid lyase (argininosuccinic aciduria), or a cofactor producer, *N*-acetylglutamate synthase (NAGS deficiency) (Summar, 2001). The outcome of a block in the urea cycle is an accumulation of precursor metabolites, including ammonia, which have no effective alternate clearance pathway. The neonate, with an immature liver and tendency toward catabolism, is poorly equipped to handle the excess metabolites and rapidly succumbs to the neurotoxic effects of high ammonia levels (Summar, 2001). Hyperammonemic encephalopathy results from osmotic swelling in the brain caused by glutamine accumulation in cerebral astrocytes, where glutamine synthesis is increased in response to high ammonia levels (Gordon, 2003).

Clinical Manifestations of UCDs
Infants with complete urea cycle enzyme defects such as OTC and CPSI deficiency are usually born at term, with no prenatal complications, because the maternal circulation prevents a buildup of toxic ammonia (Summar & Tuchman, 2001). Affected newborns are initially healthy, but shortly after receiving their first protein feedings, they begin showing signs of clinical decompensation and hyperammonemic encephalopathy. The earliest signs of ammonia toxicity are irritability,

hypotonia, hypothermia, lethargy, poor feeding, vomiting, and hyperventilation. The clinical picture mimics sepsis although the laboratory evaluation fails to confirm infection (Summar & Tuchman, 2001). A mild respiratory alkalosis with tachypnea is a common early finding that should prompt measurement of a plasma ammonia level (Burton, 2000). Neurologic deterioration is progressive, with loss of tone and reflexes, eventually leading to respiratory failure and coma. Hepatomegaly may also be present. Without treatment, most infants will die from complications such as cerebral, pulmonary hemorrhage or neurologic or cardiac problems (Leonard & Morris, 2006).

Diagnosis of UCDs
The hallmark of a UCD is an elevated blood ammonia level (>500 mcmol/L). The exception is arginase deficiency, which does not typically cause a rapid rise in plasma ammonia level. A normal ammonia level in a healthy infant is less than 65 mcmol/L. Blood sampling and handling techniques can affect results. Blood for ammonia levels should be collected by arterial or venous sampling and kept on ice, and plasma should be separated within 15 minutes of collection. Hemolysis, delayed processing, and exposure to room air can falsely elevate ammonia levels. Capillary blood is not appropriate for measurement of blood ammonia levels (Leonard & Morris, 2006; UCD Conference Group, 2001). If the ammonia level of a newborn with a suspected UCD is only modestly elevated, it should be repeated after several hours because the level can rise rapidly (Leonard & Morris, 2002).

Blood gases, electrolytes, glucose, and other routine clinical laboratory tests should be obtained. Metabolic acidosis with a normal anion gap is sometimes present in UCDs, but not as often as in disorders of organic acid metabolism. Blood urea nitrogen is low, but this is not specific or sensitive for UCDs. Liver function tests are important to rule out possible causes of hyperammonemia related to liver disorders or dysfunction (Steiner & Cederbaum, 2001).

To arrive at a more precise diagnosis, quantitative plasma and urinary amino acids are necessary. Plasma glutamine, alanine, and asparagine, which serve as waste storage forms of nitrogen, may all be elevated. Plasma arginine is low in all UCDs of neonatal onset. The amounts of citrulline, ASA, and arginine in plasma and orotic acid in urine are usually sufficient to differentiate among UCDs. Measuring enzyme activity in tissue (liver, cultured skin fibroblasts, or RBCs) at a later point in time provides a definitive diagnosis that may be desirable for genetic counseling or future prenatal testing (Burton, 2000). Molecular genetic testing using linkage analysis or mutation scanning is available for OTC and CPSI deficiencies as well as citrullinemia, allowing for diagnostic confirmation, carrier detection, and prenatal diagnosis. Three UCDs (citrullinemia, argininosuccinate lyase deficiency, and arginase deficiency) can also be detected by the amino acid panels of expanded newborn screening programs employing tandem mass spectrometry.

Differential Diagnosis of Hyperammonemia

Several other inborn errors of metabolism can cause hyperammonemia in the newborn, notably the organic acidemias propionic, methylmalonic acidemia and the fatty acid oxidation disorders medium chain acyl-CoA dehydrogenase deficiency, systemic carnitine deficiency, and long-chain fatty acid oxidation disorders, although the last group are also associated with hypoglycemia. Hyperammonemia is also a feature of pyruvate carboxylase deficiency, and pyruvate dehydrogenase deficiency. In transient hyperammonemia of the newborn (THAN), very high plasma ammonia levels, often matching those of urea cycle disorders, exist for which no underlying cause can be found. THAN is usually associated with prematurity and has no genetic basis, nor does it recur in infants who survive the initial episode (Burton, 2000). A simple algorithm can be useful to determine the cause of hyperammonemia (Figure 6-2).

Collaborative Management of UCDs

The emergency treatment of an infant with a suspected UCD includes immediate cessation of dietary protein and provision of a high-energy intake with a protein-free formula or by intravenous glucose and lipid infusion, if enteral feeding cannot be tolerated. Protein intake is stopped only temporarily, however, because failure to supply essential amino acids will eventually result in catabolism and further ammonia production. Within 48 hours, 1 to 1.5 g/kg/day of protein should be restarted, with 50% as essential amino acids. Fever, if present, must be aggressively treated. Plasma ammonia levels are monitored closely, and ammonia concentrations >500 mcmol/L must be reduced promptly with hemodialysis, extracorporeal membrane oxygenation (ECMO), or hemofiltration (Leonard & Morris, 2002). Peritoneal dialysis is much less effective in clearing ammonia from the body. For this reason, it is recommended that neonates with symptomatic hyperam-

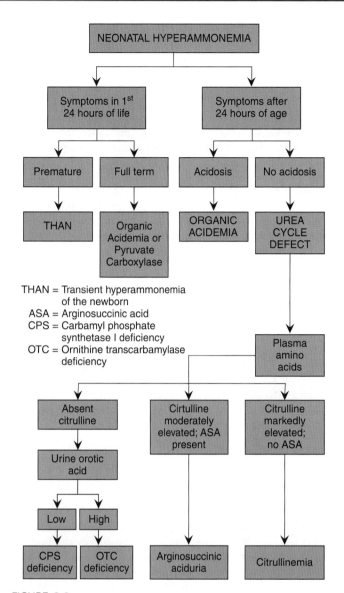

THAN = Transient hyperammonemia of the newborn
ASA = Arginosuccinic acid
CPS = Carbamyl phosphate synthetase I deficiency
OTC = Ornithine transcarbamylase deficiency

FIGURE **6-2**
Algorithm to differentiate among conditions that produce neonatal hyperammonemia. Redrawn from Burton BK (2000). Urea cycle disorders. *Clinics in liver disease* 4:815-830.

monemia be transferred without delay to a neonatal facility capable of providing hemodialysis (Wilcken, 2004).

Compounds that conjugate to amino acids, providing an alternate route for the excretion of nitrogen, can be given to lower the nitrogen burden, and therefore the ammonia burden, of an infant with a UCD. These agents (called "scavenger drugs" or diversion therapy) include sodium benzoate, which is conjugated with glycine to form hippurate, and sodium phenylbutyrate, which is oxidized in the liver to phenylacetate and then conjugated with glutamine and excreted in the urine. Serum potassium levels must be monitored closely when these drugs are used (Wilcken, 2004). A preparation combining both sodium phenylbutyrate and sodium benzoate is also available. In babies with citrullinemia and argininosuccinic aciduria, nitrogen can be excreted by increasing losses of citrulline and argininosuccinic acid, respectively. Arginine supplementation boosts the excretion of these metabolites by replenishing the supply of ornithine (Leonard & Morris, 2002). However, high doses of the intravenous preparation L-arginine-HCl can cause metabolic acidosis and must be administered via central line because it can cause tissue necrosis if extravasation occurs.

A neonate in acute hyperammonemic coma caused by a suspected UCD should be given loading doses followed by continuous infusions of the ammonia-scavenging drugs L-arginine-HCl, sodium benzoate, and sodium phenylacetate, and drug levels should be monitored to reduce the risks of toxicity. Dietary protein is reintroduced in low amounts (0.5 g/kg/day) to encourage an anabolic state, while continuing diversion therapy to control ammonia levels. Alternative therapies that have been used with variable success for neonatal UCDs include liver and hepatocyte transplantation (Wilcken, 2004).

Prognosis

Even with the most vigorous intervention, UCDs of neonatal onset are often fatal, and the few survivors have a high rate of neurologic disability (Nyhan et al, 2005). The overall mortality rate of 121 neonates with early-onset UCDs was 84% in one series (Nassogne et al, 2005). OTC deficiency was the most severe and lethal defect, particularly among males. The extent of permanent neurologic impairment in survivors is related to the duration of the hyperammonemic coma (Burton, 2000), plasma ammonia level at diagnosis, and other unidentified factors (Gordon, 2003).

DISORDERS OF AMINO ACID METABOLISM

Amino acids play a role in literally all metabolic and cellular functions. As the constituents of protein, amino acids are used for the synthesis of new protein and as a source of carbon skeletons for generating glucose and ketone bodies (Leonard, 2005b). Amino acids are classified as nonessential or essential, depending on whether they can be synthesized by the body or must be obtained from dietary sources.

The disorders of amino acid metabolism, also called aminoacidopathies, arise from deficiencies of enzymes required to metabolize specific amino acids or amino acid transporters. The effects of the aberrant metabolism are highly disease-specific. In some aminoacidopathies, clinical symptoms are caused by the relatively rapid accumulation of toxic metabolites that are substrates for the dysfunctional enzyme (Leonard, 2005b). In other amino acid disorders, damaging effects of the enzyme deficiency are more gradual and chronic in nature.

The most well-known disorder of amino acid metabolism, perhaps of all the inborn errors of metabolism, is phenylketonuria, or PKU. The clinically and biochemically heterogeneous disorders of amino acid metabolism are inherited primarily as autosomal recessive traits.

Nonketotic Hyperglycinemia (NKH)
Pathophysiology

NKH (also known as glycine encephalopathy) is a disorder of glycine metabolism that is generally fatal in its neonatal form (Leonard, 2005b). Glycine, a glucogenic amino acid, is normally metabolized by a complex of enzymes known as the glycine cleavage complex (GCS). GCS is a complex of four proteins encoded on four different chromosomes. A defect in any of these enzymes interferes with the cleavage of glycine,

resulting in a steep rise in glycine concentration in the blood and cerebrospinal fluid. Glycine potentiates firing of the N-methyl-D-aspartate (NMDA) receptors in the cerebral cortex, an effect which may be inappropriately activated in NKH. This disturbance in the function of brain glutamate receptors leads to seizures and brain damage (Payan et al, 2005).

Clinical Manifestations

In classic neonatal NKH, symptoms usually start soon after birth and are not related to feedings. The clinical picture is dominated by neurologic decompensation: rapidly increasing stupor, lethargy, unresponsiveness, respiratory distress, and sustained seizures that are difficult to control (Payan et al, 2005). Myoclonic jerking and hiccupping are also common. Within 1 to 3 days, the infant becomes comatose and death ensues. Babies who survive have intractable seizures and uniformly poor neurologic outcomes.

Diagnosis

Glycine is elevated in plasma, urine, and CSF. The CSF-to-plasma glycine concentration ratio of affected infants is >0.09. The diagnostic workup fails to find evidence such as metabolic acidosis, ketosis, hyperammonemia, or abnormal organic acids in blood or urine suggestive of another IEM. Electroencephalographic (EEG) tracings typically show a burst suppression pattern with hypsarrhythmia (random, high-voltage slow waves and spikes that arise from multiple foci and spread to all cortical areas). Confirmation of the exact enzyme deficiency causing NKH requires analysis of a liver sample.

Collaborative Management

No consistently effective therapy has been discovered for classic neonatal onset NKH. Medications to reduce seizures by blocking the NMDA receptor channel complex have had limited success (Chien et al, 2004).

Hereditary Tyrosinemia
Pathophysiology

Hereditary tyrosinemia type I, also called hepatorenal tyrosinemia or fumarylacetoacetate hydrolase (FAH) deficiency, is a severe autosomal recessive metabolic disorder affecting the liver, kidney, and nervous system (Leonard, 2005b). It is caused by a deficiency of fumarylacetoacetate hydrolase, the last enzyme in the tyrosine catabolic pathway. The offending compounds in tyrosinemia type I are fumarylacetoacetate and maleylacetoacetate, both of which accumulate in the cells and cause cell death by apoptosis. Although hepatocytes are quickly regenerated, liver function can deteriorate rapidly in babies with tyrosinemia type I. Hepatocellular disease in tyrosinemia is also associated with renal Fanconi syndrome.

Clinical Manifestations

Patients with hereditary tyrosinemia type I may come to clinical attention in the newborn period, or within the first 3 weeks of life (Clayton, 2002). Newborns present with evidence of liver dysfunction including hepatomegaly, bleeding from coagulation defects, and jaundice. Ascites may be present.

Diagnosis

The diagnostic workup includes liver function tests, which typically show elevated transaminases, direct and indirect bilirubin, and prolonged PT and PTT. Plasma tyrosine and methionine may be elevated. The urine organic acid analysis reveals increased excretion of succinylacetone. Enzyme analysis of lymphocytes confirms the diagnosis. Currently, 34 states offer or mandate screening of newborns for hereditary tyrosinemia, and it is included on all expanded newborn screening panels (NNSGRC, 2005).

Collaborative Management

Infants with tyrosinemia usually respond to treatment with 2-(2-nitro-4-trifluoromethylbenzoyl)-1,3-cyclohexanedione (NTBC), which inhibits the conversion of p-hydroxyphenylpyruvate, the transamination product of tyrosine, to fumarylacetoacetate, slowing the synthesis and accumulation of toxic metabolites. Dietary management involves feeding the infant a phenylalanine- and tyrosine-free formula, or breastfeeding, with phenylalanine supplementation as needed (Clayton, 2002). Most infants with tyrosinemia type I will require a liver transplant because of the development of hepatocellular carcinoma.

Transient Tyrosinemia
Pathophysiology

Elevated tyrosine is most likely caused by decreased activity of 4-hydroxyphenylpyruvic acid dioxygenase (4HPPD), a vitamin C–dependent enzyme in the tyrosine degradation pathway (Berry & Yudkoff, 2001). Risk factors include prematurity (hepatic immaturity), low vitamin C intake, and excessive protein intake. In some infants, transient tyrosinemia may be precipitated by endogenous catabolism. Tyrosinemia peaks in the first 14 days of life and resolves by 1 month of life.

Clinical Manifestations

Lethargy and poor feeding may be seen in neonates with hypertyrosinemia, particularly in preterm infants.

Diagnosis

Transient hypertyrosinemia is identified by positive newborn metabolic screen.

Collaborative Management

All infants with an elevated tyrosine on initial newborn screen should have a repeat screen done; with confirmatory testing for those who remain abnormal (see Hereditary Tyrosinemia). This is usually a self-limited disorder that does not require therapy (McCandless, 2004). Therapies include a low protein diet and supplemental vitamin C to increase the activity of 4HPPD and promote the metabolism of both tyrosine and phenylalanine (Berry & Yudkoff, 2001).

Phenylketonuria

Classical phenylketonuria, or PKU, is an autosomal recessive disorder caused by mutations in both alleles of the gene for phenylalanine hydroxylase, found on chromosome 12. Classic PKU occurs in about 1:12,000 live births. Although PKU rarely manifests clinically in the newborn period, it will be discussed here because it is important for neonatal caregivers to be able to provide accurate information to parents about key genetic conditions for which their newborn infants are being screened.

Pathophysiology

The effect of the inactive phenylalanine hydroxylase enzyme is an inability to metabolize phenylalanine, resulting in hyperphenylalaninemia. Following ingestion of adequate amounts of breast milk or formula, blood phenylalanine level gradually increases. Phenylketonuric compounds are excreted in the urine, one of which (phenylacetic acid) imparts the musty or mousy odor characteristic of PKU. If dietary therapy is not implemented at birth, mental retardation can occur.

Clinical Manifestations

Biochemical manifestations of PKU are present in the newborn, but no outward clinical signs or symptoms. A musty odor may be detectable in the infant's urine around the end of the first week of life, if plasma phenylalanine levels reach 10 to 15 mg/dl (Berry, 2004).

Diagnosis

Early diagnosis is critical because PKU is a preventable cause of mental retardation. Plasma phenylalanine in the normal infant is <2 mg/dl. In infants with PKU, the plasma phenylalanine level usually exceeds 4 mg/dl by 24 hours of age and is 20 to 40 mg/dl by the end of the first week of life (Berry, 2004). PKU is a pioneer of sorts among metabolic disorders: it was the first disorder for which a screening test was developed in 1961 (the Guthrie test, a bacterial inhibition assay), and the first disorder to be screened for using tandem mass spectrometry. MS/MS has dramatically decreased the number of false positive screening results, as well as further clarifying the prevalence of variants of hyperphenylalaninemia in the population (Banta-Wright & Steiner, 2004).

Collaborative Management

Phenylketonuria is currently treated with a low-phenylalanine diet; however, compliance can be a long-term problem and dietary treatment can be associated with other nutritional deficiencies. Enzyme substitution with recombinant phenylalanine ammonia lyase is being explored as an alternative form of therapy (Sarkissian & Gamez, 2005).

DISORDERS OF ORGANIC ACID METABOLISM

The organic acid disorders are disorders of intermediary metabolism resulting from a deficient enzyme or transport protein, the lack of which causes a block in a metabolic pathway. The block occurs in a step after deamination of the amino acid, and the resulting metabolites are organic acid derivatives. An organic acid is distinguished from an amino acid in that it contains no nitrogen. Because these disorders lead to an accumulation of organic acids in the urine, they are often referred to as "organic acidurias."

Maple Syrup Urine Disease

Maple syrup urine disease (MSUD), a branched-chain organic aciduria, is a disorder resulting from one or more mutations in the gene encoding the enzymes that catalyze the branched-chain amino acids (BCAA) leucine, isoleucine, and valine. The name *maple syrup urine disease* refers to the intensely sweet, maple sugar odor of the cerumen, skin, and urine that accompanies the disorder (Box 6-2). The incidence of MSUD is about 1 in 200,000 in the general population, but in the Old Order Mennonites of southeastern Pennsylvania the frequency is 1 in 358 births (Puffenberger, 2003).

BOX **6-2**

Unusual Odors Associated with Inborn Errors of Metabolism

Disorder	Odor
Maple syrup urine disease	Maple syrup—burnt sugar
Tyrosinemia type I	Cabbage or rancid butter
Multiple acyl-CoA dehydrogenase deficiency	Sweaty socks—rancid cheese
Phenylketonuria	Mousy—musty
Propionic acidemia	Cat urine
Isovaleric acidemia	Sweaty socks—rancid cheese
Ketoaciduria	Fruity
3-Methylglutaconic aciduria	Tomcat urine
Trimethylaminuria	Fish

Pathophysiology

The second common step in the degradation of a BCAA involves the enzyme branched-chain ketoacid dehydrogenase complex. This enzyme has three components: a decarboxylase that requires thiamine as a coenzyme, a dihydrolipoyl acyl-transferase, and a dihydrolipoamine dehydrogenase (Ogier de Baulny & Saudubray, 2002). A deficiency of any of these components can cause MSUD. The enzyme defect results in marked increases of branched-chain ketoacids (BCKA) in plasma, urine, and CSF, and owing to the reversibility of the initial step, a concomitant accumulation of the three BCAAs (Ogier de Baulny & Saudubray, 2002).

The neurotoxicity of MSUD is secondary to the accumulation of leucine in the plasma and organs. Leucine intoxication impairs the volume-regulating mechanisms in the brain, liver, muscle and pancreatic cells (Morton et al, 2002). A fall in serum sodium precipitates a redistribution of water in the intracellular spaces of the brain, causing cerebral edema. The brains of children with MSUD show severe cerebral edema and delayed myelination (Chuang & Shih, 2001).

Clinical Manifestations

The neonate with classical MSUD is usually born at term after an uncomplicated pregnancy and delivery. A short symptom-free interval occurs after birth. During this time, the usual postnatal endogenous protein catabolism causes a progressive rise in BCAA levels (Morton et al, 2002).

By about 48 hours of age, the untreated infant begins to show signs of the disorder. The earliest and most specific sign is the unique maple syrup odor of the cerumen. Other early signs and symptoms of MSUD are feeding difficulties, irritability, lethargy, and dystonia. Over the ensuing hours, neurologic deterioration predominates, as drowsiness and lethargy progress to coma. Distinctive hypertonic episodes with opisthotonus and slow athetoid limb movements with pedaling occur either spontaneously or with stimulation, but stop during sleep. Rigidity of the jaw is associated with dysphagia. Axial hypotonia and limb hypertonia with large-amplitude tremors and myoclonic jerks are often mistaken for convulsions (Ogier de Baulny & Saudubray, 2002).

Diagnosis

Early diagnosis and management are essential to prevent permanent brain damage. MSUD is diagnosed by plasma amino acid assay. An elevated leucine level and a high leucine-to-alanine ratio are diagnostic of MSUD. The leucine level may not rise above normal in the first 24 hours, but an increasing leucine level indicates MSUD, and valine is also elevated. A dinitrophenylhydrazine (DNPH) test of the urine, which screens for the presence of α-ketoacids, will be positive. Urine should also be tested for ketones, which are typically present. Ketonuria is never normal in the neonate and should always suggest the possibility of an inborn error of metabolism. Urinary organic acid analysis should also be performed.

By the time of diagnosis on clinical grounds, many infants with MSUD are severely encephalopathic and require emergency therapy to lower the BCAA levels (Morton et al, 2002). Newborn screening by tandem MS allows for detection of elevated BCAA concentrations in blood in patients with classical MSUD before the onset of severe encephalopathy. Newborn screening programs in 44 states now test for MSUD on newborn screening panels (NNSGRC, 2005). Unfortunately, these specimens are often collected after 24 hours of age, and results are not reported until infants are 6 to 10 days of age. An infant with classic MSUD would already be seriously ill by this time (Morton et al, 2002).

Collaborative Management

The aims of treatment of MSUD are to rapidly lower the plasma leucine level and achieve stable, long-term metabolic control with a carefully monitored low-BCAA diet. Hemodialysis or hemofiltration are used to remove toxins. High-energy enteral or parenteral nutrition, with close monitoring of BCAA levels, is the dietary therapy used in the newborn period to augment toxin removal. Even after the infant is in good metabolic control, however, common infections and injuries can rapidly induce biochemical disturbances requiring prompt changes in management to prevent a metabolic crisis (Morton et al, 2002).

Isovaleric Acidemia

Isovaleric acidemia (IVA) is a disorder of leucine metabolism caused by mutations in the gene encoding the enzyme isovaleryl-CoA dehydrogenase, mapped to chromosome 15. IVA has an incidence of about 1 in 60,000 to 250,000 live births. The disorder has both an acute and chronic form; the acute form manifests in the neonatal period as catastrophic disease (Berry, 2004).

Pathophysiology

Isovaleryl-CoA dehydrogenase catalyzes the third step in the catabolism of the branched-chain amino acid leucine in the inner mitochondrial matrix. A deficiency of isovaleryl-CoA dehydrogenase leads to accumulations of highly toxic free isovaleric acid, 3-hydroxyvaleric acid, and N-isovalerylglycine. Conjugation with carnitine allows the formation of iso-valerylcarnitine, a nontoxic by-product that can be excreted in the urine. Excess organic acids in the bloodstream inhibit gluconeogenesis and ureagenesis, predisposing the infant to both hypoglycemia and hyperammonemia. Hypoglycemia stimulates the release of free fatty acids, which are transported into the mitochondria where they are β-oxidized to produce ketones, the source of ketosis in infants with IVA and other organic acidemias. These organic acids also arrest maturation of hematopoietic precursors, leading to leukopenia and thrombocytopenia (Payan et al, 2005).

Clinical Manifestations

Infants with IVA become extremely ill in the first week of life. Early symptoms are poor feeding, vomiting, lethargy, and hypothermia. Clinical evidence of dehydration is often present. Untreated infants progress to coma, and less than half survive the initial metabolic crisis. Isovaleric acidemia can be recognized by the unpleasant "sweaty feet" or "rancid cheese" odor of body fluids. Hepatomegaly is present in some infants.

Diagnosis

The diagnosis of IVA is based on the presence of isovaleryl-glycine and its metabolites in urine, and of isovalerylcarnitine in plasma. Plasma organic acid analysis also reveals markedly elevated *N*-isovalerylglycine and 3-hydroxyvaleric acid, which can be conjugated with carnitine to create nontoxic, excretable by-products (Ogier de Baulny & Saudubray, 2002). A secondary carnitine deficiency can develop. Both ketosis and metabolic acidosis, with an elevated anion gap, are present. Secondary derangements include hyperammonemia, thrombocytopenia, neutropenia, and anemia. IVA can be detected by MS/MS using filter-paper blood-spot samples and is included on expanded newborn screening panels. Enzyme analysis can be performed on cultured amniocytes, leukocytes, and fibroblasts.

Collaborative Management

Infants who are extremely ill as a result of accumulation of isovaleric acid will need exogenous toxin removal with hemodialysis, peritoneal dialysis, or hemofiltration (Ogier de Baulny & Saudubray, 2002). Supplementation with L-glycine is another therapy effective for IVA. Glycine promotes the formation of isovalerylglycine, which is excreted more efficiently than free isovaleric acid (Payan et al, 2005). L-Carnitine is given to replace lost carnitine and to provide substrate for the formation of isovalerylcarnitine. If metabolic acidosis is severe, bicarbonate therapy is indicated. Adequate fluids are mandatory to promote excretion of isovaleric acid because the primary route of elimination is the kidney. Urine output must be carefully monitored. Initially, until the diagnosis is confirmed, protein is removed from the diet and a high-energy intake of glucose and intralipid is administered. Nutritional support is subsequently provided in the form of leucine-free amino acid mixtures followed by a reduced leucine diet. It is important to reintroduce a balanced nutritional intake, including protein, as soon as possible to promote an anabolic state in these infants.

Propionic Acidemia

Propionic acidemia (PA) is a severe autosomal recessive disorder caused by mutations in the genes that encode the two nonidentical subunits (α and β) of the propionyl-CoA carboxylase enzyme (Berry, 2004). Its estimated incidence is less than 1 in 100,000 births.

Pathophysiology

Propionyl-CoA carboxylase is involved in the metabolism of branched-chain amino acids, odd-chain fatty acids, and cholesterol. A deficiency of propionyl CoA results in an accumulation of toxic organic acid metabolites causing severe ketoacidosis. (See also Isovaleric Acidemia.) Propionate production comes from catabolism of amino acids (isoleucine, valine, threonine, and methionine), oxidation of odd-chain fatty acids, and gut bacterial activity.

Clinical Manifestations

The clinical features of PA typically manifest shortly after birth, beginning with poor feeding, vomiting, lethargy, and hypotonia (Berry, 2004). Ketonuria and metabolic acidosis develop in most infants, and severe intracellular dehydration may develop. Seizures often follow. Hepatomegaly may stem from steatosis. Infants with PA are susceptible to bacterial infections as a result of neutropenia and thrombocytopenia. The odor imparted to body fluids by propionic acid has been likened to "cat urine." Cardiomyopathy of uncertain pathogenesis is associated with PA and is a likely cause of rapid deterioration and death in infants with this disorder (Ogier de Baulny & Saudubray, 2002). A neuropathologic sequela of PA in the neonate is white-matter spongiosis.

Diagnosis

In most cases, there is a marked elevation of free propionate in the blood and urine. However, these findings are occasionally absent (Ogier de Baulny & Saudubray, 2002). In those instances, significant elevations of other propionate metabolites, such as propionyl-carnitine, β-hydroxypropionate, and methylcitrate, help to reach the diagnosis. Plasma glycine is also increased, but plasma carnitine is low. The diagnosis of PA can be confirmed either with analysis of enzyme activity in leukocytes or fibroblasts, or with specific mutation analysis. PA can be detected by MS/MS using filter-paper blood-spot samples and is included on expanded newborn screening panels, allowing presymptomatic diagnosis for some infants.

Collaborative Management

Propionic acidemia is unique in that the urinary excretion of the toxin, propionic acid, is negligible, and no alternate route can adequately remove the toxin from affected newborns (Ogier de Baulny & Saudubray, 2002). Emergency treatment to remove toxins using hemodialysis or hemofiltration is imperative. Initially, protein intake is stopped and a high-calorie intake of glucose and intralipid or nonprotein formula is substituted to suppress catabolism. Protein is reintroduced in small quantities after a few days of protein restriction (Burton, 2000). Secondary hyperammonemia may require administration of sodium benzoate, sodium phenylacetate, or a combined preparation to provide an alternate route for excretion of nitrogen. Blood ammonia levels should be followed closely. Carnitine supplementation, to prevent carnitine deficiency and to augment excretion of propionate, has also been used in the early management of infants with PA. In addition, because propionyl CoA is a biotin-containing enzyme, biotin and cobalamin are given to evaluate for a vitamin-responsive disorder.

Antimicrobial therapy with oral broad-spectrum antibiotics, such as metronidazole or neomycin, inhibits anaerobic colonic flora, thereby suppressing propionate production in the gut. Infants with PA are immune-compromised and easily susceptible to infection; therefore, strict measures to avoid exposure to microbes must be observed. Laboratory indicators of infection must be monitored closely. Infants with PA should also be assessed for evidence of cardiac failure secondary to cardiomyopathy. Long-term dietary management consists of a low-protein, high-energy diet centered on the proportion of valine, a direct precursor to propionyl CoA. Discharge teaching should include the importance of seeking medical attention immediately for any sign of illness or infection, because even a minor illness can lead to rapid deterioration in an infant with PA.

Methylmalonic Acidemia

Methylmalonic acidemia (MMA) is really a group of disorders representing inherited deficiencies of the activity of methylmalonyl-CoA mutase, a vitamin B_{12}–dependent enzyme. MMA is one of the more common organic acidemias, occurring in about 1 in 48,000 infants. About half of the mutations causing MMA are in the genes encoding this enzyme; the others have mutations in genes required for provision of cobalamin cofactors (Ogier de Baulny & Saudubray, 2002). In the most severe form of MMA, enzyme activity is completely absent.

Pathophysiology

Methylmalonyl-CoA mutase is normally responsible for the conversion of methylmalonyl CoA to succinyl CoA, a Krebs cycle intermediate. The lack of methylmalonyl-CoA mutase activity results in an intracellular accumulation of methylmalonic acid. This causes a secondary inhibition of propionyl CoA and also an accumulation of propionic acid and its metabolites. These compounds have inhibitory effects on many intermediary metabolic pathways, leading to hypoglycemia, hyperammonemia, and hyperglycinemia. Conjugation with carnitine results in a relative carnitine deficiency.

Clinical Manifestations

Most infants with MMA begin showing symptoms before the end of the first week of life. Lethargy, hypotonia, and vomiting with signs of dehydration are followed by respiratory distress, acute encephalopathy, and eventual coma. Untreated infants develop hypoglycemia, hyperammonemia, metabolic acidosis, and ketosis. MMA is similar to PA in that many infants become neutropenic and thrombocytopenic.

Diagnosis

Plasma methylmalonic acid and propionylcarnitine are increased in MMA. The presence of C4-dicarboxylic acylcarnitine distinguishes MMA from PA. Urine organic acid analysis demonstrates greatly increased methylmalonic acid and its precursors, methylcitric acid and β-hydroxypropionate. MMA can be rapidly detected by MS/MS using filter-paper bloodspot samples and is included on expanded newborn screening panels. Among the many other nonspecific laboratory findings in MMA are metabolic acidosis, hyperammonemia, hyperglycinemia, leukopenia, anemia, thrombocytopenia, and ketonuria. Molecular genetic testing is available for prenatal diagnosis.

Collaborative Management

Infants who are severely moribund and those with extreme hyperammonemia (>600 mcmol/L) are likely to have very high levels of toxic organic acids that must be removed expeditiously with hemodialysis or hemofiltration. Severe hyper-ammonemia can also be treated with sodium benzoate or sodium phenylacetate or a combined preparation to provide an alternate pathway for nitrogen removal. The acute metabolic crisis of MMA is further managed with protein restriction and administration of IV glucose and intralipid. Adequate fluid intake will enhance the elimination of methylmalonic acid, which is relatively efficiently removed from the body by the kidneys (Ogier de Baulny & Saudubray, 2002). Blood gases should be monitored to evaluate the degree of metabolic acidosis, and sodium bicarbonate may be required to control severe metabolic acidosis. In the event that the infant has a cofactor-responsive disease, pharmacologic doses of vitamin B_{12} are given. Since excess propionate is also a problem in MMA, broad-spectrum antibiotics are given to inhibit anaerobic flora and reduce intestinal propionate production (Ogier de Baulny & Saudubray, 2002). Supplemental carnitine is used to replace carnitine depletion and promote urinary propionylcarnitine elimination.

Like infants with PA, those with MMA are at high risk for infection owing to compromised immunity reflected by neutropenia and thrombocytopenia. Close monitoring of clinical and laboratory indicators of infection is warranted. These infants must also be monitored for evidence of cardiac failure related to cardiomyopathy. The discharge planning needs of infants with MMA are similar to those of infants with PA. Parents or other caretakers must be aware that even a minor illness or infection in their baby with MMA can represent a potential metabolic crisis and requires prompt medical attention.

3-Hydroxy-3-Methylglutaryl-CoA Lyase Deficiency

Pathophysiology

The enzyme known as 3-hydroxy-3-methylglutaryl-CoA lyase (HMG-CoA lyase) is a mitochondrial and peroxisomal enzyme with a dual role. It catalyzes the final step of leucine degradation and plays a key role in ketogenesis. A deficiency of HMG-CoA lyase results not only in an accumulation of the metabolites of failed leucine catabolism, but also in a severe insufficiency in ketone body formation during the brief periods of fasting or stress that can occur in the transitional and newborn periods. Symptoms are caused by the near-complete lack of exogenous energy sources for the brain during these intervals (Mitchell & Fukao, 2001).

Clinical Manifestations

HMG-CoA lyase deficiency usually presents on the first day of life and is heralded by vomiting, lethargy, tachypnea, dehydration and progressive neurologic symptoms. Severe hypoketotic hypoglycemia (blood glucose may be undetectable) is the norm (Mitchell & Fukao, 2001). Hepatomegaly may be evident on examination.

Diagnosis

Newborns can be screened for HMG-CoA lyase deficiency using MS/MS analysis of the acylcarnitine profile. The diagnosis is confirmed with analysis of enzyme activity in fibroblasts or leukocytes. Supportive laboratory findings are elevated urine organic acids that reflect leucine metabolites (3-hydroxy-3-methylglutaric, 3-methylglutaconic, and 3-hydroxyisovaleric acids). Other findings include elevated transaminases, hyperammonemia, and metabolic acidosis.

Collaborative Management

There is no specific treatment for HMG-CoA lyase deficiency. Acute symptoms of HMG-CoA lyase deficiency are treated with intravenous fluids, glucose, and bicarbonate. It is essential to suppress ketogenesis by avoiding fasting, a goal best achieved during the acute phase with intravenous glucose with electrolytes. Long-term management involves frequent feedings, including night-time feedings.

FATTY ACID OXIDATION DISORDERS

Fatty acid oxidation disorders (FAODs) are a subset of organic acid disorders that are among the most common of the known inherited disorders of metabolism. Although the FAODs are considered treatable, they are often fatal. In a series of 107 patients with FAODs, 31% died in the first week of life, and 70% within the first year (Saudubray et al, 1999). An FAOD can be caused by a deficiency of any of the enzymes involved in cellular uptake, transport, and mitochondrial oxidation of fatty acids. To date, more than 20 defects and their gene mutations have been discovered (Shekhawat et al, 2005). The most common is medium-chain acyl-CoA dehydrogenase deficiency (MCAD). Short-, long-, and very-long-chain forms of this enzyme deficiency also exist (SCAD, LCAD, VLCAD), as well as carnitine transporter defects, and deficiencies of the mitochondrial trifunctional protein (MTP) complex.

Pathophysiology of Fatty Acid Oxidation Disorders

The fatty acids are the largest source of energy in the body, and are the preferred fuels of the liver, heart, and skeletal muscles. Neonatal brown fat utilizes fatty acids to sustain nonshivering

thermogenesis. When glucose levels are low during long periods between feedings, glucagon secreted by the pancreas stimulates adipose cell lipase to liberate free fatty acids. These fatty acids are oxidized to provide energy through the mitochondrial β-oxidation pathway. Fatty acid oxidation also provides the substrate for hepatic ketogenesis. Fatty acids as a source of energy are particularly critical for the neonate who has limited stores of glycogen and a high metabolic rate; thus, any perturbation in the fatty acid oxidation pathway can rapidly lead to metabolic decompensation (Shekhawat et al, 2005).

Fatty Acid Oxidation

Three subsystems are required for the production of energy in the normal fat oxidation process (Figure 6-3): (1) the carnitine cycle, (2) the mitochondrial inner membrane system, and (3) the mitochondrial matrix system (Roe, 2002). In the first step, L-carnitine and fatty acids are taken up by the cell, and fatty acids are conjugated to fatty acyl-CoAs in the cytoplasm by enzymes of the outer mitochondrial membrane. Medium and short-chain fatty acids can penetrate the inner mitochondrial membrane for β-oxidation, but longer-chain fatty acids of dietary fat (those with carbon lengths of 14 to 20) must be actively transported into the matrix via the carnitine cycle. Activated acyl-CoAs are converted to carnitine esters by carnitine palmitoyltransferase I (CPT I), transported across the mitochondrial membrane by carnitine-acylcarnitine translocase, and re-activated by carnitine palmitoyltransferase II (CPT II).

Within the mitochondrion, long-chain acyl-CoAs are degraded by enzymes in the inner membrane system in a

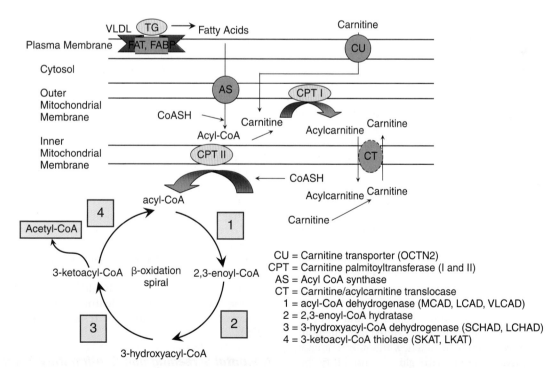

CU = Carnitine transporter (OCTN2)
CPT = Carnitine palmitoyltransferase (I and II)
AS = Acyl CoA synthase
CT = Carnitine/acylcarnitine translocase
1 = acyl-CoA dehydrogenase (MCAD, LCAD, VLCAD)
2 = 2,3-enoyl-CoA hydratase
3 = 3-hydroxyacyl-CoA dehydrogenase (SCHAD, LCHAD)
4 = 3-ketoacyl-CoA thiolase (SKAT, LKAT)

FIGURE **6-3**
The mitochondrial fatty acid oxidation pathway. This schematic representation shows the uptake of fatty acids and carnitine into the cell, transfer of fatty acid from the cytosol into mitochondria, and the fatty acid β-oxidation spiral. From Shekhawat P et al (2003). Human placenta metabolizes fatty acids: implications for fetal acid oxidation disorders and maternal liver diseases. *American journal of physiology, endocrinology & metabolism* 284:E1098-1105. Used with permission.

recurring cyclic sequence of four reactions. These are catalyzed by very-long-chain acyl-CoA dehydrogenase (VLCAD) and the mitochondrial trifunctional protein complex encompassing the three enzymes required for a single cycle of beta oxidation: enoyl-CoA hydratase, L-3-hydroxy acyl-CoA dehydrogenase (LCHAD), and thiolase. In each full cycle, the fatty acid is progressively shortened by two carbons from long, to medium, and finally to short-chain acyl-CoAs. The final system, the mitochondrial matrix, oxidizes shorter chain length fatty acids resulting from the enzymatic steps in the inner membrane system (Roe, 2002). L-Carnitine is not required for the latter process. The result of the β-oxidation system is generation of acetyl-CoA, used by the liver to produce ketone bodies and as a major source of cellular ATP.

Defective Fatty Acid Oxidation

Inborn errors of fatty acid oxidation result in a buildup of toxic metabolites both proximal and distal to the block, an insufficient yield of substrate for energy production. A deficiency of any of the enzymes required for fatty acid transport or metabolism can result in a failure of fatty acid oxidation. The primary physiologic consequence is insufficient energy production: inadequate ATP and ketone body generation. This becomes apparent during periods of increased energy demand, such as a prolonged period of fasting, fever, or other illness. When glycogen stores are depleted, free fatty acids are released as a source of energy. However, the neonate with an FAOD is unable to utilize fatty acids for fuel and rapidly becomes hypoglycemic. As a result of hypoketogenesis, the brain is without an alternate fuel source. Without early treatment, neurologic morbidity and mortality are high. A second consequence of FAODs is the accumulation of fatty acids and their derivatives, which can have toxic effects. When their oxidation is blocked, fatty acids are stored in the cytosol as triglycerides, resulting in muscular, hepatic, and cardiac lipidoses. Skeletal muscle tissue begins to break down (rhabdomyolysis), causing a skeletal myopathy characterized by muscle weakness. In defects downstream from CPT-I in the carnitine cycle, the acylcarnitine that accumulates has detergent-like properties that may disrupt the integrity of muscle membranes (Payan et al, 2005). In the heart muscle, accumulated long-chain fatty acyl-CoAs can produce electrophysiologic abnormalities including arrhythmias and cardiac arrest.

Clinical Manifestations of Fatty Acid Oxidation Disorders

Affected neonates are almost always born at term. A fasting stress sufficient to reveal the disorder can result with early breastfeeding, especially in infants who do not nurse well (Payan et al, 2005). Mitochondrial FAODs in the neonate present with three clinical phenotypes that, depending on the disorder, can be seen individually or in combination: hypoketotic hypoglycemia, cardiomyopathy, and skeletal myopathy (Roe, 2005). Neonates with MCAD, or medium-chain acyl-CoA dehydrogenase deficiency, the most common of the FAODs, usually present with glucose instability, but there have been reports of acute-life threatening episodes and even sudden death (Burton, 2000). Neonates with VLCAD, or very long-chain acyl-CoA dehydrogenase deficiency, are similarly intolerant to fasting, and develop hypoglycemia without ketosis. Additionally, with VLCAD, there may be evidence

of cardiomyopathy including cardiomegaly, ventricular arrhythmias, or unexplained cardiac arrest (Burton, 2005). Other physical findings that have been reported in neonates with disorders of fatty acid oxidation include hypotonia, seizures, irritability or lethargy (mimicking acute encephalopathy), hepatomegaly, and associated congenital malformations, such as cystic renal dysplasia.

Diagnosis of Fatty Acid Oxidation Disorders

An FAOD must be considered in any infant with an unexplained nonketotic hypoglycemia, hepatic dysfunction, isolated arrhythmia, or cardiomegaly. The initial screen for FAOD includes urine organic acid analysis, and plasma and urine free and total carnitine. A strong clue to an FAOD is urinary excretion of dicarboxylic acids, compounds not normally found in the urine (Ozand, 2000).

To reach a specific diagnosis of mitochondrial fat oxidation, a plasma acylcarnitine profile must be obtained, if this testing is available (Roe, 2005). Using whole blood samples on filter paper, the acylcarnitine intermediates formed as a result of the enzymatic block somewhere in the fat oxidation cycle are detected by electrospray or tandem mass spectrometry (MS/MS). When MS/MS screening is not available, the most useful indirect laboratory tests in neonates with suspected FAODs are glucose, electrolytes, BUN, creatinine, lactate, ammonia, transaminases, and creatine kinase (Roe, 2002).

Plasma carnitine levels are decreased, except in CPT-1 deficiency. A plasma acylcarnitine profile reveals accumulation of acyl-CoA conjugates proximal to the defect. Elevated CK levels and myoglobinuria indicate ongoing rhabdomyolysis. Additional laboratory results may show hyperammonemia, metabolic acidosis, and increased uric acid and transaminases. A liver biopsy performed during the acute phase usually reveals microvesicular and macrovesicular fatty infiltration.

Family and perinatal history can be particularly important to the diagnosis of an FAOD. Many infants diagnosed with an FAOD have a history of a sibling who died of sudden infant death syndrome (Burton, 2005). In addition, an association has been found between acute fatty liver of pregnancy (AFLP) or HELLP (hemolysis, elevated liver enzymes, low platelets) syndrome in the mother and fetal deficiency of long-chain 3-hydroxyacyl coenzyme A dehydrogenase (LCHAD), one of the enzymes in the MTP complex. When a woman heterozygous for an FAOD is carrying an affected fetus, the placenta and fetus are unable to oxidize fatty acids, leading to transfer of accumulated fatty acid intermediates to the maternal circulation (Shekhawat et al, 2005). These fatty acids overwhelm the already reduced maternal fatty acid oxidative capacity and contribute to HELLP syndrome and maternal hepatic fat deposition (AFLP).

The newborn infants of women with AFLP or those who are known carriers of FAODs should be evaluated immediately after birth with blood-spot acylcarnitine profiles, and treated as if they have an FAOD until test results are known (Jamerson, 2005).

Neonatal Screening and Confirmatory Testing for FAOD

The key to preventing the morbidity and mortality associated with FAOD is through presymptomatic diagnosis, allowing early treatment and avoidance of metabolic crisis. Neonatal screening for FAODs by tandem mass spectrometry analyzes acylcarnitines from dried blood spots and can identify 22 different abnormalities. However, an abnormal acylcarnitine profile can represent more than one FAOD, so more specific testing is required. Using cultured skin fibroblasts (or amniocytes) that have been incubated with deuterium-labeled fatty acid precursors and excess L-carnitine, MS/MS can rapidly detect any enzyme defect from translocase through SCAD (Roe, 2002). This method is possible because the enzymes of fatty acid oxidation are also expressed in the skin and other cells.

Collaborative Management of Fatty Acid Oxidation Disorders

The primary goal is to provide nutrition that will control endogenous lipolysis and prevent tissue catabolism. The newborn should feed every 3 to 4 hours, with close monitoring of blood sugar level. Breastfeeding mothers should receive lactation assistance to ensure successful breastfeeding with evidence of milk transfer. If hypoglycemia persists or the infant is unable to tolerate enteral feeding, glucose should be administered intravenously. Closely monitor for cardiac conduction disturbances.

The nurse is in a key position to prevent stressors, such as hypothermia or pain, that could precipitate a metabolic crisis, and to assess the infant for signs of intercurrent illness that might require additional therapy. Discharge teaching should emphasize the need to avoid prolonged periods of fasting and to seek medical attention if the infant shows signs of illness (fever, vomiting, diarrhea, refusal to eat, lethargy, or any other change in normal behavior). A consult should be made with a neonatal nutritionist or dietary specialist to arrange teaching for the family regarding the infant's postdischarge dietary regimen. The infant's diet will be one that is high in carbohydrate and restricted in fat and may be supplemented with L-carnitine.

Multiple Acyl-CoA Dehydrogenase Deficiency (Glutaric Aciduria Type II)

Pathophysiology

Multiple acyl-CoA dehydrogenase deficiency (MADD), formerly known as glutaric aciduria type II, is a disorder caused by a defective electron transfer flavoprotein (ETF) or electron transfer flavoprotein dehydrogenase (ETF-QO). MADD impairs both fatty acid oxidation and oxidation of branched amino acids lysine and glutaric acid. The heart, liver, and kidneys become infiltrated with fat.

Clinical Manifestations

Two different neonatal presentations have been described for MADD; both involve overwhelming illness with rapid progression to coma and death. One presentation is a neonate, often preterm, with dysmorphic facial features, polycystic kidneys, and hepatomegaly. Within the first 24 to 48 hours of life the infant develops hypotonia, metabolic acidosis, severe nonketotic hypoglycemia, and a distinctive "sweaty feet" odor of body fluids. The alternate neonatal presentation is the infant without congenital anomalies, but with similar symptoms and metabolic aberrations. Neither group lives longer than a few weeks; the few babies who survive generally succumb at a few months of age to cardiac failure.

Diagnosis

Tandem MS rapidly detects elevated acylcarnitines (C4, C5, C8, C10, and C16). Quantitative urine organic acid analysis usually reveals a pattern of elevated organic acids: lactic, glutaric, 2-hydroxyglutaric, ethylmalonic, adipic, suberic, sebacic, and other acids, some in very high amounts (Nyhan et al, 2005). The same organic acids are increased in the plasma. Volatile acid (isovaleric, acetic, isobutyric, propionic, butyric) concentrations in plasma are excessive, accounting for the characteristic odor associated with the disorder. Plasma carnitine may be low. Mutations have been identified in the genes for ETF and ETF-QO.

Collaborative Management

There is no effective treatment other than supportive care (fluids, glucose, sodium bicarbonate) for the rapid-onset, severe neonatal presentation. For the rare infant who survives the initial crisis, management involves frequent feedings with avoidance of fasting, and a diet low in fat and protein and high in carbohydrates. Some patients also respond to riboflavin. Supplementation with L-carnitine and glycine are often used as well.

CONGENITAL LACTIC ACIDOSES

The congenital lactic acidoses (also called primary lactic acidoses) are a group of disorders of lactate metabolism caused by defects in the mitochondrial respiratory or electron transport chain, the tricarboxylic acid (Krebs) cycle, or in pyruvate metabolism.

Lactic acid is the major end product of anaerobic glycolysis, accumulating when production of pyruvate exceeds utilization. The brain's dependence on oxidative metabolism makes it particularly susceptible to damage in disorders of oxidation that lead to lactic acidosis (Nyhan et al, 2005).

Pyruvate Dehydrogenase Deficiency

Pyruvate dehydrogenase (PDH) complex disorders are the most common inborn errors of pyruvate metabolism. The mutations causing PDH have an autosomal recessive inheritance pattern, except that associated with the most common $E_{1\alpha}$ subunit of the PDH enzyme. The $E_{1\alpha}$ subunit is X-linked, resulting in a preponderance of severely affected boys with PDH complex deficiency (Leonard & Morris, 2002).

Pathophysiology

Pyruvate dehydrogenase complex efficiently and irreversibly converts pyruvate, a product of glucose metabolism, to acetyl-CoA. Acetyl-CoA is one of two essential substrates needed to generate citrate for the energy-producing tricarboxylic acid cycle (also called the citric acid cycle or Krebs cycle). Thus PDH provides the link between glycolysis and the tricarboxylic acid cycle. PDH complex activity is regulated primarily by reversible phosphorylation (inactivation) of the enzyme's $E_{1\alpha}$ subunit. A deficiency in the PDH complex limits the production of acetyl-CoA, and in turn the production of citrate, blocking the tricarboxylic acid cycle and creating an energy deficit. Persistent glycolysis without pyruvate oxidation leads to the accumulation of lactate because excess pyruvate is reduced to lactate in the cytoplasm. Tissues with high energy requirements, such as those of central nervous system, are vulnerable to injury when cellular energy production is impaired.

Clinical Manifestations

The nonspecific early signs and symptoms of PDH deficiency develop soon after birth and are similar to those of other metabolic disorders. Poor feeding, lethargy, and tachypnea are followed by progressive neurologic deterioration, apnea, seizures, and coma. Fulminant lactic acidosis is present in infants with profound deficiencies of the PDH complex, and these patients often die early in the neonatal period. Infants with severe disease may have prenatal onset leading to structural brain abnormalities including microcephaly. MRI may show ventricular dilatation, cerebral atrophy, hydrancephaly, partial or complete absence of the corpus callosum, and other defects. Patients with PDH complex deficiency can also present with Leigh syndrome.

Diagnosis

Lactic acidosis is an important biochemical marker for mitochondrial dysfunction. Elevated levels of lactate and pyruvate, with or without evidence of lactic acidemia, are diagnostic indicators of inborn errors of pyruvate metabolism. Lactate and pyruvate are also elevated in the CSF of babies with this disorder. Plasma and urine amino acid analysis reveal hyperalaninemia. A definitive diagnosis of enzyme activity requires testing of leukocytes, fibroblasts, or tissue samples, or DNA analysis.

Collaborative Management

No effective treatment has been found to date for any of the PDH complex defects that manifest in the neonatal period (Berry, 2004). Therapies include alternate dietary regimens or vitamins such as thiamine that might stimulate residual enzyme activity or circumvent the enzyme defect. A ketogenic (high fat, low carbohydrate) diet has been used to provide an alternate energy source for acetyl CoA production. These diets may reduce hyperlactatemia and improve short-term neuromuscular function in infants with PDH complex deficiency. Cofactor supplementation with thiamine, carnitine, and lipoic acid is another facet of the management of babies with PDH complex deficiency.

Recently, dichloroacetate (DCA) has been used to treat PDH complex deficiency. DCA is believed to activate PDH complex activity by inhibiting PDH kinase. PDH complex is thereby "locked" in its unphosphorylated, catalytically active form (Fouquet et al, 2003).

Pyruvate Carboxylase Deficiency

Pyruvate carboxylase deficiency (PCD) is a disorder of energy metabolism that exists in three different forms. The most severe of these is a neonatal-onset form known as type B, a disorder with a high mortality rate. All forms of PCD have a frequency of about 1 in 250,000 live births and are recessively inherited.

Pathophysiology

Pyruvate carboxylase is a key regulatory enzyme in gluconeogenesis. It catalyzes the conversion of pyruvate to oxaloacetate, one of two essential substrates in the production of citrate, the first substrate in gluconeogenesis. The absence of pyruvate carboxylase activity results in malfunction of the citric acid cycle and gluconeogenesis, thereby disrupting energy metabolism in the brain. A deficiency of aspartic acid, derived from oxaloacetate, disrupts the urea cycle as well, leading to a simultaneous failure of nitrogen excretion.

Clinical Manifestations

In PCD of neonatal onset, the earliest signs and symptoms are associated with profound metabolic acidosis and include seizures, low muscle tone, abnormal eye movements, and coma. Hyperammonemia, hypoglycemia, ketosis, and ketonuria can all be present. Renal tubular acidosis can also accompany PCD.

Diagnosis

The diagnosis of PCD is based on the measurement of urinary organic acids and blood acylcarnitine profile. In type B PCD, the lactate/pyruvate ratio may be high. Plasma citrulline and lysine are elevated along with the ammonia level. Serum transaminases (SGOT, SGPT) may also be elevated. Enzyme analysis of hepatic cells or leukocytes confirms the diagnosis (Leonard, 2005b).

Collaborative Management

There is no specific therapy for this progressive disorder. Some infants have biotin-responsive disease, so pharmacologic doses of biotin are administered and the response is evaluated. A high-fat, low-carbohydrate ketogenic diet is intended to provide ketone bodies as an alternate fuel for the brain (Robinson, 2001).

DISORDERS OF CARBOHYDRATE METABOLISM
Galactosemia

Galactosemia is an inherited disorder of carbohydrate metabolism caused by a deficiency in one of the three enzymes of the galactose metabolic pathway: galactose-1-phosphate uridyl transferase (GALT), galactokinase, or UDP-galactose-4-epimerase (GALE). GALT deficiency, affecting the second step in the galactose metabolism, accounts for more than 95% of galactosemias; thus it has become synonymous with classical galactosemia.

Galactosemia has an estimated prevalence of 1 in 35,000 to 60,000 live births. At least 24 different mutations have been identified to date in the human GALT gene, located on chromosome 9 (Bosch et al, 2005).

Pathophysiology

Infants with galactosemia are unable to metabolize the sugar galactose, derived from the disaccharide lactose, the major carbohydrate of mammalian milk. In normal galactose metabolism, galactose is first converted to galactose-1-phosphate by galactokinase (GALK), which is in turn converted by the GALT enzyme to uridyl diphosphate (UDP) glucose. The severe form of galactosemia is due to almost total deficiency of GALT enzyme activity in all cells of the body. In the absence of GALT, ingestion of lactose-containing substances produces toxic levels of galactose-1-phosphate within cells. Surplus galactose is reduced to galactitol or oxidized to galactonate, metabolites that also have a direct toxic effect on the liver and other organs.

Clinical Manifestations

Most patients present in the neonatal period or in the first week or two of life. After ingestion of galactose (either cow's milk–based formula or breast milk), vomiting, diarrhea, poor weight gain, jaundice, hepatomegaly, and hypoglycemia become evident. In some infants, CNS symptoms, such as lethargy and hypotonia, predominate. Untreated infants will go on to develop cataracts secondary to the accumulation of galactitol. Sepsis, usually caused by *Escherichia coli*, is often the presenting problem, owing to low neutrophil bactericidal activity. Coagulopathy, renal tubular dysfunction, and renal Fanconi syndrome are part of a multiorgan toxicity syndrome seen after prolonged galactose exposure (Berry, 2004). Vitreous hemorrhages are a recognized complication of galactosemia that are believed to be caused by coagulopathy (Levy et al, 1996). Liver dysfunction is progressive, and many infants die during the first week of life from liver failure. In those who do survive, neurologic complications are frequent. Irreversible ovarian failure due to prenatal toxic effects of galactosemia is common in females.

Two related disorders of galactose metabolism are GALK and GALE. In galactokinase (GALK) deficiency, galactose cannot be phosphorylated into galactose-1-phosphate. The chief clinical finding in GALK deficiency is cataract formation. In GALE deficiency, most patients are asymptomatic and have normal growth and development.

Diagnosis

A galactose assay, measuring blood galactose, RBC galactose-1-phosphate, and GALT enzyme activity is used to diagnose classic galactosemia. GALT activity is low or absent. Galactose and galactose-1-phosphate are elevated. DNA analysis for the common mutations associated with GALT deficiency can also be done. Urine is positive for reducing substances. Galactosemia is included on all routine state newborn screening panels, allowing presymptomatic diagnosis.

Collaborative Management

Galactosemia is treated by feeding a formula based on sucrose rather than galactose, such as an infant soy formula. Other sources of galactose, including medications containing galactose, must also be avoided. Dietary restriction of galactose in the newborn will reverse the hepatic, renal, brain, and immune dysfunction and reduce the accumulated galactose metabolites. Additional measures to treat sepsis and correct coagulopathy are often indicated. Despite dietary treatment, long-term neurodevelopmental outcomes have not been uniformly favorable. An important part of discharge education is dietary teaching to assist the family to maintain dietary control as the infant grows and develops and help them identify occult sources of galactose in foods and other substances.

Hereditary Fructose Intolerance

Hereditary fructose intolerance (HFI) is an inherited inability to digest fructose (fruit sugar) or its precursors (sugar, sorbitol, and brown sugar). This autosomal recessive disorder has a frequency of approximately 1 in 22,000 births.

Pathophysiology

Fructose is a naturally occurring sugar that is used as a sweetener in many foods, including many baby foods. A deficiency of activity of the enzyme fructose-1-phosphate aldolase impairs the body's ability to convert fructose-1-phosphate to glyceraldehyde and dihydroxyacetone phosphate. The outcome is an accumulation of fructose-1-phosphate in the liver, kidney, and small intestine, which inhibits glycogen breakdown and glucose synthesis and causes severe hypoglycemia following ingestion of fructose. This disorder can be life threatening to infants.

Clinical Manifestations

In the neonate, the onset of clinical symptoms follows ingestion of cow's milk formula and resembles that for galactosemia.

Signs and symptoms include poor feeding, irritability, vomiting, and hypoglycemia. Jaundice, hepatomegaly, and evidence of progressive liver disease may follow. In exclusively breastfed infants, symptoms will be delayed until the time of weaning to fruits and vegetables (Steinmann et al, 2001).

Diagnosis

The diagnosis of HFI is made with assay of fructaldolase activity in a biopsy of liver or small intestine or by DNA analysis using blood leukocytes. Urine is positive for reducing substances.

Collaborative Management

Management of HFI centers on removal of all sources of fructose and sucrose from the diet. All intravenous solutions and other medications must also be free of fructose, corn syrup, and sorbitol. Supportive care includes management of liver failure, kidney dysfunction, and coagulopathy, if present. The infant's parents will benefit from consultation with a dietary specialist to learn about long-term dietary management.

Fructose-1,6-Bisphosphatase Deficiency

Fructose-1,6-biphosphatase deficiency is a rare disorder of carbohydrate metabolism.

Pathophysiology

Fructose-1,6-biphosphatase catalyzes the irreversible splitting of fructose-1,6-biphosphate into fructose-6-phosphate and inorganic phosphate. The enzyme's activity is highest in gluconeogenic tissues such as the liver and kidney (Steinmann et al, 2001). Fructose-1,6-biphosphatase deficiency is, therefore, a disorder of gluconeogenesis.

Clinical Manifestations

In fructose-1,6-biphosphatase deficiency, hypoglycemia is precipitated by fasting, not by fructose ingestion (Berry, 2005). Lactic acidosis and ketosis result from accumulating lactic, 3-hydroxybutyric, and acetoacetic acids. Hyperventilation followed by apnea may result from profound acidosis. Although the acidosis and hypoglycemia may be treated and the infant recovers from the acute attack, if the underlying disorder is not recognized, the infant can have many acute metabolic attacks and develop hepatomegaly and failure to thrive before the diagnosis is finally made.

Diagnosis

Definitive diagnosis is made by liver biopsy and assay of hepatic enzymes. Mutational analysis is available and can be used instead of biopsy (Nyhan et al, 2005).

Collaborative Management

Acute management involves glucose administration with IV solutions and correction of acidosis with sodium bicarbonate. Frequent feedings and avoidance of fasting, with limitation of fructose and sucrose in the diet, usually prevent further episodes. Dietary restriction includes the many prescription and over-the-counter medications with a syrup base containing sucrose. Stress management (e.g., during times of fever, infection, or vomiting) is critical because illness can induce a metabolic attack.

Glycogen Storage Disease

Glycogen storage disease (GSD) is a group of inherited enzyme defects that affect the glycogen synthesis and degradation cycle. Liver and muscle, having the most abundant quantities of glycogen, are usually the most severely affected tissues (Chen, 2001). More than 10 different types of GSD have been identified, with a collective incidence of about 1 in 20,000 births. Glycogen storage disease type I (GSD-I, also known as von Gierke's disease), the disorder most likely to have neonatal onset, occurs in about 1 in 100,000 births and has three subtypes (Ia, Ib, and Ic). GSD-II, known as Pompe's disease, is classified as a lysosomal storage disease (Chen, 2001).

Pathophysiology

GSD-I is the result of a deficiency of the enzyme glucose-6-phosphatase (G6Pase), an enzyme situated in the endoplasmic reticulum of the cell. Normally, G6Pase hydrolyzes glucose-6-phosphate to glucose and phosphate. An accumulation of glycogen in the liver, kidney, and intestines results from a deficiency of G6Pase. In the normal neonate, blood glucose falls during the first postnatal hours as the neonate consumes circulating glucose obtained from the mother, but then rises as endogenous glucose production begins. In the neonate with GSD-I, blood glucose continues to decline because endogenous glucose production is severely compromised (Chen, 2001). Instead, the phosphorylated intermediate compounds of glycolysis produce an excess of lactate, resulting in hyperlacticacidemia. Other secondary metabolic derangements typical of GSD-I include hyperuricemia and hyperlipidemia.

Clinical Manifestations

The neonate with GSD-I cannot cope with the normal postnatal drop in blood sugar. Despite a plentiful supply of glycogen, the neonate is unable to mobilize free glucose and becomes hypoglycemic. The abdomen may appear distended from birth as a result of an enlarged liver. Acute, nonspecific clinical deterioration is related to the buildup of lactic acid in the body. Infants with GSD-Ib are susceptible to infection as a result of neutropenia and impaired neutrophil function.

Diagnosis

Definitive diagnosis of GSD-I requires enzyme and chemical analysis of a liver sample or molecular genetic testing. Typical laboratory findings in GSD-I include increased plasma lactate and metabolic acidosis with an increased anion gap. Ketosis and ketonuria will be found during hypoglycemia. Other routine tests that should be obtained are liver function tests, plasma uric acid, triglycerides, creatinine, coagulation studies, and CBC with differential. Abdominal ultrasonography is performed to determine liver and kidney size.

Collaborative Management

The goals of treatment of GSD-I are to prevent hypoglycemia and correct secondary biochemical abnormalities. Frequent feedings or continuous gastric feedings may be necessary to maintain normoglycemia and supply the brain with a steady source of glucose, even during the night. Blood glucose levels must be monitored closely. Pharmacologic therapy to address hyperuricemia and prevent the development of gout may be necessary. Very severely affected infants will require a liver transplant. Parent teaching about long-term nutritional management, prevention of hypoglycemia, and special considerations during stress or other illnesses is critically important.

PEROXISOMAL DISORDERS

Peroxisomal disorders are complex developmental and metabolic disorders caused by defects in peroxisome biosynthesis. Two of the better known disorders, Zellweger syndrome (ZS) and neonatal adrenoleukodystrophy (NALD), are now recognized as belonging to a continuous spectrum of disorders, of which Zellweger syndrome is the most severe. Zellweger syndrome has a reported incidence of about 1 in 25,000 to 50,000 births.

Pathophysiology

Peroxisomes are subcellular organelles that synthesize bile acids, cholesterol, and plasmalogens (a type of phospholipid found in myelin sheaths of nerve fibers). Peroxisomes are also critical in the β-oxidation of very-long-chain fatty acids. Individuals with peroxisome biogenesis defects such as ZS and NALD synthesize peroxisomes normally but display defects in the import of peroxisomal enzymes into the lumen of the organelle (Baumgartner & Saudubray, 2002). Biochemical abnormalities include impaired degradation of peroxide, very long-chain fatty acids, pipecolic acid, and phytanic acid and impaired synthesis of plasmalogens, bile acids, cholesterol, and docosahexaenoic acid. In ZS, the extent of progressive multisystemic disease is profound; in NALD the systemic involvement is milder but the cerebral demyelination is more pronounced.

Clinical Manifestations

Infants with ZS present with characteristic facial dysmorphism including a high forehead, hypoplastic supraorbital ridges, flat occiput, low and broad nasal bridge, epicanthal folds, high arched palate, micrognathia, large fontanelles, wide sutures, redundant neck skin, and eye and ear abnormalities. Typically they have profound hypotonia, an absence of neonatal reflexes, and seizures. The disease affects every organ of the body, particularly the liver, kidney, and brain, resulting in hepatomegaly, renal cysts, white-matter abnormalities, and neuronal migration defects.

Diagnosis

Diagnosis of peroxisomal biosynthesis defects is based on indirect evidence of the defect. Initial tests for an infant with a suspected peroxisomal disorder include plasma very long-chain fatty acids and plasmalogens in erythrocytes (Baumgartner & Saudubray, 2002). Affected infants have elevated transaminases, bile acid intermediates, hypercholesterolemia, and increased iron and transferrin concentrations and are often hypoglycemic.

Collaborative Management

Currently, no successful treatment for the peroxisomal disorders is available. Management is supportive care and symptomatic therapy. The median life expectancy of ZS patients is less than 1 year. Milder forms of peroxisome disorders may respond to dietary therapy (Gould et al, 2001).

LYSOSOMAL DISORDERS

The lysosomal disorders are a diverse group of inherited conditions caused by dysfunctions in enzymes responsible for the degradation of complex macromolecules, such as glycogen, sphingolipids, glycoproteins, and glycosaminoglycans (Enns & Steiner, 2005). In these disorders, a complex substrate that is

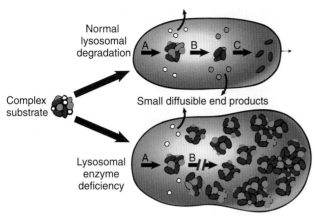

FIGURE 6-4
The pathogenesis of lysosomal storage diseases. A complex substrate is normally degraded by lysosomal enzymes A, B, and C into soluble end products. If these enzymes are deficient, catabolism is incomplete and nonmetabolized products accumulate in the lysosomes. From Kumar V et al (2004). *Robbins and Cotran: pathologic basis of disease,* ed 7 (p 160). Philadelphia: Elsevier.

normally degraded by a series of lysosomal enzymes fails to undergo degradation owing to a deficiency or malfunction of one of these enzymes (Figure 6-4). Catabolism of the substrate into soluble end products is incomplete, and insoluble intermediates that are unable to escape from the organelle accumulate within the lysosome (Wraith, 2002). More than 50 lysosomal disorders are recognized, with a collective incidence of 1 in 7000 to 10,000 births.

Niemann-Pick Type C
Pathophysiology
Niemann-Pick type C (NP-C) is a disorder of intracellular cholesterol transport that leads to an accumulation of unesterified cholesterol in lysosomes. Unesterified cholesterol, sphingomyelin, phospholipids, and glycolipids are stored in excess in the liver and spleen, and glycolipids are increased in the brain (Thomas et al, 2004).

Clinical Manifestations
Neonatal-onset NP-C is characterized by conjugated hyperbilirubinemia, ascites, hepatosplenomegaly, and hypotonia. Hydrops fetalis is a rare presentation. Respiratory failure can occur owing to lipid infiltration of the lungs.

Diagnosis
The diagnosis of NP-C requires specialized testing that must be coordinated with a metabolic laboratory. In general, the diagnosis is made on the basis of filipin staining of cultured fibroblasts and cholesterol esterification studies (Wraith, 2002). Filipin is a fluorescent probe that detects unesterified cholesterol. Biliary atresia and congenital viral infection are the chief differential diagnoses.

Collaborative Management
There is no definitive therapy for NP-C to date. Splenectomy is sometimes necessary if anemia and thrombocytopenia are severe. Liver transplantation corrects the hepatic dysfunction but not the neurodegenerative disease.

Gaucher Disease
Pathophysiology
Gaucher disease, the most common of the lysosomal storage diseases, is an inborn error of glycosphingolipid metabolism caused by the deficient activity of the lysosomal enzyme acid β-glucosidase. Widespread accumulation of glucosylceramide-laden macrophages results from the enzyme deficiency. These accumulated compounds are toxic to various tissues in the body. There are three types of Gaucher disease. Type I is the most common (95%). A subset of type II, a neuronopathic form of Gaucher disease, is the only one with neonatal onset.

Clinical Manifestations
Neonates with type II Gaucher disease can present with congenital ichthyosis or a collodion membrane (hyperkeratotic scale), hepatosplenomegaly, and/or nonimmune hydrops fetalis, hypertonicity, seizures, and other evidence of neurologic deterioration.

Diagnosis
Diagnosis is made by analysis of acid β-glucosidase activity in white blood cells or DNA analysis. Characteristic Gaucher cells (large, lipid-laden macrophages with foamy cytoplasm) can be seen in a bone marrow aspirate (Nyhan et al, 2005).

Collaborative Management
Enzyme replacement therapy for Gaucher disease is available, but has not been very effective for patients with type II disease. Splenectomy may be necessary to manage severe anemia and thrombocytopenia. Death from respiratory insufficiency or severe neurologic disease usually occurs shortly after birth or within the first year of life.

G$_{M1}$ Gangliosidosis
Pathophysiology
Gangliosides are normal components of cell membranes, particularly neurons. G$_{M1}$ gangliosidosis is a devastating lysosomal storage disease caused by a deficiency of the enzyme acid β-galactosidase, resulting in a generalized accumulation of G$_{M1}$ gangliosides, oligosaccharides, and the mucopolysaccharide keratan sulfate in both the brain and viscera.

Clinical Manifestations
Affected infants may have coarse facial features known as a "Hurler phenotype" (frontal bossing, depressed nasal bridge, maxillary hyperplasia, large ears, wide upper lip, macroglossia, and gingival hyperplasia), hirsutism of forehead and neck, a macular cherry-red spots, and corneal clouding (Figure 6-5). There is facial edema, pitting edema of the extremities or ascites; the neonate may present with hydrops fetalis and placental evidence of vacuolated cells (Nyhan et al, 2005). Neurologic examination reveals hypotonia and hypoactivity. The liver and spleen are both enlarged upon palpation.

Diagnosis
Diagnosis is made by demonstrating lack of β-galactosidase activity in white blood cells. Galactose-containing oligosaccharides can also be measured in the urine.

Collaborative Management
Currently there is no effective therapy for infants with G$_{M1}$ gangliosidosis. Enzyme therapy and gene therapy are

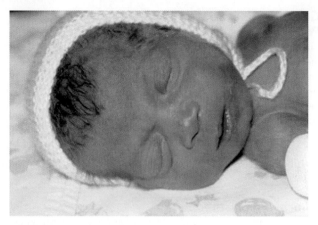

FIGURE **6-5**
The "Hurler phenotype" seen in some neonates with lysosomal storage disorders. From Wraith JE (2002). Lysosomal disorders. *Seminars in neonatology* 7:81.

being studied as potential treatments for this lethal disorder.

Mucopolysaccharidoses
Pathophysiology
The mucopolysaccharidoses (MPS) are a family of seven disorders caused by deficiency of lysosomal enzymes required for the stepwise degradation of glycosaminoglycans (polysaccharides that make up an important component of connective tissue). The undegraded glycosaminoglycans are stored in lysosomes, causing cell, tissue, and organ dysfunction. MPS VII, the type with the most prominent neonatal presentation, is caused by a deficiency of the enzyme β-glucuronidase.

Clinical Manifestations
MPS VII (Sly disease) has a well-recognized neonatal presentation with nonimmune hydrops fetalis, hepatosplenomegaly, ascites, pitting edema, hernias, skeletal abnormalities (dystosis multiplex) and corneal clouding. In the most severely affected patients, MPS I (Hurler syndrome) can present in the neonatal period with an umbilical or inguinal hernia or an excess of mongolian spots (Wraith, 2002). Hearing loss is common. Clinical evidence of heart disease is present in most patients with MPS (Neufeld & Muenzer, 2001).

Diagnosis
MPS VII is diagnosed by evaluating the activity of ß-glucuronidase in white blood cells. Urine glycosaminoglycans can also be quantitated.

Collaborative Management
Management is primarily supportive care and treatment of complications. Range-of-motion exercises are important to preserve joint function and prevent joint stiffness. Recurrent pneumonia is a frequent complication of MPS VII. Development of hydrocephalus often necessitates the insertion of a ventriculoperitoneal shunt (Neufeld & Muenzer, 2001). An ophthalmologic examination should be performed to evaluate for corneal clouding and the development of glaucoma.

Glycogen Storage Disease Type II (Pompe's Disease)
Pathophysiology
Glycogen storage disease type II (GSD II), also called acid maltase deficiency or Pompe's disease, is an inherited disorder of glycogen metabolism resulting from defects in activity of the lysosomal hydrolase acid α-glucosidase in all tissues of the body (Hirschhorn & Reuser, 2001). This enzyme is required for the degradation of a portion of the body's glycogen. Without it, excessive glycogen accumulates within the lysosomes, eventually causing cellular injury and enlarging and hindering the function of the entire organ, such as the heart. Energy production is not affected and hypoglycemia does not occur.

Clinical Manifestations
A prominent finding in infants is cardiomyopathy; progressive cardiomegaly and left ventricular thickening that eventually leads to outflow tract obstruction. Characteristic findings on ECG are large QRS complexes coupled with abnormally short PR intervals (Berry & Yudkoff, 2001). Other manifestations are hepatomegaly, striking hypotonia, macroglossia, feeding difficulties, and respiratory distress complicated by pulmonary infection.

Diagnosis
Definitive diagnosis requires the measurement of acid α-glucosidase activity in cultured skin fibroblasts or white blood cells. Serum CK is elevated (up to 10 times normal). Hepatic enzymes may also be elevated.

Collaborative Management
Until recently, no effective treatment was available for Pompe's disease, and these infants usually succumbed to cardiopulmonary failure. A recombinant version of human alpha-glucosidase, a glycoprotein enzyme needed for breakdown of glycogen in cell lysosomes, has now been developed for treatment of Pompe's disease.

DISORDERS OF CHOLESTEROL SYNTHESIS
Smith-Lemli-Opitz Syndrome
Smith-Lemli-Opitz (SLO) syndrome is a multiple congenital anomalies/mental retardation syndrome caused by an inherited defect in cholesterol biosynthesis. SLO syndrome has an estimated incidence of 1 in 60,000 births (Kelley & Hennekam, 2000).

Pathophysiology
The underlying biochemical defect in SLO syndrome is a lack of the microsomal enzyme 3 beta-hydroxysterol-delta 7 reductase (DHCR7), the final enzyme in the sterol biosynthetic pathway that converts 7-dehydrocholesterol (7DHC) to cholesterol. In the absence of DHCR7, the precursor 7DHC accumulates to potentially toxic levels, and insufficient cholesterol is produced. As cholesterol is required for the development of cell membranes and myelin, and the production of steroid hormones and bile acids, a severe deficiency of cholesterol during morphogenesis is believed to contribute to the abnormalities associated with SLO syndrome. SLO syndrome is different from other disorders of intermediary metabolism, from which the fetus is protected until after birth. Without endogenous cholesterol, the growing embryo depends

on maternal cholesterol, which may not be transported across the placenta in sufficient amounts. Thus, the fetus with SLO syndrome suffers systemic and cerebral malformations in proportion to the severity of the deficiency of cholesterol biosynthesis (Kelley & Hennekam, 2000).

Clinical Manifestations

Common findings at birth are intrauterine growth restriction, microcephaly, and hypotonia. Facial dysmorphism may feature epicanthic folds, ptosis, anteverted nares, broad nasal tip, micrognathia, and low-set ears. Associated anomalies include syndactyly of the second and third toes (>98%), postaxial polydactyly, small abnormally positioned thumbs, Hirschsprung's disease, and cataracts, and in males, hypospadias, cryptorchidism, and a hypoplastic scrotum (Thomas et al, 2004). Common clinical manifestations in the newborn include severe hypotonia, feeding difficulties with poor suck and vomiting, and excessive sleepiness with poor responsiveness (Kelley & Hennekam, 2000). Multiple defects in brain morphogenesis can be found on neuroimaging studies (Thomas et al, 2004). A severe, lethal form of SLO syndrome presents with microcephaly, lethal cardiac and brain anomalies, and ambiguous genitalia. These infants expire during the first week of life from multisystem organ failure.

Diagnosis

SLO syndrome is often recognized by its distinctive clinical features. Confirmation is made by finding elevated blood levels of its direct precursor, 7DHC. Plasma cholesterol may be normal or low. Some fetuses with SLO syndrome are identified by anomalies detected prior to birth by ultrasonography, and confirmation can be made by amniotic fluid or chorionic villus sample analysis.

Collaborative Management

Immediate management is directed toward raising body cholesterol and removing toxic precursors. Providing exogenous cholesterol not only restores low cholesterol levels but suppresses the infant's endogenous cholesterol synthesis, decreasing the production of 7DHC (Thomas et al, 2004).

DISORDERS OF METAL METABOLISM

Inborn errors of metal metabolism are genetic biochemical disorders in the way that metals are processed by the body: their synthesis, transport, absorption, storage, or utilization.

Molybdenum Cofactor Deficiency
Pathophysiology

The molybdenum cofactor is an essential component of a large family of enzymes involved in important transformations in carbon, nitrogen, and sulfur metabolism. Molybdenum cofactor deficiency is an autosomal recessive, fatal neurologic disorder, characterized by the combined deficiency of sulfite oxidase, xanthine dehydrogenase, and aldehyde oxidase.

Clinical Manifestations

Affected neonates are usually born after an uneventful pregnancy and normal delivery. Soon after birth, feeding difficulties and neurologic symptoms develop (Johnson & Duran, 2001). The neurologic picture includes intractable tonic/clonic seizures, axial hypotonia, and peripheral hypertonicity. Typical facial features include puffy cheeks, a long philtrum, and a small nose (Johnson & Duran, 2001). The neuropathologic findings are consistent with a toxic insult to the brain that causes severe neuronal loss, demyelination of white matter, reactive astrogliosis, and spongiosis. Ectopia lentis (displacement of the lens) may be noted on ophthalmologic examination.

Diagnosis

Molybdenum cofactor deficiency can be difficult to diagnose because there are no clues on routine laboratory studies (Burton, 2005). A positive sulfite dipstick of fresh urine is suggestive of the disorder; however, a negative test does not rule it out. Urinary S-sulfocysteine, thiosulfate, urothion, xanthine, and hypoxanthine levels aid in the diagnosis of molybdenum cofactor deficiency. Plasma uric acid is typically low.

Collaborative Management

There is no therapy available for molybdenum cofactor deficiency. One measure that has proved helpful is to limit the intake of sulfur-containing amino acids (cysteine and methionine). Seizures are often difficult to control.

SUMMARY

The number of known inherited disorders of metabolism has risen steadily in recent years and is likely to continue to do so. Although not all will manifest in the neonatal period, many disorders with neonatal onset are rapidly lethal if not recognized and treated without delay. Expanded newborn screening programs have saved many lives through presymptomatic diagnosis, but these programs currently screen for only a fraction of the hundreds of possible metabolic disorders. Neonatal health professionals must be vigilant and consider the diagnosis of an inborn error of metabolism in a neonate presenting with clinical manifestations resembling sepsis, or in an infant becoming ill after one or more days of normal health, particularly when the laboratory data do not fit the clinical picture. Although many neonatal metabolic disorders are not yet amenable to therapy, an exact diagnosis is important for genetic counseling and prenatal diagnostic procedures that the family may desire for future pregnancies.

Case Study

IDENTIFICATION OF THE PROBLEM

A newborn infant, just over 48 hours of age, was rooming in with his mother, who noted him to be jaundiced and unusually sleepy. His mother could not awaken him to breastfeed and she notified the nurse, who took him to the nursery to check his bilirubin level. His total serum bilirubin was 10.4. However, the infant made no response to having his heel lanced for the blood draw, and the nurse was unable to awaken him to feed. She placed a call to the infant's pediatrician and a complete blood count (CBC) with differential and blood culture were ordered. The infant was then transferred to the NICU for further evaluation. An IV of $D_{10}W$ at 100 ml/kg/day was begun, and ampicillin and gentamicin were given. However, the CBC, differential, and C-reactive protein (CRP) were all within normal limits, and subsequently, the blood culture was negative as well.

ASSESSMENT: HISTORY AND PHYSICAL EXAMINATION

The infant, a boy, was born by cesarean section to a 33-year-old G3, P2 group B streptococcus (GBS)–negative, insulin-dependent gestational diabetic mother, in satisfactory glucose control during the last trimester of pregnancy. Family history was significant for a maternal brother who died on the third day of life from unknown causes. Siblings of this infant were two healthy girls. This infant's Apgar scores were 8 and 9. Birth weight was 3790 g. The infant's blood sugar levels on day 1 were all within normal limits; he appeared healthy and roomed in with his mother, breastfeeding on demand with occasional formula supplementation. He was voiding and stooling normally.

On examination his color was pale pink with mild jaundice in room air. Respirations were regular and rapid, but there were no retractions, grunting, or flaring. His axillary temperature was 97° F, heart rate 122, respiratory rate 80, blood pressure 60/36 (mean 44). Glucose screen (point of care) was 52. An arterial blood gas was obtained and the results were pH 7.32, pO_2 71, pCO_2 30, base deficit −2. Capillary refill was 2 to 3 seconds, pulses were equal, and there was no murmur. His abdomen was rounded with mild hepatomegaly. He did not react to stimulation of any type and could not be aroused. His overall tone was decreased, he did not suck, and no Moro reflex was noted. Within 24 hours, he began having seizures requiring treatment with phenobarbital. Severe apnea and respiratory failure led to intubation and mechanical ventilation.

DIFFERENTIAL DIAGNOSIS

The chief differential diagnosis for a full-term infant becoming ill at about 48 hours of age is neonatal sepsis, although this mother was GBS negative, and the infant's laboratory data did not support this diagnosis. His serum bilirubin was not high enough to explain his somnolence and lethargy as stemming from bilirubin encephalopathy. Transient tachypnea of the newborn was unlikely because

he did not appear to be in any significant respiratory distress other than his rapid respiratory rate, and the clinical picture was more consistent with a neurologic insult. The history did not suggest an etiology for neonatal encephalopathy. The next most likely diagnostic possibilities would be inborn errors of intermediary metabolism that present with an "intoxication" syndrome and without hypoglycemia, following a symptom-free interval: organic acid disorders, amino acid disorders, and urea cycle disorders.

DIAGNOSTIC TESTS

To start differentiating between the most likely categories of metabolic disorders, a blood ammonia level is needed. Depending on this result, other important diagnostic tests might include electrolytes, blood urea nitrogen (BUN), creatinine, quantitative plasma and urine amino acids, urine organic acids, and urine orotic acid.

WORKING DIAGNOSIS

The infant's blood ammonia level was 1901 mcmol/L. This suggests a working diagnosis of a urea cycle defect. Additional testing revealed the following:

Plasma amino acids: Glutamine 1632 mcmol/L (reference range 376 to 709 mcmol/L)

Citrulline trace (reference range 10 to 45 mcmol/L)

Urine orotic acid: 852 mmol/mol creatinine (reference range 0.12 to 3.07 mmol/mol creatinine)

Following the algorithm for neonatal hyperammonemia (see Figure 6-2), these findings point to a working diagnosis of ornithine transcarbamylase (OTC) deficiency. In support of this diagnosis, the infant's symptoms began after 24 hours of age, and he had no significant acidosis.

DEVELOPMENT OF MANAGEMENT PLAN

The most urgent priority was reduction of the baby's toxic blood ammonia level. In addition, all protein intake had to be stopped temporarily until the blood ammonia level was normalized, so the baby was made NPO and no amino acids were added to the IV solution. Protein would be reintroduced within 48 hours in small yet sufficient amounts to prevent catabolism. While preparations were being made for hemodialysis, an umbilical venous catheter was inserted for administration of "scavenger drugs," or agents that supply alternatives to urea for elimination of waste nitrogen.

IMPLEMENTATION AND EVALUATION OF EFFECTIVENESS

A loading dose of sodium phenylacetate plus sodium benzoate 2.5 ml/kg was given via central catheter over 90 minutes (Ammonul, Ucyclyd Pharma, Scottsdale, AZ). In addition, a dose of arginine HCl 10% (2.0 ml/kg) was administered. Hemodialysis was initiated and after about 36 hours the infant's ammonia level was successfully reduced to less than 70 mcmol/L. He showed rapid improvement in neurologic status and was extubated. Amino acids were

Case Study—cont'd

reintroduced to the intravenous solution after another 24 hours and feedings were restarted shortly thereafter with citrulline supplementation. Following discharge, he was maintained on this regimen, plus pharmacologic diversion therapy, and he had two metabolic crises requiring hospitalization before receiving a liver transplant. An MRI of his brain at 1 year of age revealed that the neurologic prognosis remains guarded. The family also underwent genetic counseling regarding recurrence risks and prenatal genetic diagnosis for future pregnancies.

REFERENCES

Banta-Wright SA, Steiner RD (2004). Tandem mass spectrometry in newborn screening. *Journal of perinatal and neonatal nursing* 18:41-58.

Baumgartner MR, Saudubray JM (2002). Peroxisomal disorders. *Seminars in neonatology* 7:85-94.

Berry GT (2005). Inborn errors of carbohydrate, ammonia, amino acid and organic acid metabolism. In Taeusch HW et al, editors. *Avery's diseases of the newborn*, ed 8 (pp 217-226). Philadelphia: Saunders.

Berry GT, Yudkoff M (2001). Metabolism. In Polin RA, Ditmar MF, editors. *Pediatric secrets* (pp 389-407). Philadelphia: Hanley & Belfus.

Bosch AM et al (2005). Identification of novel mutations in classical galactosemia. *Human mutation* 25:502.

Burton BK (2000). Urea cycle disorders. *Clinics in liver disease* 4:815-830.

Burton BK (2005). Inherited metabolic disorders. In MacDonald MG et al, editors. *Avery's neonatology* (pp 965-979). Philadelphia: Lippincott Williams & Wilkins.

Chen Y (2001). Glycogen storage diseases. In Scriver CR et al, editors. *The metabolic & molecular bases of inherited disease* (pp 1521-1551). New York: McGraw-Hill.

Chien YH et al (2004). Poor outcome for neonatal-type nonketotic hyperglycinemia treated with high-dose sodium benzoate and dextromethorphan. *Journal of child neurology* 19:39-42.

Chuang DT, Shih VE (2001). Maple syrup urine disease. In Scriver CR et al, editors. *The metabolic & molecular bases of inherited disease* (pp 1971-2005). New York: McGraw-Hill.

Clayton PT (2002). Inborn errors presenting with liver dysfunction. *Seminars in neonatology* 7:49-63.

Enns GM, Steiner RD (2005). Lysosomal storage disorders. In Osborn LM et al, editors. *Pediatrics* (pp 1007-1011). Philadelphia: Mosby.

Fouquet F et al (2003). Differential effect of DCA treatment on the pyruvate dehydrogenase complex in patients with severe PDHC deficiency. *Pediatric research* 53:793-799.

Garganta CL, Smith WE (2005). Metabolic evaluation of the sick neonate. *Seminars in perinatology* 29:164-172.

Gordon N (2003). Ornithine transcarbamylase deficiency: a urea cycle defect. *European journal of paediatric neurology* 7:115-121.

Gould SJ et al (2001). The peroxisome biosynthesis disorders. In Scriver CR et al, editors. *The metabolic & molecular bases of inherited disease*, ed 8 (pp 3181-3217). New York: McGraw-Hill.

Hirschhorn R, Reuser AJJ (2001). Glycogen storage disease type II: acid α-glucosidase (acid maltase) deficiency. In Scriver CR et al, editors. *The metabolic & molecular bases of inherited disease* (pp 3389-3420). New York: McGraw-Hill.

Jamerson P (2005). The association between acute fatty liver of pregnancy and fatty acid oxidation disorders. *Journal of obstetric, gynecologic, and neonatal nursing* 34:87-92.

Johnson JL, Duran M (2001). Molybdenum cofactor deficiency and isolated sulfite deficiency. In Scriver CR et al, editors. *The metabolic & molecular bases of inherited disease* (pp 3163-3177). New York: McGraw-Hill.

Kelley RI, Hennekam RC (2000). The Smith-Lemli-Opitz syndrome. *Journal of medical genetics* 37:321-335.

Kenner C, Moran MB (2005). Screening and genetic testing. *Journal of midwifery and women's health* 50(3):219-226.

Leonard CO, Morris AAM (2002). Urea cycle disorders. *Seminars in neonatology* 7:27-35.

Leonard CO (2005a). Presentation and initial evaluation of metabolic disorders. In Osborn LM et al, editors. *Pediatrics* (pp 989-995). Philadelphia: Mosby.

Leonard CO (2005b). Disorders of protein metabolism. In Osborn LM et al, editors. *Pediatrics* (pp 1001-1008). Philadelphia: Mosby.

Leonard CO, Morris AA (2006). Diagnosis and early management of inborn errors of metabolism presenting around the time of birth. *Acta paediatrics* 95(1):6-14.

Levy HL et al (1996). Vitreous hemorrhage as an ophthalmic complication of galactosemia. *Journal of pediatrics* 129:922-925.

McCandless SE (2004). A primer on expanded newborn screening by tandem mass spectrometry. *Primary care clinic office practice* 31:583-604.

Mitchell GA, Fukao T (2001). Inborn errors of ketone body metabolism. In Scriver CR et al, editors. *The metabolic & molecular bases of inherited disease* (pp 2327-2356). New York: McGraw-Hill.

Morton DH et al (2002). Diagnosis and treatment of maple syrup disease: a study of 36 patients. *Pediatrics* 109:999-1008.

Nassogne MC et al (2005). Urea cycle defects: management and outcome. *Journal of inherited metabolic disease* 28:407-414.

National Newborn Screening and Genetics Resource Center (NNSGRC) (2005). National newborn screening status report. Available at: http://genes-r-us.uthscsa.edu/nbsdisorders.pdf. Retrieved September 23, 2005.

Neufeld EF, Muenzer J (2001). The mucopolysaccharidoses. In Scriver CR et al, editors. *The metabolic & molecular bases of inherited disease* (pp 3421-3452). New York: McGraw-Hill.

Nyhan WL et al (2005). *Atlas of metabolic disease*. London: Hadder Arnold.

Ogier de Baulny H, Saudubray JM (2002). Branched-chain organic acidurias. *Seminars in neonatology* 7:65-74.

Olpin SE (2004). The metabolic investigation of sudden infant death. *Annals in clinical biochemistry* 41:282-293.

Ozand PT (2000). Hypoglycemia in association with various organic and amino acid disorders. *Seminars in perinatology* 24:172-193.

Payan I et al (2005). Inborn errors of metabolism manifesting as catastrophic disease. In Spitzer AR, editor. *Intensive care of the fetus and neonate*, ed 2 (pp 1205-1220). Philadelphia: Mosby.

Puffenberger EG (2003). Genetic heritage of the old order Mennonites of southeastern Pennsylvania. *American journal of medical genetics part C: seminars in medical genetics* 121C:18-31.

Robinson BH (2001). Lactic acidemia: disorders of pyruvate carboxylase and pyruvate dehydrogenase. In Scriver CR et al, editors. *The metabolic & molecular bases of inherited disease* (pp 2275-2295). New York: McGraw-Hill.

Roe CR (2002). Inherited disorders of mitochondrial fatty acid oxidation: a new responsibility for the neonatologist. *Seminars in neonatology* 7:37-47.

Roe CR (2005). Diagnostic approach to disorders of fat oxidation—information for clinicians. Available at: http://www.fodsupport.org/dx_fod.htm. Retrieved September 16, 2005.

Sarkissian CN, Gamez A (2005). Phenylalanine ammonia lyase, enzyme substitution therapy for phenylketonuria, where are we now? *Molecular genetics and metabolism* 86(Suppl 1):S22-S26.

Saudubray JM et al (1999). Recognition and management of fatty acid oxidation defects: a series of 107 patients. *Journal of inherited metabolic disease* 22:488-502.

Saudubray JM et al (2002). Clinical approach to inherited metabolic disorders in neonates: an overview. *Seminars in neonatology* 7:3-15.

Shekhawat PS et al (2005). Fetal fatty acid oxidation disorders, their effect on maternal health and neonatal outcome: impact of expanded newborn screening on their diagnosis and management. *Pediatric research* 57:78-86.

Steiner RD, Cederbaum SD (2001). Laboratory evaluation of urea cycle disorders. *Journal of pediatrics* 138:S21-S29.

Steinmann B et al (2001). Disorders of fructose metabolism. In Scriver CR et al, editors. *The metabolic & molecular bases of inherited disease* (pp 1489-1520). New York: McGraw-Hill.

Summar M (2001). Current strategies for the management of neonatal urea cycle disorders. *Journal of pediatrics* 138:S30-S39.

Summar M, Tuchman M (2001). Proceedings of a consensus conference for the management of patients with urea cycle disorders. *Journal of pediatrics* 138:S6-S10.

Thomas JA et al (2004). Lysosomal storage, peroxisomal, and glycosylation disorders and Smith-Lemli-Opitz syndrome presenting in the neonate. In Taeusch HW et al, editors. *Avery's diseases of the newborn* (pp 258-278). Philadelphia: Saunders.

Urea Cycle Disorders (UCD) Conference Group (2001). Consensus statement from a conference for the management of patients with urea cycle disorders. *Pediatrics* 138:S1-S5.

Wilcken B (2004). Problems in the management of urea cycle disorders. *Molecular genetics and metabolism* 81:S86-S91.

Wraith JE (2002). Lysosomal disorders. *Seminars in neonatology* 7:75-83.

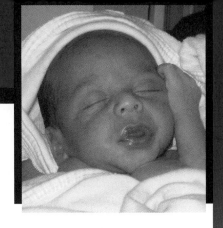

Chapter 7

Endocrine System

Laura Stokowski

Recent discoveries in fields such as genetics and cell biology have simultaneously advanced our understanding of endocrine disorders. Endocrine processes are fundamental to growth and development of the fetus and newborn. Prompt recognition of endocrine disorders in the neonate is the chief prerequisite to our ability to institute life-saving treatment and minimize long-term morbidity. This chapter will provide an overview of the clinical endocrine disorders that may be seen in the neonatal period.

THE ENDOCRINE SYSTEM

The word endocrine, from the Greek words *endo* (within) and *krinein* (to separate), describes a diverse group of ductless organs that secrete hormones directly into the bloodstream. The classic endocrine glands are the hypothalamus, pineal, pituitary, thyroid, parathyroid, thymus, pancreatic islet cells, adrenals, ovaries, and testes. Among the many roles of the endocrine system are coordination and regulation of metabolism, growth and development, and reproduction. In controlling body homeostasis, the endocrine and central nervous systems are intimately linked, forming the neuroendocrine system.

The endocrine glands are those that synthesize, store, and secrete hormones. Hormones are the chemical messengers, or signals, of the endocrine system. Secreted into the blood or extracellular fluid, hormones exert their actions on specific cells, usually in distant tissues, called target cells. Target cells respond to certain hormones because they contain receptors for those precise hormones. Hormones must first bind to these receptor sites before exerting physiologic actions. Some hormones, such as insulin, are fully active on release into the circulatory system, whereas others, such as T_4, require activation to produce their biologic effects (Kronenberg et al, 2003).

Many hormones are insoluble in water and must be bound to proteins to be transported in the circulatory system. These protein-bound hormones exist in rapid equilibrium with minute quantities of hormone that remain in the aqueous plasma. It is this "free" fraction of the circulating hormone that is taken up by the cell and represents the active hormone concentration.

Target hormone levels also serve as powerful negative feedback regulators of their own production via suppression of trophic hormones and hypothalamic releasing hormones. As the target hormone level rises, a message is sent to the anterior pituitary to reduce production of the respective trophic hormone, and also to the hypothalamus to reduce production of the respective releasing hormone. Endocrine disease can be caused by hormone overproduction, hormone underproduc-

tion, or altered tissue responses to hormones (Kronenberg et al, 2003).

Development of the fetal endocrine system is more or less independent of maternal endocrine influences (Rubin, 2004). The placenta blocks the entry of most maternal hormones into the fetal circulation, but the minute quantities that do achieve transplacental passage can have profound effects. Some of these prenatal exposures are essential to fetal growth and development; others may contribute to fetal and neonatal endocrine dysfunction.

Fetal Origins of Adult Disease

The intrauterine endocrine milieu can have powerful effects on growth and development of the fetal endocrine system. When exposed to a variety of different stressors (maternal undernutrition, uteroplacental insufficiency, or psychologic stress) the fetus releases glucocorticoids and catecholamines that, during critical periods of development, affect the development of the fetal hypothalamic-pituitary-adrenal axis. Chronic stress can also induce intrauterine growth restriction, or the so-called thrifty phenotype, in the fetus, an adaptation to the limited supply of nutrients. The way in which the fetus adapts is believed to permanently alter its physiology and metabolism, a concept known as programming. Permanent alterations in fetal metabolic programming contribute to endocrine, metabolic, and cardiovascular disease in adult life (Fowden & Forhead, 2004).

Neonatal Endocrine Disorders

Endocrinopathy in the newborn can be caused by a mutation in a single gene or by genomic imprinting, when the expression of the gene depends on which parent passed on that particular gene (Rubin, 2004). In addition to well-described neonatal endocrine disorders such as hypothyroidism and congenital adrenal hyperplasia, endocrine dysfunction can affect the preterm infant in a variety of ways as a function of maturation. Endocrinopathy is associated with a number of chromosomal anomalies that present in the newborn period, including Down syndrome and Prader-Willi syndrome. Finally, there is the question of potentially disruptive effects of agents in the environment on the development of the endocrine system (Rubin, 2004). Numerous chemicals have known estrogenic or antiandrogenic properties and have been shown to disturb sexual differentiation in animals (Toppari, 2002). It is not known to what extent these agents are responsible for increases in hypospadias and testicular dysgenesis syndrome that have been reported in some parts of the world.

PITUITARY GLAND AND HYPOTHALAMUS

The pituitary gland has two distinct structures, the anterior and posterior pituitary, with different embryologic origins. The anterior pituitary develops from oral ectoderm, a diverticulum called Rathke's pouch, and its cells differentiate into specific hormone-secreting cells. The posterior pituitary develops from neuroectoderm evaginating ventrally from the developing brain. The two tissues grow together into a single gland but remain functionally separate.

The hypothalamus, located just above the pituitary gland, secretes the releasing and inhibiting hormones that in turn influence the production of anterior pituitary hormones. Hypothalamic hormones are carried to the anterior pituitary via hypothalamic-hypophyseal portal veins where they bind to receptors on the anterior pituitary cells. Hormones produced by the anterior pituitary include growth hormone, prolactin, adrenocorticotropic hormone (ACTH), thyroid-stimulating hormone (TSH), follicle-stimulating hormone (FSH), and luteinizing hormone (LH). Hormones secreted by the posterior pituitary include oxytocin and hypothalamic-produced vasopressin (antidiuretic hormone, ADH). The hypothalamus is the interface between the endocrine and autonomic nervous systems (Rubin, 2004).

Disorders of the Anterior Pituitary
Congenital Hypopituitarism

Congenital hypopituitarism, though rare in the newborn, has a number of possible etiologies. Some cases of congenital hypopituitarism are attributed to mutations in genes encoding transcription factors involved in pituitary gland development (Palma Sisto, 2004). Congenital hypopituitarism can be caused by malformations including holoprosencephaly, septo-optic dysplasia, and other midline cerebral anomalies, the same developmental defects of the embryonic brain that lead to hypothalamic dysfunction. Infection and hypovolemic shock stemming from birth-related complications such as placenta previa and abruptio placentae are additional etiologies (Geffner, 2002).

Pathophysiology. Complete absence of the pituitary gland (pituitary agenesis) and other pituitary lesions can produce deficiencies of one or all pituitary hormones.

Panhypopituitarism is a deficiency of all pituitary hormones. In the newborn, the foremost effect of congenital hypopituitarism is hypoglycemia. Owing to the absence of growth hormone, and possibly cortisol as well, insulin acts in an unopposed manner, placing the neonate at risk for hypoglycemia (Geffner, 2002). In males, hypopituitarism can cause micropenis. Deficiency of growth hormone, and often gonadotropin, combine to stunt penile growth in utero; this is usually referred to as hypogonadotropic hypogonadism. Although fetal pituitary growth hormone is not the primary stimulus for fetal growth, growth hormone does make an important contribution to birth size.

Clinical Manifestations. Neonates may present with midline craniofacial defects such as cleft lip, cleft palate, or bifid uvula. Males may have a micropenis, defined as a normally formed and proportioned penis with a stretched penile length more than 2 SDs below the mean for age. Average penile length for preterm infants 30 weeks of age or older is 2.5 ± 0.4 cm and for term infants 3.5 ± 0.4 cm. For preterm infants 24 to 26 weeks' gestation, the following formula can be used: penile length in centimeters = 2.27 + 0.16 × (gestational age

in weeks) (Tuladhar et al, 1998). Hypoglycemia can be mild or severe and persistent. Later in the neonatal period infants may present with prolonged jaundice and direct hyperbilirubinemia, or evidence of other endocrinopathy, such as diabetes insipidus (high urine output, dehydration, hypernatremia).

Diagnosis. A pediatric endocrinologist usually coordinates the diagnostic testing and interpretation for these infants. The aim of laboratory testing is to determine which hormone deficiencies are present. Measurement of growth hormone, thyroid hormone, and cortisol are essential. Magnetic resonance imaging (MRI) of the brain is used to define the anatomy and look for a structural cause of hypopituitarism. For infants with suspected septo-optic dysplasia, an ophthalmologic examination is indicated.

Collaborative Management. The immediate goals of management are to stabilize the neonate's blood sugar and ensure that the neonate is not at risk of life-threatening cortisol insufficiency. Hypoglycemia may not resolve without growth hormone replacement. Further treatment is geared toward correcting specific hormonal deficiencies (Palma Sisto, 2004). The infant will require follow-up management by the pediatric endocrinologist throughout hospitalization and after discharge.

Disorders of the Posterior Pituitary
Diabetes Insipidus

Diabetes insipidus (DI) is a deficiency of antidiuretic hormone (vasopressin). In neonates, central or neurogenic DI can be associated with congenital midline anatomic defects (septo-optic dysplasia, holoprosencephaly), central nervous system injury such as intracranial hemorrhage or hypoxia, neoplasms, or it can be idiopathic (Saborio et al, 2000).

Pathophysiology. Normally, ADH secretion is triggered by changes in osmolality detected by supraoptic and paraventricular osmosensors in the brain. Increased osmolality stimulates the posterior pituitary to release ADH, which in turn increases the permeability of the renal collecting tubules to water, reducing urinary water loss. Damage to the osmosensors, the posterior pituitary gland, or the hypothalamic-hypophyseal axis results in a deficiency of ADH and increased urinary free water loss.

Clinical Manifestations. Neonates with diabetes insipidus may suck vigorously during feeding but vomit immediately afterward (Saborio et al, 2000). Urine output is high, in excess of 5 ml/kg/hr, with low specific gravity (<1.010). Irritability and fever may accompany evidence of dehydration (poor skin turgor, depressed anterior fontanelle, sunken eyes, mottled skin, weak pulses, low blood pressure, and constipation).

Diagnosis. Serum electrolytes, osmolality, and plasma ADH levels are the primary laboratory tests used to diagnose DI. Plasma ADH is normally elevated in the newborn following delivery, playing a role in the low urine output that is typical on the first day of life. Hypernatremia as high as 180 mEq/L may be seen in DI, with elevated serum osmolality. Urinalysis reveals inappropriately dilute urine (low urine osmolality and low specific gravity). MRI is used to visualize the pituitary gland and stalk to delineate the cause of diabetes insipidus (Saborio et al, 2000).

Collaborative Management. Diabetes insipidus in neonates requires very careful fluid management. Severe dehydration and hypernatremia are corrected primarily with intravenous fluids (Muglia & Majzoub, 2004). Insensible water losses should be minimized. Serum electrolytes and osmolality, blood glucose, accurate intake and output, and the evidence of dehydration (weight loss, blood pressure, pulses, skin turgor, etc.) should be closely monitored during treatment. Infants with severe hypernatremia must be observed for possible seizure activity. Although it is expected that serum sodium will decrease, very rapid shifts in serum sodium should be avoided. The infant's neurologic status must be monitored closely for signs and symptoms of cerebral edema during therapy to correct serum sodium (Ferry, 2005). Hyperglycemia must be avoided as this may lead to glycosuria and exaggerate the diuresis. If it is not possible to manage DI with fluids alone, the agent of choice for pharmacologic treatment is desmopressin (DDAVP), a long-acting synthetic analogue of pituitary ADH. Intranasal DDAVP can be diluted with normal saline for administration to the neonate. Subcutaneous and oral formulations of DDAVP are also available, as well as short-acting intravenous aqueous pitressin for emergency treatment of severe dehydration. Caution must be observed when using vasopressin and high fluid intake to manage DI in the neonate because this combination can result in hyponatremia (Muglia & Majzoub, 2004).

Syndrome of Inappropriate Antidiuretic Hormone (SIADH)

SIADH is an impairment of free water clearance associated with inappropriately raised secretion of antidiuretic hormone (vasopressin). SIADH is believed to be associated with central nervous system infection and injury, such as birth asphyxia, intracranial hemorrhage, and meningitis.

Pathophysiology. An uncontrolled release of ADH can occur in sick preterm and term infants, resulting in renal free water retention that is inappropriate to the level of serum osmolality. The infant becomes hyponatremic, not because of true sodium depletion, but because of a dilutional effect from the fluid that is retained. ADH levels can become elevated in infants born after fetal distress, or those with severe pulmonary disease, undergoing surgery, or experiencing pain. Raised ADH levels are common in acutely ill neonates (Modi, 1998).

Clinical Manifestations. Signs and symptoms of SIADH are oliguria, hyponatremia, low serum osmolality (<275 mOsm/L), weight gain, and edema. Patients with SIADH are euvolemic or hypervolemic.

Diagnosis. The diagnosis of SIADH should be made when circulating ADH is elevated in the absence of both osmotic and baroreceptor stimuli (Modi, 1998). Serum electrolytes and osmolality reveal hyponatremia and hypo-osmolality. Urine reveals high sodium loss. There should also be normovolemia, normal blood pressure, and normal renal, cardiac, adrenal, and thyroid functions. True SIADH fulfilling all diagnostic criteria is probably uncommon in the neonate. Apparent SIADH may be due to hypovolemia-induced baroreceptor-driven ADH secretion, a normal response to reduced blood volume in the sick neonate (Modi, 1998).

Collaborative Management. Fluid restriction, with close monitoring of intake, output, serum electrolytes, blood glucose, accurate daily weights, evidence of increasing edema, and measures of hydration are the essentials of management. It can be difficult to restrict fluids because infants receive all of their nutrition in liquid form. Diuretics, such as furosemide, are sometimes used to promote free water excretion. Comparison of intake and output is important. A careful neurologic

assessment should be performed, noting changes in relation to fluid or sodium balance.

THYROID GLAND

The thyroid gland is a butterfly-shaped structure made up of two lateral lobes connected by a thin band of tissue called the isthmus. Composed of densely packed follicular cells containing colloid, the thyroid gland also contains parafollicular cells (C-cells) that produce the calcium-lowering hormone calcitonin.

The thyroid hormones thyroxine (T_4) and triiodothyronine (T_3) are produced from the amino acid tyrosine. Essential to this process is the trapping and storage of iodide, a trace element required for thyroid hormone synthesis. Thyroglobulin (Tg), a thyroid hormone precursor, is synthesized in the follicular cell. Iodine is taken up by the Tg molecule, incorporated into its tyrosine residues, and returned to the colloid, where a coupling reaction takes place. This step, called organification, is catalyzed by the enzyme thyroid peroxidase (TPO). The coupling of two tyrosine residues produces T_4, while the coupling of diodotyrosine (DIT) with monoiodotyrosine (MIT) produces T_3. These are stored in the follicular lumens until TSH stimulates their release into the circulation.

The thyroid gland produces mostly T_4, which serves as a storage pool for T_3. T_3 is the most biologically active thyroid hormone, with greater affinity for the thyroid receptor. Circulating T_4 is metabolized by outer-ring 5' monodeiodination to T_3 in the peripheral tissues. Inner ring 5' monodeiodination of T_4 produces reverse T_3 (rT_3), an inactive metabolite. T_4 and T_3 circulate in plasma bound to thyroid-binding globulin (TBG), leaving just a small fraction in equilibrium as free hormone. It is possible for TBG, which is synthesized in the liver, to be deficient even though the free hormone levels are normal. It is the free hormone that is available to the tissues, with the bound hormone acting as a circulating reservoir. The concentration of free hormone determines the individual's metabolic state.

The hypothalamic-pituitary-thyroid (HPT) axis controls thyroid hormone secretion (Figure 7-1). The hypothalamus synthesizes thyrotropin, stimulating release of TSH from the anterior pituitary. In turn, TSH stimulates uptake of iodine by the thyroid, thyroid hormone synthesis and release, and increased size and vascularity of the thyroid gland itself. The feedback loop is responsive to changes in free hormone concentration, and TSH secretion adjusts accordingly.

Fetal and Neonatal Thyroid Development

The thyroid gland is the first endocrine organ to develop in the human embryo (Park & Chatterjee, 2005). Concurrent with development of the fetal thyroid are growth and maturation of the hypothalamus and pituitary glands. At about 10 to 12 weeks' gestation, the hypothalamus begins synthesizing TRH, the pituitary gland begins secreting TSH, and TBG is detectable in fetal serum. Maternal thyroxine is measurable in amniotic fluid before the onset of fetal thyroid function. Before 20 weeks' gestation, this transplacental passage of maternal T_4 largely provides for fetal thyroidal needs. By the start of the second trimester, however, the fetal contribution to circulating thyroid hormones is significant. The capacity of the fetal thyroid gland to trap and store iodide and synthesize thyroid hormones begins at about 11 weeks of gestation, but hormone production is limited until 18 to 20 weeks, when iodine uptake

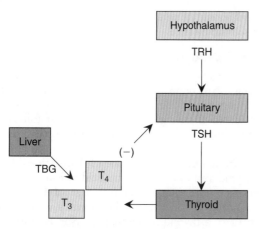

FIGURE **7-1**
The hypothalamic-pituitary-thyroid (HPT) axis. Thyroid hormone levels are regulated by a system of feedback inhibition operating along the HPT axis. The hypothalamus secretes thyrotropin-releasing hormone *(TRH)*, which stimulates the pituitary to secrete thyroid-stimulating hormone *(TSH)*. TSH, in turn, stimulates the thyroid gland to produce and secrete thyroid hormones (T_4 and T_3) into the circulation, which circulate bound to TBG synthesized by the liver. Once levels of T_4 and T_3 are adequate, further production of TSH is suppressed.

increases markedly. The only source of iodide for the fetus is transplacental passage from the maternal circulation and placenta.

As pregnancy progresses, the placenta becomes less permeable to maternal thyroid hormone. Permeability is likely to be highest during the first trimester because thyroid hormone is critical to fetal neurodevelopment, and there is no other source available to the fetus during this period. As the fetal HPT system matures, there is less dependence on maternally derived thyroid hormone for normal neurologic development. Maternal hypothyroidism during early gestation can lead to central nervous system damage in the fetus. Because the placenta is impermeable to TSH, the fetal HPT axis develops independently of maternal influence (Polk & Fisher, 2004).

During fetal life thyroid hormone is required for central nervous system maturation but not for metabolism, growth, or generation of heat. An excess of bioactive T_3 could be harmful to fetal development. For this reason, the concentration of T_3 is tightly controlled in the tissues (van Wassenaer & Kok, 2004). This is accomplished by preferential conversion of excess fetal T_4 to the bio-inactive reverse T_3 by type III deiodinase. In the event of T_4 deficiency, as in fetal hypothyroidism, T_4 is shunted to the brain where it is deiodinated to T_3 to provide a critical source of intracellular T_3 to the developing brain.

Birth represents a temporary state of hyperthyroidism for the newborn. In response to sudden exposure to a cold environment, the pituitary releases a surge of TSH that peaks at 70 to 100 munits/ml at 30 minutes after birth. This cold-stimulated TSH surge provokes rises in serum T_4, T_3, and free T_4 that peak at about 48 hours. T_4 increases in the majority of infants to 6.5 mcg/dl or more. The rise in T_4 causes the TSH to decline to 20 munits/ml or less (the cutoff used in most screening programs for congenital hypothyroidism) because of feedback inhibition. Free and total T_4 and T_3 gradually decrease over the next 1 to 2 months.

Congenital Hypothyroidism (CH)

Congenital hypothyroidism is a deficiency of thyroid function present at the time of birth. With an incidence of 1 in 3000 to 4000 births, it is the most common congenital endocrine disorder. Early diagnosis and treatment are essential to prevent permanent neurologic damage. Because the majority of affected infants are asymptomatic at birth, neonatal screening for hypothyroidism is now mandated so infants with CH are promptly identified and treated. Most of the genetic mutations that produce CH can be sorted into two groups: those that cause thyroid dysgenesis and those that lead to dyshormonogenesis (Park & Chatterjee, 2005).

Thyroid Dysgenesis

The most common cause (85%) of permanent CH is thyroid dysgenesis, which includes thyroidal ectopy, hypoplasia, and complete thyroid agenesis. The severity of thyroid dysfunction is variable, depending on the amount of functional thyroid tissue that remains. Ectopic thyroid tissue (lingual, sublingual, subhyoid) may provide adequate amounts of thyroid hormone in some infants. Occasionally, ectopia are associated with thyroglossal duct cysts. A majority of these infants have a thyroid remnant, usually found midline at the base of the tongue, as a result of failure of the gland to descend normally during embryologic development.

Thyroid dysgenesis occurs in 1 in 4000 live births; however, the incidence in black infants is 1 in 32,000 live births and in Hispanic infants, 1 in 2000. The disorder has a female:male ratio of 2:1. Only 2% of thyroid dysgenesis is due to mutations in the homeobox genes that control thyroid differentiation (TTf-1, TTf-2, or PAX-8). Down syndrome is associated with an increased prevalence of thyroid dysgenesis. No serum Tg is measurable in thyroid agenesis, distinguishing it from functional thyroid tissue, which is associated with measurable serum Tg concentrations.

Thyroid Dyshormonogenesis

About 10% of infants with congenital hypothyroidism have inborn defects of thyroid hormone metabolism. Mutations in genes coding for proteins involved in thyroid hormone synthesis result in failure of one of the steps in this process, leading to thyroid insufficiency. These biochemical defects are usually inherited as autosomal recessive traits and include TSH hormone resistance, iodide organification defects, iodide transport defects, iodotyrosine deiodinase defects, and thyroglobulin deficiency. Deficient activity of the enzyme thyroid peroxidase (TPO) is one of the most common disorders of thyroid synthesis. Although dyshormonogenesis usually results in a compensatory goiter, it is not usually apparent during the neonatal period.

Thyroid-Binding Globulin Deficiency

Infants born with congenital TBG deficiency have low TBG and total T_4 but normal TSH concentrations and are normal with respect to thyroid function. Familial congenital TBG deficiency, transmitted as an X-linked trait, occurs in 1 in 5000 newborns. The defect can be complete or partial and is usually an incidental finding on neonatal screening. A TBG level can be measured to confirm the diagnosis for the purpose of parental counseling, but no treatment is required.

Hypothalamic-Pituitary Hypothyroidism

Five to ten percent of infants with congenital hypothyroidism can be accounted for by what is called secondary-tertiary or central hypothyroidism. A deficiency of hypothalamic TRH or pituitary TSH can occur as a consequence of a developmental defect of the pituitary or hypothalamus. Central hypothyroidism is usually associated with other anomalies of the midbrain such as absence of the septum pellucidum or other midline defects, hypopituitarism, pituitary stalk interruption, or empty sella syndrome which lead to typical laboratory findings of low serum T_4, and low or inappropriately normal serum TSH.

Thyroid Hormone Resistance

An increasing number of patients are being found with resistance to the actions of endogenous and exogenous T_4 and triiodothyronine (T_3). Most patients have goiter, and levels of T_4, T_3, free T_4, and free T_3 are elevated. These findings have often led to the erroneous diagnosis of Graves' disease, although most affected patients are clinically euthyroid. The unresponsiveness may vary among tissues.

Clinical Manifestations of Congenital Hypothyroidism

Few neonates are diagnosed with congenital hypothyroidism on clinical grounds. When present, signs and symptoms of CH in the neonate are subtle and nonspecific; thus they are not immediately linked with hypothyroidism. Early diagnosis is critical, however, to ensure prompt treatment that will reduce the risk of mental retardation. The signs and symptoms of hypothyroidism in the neonate reflect the wide-ranging actions of thyroid hormones on metabolism, intestinal motility, cardiac function, temperature regulation, neurologic function, and skeletal maturation (Box 7-1). The possibility of CH must be considered in any infant presenting with prolonged jaundice, hypothermia, an enlarged (>1 cm) posterior fontanelle, failure to feed well, or respiratory distress with feeding (Polk & Fisher, 2004).

Other features traditionally associated with hypothyroidism (macroglossia, dry skin, lethargy, hoarse cry, coarse hair, and constipation) evolve over the first weeks of life. A palpable, enlarged thyroid gland (also called a goiter) can be associated with impaired thyroid hormone synthesis and hypothyroidism. Hyperplasia of the thyroid gland results from hypersecretion of TSH in response to low T_3 and T_4 levels. Infants with suspect-

ed central hypothyroidism may present with midline or cranial defects or other signs of pituitary deficiency. Central hypothyroidism should be suspected in infants presenting with septo-optic dysplasia, hypoglycemia, micropenis, or cleft lip or palate.

Diagnosis of Congenital Hypothyroidism

Neonatal Screening. Routine screening of all newborn infants for congenital hypothyroidism has greatly improved early detection and treatment of the disorder, preventing much of the mental retardation that was previously associated with CH. The incidence of congenital hypothyroidism, as detected through newborn screening, is approximately 1 per 3000 to 4000. Screening all newborns for CH is mandated in all U.S. states and throughout Canada.

Most screening programs in North America initially measure T_4 on all specimens, measuring TSH only if T_4 is low. Owing to the physiologic surge in TSH in the first hours of life as the newborn adapts to the extrauterine environment, the screening specimen must be collected when the infant is at least 24 hours of age. If blood is collected earlier, particularly in the first 3 hours of life, a false positive result can occur. In those instances, a repeat specimen must be collected within the first 7 days of life, regardless of prior test results. Protein intake is not required prior to screening for CH.

False negatives can occur with screening; as many as 5% to 8% of infants with central CH can be missed with primary T_4 testing because their initial T_4 levels are in the normal range (Polk & Fisher, 2004). A similar problem can occur with infants who have hypothyroxinemia with delayed TSH elevation and those with residual thyroid tissue, such as an ectopic thyroid gland, because their initial T_4 levels are also in the normal range. All of these infants would be detected by repeat screening at 2 to 6 weeks of age.

Certain infants are at risk for a missed or delayed diagnosis, including those born at home, those who are extremely ill in the neonatal period, and those who are transferred between hospitals at an early age. Screening errors, including incorrect specimen collection, or improper storage and transport can lead to false negative results. Thyroid medications taken by the mother during pregnancy can also produce false negative results. Blood transfusions can alter test results. Preservatives (EDTA or citrate) in blood-collection containers can result in false negative or false positive screening results.

When a low T_4 and elevated TSH level (>40 munits/L) are encountered, the neonate should be presumed to have primary hypothyroidism until proven otherwise. A thorough examination for signs and symptoms of CH is indicated, along with confirmatory serum testing. Treatment with L-thyroxine should be initiated while awaiting the results of further testing.

Laboratory Testing. Low serum total and free T_4 and T_3, along with elevated TSH levels, confirm CH in the neonate. Permanent congenital CH is highly likely in a full-term neonate with a serum T_4 less than 6 mcg/dl and a serum TSH greater than 50 munits/L. A normal T_4 (e.g., >10 mcg/dl) in combination with elevated TSH suggests that the infant has enough functional thyroid tissue to respond to excess TSH stimulation, the pattern seen in a subgroup of infants with compensated or subclinical hypothyroidism. Age-related reference norms, for both gestational age and hours of age, should be used when interpreting all thyroid test results. If maternal antibody-mediated hypothyroidism is suspected,

---

BOX 7-1

Signs and Symptoms of Hypothyroidism in the Neonate

- Birth weight >4 kg, gestation longer than 42 weeks
- Large, open posterior fontanelle (>1 cm)
- Umbilical hernia
- Abdominal distention
- Poor feeding
- Hypothermia, cool extremities
- Prolonged jaundice
- Bradycardia
- Poor muscle tone
- Mottled skin

maternal antithyroid (TSH receptor blocking, TRBAb) antibody testing should be done. Other thyroid autoantibodies that can produce hypothyroidism include thyroglobulin (TGAb) and thyroperoxidase antibodies (TPOAb). Thyroid-binding globulin levels can be measured to rule out TBG deficiency. Thyroglobulin levels in infants with possible CH can help to differentiate between thyroid agenesis and dyshormonogenesis, as an adjunct to thyroid imaging.

Imaging Studies. Infants with biochemical evidence of CH usually undergo radionuclide scanning studies using iodine-123. Uptake of radioisotopes aids in detection of an ectopic (lingual or sublingual) or missing gland. A normal or enlarged gland on radioisotope scan suggests a defect in thyroxine synthesis as the source of CH. Thyroid ultrasound can also be useful initially to demonstrate presence or absence of a gland. Lateral radiographs of the knee and foot reveal bone age, indicating the degree of intrauterine hypothyroidism experienced by the fetus. Ossification of the distal femoral epiphysis usually appears at 36 weeks' gestation; its absence in a term or post-term infant suggests delayed bone maturation from long-standing hypothyroidism.

Collaborative Management of Hypothyroidism

Early, adequate treatment of permanent CH is critical for optimal neurologic development. The goal of hormone replacement therapy is to rapidly normalize the infant's serum T_4 level, and maintain it in the upper half of the normal range (Polk & Fisher, 2004). The agent of choice is sodium-L-thyroxine (NaT_4) because it is substantially converted to T_3 within the brain. Infants receiving thyroid replacement therapy must be monitored closely for adequacy of treatment and evidence of thyrotoxicosis (irritability, tachycardia, poor weight gain). Serum T_4 should normalize in 1 to 2 weeks; serum TSH can take longer to normalize.

Transient Disorders of Thyroid Function
Transient Hypothyroxinemia of Prematurity

Preterm infants have the same incidence of permanent congenital hypothyroidism as full-term infants. In addition, about 50% of infants born at less than 30 weeks' gestation exhibit transiently low thyroxine levels when compared to their full-term counterparts. This relative hypothyroxinemia is primarily a function of HPT axis immaturity, a physiologically normal stage of thyroid system development. However, many other factors influence thyroid function, particularly in the extremely preterm infant. The abrupt cessation of maternal T_4 supply, occurring at the time of birth when demand for thyroid hormone is high, contributes to low thyroid hormone levels. Other factors include immature ability to concentrate iodine and to synthesize and iodinate thyroglobulin. Preterm infants may also suffer from insufficient iodine intake during the early weeks after birth before full enteral feeding is established. In addition, iodine excess related to the use of iodine-containing antiseptics and radiopaque agents can interfere with thyroid function by blocking thyroid hormone release from the thyroid gland.

Pathophysiology. The postnatal TSH surge of the preterm infant is similar, yet quantitatively lower, than that of the more mature infant. Likewise, the corresponding rise in T_4 that occurs in preterm infants is blunted in comparison to term infants. It takes approximately 4 to 8 weeks, depending on the gestational age at birth, for normal term hormone levels to be reached (Polk & Fisher, 2004). The more severe the hypothyroxinemia, the more preterm the infant is. Infants with transiently low thyroxine need follow-up testing to ensure that the low T_4 levels rise into the normal range over time.

Extremely preterm infants (24 to 27 weeks' gestation) are at an even greater disadvantage, having a distinct and more ineffective pattern of postnatal thyroid function (Murphy et al, 2004). In these very immature infants, the TSH surge is significantly reduced, and TSH levels continue to fall after birth to less than cord blood values by 7 hours of age. Such very low TSH levels fail to stimulate a postnatal rise in T_4 at all. T_4 levels in extremely immature infants remain quite low after birth and are even slightly lower than cord blood values at 24 hours of age.

Clinical Manifestations. Hypothyroxinemia of prematurity is a subtle condition; there are no overt signs and symptoms of hypothyroidism. Many classic signs and symptoms of hypothyroidism are common clinical findings in the preterm infant (slow intestinal motility, distention, prolonged jaundice, low muscle tone, mottled skin, etc.).

Diagnosis. Hypothyroxinemia of prematurity is identified by routine newborn screening. T_4 and free T_4 are low, but TSH is not elevated above the cutoff of 20 munits/L. This is the critical difference between transient hypothyroxinemia of prematurity and congenital hypothyroidism. A repeat test is conducted after several weeks to recheck T_4 and monitor for a possible delayed rise in TSH.

Collaborative Management. Although hypothyroxinemia of prematurity is associated with higher mortality and neurodevelopmental deficits, cumulative evidence to date has not been able to demonstrate clear benefits of routinely supplementing these infants with thyroxine during early infancy (van Wassenaer & Kok, 2004). The exception is the infant with an elevated TSH level; these infants require treatment. Thyroid function tests should be followed carefully in preterm infants at risk for hypothyroxinemia, and treatment should be instituted promptly when indicated. It is a good idea to flag or highlight the low thyroid results from the initial newborn screen to ensure that repeat thyroid testing is not overlooked.

Nonthyroidal Illness

In some ill preterm infants, T_4 is preferentially converted to rT_3 instead of T_3, possibly as an adaptive response to lower the metabolic rate during times of severe illness (Ogilvy-Stuart, 2002). The outcome is low serum concentrations of both T_4 and T_3. Reverse T_3 is elevated and TSH is normal. This condition, also known as low T_3 syndrome or euthyroid sick syndrome, occurs in infants who have immature lungs or infections, because the cytokines produced in response to illness or inflammation are believed to inhibit thyroid function, metabolism, or thyroid hormone action (van Wassanaer & Kok, 2004). The low T_4 from nonthyroidal illness reverses spontaneously when the infant's condition improves, and no treatment is required. Similar effects are also seen in infants who are receiving dopamine or glucocorticoids, both of which can lower serum T_4 concentrations.

Transient Primary Hypothyroidism

Hypothyroidism is defined as transient when a low T_4 and elevated TSH in apparently healthy full-term infants revert to normal spontaneously or after several months of thyroxine supplementation. About 5% to 10% of the infants identified by newborn screening programs as having congenital hypothyroidism eventually are recognized as having a transient condition. Initial management is the same as for CH.

Transplacental Passage of Drugs or Antibodies

One cause of transient hypothyroidism in the newborn is transplacental passage of antithyroid agents taken during pregnancy for the treatment of maternal Graves' disease. Medications such as propylthiouracil (PTU), methimazole, radioiodine, and amiodarone can inhibit fetal thyroid production. A similar inhibitory effect can occur if the fetus is exposed to excess iodine in utero. If the mother has a history of autoimmune thyroid disease, maternal TSH receptor–blocking antibodies (TRBAb, also termed thyrotropin binding inhibitor immunoglobulin, or TBII) readily cross the placenta and block the fetal thyroid, producing hypothyroidism. These TRBAbs can persist in the infant's circulation for 2 to 3 months after birth before they are completely metabolized and disappear. However, it can be difficult to predict the effects of these antibodies because some mothers will simultaneously produce TSH-receptor stimulating antibodies that will offset the effects of the TRBAbs.

Clinical Manifestations. Like congenital hypothyroidism, transient hypothyroidism is usually asymptomatic in the newborn. If present, the signs and symptoms are the same as for congenital hypothyroidism. Transient hypothyroidism caused by antithyroid drugs (goitrogens) can cause a goiter in the neonate. Iodine deficiency or excess has a similar effect.

Diagnosis. Transient hypothyroidism is usually detected by routine neonatal screening, or based on maternal history. The neonate displays the thyroid profile of low T_4 and elevated TSH that is characteristic of hypothyroidism. When the maternal history is positive for autoimmune thyroid disease, TRBAb and TRSAb levels (as indicated) are also obtained for baseline purposes. Thyroid imaging tests may also be conducted.

Collaborative Management. Transient hypothyroidism caused by maternal antithyroid medication will resolve spontaneously when the medication is cleared from the infant's circulation, usually within a day or two after birth. The infant's serum T_4 and TSH should be monitored to ensure that they return to normal. Supplementation with L-thyroxine is not usually necessary. Transplacentally acquired TSH receptor–blocking antibodies can be slow to degrade completely; therefore most infants will require supplementation for several months. TRBAb levels in the infant can be monitored to determine when to discontinue therapy. Breastfeeding is not contraindicated in neonates whose mothers who continue their antithyroid medication in the postpartum period, as very little transfers into the breast milk (Polk & Fisher, 2004).

Hyperthyroidism (Neonatal Graves' Disease)

Pathophysiology. The transient condition neonatal Graves' disease occurs in infants born to mothers with active or inactive Graves' disease, or to those who have undergone thyroidectomy or radioiodine ablation of the thyroid gland. Maternal TSH-receptor stimulating antibodies (TRSAb or TSA) cross the placenta readily and stimulate the fetal thyroid gland, causing an overproduction of thyroid hormone and in some cases development of a goiter. Usually the higher the

TRSAb level in the mother, the more severely affected the infant.

Hyperthyroidism in the neonate is usually transient, lasting approximately 3 to 12 weeks. The clinical course varies depending on characteristics of the mother's disease and treatment. The onset of hyperthyroidism may be delayed for a week or longer in neonates whose mothers produce not only TRSAb but TSH receptor-blocking antibodies as well. Similarly, if the mother took antithyroid medication during pregnancy, the neonate might not exhibit evidence of hyperthyroidism for several days until the drugs are metabolized (and, in fact, may be hypothyroid during that time). Occasionally, the hyperthyroidism persists beyond the expected recovery period and becomes true, permanent Graves' disease.

Clinical Manifestations. Neonates may be born preterm with evidence of intrauterine growth restriction. Common clinical signs of thyrotoxicosis include tachycardia, arrhythmias, hypertension, tachypnea, poor feeding, vomiting, sweating, hyperthermia, flushing, diarrhea, restlessness, tremors, irritability, and hyperalertness. In severe cases of untreated maternal Graves' disease, advanced bone age, craniosynostosis, and microcephaly may be evident in both the fetus and newborn. The infant should be examined for a goiter, which can be very small or large enough to compress the trachea and cause respiratory distress in the newborn. A goiter is a symmetrical, smooth enlargement of the gland and can be recognized as a swelling in the anterior neck of the neonate (Figure 7-2). It is important to appreciate that a goiter can increase in size during the early neonatal period.

Diagnosis. Serum T_4, free T_4, and T_3 are elevated, and serum TSH is low, all relative to age-appropriate norms. A TRSAb titer in the neonate will give an indication of the severity of the expected course of the disease. Infants at risk (e.g., high maternal titer of TRSAb) for severe thyrotoxicosis require frequent monitoring of free T_4 and TSH. A good maternal history is essential (e.g., history of radioablation therapy, antithyroid drugs taken during pregnancy and when they were taken, and maternal symptoms, if any).

Collaborative Management. The mainstays of treatment of hyperthyroidism in the neonate are iodine, antithyroid medication, sedation, and β-adrenergic blockers, if needed. Treatment is tailored to the severity of the infant's symptoms. Lugol's iodine solution (potassium iodide), given in

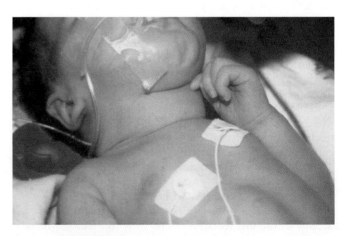

FIGURE **7-2**
Newborn infant presenting at birth with goiter.

a single drop three times daily, acutely inhibits the release of thyroxine from the thyroid gland. Other preparations include iodine-based contrast agents (ipodate), PTU, and methimazole. Propranolol can be used to manage cardiovascular symptoms. The infant's serum T_4 must be followed closely during treatment to monitor for possible iatrogenic hypothyroidism. TRSAb levels are also followed to monitor the infant's recovery and aid in determining the appropriate time for weaning antithyroid medication.

ADRENAL GLAND

The highly vascular adrenal glands are located at the superior poles of the kidneys. Each gland is composed of two distinct, independently functioning organs: the outer cortex, which produces steroid hormones (mineralocorticoids, glucocorticoids, and androgens), and the inner medulla, which produces catecholamines. Adrenal steroid production and regulation require a functional hypothalamic-pituitary-adrenal (HPA) axis. Cortisol is also released in response to stress, hypoglycemia, surgery, extreme heat or cold, hypoxia, infection, or injury.

Aldosterone, the most important mineralocorticoid, regulates renal sodium and water retention and potassium excretion. Aldosterone affects not only electrolyte balance but blood pressure and intravascular volume as well. Aldosterone is regulated by the plasma renin-angiotensin system, which in turn stimulates production of aldosterone.

Adrenal androgens include dehydroepiandrosterone (DHEA), DHEA sulfate, and androstenedione and are regulated by ACTH. These steroids have minimal androgenic activity but are converted in the peripheral tissues to two more potent androgens, testosterone and dihydrotestosterone (DHT).

Fetal Adrenal Gland

The fetal adrenal is evident from 6 to 8 weeks of gestation and rapidly increases in size. Early in gestation, the fetal adrenal cortex differentiates into three regions: an inner prominent fetal zone, an outer definitive zone, and a transitional zone. After birth, the fetal zone involutes and the definitive zone forms the mature gland. Cortisol maintains intrauterine homeostasis and influences the development of a wide variety of fetal tissues. Cortisol is essential for prenatal maturation of organ systems including lungs, GI tract, liver, and the CNS which are vital for neonatal survival.

The fetal adrenal gland and the placenta are an integrated endocrine system known as the fetoplacental unit. The fetal zone of the developing adrenal gland produces DHEA and DHEA sulfate, precursors for placental estrogen, which is critical to maintenance of the pregnancy and fetal well-being. In turn, the placenta regulates fetal exposure to maternal cortisol by oxidizing cortisol to the biologically inactive cortisone, protecting the fetus from excessive cortisol levels. The placenta also releases corticotropin releasing hormone (CRH), which heightens activity of the fetal HPA axis and stimulates fetal cortisol production. All of this contributes to the prenatal cortisol surge that prepares the fetus for the stress of birth and adaptation to the extrauterine environment.

Neonatal Adrenocortical Function

Plasma cortisol levels are elevated at the time of birth but decline in the first few days of life. In term infants, a nadir is seen on day 4 of life. Likewise, levels of cortisol precursors such as 17-hydroxyprogesterone (17-OHP) are high at birth but decrease to normal neonatal levels by 12 to 24 hours of age. Cortisol is regulated by pituitary ACTH, which in turn is controlled by hypothalamic CRH via a negative feedback loop.

Aldosterone and plasma renin activity are elevated in neonates compared with values for older infants, allowing for positive sodium balance until the kidneys fully mature. The hyponatremia and urinary sodium losses often seen in preterm infants during the early postnatal weeks are due to a relative mineralocorticoid deficiency as a consequence of immaturity of both the kidneys and the adrenal glands.

Adrenal Disorders in the Neonate
Transient Adrenocortical Insufficiency of Prematurity

A limited ability of the adrenal glands to maintain cortisol homeostasis in the early days of life has been observed in some preterm newborns. Manifestations are a low serum cortisol, normal or exaggerated pituitary response, and good recovery of adrenal function by day 14 of life. A proportion of very low birth weight infants with inotrope and volume-resistant hypotension show an inadequate adrenal response to stress in the immediate postnatal period (Ng et al, 2004).

Adrenal Hemorrhage

Adrenal hemorrhage in the neonate can occur as a result of traumatic delivery, breech presentation, macrosomia, or defective coagulation. The large size and vascularity of the fetal adrenal gland may predispose it to injury and rupture during the birth process. Classic findings include a flank mass on either side, with discoloration and purpura of the overlying skin. In severe cases, the infant may exhibit signs of adrenal insufficiency and anemia.

Congenital Adrenal Hyperplasia

Congenital adrenal hyperplasia (CAH) is a group of autosomal recessive disorders resulting from a deficiency of one of the five enzymes required to synthesize cortisol from cholesterol in the adrenal cortex. Each enzyme is encoded by its own gene, and mutations in the 21-hydroxylase gene, CYP21, are the most frequent. 21-Hydroxylase (21-OHD) deficiency accounts for 95% of CAH and is the most common cause of ambiguous genitalia of the neonate.

Pathophysiology. A lack of 21-hydroxylase prevents conversion of progesterone to its two end products: cortisol and aldosterone (Figure 7-3). By reduced negative feedback regulation, the absence of cortisol causes oversecretion of ACTH, which chronically stimulates the adrenal cortex, resulting in hyperplasia of the gland. The precursor steroids proximal to the blocked step accumulate and are shunted into other metabolic pathways such as androgen biosynthesis. In a female fetus, these superfluous yet potent systemic androgens cause virilization of the developing external genitalia. Also important may be the effects of this androgen exposure on the developing central nervous system (Berenbaum, 2004). Internal reproductive organs (ovaries, fallopian tubes, and uterus) are not affected by androgen exposure and develop normally.

Classic 21-OHD has a worldwide incidence of about 1 in 15,000 live births (Therrell, 2001). Two-thirds of those have a severe form known as salt-wasting or salt-losing in which there is a concurrent inability to produce aldosterone. High sodium excretion leads to profound hyponatremia, dehydration, and hyperkalemia. Glucocorticoid deficiency impairs carbohydrate

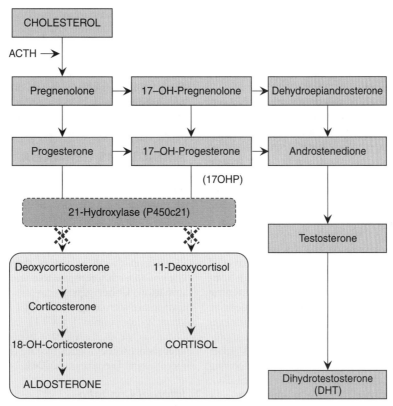

FIGURE **7-3**
Pathophysiology of congenital adrenal hyperplasia caused by 21-hydroxylase deficiency. A deficiency of the enzyme 21-hydroxylase prevents the normal conversion of cholesterol to aldosterone and cortisol. Precursor steroids including 17-hydroxyprogesterone proximal to the blocked step are shunted into the androgen synthesis pathway, resulting in an excess production of androgens.

metabolism, resulting in hypoglycemia and leading to hypotension, shock, and cardiovascular collapse from adrenal insufficiency. The remaining one-third has a simple virilizing form. These infants have an incomplete enzymatic block, with enough aldosterone biosynthesis to maintain fluid and electrolyte homeostasis.

Clinical Manifestations. Affected female infants are usually recognized at birth by their nontypical genitals. A range of findings is possible, including clitoromegaly, posterior fusion of the labia majora, and a single perineal orifice instead of separate urethral and vaginal openings (Merke & Bornstein, 2005). In the last instance, the vagina joins the urethra above the perineum, forming a single urogenital sinus. In severe cases, clitoral hypertrophy is so marked that it resembles a penile urethra (Figure 7-4). These infants can be mistaken for boys with bilateral cryptorchidism and hypospadias. There may also be hyperpigmentation of the genital skin resulting from excessive pituitary ACTH secretion. Male infants with 21-OHD are phenotypically normal and may not be identified in the immediate neonatal period, because the onset of adrenal symptoms is delayed until 7 to 14 days of life. Undetected infants may present to the emergency room with signs and symptoms of impending adrenal collapse: vomiting, weight loss, lethargy, dehydration, hyponatremia, hyperkalemia, hypoglycemia, hypovolemia, and shock.

Diagnosis. A markedly elevated 17-hydroxyprogesterone (17-OHP) level is diagnostic for classic 21-hydroxylase deficiency. Random 17-OHP levels in affected infants can reach

10,000 ng/dl (normal is <100 ng/dl) (Speiser & White, 2003). However, such high 17-OHP levels may not be reached until the second or third day of life, so a specimen drawn too early could lead to false reassurance that the infant does not have

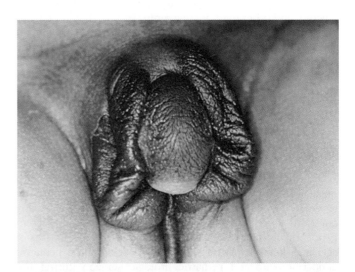

FIGURE **7-4**
External genitalia of 46XX neonate with congenital adrenal hyperplasia. Note clitoromegaly with rugosed, hyperpigmented, and partly fused labioscrotal folds. From Stokowski L (2004). Endocrine disorders. In Verklan MT, Walden M, editors. *Core curriculum for neonatal intensive care nursing* (p 723). Philadelphia: Elsevier.

CAH. Biochemical support for the diagnosis of CAH also includes elevated serum DHEA and androstenedione levels in males and females, and elevated serum testosterone in females. Molecular genetic analysis is not usually essential for the diagnosis but may be helpful to confirm the exact type of defect and to aid in genetic counseling.

Part of the evaluation of every newborn with ambiguous genitalia is a karyotype or FISH test for sex chromosome material, and this is also true when the suspected diagnosis is CAH. Some infants are so externally virilized that it might be difficult for parents to believe the infant is genetically female without the proof presented by chromosome testing. Imaging studies, including pelvic and abdominal ultrasound, will determine the presence or absence of a uterus, evaluate adrenal size, and more rapidly identify the gender of the infant.

The increased serum 17-OHP levels in affected infants permit screening for the disorder using blood filter specimens on routine newborn screening panels. The major objectives of newborn screening for CAH are the presymptomatic identification of infants at risk for the development of life-threatening adrenal crises and prevention of incorrect sex assignment of affected female infants with ambiguous genitalia. The former is particularly important for affected boys whose initial manifestation may be adrenal crisis. Currently 42 of 50 states either have programs already in place or have mandates for screening newborns for congenital adrenal hyperplasia (NNSGRC, 2005). False positives can occur in preterm infants or sick infants, both of whom have higher levels of 17-OHP.

Collaborative Management. The newborn with CAH requires urgent expert medical attention. When the diagnosis of CAH is confirmed, physiologic replacement dosing of cortisol is begun in order to suppress ACTH and androgen overproduction, but not enough to completely suppress the HPA axis (Merke & Bornstein, 2005). Aldosterone replacement maintains fluid and electrolyte homeostasis. Agents of choice in the newborn are hydrocortisone, a glucocorticoid, plus fludrocortisone, a mineralocorticoid. Further clinical management is guided by daily weights, adrenal steroid concentrations, plasma renin activity (PRA), electrolytes, blood glucose, and other data. Plasma renin activity should be compared to age-specific norms, because basal PRA is higher in the newborn than in older infants. Dietary sodium chloride supplementation is often necessary.

The overwhelming majority of 46XX individuals with CAH develop a female gender identity, regardless of the degree of genital virilization present at birth, according to currently available evidence (Berenbaum, 2004). Therefore, even in cases where babies are initially "misassigned" as boys, it is still generally recommended that these genetic females with CAH be raised as females (Berenbaum, 2004; Brown & Warne, 2005). Hypertrophy of the clitoris will gradually abate with medical therapy; however, severe virilization will not be reversed. Parents of virilized female infants may have many questions about possible genital surgery. Although such surgery is not usually performed until the infant is 2 to 6 months of age, it is helpful for the parents to meet with the pediatric endocrinologist and pediatric urologic surgeon during the initial hospitalization or shortly afterward to discuss available options, one of which is to delay surgery performed for cosmetic purposes until the child is old enough to participate in the decision (Crouch & Creighton, 2004). The goals of genital surgery for virilized girls with CAH are to achieve genital appearance compatible with gender, unobstructed urinary emptying without incontinence or infections, and good adult sexual and reproductive function. Surgery may not be necessary in infants with lesser degrees of virilization (LWPES/ESPE, 2002). After discharge, infants with CAH must be closely followed by a pediatric endocrinologist for assessments of hormone levels, blood sugar, blood pressure, growth, skeletal maturation, and other parameters necessary to guard against over- or undertreatment.

AMBIGUOUS GENITALIA
Sexual Differentiation of the Fetus
The first events in sexual differentiation are directed by genes. During the early weeks of development, all embryos have bipotential gonads and structures for both male and female internal and external genitalia. Male-specific development requires the expression of the testis-determining gene (SRY) located on the short arm of the Y chromosome. This directs the gonad to differentiate to a testis, the key event in sex determination. Other genes that are important to testis differentiation are steroidogenic factor 1 (SF-1), the tumor-suppressor gene Wilms' tumor 1 (WT1), and the SOX9 gene. If the Y chromosome is absent, the gonad differentiates to an ovary; there is no firm evidence to date that an ovarian differentiation factor exists (Federman, 2004).

Internal Genitalia
The next events in sexual development are hormonally mediated. By 7 weeks of gestation, the fetus has two sets of primitive ducts that will become the internal reproductive tracts: the müllerian (female) and wolffian (male). In the XY fetus, the testis differentiates by the end of week 7. The embryonic testis develops two types of hormone-producing cells: the Sertoli and the Leydig cells. The Sertoli cells begin secreting müllerian-inhibiting factor (MIF), causing the müllerian ducts to regress. By the 9th week, testicular Leydig cells are secreting the androgens necessary for further virilization of the male fetus.

Testosterone, the major androgen produced by the testes, acts locally in high concentrations to induce development of the wolffian ducts into the epididymis, vas deferens, and seminal vesicles. In the absence of testosterone, the wolffian ducts regress at 11 weeks' gestation. Müllerian ducts require no ovarian hormonal inducement to develop into Fallopian tubes, uterus, and upper vagina. This occurs in fetuses with a normal ovary or on any side lacking a gonad.

External Genitalia
The primitive external genital structures are identical in both sexes (Figure 7-5). In this indifferent stage, a genital tubercle forms and elongates to form a phallus and urogenital sinus, surrounded by inner urogenital folds and labioscrotal swellings. Between the 8th and 14th weeks of gestation, male differentiation of the external genitalia takes place. Central to this development is availability of dihydrotestosterone (DHT), a potent metabolite produced from testosterone by the enzyme 5-α reductase-2. With 10 times the binding affinity of testosterone, DHT binds to androgen receptors in the genital tissues, stimulating fusion of the urethral folds to form the penile shaft, and the labioscrotal swellings to form the scrotum (Federman, 2004). The urogenital sinus becomes the urethra. Penile growth continues throughout gestation, and migration of the

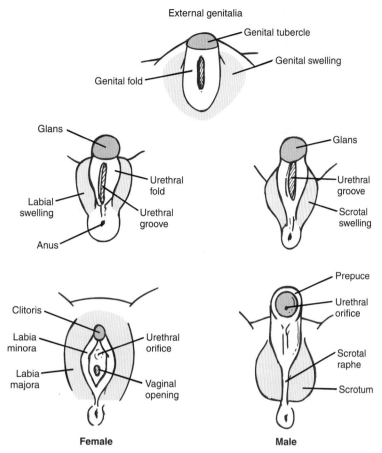

External genitalia

Genital tubercle

Genital swelling

Genital fold

Glans

Urethral fold

Labial swelling

Urethral groove

Anus

Glans

Urethral groove

Scrotal swelling

Clitoris

Labia minora

Labia majora

Urethral orifice

Vaginal opening

Prepuce

Urethral orifice

Scrotal raphe

Scrotum

Female

Male

FIGURE **7-5**
Development of the external genitalia. From Houk CP, Lee PA (2005). Intersexed states: diagnosis and management. *Endocrinology and metabolism clinics of North America* 34:791-810.

testes from the abdominal cavity to the scrotum does not occur until 25 to 35 weeks' gestation.

In the absence of DHT, feminization of the external genitalia occurs. The phallus becomes a clitoris, and the labioscrotal swellings remain unfused to form the labia majora and minora. The urogenital sinus develops into the lower vagina and urethra. Feminine external genital development is complete by 11 weeks' gestation. Androgen exposure after this critical period can promote growth of the clitoris but does not cause labial fusion or the development of a penile urethra (Houk & Lee, 2005).

Disorders of Sexual Development

A disorder of sexual development (DSD) is a congenital disorder with atypical development of chromosomal, gonadal, or anatomic sex (Lee et al, 2006). The majority of DSDs result from one of two conditions: either a failure in one of the steps of the male developmental pathway, or the exposure of an XX fetus to androgens during a sensitive period of development.

46XX DSD

The most frequently encountered intersex condition in the neonate is the virilized female, or the 46XX infant with ambiguous external genitalia but normal female internal structures (Forest et al, 2004). The most common etiology is congenital adrenal hyperplasia, caused by 21-hydroxylase deficiency (21-OHD). This enzyme deficiency results in an overproduction of androgens at a critical stage of development, causing masculinization of the external, but not the internal (ovaries, uterus, fallopian tubes), genitalia. In the most severe cases, the excess androgens also prevent the vagina from fully descending into the perineum, leaving a common urogenital canal. (See previous section, Adrenal Disorders.)

Other possible, yet rare, causes of virilization of external genitalia in the 46XX infant are placental aromatase deficiency, maternal androgen-producing or adrenal tumors, and maternal medications with androgenic action taken during pregnancy.

46XY DSD

The combination of a 46XY karyotype with ambiguous genitalia results from a failure in one of the steps involved in the synthesis or response to testosterone during sexual differentiation and penile growth. These infants have bilateral testicular development, but incomplete virilization of the internal or external genitalia. This results in an external phenotype ranging from completely female to isolated hypospadias or cryptorchidism. Another condition associated with incomplete virilization in the XY male is cloacal exstrophy, a defect of embryogenesis involving exstrophy of the bladder. Although not a DSD, significant ambiguity of external genitalia may be present.

Androgen Insensitivity Syndrome (AIS)

Pathophysiology. AIS is caused by a loss-of-function mutation in the androgen receptor gene located on the long arm of the X chromosome. Both testosterone and its target tissue metabolite, DHT, must bind to androgen receptors in order to masculinize the genital tissues. When androgen receptor activity is impaired, androgen binding is insufficient. One variant of AIS is receptor negative: cytosol receptors are incapable of binding DHT. Another variant is receptor positive: receptors are able to bind DHT but this does not result in normal differentiation. Both internal wolffian structures and external genitalia fail to respond to high levels of testosterone and DHT. There are partial and complete forms of the disorder, resulting in different degrees of undervirilization. In partial androgen insensitivity syndrome (PAIS) the clinical phenotype varies considerably and often parallels the severity of androgen resistance.

Clinical Manifestations. Infants with PAIS have undervirilization ranging from simple hypospadias to microphallus with a labia majora-like bifid scrotum, undescended testes, and a urogenital sinus. No visible features distinguish PAIS from other causes of incomplete masculinization. Infants with complete androgen insensitivity (CAIS) are born with apparently female genitalia. However, these neonates may have palpable inguinal or labial masses, which further testing will reveal to be testes. Some may also have a short, blind-ending vagina.

Diagnosis. The diagnosis of CAIS is missed in the newborn period unless the infant presents with bilateral masses in the labia or inguinal canals or a boy was expected based on a prenatal karyotype. CAIS might also be discovered at the time of inguinal hernia repair (Hyun & Kolon, 2004), or there may be a history of similarly affected family members. Important investigations include a karyotype, levels of testosterone, DHT and LH, and genital skin fibroblasts for androgen-binding testing. In PAIS, the ratio of androstenedione to testosterone is normal. Testosterone, estradiol and LH are normal or high; FSH is usually normal. Less than half of infants with suspected PAIS have abnormal androgen binding; those with normal binding may have a defect in DNA binding or transcriptional activation (Misra & Lee, 2005). Molecular genetic testing can identify mutations in the AR gene by direct sequence analysis. Imaging studies reveal the absence of female internal reproductive structures (uterus, fallopian tubes). Two normal testes are present.

Collaborative Management. Infants with CAIS have unambiguously female external anatomy and are raised in the female gender. Testes are removed (usually after puberty) to prevent later malignancy. The gender assignment of infants with PAIS can be more complex and is often based on the severity of the phenotype (Misra & Lee, 2005). When the phenotype is predominantly male, a male sex of rearing is recommended. However, there are no consensus guidelines for the management of infants with severe perineoscrotal hypospadias and microphallus. The detection of somatic mutations in AIS is of importance for correct sex assignment because the presence of a functional wild-type AR receptor can induce virilization at puberty (Kohler et al, 2005). When a male sex of rearing is contemplated, a therapeutic trial with pharmacologic doses of androgen, especially in those with an identified AR mutation, is often used to predict potential androgen responsiveness at puberty. If there is no phallic growth in response to testosterone, some have recommended consideration of a female gender assignment. However, many experts now believe that, given the putative influence of prenatal androgen exposure on the developing central nervous system, and the possibility that the child will develop a male gender identity, it is more prudent to raise these infants as boys.

Testosterone Biosynthetic Defects

Pathophysiology. Defects in the chain of steroidogenic enzymes involved in the testosterone biosynthesis pathway result in insufficient androgen concentrations during fetal development. Disorders include congenital lipoid adrenal hyperplasia (CLAH), 3β-HDD, 17α-hydroxylase/lyase deficiency, and 17β-hydroxysteroid dehydrogenase deficiency (17β-HSD). CLAH is caused by a defect in the steroidogenic acute regulatory (StAR) protein, responsible for transporting cholesterol to the inner membrane of the mitochondria. Insufficient testosterone in affected males leads to underdeveloped wolffian duct structures and external male anatomy. Müllerian structures are absent because there is normal testicular MIF production.

Clinical Manifestations. Male infants with CLAH present with complete adrenal insufficiency: vomiting, weight loss, and hypotension. Genital appearance is primarily female. Infants with 3β-HDD can present with varying degrees of genital ambiguity and evidence of salt-losing crisis (see 21-OHD). Infants with 17α-hydroxylase/lyase deficiency have genital ambiguity; with primary 17α-hydroxylase deficiency patients also have hypertension. These male infants with 17β-HSD present with what appears to be external female genitalia that may include mild clitoral enlargement. An inguinal hernia may be present, possibly the only finding that will bring the infant to medical attention.

Diagnosis. General laboratory investigations in suspected testosterone biosynthetic defects include chromosomes, baseline levels of testosterone, androgen precursors and DHT, and levels of steroids and steroid precursors. An hCG stimulation test can be performed to measure the ratio of androstenedione to testosterone; an elevated ratio suggests 17β-HSD deficiency.

Collaborative Management. Acute management of these disorders requires full steroid replacement with both glucocorticoids and mineralocorticoids. In CLAH and 3β-HDD, general supportive measures may be necessary, as severe adrenal insufficiency can cause rapid metabolic decompensation if the disorder is not recognized at birth (Misra & Lee, 2005). Genetic XY infants with CLAH are raised in the female gender. Children with 17β-HSD often virilize significantly at puberty owing to increased peripheral conversion of androstenedione to testosterone by 17β-HSD isoenzymes, making gender assignment of those diagnosed as neonates a less straightforward decision.

5-α Reductase-2 Deficiency (5-ARD-2)

Pathophysiology. 5-ARD-2 deficiency is an autosomal recessive disorder caused by more than 20 different mutations of the 5-ARD gene. 5-ARD-2 is an enzyme found in the genital skin and fibroblasts of the developing fetus, without which testosterone is not converted to DHT, and fetal external genitalia do not virilize. Development of the internal structures is unaffected because DHT is not required, so the wolffian ducts differentiate normally in response to testosterone and the müllerian ducts regress. At puberty, the external genitalia become virilized and fertility is possible (Misra & Lee, 2005).

Clinical Manifestations. The spectrum of findings ranges from mild undervirilization (isolated micropenis or hypospadias) to severe undervirilization (a female phenotype with clitoromegaly, mild rugation, or pigmentation) (Figure 7-6). Testes are intact and are found in the inguinal canals or labioscrotal folds, or are retained in the abdomen. The uterus and fallopian tubes regress because of normal secretion of MIS. Wolffian duct differentiation is not affected because DHT is not required. Male internal ducts terminate either in a blind pseudovaginal pouch or on the perineum.

Diagnosis. Diagnosis is made by assessing the ratio of testosterone to DHT following an hCG stimulation test. A normal T/DHT ratio is less than 10:1. In 5-ARD-2 deficiency, this ratio is elevated. The hCG stimulation test also rules out other causes of undervirilization, such as Leydig cell hypoplasia and testosterone biosynthetic defects. Analysis of 5-ARD-2 activity in genital skin fibroblasts provides a definitive diagnosis.

Collaborative Management. Boys with 5-ARD-2 respond to endogenous testosterone and undergo virilization and penile growth at puberty. The mechanism behind this late virilization may be extraglandular DHT formation due to peripheral conversion of increased testicular testosterone by unaffected isoenzymes (Sultan et al, 2002). For this reason, it is recommended that when the diagnosis is made in the newborn period, a male sex assignment should be made (Goodwin & Caldamone, 2004).

Gonadal Dysgenesis

This group of disorders is usually associated with chromosomal anomalies or mutations or deletions of genes responsible for sexual differentiation. Karyotypes producing gonadal dysgenesis include 46XY, 46XX, 46XY/46X, and mosaic forms including the Y chromosome. Gonadal dysgenesis can occur as an iso-

lated condition or as part of a complex syndrome such as Fraser, Denys-Drash, or campomelic dysplasia (Brown & Warne, 2005).

Pathophysiology. A dysgenetic testis either fails to produce testosterone at all or produces insufficient testosterone, resulting in varying degrees of undervirilization of the fetus. The most likely cause of gonadal dysgenesis is a mutation in the sex-determining gene (Palma Sisto, 2004). Gonadal dysgenesis is considered partial or incomplete when the testes are dysgenetic or incompletely formed, and complete when the gonads are streaks containing only stromal tissue. Mixed gonadal dysgenesis occurs when one gonad is a streak and the other is a well-formed testis. The internal ducts correlate with the ipsilateral gonad. On the side of a streak gonad, a fallopian tube and a hemiuterus will develop, and on the side of a normal testis, the vas deferens and epididymis will form.

Clinical Manifestations. The external genitalia are highly variable depending on how much testosterone is produced. In mixed gonadal dysgenesis, the external genitalia are asymmetric, appearing male on one side and female on the other. A vagina and uterine cavity may be present. Complete (or pure) gonadal dysgenesis is a form of sex reversal that results in unambiguously female genitalia with features of Turner's syndrome. These infants might not be identified in the newborn period unless a discrepancy is noted between a prenatal karyotype (46XY) and appearance of the genitals.

Diagnosis. Determining the sex chromosome complement by FISH testing is the most important diagnostic test. Imaging studies, genitography, or laparoscopy is used to define the internal anatomy. Gonadal histologic analysis is necessary to differentiate gonadal dysgenesis from true gonadal intersex, a condition wherein elements of both testes and ovaries are present in the same individual (see later discussion).

Collaborative Management. Determining the sex of rearing for the infant with partial or mixed gonadal dysgenesis can be a difficult decision, one that is usually based on the degree of virilization and details of the internal anatomy (Goodwin & Caldamone, 2004). When a uterus is present, the female sex assignment may be preferred. Most infants with complete gonadal dysgenesis are raised as females.

Ovotesticular DSD

In ovotesticular DSDs both ovarian and testicular components are present in the same individual (Houk et al, 2005). Possible combinations include an ovary on one side and a testis on the other, an ovary or testis with an ovotestis, or two ovotestes. More than half of affected babies will have an XX karyotype. This condition was formerly known as true hermaphroditism, a label that is considered outdated.

Pathophysiology. The amount of testosterone produced by the testicular tissue that is present determines the degree of differentiation of wolffian ducts, regression of müllerian ducts, and virilization of external genitalia. The internal ducts usually parallel the ipsilateral gonadal histology. Ovarian tissue can be normal.

Clinical Manifestations. Asymmetry of the external genitalia is common. Genital ambiguity ranges from a female phenotype with slight clitoromegaly to a mildly undervirilized male phenotype. The most common presentation is marked genital ambiguity: microphallus with penoscrotal or perineoscrotal hypospadias, fusion of labioscrotal folds, and cryptorchidism (Misra & Lee, 2005).

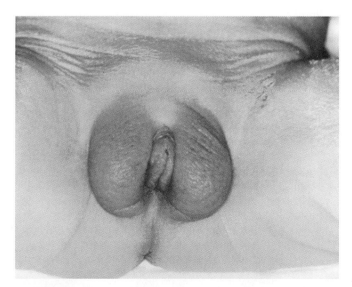

FIGURE 7-6
External genitalia of 46XY neonate with 5-α reductase deficiency. Undervirilization is so severe in this infant that the phenotype is almost completely female, with labia majora–like bifid scrotum and severe microphallus. From Stokowski L (2004). Endocrine disorders. In Verklan MT, Walden M, editors. *Core curriculum for neonatal intensive care nursing* (p 723). Philadelphia: Elsevier.

Diagnosis. FISH testing is used to determine sex chromosome complement. Imaging studies are used to define the internal anatomy. To diagnose true gonadal intersex, the presence of functional ovarian tissue containing follicles and testicular tissue with distinct seminiferous tubules must be established (Misra & Lee, 2005). Laparoscopy with gonadal biopsy is necessary at some point to confirm the diagnosis.

Collaborative Management. Principles of management for infants with true gonadal intersex are similar to those of gonadal dysgenesis.

General Principles of Management of DSDs

The fact that doctors and nurses are not quite sure if one's long-awaited newborn baby is a boy or a girl must surely be one of the most incomprehensible things that parents can hear in the delivery room. This situation requires a high degree of sensitivity and tact. Many infants are identified prenatally following ultrasound recognition of genital ambiguity or a karyotype/phenotype discordance, and these families will be prepared, to some degree, for the experience of having a baby of uncertain sex. Others will be taken completely by surprise. In spite of the family's desire for a quick answer, no attempt should be made by medical professionals at the time of birth to guess the sex of the baby (Ogilvy-Stuart & Brain, 2004). The extreme phenotypic heterogeneity seen in DSDs makes it impossible to accurately predict either the diagnosis or the karyotype from a brief genital examination (Houk & Lee, 2005).

The Lawson Wilkins Pediatric Society and the European Society for Paediatric Endocrinology recently established an International Consensus Conference on Intersex. The result was a consensus statement on management of intersex disorders (Lee et al, 2006). That document represents the first agreed-on set of guiding principles for approaching and managing the newborn with a DSD.

Clinical Manifestations. Essential to the evaluation of the neonate with genital ambiguity is obtaining a detailed family history. Any of the following might suggest a congenital or inherited DSD: maternal virilization or ingestion of hormones or oral contraceptives during pregnancy; consanguinity; history of urologic abnormalities, infertility, or genital ambiguity in other family members; or previous neonatal deaths that might suggest an undiagnosed adrenal crisis. Dysmorphic features suggest the possibility of a syndrome.

A detailed assessment of the genitalia should be conducted. This and all subsequent examinations should respect the privacy of the infant and the family as much as possible, avoiding overexposure of the infant even for educational purposes (Houk & Lee, 2005). Although the physical assessment alone does not permit a firm diagnosis, some assessment findings can guide the diagnostic process in one direction or another. A precise description of the anatomy is more useful than simple staging classifications. If preferred, however, the degree of virilization can be documented by Prader staging from a phenotypic female with mild clitoromegaly (Prader stage II) to phenotypic male with glandular hypospadias (Prader stage V) (Figure 7-7). Look for symmetry or asymmetry of the genitalia. The presence of a uterus can be determined by digital rectal examination as an anterior midline cordlike structure (Hyun & Kolon, 2004).

Gonads. Determine whether gonads are palpable. Presence or absence of palpable gonads helps to differentiate the major categories of DSDs. An apparent male infant with bilateral or a single impalpable testis with hypospadias should be regarded as having a potential DSD until proven otherwise. A palpable gonad excludes the diagnosis of virilized genetic female (46XX) with CAH. A gonad palpated below the external inguinal ring is presumed to contain testicular tissue. Because ovaries are rarely palpable, a unilateral gonad is usually a testis or occasionally an ovotestis. To palpate testes, place finger flat from internal ring, and milk down into the labioscrotal folds. Gonads may be situated high in the inguinal canal, requiring a careful examination. Sweep the fingers down along the line of the inguinal canal on each side, beginning well above the site of the internal inguinal ring. A gonad milked down by this maneuver is gently grasped by the other hand and its size and consistency noted. Ovotestes are softer and less homogenous than testes (Brown & Warne, 2005). Bilateral absence of the testes is known as cryptorchidism.

Phallus. Phallic size should be measured with a straightedge ruler, depressing the fat pad and measuring the stretched length from pubic tubercle to tip of penis, not including the foreskin. Both length and diameter of the penis should be noted. Chordee (ventral curvature of the penis) should

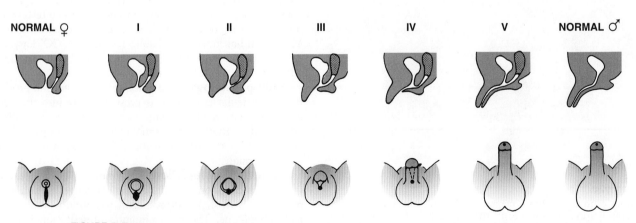

FIGURE **7-7**
Degrees of genital virilization according to the stages of Prader. The *upper panel* shows sagittal view and the *lower panel* shows perineal view. From Sperling M, editor. *Pediatric endocrinology*, ed 2 (p 406). Philadelphia: Saunders.

be noted as it may decrease the apparent length of the penis. The actual position of the urethral meatus should be determined. Clitoral size should also be measured when clitoromegaly is present. Clitoral length greater than 9 mm in term infants is considered excessive. Clitoral size often appears large in preterm infants because breadth remains constant from 27 weeks onward. A prominent, but not truly enlarged, clitoris, or a normally sized penis concealed by an abundance of prepubic fat are two normal assessment findings that sometimes prompt referrals for genital ambiguity (Houk & Lee, 2005).

Labioscrotal Folds. Labial fullness, a benign finding, is another feature occasionally mistaken for genital ambiguity. The labioscrotal folds are examined for fusion, which starts posteriorly and moves anteriorly, increasing the anogenital distance. The perineum is inspected by gently separating the labia and using an exam light to confirm the presence of separate urethral and vaginal openings or a single urogenital orifice (an opening connected to both urinary and genital systems). If skin tags with slightly bluish hue are seen, a hymen and vagina are present. Note rugosity or hyperpigmentation of the labioscrotal fold, signifying hypersecretion of ACTH associated with CAH.

Diagnostic Studies. DSDs are diagnosed with a combination of biochemical, hormonal, and genetic testing. The principal aim of an initial investigation is to rule out a life-threatening illness such as congenital adrenal hyperplasia, which can precipitate an adrenal crisis. Such testing includes serum 17-hydroxyprogesterone (17-OHP) level (after 24 to 48 hours of age), electrolytes, glucose, baseline levels of testosterone, DHT, and other steroid precursors (progesterone, dehydroepiandrosterone, Δ^4-androstenedione, and 17α-hydroxypregnenolone). A karyotype with X- and Y-specific probe detection is obtained from all infants, even if a prenatal karyotype is available (Lee et al, 2006).

A urinary steroid profile is helpful in the diagnosis of disorders of steroid biosynthesis. Other investigations that may be warranted include ACTH stimulation test, plasma renin activity, and serum MIF, LH, and FSH. An hCG stimulation test is undertaken to delineate a block in testosterone biosynthesis from androstenedione (17β-hydroxysteroid dehydrogenase deficiency) or conversion of testosterone to DHT (5α-reductase deficiency). An hCG test involves measuring baseline levels of testosterone and its precursors DHEA or DHEA sulfate and androstenedione and its metabolite DHT. One to three intramuscular injections of high-dose hCG are given at 24-hour intervals, and repeat testosterone levels are drawn at 72 hours or 24 hours after the last injection (Ogilvy-Stuart & Brain, 2004).

Imaging studies include pelvic ultrasound to determine presence or absence of gonads in the inguinal region and to assess the müllerian anatomy, pelvic MRI, and urogenital sinugram (retrograde injection of contrast into urogenital sinus opening to confirm presence of and delineate anatomy of lower vagina). Laparoscopic exploration with gonadal biopsy may be necessary to evaluate gonadal histology. Finally, molecular genetic analysis may be required to arrive at a definitive diagnosis for some disorders.

Interpretation of Findings. The most common cause of genital ambiguity in the newborn is 21-hydroxylase deficiency. This form of congenital adrenal hyperplasia, responsible for over 90% of cases of ambiguous genitalia, presents with a virilized XX (female) infant. Among the remainder of cases of ambiguous genitalia, the most common diagnoses are gonadal

TABLE 7-1	Diagnostic Groupings of DSDs, Based on Initial Examinations
Findings	**Disorder(s) Suggested**
Presence of uterus Absence of palpable gonads Hyperpigmentation	Congenital adrenal hyperplasia (21-OHD) in a virilized female
Presence of uterus Asymmetric external genitalia Palpable gonads	Gonadal dysgenesis with Y chromosome or true hermaphroditism
Symmetric external genitalia Palpable gonads Absent uterus	Undervirilized XY male (PAIS or testosterone biosynthetic defect)

From Brown J, Warne G (2005). Practical management of the intersex infant. Journal of pediatric endocrinology & metabolism *18:3-23.*

dysgenesis, followed by partial androgen insensitivity syndrome, and testosterone biosynthetic disorders (Brown & Warne, 2005). It is not always possible to reach a diagnosis in the undervirilized male infant. In a study of 67 XY infants with external sexual ambiguity, testicular tissue, and/or a XY karyotype, in 52% of cases, no diagnosis could be reached, despite an exhaustive clinical and laboratory workup, including sequencing of the androgen receptor (Morel et al, 2002). Provisional diagnostic groupings can be determined based on presence or absence of a uterus, symmetry of the external genitalia, and presence of gonads (Table 7-1), providing a basis for more focused additional investigations (Brown & Warne, 2005).

Talking with Families. Optimal care of the infant with a DSD involves a well-coordinated team approach. The team comprises at minimum the attending neonatologist, neonatal nurse, endocrinologist, pediatric surgeon/pediatric urologic surgeon, social worker, counselor or other mental health professional, and in some instances, geneticist. The initial contact with parents of a newborn with a DSD is extremely important. This interaction should emphasize that a DSD is not a shameful condition and does not preclude the child from becoming a well-adjusted, functional adult (Lee et al, 2006). A single person should be identified to communicate diagnostic findings and plans with the family. When discussing possible diagnoses with the family, language must be carefully chosen. The terms "hermaphrodite" and "pseudohermaphrodite" are outdated, confusing, and perceived as distasteful by many (Houk et al, 2005). These words should be avoided, and instead, accurate, informative terms that describe the infant's diagnosis should be used. A clear explanation of sexual development in the fetus will help parents understand how an infant can be born with atypical genitalia, an important component of parental coping (Houk & Lee, 2005).

It is the parents who have the responsibility to make or defer decisions about care for their infant with a DSD, including gender-of-rearing (Houk & Lee, 2005). The role of the health care team is to provide information, to share and explain all diagnostic findings, to inform parents of all available options, and to support the parents in the decision-making process. The approach should be family-centered as well as culturally sensitive (Thyen et al, 2005). Family concerns must be respected and addressed in strict confidence (Lee et al,

2006). Communication should be open and honest, including candid discussion of the controversies and dilemmas concerning gender assignment and early genital surgery. Parental acceptance of the child with a DSD and condition are key determinants of a favorable outcome (Houk & Lee, 2005).

Gender Assignment. Parents are naturally anxious to find out their baby's gender so that they can name the baby and announce the birth to family and friends. Nevertheless, it must be sensitively communicated that although their distress is acknowledged, when gender is in doubt, a gender-of-rearing decision is one with lifelong implications and cannot be made in haste. Gender assignment must be deferred until expert evaluation of the newborn takes place and sufficient data are available for a fully informed decision (Lee et al, 2006). Unfortunately, some tests required for evaluation of a DSD must be sent out to referral laboratories, and the long wait for results can be frustrating for the parents. It is helpful if an experienced mental health professional can meet very early with the parents to help them formulate what to tell family and friends in the interim (Ogilvy-Stuart & Brain, 2004). All infants should receive a gender assignment as soon as the best course is reasonably determined (Lee et al, 2006).

PANCREAS

The pancreas is both an exocrine and endocrine gland. The endocrine pancreas is responsible for hormonal regulation of blood glucose levels. The endocrine functions are performed by clusters of cells called islets of Langerhans that include alpha, beta, and delta cells. Hormones secreted by the endocrine pancreas include glucagon, insulin, amylin, and somatostatin.

Fetal insulin, present by 8 to 10 weeks' gestation, is secreted in response to both glucose and amino acids. The fetus is critically dependent for growth on its own supply of insulin, which does not cross the placenta. Insulin stimulates uptake of glucose by muscle and adipose tissue. The fetal pancreas becomes progressively more responsive to glucose late in gestation, and β-cell mass increases markedly (Dunne et al, 2004). At birth, when maternal glucose supply ceases, the neonate's blood glucose level declines, along with plasma insulin. A concomitant surge in counter-regulatory hormones epinephrine and glucagon sets in motion the production of glucose that will sustain the neonate until milk feeding is established.

The exocrine portion of the pancreas constitutes 80% of the total gland. Acinar cells secrete digestive enzymes including trypsin, lipase, and amylase into the duodenum. Epithelial cells along the pancreatic ducts secrete bicarbonate and water that neutralize gastric acid.

Disorders of the Pancreas

Rare pancreatic disorders in the newborn include congenital anomalies such as pancreatic agenesis, pancreatic hypoplasia, and annular pancreas. Disorders of the endocrine pancreas include neonatal diabetes mellitus and hyperinsulinism, as well as the developmental disorder of the pancreas seen in the infant of the diabetic mother. The most common newborn disorder of the exocrine pancreas is cystic fibrosis.

Infant of a Diabetic Mother (IDM)

Pathophysiology. If maternal glycemic control is poor in the third trimester, high circulating maternal glucose levels chronically stimulate the fetal pancreas to release insulin,

leading to fetal fat deposition. At birth, the neonatal β-cells take time to adjust to the lower circulating glucose level, and continue to secrete insulin, preventing the mobilization of glycogen and fat as sources of glucose. This failure of normal metabolic adaptation places the baby at risk of hypoglycemia.

Excess fetal insulin may also be the cause of delayed maturation of type II alveolar cells and pulmonary surfactant deficiency seen in some IDMs. Transient functional anomalies of the heart, including cardiomyopathy and intraventricular septal hypertrophy, begin in utero with glycogen loading of the septum (Nold & Georgieff, 2004). A delayed adaptation in parathyroid regulation after birth is the source of hypocalcemia and hypomagnesemia of the IDM. An increase in fetal erythropoiesis leading to polycythemia in the IDM is common but its etiology is unknown. Hyperbilirubinemia results from the presence of an excess hemoglobin, in turn, resulting in a larger than normal bilirubin load.

The higher rate of congenital anomalies associated with diabetic pregnancy is related to maternal glycemic control at the time of conception and during early gestation, when organogenesis is taking place. Congenital malformations associated with maternal diabetes include those of the central nervous system (anencephaly, meningomyelocele, encephalocele, caudal dysplasia), the heart (transposition of the great vessels, coarctation of the aorta, ventricular septal defects, atrial septal defects), the kidneys (hydronephrosis, renal agenesis), and the gastrointestinal tract (duodenal atresia, small left colon syndrome).

Clinical Manifestations. As a result of fat accumulation in late gestation, affected fetuses can develop macrosomia, with birth weights that are not in proportion with their length and head circumference measurements. Intrauterine growth restriction is a less common presentation, seen in advanced maternal diabetic vascular disease. Skin tones may be ruddy with sluggish capillary refill. The neonate may present in respiratory distress. If there is a history of difficult vaginal delivery with shoulder dystocia, the infant may present with musculoskeletal or peripheral nerve findings, suggesting fractured clavicle or humerus or brachial plexus palsy. With the latter condition, the affected arm is held limply at the side, and movements, including Moro responses, are asymmetric. Deep tendon reflexes are absent. Crepitus may be palpated along the clavicle if a fracture is present.

Diagnosis. Macrosomia at birth is a good marker for detecting the infant at risk for neonatal morbidities related to maternal diabetes (Nold & Georgieff, 2004). In spite of the IDM's size, it is also important to determine gestational age to assess the risk of problems related to prematurity. The IDM must be monitored for hypoglycemia, which usually occurs within an hour or two of birth. Objective measurements of blood and plasma glucose should be used rather than relying on symptoms of hypoglycemia, because the latter are nonspecific and unreliable. Point-of-care blood glucose test results indicating hypoglycemia (<40 mg/dl in the newborn) should be verified with a serum laboratory glucose; however, treatment should not be delayed while awaiting the results of the laboratory test. If no treatment is initiated and the serum glucose confirms hypoglycemia, valuable time is wasted, but if treatment is begun and the serum glucose is actually higher than the point-of-care glucose, the treatment is relatively benign.

Additional testing required for the IDM is a serum calcium concentration and, if this is low, a serum magnesium.

Hemoglobin level should be measured with a venous, rather than a capillary, blood sample. Additional diagnostic tests will depend on findings of the initial physical examination.

Collaborative Management. Prevention of hypoglycemia is usually the primary concern in the management of the IDM. Early, frequent milk feedings in stable infants are ideal, if tolerated. Infants born preterm may display immature feeding skills, despite their large size, and require gavage feedings. Severe or persistent hypoglycemia is managed with intravenous glucose boluses, followed by continuous glucose infusion starting at 6 to 8 mg/kg/min. Glucose infusions must be weaned slowly, with close monitoring of blood glucose levels, as the neonate acquires the ability to sustain a normal blood sugar level between feedings.

Neonatal Diabetes Mellitus

Neonatal diabetes mellitus (NDM) is a rare disorder manifested by persistent, insulin-sensitive hyperglycemia occurring as early as the first week of life and lasting more than 2 weeks (Sperling, 2005). About half of all cases of NDM are of the transient form (TNDM), and half the permanent form (PNDM).

Pathophysiology. The fundamental problem in neonatal diabetes mellitus is a failure of the pancreas to release sufficient insulin in response to high blood glucose levels. NDM is unrelated to the presence of anti-insulin or anti-islet cell antibodies. In TNDM, diabetes develops within days of birth and resolves again within weeks or months, before recurring, in a milder form, in late childhood. PNDM develops within days to months after birth and persists throughout life. Most cases of PNDM are caused by transcription factors involved in β-cell development and in insulin secretion, the glucose-sensing enzyme glucokinase, and a gene-regulating immune response. The most common genetic causes are activating mutations of the K_{ATP} channel. Most cases of TNDM are caused by one of three genetic mechanisms: a paternal uniparental isodisomy of chromosome 6, a paternally inherited duplication of 6q24, or a maternal methylation defect within the same region (Sperling, 2005).

Clinical Manifestations. A common feature of NDM is intrauterine growth restriction, a result of insufficient insulin secretion and subsequent failure to thrive in utero. Intrauterine growth restriction in infants with deficient insulin secretion in utero highlights the importance of insulin as a growth hormone. In addition to being small for gestational age, infants with NDM exhibit hyperglycemia, glycosuria, osmotic polyuria, dehydration, and minimal ketoacidosis.

Diagnosis. The diagnosis is made by demonstrating hyperglycemia with low levels of insulin, insulin-like growth factor-1, and C-peptide. The hyperglycemia responds to insulin infusion. Antibodies to insulin or islet cells are absent. If there are signs and symptoms of malabsorption, pancreatic agenesis should be ruled out by abdominal ultrasound. Transient and permanent NDM cannot be differentiated, based on clinical course, in the neonatal period; genetic testing for chromosome 6 anomalies is required (Polak & Shield, 2004).

Collaborative Management. Insulin therapy is necessary to manage hyperglycemia and achieve adequate growth, initially by continuous drip and transitioning to subcutaneous injection of an intermediate-acting insulin preparation when condition permits. A high caloric intake can be difficult to maintain. In some infants, insulin therapy can be withdrawn

after a period of time when it is observed that exogenous insulin induces hypoglycemia. The course of disease in NDM is highly variable. Some infants with transient NDM will have spontaneous recovery with no further disease recurrence, whereas others will have apparent remission with recurrence of permanent disease in late childhood. Infants with permanent NDM have no remission of their disease.

The opportunity for parents to speak with the pediatric endocrinologist and geneticist should be provided, if possible, for information and guidance about both the cause of NDM and the plans for continuing care for their infant. Close follow-up is essential even if the diabetes has resolved because of the high rate of recurrence later in childhood.

Congenital Hyperinsulinism

Congenital hyperinsulinism is the most frequent cause of severe, persistent hypoglycemia in the newborn. Synonyms for this heterogeneous disorder are hyperinsulinemic hypoglycemia (HH) and persistent hyperinsulinemic hypoglycemia of infancy (PHHI). Several different genetic forms have been described. About 10% to 15% of congenital hyperinsulinism is transient and will spontaneously resolve at 1 month of age (deLonlay et al, 2002). Beckwith-Wiedemann syndrome is a congenital overgrowth syndrome with hyperinsulinism caused by β-cell hyperplasia.

Pathophysiology. Hyperinsulinism is due to unregulated insulin release from either the entire pancreas (diffuse β-cell hyperfunction) or from confined areas of the pancreas (focal adenomatous islet-cell hyperplasia). Insulin lowers circulating glucose, suppressing lipolysis and ketogenesis and decreasing the availability of free fatty acids and ketone bodies. Since these are alternative energy substrates for the brain during hypoglycemia, hyperinsulinemia places the infant at risk of severe neurologic dysfunction and seizures as consequences of neuroglycopenia.

Clinical Manifestations. Most infants with congenital hyperinsulinism present within the first postnatal days. Generally they are born at term and are normal or large for gestational age. Many are macrosomic with a characteristic facial appearance.

Neonates with Beckwith-Wiedemann syndrome present with a constellation of findings including macroglossia, abdominal wall defects, Wilms' tumors, renal abnormalities, and facial nevus.

Diagnosis. Congenital hyperinsulinism is recognized by severe hypoglycemia with an insulin level that is inappropriate to the level of blood glucose that is present (e.g., an insulin level >5 microunits/ml with a plasma glucose level <50 mg/dl).

Diagnostic criteria are a high glucose requirement (>6 to 8 m/kg/min) needed to maintain normoglycemia, low serum blood glucose by laboratory analysis, measurable insulin, raised C-peptide, low free fatty acids, and low ketone body concentrations. Blood sampling must take place during hypoglycemia to be of diagnostic value (Lindley & Dunne, 2005). The administration of glucagon during hypoglycemia results in a glycemic response.

Collaborative Management. The cornerstones of management are a high caloric intake and pharmacologic therapy to inhibit insulin secretion by the pancreas. A central venous catheter is required for reliable and safe administration of high glucose infusates during the acute phase. Glucose infusion rates of 10 to 15 mg/kg/min or higher may be required.

Drugs include diazoxide, which inhibits insulin secretion by blocking the sulfonylurea receptor of the β-cell, and octreotide, which is a somatostatin analogue. Diazoxide must be used with caution in the presence of hyperbilirubinemia because it is highly protein bound and will displace bilirubin from albumin binding sites. Glucagon to mobilize hepatic glucose can be added if needed as a short-term adjunct to therapy (Katz & Stanley, 2005).

Unfortunately, the responsiveness of infants with hyperinsulinism to these agents is inconsistent and variable. Babies who do not show an adequate and immediate response may require pancreatectomy to prevent recurrent neuroglycopenia. Preoperative localization procedures and intraoperative biopsies will determine the exact nature of the lesion and how much of the pancreas must be removed. Focal disease may require only a partial pancreatectomy, but a near-total (>95%) removal of the pancreas is indicated for diffuse congenital hyperinsulinism. Loss of the pancreas can pose additional risks such as pancreatic insufficiency and diabetes mellitus.

Cystic Fibrosis

Cystic fibrosis (CF) is an autosomal recessive disorder caused by mutations in the gene encoding for the cystic fibrosis transmembrane conductance regulator (CFTR) protein. Data from newborn screening programs in the United States reveal that CF occurs in 1 of 2500 to 3700 births overall and is most common among non-Hispanic whites (Grosse et al, 2004).

Pathophysiology. Mutations in the CFTR gene affect the cyclic adenosine-5'-monophosphate (AMP)-mediated signals that stimulate chloride conductance in the epithelial cells of the exocrine ducts. Deficient chloride transport and the associated water-transport abnormalities result in the production of abnormally viscid mucus. Nearly all organs and systems of the body are affected, including the lungs and upper respiratory tract, gastrointestinal tract, pancreas, liver, sweat glands, and genitourinary tract. In the neonate, hyperviscous secretions in the intestines and a deficiency of pancreatic enzymes can combine to create a sticky plug of meconium, a condition known as meconium ileus. The meconium has a higher protein and lower carbohydrate concentration, making it more viscid than normal meconium (Irish, 2003).

Clinical Manifestations. Without a family history or prenatal screening, CF is not recognized at the time of birth in most affected neonates unless a meconium ileus is present. A simple meconium ileus is usually identified at 24 to 48 hours of age (occasionally earlier) when there are signs of intestinal obstruction: abdominal distention, bilious vomiting, and either failure to pass meconium or passage of gray-colored stools. On examination, the dilated loops of bowel have a doughy character that indent on palpation. A complicated meconium ileus has a more dramatic presentation with severe abdominal distention, signs of peritonitis such as tenderness, erythema, and clinical evidence of sepsis. The neonate may be acutely ill and require urgent surgical attention. Although not always present in the neonatal period, most patients with CF have pancreatic enzyme insufficiency and present with digestive symptoms or failure to thrive early in life.

Diagnosis. The possibility of CF is raised in the neonate with meconium ileus, and the diagnosis can be confirmed with DNA testing. A sweat test can also be performed after the first 48 hours of life, if the infant is not edematous (Irish, 2003). A sweat test uses electrical-chemical stimulation of the skin to induce sweat, which is collected and analyzed for chloride content. Newborn screening for CF can be accomplished by measuring immunoreactive trypsinogen in dried blood samples. Screening for CF is now universally offered or mandated in 17 states. CF was named as one of 29 conditions that should be included on all state-mandated newborn screening panels (American College of Medical Genetics, 2004). Sometimes a meconium ileus is identified on prenatal ultrasound as a hyperechoic mass in the terminal ileum, representing inspissated meconium, and dilated bowel loops. Postnatal abdominal radiographs show unevenly dilated bowel and, occasionally, a characteristic "soap bubble" pattern, or small bubbles of gas that are caused by air mixing with the tenacious meconium (Irish, 2003).

Collaborative Management. A meconium ileus requires prompt attention to prevent complications such as volvulus, bowel necrosis, or intestinal perforation. Treatment for simple meconium ileus is a therapeutic Gastrograffin (meglumine diatrizoate) enema performed under fluoroscopy. Gastrograffin is a hyperosmolar, radiopaque solution that evacuates the inspissated meconium from the intestine. Gastrograffin is not used in infants with evidence of volvulus, gangrene, perforation, peritonitis, or atresia of the small bowel. The risks of the procedure are ischemia, hypovolemic shock, and perforation. It is essential to provide adequate hydration to compensate for the rapid fluid losses that can occur with the Gastrograffin enema. It usually takes 24 to 48 hours to evacuate the softened meconium, and serial radiographs are usually ordered to monitor the evacuation. Feedings are started when signs of obstruction have subsided (Irish, 2003). An infant who has undergone a Gastrograffin enema should be observed closely for at least 48 hours for signs and symptoms of perforation of the bowel; late perforation is a rare but possible complication as long as 48 hours after the procedure (Irish, 2003).

Cystic fibrosis is also managed with a diet high in energy and fat to compensate for malabsorption and the increased energy demand of chronic inflammation. In addition to vitamin and mineral supplementation, a hydrolyzed protein formula containing medium-chain triglycerides is used. Medium-chain triglycerides do not require digestion by pancreatic enzymes for absorption. Pancreatic enzyme supplements are also needed to improve fat absorption. Meticulous care of the perianal area must be taken because these enzymes can cause severe perianal dermatitis. Finally, of utmost importance, the care of the neonate with cystic fibrosis requires a team approach, in order to provide the family with the necessary resources and anticipatory guidance to manage this disorder and prevent complications for the best possible outcome.

SUMMARY

Some neonatal endocrine disorders are quite rare, and recognizing them requires a high index of suspicion (Palma Sisto, 2004). In recent years, neonatal screening programs have permitted the presymptomatic diagnosis of some of these disorders. This has led to earlier treatment and reduced morbidity, although most endocrine disorders still imply lifelong therapy for the affected infant.

Case Study

IDENTIFICATION OF THE PROBLEM

A 34-week gestation, 1.33-kg male infant was admitted to the NICU for small size and prematurity. Admission vital signs were HR 128, RR 72, BP 42/23 (mean 30), axillary temperature 97.4° F. Blood glucose screen (point of care) was 104.

A peripheral IV was started with $D_{10}W$ at 80 ml/kg/day (GIR 5.5 mg/kg/min) and the infant was made NPO. A repeat blood glucose screen on $D_{10}W$ was 545. In the belief that this was an error, it was repeated, and the result was 550. A serum glucose level was drawn, and the IV fluids were changed to D_5W. The serum glucose was 535. The initial $D_{10}W$ fluid bag was sent to the lab for analysis.

A repeat blood glucose screen on D_5W was 550 (serum 632). IV fluids were changed to normal saline, and the repeat blood glucose was 443 (serum 635). An insulin drip was started at 0.05 units/kg/hr and titrated to maintain blood glucose level <250.

ASSESSMENT: HISTORY AND PHYSICAL EXAMINATION

The infant was born by cesarean section to a 25-year-old G_1P_0 mother following a pregnancy complicated by oligohydramnios. Apgar scores were 7 and 9 and the arterial cord pH was 7.27. Length was 38.5 cm, and head circumference 28 cm, placing him below the 10th percentile for all growth parameters.

Arterial blood gas taken in room air: pH 7.30, pCO_2 35, PO_2 128, base excess –7.7

Following this, 10 ml/kg of normal saline was given for metabolic acidosis.

Examination revealed a small but healthy-appearing male infant, without evidence of respiratory distress.

DIFFERENTIAL DIAGNOSIS

The initial suspected "diagnosis" for the extremely elevated blood glucose in this case was operator error; when the same result was obtained with a repeat specimen and confirmed by serum glucose, it was still viewed with a high degree of suspicion and the intravenous fluids were sent to the laboratory for analysis. The differential diagnosis of hyperglycemia in neonates includes iatrogenic causes, poor insulin sensitivity of the very low birth weight or growth-restricted infant, sepsis, pancreatic agenesis, insulin resistance, transient or permanent neonatal diabetes mellitus, and side effects of medications such as glucocorticoids and theophylline. Several of these were ruled out as they did not apply (the infant was not extremely premature, nor had he received any medications known to cause blood glucose elevation). Furthermore, the problem persisted after changing the IV fluids, ruling out an iatrogenic cause. Insulin resistance was ruled out because the infant responded promptly to an infusion of insulin. He did show evidence of intrauterine growth restriction but it was believed more likely that this was a consequence, rather than a cause, of his primary problem.

DIAGNOSTIC TESTS

The following tests were ordered to further hone in on the cause of hyperglycemia:

CBC: Hct 42%; WBC 4.4; Segs 20; Bands 8; platelets 274,000

Blood cultures were negative at 24 and 48 hours.

Abdominal ultrasound (to rule out pancreatic agenesis): The organ appeared normal.

Insulin autoantibodies were negative. The insulin drip was stopped for 2 hours and insulin and C-peptide levels were drawn.

Results: Insulin level <2 micro–international units/ml
C-peptide <0.5 ng/ml (reference range 0.8 to 3.1 ng/ml)
Concurrent plasma glucose was 412

WORKING DIAGNOSIS

The infant's presentation at birth and clinical course were most consistent with a diagnosis of neonatal diabetes mellitus. He was intrauterine growth restricted, indicating a prenatal onset of the condition, and he had a mild metabolic acidosis. He had no evidence of autoimmune or structural pancreatic disease. He did not have septicemia or evidence of other infection. Furthermore, his laboratory studies revealed severe insulinopenia. The low level of C-peptide, a single-chain amino acid normally released with insulin in equal amounts, supports this diagnosis. It was not known whether his NDM was transient or permanent; this would require molecular genetic analysis, a test that was not done during the initial hospitalization.

DEVELOPMENT OF MANAGEMENT PLAN

The management plan was to reintroduce glucose while continuing the insulin infusion, advancing to total parental nutrition as tolerated. Glucose levels would be monitored at least every 2 hours, with the goal of keeping the blood glucose <250. The plan included the introduction of feedings as early as feasible to improve control of blood glucose. Continuous insulin would be weaned as tolerated. If his diabetes showed no signs of resolution, subcutaneous insulin would be started for long-term management. The infant would continue to be followed by the pediatric endocrinologist.

IMPLEMENTATION AND EVALUATION OF EFFECTIVENESS

Over the first few days, stabilization of the blood glucose level proved difficult. On TPN, the infant fluctuated between hyperglycemia and hypoglycemia. Feedings were introduced and this provided a measure of stability, although weight gain remained slow. The infant was eventually successfully managed with and discharged on subcutaneous insulin.

REFERENCES

American College of Medical Genetics (2004). Newborn screening: toward a uniform screening panel and system. Available at: http://mchb.hrsa.gov/screening. Retrieved August 14, 2005.

Berenbaum SA (2004). Androgens and behavior: implications for the treatment of children with disorders of sexual differentiation. In Pescovitz OH, Eugster EA, editors. *Pediatric endocrinology: mechanisms, manifestations, and management* (pp 275-284). Philadelphia: Lippincott Williams & Wilkins.

Brown J, Warne G (2005). Practical management of the intersex infant. *Journal of pediatric endocrinology & metabolism* 18:3-23.

Crouch NS, Creighton SM (2004). Minimal surgical intervention in the management of intersex conditions. *Journal of pediatric endocrinology & metabolism* 17:1591-1596.

deLonlay P et al (2002). Heterogeneity of persistent hyperinsulinemic hypoglycemia. A series of 175 cases. *European journal of pediatrics* 161:37-38.

Dunne MJ et al (2004). Hyperinsulinism in infancy: from basic science to clinical disease. *Physiological reviews* 84:239-275.

Federman DD (2004). Three facets of sexual differentiation. *New England journal of medicine* 350:323-324.

Ferry RJ (2005). Hormonal control of fluid and electrolytes. In Moshang T, editor. *Pediatric endocrinology* (pp 269-274). St Louis: Elsevier.

Forest MG et al (2004). The virilized female: endocrine background. *BJU international* 93(Suppl 3):35-43.

Fowden AL, Forhead AJ (2004). Endocrine mechanisms of intrauterine programming. *Reproduction* 127:515-526.

Geffner ME (2002). Hypopituitarism in childhood. *Cancer control* 9:212-222.

Goodwin G, Caldamone A (2004). Ambiguous genitalia in the newborn. In Taeusch W et al, editors. *Avery's diseases of the newborn* (pp 1378-1394). Philadelphia: Elsevier.

Grosse SD et al (2004). Centers for Disease Control and Prevention. Newborn screening for cystic fibrosis: evaluation of benefits and risks and recommendations of state newborn screening programs. *MMWR: recommendations and reports* 53:1-36.

Houk CP, Lee PA (2005). Intersexed states: diagnosis and management. *Endocrinology and metabolism clinics of North America* 34:791-810.

Houk CP et al (2005). Intersex classification scheme: a response to the call for change. *Journal of pediatric endocrinology & metabolism* 18:735-738.

Hyun G, Kolon TF (2004). A practical approach to intersex in the newborn period. *Urologic clinics of North America* 31:435-443.

Irish M (2003). Surgical aspects of cystic fibrosis and meconium ileus. *eMedicine*. Available at: http://www.emedicine.com/ped/topic2995.htm. Retrieved August 31, 2005.

Katz LL, Stanley CA (2005). Disorders of glucose and other sugars. In AR Spitzer, editor. *Intensive care of the fetus and neonate* (pp 1167-1179). Philadelphia: Mosby.

Kohler B et al (2005). Androgen insensitivity syndrome: somatic mosaicism of the androgen receptor in seven families and consequences for sex assignment and genetic counseling. *Journal of clinical endocrinology & metabolism* 90:106-111.

Kronenberg H et al (2003). Principles of endocrinology. In Laresen PR, editor. *Williams textbook of endocrinology* (pp 1-9). St Louis: Saunders.

Lawson Wilkins Pediatric Endocrine Society and European Society for Paediatric Endocrine Society (LWPES/ESPE) (2002). Consensus statement on 21-hydroxylase deficiency. *Journal of clinical endocrinology & metabolism* 87:4048-4053.

Lee PA et al (2006). International Consensus Conference on Intersex organized by the Lawson Wilkins Pediatric Endocrine Society and the European Society for Paediatric Endocrinology. Consensus statement on management of intersex disorders. *Pediatrics* 118:e488-e500.

Lindley KJ, Dunne MJ (2005). Contemporary strategies in the diagnosis and management of neonatal hyperinsulinemic hypoglycemic. *Early human development* 81:61-72.

Merke DP, Bornstein SR (2005). Congenital adrenal hyperplasia. *Lancet* 365:2125-2136.

Misra M, Lee MM (2005). Intersex disorders. In Moshang T, editor. *Pediatric endocrinology*. St Louis: Elsevier.

Modi N (1998). Hyponatremia in the newborn. *Archives of disease in childhood fetal neonatal edition* 78:F81-F84.

Morel Y et al (2002). Aetiological diagnosis of male sex ambiguity: a collaborative study. *European journal of pediatrics* 161:49-59.

Muglia LJ, Majzoub JA (2004). Disorders of the posterior pituitary. In Pescovitz OH, Eugster EA, editors. *Pediatric endocrinology: mechanisms, manifestations, and management* (pp 289-322). Philadelphia: Lippincott Williams & Wilkins.

Murphy N et al (2004). The hypothalamic-pituitary-thyroid axis in preterm infants; changes in the first 24 hours of postnatal life. *Journal of clinical endocrinology & metabolism* 89:2824-2831.

National Newborn Screening and Genetics Resource Center (NNSGRC) (July 28, 2005). U.S. national newborn screening status report. Available at: http://genes-r-us.uthscsa.edu/nbsdisorders.pdf. Retrieved August 8, 2005.

Ng PC et al (2004). Transient adrenocortical insufficiency of prematurity and systemic hypotension in very low birthweight infants. *Archives of disease in childhood fetal neonatal edition* 89:F119-F126.

Nold JL, Georgieff MK (2004). Infants of diabetic mothers. *Pediatric clinics of North America* 51:619-637.

Ogilvy-Stuart AL (2002). Neonatal thyroid disorders. *Archives of disease in childhood fetal neonatal edition* 87:F165-F171.

Ogilvy-Stuart AL, Brain CE (2004). Early assessment of ambiguous genitalia. *Archives of disease in childhood* 89:401-407.

Palma Sisto PA (2004). Endocrine disorders in the neonate. *Pediatric clinics of North America* 51:1141-1168.

Park SM, Chatterjee VKK (2005). Genetics of congenital hypothyroidism. *Journal of medical genetics* 42:379-389.

Polak M, Shield J (2004). Neonatal and very-early-onset diabetes mellitus. *Seminars in neonatology* 9:59-65.

Polk DH, Fisher DA (2004). Disorders of the thyroid gland. In Taeusch W et al, editors. *Avery's diseases of the newborn* (pp 1399-1410). Philadelphia: Elsevier.

Rubin L (2004). Embryology, developmental biology, and anatomy of the endocrine system. In Taeusch W et al, editors. *Avery's diseases of the newborn* (pp 1335-1343). Philadelphia: Elsevier.

Saborio P et al (2000). Diabetes insipidus. *Pediatrics in review* 21:122-129.

Speiser PW, White PC (2003). Congenital adrenal hyperplasia. *New England journal of medicine* 349:776-788.

Sperling MA (2005). Neonatal diabetes mellitus: from understudy to center stage. *Current opinion in pediatrics* 17:512-518.

Sultan C et al (2002). Ambiguous genitalia in the newborn. *Seminars in reproductive medicine* 20:181-188.

Therrell BL (2001). Newborn screening for congenital adrenal hyperplasia. *Endocrinology and metabolism clinics of North America* 30:15-29.

Thyen U et al (2005). Deciding on gender in children with intersex conditions. *Treatments in endocrinology* 4:1-8.

Toppari J (2002). Environmental endocrine disrupters and disorders of sexual differentiation. *Seminars in reproductive medicine* 20:305-311.

Tuladhar R et al (1998). Establishment of a normal range of penile length in preterm infants. *Journal of paediatric and child health* 35:471-473.

van Wassenaer AG, Kok JH (2004). Hypothyroxinaemia and thyroid function after preterm birth. *Seminars in neonatology* 9:3-11.

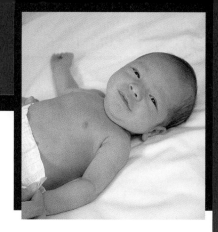

Chapter 8

Genitourinary System

Leslie Parker

Comprehensive nursing care of infants with renal or genital disorders requires a thorough understanding of normal anatomy and physiology. Because the development of the renal and genital systems arises from shared structures, abnormalities in one system can affect the development of the other. Because nurses provide hands-on care to infants in both the newborn nursery and the neonatal intensive care unit, they are often the first to recognize abnormalities in the renal and genital systems. To readily identify such disorders and participate in their collaborative management, nurses need a clear understanding of the normal anatomy and physiology of the genital and renal systems and the pathologic processes that may be present in the neonatal patient.

The kidneys function to maintain fluid, electrolyte, and acid-base balance as well as to rid the body of nitrogenous waste. Perinatal depression, medical management for common neonatal conditions, and dehydration are only a few of many factors that place the newborn at risk for renal compromise. Timely, accurate nursing assessment and intervention is of utmost priority to ensure optimal outcome for the infant and their families.

This chapter outlines the anatomy, physiology, and assessment of the genitourinary system. It also describes various abnormalities and disease processes commonly identified in the neonatal period—including pathophysiology, diagnosis, and treatment.

THE URINARY SYSTEM

The urinary system consists of the kidneys, ureters, urinary bladder, and the urethra (Figure 8-1). In utero, the placenta regulates fluid and electrolyte balance and acid-base homeostasis and functions as the excretory organ for the fetus. Functional kidneys are therefore not necessary for fetal homeostasis. Consequently, pathologic conditions such as aplastic, hypoplastic, and otherwise nonfunctioning kidneys may not be detected until after birth. Fetal urination, swallowing, and breathing affect amniotic fluid volume. Excretion of fetal urine contributes significantly to amniotic fluid volume, especially during the third trimester. A reduction in fetal urine excretion results in potentially severe oligohydramnios.

A balance among genetic influences, cellular mediators, and the interaction of various molecular mechanisms is necessary for the initiation and development of the kidney. Depending on the timing of development, insult or failure of the primitive structures to grow or to branch appropriately may result in a variety of uropathies—including dysplasia and renal agenesis.

PHYSIOLOGY OF KIDNEY FUNCTION

The structure of the kidney includes the cortex, the major and minor calices, and the renal pelvis (Figure 8-2). The functions of the kidney include regulation of fluid and electrolyte balance, regulation of arterial blood pressure, and excretion of toxic and waste substances. These regulatory mechanisms are all intimately tied to the formation of urine. Three basic processes are involved in the formation of urine: ultrafiltration of plasma by the glomerulus, reabsorption of water and solutes from the ultrafiltrate, and secretion of certain solutes into the tubular fluid (Koeppen & Stanton, 2001). The kidney is divided into two sections, the outer renal cortex and the inner medulla.

The nephron, which is the site of urine formation, is the functional unit of the kidney. It consists of a glomerulus (Bowman's capsule and glomerular capillaries), and a renal tubule that has three sections: a proximal convoluted tubule, the loop of Henle, and a distal convoluted tubule (Figure 8-3). After urine is produced by the kidney, it drains into the minor and major calyces, which are cuplike structures. Urine then drains into a single large cavity called the renal pelvis, out through the ureter, and into the bladder. The process of nephron formation—nephrogenesis—begins during the 2nd month of gestation and is anatomically complete by approximately 35 weeks' gestation. Functional immaturity of the nephrons continues throughout infancy. Renal development will progress at the same rate regardless of gestational age at birth. At the completion of nephrogenesis, each kidney contains approximately 1 million nephrons.

Nephrogenesis begins deep within the renal cortex near the medulla in the juxtamedullary region and continues outwardly (Koeppen & Stanton, 2001). The juxtamedullary nephrons differ from the superficial cortical nephrons in that their glomeruli are larger; the loop of Henle is longer; and the efferent arteriole forms a more complex vascular system. The less mature superficial cortical nephrons make up the majority of nephrons; the more mature juxtamedullary nephrons account for a very small percentage of the total number (Nafday et al, 2005). Altered renal function in the premature infant may therefore be caused by anatomic as well as physiologic immaturity.

Renal Blood Flow

Urine formation begins with blood flow. The pressure-driven process of ultrafiltration depends on optimal arterial pressure and is regulated by the dilatation and constriction of afferent and efferent arterioles (Koeppen & Stanton, 2001). Adequate renal blood flow is therefore essential to kidney function.

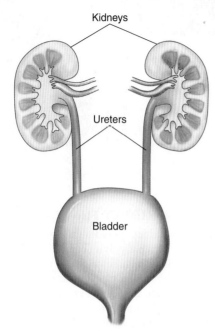

FIGURE **8-1**
The renal system.

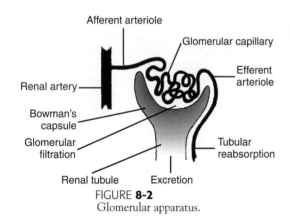

FIGURE **8-2**
Glomerular apparatus.

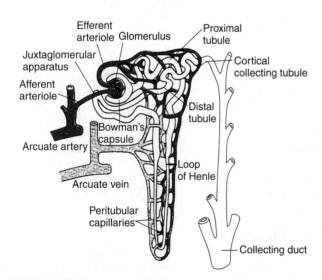

FIGURE **8-3**
The nephron. From Guyton AC, Hall JE (1997). *Human physiology and mechanisms of disease*, ed 6. Philadelphia: Saunders.

During the first 12 hours of life, 4% to 6% of the cardiac output goes to the kidney; this increases to 8% to 10% over the next few days. This is compared to 25% in the adult. Renal blood flow not only provides oxygen and nutrients to the kidneys but also affects the rate of solute and water reabsorption by the proximal tubule, participates in the concentration and dilution of the urine, and delivers substrates for excretion in the urine.

The left and right renal arteries arise from the aorta. After entering the kidneys, they divide and branch several times to eventually give rise to the afferent arterioles. Each nephron receives one afferent arteriole, which after dividing forms the glomerulus. The distal ends of the glomerular capillaries merge to form the efferent arterioles, which carry blood away from the glomerulus. The efferent arterioles divide to form the peritubular capillaries, which surround the tubular parts of the nephron in the renal cortex. Other vessels called the vasa recta also arise from the efferent arterioles to surround the tubular parts of the nephron in the renal medulla. The peritubular capillaries empty into the venous system and eventually leave the kidneys in the form of the renal vein. The fetus and infant have a decreased renal blood flow due to increased renal vascular resistance and decreased mean arterial pressure. The renal vascular resistance is elevated in the fetus because fetal renal function is required only for production of amniotic fluid (Blackburn, 2003). Renal blood flow increases with advancing gestational and chronologic age.

Glomerular Filtration

As blood flows into the kidney via the renal artery, it is directed into the afferent arteriole that carries it into the glomerulus, which consists of the glomerular capillaries and Bowman's capsule. Plasma that is driven through the glomerular capillaries is filtered through the filtration barrier, and the protein-free plasma, or ultrafiltrate, is forced into Bowman's capsule or leaves via the efferent arteriole and enters into the renal vein. To produce this ultrafiltrate, the glomerulus functions as a filtering site. Glomerular capillaries are lined with epithelial cells that are called podocytes. These podocytes form one of the layers of Bowman's capsule (see Figure 8-3). The endothelial cells of the glomerular capillaries are covered by a basement membrane that is also surrounded by podocytes. The basement membrane, podocytes, and the endothelial cell of the glomerular capillaries form the filtration barrier. The epithelial cells of this filtration barrier express negatively charged glycoproteins and contain many small openings that are called fenestrations. The size of the fenestrations inhibits passage of large proteins such as blood cells and platelets but is highly permeable to passage of water, small solutes, urea, and glucose. In addition, positively charged large proteins are repelled by the cationic cell membrane (Koeppen & Stanton, 2001).

The glomerular filtration rate (GFR) is the rate at which fluid is filtered through the glomerulus. Because it is equal to the sum of all filtration rates of all nephrons in both kidneys, the GFR reflects kidney function, with a decrease in GFR signaling renal disease. Oncotic and hydrostatic pressures (Starling forces) drive the ultrafiltration process. Oncotic pressure is osmotic pressure generated by large proteins or colloids. Hydrostatic pressure, on the other hand, is pressure exerted by fluids in equilibrium and depends on arterial pressure and vascular resistance (Koeppen & Stanton, 2001).

Oncotic pressure in Bowman's space is very near zero because ultrafiltrate is nearly protein-free. Filtration at this level is therefore driven by hydrostatic pressure across the glomerular capillaries. Hydrostatic pressure within Bowman's space and glomerular oncotic pressure oppose glomerular hydrostatic pressure in the capillaries. The GFR is proportional to the sum of hydrostatic and oncotic pressures that exist along the renal capillaries multiplied by the ultrafiltration coefficient. The difference between the permeability of the glomerular capillary and the glomerular surface area available for filtration is the ultrafiltration coefficient (Koeppen & Stanton, 2001). GFR is therefore affected by changes in arterial blood pressure, vascular resistance, concentration of plasma proteins, and glomerular capillary permeability. Alteration in the permeability of the glomerular capillaries may result from inherent damage to the capillary, thus altering the pore size or changing the electrical charge within the membrane. GFR may also be affected by urinary system obstruction.

GFR in the fetus is relatively low because of increased renal vascular resistance and decreased renal blood flow. It increases rapidly in the first few hours following birth. The filtration rate increases with increasing gestational age and continues after birth because of an increase in number and growth of the nephrons (Blackburn, 2003). The GFR reaches full-term levels by 32 to 35 weeks' gestation. In the preterm infant functional maturation is determined by conceptional age, not by postnatal age (Solhaug et al, 2004). When corrected for body surface area, GFR is reportedly 10 ml/min/1.73 m^2 at 28 weeks' gestation and rises to 30 ml/min/1.73 m^2 at term. The GFR, even in the term infant, is low compared to that in the older infant or child. This low GFR is adequate in normal circumstances, but in adverse conditions such as sepsis, hypoxia, or the administration of nephrotoxic medications, the GFR may not meet the physiologic needs of the infant (Toth-Heyn et al, 2000). The rise in GFR is not caused by an increase in nephrons; rather it is believed to reflect a decrease in vascular resistance and an increase in glomerular surface area (Riccabona, 2004). Medications given to control various maternal conditions have had detrimental effects on fetal GFR and subsequent neonatal renal function. Examples of these drugs have included beta-adrenergic antagonists (ritodrine hydrochloride), prostaglandin inhibitors (indomethacin), nonsteroidal anti-inflammatories, and angiotensin-converting enzyme inhibitors (Benini et al, 2004; Itabashi et al, 2003; Tabacova & Kimmel, 2001).

Assessment of GFR is important in evaluating renal function. One method of assessing GFR is measurement of the renal clearance of a substance. Renal clearance represents a volume of plasma completely cleared of a substance by the kidneys over a specified period of time (Koeppen & Stanton, 2001). Various substances are used as markers for measuring GFR. Marker substances must do the following: (1) freely filter across the glomerulus into Bowman's space; (2) not be reabsorbed or secreted by the nephron; (3) not be metabolized or produced by the kidney; and (4) not alter GFR (Koeppen & Stanton, 2001). Para-aminohippurate (PAH) is a substance that the body does not produce, that is secreted by the proximal tubules, and that meets the marker criteria. PAH, which is nearly completely cleared, moves through the renal tubules so that it is effectively cleared via plasma movement within the kidney. Therefore measurement of the renal clearance of PAH can determine the effective renal plasma flow.

This is significant because measurement of the effective renal plasma flow is a direct way of determining the renal functioning. However, this measurement is only accurate at low plasma concentrations of PAH. PAH is not produced by the body; therefore, it must be administered by infusion. Insulin also may be used as a tag substance for testing the intactness of the kidney's filtering system and glomerular filtration rate (Koeppen & Stanton, 2001). However, it too must be administered via infusion.

Creatinine, a by-product of muscle metabolism, also meets the marker criteria. Measurement of serum creatinine levels is clinically the most useful method of estimating renal function in neonates. Because creatinine readily crosses the placenta, levels obtained during the first week reflect maternal levels. After birth, the GFR in term infants increases as renal blood flow increases and vascular resistance decreases. This increase in function usually occurs over the first week of life and results in a drop in creatinine levels to nearly 0.4 mg/dl, depending on clinical status and gestational age. GFR does not increase as drastically until the completion of nephrogenesis. Therefore premature infants do not demonstrate the same decline in serum creatinine levels as infants born after 36 weeks' gestation. Small increases in serum creatinine levels may indicate a significant decrease in GFR. Monitoring trends in serial creatinine levels may therefore render a more accurate evaluation of renal function.

Regulation of renal blood flow—and consequently GFR—is achieved by hormonal and sympathetic nervous system (SNS) influences. The renal vessels, including the afferent and efferent arterioles, are highly innervated by sympathetic nerve fibers. Mild stimulation of the SNS does not cause a change in renal vascular tone. However, under severe physiologic stress such as that caused by significant fluid loss, activation of the renal sympathetic nerve fibers causes vasoconstriction of the renal arteries, which in turn decreases GFR.

Hormonal control is exerted mainly via activation of the renin-angiotensin-aldosterone system (RAS). The RAS plays a significant role in blood pressure regulation and sodium homeostasis. Renin is an enzyme that is found in high levels in the plasma and is produced and stored in the specialized cells of the juxtaglomerular apparatus. It is found in the fetus, beginning at about 3 months' gestation. Newborns have a significantly higher renin level than adults. This high level may be related to the neonate's altered glomerular filtration rate, vascular resistance, and renal blood flow.

When renal blood flow is diminished as the result of a decrease in arterial pressure, the vessel walls of the afferent arterioles are less stretched and the release of renin is stimulated. Renin then leads to the production of angiotensin I from angiotensin that is synthesized in the liver, which is then converted by angiotensin-converting enzyme to angiotensin II. Angiotensin II then stimulates secretion of aldosterone by the adrenal cortex. Aldosterone in turn triggers the increased reabsorption of sodium and water, thereby increasing extracellular fluid volume and renal perfusion (Figure 8-4). The ultimate goal of the renin-angiotensin cycle is to maintain adequate systemic blood flow to supply the body's vital organs (Tortora & Grabowski, 2003).

Renal prostaglandins are very potent vasoactive hormones. They are manufactured in the renal medulla and act to balance the RAS via vasodilatation, natriuresis, and diuresis. This action opposes the hormone angiotensin II, which acts as a vasoconstrictor and stops or reduces renin secretion.

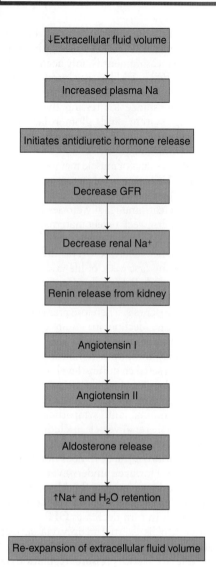

FIGURE 8-4
The renin-angiotensin-aldosterone regulation of extracellular fluid.

Similar to other organs, the renal blood flow and GFR are maintained fairly constantly over a range of arterial blood pressures, mainly via autoregulation. Renal autoregulation is accomplished by at least two mechanisms: the pressure-sensitive myogenic mechanism and the flow-dependent tubuloglomerular feedback mechanism. The myogenic mechanism functions by dilation or constriction of the afferent arterioles. When smooth vascular muscles are stretched, they tend to contract. When arterial pressure increases, the renal afferent arteriole stretches, thus causing the smooth muscle to contract. The increase in resistance within the arteriole offsets the increase in pressure, and thus this myogenic mechanism maintains renal blood flow and GFR at a relatively constant state. Although the myogenic mechanism may be intrinsic to all organ systems, the tubuloglomerular feedback mechanism is unique to the renal system. The tubuloglomerular feedback mechanism causes an increase or decrease in GFR and renal blood flow in response to the flow of tubular fluid within the nephrons. A key component of the tubuloglomerular feedback mechanism is the juxtaglomerular apparatus (JGA). The JGA consists of the macula densa, the extraglomerular mesangial

cells, and the granular cells of the afferent and efferent arterioles that produce rennin (Koeppen & Stanton, 2001). A change in the flow of tubular fluid is sensed by the macula densa, which in turn triggers a signal that causes a change in afferent artery resistance. The change in resistance in the afferent arteriole then either increases or decreases GFR and renal blood flow.

Secretion and Reabsorption
The kidneys control fluid and electrolyte balance by reabsorption and secretion of sodium and water. The four segments of the nephron—the proximal tubule, loop of Henle, distal tubule, and the collecting duct—determine the composition and volume of urine.

In the neonate the thin, ascending portion, which controls reabsorption, is not fully formed, because nephron formation starts in the medullary area. By birth, it has extended from the medullary to the juxtamedullary area. The descending portion of the tubular system, which controls urine secretion, thus is more fully developed than the ascending segment at birth. The ability to concentrate urine is decreased in the newborn because although urine secretion occurs readily, reabsorption is limited. The infant is more likely to lose sodium, glucose, and other solutes in the urine. This process is further reduced in the preterm infant and may result in significant fluid and electrolyte disturbances.

Tubular reabsorption, secretion, and excretion are tied closely together. These processes are concerned with the maintenance of the internal homeostasis. This maintenance depends on a flexible and dynamic reabsorption pattern that responds to other body systems.

Tubular reabsorption is the process where substances from the tubular lumen move into the capillary system. It occurs by simple diffusion and active transport (Tortora & Grabowski, 2003). Many of the body's nutrients, electrolytes, and 99% of the filtered water are reabsorbed, thus achieving a balance for continued growth and normal physiologic function. Simple diffusion involves movement of substances down a gradient—from an area of higher to an area of lower concentration. Active transport requires energy derived directly from adenosine triphosphate because the net movement of substances is against a gradient. Molecular structures may link together to piggyback—or carry one another—across the membrane. Sodium first undergoes simple diffusion across the tubular membrane and then is transported via this mechanism of active transport by the sodium pump into the interstitial fluid. Sodium filtration depends on the glomerular filtration rate. Thus a higher glomerular filtration rate results in an increase in sodium reabsorption into the vascular space. If the extracellular fluid volume increases, sodium reabsorption is decreased. Thus the regulation of fluids and electrolytes is highly complex because sodium, in turn, influences other substances to move against their gradients.

Water follows the sodium ion across the membrane and into the capillary bed. This type of transport of a second substance is often referred to as secondary active transport. Simple facilitated diffusion is similar to active transport in that a carrier substance is used, but the net movement is not against a gradient. Glucose is one secondary substance that secondary active transport carries along with sodium across the membrane. Glucose is reabsorbed by the proximal tubules, thus appearing in the urine only when the renal threshold or the maximal tubular transport capacity has been exceeded or when the permeability of the filtering capillaries has been altered. Amino acids, water-soluble vitamins, albumin, and lactate are also transported in this fashion.

Tubular secretion moves substances from the epithelial lining of the tubules' capillaries into the interstitial fluid and finally into the lumen. Thus the substances are secreted into the tubular lumen. Potassium and hydrogen undergo tubular secretion. Tubular excretion—the process by which substances enter into the filtrate that will eventually exit the body as urine—is linked with the secretion just described. Ions such as potassium, which are secreted in the distal tubule (a portion is also reabsorbed in the proximal tubule), find their way into the urine when the body has no need for higher concentration levels. The movement of hydrogen ions influences the excretion of potassium; thus metabolic acidosis and alkalosis affect potassium levels. Hormones and drugs, especially diuretics, affect potassium movement. In the presence of aldosterone, potassium is secreted; thiazides, in contrast, result in potassium excretion. Other filtrates that present in the urine include urea, creatinine, and other ions that are not needed by the body.

The regulation of fluids and electrolytes is an important function of the processes of tubular secretion, reabsorption, and excretion. Excretion of toxins, drugs, and other by-products of metabolism is also important and has been previously mentioned.

ASSESSMENT OF THE GENITOURINARY SYSTEM
History
Having a thorough familial history on record for neonates suspected of having urogenital abnormalities is imperative. Many urogenital problems have an inheritance pattern, which suggests genetic predisposition. The history should focus on any family members who have renal transplants or have undergone dialysis, those with a history of renal failure, and those with cystic kidney disease or anomalies of the GU system. A review of the history should also include any prior fetal or neonatal deaths. Are there any abnormalities of the external genitalia, such as hypospadias, ambiguous genitalia, or undescended testicles? Do any members have low-set ears, or were they born with a single umbilical artery? Prenatal histories should be reviewed for antepartal factors that may predispose the infant to renal problems. Were oligohydramnios or abdominal distention present on prenatal ultrasonography? Was there a history of perinatal depression?

Neonatal history should include the following questions:
1. Has micturition taken place? If so, at what age? (The first voiding may occur in the delivery room and should be documented by 24 hours of life.)
2. Has the infant undergone any significant hypoxic episodes that may result in decreased renal blood flow?
3. Is the fluid intake sufficient relative to clinical status, gestational age, and immediate environment (radiant warmer or humidified isolette)? The radiant warmer increases insensible water loss.
4. Is the infant under treatment for jaundice? (Phototherapy increases fluid losses.)
5. Is the infant experiencing any bleeding or increased GI losses from nasogastric suctioning, vomiting, diarrhea, or increased ostomy output?
6. What is the specific gravity of urine? (Normal range is 1.003 to 1.015.)
7. What is the infant's age?
8. Has the infant received any nephrotoxic medications?
9. What is the infant's blood pressure? (Hypotension can indicate volume depletion, whereas hypertension [HTN] is associated with an underlying renal abnormality.)

Physical Assessment
Physical examination should include inspection, palpation, and percussion. Auscultation is not generally useful for the renal system.

Inspection
Observation of the abdominal region is an important place to start. Is distention present? If so, is it unilateral or generalized? Mild abdominal protuberance in the neonate may be a normal finding because the abdominal musculature is relatively weak at birth in comparison to the eventual state of the musculature several months after birth. Absence of muscle tone is a characteristic finding in prune-belly syndrome. Abdominal asymmetry is an abnormal finding. Is drainage coming from the umbilicus? Does the bladder appear distended?

Next, the genital area is inspected. Peritoneal tissue that leads to the anal opening should be intact and smooth in appearance. Any abnormal openings, depressions, or swellings should be noted. The anus is normally located midline and should be tested for patency by gentle insertion of a gloved, well-lubricated small finger. Gentle stroking of the anal tissue and observation for anal sphincter constriction may test the anal wink, which indicates muscle tone. Inspection is also made for meconium or stool.

Male. Inspect the skin over the scrotum for color, rugae, edema, or ecchymosis. If the infant is a full-term male, the scrotal sac should be full, and rugae should be present. The premature male infant exhibits a generally flaccid, smooth scrotal sac. The scrotum is generally darkly pigmented, without bluish discoloration. A blue color may denote disruption of circulation to the area indicating the presence of a possible testicular torsion. The scrotum that is enlarged or edematous may accompany a hydrocele (a trapping of fluid in the tunica vaginalis), or it may result from pressure on this tissue during the birth process, especially during a breech delivery. If a hydrocele is suspected, transillumination of the scrotum with a good light source, such as a transilluminator or a flashlight, helps determine the presence of fluid. On transillumination, fluid allows light to pass through it and shows as a highly lightened area.

Penile size, resting position, and position of the urinary meatus should be assessed. If the penile structure is abnormally large or small in proportion to the gestational age and the rest of the body parts, a genital problem may be present. Micropenis—penile hypoplasia with an otherwise normal appearance—is associated with a number of clinical syndromes or chromosomal aberrations. The penis is generally straight. Downward incurvation, bowing, or chordee is most often associated with hypospadias. Priapism, or a constantly erect penis, is also an abnormal finding. The urinary meatus should be located midline on the ventral portion of the glans penis. Alterations of position result in dorsal or ventral placement anywhere along the shaft of the penis. This condition is known as epispadias if the urinary meatus is on the dorsum of the penis or as hypospadias if the opening is displaced along the ventral penile surface. The foreskin of the uncircumcised male is gently retracted for accurate observation and then should be returned to its unretracted state after inspection; otherwise, swelling with associated decreased circulation to the glans penis may occur.

Female. Inspect the female infant's labia, clitoris, urinary meatus, and external vaginal orifice. The labia minora in the term infant should be well formed. The labia majora should be present and should extend beyond the labia minora. The labia minora in the premature female infant may be larger than the labia majora. The less mature the female infant, the smaller the labia majora. The labia may have a dark pigmentation. This is of no clinical significance. Clitoral tissue should be present. The clitoris may be enlarged in both full-term and preterm infants. Because the labia may not be fully developed, the clitoris of preterm infants may be quite prominent. The urinary meatus should be patent and anterior to the vaginal orifice. The vagina should be inspected for patency, and any vaginal secretions should be noted. A white, milky vaginal secretion in the first few days of life, followed by pseudomenses or slight vaginal bleeding, is a normal finding. A hymenal tag may be present. The hymenal tag usually disappears within a few weeks and is a normal finding with no clinical significance.

Both Sexes. Bruising and related swelling of the genitalia following breech delivery should be appropriately documented. Ecchymosis and sometimes hematomas may also be observed after traumatic delivery. These birth-related findings are transient and should resolve within several days. Although inguinal hernias may be found in either sex, they occur less often in females. The urinary stream should be continuous and straight. The genital and peritoneal regions must be observed to ensure that a clear differentiation of the sexes is possible. If it is not, ambiguous genitalia must be considered (see Chapter 7).

Palpation

This portion of the physical examination may be upsetting to the neonate and thus is best left until last. Place the infant in the supine position with the knees and hips flexed and provide a means of nonnutritive sucking for the infant. This position usually puts the infant at ease and facilitates relaxation of the abdominal muscles. The abdomen is then gently palpated with a gradual downward movement, anteriorly to posteriorly. The kidneys may be felt on deep palpation. Another technique that is sometimes successful is placing the infant again in the supine position and then placing the fingers of one hand along the flank with the thumb while palpating the abdomen. This technique allows the examiner to possibly trap the kidney's pole between the fingers and the thumb (ballottement). The kidneys are only reliably palpated in the first 1 to 2 days of life (Hernandez & Glass, 2005).

On palpation, the kidneys should be bilaterally equal in size. The right kidney may be slightly lower than the left kidney because of the position of other abdominal organs. No masses should be felt during abdominal palpation. However, if one is encountered, its position, mobility on palpation, and contour (flat, lumpy, or depressed) must be accurately described. The majority of abdominal masses involve the kidney. The most common cause of an enlarged kidney in the neonate is hydronephrosis, and the second is multicystic kidney disease (Vogt & Avner, 2002). Bladder distention or ureterocele may present as a mobile mass. If Wilms' tumor is suspected, palpation is contraindicated. Palpation in this instance may break the tumor into small fragments, thus leading to tumor seeding.

Male. Palpate the scrotal sac for each testis and cord. If the testis is absent, palpate along the canal to assess location. The scrotal sac may be palpated by gentle pressing of the tissue between two fingers—one on the anterior surface and the other on the posterior surface. Gentle movement of the fingers upward over the scrotum until the testes are detected bilaterally indicates whether one or both testes are descended and their location in relationship to the internal ring in the inguinal canal. Until 28 weeks' gestation, the testes are abdominal organs. Between 28 and 30 weeks, they begin to descend into the inguinal canal. The cremasteric reflex, recoil of the testes toward the inguinal canal, may be elicited by gentle stroking of the upper thigh or scrotal sac.

Percussion

If bladder distention is palpated or observed, percussion should be performed. This technique is useful in determining whether fluid is filling the bladder, a situation denoted by a somewhat tympanic sound; if a solid mass is present, dullness is noted. Percussion may also be used over the entire abdominal region. Examination of the abdomen and intestinal area is discussed in depth in Chapter 5.

Related Findings

Neonates should be inspected for general characteristics that strongly suggest renal abnormalities. Potter's facies (flattened, beaklike nose; wide-set eyes; micrognathia; disproportionately large ears; short neck) accompanied by abnormal positioning of the hands and feet and pulmonary hypoplasia are all associated with oligohydramnios. These characteristics may indicate the presence of a renal disorder. One should assess for characteristics consistent with the presence of a genetic syndrome. Syndromes commonly have associated renal anomalies. Presence of a single umbilical artery is also a common finding when renal problems are present. The ears should be assessed for abnormalities; preauricular ear tags have been associated with urinary tract abnormalities (Kugelman et al, 2002; Srinivasan & Arora, 2005).

Meningomyelocele and other neural tube defects may result in decreased or absent innervation to the bladder. The result may be a neurogenic bladder characterized by bladder distention. If untreated, the urinary stasis ultimately leads to urinary and cystic infection.

Various syndromes that have associated renal and genital problems are listed in Table 8-1.

RISK FACTORS

Table 8-2 lists maternal, neonatal, and other risks associated with urogenital disorders. Specific risk factors for each of the urogenital dysfunctions are addressed in the appropriate sections.

DIAGNOSTIC WORKUP

The diagnostic workup for potential renal problems includes several diagnostic screening tests.

Urine Collection

Urine collection is a relatively simple procedure in the neonate. Several adhesive-backed collection bags are available. Care should be taken not to include the rectum or scrotum within the opening of the bag. The penis should not be left in urine because infection and skin irritation may occur. Skin irritation

TABLE 8-1	Syndromes Associated with the Development of Urogenital Disorders	
Syndromes	**Renal Component**	**Genital Component**
Potter's association	Renal agenesis	Absence of vas deferens, seminal vesicle, upper vagina, uterus
Meckel's syndrome	Polycystic kidneys	Ambiguous genitalia
		Hypoplastic phallus
		Cryptorchidism
Trisomy 21	Cystic kidneys and other renal anomalies	Hypoplastic penis and scrotum
		Cryptorchidism
Trisomy 18	Dysplastic renal system	Hypoplastic clitoris and labia minora
		Cryptorchidism
Turner's syndrome	Horseshoe kidney	Infantile genitalia
	Duplications of the collecting system	
Prune-belly syndrome	Urinary tract dysplasia	
	Bladder and ureter dilation	
	Patent urachus	Cryptorchidism
Errors of metabolism	Renal tubular dysfunction	
Galactosemia		
Tyrosinemia		
Glycogen storage		
(Gierke's) disease		
Adrenogenital syndrome		Masculinization of the female
		Incomplete masculinization of the male
		Clitoral hypertrophy
Hypospadias		
Hypoplastic penis		
Cryptorchidism		

with the use of these bags is possible; therefore care should be taken to maintain skin integrity. Alternative collection systems can be used if sterile specimens are not required and accurate measurement of output is not needed. Cotton balls can be placed inside diapers to catch a small specimen for dipstick analysis or for measurement of specific gravity. Many institutions now use superabsorbency disposable diapers. The super-absorbent material can potentially alter the results of the urine test. Further nursing research is needed to evaluate accuracy of laboratory values in these newer products. In male infants, test tubes or syringe barrels may be secured to the penis to collect small specimens.

When sterile urine specimens are required for culture, a suprapubic bladder tap or urethral catheterization should be performed. The performance of the suprapubic tap requires minimal equipment and time. The lower abdomen is prepared with an antimicrobial solution and allowed to dry. If the infant has voided within the previous hour, the attempt should be delayed until the infant has a full bladder. If severe dehydration, abdominal congenital anomalies, or distention are present, a suprapubic tap may not be indicated. The procedure is usually performed with a 3-ml syringe with a 23- to 25-gauge straight needle. The needle is placed midline, 1 to 1.5 cm above the symphysis pubis, and is inserted perpendicularly or at a slight angle, pointing toward the head. Entry into the bladder is determined when resistance decreases as the needle is inserted. A slight traction on the plunger facilitates aspiration of urine into the syringe. If no urine is obtained on the first attempt, a second attempt should be delayed until sufficient urine buildup has occurred. At the completion of the procedure, pressure should be applied over the puncture site until all evidence of bleeding has ceased.

This procedure may have complications such as uterine and bowel perforations, trauma to other portions of the renal system, and infection. The procedure is not recommended for any neonate with clotting disorders or disseminated intravascular coagulation. Urethral catheterization may also be performed to obtain sterile urine specimens. After prepping with an antimicrobial solution, a 3.5 French or 5 French feeding tube is coated with lubricant and inserted into the urethra until urine returns. Discarding the initial 1 to 2 ml of urine obtained will increase the accuracy of the culture results (Peniakov et al, 2004). Because bagged specimens often have a significant risk of contamination, they are not recommended for Gram stain or culture.

Urinalysis

One of the first steps in a urogenital workup is urinalysis. Variables normally assessed in urinalysis include color, pH, specific gravity, white blood cells, blood, and protein. Urinalysis includes gross assessment as well as dipstick and microscopic evaluation. The urine is most often straw-colored, but this may be altered by the type and amount of solutes. Dipstick testing of urine can provide a wide range of information. This test requires that only one to two drops of urine be placed on the dipstick, or the stick may be dipped into a specimen of urine. The results are obtained within 30 seconds to 1 minute after the stick is wet with urine. The exact timing for the most accurate reading is found on the bottles of the dipstick materials, based on the manufacturer's suggested clinical timing cycle. In addition to pH, specific gravity, protein, and blood, the dipstick test may also assess the presence of leukocytes, nitrites, glucose, bilirubin, and ketones in the urine.

TABLE 8-2	Risk Factors Associated with Genitourinary Dysfunction	
Risk Factor	**Urogenital Defect**	
MATERNAL		
Fetal alcohol syndrome	Hydronephrosis	
	Hypospadias	
	Small, rotated kidneys	
Maternal cocaine use	Genitourinary anomalies	
Rubella	Renal artery stenosis	
Oligohydramnios	Renal agenesis	
Positive familial history:	Other similar renal anomalies	
Polycystic kidneys		
Renal transplants		
Medullary cystic disease		
Nephritis		
Tubular acidosis		
Renal tubular necrosis		
NEONATAL		
Asphyxia	Renal tubular necrosis	
Resuscitation	Renal tubular necrosis	
Vascular catheterization	Renal vessel thrombosis	
Birth and other trauma	Renal tubular necrosis	
	Physical renal damag	
	Renal hemorrhage	
	Peritoneal lacerations	
Polycythemia; dehydration	Renal vessel thrombosis	
	Renal necrosis	
Nephrotoxic drugs		
Gentamicin		
Hyperosmotic fluids		
Metabolic buffers		
Disseminated intravascular coagulation		
OTHER DEFECTS		
Spina bifida	Urinary stasis	
Meningomyelocele	Urinary stasis, infection	
Compression of aorta	Acute renal failure	
Abdominal wall defects	Multiple urogenital deformities	

Renal regulation of acid-base balance has previously been discussed. Urinary pH values range from 4.5 to 8 and reflect the kidney's attempt to maintain acid-base balance. The newborn initially excretes alkalotic urine with a pH of 6. Urine pH values in the newborn should be evaluated in relation to the serum bicarbonate values. Production of alkaline urine with documented metabolic acidosis may indicate renal pathology.

Specific gravity indicates the kidney's ability to concentrate and dilute urine. Specific gravity measurement in the newborn can be misleading in its interpretation. Normal levels often range from 1.001 to 1.015. A low specific gravity may appear normal but may not be an accurate reflection of renal functioning because the infant has a decreased ability to concentrate urine. High specific gravities often reflect dehydration vs high solute excretion. Excretion of glucose and protein in the urine may artificially increase the specific gravity in the newborn. Urine osmolality is a more accurate measure of the kidney's urine concentrating ability. It is the measure of the number of solute particles dissolved in a given volume of solution.

Small amounts of protein may be found in the urine. Glomerular filtrate is nearly protein-free, and the majority of the protein that is filtered is reabsorbed along the nephron's tubular system. Glomerular and tubular damage can result in excessive proteinuria. Extrarenal pathology may also result in proteinuria. The source of persistent, large quantities of proteinuria must therefore be evaluated.

Sources of hematuria include sepsis, urinary obstruction, urinary tract infection, acute tubular necrosis, renal thrombosis, trauma, or administration of nephrotoxic drugs (Vogt & Avner, 2002). Because of the various sources of red blood cells in urine, the source should be quickly determined. Blood is a protein; therefore if blood is present, a positive protein test result should also be expected.

Trace amounts of glucose may occasionally be detected in the term infant's urine but is found more often in the premature infant's urine. Glucosuria occurs in when the renal tubules have reached their threshold for reabsorption of glucose, thus resulting in excretion. Glucosuria also occurs with increased glucose loads that may be administered via parenteral nutrition. This increases glucose load and can lead to osmotic diuresis.

Urine Chemistries

Urine chemistries are helpful in determining fluid and electrolyte balance when evaluated in comparison to serum electrolyte levels.

Sodium excretion is very high in the fetus and premature infant but decreases with increasing gestational age. The term infant conserves renal sodium, and renal sodium loss is small. Increasing GFR, combined with impaired reabsorption of sodium in the renal tubules, is thought to cause the high level of excretion in the premature neonate. In addition, kidneys of premature infants display a relative unresponsiveness to aldosterone. Sodium is regulated by extracellular fluid volume and hormonal influences.

Potassium is freely filtered by the glomerulus. Urinary potassium levels are low, however, because the majority of filtered potassium is reabsorbed by the proximal tubule and, to a lesser extent, the loop of Henle. Urinary potassium levels reflect the amount secreted by the collecting tubule. As a result, increased potassium load can significantly increase serum potassium levels.

Serum Chemistries

The measurement of serum chemistries plays a large role in assessing renal functioning. In the premature or compromised infant, serum electrolyte levels may indicate a wider range of problems than occurs in the term healthy newborn. Dehydration, fluid overload, metabolic disorders, fluid-losing and electrolyte-losing disorders, and respiratory compromise all lead to alterations in serum electrolyte levels. High serum sodium levels may reflect dehydration, excessive fluid loss, or administration of high solute loads. Low sodium levels can occur with overhydration or possibly with inappropriate antidiuretic hormone secretion. Potassium losses are apparent with diuretic use and with episodes of diarrhea. Hyperkalemia may occur with excess administration or decreased renal function.

Blood Urea Nitrogen and Creatinine

Another indication of renal functioning is the determination of blood urea nitrogen (BUN) and creatinine levels. Although these indices are not absolute indicators of long-term renal problems, these values can be used to identify and treat acute problems. During the first few days of life, BUN levels should not be greater than 20 mg/dl. Elevated levels of BUN can be caused by significant dehydration and by ingestion of high protein loads (Friedlich et al, 2004). Assessment of creatine level is the most important indicator of neonatal renal function (Kemper & Muller-Wiefel, 2001). Creatinine levels at birth reflect maternal levels, gestational age, and the infant's GFR. Levels should begin to decrease gradually over the first 10 days as GFR increases. The more immature the infant, the higher the initial creatinine level and the longer it takes to fall (Gallini et al, 2000). Serial levels should be obtained to better evaluate renal function. Table 8-3 provides a summary of blood and urine chemistries in term and preterm infants.

Urine Culture

Urine culture in the newborn is used as an assessment for urinary tract infection. Urine infections are common in the infant and can occur when urinary tract deformities are present or when organisms have been introduced via invasive procedures. Urine cultures should be obtained by either in-and-out catheterization or suprapubic tap to maintain sterility of the specimen.

Radiologic Examination

Radiologic examination includes a range of tests available for determining anatomic and physiologic function.

Renal Ultrasonography

The safest and one of the most useful tests to determine renal anomalies is ultrasonography (Mercado-Deane et al, 2002).

TABLE 8-3	Differences in Renal Function Between Full-Term and Preterm Infants	
	Preterm	**Full-Term**
Creatinine clearance 1 wk after birth (ml/min/1.73 m²)	11 ± 5 (GA 25 to 28 wk) 15 ± 6 (GA 29 to 34 wk)	46 ± 15
Plasma creatinine 1 wk after birth (mg/dl)	1.4 ± 0.8 (GA 25 to 28 wk)	0.5 ± 0.1
Maximum urine osmolality (mOsm/kg H₂O)	400 to 700	600 to 900
Proteinuria (mg/m²/day)	88 to 377	68 to 309
Plasma bicarbonate (mEq/L)	19.5 ± 2.9	21.0 ± 1.8
Mean fractional excretion of sodium (%)	4 (GA <30 wk)	<2

From Springate JE et al (1987). Assessment of renal function in newborn infants. Pediatrics in review 9(2):56. Reprinted with permission from Pediatrics in review.
GA, *Gestational age.*

Ultrasound is readily available, is inexpensive, and can detect most structural renal abnormalities (Caty & Wright, 2003). The two-dimensional mode and Doppler imaging are the usual techniques. The two-dimensional mode may be used to illustrate kidney structure, and Doppler imaging provides information relative to flow in the renal arteries and veins. Analysis can often determine differences in normal vs cystic tissue. Solid tumors and masses may be readily apparent. In most institutions, ultrasound examinations are performed before invasive studies. In many cases, accurate and specific diagnosis may be determined from ultrasonography alone. If the infant is stable, it is recommended one wait 3 to 5 days following birth to perform the initial renal ultrasound in order to avoid false negative results due to the decreased urine production during the first few days of life (Riccabona, 2004). Ultrasonography is useful in identifying renal obstruction, hydronephrosis, presence of calculi, and in some cases, advanced parenchymal disease (Lewis, 2003; Caty & Wright, 2003).

Over the past two decades, the use of prenatal ultrasound has dramatically increased the number of prenatally diagnosed renal anomalies. Genitourinary anomalies are the most commonly anomaly diagnosed via prenatal ultrasound (Hrair-George et al, 2004; Mesrobian et al, 2004). The kidney, bladder, and amniotic fluid can be visualized as early as 12 weeks. The kidney may be visualized after 16 to 17 weeks in most fetuses. The majority of renal anomalies are now diagnosed with prenatal ultrasound. The presence of abnormally sized kidneys, renal cysts, hydronephrosis, abnormal bladder size, and oligohydramnios suggest significant renal or urinary tract abnormality (Vogt & Avner, 2002). This has drastically changed the management of neonatal renal abnormalities.

The treatment of neonatal renal disease can now be initiated prior to the onset of symptoms, thus improving long-term prognosis. Prenatal ultrasound also provides an opportunity for in utero treatment of certain disorders and allows the opportunity for family counseling; if the renal anomaly is incompatible with life, elective termination of the pregnancy may be considered.

Voiding (Micturating) Cystourethrogram (VCUG)

A VCUG is used primarily to assess for reflux. It also assesses bladder anatomy and function of the urethral anatomy (Riccabona, 2002). To perform this procedure, a urinary catheter is placed and contrast material is instilled into the bladder (Gordon & Riccabona, 2003). Fluoroscopy is then used to monitor filling and voiding mechanisms and to assess for the presence of reflux.

Radionuclide Renal Imaging. Radionuclide renal imaging is the most sensitive technique to assess renal parenchyma. It is usually performed to assess renal function and renal damage (Dillon, 2002). A small amount of an actively labeled substance (radioisotope) is injected. The most commonly used radioisotope is technetium-99m mercaptoacetyltriglycine (99mTC-MAG-3). The 99mTC-MAG-3 is eliminated by tubular secretion and assesses renal function. It can also be used to visualize kidney mass as well as ureter and bladder outline. In the premature infant, contrast material should be used selectively because the solution is hyperosmolar and may lead to further renal compromise.

Another radionuclide test is diuretic renography, which is used most often to differentiate between obstructive and nonobstructive uropathies. A radioisotope injection is given, followed 15 to 30 minutes later by a diuretic injection. The diuretic facilitates the movement of the radioisotope through the renal system. A gamma computer tracks the isotope's movement. If a urinary obstruction is present, the isotope's progress is slowed or impeded, thus showing retention of the radioactive substance. If dilation exists along the renal system, urine is retained at the uteropelvic junction until overflow occurs with diuretic action. The stretching of the muscle fibers at this point causes strong contractions to begin. Soon, the urine is released, thus rapidly moving the isotope along (about 10 to 15 minutes) and showing a sharp, immediate decline in isotope concentration. In a normal kidney, the isotope takes about 25 minutes to clear the system, and the isotope concentration gradually declines.

Computed Tomography (CT) and Magnetic Resonance Imaging (MRI)

CT and MRI provide high-resolution cross-sectional imaging. There is little advantage to the use of these modalities over other renal imaging techniques, and their use is limited to situations where other tests are inconclusive (Friedlich et al, 2004).

MANAGEMENT

Fluid, Electrolytes, and Nutrition

When renal failure is suspected, serum electrolytes, phosphorus, and calcium levels should be monitored serially, to prevent derangement. Urine and serum chemistries should be monitored as frequently as clinically indicated. Fluids should be carefully managed relative to clinical presentation and response to therapy.

Abnormalities in fluid status are common and must be carefully monitored. Nursing management involves the ongoing assessment and reporting of aberrant signs and symptoms. Daily or twice-daily weights may be required for a baseline determination of excessive fluid retention or loss. Accurate intake and output must be measured. Urine specific gravity should be frequently monitored. Potassium and phosphorus restrictions may also be imposed, although if the infant is asymptomatic, such electrolyte restrictions may not be necessary.

Hyperkalemia is a consequence of renal failure and, if associated with ECG changes, is considered a medical emergency. Maintenance of appropriate potassium levels is most important in the management of renal failure. Careful cardiac monitoring is essential to detect any abnormal rhythms or patterns that result from alterations in potassium levels. Potassium should not be added to parenteral fluids until an appropriate urine output has been established. The goals of hyperkalemia management are to decrease myocardial excitability, enhance cellular potassium uptake, and facilitate potassium excretion. Administration of intravenous calcium gluconate aids in decreasing myocardial excitability. Cellular uptake of potassium can often be achieved through combined administration of glucose and insulin, administration of sodium bicarbonate (1 mEq/kg), and exchange transfusion. These measures are only temporary solutions to the problem. They do not remove the excess potassium from the body. The administration of a cation-exchange resin such as Kayexelate binds the serum potassium and actively removes it from the body. Each gram per kilogram administered will decrease the potassium level by 1 mEq/L (Karlowicz & Adelman, 2005). Since the mechanism of action is exchange of a sodium ion for a potassium ion,

hypernatremia, fluid overload, and congestive heart failure are potential side effects (Karlowicz & Adelman, 2005). This therapy is not an immediate solution since it takes several hours to take effect. Dialysis may be necessary to return the body to normal potassium levels (Vogt & Avner, 2002).

Renal disease may also lead to elevated phosphorus levels. Use of aluminum hydroxide to bind phosphorus in the intestines may be helpful if management is warranted. However, dialysis is usually indicated for treatment of hyperphosphatemia in the neonatal patient (Friedlich et al, 2004). A formula that is low in phosphorus may be given in the form of Similac PM 60/40 (Ross Laboratories, Columbus, OH) or SMA (Wyeth, Madison, NJ). Hypocalcemia is common and if symptomatic may be treated with calcium supplements, which can be used after the phosphorus level has been normalized. Calcium supplementation may also be required because the phosphorus level affects the calcium level. These levels are inversely proportional; as one increases, the other decreases. Caution should be practiced during intravenous administration of calcium. Rapid administration can precipitate a cardiac arrest; thus, administration of this agent requires close nursing observation. Vitamin D supplementation is also a useful adjunct for the correction of calcium levels because it facilitates the absorption of calcium from the gut during enteral feedings. Metabolic acidosis is common because of an inability to excrete hydrogen ions and an increased rate of production. Sodium bicarbonate should be used for a pH less than 7.2 (Friedlich et al, 2004).

Hyponatremia is common and is usually related to fluid overload and increased ADH production (Karlowicz & Adelman, 2005). A sodium level less than 120 mEq/L can result in seizures and must be treated with sodium replacement therapy. Careful monitoring of fluid status and restricting fluid intake to insensible water loss plus urinary output is imperative to prevent hyponatremia.

Fluid shifts may occur secondarily to fluid overload or to a change in electrolyte balance, thus resulting in edema. Assessment for the presence of edema includes observation of the periorbital area and observation of dependent surfaces, including examination of the hands, feet, labia, and scrotum. Pitting should be determined by gentle depression of a fingertip into the suspected edematous site. Caution should be taken around the ocular area because direct pressure on the eyeball may precipitate bradycardia. A late manifestation of renal disease is ascites.

Positive growth and nutrition may be compromised because of protein and fluid restriction. Optimal nutritional status should always be an integral part of management. Adequate nutritional status positively affects the outcome of infants who experience renal compromise. If fluid restriction has been imposed, the caloric consumption must be increased without increasing fluid volume. Hyperalimentation may be initiated in infants who are not capable of receiving enteral feedings. The overall goal of nutritional therapy is the preservation of a positive nitrogen balance and the avoidance of increases in nitrogenous waste products that can lead to further increases in urea nitrogen levels and uremia. Protein intake should be determined by overall caloric intake and BUN levels. Recommended protein intake is 1 to 2 g/kg/day (Drukker & Guignard 2002).

Skin Management

Skin integrity is a concern, especially when pitting edema is present. The infant's position should be changed every 2 hours to decrease effects of dependent edema. Skin around any operative site should be inspected with every dressing change for signs of irritation or infection. The skin must be kept dry and clean to prevent skin breakdown and infection.

Respiratory Management

Respiratory compromise is common in the infant who is experiencing alterations in urinary elimination. During fetal life, insufficient amniotic fluid is linked to decreased development of the respiratory tree (see discussion on Potter's association). Varying degrees of lung hypoplasia may exist, resulting in potentially significant respiratory distress.

Before extensive therapy is initiated for the treatment of renal anomalies, careful evaluation of respiratory status should be performed (see Chapter 1). Measures to improve renal function should not be undertaken if respiratory capacity is insufficient to support life.

General Preoperative Management

If surgical intervention is indicated, preoperative care is directed toward achieving and maintaining the stability of the fluid and electrolyte balance and the hemodynamic status of the infant. Assessment for any signs of urinary tract infection—such as poor feeding, temperature instability, cyanosis, and any other detectable subtle change from the infant's baseline norm—should be ongoing. Surgery should be delayed until the infant is free from any possible urinary tract infections (Riccabona, 2004).

General Postoperative Management

Postoperatively, nursing management is again focused on careful assessment and monitoring of the fluid and electrolyte status as well as the hemodynamic system—including blood pressure, pulse, and respiration of the infant. Accurate measurement of fluid intake and output is critical. If renal function is at risk due to a blockage at the level of the ureter, surgical placement of a nephrostomy tube may be indicated. The insertion site should be covered with a sterile dressing.

Because the renal system is a highly vascular system, the chance for bleeding or infection is great. After the insertion of a nephrostomy tube or tubes, pink-tinged urine or even urine with visible bloody streaks is common. Because they are located within the renal pelvis, these tubes should not be irrigated. The tubes should be connected to a closed drainage system to maintain sterility. A clean dressing surrounding the tube should be used to maintain the position and protect the underlying skin. On removal of such tubes, urine leakage for as long as 48 hours is not unusual.

Maintenance of an aseptic suture line is important. Any dressings, especially over a nephrostomy site, should be closely observed for bleeding or drainage. An infant with a nephrostomy tube or who has undergone other renal surgery is at risk for infection. Broad-spectrum antibiotics are indicated.

Fetal Surgery

Fetal surgery may be performed to place a vesicoamniotic shunt (Figure 8-5). This is a shunt that is placed in the bladder to drain urine from the bladder into the amniotic fluid. This technique has been utilized to reduce oligohydramnios and its associated complications (Chandler & Gauderer, 2004). The goals of in utero shunting include restoration of adequate

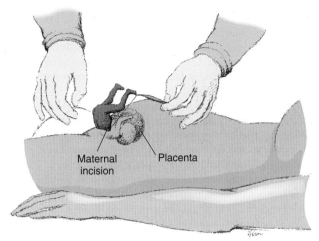

FIGURE **8-5**
Fetal surgery to prevent hydronephrosis.

amniotic volume for lung development and preservation of renal function by relieving obstruction (Karlowicz & Adelman, 2005).

Recent literature suggests that this procedure generally results in minimal improvement in outcome (Gordon et al, 2001; Thomas, 2001). The one condition in which it may prove beneficial is posturethral valves, but even this remains controversial (Agarwal & Fisk, 2001; Holmes et al, 2001). Complications of vesicoamniotic shunt placement include dislodgement, premature labor, urinary ascites, and chorioamnionitis.

Parental Support

The parents' response to their infants' conditions will vary and must be addressed individually. Consenting to a major surgical procedure on their infant so early in life may be very difficult. The parents must be given accurate information as to the prognosis for their infant and should be encouraged to express their concerns. Use of the interdisciplinary team is essential. Collaboration among the neonatologist, pediatric urologist, nurse, clergy, and social worker helps the parents adjust to this frightening situation. If the infant's clinical status is terminal, early identification and involvement of their support network—other parents, family, or friends—or the clergy can assist the parents in coping with the reality that their child may not survive. When the bedside nurse anticipates this need and responds early, the optimal possible outcome is ensured.

The general principles of collaborative management have been outlined. The remainder of the chapter addresses the most common GU neonatal problems.

URINARY TRACT INFECTION
Pathophysiology

Both full-term and premature infants are at risk for developing any type of infection because of their immature immune status. In the newborn, the specific and the nonspecific immunity as well as the complement system are diminished, resulting in a vastly increased incidence of infection including infection of the bladder and kidney. Urinary tract infections are commonly associated with neonatal sepsis and it is often unknown whether the sepsis led to the UTI or visa versa (see Chapter 9).

The incidence of urinary tract infections (UTIs) in the neonates is 1% in term infants and 3% to 10% in preterm infants (Long & Klein, 2001). During infancy, UTIs are more common in male infants possibly due to an increased risk of UTI in the uncircumcised male (Nese et al, 2004; Bonacorsi et al, 2005). Neonatal UTI's are often associated with renal malformation or urinary obstruction including vesicoureteral reflux (Nese et al, 2004).

Obstruction typically causes urinary flow to be impeded, resulting in urinary stasis and retrograde flow of urine from the bladder to the kidney, predisposing the neonate to bacterial colonization and ultimately UTI. A neurogenic bladder lacks innervation and is unable to properly and completely empty. It often accompanies spinal or neural tube deformities such as spina bifida or meningomyelocele. The resulting urinary stasis predisposes the infant to UTI.

Most UTIs are caused by *Escherichia coli*; however, *Klebsiella*, *Pseudomonas*, *Proteus*, *Enterococcus*, *Staphylococcus*, and *Candida* are becoming more common as causative agents, especially as a result of nosocomial infection (Nese et al, 2004; Long & Klein, 2001; Langley et al, 2001).

Diagnosis

Because neonates have immature nonspecific and specific immune systems, localization of infection is not usually possible. The clinical manifestations of a UTI are often subtle, and many infants affected with a UTI are asymptomatic. General signs and symptoms of infection are commonly present including temperature instability, poor feeding, cyanosis, abdominal distention, poor weight gain, hepatomegaly, jaundice, and fever (Biyikli et al, 2004; Long & Klein, 2001; Garcia & Nager, 2002). Urinalysis may show proteinuria, hematuria, and the presence of leukocytes or bacteria. The nurse should report these signs to the medical team for further diagnostic workup.

Initial examination of the infant suspected of having a UTI should include a thorough family and perinatal history. Any positive familial history of pyelonephritis or nephritis or maternal infections, especially of the genital tract, should be noted. Neonatal procedures such as suprapubic bladder taps or bladder catheterization should be noted along with the dates the procedures were performed. These dates estimate the incubation time for possible pathogens. A urine Gram stain and culture should be obtained using either suprapubic aspiration or sterile bladder catheterization. Bagged urine specimens should never be used for culture purposes because of the likelihood of perineal contamination (Biyikli et al, 2004). False positive cultures obtained from bagged specimens can lead to misdiagnosis and inappropriate treatment. Any bacteria obtained from a suprapubic aspiration must be considered diagnostic, whereas urine obtained via catheterization can have up to 10^3 CFUs (colony-forming units) before a UTI is diagnosed. Because of the strong possibility of systemic infection, a blood culture should also be obtained.

Treatment

Prompt treatment of any suspected UTI is imperative to prevent permanent renal damage, which can result in hypertension or end-stage renal disease (Biyikli et al, 2004; Wald, 2004). Empiric broad-spectrum antibiotic therapy should be initiated when the initial workup is complete. Antibiotic coverage may be adjusted after the infecting bacteria has been identified on Gram stain or urine culture and sensitivities are obtained. Antibiotic therapy generally continues for a minimum of 7 to 10 days. A repeat urine culture should be obtained 48 to 72 hours after initiation of treatment. It is estimated that 30% to 50% of infants diagnosed with a UTI have urinary tract abnormalities (Biyikli et al, 2004). Any infant who has been diagnosed with a UTI should have imaging studies performed to assess for the presence of an underlying abnormality that may predispose the infant to future infections and subsequent renal parenchymal damage (Zamir et al, 2005). The current recommended studies include a renal ultrasound to assess the upper urinary tract for abnormalities such as hydronephrosis and a VCUG (voiding cystourethrogram) to detect abnormalities of the lower urinary tract such as vesicoureteral reflux and to ensure that no damage to the urinary tract exists (Gordon & Riccabona, 2003). If the infection results from a suspected urinary or renal obstruction, further diagnostic studies should be performed. Prophylactic antibiotic therapy should be prescribed until the presence of reflux has been eliminated.

With prompt diagnosis and treatment, the prognosis is generally good for an isolated urinary tract infection. However, the potential for serious complications, including severe damage to the renal system, exists.

CIRCUMCISION

The practice of circumcision has been the source of a great deal of controversy over the past several decades. Circumcision is defined as the removal of the prepuce from the glans of the penis. It is assumed that the function of the prepuce is protection of the glans. There are currently three commonly utilized methods of circumcision. These include the use of the Gomco clamp, the plastibell device, and the Mogen clamp.

In 1971, 1975, and 1983, the American Academy of Pediatrics (AAP) recommended against routine circumcision based on lack of medical indication for the procedure (American Academy of Pediatrics, 1971, 1975, 1983). In 1989, a multidisciplinary Task Force on Circumcision established by the AAP summarized the pros and cons of circumcision but did not make a specific recommendation whether routine circumcision was necessary (AAP, 1989). In 1999, this task force again summarized the existing scientific evidence. They acknowledged that although there were potential benefits to circumcision, there was insufficient data to recommend routine circumcision. Therefore parents should be provided with accurate and unbiased information and allowed to make the decision whether to circumcise their child (AAP, 1999).

Numerous studies have shown an association between UTIs and an uncircumcised status (Singh-Grewal et al, 2005). These studies found a three to seven times higher risk of UTI in uncircumcised vs circumcised males. The theory behind this increased incidence is colonization of the prepuce with bacteria that are subsequently introduced into the urethral opening.

Other health concerns that been reported to increase in the noncircumcised male include cancer of the penis, sexually transmitted diseased, and HIV (Agot et al, 2004; Lerman & Liao, 2001; Baldwin et al, 2004; Schoen et al, 2000).

The controversy related to circumcision arises when one analyzes whether the risks of the procedure outweigh the benefits. The complication rate associated with circumcision is between 0.2% and 3% (Singh-Grewal et al, 2005). In most cases complications are minor and include bleeding and mild infection. More serious complications are rare and include amputation of the glans, acute renal failure (ARF), and sepsis.

It is clear that neonatal circumcision without analgesia produces significant pain and physiologic stress. Infants undergoing circumcision have been shown to have changes in heart rate, blood pressure, oxygen saturation, and cortisol levels. If neonatal circumcision is performed, appropriate procedural analgesia such as dorsal penile blocks should be provided.

Nursing care following circumcision includes assessment for symptoms of bleeding every 30 minutes for at least 2 hours (Kaufman et al, 2001). The first void after circumcision must be assessed and documented to evaluate for urinary obstruction related to penile injury or edema. A petroleum gauze should be applied to the circumcision site to prevent bleeding and to protect the site.

ACUTE RENAL FAILURE
Pathophysiology
Acute renal failure (ARF) occurs when GFR severely decreases abruptly or stops completely with a subsequent decrease in fluid and electrolyte regulation and acid-base homeostasis (Barletta & Bunchman, 2004; Andreoli, 2004). It is a common problem in the newborn and is estimated to affect as many as 24% of all neonates admitted to an intensive care unit (Drukker & Guignard, 2002). This estimate does not accurately reflect the true incidence of ARF since cases of nonoliguric

renal failure are not included (Drukker & Guignard, 2002). Acute renal failure in the neonate is suspected when urinary output falls below 1 ml/kg/hr and is accompanied by serum creatinine levels greater than 1.5 mg/dl. Any condition that interferes with kidney function can lead to acute renal failure (Table 8-4).

Acute renal failure may be classified as prerenal, intrinsic, and postrenal. Prerenal failure is by far the most common form and results from inadequate renal perfusion to a normal kidney (Agras et al, 2004). Perfusion may be inadequate because of increased fluid losses from hemorrhage, increased insensible water loss, or fluid loss due to third spacing. Perfusion may also be adversely affected by decreased flow to the kidney due to congestive heart failure or hypoxia (Andreoli, 2004). Persistent hypoxia leads to shunting of blood away from the kidneys toward the more critical organs of the body. This results in hypoperfusion of the kidney and a subsequent decrease in GFR. Failure to adequately recognize and treat prerenal failure can result in progression of renal failure ultimately leading to intrinsic renal failure.

Intrinsic renal failure is a result of damage to the actual renal parenchyma. It can result from progression of prerenal and postrenal failure, infection, renal vein thrombosis, and nephrotoxicity from medications such as aminoglycosides,

TABLE 8-4	Major Causes of Acute Renal Failure in the Newborn	
Prerenal Failure	**Intrinsic Renal Failure**	**Postrenal Failure**
Systemic hypovolemia	Acute tubular necrosis	Congenital malformations
Fetal/neonatal hemorrhage	Congenital malformations	Imperforate anus
Septic shock	Bilateral agenesis	Urethral stricture
Necrotizing enterocolitis	Renal dysplasia	
Polycystic kidney disease	Posterior urethral valves	
Dehydration		Urethral diverticulum
Renal hypoperfusion	Glomerular immaturity	Primary vesicoureteral reflux
Perinatal asphyxia	Infection	
	Congenital syphilis	
Congestive heart failure	Toxoplasmosis	Ureterocele
		Megacystis megaureter
Cardiac surgery	Pyelonephritis	
Respiratory distress syndrome	Renal vascular	Eagle-Barrett syndrome
	Renal artery thrombosis	(Prune-belly syndrome)
Pharmacologic	Renal venous thrombosis	
Tolazoline	Disseminated intravascular coagulation	Ureteropelvic junction obstruction
Captopril		
Indomethacin		Extrinsic compression
	Nephrotoxins	
	Aminoglycosides	Sacrococcygeal teratoma
	Indomethacin	
	Amphotericin B	Hematocolpos
	Contrast media	Intrinsic obstruction
	Intrarenal obstruction	
		Renal calculi
	Uric acid nephropathy	Fungus balls
		Neurogenic bladder
	Myoglobinuria	
	Hemoglobinuria	

Modified from Vogt BA et al (2006). The kidney and urinary tract. In Fanaroff AA et al, editors. Neonatal-perinatal medicine: diseases of the fetus and infant, ed 8. Philadelphia: Mosby.

indomethacin, and amphotericin B (Andreoli, 2004; Itabashi et al, 2003).

Acute tubular necrosis (ATN) is the most common cause of intrinsic renal failure. ATN is renal tubular cellular injury due to severe hypoxia, dehydration, sepsis or blood loss (Andreoli, 2004; Mercado-Deane, 2002). Other causes of intrinsic renal failure include structural abnormalities of the kidney such as renal dysplasia and polycystic or multicystic kidney disease.

Postrenal failure is caused by obstruction of the urinary tract (Haycock, 2003). Anomalies that can cause postrenal failure include posturethral valves, ureteropelvic and ureterovesical junction obstruction, prune-belly syndrome, and neurogenic bladder. A backup of urine into the kidney pelvis inhibits the ability of the kidneys to function. If this condition persists, fluid permanently fills the tissue spaces, with resultant hydronephrosis and renal damage.

Diagnosis

Acute renal failure may be a manifestation of many other problems, and diagnosis must be aimed at identifying the causative agent and not simply limited to determining the presence of acute renal failure. The specific diagnostic tests are determined by the contributing process suspected by the practitioner. This hypothesis requires a thorough nursing assessment in conjunction with an aggressive medical workup. Table 8-5 provides a list of diagnostic indices for neonatal acute renal failure.

A careful prenatal, perinatal, and postnatal history is necessary in evaluating an infant with symptoms of renal failure.

Family history and prenatal history including ultrasound results and amniotic fluid measurements should be examined in any infant with signs of acute renal failure. Other important history includes the presence of perinatal depression or conditions associated with decreased renal blood flow and administration of nephrotoxic medications. Physical exam may reveal a flank mass, abnormal genitalia, or the presence of other congenital anomalies.

Decreased urine output, edema, and lethargy are clinical signs that may point to acute renal failure. Oliguria is the most significant sign of acute renal failure, but a high-output failure also occurs. Edema is usually caused by fluid overload rather than by the condition itself. Hematuria and proteinuria are common signs of failure. Some neonates also present with abdominal distention or a flank mass. Serum BUN and creatinine levels will also increase. Because hypoperfusion of the kidneys may be common in the neonate, efforts should be made to determine the cause of the oliguria. With intrinsic renal failure, hematuria and hemoglobinuria may occur. Urine-to-plasma osmolality ratio of 1:1 or less may indicate renal failure. Renal compromise can be detected even in utero through evaluation of fetal urine samples. The maximum fetal urine electrolyte levels considered within normal limits are sodium, 100 mEq/L; chloride, 90 mEq/L; and osmolality, 210 mOsm/kg. Levels greater than the values given here are indicative of renal failure and poor prognosis.

Urine output should be at least 1 ml/kg/hr. Urine output, at least initially, may be within normal limits. The use of diuretics may alter the results of urine tests, thus causing decreased

TABLE 8-5	Diagnostic Indices in Neonatal Acute Renal Failure	
	Prerenal Oliguria Without Renal Failure	**Prerenal and Intrinsic Renal Failure**
SERUM FINDINGS		
Na	Normal or elevated	Low normal or elevated
K	Normal or elevated	Normal or elevated
BUN	Normal or elevated	Elevated
Creatinine	Normal or elevated	Elevated
Ca	Normal	Low
P	Normal	Normal or elevated
URINE FINDINGS		
RBC, protein, casts, and tubular cell casts	Usually absent	Present
Specific gravity	Increased	Low
Urine volume	Low	Low in 60% to 80% (1 ml/kg/hr), normal or high in 40% (>2.4 ml/kg/hr)
Urine osmolarity (mOsm/kg water)	Increased >300 to 400	Decreased <300
Urine Na (mEq/L)	<30 mEq/L (preterm infant) <20 mEq/L	>30 mEq/L
Creatinine clearance	Normal or decreased	Decreased
U/P creatinine	>20:1	<10:1
U/P urea	>20:1	<10:1
U/P osmolarity	<1.5:1	>1.5:1
FE_{Na}%	<1% (term infant) <3% (preterm infant)	>2% (term infant) >3% (preterm infant)
RFI	<3%	>3%

Modified from John EG, Yeh TF (1985). Renal failure. In Yeh TF, editor. Drug therapy in the neonate and small infant. Chicago: Year Book Medical Publishers. Reprinted with permission.
U/P, Urine/plasma ratio; RFI, renal failure index; BUN, blood urea nitrogen.

specific gravity (dilute urine) and changes in urine electrolytes (increased loss of potassium with loop or thiazide diuretics and increased loss of chloride ions). Diuretic use should be documented when renal function studies are performed. Shock and volume depletion should always be evaluated when oliguria results. In the presence of open or draining congenital anomalies, hidden fluid losses may occur. Surgery to repair defects can lead to third-spacing of fluids, leaving the infant further fluid-compromised.

The blood pressure may at first decrease and then rebound to an above-normal level. Hypertension, or a blood pressure of greater than 90/65 mm Hg in full-term infants, is often the result of fluid overload or increased secretion of renin and aldosterone.

Serum electrolytes may indicate an elevated creatinine, BUN, and phosphorus level as well as hyponatremia. Urine should be sent for sodium and creatinine levels. The fractional excretion of sodium and the renal failure index may be calculated, which may help determine whether the renal failure is prenal or intrinsic renal failure. A renal ultrasound should be performed to look for structural changes in the kidney.

Treatment

The treatment aims to prevent the long-term complications of acute renal failure. Symptomatic treatment is administered until a definitive cause is determined and treated. Once absence of a urinary obstruction is established, a fluid challenge of intravenous isotonic solution, 10 to 20 ml/kg given over 1 hour, is helpful in differentiating prenal from intrinsic failure. If urine output is at least 1 ml/kg/hr within 2 hours of the fluid infusion, the cause of the renal failure is probably related to hypoperfusion. Use of a diuretic after the fluid challenge may be necessary if urine output does not increase immediately after the fluid challenge. To treat prerenal renal failure, administration of low-dose dopamine may be attempted to increase renal perfusion.

Fluid replacement depends on the type of renal failure the infant exhibits. If intrinsic failure exists, fluid replacement is limited to insensible loss and replacement of renal output. Acidosis is common with renal failure because the kidney functions to excrete excess acid from the blood. Acidosis may be treated with either sodium acetate in IV solutions or the administration of sodium bicarbonate. Sodium bicarbonate should be used with caution because it is hypertonic and has been found to increase intracranial pressure and resultant intraventricular hemorrhage in the preterm infant. It may also cause hypercarbia if inadequate ventilation exists.

Hyponatremia is common and may be due to either fluid overload or increased renal losses of sodium. Sodium supplementation may be required (Haycock, 2003). Since the kidneys are responsible for excreting excess phosphorus, hyperphosphatemia often occurs. Treatment includes dietary restriction and the use of oral calcium carbonate, which binds to phosphate and prevents absorption (Haycock, 2003). Hypocalcemia is also common, requiring additional calcium supplementation.

Accurate calculation of fluid intake and output is vital in guarding against fluid overload and resultant hypertension and edema. Nurses should also remember that potassium affects cardiac conduction. Therefore, because these neonates may experience hyperkalemia, all intake of potassium must be eliminated. This measure includes the use of only fresh blood

for transfusions because the older the blood, the more likely the cells are to have broken down and released potassium. Treatment of hyperkalemia includes administration of sodium bicarbonate with dextrose and insulin. This is only a temporary solution. These measures drive the potassium from the intracellular space into the extracellular space. Calcium may be used to protect the heart muscle from the adverse effects of hyperkalemia. Kayexelate will eliminate potassium from the body but may be ineffective in infants less than 29 weeks' gestation and has been associated with necrotizing enterocolitis (Karlowicz & Adelman, 2005). These treatments may be used as a bridge until dialysis can be initiated.

Anemia is a potential consequence of renal failure due to decreased erythropoietin released from the kidney. Careful monitoring of the infant's hematocrit is essential. Treatment with Epogen or packed red blood cell transfusion may be necessary. Changes in the vital signs, activity level, or color should be assessed so that subtle changes indicating anemia may be detected.

Hypertension secondary to fluid overload or increased renin secretion may be treated by sodium and fluid restriction. Antihypertensive agents such as hydralazine, nicardipine, and nitroprusside may also be required (Karlowicz & Adelman, 2005). Infants with renal failure are prone to infections due to multiple invasive procedures and extended length of hospitalization. The infant should be monitored for signs of infection and any abnormality reported so that treatment is begun immediately.

Because the kidney is the clearinghouse for certain drugs, the metabolism of many drugs is altered when renal failure occurs. Aminoglycosides, penicillins, cephalosporins, theophylline, indomethacin, tolazoline, amphotericin, and magnesium should all be used with caution and levels should be carefully monitored.

Adequate nutrition is critically important to prevent catabolism and malnutrition but difficult to attain because of protein and fluid restriction. If the infant is taking enteral nutrition, some experts recommend feedings with breast milk, Similac PM 60/40 (Ross Laboratories, Columbus, OH), and SMA (Wyeth, Madison, NJ) because of their decreased sodium, potassium, and phosphorus loads.

If the infant's condition continues to deteriorate and high BUN and creatinine levels coupled with increasing ammonia levels are present, dialysis may be necessary. Renal replacement therapy is indicated when maximal medical therapy has failed. Specific indications include hyperkalemia, severe hyponatremia, acidosis, hypocalcemia, hyperphosphatemia, volume overload, and malnutrition (Karlowicz & Adelman, 2005). Renal replacement therapy is a challenge at any age, but in the neonatal patient can be especially difficult.

There are currently two types of dialysis that are typically used in the neonatal patient. These include peritoneal dialysis and hemofiltration. Either method can be used within the neonatal intensive care unit; however, expert professionals must be in charge of this procedure because close monitoring of the infant's status is necessary.

Peritoneal dialysis is the most common type of dialysis performed in the neonatal population. During peritoneal dialysis, hyperosmolar dialysate is infused into the peritoneal cavity through a surgically placed Silastic Tenckhoff catheter. Following dialysis, the fluid is drained from the cavity. Depending on the need for solute and fluid removal, cycle time, dwell time, volume, and the osmolar concentration of the fluid can be adjusted.

Hemofiltration is a continuous filtration process. Continuous arteriovenous hemofiltration (CAVM) involves cannulation of both an artery and a vein. Blood is removed via the artery driven across a filter and replaced via the vein. Continuous venovenous hemofiltration involves either cannulation of two veins or placement of a double-lumen venous line. A pump is used to draw blood into the filtration circuit. Care responsibility includes monitoring the equipment, monitoring the cycles if performed manually, performing clotting studies, and administering heparin and other drugs via the dialysis setup. Catheter care includes maintenance of aseptic technique, prevention of hemorrhage and clotting, and observation of the insertion site for signs of infection or dislodgment.

The infant should be observed for signs and symptoms of chemical imbalances during the entire dialysis procedure. Accurate measurement of fluid intake and output and electrolyte levels is critical. Fluid shifts affecting blood pressure and electrolyte balance can occur rapidly and cause cardiac arrhythmias, muscle spasms, seizures, and shock.

Complications of renal failure include hyperkalemia, volume overload, hyponatremia, hypertension, acidosis, hypocalcemia, hyperphosphatemia, sepsis, anemia, azotemia (increased level of nitrogenous waste products in the blood), and nutritional compromise.

The prognosis of acute renal failure depends solely on the ability to treat the underlying problem. Early detection—sometimes even in utero—and treatment of acute renal failure guide the treatment course, possibly preventing life-threatening complications.

POTTER'S SYNDROME
Pathophysiology

Potter's syndrome occurs in approximately 1 in 10,000 births with an increased incidence occurring in male infants. It is an association of defects that begins with bilateral renal agenesis. Renal agenesis occurs when the ureteric bud fails to divide and develop, culminating in the complete absence of the kidney. The developing fetus continuously swallows amniotic fluid. This amniotic fluid is absorbed by the GI system and is then secreted into the amniotic cavity by the kidney. When there is little to no urinary output, severe oligohydramnios occurs, which causes the various deformities associated with Potter's syndrome (Potter, 1965). The presence of adequate amounts of amniotic fluid is necessary for normal pulmonary development. When severe oligohydramnios is present, normal pulmonary development does not occur and the lungs become hypoplastic. Potter's sequence is a less severe form usually associated with less dramatic oligohydramnios. Etiology may include autosomal recessive polycystic kidney disease, dysplastic kidneys, renal hypoplasia, and obstructive uropathies. Although no strong genetic predisposition exists, a multifactorial inheritance pattern has been suggested.

Diagnosis

Infants are often premature, small for gestational age, and are in the breech position. Many are stillborn. Clinical manifestations are due to the effects of severe oligohydramnios. A typical appearance of the facies includes low-set, malformed ears and micrognathia, "senile" appearance, wrinkled skin, parrot-beak nose, and eyes that are wide-set with obvious epicanthal folds. Variable degrees of respiratory distress due to pulmonary hypoplasia are present. Severity depends on the degree of oligohydramnios. Contractures of the limbs are typically present due to intrauterine compression (Potter, 1965).

Potter's syndrome is usually readily identifiable on direct observation because of its characteristic features. Prenatal history includes severe oligohydramnios and bilateral renal agenesis or other renal disorders. Regardless of the results of the prenatal ultrasound, an abdominal ultrasound following birth is indicated to reinforce the diagnosis of renal agenesis.

Treatment

Potter's syndrome is almost universally fatal because of pulmonary hypoplasia and subsequent respiratory failure. Because of this irreversible pulmonary hypoplasia, current treatment of neonates with Potter's syndrome does not include renal transplantation or long-term dialysis.

Assisting the family to cope during and after the death of their infant is the primary aspect of nursing care in the infant with Potter's syndrome. The nurse should encourage parents to visit and hold their infant. Support from pastoral services or social work is imperative during this difficult time.

RENAL APLASIA
Pathophysiology

When one of the ureteric buds fails to form in utero, unilateral renal aplasia, or absence of the kidney occurs. The rate of occurrence may be as high as 1 in 500 births. It is most often associated with other structural defects, such as VACTLRL association (vertebral anomalies, tracheoesophageal atresia, esophageal atresia, renal agenesis, renal dysplasia, and limb defects), caudal regression syndrome, many chromosomal defects, and other associated anomalies (Durson et al, 2005). No specific inheritance pattern is noted.

Diagnosis

The infant may be asymptomatic if renal disease is absent in the unaffected kidney. Renal function of a single kidney is sufficient to support life. However, the remaining kidney is often affected with vesicourethral reflux, ureteropelvic junction obstruction, renal dysplasia, and ureterocele. The exact symptoms exhibited are directly associated with the infant's particular renal abnormality. If the contralateral kidney is significantly affected, the infant may exhibit signs of renal failure.

The differential diagnosis centers on the confirmation of the presence of a single kidney and investigation of the contralateral kidney for abnormalities. This determination is best made by renal ultrasonography and VCUG.

Treatment

The major focus of care is preparation of the infant and family for preliminary testing. If kidney function is not compromised, no nursing care beyond normal newborn care may be necessary. The sections on the specific disorders contain more information on nursing management to be implemented if kidney disease is found. This condition often goes undetected in the newborn period and may be an incidental finding later in life.

The prognosis for survival with a single kidney is excellent if the remaining kidney is disease-free.

CYSTIC KIDNEY DISEASE

Cystic disease of the kidney involves replacement of normal kidney mass with cysts. The amount of cystic formation within each or both kidneys determines the severity of the disease. If the kidney is severely affected, ureteral agenesis may also exist. Cystic disease includes polycystic kidney disease and multicystic kidney disease.

Polycystic Kidney Disease

Polycystic kidney disease is a bilateral process that involves micro- or macroscopic cysts which are distributed throughout the renal parenchyma (Thomas, 2002a). There are two types of polycystic kidney disease: autosomal dominant polycystic kidney disease (ADPKD) and autorecessive polycystic kidney disease (ARPKD). ADPKD is rarely evident in the neonatal period, with symptoms presenting in the fourth to fifth decade of life.

In contrast, ARPKD presents in the neonatal period. The kidneys are enlarged with a normal pelvis, calyces, and ureter. The parenchyma of the kidney is replaced by cysts (Figure 8-6). Liver involvement including hepatic fibrosis is nearly universal, but hepatic symptoms are rarely significant in the neonatal period. The incidence of ARPKD is 1:10,000 to 40,000 births, with the majority presenting as a sporadic anomaly, but an association with other syndromes has been reported (Vogt & Avner, 2002; Rizk & Chapman, 2003).

Diagnosis

Prenatal ultrasound may show enlarged kidneys with increased echodensity. The neonate may present with bilateral abdominal masses and hypertension (Guay-Woodford & Desmond, 2003; Zerres et al, 2003). Severe respiratory distress may be present due to the large kidney pressing on the diaphragm or due to pulmonary hypoplasia (Mesrobian et al, 2004). Diagnosis is via ultrasound showing small cysts in the collecting ducts. A positive family history is often present.

Treatment

Treatment of ARPKD is mainly supportive and includes ventilatory support if respiratory distress is present. Hypertension can often be difficult to control and may require treatment with fluid restriction and possibly antihypertensive medications (Thomas, 2002a).

The prognosis for ARPKD is improving with advancements in neonatal care. Of affected infants, 6% to 30% die in the neonatal period, usually as a result of respiratory failure from pulmonary hypoplasia (Capisonda et al, 2003). In those who survive the neonatal period, 70% to 87% are alive at 1 year and 70% to 88% are alive at 5 years (Capisonda et al, 2003). Fifty percent of infants will advance to end-stage renal disease and will require dialysis and renal transplantation. Hepatic complications are common and include portal hypertension and biliary disease (Shneider & Magid, 2005). Nephrectomy may be indicated due to respiratory distress from compression on the diaphragm and lung by the enlarged kidney (Mesrobian et al, 2004).

Multicystic Kidney Disease

Since the general acceptance of routine prenatal ultrasound, the incidence of unilateral multicystic kidney disease (MKD) has increased dramatically. The incidence is 1:2400 to 1:4300 (Dell & Avner, 2003). It occurs due to early obstruction of the ureter that leads to maldevelopment of the kidney. With MKD, there is a collection of noncommunicating cysts (Figure 8-7). The cysts are of different sizes and have been referred to having a "bunch of grapes" appearance (Thomas, 2002a). The majority of MKD cases are unilateral. Ten percent are bilateral, which carries a grim prognosis as a result of respiratory failure due to pulmonary hypoplasia.

Diagnosis

Unilateral cases of MKD are most often asymptomatic. If symptoms do exist, it typically presents with a palpable flank mass in an otherwise normal infant (Chandler & Gauderer, 2004). Diagnosis is via ultrasound showing multiple noncommunicating cysts (Chandler & Gauderer, 2004). Radionuclide renal scan shows no function of the affected kidney (Kuwertz-Broeking et al, 2004).

Treatment

If urine output is normal, careful consideration of fluid intake and output may not be necessary; if renal function is compromised, strict attention must be paid to fluid balance. Electrolyte status should be monitored at least daily.

The treatment for unilateral MKD is controversial. Historically, management included nephrectomy due to the

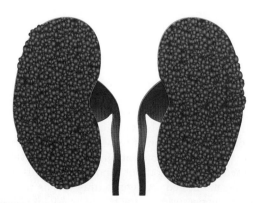

FIGURE **8-6**
Autosomal recessive polycystic kidney disease. From Thomas DFM (2002). Cystic renal disease. In Thomas DFM et al, editors. *Essentials of paediatric urology* (p 98). London: Martin Dunitz.

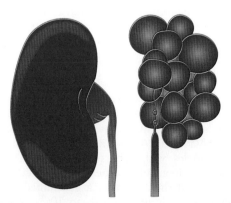

FIGURE **8-7**
Unilateral multicystic kidney disease. From Thomas DFM (2002). Cystic renal disease. In Thomas DFM et al, editors. *Essentials of paediatric urology* (p 99). London: Martin Dunitz.

increased risk of hypertension and malignancy in the affected kidney (Ylinen et al, 2004b). Recent evidence indicates that these kidneys generally spontaneously involute and that the risk of either hypertension or malignancy is relatively low (Al-Ghwery & Al-Asmari, 2005; Ylinen et al, 2004a). Many nephrologists are now recommending conservative treatment with yearly ultrasound examinations and nephrectomy only if complications such as infection or hypertension occur. Since vesicoureteral reflux and ureteropelvic junction obstruction are common in the contralateral kidney, some experts recommend routine VCUGs (Thomas, 2002a). Others report that ultrasound follow-up is adequate to rule out any abnormalities of the contralateral kidney (Ismaili, 2005; Kuwertz-Broeking et al, 2004). Infants should have long-term follow-up with renal ultrasound and blood pressure measurements (Rabelo et al, 2004).

If the infant undergoes a complete nephrectomy, strict adherence to aseptic technique must be followed. Because the infant is prone to infection, vital signs should be monitored at least every 2 to 4 hours after the immediate postoperative period. Any dressings should be inspected for the presence of bloody drainage or secretions. Initially, a small amount of bleeding at the site is common, but it should be short-lived. No urine drainage should be noted on the dressing because the entire kidney has been removed. Abdominal decompression is often necessary to prevent distention that could cause pressure and pull the suture line apart. Feedings may be resumed once bowel sounds can be auscultated and the nasogastric tube has been removed. Feedings are usually tolerated 2 to 3 days after surgery.

PRUNE-BELLY SYNDROME (EAGLE-BARRETT SYNDROME)
Pathophysiology

An infant born with prune-belly syndrome has a triad of anomalies including lack of appropriate abdominal musculature, undescended testicles, and urinary tract malformations (Smith & Woodard, 2002) (Figure 8-8). The abdominal muscles may be so weakened that the abdominal region actually appears wrinkled, much like a prune's surface. It predominantly affects males rarely occurring in females (Keating & Rich, 2000). The incidence rate is approximately 1 in every 35,000 to 50,000 births (Keating & Rich, 2000). The associated urinary abnormalities include an enlarged, poorly functioning bladder, vesicoureteral reflux, and urethral obstruction. The ureters may be tortuous and severely dilated. The kidneys may be dysplastic due to urinary tract obstruction with reflux of urine into the kidneys. A patent urachus may also be present. Other associated problems include orthopedic deformities, respiratory insufficiency, imperforate anus, and cardiac anomalies (Denes et al, 2004; Salihu et al, 2003).

There are presently two theories related to the etiology of prune-belly syndrome. One theory is that in utero urethral obstruction causes backup of urine into the bladder resulting in extreme bladder dilation. This leads to pressure on the abdominal muscles with subsequent abnormal abdominal wall muscle development (Leeners et al, 2000). Presently the most accepted theory is that a generalized mesodermal abnormality occurs during the 4th to 10th weeks of fetal development (Strand, 2004). During this time the bladder is taking shape and being separated from the allantois, and the abdominal wall is forming. This abnormal mesodermal

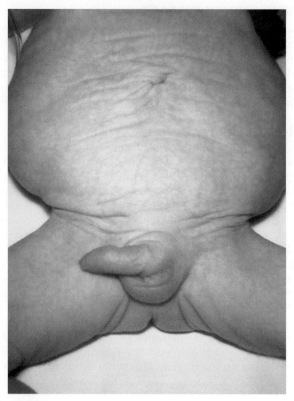

FIGURE **8-8**
Prune-belly syndrome. From Clark DA (2000). *Atlas of neonatology* (p 189). Philadelphia: Saunders.

development leads to the triad of defects seen with prune-belly syndrome.

Diagnosis

Prenatal ultrasound may reveal oligohydramnios if fetal renal function is compromised. The presence of a distended bladder, dilated ureters, and an abnormal abdominal wall is highly suggestive of a prenatal diagnosis of prune-belly syndrome (Leeners et al, 2000). The diagnosis of prune-belly syndrome can be made as early as 13 weeks' gestation.

Woodard classified patients with prune-belly syndrome into three groups. The first group accounts for 20% of all cases of prune-belly syndrome. These patients have severe renal dysplasia with pulmonary hypoplasia. This category is almost universally fatal. Group two accounts for 40% of patients and presents with significant urinary tract abnormalities but have adequate renal function. Future renal compromise occurs as a result of obstruction or infection. The last group, which accounts for 40% of patients, has mild urinary tract abnormalities and normal kidney function (Smith & Woodard, 2002; Denes et al, 2004; Fusaro et al, 2004).

The diagnosis of prune-belly syndrome is usually obvious on observation. Determination of renal function is necessary. An electrolyte panel including creatinine and BUN levels should be obtained. Urinary output and fluid status must be meticulously monitored. A renal ultrasound is indicated to evaluate the upper urinary tract, and a VCUG should be performed to evaluate the bladder size and assess for the presence of vesicoureteral reflux. Radionuclide renal scan should be done to determine the amount of renal function.

Treatment

This triadic anomaly leads to severe urinary tract complications. The bladder in infants with prune-belly syndrome is large, distended, and often has a large postvoid residual. Bladder decompression may be necessary for the prevention of stasis and resultant reflux of urine into the kidney. This may be accomplished by either catheterization or Credé's method. This method involves the practitioner's placing both hands under the infant's flank area and bringing the thumbs together at the umbilicus. Pressure is gently applied, and the thumbs are rolled downward from the umbilicus to the symphysis pubis, which should allow bladder emptying. A nephrostomy, ureterostomy, or vesicostomy diversion may be required if urine drainage is compromised until the infant can tolerate extensive surgical intervention. To correct the severe bladder distention, reduction cystoplasty may be necessary. Prenatal placement of a vesicoamniotic shunt has been used to decrease oligohydramnios and its associated defects and to improve renal function (Leeners et al, 2000; Perez-Brayfield et al, 2001).

Abdominoplasty to improve the appearance of the abdomen has been shown to increase self esteem and improve abdominal strength (Denes et al, 2004). An increase in abdominal strength may decrease the constipation that may occur because the individual is unable to perform the Valsalva maneuver. It can also improve posture. Strengthening the abdominal muscles may also decrease the respiratory infections that are due to lack of abdominal support (Smith & Woodard, 2002).

Undescended testes are present in all affected males. Orchiopexy is recommended prior to 6 months of age.

There are currently differences of opinion as to the timing of surgical intervention. Some urologists recommend a nonoperative approach unless significant renal compromise occurs. Others recommend early urinary reconstruction to eliminate urinary stasis, correct reflux, and improve bladder drainage. Recent evidence suggests that concurrent early urinary reconstruction, bilateral orchiopexy, and abdominoplasty is associated with improved results (Denes et al, 2004).

Urinary stasis, reflux, and infection can lead to progressive deterioration in renal function. Careful follow-up is critical to identify and monitor for these complications and to avoid further renal damage (Denes et al, 2004). The effects of renal damage that occur in the early stages of life require careful attention to fluid and electrolyte balance, removal of wastes, and adequate nutrition for growth and development. Frequent hospitalizations may be necessary during childhood. Parents need to be prepared for this and need to be assisted with financial as well as psychosocial support.

If bladder distention and urinary retention continue to occur until the infant is discharged, parents must be taught a method of emptying the bladder. This may involve Credé's method or intermittent catheterization. Parents must be taught the signs and symptoms of a UTI—including increased irritability with urination, temperature instability, increase or decrease in urine output, and cloudy or foul-smelling urine. They must understand the importance of early detection and intervention to prevent long-term renal compromise. If a vesicostomy or other urinary diversion has been performed, specific instructions are necessary to prevent bladder contamination.

Consideration for parental feelings must also center on the physical appearance of their baby. Because the American culture places great value on appearance, it may be difficult for parents to accept the loss of their "perfect" dream baby. Parental support is a must. A good strategy for increasing the parent-infant interaction is to include them as much as possible in the daily care of their infant.

The prognosis is directly related to the degree of severity of the underlying renal dysfunction. Pulmonary hypoplasia due to oligohydramnios is an important determinant for survival (Leeners et al, 2000). Twenty percent of infants with prune-belly syndrome will die in the first 2 months of life. Chronic renal dysfunction develops in 30% of surviving infants (Fusaro et al, 2004).

EXSTROPHY OF THE BLADDER
Pathophysiology

In exstrophy of the bladder, the anterior abdominal wall fails to close at the point of the bladder. During the first 4 weeks of gestation, the abdominal wall begins to fuse. Exstrophy results when the mesenchymal cells fail to migrate over the abdomen, and a thin membrane forms over the abdominal contents. This membrane later ruptures and leaves the bladder exposed. Exstrophy of the bladder is the most common condition in a spectrum of anomalies ranging from simple epispadias to cloacal exstrophy (Hrair-George et al, 2004). All the anomalies are due to abnormal development of the cloacal membrane.

The incidence of this defect is 1 in 24,000 to 40,000 live births, with males being affected more than females (Huether, 2004). No risk factors or causative agents are known.

Diagnosis

Prenatal ultrasound may suggest the presence of bladder exstrophy, but definitive diagnosis does not occur until after birth, when the defect is obvious on visual inspection (Figure 8-9). The bladder region appears open or uncovered. Because of the failure of the abdominal and anterior bladder wall to close, the posterior wall of the bladder is exposed. The implantation of the ureters may be visible as urine continues to pass from the orifices. A concomitant defect exists in the genitalia. In the male, the penis may be short, flat, and angulated. Epispadias is present. In the female, the labia do not meet in the midline, and a divided clitoris exists. Exstrophy of the bladder is generally not associated with any other anomalies, and the kidneys are generally normal. Prolapse of the rectum may also be evident prior to surgical correction. The failure of the pubic bones to meet anteriorly causes the hips to rotate outward (Kiddoo et al, 2004). Cloacal exstrophy is the most severe expression in this spectrum of anomalies. Not only does it have all the features of classic bladder exstrophy, infants also present with exstrophy of the bowel, a poorly developed hindgut, and absence of the anus and anal canal. The bladder is split into two halves and the penis is also split. Other anomalies such as neural tube defects and spinal dysraphisms are common.

Treatment

Immediately following birth, the exposed bladder should be covered with plastic wrap or a similar material to protect it from injury. Petrolatum or gauze should not be used, because they can become dry and adhere to the tissue. A tie instead of an umbilical clamp should be used to prevent injury to the bladder. Dressings should be changed as needed to prevent skin

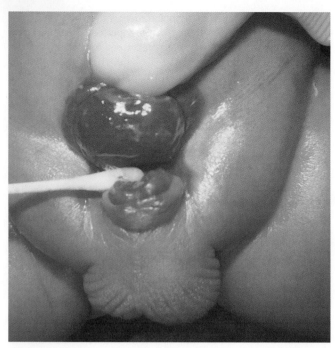

FIGURE **8-9**
Exstrophy of the bladder. From Clark DA (2000). *Atlas of neonatology* (p 201). Philadelphia: Saunders.

irritation. Incubator humidification helps to prevent excess drying. Diapers should be kept folded well below the defect if wound infections are to be avoided. The infant should be transported to a tertiary care facility experienced with care of the infant with exstrophy of the bladder.

Because bladder exstrophy exposes the urinary tract to the environment, careful attention should be given to prevention of infection in these infants before and after surgical correction of the defect. Broad-spectrum antibiotic therapy is initiated prior to surgery and continued for at least 7 days after surgery because 42% of wound dehiscence is caused by infections. Strict observation of aseptic technique is essential. If infection is suspected, aggressive treatment should be initiated.

Two types of repair are currently performed for correction of bladder exstrophy. In the staged repair, the bladder is closed within 48 to 72 hours following birth. Epispadias repair is delayed until the infant is 12 to 18 months of age, and bladder neck pexy is usually required at 3.5 to 5 years of age to improve continence (Kiddoo et al, 2004).

In a complete repair procedure, the repair may be delayed up to 6 weeks. The child may go home during this time, and the parents must be taught the principles of skin management and the importance of the regularity of dressing changes as a method of preventing infection. Surgical correction involves concurrent bladder and epispadias repair. The bladder neck is reapproximated in an attempt to encourage continence (Kiddoo et al, 2004; Hammouda & Dotb, 2004).

In both procedures, a suprapubic catheter and bilateral ureteral stents are placed to allow drainage of urine while the bladder heals. The infant is immobilized for 4 weeks following surgery with traction to facilitate wound healing.

Prognosis is generally favorable with most children leading nearly normal lives (Hammouda & Dotb, 2004). Possible long-term complications include incontinence and postoperative hydronephrosis.

RENAL VEIN THROMBOSIS
Pathophysiology

Renal vein thrombosis (RVT) occurs in approximately 2.2 of 100,000 term infants, with preterm infants having a sixfold increase in incidence. Risk factors include male gender, hyperviscosity, polycythemia, umbilical catheterization, perinatal asphyxia, and conditions associated with decreased blood flow (Vogt & Avner, 2002). Hypercoagulation disorders such as protein C deficiency, homocystinuria, and factor V Leiden increase the likelihood of RVT formation (Zigman et al, 2000; Marks et al, 2005).

Diagnosis

Clinical manifestations include hematuria, decreased urinary output, decreased renal function, enlarged palpable kidneys, anemia, and thrombocytopenia (Vogt & Avner, 2002; Anochie & Eke, 2004). Diagnosis includes Doppler ultrasound studies, which indicate enlarged kidneys and provide information on renal blood flow. It may also reveal the thrombosis located in the renal vein. A renal venography may be more sensitive, especially in the detection of asymptomatic thrombi (Roy, 2002). A radionuclide renal scan may be performed to assess function of the affected kidney.

Treatment

Treatment includes fluid and electrolyte therapy and treatment of associated renal failure. Treatment options for resolution of the thrombus range from observation to treatment with thrombolytic agents such as urokinase, streptokinase, or tissue plasminogen activator (Vogt & Avner, 2002). Systemic heparinization with low-molecular-weight heparin can also be used. When using thrombolytic agents, careful monitoring of coagulation status is imperative. Extreme caution needs to be taken when using these agents in low-birth-weight infants because of the risk of intraventricular hemorrhage (Weinschenk, 2001).

Prognosis depends on the extent of the thrombus and whether the lesion is unilateral or bilateral. Hypertension and chronic renal failure are long-term complications and must be monitored on a regular basis (Zigman et al, 2000; Marks et al, 2005).

HYDRONEPHROSIS
Pathophysiology

Hydronephrosis is the accumulation of urine within the renal pelvis and calices to the point of overdistention. If left untreated, this buildup of fluid can result in irreversible damage to the kidney. Hydronephrosis often follows obstruction of urine flow at the junction of the ureteropelvis, the ureterovesical valve, or the urethrovesical valve. Nonobstructive abnormalities such as vesicourethral reflux and prune-belly syndrome can also cause hydronephrosis. The degree of hydronephrosis is classified from grade I to grade V depending on severity.

Hydronephrosis is the most common renal abnormality detected prenatally. The diagnosis of antenatal hydronephrosis has greatly increased since the routine use of prenatal ultrasound (Cheng et al, 2004). It is estimated that fetal hydronephrosis is present in 2.3% of all pregnancies (Sairam et al, 2001). Many of these cases resolve spontaneously without treatment.

Diagnosis

The majority of hydronephrosis is diagnosed via prenatal ultrasound showing a dilated renal pelvis. This can be performed as early as 12 weeks' gestation. If bilateral hydronephrosis is present, oligohydramnios may be detected. In the newborn, hydronephrosis may be detected as a large, smooth, solid, palpable abdominal mass at the region of the kidney. Because many different forms of abdominal masses may occur, determination of the origin of the mass is essential. This condition must be differentiated from cystic kidney disease, urogenital tumors, and renal vein thrombosis.

Urine output may be decreased or normal, depending on the amount of functioning kidney mass. If only one kidney is involved, urine output may be normal because a single kidney is sufficient for adequate removal of water and waste. UTI often accompanies hydronephrosis and makes fever and discomfort observable signs. Urinalysis may show hematuria, proteinuria, and the presence of white blood cells. If hydronephrosis is bilateral, features consistent with Potter's syndrome including pulmonary hypoplasia due to oligohydramnios may be evident.

The first diagnostic study indicated is a renal ultrasound. If the infant is clinically stable, this test should not be done prior to 24 to 72 hours of age because of the infant's relative dehydration, which may mask the presence of hydronephrosis (Riccabona, 2004). A VCUG should then be performed to assess for the presence of reflux (Riccabona, 2002, 2004). Some clinicians also recommend a radionuclide renal scan at approximately one month of age to assess renal function (Peppas, 2003; Riccabona, 2004). When diagnosed antenatally, it is necessary to confirm the diagnosis with a postnatal ultrasound (Riccabona, 2004).

Treatment

Treatment is dependent on the severity of the hydronephrosis. Mild to moderate hydronephrosis is usually managed conservatively with close ultrasound monitoring. A VCUG is generally indicated regardless of ultrasound results to rule out vesicorenal reflux. Although severe hydronephrosis may also be managed with conservative treatment, a number of these infants will require pyeloplasty later in childhood because of deterioration in renal function. If reflux is present, prophylactic antibiotics are generally prescribed to prevent UTIs and subsequent renal damage. When severe hydronephrosis is diagnosed prenatally, vesicoamniotic shunting (placement of a catheter into the bladder to drain urine) has been utilized in an attempt to reduce oligohydramnios and its associated complications (Chandler & Gauderer, 2004). After birth, definitive surgery is performed to correct the obstructive defect or to provide a diversion of urine flow. Early detection is necessary because damage to the kidneys may occur as early as the 4th month of gestation.

Careful assessment is necessary for any infant with hydronephrosis. Vital signs, including blood pressure, must be monitored at least every 4 hours—more frequently if they are unstable. The blood pressure is especially important because hypertension is common in infants with hydronephrosis. Fluid and electrolyte status must be carefully monitored. Fluid intake and output should be recorded at least every 2 to 4 hours. Urine specific gravity may be checked every 4 to 8 hours. Electrolytes, including serum creatinine and BUN, should be monitored closely. A urine dipstick assessment may be useful for determining the presence of protein or blood in the urine.

Assessment of hydration status is important. The fontanelles should be observed to determine whether they are sunken or bulging. Assessment for the presence of any dependent or pitting edema should be performed and recorded. Skin turgor should demonstrate instant recoil.

Prognosis depends on the underlying causative factor and on the degree of severity of any permanent renal damage. Complications include hypertension, urinary tract infection, and progressive renal damage.

OBSTRUCTIVE UROPATHY
Pathophysiology

Urinary obstruction occurs when there is obstruction to the urinary flow. This causes reflux of urine back into the kidney with resultant hydronephrosis. The increased pressure in the kidney can lead to irreversible kidney damage (Postlethwaite & Dickson, 2003). Obstruction can be unilateral or bilateral. Obstruction can occur at the ureterovesical junction, the ureteropelvic junction, or due to posturethral valves (Chevalier, 2004) (Figure 8-10).

The most common cause of urinary obstruction is ureteropelvic junction obstruction (UPJ). UPJ occurs when there is obstruction of urinary flow from the pelvis of the kidney into the ureter. It can be due to stenosis of the ureter or its associated valves or can be due to an insertion anomaly of the ureter. Ureterovesical junction obstruction is caused by obstruction of flow from the ureter into the bladder. Posterior urethral valves (PUV) can cause severe obstruction uropathy and occur exclusively in males. PUV occurs when urine is obstructed at the level of the bladder outlet due to the presence of enlarged valves.

Diagnosis

Urinary obstruction is frequently diagnosed on prenatal ultrasound and may be apparent as early as 16 to 17 weeks' gestation. Findings can range from mild hydronephrosis to extreme obstruction with oligohydramnios. A distended, thickened bladder may be seen with PUVs (Mesrobian et al, 2004).

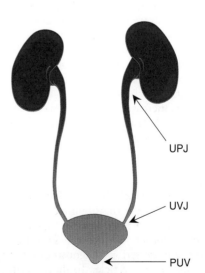

FIGURE **8-10**
Location of most common sites of congenital urinary tract obstruction. *UPJ*, Ureteropelvic junction; *UVJ*, ureterovesical junction; *PUV*, posterior urethral valves. From Chevalier RL (2004). Perinatal obstructive nephropathy. *Seminars in perinatology* 28:124-131.

Neonates may present with symptoms of a UTI or, if significant hydronephrosis is present, an abdominal mass. Infants with PUV may present with a poor urinary stream and an enlarged bladder on exam. Diagnosis is via renal ultrasound followed by VCUG to assess for reflux. A radionuclide renal scan is also recommended to assess renal function.

Treatment

Treatment depends on the severity of the obstruction and whether the obstruction is unilateral or bilateral. If mild, conservative management is appropriate with frequent renal assessment. Prophylactic antibiotics may be indicated to prevent urinary tract infections, which can increase the possibility of poor renal function.

If the obstruction is severe, surgical intervention may be indicated. A urinary diversion such as a pyelostomy tube that is inserted into the renal pelvis is placed following surgery to allow any postoperative edema to resolve. A pyelostomy tube may also be necessary if surgery is contraindicated because of the infant's clinical instability.

The initial treatment of posturethral valves is urinary diversion with bladder catheterization or suprapubic diversion. If the obstruction is severe, significant diuresis may follow urinary diversion and meticulous monitoring of fluid and electrolytes and replacement of losses is critical to avoid dehydration. Posturethral valves are corrected by endoscopic ablation (rupture) of the enlarged valves.

Prognosis depends directly on the presence of renal damage and whether the obstruction was unilateral or bilateral. Infants with PUV often have significant bladder dysfunction. Long-term follow-up is essential for the early detection of chronic renal problems (Holmdahl & Sillen, 2005; Ylinen et al, 2004a). The parents should be educated about the need for follow-up care.

HYDROCELE
Pathophysiology

A hydrocele, the collection of fluid in the scrotal sac, is a common finding in the neonate. This fluid originates from the peritoneal cavity, which communicates with the scrotum through the processus vaginalis. The presence of a hydrocele is closely related to an inguinal hernia. The only difference is the size of the process vaginalis (Madden, 2002). If it is small in diameter, only fluid can flow into the scrotum. Larger passageways may allow escape of a segment of bowel into the scrotum resulting in an inguinal hernia.

Several factors increase the likelihood of a patent processus vaginalis. These include increased abdominal pressure secondary to ventriculoperitoneal shunt or high ventilatory pressures (Madden, 2002).

Diagnosis

Clinical manifestations include the presence of painless scrotal swelling. It can be readily transilluminated with the use of a good light source. The most critical aspect of diagnosis is differentiating whether the scrotal swelling is due to a hydrocele or the more serious diagnosis of either an inguinal hernia or torsion of the testicle. To differentiate between an inguinal hernia and a hydrocele, palpitation is necessary. Inguinal hernias are generally reducible, whereas hydroceles are not. A rectal examination with simultaneous palpation of the inguinal canal may also be necessary. If the examiner

encounters loops of intestine near the vas deferens or the ductus deferens within the scrotal sac, an inguinal hernia is present.

Treatment

Treatment is rarely indicated for hydroceles. Ninety percent will spontaneously resolve in the first year of life due to closure of the processus vaginalis. Indications for surgical correction include failure to resolve in one year or symptoms including pain. Surgery entails drainage of fluid from the scrotal sac and closure of the processus vaginalis (Madden, 2002). Until the hydrocele has resolved, the infant should be closely assessed for signs of intestinal herniation. If an inguinal hernia is suspected, surgical intervention is indicated.

Parents should be taught the signs of herniation and incarceration before discharge. These signs are the presence of a lump in the groin (this lump is especially noticeable when the infant is crying) and increased irritability on the part of the infant. They must understand the need to seek immediate medical attention if either of these symptoms appears. Careful attention must be paid to skin care of the edematous scrotum.

INGUINAL HERNIA
Pathophysiology

Inguinal hernia is one of the most common surgical problems in the infant with an incidence of 16% in VLBW infants (Rajput et al, 1992). An inguinal hernia occurs when the small intestines pass through the open processus vaginalis (Figure 8-11). The testes usually descend into the processus vaginalis at 28 weeks' gestation. The processus vaginalis obliterates between 38 and 48 weeks' postconceptional age. When the processus vaginalis is open, fluid or intestines can pass through the opening, resulting in either a hydrocele or an inguinal hernia.

The premature infant is at a very high risk of inguinal hernias because of the increased intra-abdominal pressure that occurs following birth. The incidence of inguinal hernias is inversely related to gestational age and birth weight. Infants with a birth weight of 500 to 1000 g have a 42% incidence; infants with a birth weight of 1000 to 1500 g have a 10% risk; and those with a birth weight of 1500 to 2000 g have only a 3% incidence of inguinal hernia (Peevy et al, 1986). Right-sided hernias occur more often than left-sided ones, and bilateral hernias make up only a small percentage of occurrences. Males are commonly affected more than females. Other risk factors include cystic fibrosis, congenital hip dysplasia, the presence of a ventriculoperitoneal shunt, and abdominal wall defects (Berseth & Poenaru, 2004).

Diagnosis

The most common manifestation is the presence of an inguinal bulge or mass as the omentum of the small intestine slides through the open processus vaginalis (Pulsifer, 2005; Sheldon, 2001). In many cases, crying or increased abdominal pressure can exaggerate the hernia. In reducible hernias, the intestine can be gently manipulated back into the abdomen. The most important aspect in diagnosis is differentiating between an inguinal hernia and other scrotal masses including hydroceles and testicular torsion. If the scrotum can be transilluminated, the mass could be either a hydrocele or an inguinal hernia (Benjamin, 2002). Testicular torsion is suspected if the scrotum has a hard, solid mass. This is a surgical emergency and

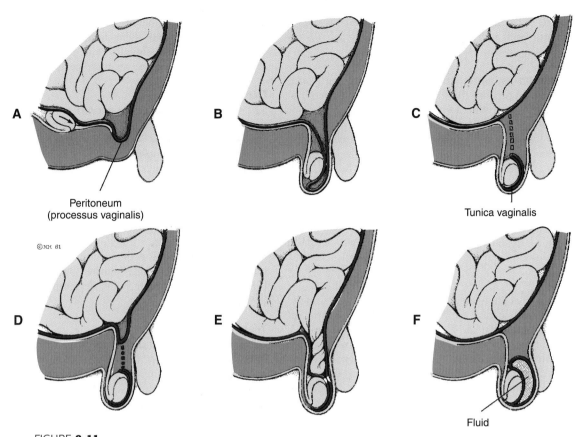

FIGURE 8-11
Development of inguinal hernias. **A** and **B,** Prenatal migration of processus vaginalis. **C,** Normal. **D,** Partially obliterated processus vaginalis. **E,** Hernia. **F,** Hydrocele. From Hockenberry MJ (2003). *Wong's nursing care of infants and children,* ed 7 (p 478). St Louis: Mosby.

must be immediately reported to the surgical team (Benjamin, 2002). If it is not possible to distinguish between an inguinal hernia or a hydrocele, a rectal examination and palpating the scrotum simultaneously may reveal whether an intestinal loop is present in the scrotal sac rather than a fluid-filled hydrocele.

Treatment

Inguinal hernias should be reduced daily and as needed to assess for the presence of an incarcerated hernia. Inguinal hernias may be reduced by gently applying pressure to the hernia. When the hernia is easily reducible, there is no need for immediate repair. An incarcerated hernia occurs when the intestines are caught within the processus vaginalis. Vomiting and abdominal distention may indicate obstruction of the herniated intestine. Strangulation of the bowel and gonads occurs when the circulation becomes compromised. Necrosis may follow a few hours later.

When the hernia is difficult to reduce or if there are other symptoms of incarceration such as a firm tense mass and inconsolable crying, incarceration must be considered, and an immediate surgical consult is indicated (Benjamin, 2002).

If signs of incarceration without strangulation are present, the surgical team may attempt reduction. After the infant is well sedated and placed in the Trendelenburg position, ice packs are placed on the hernia to reduce intestinal edema. If gentle reduction is successful, surgery may be delayed for 24 to 48 hours.

Because 69% of hernias become incarcerated, usually within the first year of life, surgery is indicated in all infants diagnosed with inguinal hernias. Surgical correction involves repair of the hernia and separation of the hernia from the inguinal canal. Because of the increased incidence of herniation in the contralateral testis, both testicles are commonly explored. Inguinal hernias are generally repaired prior to discharge to avoid the risk of incarceration at home. The most common complication following surgery is postoperative apnea. All premature infants require 24 hours of observation prior to discharge.

The focus of postoperative nursing care is on adherence to aseptic technique with regard to suture line maintenance. The infant should be placed in a side-lying or supine position with the head turned to the side to prevent disruption of the suture line. Operative dressings should be observed for any drainage and bleeding. They should be kept dry, and the underlying skin should be inspected for irritation or breakdown. Pain should be assessed every 4 hours, and appropriate pain management should be initiated when indicated.

TORSION OF THE TESTICLE
Pathophysiology

Torsion of the testicle occurs when the testis and coverings twist inside the scrotum. Blood flow to the testicle is compromised, which frequently results in a nonviable testicle. In the newborn, testicular torsion is often an antenatal event with nearly universal necrosis of the testicle.

Diagnosis

Testicular torsion presents with unilateral acute pain and scrotal swelling. In torsion, the scrotum is firm to the touch, is very tender, and is often discolored. The surrounding abdomen may also show significant discoloration and be either plethoric or cyanotic. The mass itself cannot be transilluminated. The clinical presentation of testicular torsion is similar to other scrotal abnormalities such as hydrocele, inguinal hernia, and trauma. The diagnosis of testicular torsion must be considered in any infant with scrotal swelling because of the emergent need for surgical intervention. The presence of scrotal discoloration strongly supports the diagnosis. Information related to testicular blood flow can be obtained via the use of color Doppler ultrasound (van der Sluijis et al, 2004).

Treatment

The treatment of acute testicular torsion is immediate surgery to untwist the testicle and restore blood supply. The timing of the intervention is critical. If surgery does not take place within 4 to 6 hours following initiation of symptoms, there is little to no chance of testicular survival. If the torsion occurs antenatally, the chance for testicular survival is nearly nonexistent and surgery would be futile. The most important determinant in the decision to perform surgery is the appearance of the scrotum in the delivery room. If the scrotum appears normal initially and then becomes acutely painful, swollen, and discolored, immediate surgery is indicated in an attempt to salvage the testicle. If the scrotum appears blue, hard, and painless immediately after birth, the torsion occurred prenatally and the testicle has already necrosed.

Controversy exists regarding the treatment of antenatally occurring testicular torsion. Some advocate conservative treatment with regular ultrasounds to monitor atrophy (Ricci et al, 2001; Thomas, 2002b; van der Sluijis et al, 2004). Others suggest that orchiopexy on the contralateral testis is indicated as soon as possible to prevent the possibility of torsion of both testes (Fuhrer et al, 2005; Sorensen et al, 2003; Yerkes et al, 2005).

The focus of nursing care is on keeping the infant comfortable and as quiet as possible. The abdominal girth should be measured every 4 hours for any signs of distention. Positioning of the infant should be only on the back with head turned to the side or in a side-lying position so as to avoid too much pressure being placed on the abdominal and scrotal areas.

If surgery is required, nursing care is centered on stability of the vital signs and prevention of infection. The suture line is generally small but still requires aseptic technique. The site should be assessed for the presence of edema, drainage, or discoloration. A urinary drainage bag may be necessary to protect the skin and to prevent infection if excessive drainage is present.

NEPHROBLASTOMA (WILMS' TUMOR)
Pathophysiology

Wilms' tumor is a well-encapsulated heterogeneous tumor of the kidney. The incidence is 0.2% of neonates, but the tumor does occur more frequently in the young infant. Associated conditions include aniridia (lack of development or absence of

the iris), GU tract anomalies, and Beckwith-Wiedemann syndrome. The presence of these signs in the neonate should alert the health care professional to the potential development of Wilms' tumor beyond the neonatal period.

Diagnosis

The typical presentation is a smooth, solid abdominal or flank mass that rarely crosses the midline (Lin, 2003). The infant otherwise appears well. Microscopic hematuria may be present (Duffy, 2002). Hypertension may occur because of the possibility of renal artery stenosis or increased renin secretion (Leclair et al, 2005; Hartman & MacLennan, 2005). Wilms' tumor can be diagnosed on prenatal ultrasound. Fetuses diagnosed with Wilms' tumor have an increased incidence of fetal distress, hydrops, and prematurity (Leclair et al, 2005). Postnatally, the initial diagnostic procedure is usually an abdominal ultrasound to determine the origin of the abdominal mass. This is generally followed by computed tomography (CT) to detect the tumor and to determine the stage of cancer (Duffy, 2002).

Treatment

Because the encapsulated tumor may rupture and seed the tumor to other areas of the body, repeated abdominal examinations should be avoided. Treatment of Wilms' tumor includes removal of the affected kidney, chemotherapy, and possibly radiation. Occasionally the tumor may affect both kidneys, requiring initial chemotherapy to shrink the tumor followed by resection of the tumors (Duffy, 2002).

Prognosis is related to stage of the disease and the size of the tumor. Children younger than 2 years of age generally have a more favorable prognosis than older children.

The diagnosis of cancer in a young infant can be devastating to the family. Clear, easy-to-understand information related to treatment and prognosis is required to assist parents to have realistic expectations related to their infant's diagnosis.

SUMMARY

The infant who presents with genitourinary abnormality presents unique challenges to the neonatal care team. Although aberrations in the genital system are not life-threatening, their appearance can be traumatic for the parents. Urinary tract pathology, on the other hand, can result in emergent life-threatening events at any age. Renal abnormality and diseases that manifest in the neonatal period can have lifelong consequences. The neonatal nurse must be able to accurately assess and respond to alterations in renal function. Astute nursing care of the infant and parents is paramount to optimal management and outcome. The neonatal nurse is in the position to be the first member of the health care team to detect the minor changes in neonatal physiologic functions that could signal onset of significant compromise. To do this, the neonatal nurse must have knowledge of normal renal physiology.

Parental support is another aspect of nursing care that is of major importance when caring for the infant with GU conditions. Timely assessment of parental coping mechanisms, alterations in parent-infant attachment, and evaluation of the parents' response to teaching provides vital information that will ultimately affect the infant's overall well-being.

Case Study

IDENTIFICATION OF THE PROBLEM

Infant with an average urinary output of 0.4 ml/kg/hr for the last 24 hours.

ASSESSMENT: HISTORY AND PHYSICAL EXAMINATION:

Child is a 3-day-old, 900-g, 28 weeks' gestational age infant born to a 28-year-old gravida 1, para 0 mother. Blood type is A+ and all serologies including VDRL, HbsAg, GC, and HIV are negative. The mother received good prenatal care during this pregnancy. No smoking or drug or alcohol use reported. Delivery was via cesarean section due to placental abruption at 28 weeks' gestation. No antibiotics or prenatal steroids were administered prior to delivery. Infant required intubation at delivery because of apnea and low heart rate. Apgar scores were 4 at 1 minute and 8 at 5 minutes. Infant was transferred to the level three NICU. His problems included the following:

Fluid, electrolytes, and nutrition: He is currently on minimal enteral feedings of 1 ml every 12 hours and tolerating these well. His total fluid volume is 120 ml/kg/day of total parenteral nutrition.

Respiratory: Received two doses of artificial surfactant for a chest radiograph consistent with hyaline membrane disease. He remains intubated on moderate ventilatory settings.

Cardiovascular: Infant has had several episodes of hypotension that have resolved spontaneously without treatment. Heart rate is 175. Current blood pressure has a mean arterial pressure of 28.

Infectious disease: Receiving ampicillin and gentamicin for suspected sepsis. No culture proven sepsis.

Hematologic: Hematocrit is 35%. Under phototherapy for hyperbilirubinemia.

Neurologic: A cranial ultrasound has been ordered for 1 week of life.

Social: Parents are married. This is their first child. They are appropriately concerned and have been updated at the bedside daily.

Physical Assessment

General: No obvious anomalies noted.

HEENT: Anterior fontanelle soft and flat. Eyes clear without drainage, red reflex present. Pupils equally reactive to light. Nares patent bilaterally. No clefts or abnormalities of mouth noted. Ear canals patent bilaterally.

Chest and lungs: Heart rate regular without murmur. Pulses equal in all four extremities. Quiet precordium. Capillary refill time is 2 seconds. Lungs equal with fine crackles bilaterally.

Abdomen: Soft and nondistended. Positive bowel sounds auscultated in all four quadrants. No masses felt. Umbilical cord normal. Liver felt 2 cm below right intercostal margin.

GU: Normal female infant. Genitalia appropriate for gestational age.

Skeletal: Moves all extremities well. No obvious anomalies noted.

Neurologic: All reflexes present. Tone appropriate for gestational age.

DIFFERENTIAL DIAGNOSIS

The differential diagnosis of oliguria in this infant includes:

Prerenal failure associated with decreased renal blood due to low systemic blood pressure or inadequate fluid intake.

Intrinsic renal failure due to the administration of nephrotoxic medications (gentamicin) or acute tubular necrosis due to perinatal depression related to the placental abruption and as evidence by the low Apgar scores.

Postrenal obstruction due to a neurogenic bladder related to fentanyl administration.

DIAGNOSTIC TESTS

Palpate the abdomen for the presence of a distended bladder and perform an in-and-out catheterization.

Electrolytes: sodium 148, potassium 3.5; creatinine 0.4; BUN 10.

Weight is 780 g.

Gentamicin trough is 0.4 mg/L.

Urine specific gravity is 1020. No protein, blood, or WBCs are present in the urine.

The next step should be administration of 10 to 20 ml/kg of normal saline via IV. Use of a diuretic after the fluid challenge may be necessary if urine output does not increase immediately after the fluid challenge.

WORKING DIAGNOSIS

The bladder is not distended. No urine is obtained via in-and-out catheterization, thus ruling out postrenal failure.

Physical assessment is impressive for lack of abdominal masses that would possibly indicate an enlarged kidney and associated intrinsic renal failure. Tachycardia is present, possibly indicating mild dehydration. A borderline mean arterial pressure may indicate decreased intravascular volume or decreased systemic blood flow.

Infant has lost 120 g over the past 3 days.

Gentamicin level is normal and does not support the presence of intrinsic renal failure.

The sodium level and specific gravity are elevated, which are both consistent with prerenal failure.

The creatinine and BUN are normal. If elevated, they would support a diagnosis of intrinsic renal failure.

There is no blood or protein in the urine. The presence of these substances would also support a diagnosis of intrinsic renal failure.

Continued

Case Study—cont'd

The administration of a fluid challenge produced a urine output of over 1 ml/kg/hr, thus indicating a diagnosis of prerenal failure.

No other workup such as a renal ultrasound would be indicated at this time.

DEVELOPMENT OF MANAGEMENT PLAN

Ensure administration of an adequate fluid volume by increasing fluid volume appropriately to ensure a urine output over 1 ml/kg/hr. Compensate for fluid losses due to insensible water losses including losses from phototherapy.

Low-dose dopamine may increase renal blood flow.

Ensure appropriate renal blood flow by increasing mean arterial pressure. If increase in fluid volume does not increase blood pressure sufficiently, inotropes such as higher dose dopamine or dobutamine may be administered.

IMPLEMENTATION AND EVALUATION OF EFFECTIVENESS

Monitor skin turgor and fontanelles for signs of dehydration.

Monitor serum electrolytes closely to ensure normalization of sodium levels.

Monitor vital signs every 3 to 4 hours to ensure normalization of blood pressure and heart rate.

Carefully monitor intake and output to ensure that infant is receiving adequate volume to result in a urine output of over 1 ml/kg/hr.

Daily or twice daily weights.

Monitor specific gravity to ensure resolution to a normal range.

REFERENCES

Agarwal SK, Fisk NM (2001). In utero therapy for lower urinary tract obstruction. *Prenatal diagnosis* 21:970-971.

Agot KE et al (2004). Risk of HIV-1 in rural Kenya: a comparison of circumcised and uncircumcised men. *Epidemiology* 15:157-163.

Agras PL et al (2004). Acute renal failure in the neonatal period. *Renal failure* 26:305-309.

Al-Ghwery A, Al-Asmari A (2005). Multicystic dysplastic kidney: conservative management and follow-up. *Renal failure* 27:189-192.

American Academy of Pediatrics (AAP): Committee on the Fetus and Newborn (1971). *Standards and recommendations for hospital care of newborn infants.* Evanston, IL: Author.

American Academy of Pediatrics (AAP): Committee on the Fetus and Newborn (1975). Reports of the Ad Hoc Task Force on Circumcision. *Pediatrics* 56:610-611.

American Academy of Pediatrics (AAP): Committee on the Fetus and Newborn (1983). *Guidelines for perinatal care.* Elk Grove Village, IL: Author.

American Academy of Pediatrics (AAP) (1989). Report of the Task Force on Circumcision. *Pediatrics* 84:388-391.

American Academy of Pediatrics (AAP) (1999). Report of the Task Force on Circumcision. Circumcision policy statement. *Pediatrics* 103:686-693.

Andreoli SP (2004). Acute renal failure in the newborn. *Seminars in perinatology* 28:112-123.

Anochie IC, Eke F (2004). Renal vein thrombosis in the neonate: a case report and review of the literature. *Journal of the National Medical Association* 96(12):1648-1652.

Baldwin SB et al (2004). Condom use and other factors affecting penile human papillomavirus detection in men attending a sexually transmitted disease clinic. *Sexually transmitted diseases* 31:601-607.

Barletta GM, Bunchman TE (2004). Acute renal failure in children and infants. *Current opinions in critical care* 10:499-504.

Benini D et al (2004). In utero exposure to nonsteroidal anti-inflammatory drugs: neonatal renal failure. *Pediatric nephrology* 19:232-234.

Benjamin K (2002). Scrotal and inguinal masses in the newborn period. *Advances in neonatal care* 2:140-148.

Berseth CL, Poenaru D (2004). *Abdominal wall problems.* In Tausch HW et al, editors. *Avery's diseases of the newborn.* Philadelphia: Elsevier.

Biyikli NK et al (2004). Neonatal urinary tract infections: analysis of the patients and recurrences. *Pediatrics international* 46:21-25.

Blackburn ST (2003). *Maternal, fetal and neonatal physiology: a clinical perspective.* Philadelphia: Saunders.

Bonacorsi S et al (2005). *Escherichia coli* strains causing urinary tract infection in uncircumcised infants resemble urosepsis-like adult strains. *Journal of urology* 173:195-197.

Capisonda R et al (2003). Autosomal recessive polycystic kidney disease: outcomes from a single-center experience. *Pediatric nephrology* 18:19-26.

Caty H, Wright N (2003). Imaging in paediatric nephrology. In Webb N, Postlethwaite R, editors. *Clinical paediatric nephrology.* New York: Oxford University Press.

Chandler JC, Gauderer MW (2004). The neonate with an abdominal mass. *Pediatric clinics of North America* 51:979-997.

Cheng AM et al (2004). Outcome of isolated antenatal hydronephrosis. *Archives of pediatric and adolescent medicine* 158:38-40.

Chevalier RL (2004). Perinatal obstructive nephropathy. *Seminars in perinatology* 28:124-131.

Dell KM, Avner ED (2003). Clinical presentation and evolution of cystic disease. In Webb N, Postlethwaite R, editors. *Clinical paediatric nephrology.* New York: Oxford University Press.

Denes FT et al (2004). Comprehensive surgical treatment of prune belly syndrome: 17 years' experience with 32 patients. *Urology* 64:790-794.

Dillon HK (2002). Prenatal diagnosis. In Thomas DFM et al, editors. *Essentials of paediatric urology.* London: Martin Dunitz.

Drukker A, Guignard JP (2002). Renal aspects of the term and preterm infant: a selective update. *Current opinions in pediatrics* 14:175-182.

Duffy PG (2002). Genitourinary malignancies. In Thomas DFM et al, editors. *Essentials of paediatric urology.* London: Martin Dunitz.

Durson H et al (2005). Associated anomalies in children with congenital solitary functioning kidney. *Pediatric surgery international* 21:456-459.

Friedlich PS et al (2004). Acute and chronic renal failure. In Taeusch HW et al, editors. *Avery's diseases of the newborn.* Philadelphia: Saunders.

Fuhrer S et al (2005). Intrauterine torsion of a testicular teratoma: a case report. *Journal of perinatology* 25:220-222.

Fusaro F et al (2004). Renal transplantation in prune-belly syndrome. *Transplant international* 17:549-552.

Gallini F et al (2000). Progression of renal function in preterm infants < or = to 32 weeks, *Pediatric nephrology* 15:119-124.

Garcia FJ, Nager AL (2002). Jaundice as an early diagnostic sign of urinary tract infection in infancy. *Pediatrics* 109:846-851.

Gordon I, Riccabona M (2003). Investigating the newborn kidney: update on imaging techniques. *Seminars in neonatology* 8:31-39.

Gordon M et al (2001). Outcome analysis of vesicoamniotic shunting in a comprehensive population. *Journal of urology* 166:1036-1040.

Guay-Woodford LM, Desmond RA (2003). Autosomal recessive polycystic kidney disease: the experience in North America. *Pediatrics* 111:1072-1080.

Hammouda HM, Dotb H (2004). Complete primary repair of bladder exstrophy: initial experience with 33 cases. *Journal of urology* 172:1441-1444.

Hartman DJ, MacLennan GT (2005). Wilms' tumor. *Journal of urology* 173:2147.

Haycock GB (2003). Management of acute and chronic renal failure in the newborn. *Seminars in neonatology* 8:325-334.

Hernandez JA, Glass SM (2005). Physical assessment of the newborn. In Thureen PJ et al, editors. *Assessment and care of the well newborn*. St Louis: Saunders.

Holmdahl G, Sillen U (2005). Boys with posterior urethral valves: outcome concerning renal function, bladder function and paternity at ages 31–44 years. *Journal of urology* 174:1031-1034.

Holmes N et al (2001). Fetal surgery in post urethral valves: long-term postnatal outcomes. *Pediatrics* 108:E7.

Hrair-George O et al (2004). Urologic problems of the neonate. *Pediatric clinics of North America* 51:1051-1062.

Huether SE (2004). Alterations of renal and urinary tract function in children. In McCance KL, Huether SE, editors. *Pathophysiology: the basis for disease in adults and children*. St Louis: Mosby.

Ismaili K et al (2005). Routine voiding cystourethrography is of no value in neonates with unilateral multicystic dysplastic kidney. *Journal of pediatrics* 46:759-763.

Itabashi K et al (2003). Indomethacin responsiveness of patent ductus arteriosus and renal abnormalities in preterm infants treated with indomethacin. *Journal of pediatrics* 143:203-207.

Karlowicz MG, Adelman RD (2005). Acute renal failure. In Spitzer AR, editor. *Intensive care of the fetus and neonate*. Philadelphia: Mosby.

Kaufman MW et al (2001). Neonatal circumcision: benefits, risks and family teaching. *American journal of maternal child nursing* 26:197-201.

Keating MA, Rich MA (2000). Prune-belly syndrome. In Ashcraft KW, editor. *Pediatric surgery*. Philadelphia: Saunders.

Kemper MJ, Muller-Wiefel DE (2001). Renal function in congenital anomalies of the kidney and urinary tract. *Current opinions in urology* 11:571-575.

Kiddoo DA et al (2004). Initial management of complex urological disorders: bladder exstrophy. *Urologic clinics of North America* 31:417-426.

Koeppen B, Stanton B (2001). *Renal physiology*. St Louis: Mosby.

Kugelman A et al (2002). Pre-auricular tags and pits in the newborn: the role of renal ultrasonography. *Journal of pediatrics* 141:388-391.

Kuwertz-Broeking E et al (2004). Unilateral multicystic dysplastic kidney: experience in children. *British journal of urology international* 93:388-392.

Langley JM et al (2001). Unique epidemiology of nosocomial urinary tract infection in children. *American journal of infection control* 29:94-98.

Leclair MD et al (2005). The outcome of prenatally diagnosed renal tumors. *Journal of urology* 173:186-189.

Leeners B et al (2000). Prune-belly syndrome: therapeutic options including in utero placement of a vesicoamniotic shunt. *Journal of clinical ultrasound* 28:500-507.

Lerman SE, Liao JC (2001). Neonatal circumcision. *Pediatric clinics of North America* 48:1539-1557.

Lewis MA (2003). Antenatal detection of renal anomalies. In Webb N, Postlethwaite R, editors. *Clinical paediatric nephrology*. New York: Oxford University Press.

Lin YC (2003). Early recognition of infant malignancy: the five most common infant cancers. *Neonatal network* 22:11-18.

Long SS, Klein JO (2001). Bacterial infections of the urinary tract. In Remington JS, Klein JO, editors. *Infectious diseases of the fetus and newborn infant*. Philadelphia: Saunders.

Madden NP (2002). Testis, hydrocoele and varicocoele. In Thomas DFM et al, editors. *Essentials of paediatric urology*. London: Martin Dunitz.

Marks SD et al (2005). Neonatal renal venous thrombosis: clinical outcomes and prevalence of prothrombotic disorders. *Journal of pediatrics* 146:811-816.

Mercado-Deane MG et al (2002). US of renal insufficiency in neonates. *Radiographics* 22:1429-1438.

Mesrobian HG et al (2004). Urologic problems of the neonate. *Pediatric clinics of North America* 51:1051-1062.

Nafday SM et al (2005). Renal disease. In MacDonald MC et al, editors. *Avery's neonatology: pathophysiology and management of the newborn*. Philadelphia: Lippincott Williams & Wilkins.

Nese K et al (2004). Neonatal urinary tract infections: analysis of the patients and recurrences. *Pediatrics international* 46:21-25.

Peevy KJ et al (1986). Epidemiology of inguinal hernias in preterm infants. *Pediatrics* 77:246-247.

Peniakov M et al (2004). Reduction in contamination of urine samples obtained by in-out catheterization by culturing the later urine stream. *Pediatric emergency care* 20:1-3.

Peppas DS (2003). Pediatric urologic emergencies. In Gearrhart JP, editor. *Pediatric urology*. Totowa, NJ: Humana Press.

Perez-Brayfield MR et al (2001). In utero intervention in a patient with prune-belly syndrome and severe urethral hypoplasia. *Urology* 57:1178vii-1178ix.

Postlethwaite RJ, Dickson A (2003). Common urologic problems. In Webb N, Postlethwaite R, editors. *Clinical paediatric urology*. New York: Oxford University Press.

Potter EL (1965). Bilateral absence of ureters and kidneys: a report of 50 cases. *Obstetrics & gynecology* 25:3-12.

Pulsifer A (2005). Pediatric genitourinary examination: a clinician's reference. *Urology nurse* 25:163-168.

Rabelo EA et al (2004). Natural history of multicystic kidney conservatively managed: a prospective study. *Pediatric nephrology* 19:1102-1107.

Rajput A et al (1992). Inguinal hernia in very low birth weight infants: incidence and timing of repair. *Journal of pediatric surgery* 27:1322-1324.

Riccabona M (2002). Cystography in infants and children: a critical appraisal of the many forms with special regards to voiding cystourethrography. *European radiology* 12:2910-2918.

Riccabona M (2004). Assessment and management of newborn hydronephrosis. *World journal of urology* 22:73-78.

Ricci P et al (2001). Prenatal testicular torsion: sonographic appearance in the newborn infant. *European radiology* 11:2589-2592.

Rizk D, Chapman AB (2003). Cystic and inherited kidney disease. *American journal of kidney diseases* 42:1305-1317.

Roy M et al (2002). Accuracy of Doppler echocardiogram for the diagnosis of thrombosis associated with umbilical venous catheter. *Journal of pediatrics* 140:131-134.

Sairam S et al (2001). Natural history of fetal hydronephrosis diagnosed on mid-trimester ultrasound. *Ultrasound in obstetrics and gynecology* 17:191-196.

Salihu HM et al (2003). Prune belly syndrome and associated malformations. A 13-year experience from a developing country. *West Indian medical journal* 52:281-284.

Schoen EJ et al (2000). The highly protective effect of newborn circumcision against invasive penile cancer. *Pediatrics* 105:E36.

Sheldon CA (2001). The pediatric genitourinary examination: inguinal, urethral and genital disease. *Pediatric urology* 48:1339-1367.

Shneider BL, Magid MS (2005). Liver disease in autosomal recessive polycystic kidney disease. *Pediatric transplantation* 9:634-639.

Singh-Grewal D et al (2005). Circumcision for the prevention of urinary tract infection in boys: a systematic review of randomized trials and observational studies. *Archives of diseases in childhood* 90:853-858.

Smith EA, Woodard JR (2002). Prune-belly syndrome. In Walch PC et al, editors. *Campbell's urology*. Philadelphia: Saunders.

Solhaug MJ et al (2004). The developing kidney and environmental toxins. *Pediatrics* 113:1084-1091.

Sorenson MD et al (2003). Prenatal bilateral extravaginal testicular torsion—a case presentation. *Pediatric surgery international* 20:892-893.

Srinivasan R, Arora RS (2005). Do well infants born with an isolated single umbilical artery need investigation? *Archives of disease in childhood* 90:100-101.

Strand WR (2004). Initial management of complex pediatric disorders: prune-belly syndrome, posterior urethral valves. *Urologic clinics of North America* 31:399-415.

Tabacova SA, Kimmel CA (2001). Enalapril: pharmacokinetics/dynamic inferences for comparative developmental toxicity. *Reproductive toxicology* 15:467-478.

Thomas DFM (2001). Prenatal diagnosis: does it alter outcome? *Prenatal diagnosis* 21:1004-1011.

Thomas DFM (2002a). Cystic renal disease. In Thomas DFM et al, editors. *Essentials of paediatric urology*. London: Martin Dunitz.

Thomas DFM (2002b). The acute scrotum. In Thomas DFM et al, editors. *Essentials of paediatric urology*. London: Martin Dunitz.

Tortora GJ, Grabowski SR (2003). *Principles of anatomy and physiology*. New York: Wiley.

Toth-Heyn P et al (2000). The stressed kidney: from pathophysiology to clinical management of neonatal vasomotor nephropathy. *Pediatric nephrology* 14:227-239.

van der Sluijs JW et al (2004). Prenatal testicular torsion: diagnosis and natural course: an ultrasonographic study. *European radiology* 14:250-255.

Vogt BA, Avner ED (2002). The kidney and urinary tract. In Fanaroff AA et al, editors. *Neonatal-perinatal management*. Philadelphia: Mosby.

Wald E (2004). Urinary tract infections in infants and children: a comprehensive overview. *Current opinion in pediatrics* 16:85-88.

Weinschenk N et al (2001). Combination thrombolytic and anticoagulant therapy for bilateral renal vein thrombosis in a premature infant. *American journal of perinatology* 18:293-297.

Yerkes EB et al (2005). Management of perinatal torsion: today, tomorrow or never? *Journal of urology* 174:1579-1582.

Ylinen E et al (2004a). Prognostic factors of posterior urethral valves and the role of antenatal detection. *Pediatric nephrology* 19:874-879.

Ylinen E et al (2004b). Nephrectomy for multicystic dysplastic kidney: if and when? *Urology* 63:768-772.

Zamir G et al (2005). Urinary tract infection: is there a need for routine renal ultrasonography? *Archives of diseases in children* 89:466-468.

Zerres K et al (2003). Autosomal recessive polycystic kidney disease (ARPKD). *Journal of nephrology* 16:453-458.

Zigman A et al (2000). Renal vein thrombosis: a 10-year review. *Journal of pediatric surgery* 35:1540-1542.

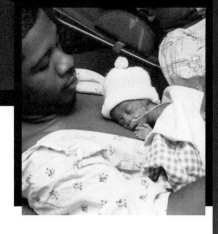

Chapter 9

Immune System

Judy Wright Lott

The primary function of the immune system is to protect the body from invading microorganisms such as bacteria, viruses, fungi, protozoa, and parasites. The uncompromised mother's uterus provides a safe environment for the healthy fetus. During and after delivery, the newborn is exposed to a wide variety of microorganisms. Immune system development begins in early gestation; however, the immune system cannot function as efficiently at the time of birth—even in the term newborn—as in older infants, children, or adults. The immaturity of the immune system is responsible for the relatively high prevalence of infectious disease during the neonatal period, as well as the occurrence of neonatal infection from microorganisms that do not generally cause infection in older individuals. The diagnosis and treatment of the most common causes of newborn infection will be discussed in this chapter.

The susceptibility and high mortality and morbidity make early identification and treatment of infection in a newborn a critical component of care. Identifying and caring for a newborn with an infection can be one of the greatest challenges in nursing. Nurses are often the first to recognize that there is something "wrong" with an infant, and this often leads to investigation of the signs. Generally, treatment is begun once a presumptive diagnosis of infection is made because the benefits of early treatment outweigh risks of unnecessary treatment.

INCIDENCE OF NEONATAL INFECTION

The incidence of infection varies according to the level of perinatal care available, economic standards, and other perinatal risk factors in term newborns. In the United States, the incidence in term newborns has been approximately 2% to 4% per 1000 live births since 1980. The worldwide range has been 1% to 8% per 1000 live births, with lower rates in developed countries. The highest prevalence of neonatal infection occurs in males and low-birth-weight infants. The lower the birth weight, and consequent lower gestational age, the higher the risk for infection (Baltimore, 2003). Infection case fatality rates range from less than 10% to greater than 50%, with the highest mortality rates for preterm infants and infants with early-onset infection. Improved knowledge and technology to care for less mature and smaller newborns has led to an increased population of newborns at higher risk for bacterial infection. Neonatal infection rates are much higher in developing countries than in the United States, however. As many as 20% of, or 30 million, newborns in developing countries contract infection in the neonatal period and more than 1.5 million of them die (Stoll, 2005). Fifty percent of all neonatal deaths that occur on the first day of life are caused by infection. Even with aggressive therapy, the mortality rate for early-onset group B streptococcal (GBS) infection is high. Major complications of infection include respiratory distress, shock, acidosis, disseminated intravascular coagulation (DIC), and meningitis.

CLINICAL SIGNS OF INFECTION

Signs and symptoms of infection are listed in Box 9-1. Temperature instability or hypothermia, the inability of the neonate to maintain temperature in the neutral thermal zone (usually between 97.7° F and 99° F axillary), is a frequent indication of serious infection. Newborns traditionally do not have well-developed febrile mechanisms; thus, the absence of fever does not indicate the absence of infection. Premature infants more often present with a low body temperature. Hyperthermia may occur in term newborns, with temperatures of more than 100.1° F, but it is relatively rare in preterm infants.

An infected infant may present with lethargy, poor feeding, decreased reflexes, abdominal distention, delayed gastric emptying time, and perhaps diarrhea or loose green or brown stools. Hypoglycemia or hyperglycemia, as well as glycosuria, may result from the inability to maintain normal metabolic processes and impaired glucose metabolism.

Vascular perfusion is typically decreased; the infected neonate may appear gray, mottled, or ashen in color with poor perfusion, prolonged capillary filling time, and hypotension. Skin changes include cyanosis and petechiae. Thrombocytopenia is often present. Infections can cause DIC, resulting in altered prothrombin time, partial thromboplastin time, and split fibrin product laboratory values. Hemolytic anemia may occur as a part of the inflammatory process, which can significantly decrease oxygen-carrying capacity, especially in the preterm infant.

Apnea in a term (nonsedated) newborn in the first few hours of life should be considered a serious sign of inability to regulate the brain's respiratory center. Apnea in the first 24 hours of life in a preterm newborn is a common sign of infection. Respiratory distress can be an early sign of pneumonia and must be considered carefully. Cardiovascular shock can be a sudden clinical sign of fulminant infection that requires immediate and aggressive intervention to restore adequate circulation. Unexplained bradycardia, sclerema, and sudden purpura, rash, or petechiae are other signs of systemic infection.

A complete blood count (CBC) is often the first step in identifying infection. The CBC of an infected infant may reveal leukopenia, especially neutropenia with a cell count of polymorphonuclear (mature) leukocytes less than 5000/mm^3,

BOX 9-1

Signs and Symptoms of Neonatal Infection

Clinical
- General
- Poor feeding
- Irritability
- Lethargy
- Temperature instability

Skin
- Petechiae
- Pustulosis
- Sclerema
- Edema
- Jaundice

Respiratory
- Grunting
- Nasal flaring
- Intercostal retractions
- Tachypnea/apnea

Gastrointestinal
- Diarrhea
- Hematochezia
- Abdominal distention
- Emesis
- Aspirates

CNS
- Hypotonia
- Seizures
- Poor spontaneous movement

Circulatory
- Bradycardia/tachycardia
- Hypotension
- Cyanosis
- Decreased perfusion

Laboratory Values
White blood cell count
- Neutrophils
  <5000 cells/mm^3, neutropenia
  >25,000 cells/mm^3, neutrophilia
- Absolute neutrophil count (neutrophil and bands)
  <1800 cells/mm^3 (during first week)
- Immature: total neutrophil ratio
  ≥0:2
- Platelet count
  <100,000, thrombocytopenia
Cerebrospinal fluid
- Protein
  150 to 200 mg/L (term)
  300 mg/L (preterm)
- Glucose
  50% to 60% or more of blood glucose level

Adapted with permission from Lott JW, Kilb JR (1992). The selection of antibacterial agents for treatment of neonatal infection. *Neonatal pharmacology quarterly* 1(1):19-29.

or the infant may have a large number of immature leukocytes (>25,000 cells/mm^3), in particular, bands (immature neutrophil), with the immature-to-mature cell ratio greater than 0.2. Jaundice, hepatosplenomegaly, and irritability may also be found in infants with infection. The wide variability of signs of infection warrants inclusion of infection as part of the differential diagnosis in any ill infant.

Risk Factors

Prematurity is the most prevalent risk factor for infection. Premature infants are far more susceptible to the invasion of foreign microorganisms. Preterm infants have decreased maternal antibodies (passive immunity). The maternal antibodies, developed by exposure to antigens and subsequent creation of an antibody defense system, provide temporary protection to the newborn, but preterm newborns are born before the majority of maternal antibodies are transferred from the maternal circulation. Also, the cellular immune system is not well developed in the preterm newborn, thus there is decreased phagocytic cellular defenses.

Prolonged rupture of the fetal membranes (PROM) is a well-known risk factor for the development of infection. The fetus is at increased risk because the break in the amniotic sac provides a pathway for the migration of microorganisms up the vaginal vault to the fetus. Delaying delivery in a pregnancy in a mother with PROM and a preterm fetus until pulmonary maturity is achieved creates the potential environment for bacterial proliferation and subsequent newborn infection. The benefit in promoting maturity of the immature lungs is weighed against the risk of overwhelming infection in the baby. PROM lasting longer than 24 hours is considered a risk factor in the evaluation of infants for potential for infection.

Although the most common cause of fever in labor is decreased fluid volume, a fever may indicate maternal infection. A mother with an infection before or during delivery may transmit it to the infant. If maternal temperature is 101° F at delivery, evaluation for infection in the newborn is warranted. Maternal cervical or amniotic fluid cultures may identify the causative microorganism. If the maternal illness suggests viral infection, newborn viral cultures should be obtained. Early identification of causative agents in the mother may help in the management of the newborn by allowing faster identification of the microorganism and initiation of appropriate antimicrobial therapy.

Foul-smelling amniotic fluid is an indication for newborn antimicrobial therapy in symptomatic infants. Routine blood cultures and a CBC with differential are indicated for identification of newborn infection. Under these circumstances, the placenta should be sent for pathologic evaluation. Other risk factors associated with newborn infection are antenatal or intrapartal asphyxia, iatrogenic complications of treatment, and invasive procedures.

Stress inhibits the ability to fight infection by increasing the metabolic rate, which requires more oxygen and energy. A severely compromised hypoxemic newborn may have regional tissue damage. Ischemic or necrotic areas in the lungs, heart, brain, or gastrointestinal system promote colonization and overgrowth of normal bacterial flora. This overgrowth of bacteria is one of the most common sources of newborn infection. Tissue damage can be prevented or repaired only if the infectious process is reversed and adequate tissue perfusion is restored.

There are several known maternal factors associated with newborn infection: low socioeconomic status, malnutrition, inadequate prenatal care, substance abuse, PROM (before 37 weeks of gestation or at the start of labor), presence of a urinary tract infection at delivery, peripartum infection, clinical amnionitis, and general bacterial colonization.

Newborn risk factors include antenatal stress, intrapartal stress (perinatal asphyxia), congenital anomalies, male sex, multiple gestations, concurrent neonatal disease processes, prematurity, immaturity of the immune system, invasive admission procedures, and antimicrobial therapies.

Differential Diagnosis

The microorganisms responsible for newborn infection have changed over the past 60 years, and there are marked regional variations. Microorganisms commonly responsible for early-onset infection include *Streptococcus*, *Listeria monocytogenes*, and the gram-negative enteric rods. Late-onset infections are most often caused by *Staphylococcus*, *Pseudomonas*, or *Bacteroides fragilis* (anaerobes) (Table 9-1). After day 7, nosocomial microorganisms should be considered. These microorganisms include *Staphylococcus epidermidis*, particularly when invasive medical devices have been used; *S. aureus* (common skin contaminant); and the spectrum of gram-negative enteric rods, including *Klebsiella*, *Pseudomonas*,

Serratia, and *Escherichia coli*. Hospitalized preterm newborns are often affected by repeated episodes of infection. Many of these episodes are termed presumed, suspected, or clinical infection because no microorganism is recovered and cultured, despite clinical evidence of infection that responds to antimicrobial agent therapy.

A high index of suspicion of infection, early identification of the microorganism, and institution of appropriate therapy provide the best outcome. The evaluation for infection generally includes a CBC with differential, platelet count, and blood, urine, and cerebrospinal fluid (CSF) cultures. Gram stain of the CSF or urine can give an early indication of the type of microorganism responsible for the infection. Cell count and protein and glucose levels of the CSF may also indicate the presence of infection. A chest radiograph can identify the presence of pneumonia. Other tests that may be useful include latex agglutination (LA) or counterimmunoelectrophoresis (CIE) of urine or CSF or other body cavity fluids, erythrocyte sedimentation rate (ESR), and acute phase proteins. Other nonspecific findings, such as hypoglycemia, hypocalcemia, thrombocytopenia, hyponatremia, and metabolic acidosis, may also be present. Definitive diagnosis is based on recovery of a microorganism in blood, CSF, urine, or other body fluids.

Prognosis

The introduction of broad-spectrum antimicrobial agents dramatically improved the prognosis for infection, and there has been a decline in infection-associated neonatal and infant deaths in the United States (Baltimore, 2003). However, infection still accounts for significant morbidity and mortality in the neonatal period. Consequences of bacterial infection include prolonged hospitalization, increased hospital costs, and increased mortality.

Management

Management of a newborn with infection is aimed at the traditional "ABCs": airway, breathing, circulation, including oxygen, ventilation, correction of acidosis, volume expansion, extracorporeal membrane oxygenation (ECMO) (if persistent pulmonary hypertension [PPHN] is present), antimicrobial agents, and immune therapy. The exact management plan is based on an assessment of clinical signs, careful history, and appropriate laboratory findings.

Antimicrobial Agents

The selection of antimicrobial agents is based on identification of the microorganism and the infant's response to therapy. Infectious microorganisms are divided into two broad classes, based on Gram-stain results: gram-positive and gram-negative. The shape of the microorganism categorizes it as either a coccus or a rod. Generally, the gram-positive organisms respond to broad-spectrum antibiotics, such as penicillin analogues and first-generation cephalosporins (beta-lactamases), and the beta-lactamase penicillins. The gram-negative microorganisms are most often susceptible to aminoglycosides and cephalosporins. Tests must be run to determine the specific sensitivity of a microorganism to the antimicrobial agent selected to ensure that the appropriate agent is prescribed.

Gram-positive cocci generally respond to penicillin, unless the microorganism produces beta-lactamase (or penicillinase). The beta-lactamase destroys the penicillin. *S. aureus* is a beta-

TABLE 9-1	Common Microorganisms Causing Neonatal Infection	
Gram-Positive		**Gram-Negative**
Cocci	**Streptococcus**	**Neisseria meningitidis**
	Group A	**Neisseria gonorrhoeae**
	Group B	
	Group D	
	Pneumococci	
	Staphylococcus aureus (coagulase⁺)	
	Staphylococcus epidermidis (coagulase⁻)	
Rods	**Listeria monocytogenes**	**Enterobacteriaceae**
	Anaerobes	*Escherichia coli*
	Clostridium difficile	*Klebsiella*
	Clostridium perfringens	*Shigella*
	Clostridium botulinum	*Proteus*
	Clostridium tetani	*Salmonella*
		Serratia
		Citrobacter
		Haemophilus influenzae
		Pseudomonas
		Anaerobes
		Bacteroides fragilis

lactamase–producing microorganism and is therefore not responsive to penicillin. A group of semisynthetic penicillins with added side chains are used for treatment of *S. aureus* infection. Of this group, nafcillin and oxacillin are most often used. Other similar drugs are methicillin, dicloxacillin, and cloxacillin. First-generation cephalosporins, such as cefazolin, cephalexin, and cephalothin, are also resistant to beta-lactamase.

S. epidermidis and *S. aureus* strains may be resistant to penicillin, semisynthetic penicillins, and cephalosporins. Methicillin-resistant *S. aureus* is unresponsive to the semisynthetic penicillins. In this case, vancomycin is the drug of choice. It may also be used for *S. epidermidis* and infection related to foreign bodies or invasive procedures. The emergence of resistant strains to available antimicrobial agents is an increasing problem, due to the lack of other safe and effective antimicrobial agents to treat the infection.

Third-generation cephalosporins are used to treat gram-negative cocci that are penicillin- and methicillin-resistant. *Listeria monocytogenes*, a gram-positive rod, generally responds to ampicillin therapy. Aminoglycosides or third-generation cephalosporins are the drugs of choice for gram-negative enteric rods. Some gram-negative rods are classified according to their lactose fermentation ability. The lactose fermenters, *E. coli* and *Klebsiella*, are sensitive to aminoglycosides and third-generation cephalosporins. *Shigella* and *Salmonella* are non–lactose fermenters, which respond well to ampicillin and third-generation cephalosporins.

Haemophilus influenzae is usually sensitive to ampicillin and third-generation cephalosporins, although some strains are ampicillin-resistant. *Pseudomonas* requires the following combination therapy: aminoglycoside and an anti-pseudomonas penicillin such as azlocillin, carbenicillin, imipenem, mezlocillin, piperacillin, and ticarcillin.

Two anaerobic microorganisms, *Bacteroides fragilis* (gram-negative) and *Clostridium* (gram-positive), are sometimes the cause of newborn infections. *B. fragilis* is susceptible to metronidazole (Flagyl), clindamycin, chloramphenicol, and some of the newer beta-lactamases, such as imipenem and ampicillin with sulbactam. *Clostridium* is usually susceptible to penicillin.

A combination of ampicillin or penicillin and gentamicin is useful for antibacterial action against *Streptococcus*, *L. monocytogenes*, and gram-negative enteric rods. This combination of antimicrobial agents has a synergistic effect (in vitro), increasing the efficacy of either drug therapy used alone. Additional therapy or selection of other agents is necessary if staphylococcal infection is suspected, if *Pseudomonas* or *Bacteroides* (most often iatrogenically acquired) is present, if there is an outbreak of resistant organisms, or if prolonged ampicillin and gentamicin therapy has been used. Antimicrobial agents must be re-evaluated after completion of cultures and sensitivity testing. Tables 9-2 and 9-3 show generally recommended antimicrobial choices for infections caused by gram-positive and gram-negative microorganisms.

TYPES OF NEONATAL INFECTION

This section briefly describes the types of microorganisms that typically cause neonatal infection and their clinical manifestations, diagnosis, and collaborative management. The discussion includes both congenitally acquired and nosocomially acquired infections caused by bacterial, viral, fungal, and protozoal organisms.

TABLE 9-2	General Antimicrobial Selection Guidelines for Gram-Positive Microorganisms
Microorganism	**Antimicrobial**
Streptococcus	Penicillin or ampicillin
Staphylococcus aureus	Semisynthetic penicillins, such as methicillin (or methicillin-type) nafcillin, oxacillin, dicloxicillin, cephalin, cephalothin
Methicillin-resistant *Staphylococcus aureus* (MRSA)	Vancomycin
Staphylococcus epidermidis	Vancomycin
Listeria monocytogenes	Ampicillin
Clostridium difficile	Penicillin

TABLE 9-3	General Antimicrobial Selection Guidelines for Gram-Negative Microorganisms
Microorganism	**Antimicrobial**
Escherichia coli	Aminoglycosides or third-generation cephalosporins
Klebsiella	Aminoglycosides or third-generation cephalosporins
Shigella	Ampicillin and third-generation cephalosporins
Salmonella	Ampicillin and third-generation cephalosporins
Haemophilus influenzae	Ampicillin and third-generation cephalosporins; some strains are ampicillin-resistant
Pseudomonas	Aminoglycoside plus an anti-pseudomonas penicillin
Bacteroides fragilis	Metronidazole, clindamycin, some beta-lactamases such as imipenum and ampicillin with sulbactim; and chloramphenicol

Bacterial Infections
Group B Streptococcus

Group B beta-hemolytic streptococci were unknown to the perinatal scene until the early 1970s when they replaced *E. coli* as the single most common agent associated with bacterial meningitis during the first 2 months of life. The incidence of infection with group B streptococci has increased over the past 10 years, and they frequently cause postpartum infections in otherwise normal mothers (Edwards et al, 2005). Use of a rapid screening test to identify colonized mothers and intrapartum treatment with ampicillin has been shown to reduce vertical transmission (Lim et al, 1986).

born deaths associated with either early
t week of life) or late onset continues to
n high-risk urban centers. Potential for
sequelae for infant survivors of meningeal
infections is approximately 15% (Edwards et al, 2005). The
mortality rate of infected newborns varies according to time
of onset. Early onset infection (within the first week of life) has
a mortality rate between 5% and 50%; late-onset (after first
week of life) mortality is approximately 2% to 6% (Palazzi
et al, 2005).

Pathophysiology. *Streptococcus* is a gram-positive diplo-
coccus with an ultrastructure similar to that of other gram-
positive cocci. It was classified as hemolytic because of its
double zone of hemolysis surrounding colonies on blood agar
plates. Culture of body fluids, such as blood, urine, CSF, and
other secretions, is the most common method of identifying
group B streptococci. Counterelectrophoresis and latex agglutination are rapid assays that enable a presumptive diagnosis
before cultures are returned. Rapid identification of the group
B streptococcus organism is important in treating colonized
pregnant women and in the early diagnosis and treatment of
infection in the sick, unstable septic infant. To accurately
predict maternal colonization with group B streptococci, both
vaginal and rectal areas should be cultured on more than one
occasion (Adair et al, 2003; Benedetto et al, 2004). Newer
techniques using the LightCycler Strep B analyte-specific
reagents (Roche Diagnostics Corp.; Indianapolis, IN) gives
results more rapidly than traditional cultures thus decreasing
time to diagnosis (Uhl, et al, 2005).

Clinical Manifestations

Group B streptococcus has been identified as a relatively
common cause of mid-gestational fetal loss in women who
experience vaginal hemorrhage, PROM, fetal membrane
infection, and spontaneous abortion. The rate of stillbirth is
reported to be as high as 61% in association with these
bacteria. Early-onset neonatal infections with group B
streptococcus can be asymptomatic or can manifest with severe
symptoms of respiratory distress and shock, which can rapidly
progress to death (Edwards et al, 2005).

Early-Onset Group B Streptococcus

Early-onset group B streptococcus infection usually appears
within the first 24 hours of life and is most common in premature infants. Congenital pneumonia is a more common
presentation sign in infants who weigh 1000 g or less. The
most common presentations are pneumonia and meningitis.
Signs of respiratory distress, apnea, grunting, tachypnea, and
cyanosis are common. Hypotension is found in 25% of newborns with group B streptococcus infection; these infants are
at risk for cardiopulmonary collapse. Nonspecific signs of
infection include lethargy, poor feeding, temperature instability,
abdominal distention, pallor, tachycardia, and jaundice.
Experienced nurses may observe that the neonate "just doesn't
look right," which is sometimes a critical point for early
detection and implementation of therapy.

Overwhelming group B streptococcal septicemia is often
compounded by meningitis. Lumbar puncture and examination of the CSF is the only way to exclude meningeal
involvement and therefore is an important part of the workup.
Seizures may occur in infants with group B streptococcal
meningitis. Low-birth-weight infants have been identified as

particularly vulnerable, but a study in Texas revealed a high
incidence of infection in term newborns (Edwards et al, 2005).
These infants had no risk factors for infection; therefore, there
was a delay in identification and treatment. The mortality rate
in these term newborns was 14% (Edwards et al, 2005).

Late-Onset Infection

Late-onset infection with group B streptococcus usually occurs
in term newborns 7 days to 12 weeks of age. The fatality rate is
less than that with early-onset infection, but meningitis may
lead to permanent neurologic damage, varying in severity from
mild handicaps to severe impairment. Complications include
global or profound mental retardation, spastic quadriplegia,
cortical blindness, deafness, uncontrolled seizures, hydrocephalus,
and diabetes insipidus. Thus, early treatment is an important
part of the prevention of long-term serious sequelae. An infant
with a positive blood culture can often be asymptomatic
initially. The diagnosis of group B streptococcal infection is
complicated because signs and symptoms of neonatal infection
are not specific and symptoms may represent other conditions
of the neonate. For example, apnea may be a symptom of
central nervous system immaturity in the preterm neonate, but
it is also associated with infection. The caregiver must have a
high index of suspicion for infection in all conditions
involving the neonate. Infection should be considered in the
differential diagnosis of most newborn illnesses. Screening
tests, such as complete blood count with differential, are often
used to identify the need for further evaluation for infection.
Abnormal results indicate the necessity for definitive testing
and implementation of antimicrobial therapy.

Management. Regional and hospital differences in infectious agents must be considered in the selection of antimicrobial therapy. Before culture results are returned, administration
of a broad-spectrum penicillin and an aminoglycoside provides
coverage for the most prevalent microorganisms. Generally,
ampicillin and gentamicin are selected until culture results and
sensitivities are available. Group B streptococcus is generally
very sensitive to penicillin G, and, in many institutions,
penicillin G is substituted for ampicillin once the diagnosis is
made. Therapy is maintained for 7 to 10 days for infection and
14 to 21 days for meningitis. The lumbar puncture may be
repeated midway or at the end of therapy to ensure that there
are no microorganisms remaining in the CSF.

Fluid management, volume expansion, and appropriate
antimicrobial therapy are the key components of nursing care.
Infants with group B streptococcal infection are often very
labile and do not tolerate frequent interventions. Minimal
handling is sometimes required for their care.

Edwards et al (2005) suggest that the most potentially
lasting method for prevention of early- and late-onset infections, as well as maternal morbidity associated with GBS, is the
active immunization of all women of childbearing age, either
before pregnancy or late in pregnancy (at approximately
7 months' gestation). Passive transmission of antibodies to
the newborn occurs via the placenta; however, women often
deliver infants prematurely, before the successful transmission
of appropriate protective antibodies. Edwards et al (2005) state
that because 65% to 85% of all infants with GBS disease are
born at term, vaccines given to women early in the third
trimester could prevent up to 95% of these infections. The
cost of developing a suitable vaccine would probably be less
than the cost of the care required by the critically ill newborn

and the chronically ill, debilitated, severely handicapped newborn.

Staphylococcus

From the 1950s to the 1970s, coagulase-positive S. aureus was the main organism identified as a pathogen in hospitals. In the 1980s, coagulase-negative organisms, in particular S. epidermidis, were discovered to be equally important. These organisms have caused many serious and even fatal infections in newborns.

Critically ill and preterm newborns are already immuno-compromised and therefore are especially vulnerable to infections. Open skin lesions, surgical incisions, or puncture wounds caused by diagnostic tests or procedures are conducive to bacterial growth, especially S. aureus or S. epidermidis (Orschein et al, 2005). Nosocomial infections may also be transmitted to the neonate through contaminated articles or from the hands of health care providers. Overgrowth of S. epidermidis may occur in nurseries where an attempt has been made to reduce colonization of S. aureus. Development of resistant organisms is a risk for critically ill or preterm infants who require extensive invasive treatments. Coagulase-negative staphylococci or methicillin-resistant S. aureus have a potential for causing rapid decompensation (Healy et al, 2004). Staphylococci release endotoxins that have systemic effects, including alteration of the skin's protective layer. Scalded skin syndrome is one of the most common examples of this effect.

Management. Management and supportive therapy for staphylococcal infection are initially the same as for infection with group B streptococci. Antimicrobial therapy begins with ampicillin and gentamicin. Once definitive cultures and sensitivities are available and if the organism is ampicillin resistant, the drug of choice is one of the synthetic penicillins: oxacillin, methicillin, cloxacillin, dicloxacillin, or nafcillin. If the organism is methicillin resistant, the best available drug is vancomycin. It is essential that the choice of antimicrobial agent be carefully made and reconsidered when culture results are available.

Escherichia coli

E. coli is a gram-negative, non–spore forming motile rod. It is a normal inhabitant of the gastrointestinal tract and the most common cause of gram-negative infection in the newborn. Colonization of the gastrointestinal tract with E. coli occurs postnatally through environmental exposure and enteral feedings (Kitajima, 2003).

Listeria monocytogenes

L. monocytogenes has been recognized as a cause of perinatal complications since the early 1900s. It is found in birds and mammals, including domestic and farm animals. It is found in unpasteurized milk, soil, and fecal material. Listeria infection appears to be underdiagnosed and an underreported cause of congenital infection. A study done at the University of Southern California looked at 20 mother-infant pairs from whom Listeria was isolated in the prior 10 years. Antepartum factors, such as high maternal leukocyte count, fetal tachycardia, decreased fetal heart rate variability, and absence of intrapartum fetal heart rate accelerations, were identified in the history of the newborns diagnosed with congenital Listeria infection (Bortolussi & Mailman, 2005; Ichiba et al, 2000).

The incidence of Listeria infection in the United States is unknown, and the route of transmission is unclear. Investigators of recent outbreaks, however, have shown that the infection can be foodborne. In a study that examined United States hospital discharge data from 1980 to 1982, it was determined that the incidence of listeriosis in newborns was 568 per 1 million of the population per year (Bortolussi & Mailman, 2005; Ichiba, 2000). The number of fetal deaths caused by Listeria is unknown.

Clinical Manifestations. A mother infected with Listeria commonly has flulike symptoms, including malaise, fever, chills, diarrhea, and back pain. It is also possible to contract the infection and remain asymptomatic or have only minor symptoms. This organism has been identified as a cause of spontaneous abortion (Dimpfl & Gloning, 1995).

If contracted between 17 and 28 weeks' gestation, Listeria can cause fetal death or premature birth of an acutely ill newborn who may die hours later. However, early maternal treatment with intravenous ampicillin and gentamicin has been associated with normal newborn outcome (Bortolussi & Mailman, 2005; Ichiba et al, 2000). Infection late in pregnancy may cause the infant to be born with a congenital infection, usually pneumonia. Mortality rates are high but are usually related to the amount of prematurity. Late-onset listeriosis, which can occur up to 4 weeks after delivery, can easily result in meningitis. A term newborn with listeriosis has less chance of dying but often suffers complications of hydrocephalus and mental retardation (Visintine et al, 1977). However, in either preterm or term neonates in whom meningitis develops, there is a 70% mortality rate if treatment is delayed.

Newborns infected with Listeria may be born prematurely and be meconium stained, exhibit apnea and flaccidity, have a papular erythematous skin rash and hepatosplenomegaly, and be poor feeders (Visintine et al, 1977). Preterm birth associated with meconium staining should always be considered suspicious for listeriosis.

Management. Intrapartum administration of antibiotics may decrease fetal morbidity and mortality rates. Ampicillin in combination with an aminoglycoside is the most common treatment. Investigators have shown that newborn survival rates are significantly different if the mother as well as the infant receives treatment (71% vs 29%) (Bortolussi & Mailman, 2005; Ichiba et al, 2000).

Careful handwashing is a very important aspect of caring for the infant infected with Listeria. Institutional policy may require that the infant be isolated for the first 24 hours of life, until the antibiotics are on board. The mother's urine, stool, and lochia should be cultured, and if positive, she should be given ampicillin. Listeriosis often presents suddenly in the last trimester of pregnancy, precipitating an unexpected preterm delivery. Extensive emotional support may be necessary for the mother and family.

Neonatal Meningitis

Pathophysiology. Meningitis can be a sequelae of newborn infection. The incidence of meningitis associated with newborn infection is thought to be approximately 25% of those presenting with infection. Meningitis is more common as a complication of late-onset infection. The morbidity rate is higher for preterm infants than for term infants. Morbidity of survivors of infection with gram-negative bacilli or group B streptococci approaches 20% to 50%. These complications include mental and motor problems, seizure disorders, hydrocephalus, hearing loss, blindness, and abnormal speech patterns (Palazzi et al, 2005).

CSF fluid should be prepared and other appropriate cultures obtained. High CSF protein and low glucose levels are also indicators of meningitis. As with all procedures in the neonate, the lumbar puncture (LP) presents risks, which must be weighed against the benefit of having a CSF culture. Often the preterm infant may be considered so critically unstable that the LP is deferred. Stoll et al (2004) evaluated the epidemiology of meningitis in very-low-birth-weight infants and compared the CSF and blood culture results. In their review of 9641 infant records, they found that one-third of the infants who had meningitis had negative blood cultures. They cautioned that the discordance in the CSF and blood culture results could lead to underdiagnosis of meningitis in low-birth-weight infants.

Clinical Manifestations. Initially, the infant with meningitis presents with signs and symptoms of generalized infection. In addition, the meningeal irritation results in increased irritability, crying, increased intracranial pressure leading to bulging fontanelles, lethargy, tremors or twitching, seizure activity, vomiting, alterations in consciousness, and diminished muscle tone. Focal signs include hemiparesis, horizontal deviation of the eyes, and some cranial nerve involvement (Palazzi et al, 2005).

Risk Factors. About one fourth of infants with infection will develop meningitis. Although the overall incidence of bacterial meningitis in newborns is less than 1%, the incidence is much higher in preterm newborns (Palazzi et al, 2005). Male infants are more vulnerable to infection and, consequently, meningitis. Female infants have lower rates of respiratory distress syndrome and lower rates of most congenital infections. Geography and socioeconomic factors are influential in patterns of neonatal disease. These differences probably reflect populations served, including unique cultural activities and sexual practices, as well as local customs. It probably also reflects different treatment patterns in local nurseries and variations of antimicrobial selections.

Prognosis. Brain abscess is associated with a poor prognosis; approximately 50% of affected patients die. Destruction of brain tissues, hemorrhages, and infarcts causing necrosis to vital brain cells may cause extensive brain damage, leading to death or poor neurologic outcomes. With the introduction of ultrasonography and computerized tomography, brain abscesses are being identified earlier.

Management. The selection of antimicrobial therapy for meningitis is based on the causative microorganism. Supportive therapy is necessary for the newborn with meningitis. Acute observation and monitoring of vital signs and activity level are crucial. Infants who become critically ill with meningitis may deteriorate quickly and need rapid, acute interventions. Infants often require long-term antibiotic therapy, and often, venous access is a problem. Placement of a percutaneous line for parenteral nutrition may be necessary. Families need educational and emotional support during the long-term hospitalizations, particularly if complications develop.

Congenital Infections

The microorganisms most often responsible for congenitally acquired infections have been grouped together as the microorganisms implicated in congenital infections has grown, so the acronym is no longer inclusive. It is still used when discussing infections acquired by the fetus in utero.

Toxoplasmosis

The importance of the parasite *Toxoplasma gondii* was discovered by perinatal health care workers in the 1980s. Toxoplasma is a pathogen that is ever-present in nature. Perinatal transmission takes place when the mother contracts the protozoa and the subsequent protozoemia transmits the organism transplacentally to the fetus. The microorganisms then invade and multiply within the placenta and eventually enter the fetal circulation. The life cycle of *Toxoplasma* is complicated. The predominant host of this organism is the ordinary house cat; however, other animals, such as camels in the Middle East, can serve as hosts. There are significant differences in the prevalence rates of this microorganism throughout the world (Remington et al, 2005). The tissue cyst form of the microorganism persists in the flesh of animals, such as cattle and sheep. The oocyte form of the parasite persists in soil contaminated by cat feces. Thus, congenital toxoplasmosis is known to be transmitted from undercooked meat or food or from fomites in cat feces. In the United States, approximately 20% to 70% of the population has been exposed to this protozoan. There is wide variability of the prevalence of seropositive women of childbearing age among countries, geographic regions of the same country, and ethnic origin; different cultural practices regarding food are probably the major cause of this difference. Since meat is the main vector for transmission, areas where there is less *T. gondii* present in meat because of improved methods for processing or cooking meat have lower prevalence rates (Remington et al, 2005).

The greatest risk is when a nonimmune pregnant woman is exposed to *T. gondii* during fetal organogenesis (weeks 4 to 8 of gestation), when the risk for congenital anomalies is high (Remington et al, 2005).

Clinical Manifestations. Acute toxoplasmosis in a pregnant woman often goes undetected and undiagnosed because the signs and symptoms are not severe. Clinical questioning after the identification of an infected newborn or infant often leads to reflection and memories of a period of enlarged lymph nodes and fatigue without fever. Women sometimes report a mononucleosis-like or flulike syndrome that may have a febrile course, with malaise, headache, fatigue, sore throat, and sore muscles. These symptoms may persist up to 6 months; however, that duration is unusual. A newborn with congenital toxoplasmosis can present with hydrocephalus, chorioretinitis, and intracranial calcifications. There is a wide variety of clinical signs in the scope of the disease. The newborn can appear normal at birth, or exhibit severe erythroblastosis, hydrops fetalis, and other clinical signs (Remington et al, 2005).

Neurologic signs similar to encephalitis (e.g., convulsions, bulging fontanelles, nystagmus, and increased head circumference) may be the only significant presentation of this clinical problem. If the newborn receives treatment, signs may disappear, allowing normal cerebral growth and development, if there was no permanent neurologic damage.

Mild cases of the disease may not be recognized in the newborn period. Signs of delayed onset of disease in premature newborns include severe central nervous system or eye lesions appearing at 3 months of age. In term newborns, delayed disease may occur in the first 2 months of life and is usually mild. Clinical signs include generalized infection, enlarged liver and spleen, late-onset jaundice, enlarged lymph nodes, or late-onset central nervous system problems, including hydrocephalus and eye lesions. Infants with congenital toxoplasmosis may have new lesions appearing until age 5 years (Remington et al, 2005).

Management. The best and most effective treatments are prevention and early recognition. The cost effectiveness of pregnancy serology screening depends on the costs of the tests and the estimated cost of treating the infection, if identified early. At present in the United States, screening is done erratically and there are no particular screening standards. Counseling education for the prevention of toxoplasmosis should focus on avoidance of raw meat and use of gloves during feline litter box handling and during gardening in what may be contaminated soil. Toxoplasmosis cannot be contracted by merely handling or being around a cat, so it is not necessary for the family cat to be banished. Pregnant women who are seronegative should exercise caution to avoid the risk of contracting *T. gondii* during pregnancy by avoiding cat litter, digging in the soil, and handling or eating undercooked meat. They should inform their health care provider if they experience any signs that could be attributed to *T. gondii* infection.

Treatment for congenital toxoplasmosis is pyrimethamine plus sulfonamides. The suggested dose is 2 mg/kg/day orally for 2 days followed by 1 mg/kg/day for 2 or 6 months, then 1 mg/kg/day every Monday, Wednesday, and Friday for 1 year. The medication is given in doses of 100 mg/kg/day in two divided oral doses for 1 year. Leucovorin 10 mg is given three times weekly during and for 1 week after pyrimethamine therapy. These drugs are potentially toxic and need close monitoring. Corticosteroids are given in the form of prednisone at 1 mg/kg/day in two divided doses until there is resolution of elevated protein in cerebrospinal fluid (CSF) or active chorioretinitis (Remington et al, 2005). Toxoplasmosis is one of the most common causes of deafness. The Collaborative Perinatal Project found a doubling in the frequency of deafness in infants of mothers with the antibody for toxoplasmosis. There was a 60% increase in microcephaly and a 30% increase in low intelligence quotients (<70) in relation to high antibody levels in mothers (Remington et al, 2005).

Nursing Management. Nursing management is supportive and dependent on the severity of the infection. Neurologic impairment at birth can be significant, requiring ventilation and seizure control. Documented positive infants should be cared for by nonpregnant personnel to prevent risk of transmission.

Rubella

In 1941, N. McAlister Gregg described 78 patients with congenital cataracts. These patients were small for gestational age and had feeding difficulties and congenital heart problems. A history of German measles during pregnancy was found in 68 of the cases (87%). Much of the current knowledge about the effects of congenital rubella was established by Gregg's report on these patients (Gregg, 1941). It has been further established that the rubella virus can be responsible for other abnormalities. The most important consequences of rubella are the miscarriages, stillbirths, fetal anomalies, and therapeutic abortions that result when rubella infection occurs during early pregnancy, especially during the first trimester. An estimated 20,000 cases of congenital rubella syndrome (CRS) occurred during 1964 and 1965 during the last U.S. rubella epidemic before rubella vaccine became available.

The largest number of cases of rubella occurred in 1969, with 57,686 reported cases. With the advent of vaccination in 1969, the number of cases began to decline rapidly; since 1992, fewer than 500 cases have been reported annually. The majority of these cases occurred in populations that do not accept conventional medicine and do not immunize their children. However, the proportion of cases of adults older than 20 years has increased from 29% in 1991 to 74% in 1999. In 1989, a second dose of rubella vaccine was added to the immunization schedule to be given prior to school entry or in the prepubertal period (Cooper & Alford, 2005). Since 1992 about six cases of CRS have been reported annually; these cases were seen in infants whose mothers were from countries where rubella vaccine is not normally given (CDC, 2001).

Since 1992, reported indigenous rubella and CRS have continued to occur at a low but relatively constant endemic level with an annual average of fewer than 200 rubella cases (128 cases in 1995 and 213 cases in 1996). However, in the United States, surveillance for CRS relies on a passive system. Consequently, the reported annual totals of CRS are regarded as minimum figures, representing an estimated 40% to 70% of all cases. Failure to immunize many young children has resulted in an increase in rubella incidence. Therefore, despite a national immunization program, at least 10% of women of childbearing age are vulnerable to the virus, particularly the wild virus, because either they have not been immunized or they have not acquired immunity from the infection themselves. Small rubella outbreaks have been reported all over the United States. Although there has been a change in the epidemiology of the infection over the past 25 years and a significant decrease in the incidence, rubella has not been eradicated. Prevention of rubella in postpubertal women and CRS continues to be a major goal of the CDC (Cooper & Alford, 2005).

Clinical Manifestations

The abnormalities most commonly associated with CRS are auditory (e.g., sensorineural deafness), ophthalmic (e.g., cataracts, microphthalmia, glaucoma, chorioretinitis), cardiac (e.g., patent ductus arteriosus, peripheral pulmonary artery stenosis, atrial or ventricular septal defects), and neurologic (e.g., microcephaly, meningoencephalitis, mental retardation). In addition, infants with CRS frequently exhibit both intrauterine and postnatal growth retardation. Other conditions sometimes observed among babies who have CRS include radiolucent bone defects, hepatosplenomegaly, thrombocytopenia, and purpuric skin lesions. Newborns who are moderately or severely affected by CRS are readily recognizable at birth, but mild CRS (e.g., slight cardiac involvement or deafness) may be detected months or years after birth, or not at all (Cooper & Alford, 2005; Neto et al, 2004).

Although CRS has been estimated to occur among 20% to 25% of infants born to women who acquire rubella during the first 20 weeks of pregnancy, this figure may underestimate the risk for fetal infection and birth defects. When infants born to mothers who were infected during the first 8 weeks of gestation were followed for 4 years, 85% were found to be affected. The risk for a defect decreases to about 52% for infections that occur during the 9th to 12th weeks of gestation. Infection after the 20th week of gestation rarely causes defects. Subclinical maternal rubella infection can also cause congenital malformations. Fetal infection without clinical signs of CRS can occur during any stage of pregnancy (Cooper & Alford, 2005; Neto et al, 2004).

The typical presentation of the rubella virus is mild, with malaise, low-grade fever, headache, and conjunctivitis. In 1 to 5 days, a macular rash appears on the face and usually disappears after 3 to 4 days. Natural viremia is necessary for placental and fetal rubella infection. Most cases occur following primary disease. Frequently, skin rashes that resemble rubella may occur as a result of adenovirus, enterovirus, or other respiratory virus infections. Laboratory titers are recommended to confirm the diagnosis of rubella infection (Cooper & Alford, 2005).

A fetus infected with rubella often has cardiac defects and deafness. The central nervous system seems particularly vulnerable to the rubella virus, especially if the virus is acquired before the first 16 weeks of gestation. Congenital rubella syndrome is described by the CDC as hearing loss, mental retardation, cardiac malformations, and eye defects.

The rubella virus can slow cell replication. This causes intrauterine growth restriction and a failure of cell differentiation during fetal organ formation. Tissue damage also seems to occur from the inflammatory response to the infection or is even possibly an autoimmune reaction. Myocarditis, pneumonitis, hepatosplenomegaly, and vascular stenosis can also be present because of these processes. As is seen with other severe congenital infections, signs and symptoms may continue to develop until the patient is 10 to 20 years of age. Late clinical signs of this disease include insulin-dependent diabetes, thyroid abnormalities, hypoadrenalism, hearing loss, and eye damage (Cooper & Alford, 2005; Neto et al, 2004).

Differential Diagnosis

The possibility of subclinical infection with rubella highlights the need for laboratory confirmation. Clinical confirmation of rubella isolation is obtainable in approximately 4 to 6 weeks. The detection of rubella antibody confirms the presence of the infection. Rubella-specific IgG persists for life and can be detected by enzyme immunoassay. With confirmed serologic results, the risk of fetal damage after 16 weeks' gestation appears to be small.

Demonstration of rubella-specific IgM in fetal blood obtained by cordocentesis has been used to establish diagnosis in utero. Chorionic villus sampling has also demonstrated recovery of the virus during the first trimester (Cooper & Alford, 2005; Neto et al, 2004).

Management

Infants should be vaccinated against rubella at 15 months of age and again prior to school entry. Women who do not have detectable IgG rubella antibody and are of childbearing age (and not pregnant) should be immunized. They should avoid pregnancy for at least 3 months after immunization to decrease the risk for development of rubella syndrome in the fetus. Health care workers who may be inadvertently exposed to rubella should be immunized if they do not have immune titers. If a woman receives rubella vaccine and has recently received blood products or RhoGAM (RhIG), the vaccine may not trigger an immune response because blood products and RhoGAM have pooled sera that may contain antibodies against rubella. Thus, the woman's body does not produce antibodies. These women should have titers drawn 6 weeks after vaccination or at most 3 months after vaccination (CDC, 2001; Cooper & Alford, 2005).

In more than 500 women who were accidentally immunized against rubella while pregnant, there were no cases of congenital rubella syndrome. Rubella vaccination is not recommended during pregnancy, yet the risks to the fetus have been determined to be negligible and an inadvertent rubella vaccination by itself is not considered an indication for termination of pregnancy.

Currently, treatment in the nursery of the rubella-infected infant is rare. Therapy for identified problems, such as respiratory, cardiac, or neurologic deficits, is supportive and there is no specific recommended therapy. Caretakers should have known immune titers and not be pregnant. Rubella-specific IgM can usually accurately identify these infants. Persistent shedding of the virus may last until 1 year of life; thus, pregnant women should avoid contact with these patients. Follow-up care for surgical corrections of heart defects and cataracts as well as special schooling may be needed for these infants.

Cytomegalovirus

Infection with cytomegalovirus (CMV), a member of the herpes family, is common. CMV is a DNA virus covered with a glycoprotein coat that closely resembles the herpes and varicella-zoster viruses. By adulthood, most people have been exposed to CMV and antibodies have developed to it. CMV infection is more prevalent in lower socioeconomic groups and is especially common in developing countries. In the United States, women of childbearing age from lower socioeconomic groups have an incidence of infection of approximately 6%, whereas those from higher socioeconomic groups have an incidence of approximately 2%. CMV may lie dormant, with periods of exacerbation followed by remission. During remission, the patient is asymptomatic, but the virus is shed (Stagno & Britt, 2005). The virus is usually transmitted person to person through body fluids and secretions. Blood, urine, breast milk, cervical mucus, semen, and saliva harbor CMV. The virus can cause an infectious mononucleosis–like syndrome, with general malaise, liver complications, fever, and general fatigue. Perinatal transmission can occur within 2 to 3 days of infection by transplacental crossing of the organism. The fetus can also contract the virus intrapartally from infected maternal cervical secretions while descending through the birth canal. CMV can also be transmitted through infected breast milk (Stagno & Britt, 2005).

Clinical Manifestations

More damage occurs to the fetus when the exposure to and acquisition of CMV occur from a primary lesion. Congenital CMV occurs in approximately 0.2% to 2.2% of all newborn infants. Primary lesions cause intrauterine growth restriction, microcephaly, periventricular calcifications, deafness, blindness, congenital cataracts, profound mental retardation, hepatosplenomegaly, and jaundice. A characteristic pattern of petechiae, called "blueberry muffin" syndrome, is associated with congenital CMV. Approximately 26% of severely infected infants die. Severe complications at birth are seen in approximately 5% of congenital infections. Sequelae develop in 5% to 15% of asymptomatic infected infants and in 90% of symptomatic infected infants (Stagno & Britt, 2005). Recurrent CMV infections are not as severe because of partial antibody protection from previous exposure. The incidence of neonatal complications is reported to be from 5% to 10% for hearing loss, 2% for chorioretinitis, and less than 1% for mental retardation (Stagno & Britt, 2005).

Diagnosis

Suspicious clinical findings or obstetric history warrant further investigation for CMV infection. Urine culture for CMV is the most rapid and sensitive indicator of infection. IgG and IgM antibody titers should also be measured. Elevated IgM levels alone denote exposure to CMV but are not diagnostic because there is no method to determine the timing of the exposure. Elevated neonatal IgG titers indicate perinatally acquired CMV infection. A negative maternal IgG titer and a positive neonatal IgG titer indicate postnatal transmission. Experimentally, elevated rheumatoid factors may provide evidence to support the diagnosis of CMV in subclinical cases (Stagno & Britt, 2005).

Prevention

Transmission of CMV via infected blood products has been significantly decreased through the use of CMV-negative donors or irradiation of blood products. Premature and low-birth-weight infants are especially vulnerable to the infusion of this virus in blood products. The best method of prevention is the institution of universal precautions, including good handwashing techniques.

Management

Newborns infected with CMV display a wide range of signs. General supportive therapy is based on the presence of these clinical manifestations. Specific therapy for CMV is still in the experimental stage but includes immunoglobulin therapy, vaccines, and chemotherapy. Intravenous immunoglobulin therapy provides passive immunity to at-risk infants but not to those already infected. Two live attenuated vaccines for CMV have been developed and tested on renal transplant patients. Theoretically, these vaccines would be useful preconceptionally or perinatally to prevent vertical transmission; however, only limited research has been done with this population. Chemotherapy offers the most promise for treatment of neonatal CMV infection; however, clinically, it has not been shown to be effective in improving long-term outcome (Stagno & Britt, 2005).

Syphilis

The microorganism *Treponema pallidum* has persisted as a threat to perinatal patients for over 400 years. Many women do not receive adequate treatment for primary or secondary infections, despite the availability of effective therapy for more than 40 years. The virus can be dormant for years, much like the herpes family of viruses. The incidence of syphilis is increasing because of increased substance abuse, sexual practices involving multiple partners, and increased numbers of human immunodeficiency virus (HIV)-positive immunocompromised individuals, who act as reservoirs for *T. pallidum*. Consequently, there has been a resurgence of congenital infections. Recent worldwide concern regarding the role of genital ulcers in conjunction with HIV infection has created great concern for eradication of sexually transmitted diseases (Ingall et al, 2005).

The diagnosis of antepartum syphilis is most often made by screening at the first prenatal visit. Screening usually involves the use of the Venereal Disease Research Laboratory (VDRL) test or rapid plasma reagin (RPR) test, each of which measures anticardiolipin antibody. These tests are reactive in almost 80% of patients with secondary or early latent (<1 year duration) primary syphilis. A definitive diagnosis can be made with an elevated VDRL or RPR accompanied by a positive *T. pallidum* fluoroantibody test or a reactive serologic test for *T. pallidum* in the CSF. Condylomata lata, bony changes, or snuffles in the presence of a positive serologic test are diagnostic (Ingall et al, 2005). Untreated syphilis adversely affects pregnancy outcome. Vertical transmission of treponemas can occur at any time during pregnancy. The microorganisms can cause preterm labor, PROM, stillbirth, congenital infection, or neonatal death. Current untreated secondary infection causes the greatest risk of damage to the fetus, particularly if infection occurs during the period of organogenesis. Late untreated syphilis in the mother usually results in delivery of an asymptomatic infant who needs treatment in the newborn nursery.

Reports state that, between 1983 and 1985, 437 infants in the United States were delivered with congenital syphilis. The mean age of acquiring prenatal care was 22 weeks' gestation, and at least half of the cases were preventable because they were results of failure of initial or third-trimester screening (Ingall et al, 2005). A study by Ogunyemi and Hernández-Loera (2004) found that maternal use of cocaine led to a greater risk for untreated maternal syphilis and consequent congenital syphilis.

Clinical Manifestations

When newborns acquire syphilis from hematogenous spread across the placenta, the effects are on the major organ systems of the fetus, especially the central nervous system. Common presentations of the infected infant are hepatosplenomegaly, jaundice, low birth weight, intrauterine growth restriction, anemia, and osteochondritis. There is often a bilateral superficial peeling of the skin (desquamation) on the neonatal palms and soles. Nonimmune hydrops is a common presentation in congenital syphilis. The symptoms of perinatal syphilis are similar to those of any other viral infection that spreads hematogenously from the mother to the placenta and on to the developing fetus (Ingall et al, 2005; Peihong et al, 2001).

Differential Diagnosis

A lumbar puncture for CSF analysis and radiographs of the long bones facilitate the definitive diagnosis of syphilis in the neonate. Congenital neurosyphilis is always a consideration, and the CSF should be examined for the presence of spirochetes. Radiologic changes such as osteochondritis (a blurring of the epiphyseal borders) demonstrate recent fetal infection (within 5 weeks), and periostitis represents prolonged involvement, probably within 16 weeks or second-trimester infection.

Stillborn infants should be examined by whole-body radiographic study and autopsy if possible. Spirochetes can be visualized by special staining techniques (Ingall et al, 2005). Interpretation of serologic tests for syphilis on serum obtained from cord blood is complicated because of the transplacental transfer of maternal IgG antibody. VDRL titers at least two dilutions higher than maternal VDRL titers indicate probable fetal infection.

Prognosis

Infants with syphilis should receive the same amount of follow-up as normal infants. Serologic measurements can be made at follow-up visits at 1, 2, 3, 6, and 12 months of age. The infection can be effectively treated, but the physiologic and developmental prognosis depends on the degree of organ damage sustained during fetal development.

Management

The recommended treatment for a newborn presumed to be infected with congenital syphilis is aqueous penicillin G. In many perinatal centers, the presence of a positive VDRL in a neonate dictates treatment as if positive for syphilis. If neonatal clinical manifestations are highly suspicious for syphilis and there is a positive VDRL but the titer is not significantly higher than the maternal titer, syphilis treatment should be instituted. A newborn with an antibody titer four times or more higher than the maternal level should be treated as if a definitive diagnosis has been obtained. To prevent neurosyphilis, the infant should be given aqueous penicillin G, 100,000 to 150,000 units/kg intravenously in two or three divided doses for at least 10 to 14 days, or 50,000 units/kg/day of procaine penicillin in a daily dose for 10 to 14 days.

For asymptomatic infants whose mothers were treated adequately during pregnancy, treatment is not necessary unless follow-up cannot be ensured. Some clinicians recommend a single dose of benzathine penicillin, 50,000 units/kg intramuscularly, if the infant is not likely to be followed up. If maternal treatment did not include penicillin and if neonatal follow-up is likely to be unreliable, the neonate is given a full 10-day course (Ingall et al, 2005).

Isolation of an infant with suspicious symptoms may be necessary until appropriate treatment is given. There is a definite role for nursing education and support in the treatment of an infant exposed to syphilis. The 10- to 14-day course of penicillin treatment may lead to the establishment of a trusting relationship between the nurse and family, thus providing opportunity to give more information regarding sexual risk factors. Families often need encouragement and support to get treatment for other sexual partners and to obtain other necessary medical evaluations (such as HIV screening or drug counseling).

Herpes Simplex Virus

Herpes simplex virus (HSV) is a member of a family of large DNA viruses. They contain linear, double strands of DNA. The herpes family also includes CMV, varicella-zoster, and Epstein-Barr virus. HSV possesses the quality of "latency," whereby the virus can persist in a latent state for a period of time and then be reactivated by certain stimuli. A strand of the viral DNA persists in an infected individual for a lifetime; thus, the virus maintains a "foothold" in its host. Clinical experiences demonstrate that, after primary HSV infection, at the site of the infection (perhaps an oral or genital site) the microorganism invades the sensory nerve endings and remains there. The more severe the primary infection, as determined by the size and extent of the skin lesion, the more likely are frequent recurrences.

Potential stimuli for HSV reactivation include periods of stress, emotional trauma, and prolonged exposure to the sun. Maintenance of the latency state and recurrence of the virus are topics of intense current research. There are many unanswered questions about what triggers latency and about the cofactors for reactivation of the virus.

Maternal HSV is usually the source of neonatal infection. The risk of neonatal infection is estimated to be 5% if it is recurrent herpes and higher if it is a primary infection (Arvin et al, 2005; Langlet et al, 2003).

Recurrent infections are the most common problem in pregnancy. Transmission of the infection to the fetus can be caused by passage through infected genital secretions in the intrapartum period or by ascending infection from the vaginal vault via ruptured (or not) membranes. Many women can be asymptomatic and still be shedding HSV. Although primary infection is less common, it causes the most severe neonatal disease, most likely including central nervous system problems, disseminated disease into other organ systems, and probable death. The incidence of intrapartum transmission with a primary infection is approximately 40% to 50%. Many neonatal complications such as prematurity, intrauterine restriction, and respiratory distress syndrome can potentiate the neonate's illness, limiting the ability to fight off HSV. There is a broad range of severity of neonatal infection, from severe to benign and asymptomatic. In the United States, there are from 11 to 33 cases of neonatal herpes infection per 100,000 live births. With approximately 4 million deliveries per year in the United States, that results in from 520 to 1320 neonates with HSV (Arvin et al, 2005). Susceptibility of the newborn to HSV is increased because there is a lack of passively acquired maternal antibody in some infants.

Clinical Manifestations

Acquisition of HSV in utero can result in spontaneous abortion, preterm birth, or a normal baby. Manifestations of the disease are broad; the clinical presentation of the congenital acquisition of the infection includes skin vesicles or scarring, hypopigmentation, chorioretinitis, microcephaly, and hydranencephaly. There are three categories of neonatal patients. The first category includes patients with localized infections of the skin, eyes, or mouth. The second category includes patients with encephalitis. In this group, neurologic sequelae occur in approximately 50%. Approximately one third of these patients do not have skin vesicles, and they are identified by history alone. CSF is positive for the virus in 25% to 40% of these cases. Presence of cells and increased protein are very common in the CSF of patients with encephalitis, and they die if not treated. The third category of neonatal patients includes those with disseminated disease characterized by irritability, seizures, respiratory distress, jaundice, DIC, shock, and other symptoms of viral and bacterial infection. All major neonatal organs may be involved. Liver and the adrenals are the most common reservoirs for the virus. The central nervous system is involved in 70% to 90% of affected neonates. In more than 20% of the newborns with disseminated disease, skin vesicles do not develop, making identification of positive infants more difficult (Arvin et al, 2005; Neto et al, 2004).

Differential Diagnosis

Laboratory tests can differentiate HSV infection from other bacterial and viral infections. The most rapid method employs cytologic examination. Routine cultures should be obtained from any vesicle on the skin, oropharyngeal or eye secretions, or stool. Viral typing is done for epidemiologic purposes only. HSV types I and II are the most commonly known. Type I has been most closely associated with any herpes found outside the genital area; type II is commonly referred to as genital herpes. However, either type can occur almost anywhere in the body. Treatment does not differ for these different viral types (Arvin et al, 2005).

Risk Factors

Intrapartal transmission is more likely to occur in the presence of ruptured membranes. Other risk factors include intrauterine fetal monitoring and fetal scalp sampling. It is not recommended that women infected with HSV be monitored by these methods. Transmission from mother to infant from an infected breast lesion has been reported. Transmission has also been documented from oral lesions.

Prevention

Presence of maternal active HSV genital lesions is a contraindication to vaginal delivery. If the membranes have been ruptured 4 hours or longer, cesarean section may or may not prevent transmission to the neonate. Postnatal nosocomial transmission is greatly reduced with good handwashing techniques and universal precautions.

Management

The most recent methods of treatment include the antiviral drugs acyclovir and vidarabine. The results of these methods of therapy and treatment are reported in the National Institute of Allergy and Infectious Diseases (NIAID) Joint Collaborative Antiviral Study. These drugs have potentially influenced neonatal morbidity and mortality from disseminated disease and encephalitis.

Vidarabine is usually given intravenously in dosages of 15 to 30 mg/kg/day over a 12-hour period for 10 to 14 days. It has been reported that newborns receiving the higher dosages of 30 mg/kg/day seem to progress to less serious forms of the disease. In some circumstances, longer periods of treatment may be necessary, because infants can have either a clinical recurrence or a clinical progression of the disease (Arvin et al, 2005).

Acyclovir, a relatively new antiviral agent undergoing clinical study, is the recommended mode of therapy at this writing. Acyclovir appears to be very helpful in decreasing the frequency of the reactivation of the virus, particularly in the treatment of herpes simplex encephalitis. Acyclovir is a selective inhibitor of viral replication and thus has few side effects. The recommended dosage is 30 mg/kg/day intravenously divided over 8 hours. Duration of therapy is 10 to 14 days (Arvin et al, 2005).

Early identification and intervention are essential, because early institution of antiviral therapy has been shown to improve outcome and decrease sequelae (Arvin et al, 2005). Newborns with eye involvement should be given topical antiviral agents such as trifluridine, one drop every 2 hours, as well as intravenous therapy. Vidarabine and acyclovir are potent drugs with a potential for toxicity. Neonatal therapeutic ranges for these drugs have not been established. Monitoring of the infant's physiologic status is necessary to detect potential side effects. Infected infants must be isolated because viral shedding provides a reservoir for infecting other infants in the nursery.

HSV continues to be a life-threatening neonatal infection in the United States. There is growing concern about transmission of the virus to unborn children with the concomitant increase in genital herpes as a sexually transmitted disease. It is important for all health care providers in the perinatal arena to maintain a high index of suspicion in infants whose symptoms may be compatible with HSV infection. Early identification allows prompt treatment or necessary continued observation or both. Continued research may produce a more rapid method of virus identification and perhaps a safe and effective vaccine. Prevention of neonatal HSV depends on improved knowledge regarding the factors of virus transmission between mother and infant. Appropriate use of cesarean section in women with active genital herpes is an important management step (Arvin et al, 2005).

Primary nursing responsibilities in the management of a family with HSV infection are education and support. Mothers should be educated as to the mode, methods, and possible origins of the HSV, and concerns should be addressed regarding potential transmission to newborns. Nurses are often the first to document a mother's comment that she "had a small bump or blister and fever" right before her infant was born. Careful history taking and thorough questioning can often identify potentially infected patients early. With the diagnosis of genital herpes and subsequent monitoring procedures, families often feel stigmatized as well as anxious. Parents and responsible family members need education and support. Mothers with a history of genital HSV should be investigated for findings of active infection during the prepartum period. The definition of an active lesion includes one of the following at birth:

1. Positive viral culture of a lesion
2. Positive fluorescent antibody test
3. Presence of skin vesicles or lesions
4. Cytologic screen with identified HSV markers

All family members with active lesions anywhere on the body should be taught careful handwashing techniques to use before handling the baby. Any person with an oral HSV infection who handles the infant must wash well, wear a mask, and not kiss the infant anywhere until the lesions are completely crusted over and healed (Arvin et al, 2005).

A common nursery issue that arises when a mother has active genital herpes is whether isolation is required and what form of isolation is indicated. Transmission occurs through direct contact with the infected lesion. There must be thorough handwashing before handling the infant and after touching the genital area. The risks for transmission are unknown, but they are low. Hospital personnel usually gown and glove until viral status is known. Positive cultures at birth may just reflect colonization; cultures should be repeated at 24 to 48 hours. If cultures are positive, the infant is considered to be infected. Breastfeeding is contraindicated if the mother has a lesion on her breast. Infants are not isolated unless they themselves are infected. Many nurseries have guidelines regarding a 24- to 48-hour observation period to check cultures on an infant who was delivered vaginally through an infected genital area. An uninfected child does not require prolonged hospitalization, and, on discharge, the family needs information and education. Families should be informed that immediate medical consultation should be obtained with the development of major findings, including malaise, irritability, fever, temperature instability, respiratory distress, apnea, large abdomen or liver, sudden changes in skin color, new skin vesicles, lesions on the mucous membranes, or conjunctivitis. Sudden onset of systemic disease in a small, recovering preterm infant can include DIC and shock. Skin lesions are often absent in these severe cases, which may delay diagnosis (Arvin et al, 2005; Langlet et al, 2003).

Varicella

Varicella is the member of the herpesvirus family that commonly causes chickenpox as well as varicella zoster. Most women of childbearing age in the United States have been exposed to or have contracted this virus, yet women from other parts of the world may not be seropositive. Incidence of this virus in pregnant women is very low, probably approximately 0.5 in 10,000 pregnancies (Gershon, 2005).

Symptoms of varicella are usually present 10 to 20 days after exposure and include fever, malaise, and an itchy rash. The maculopapular rash eventually forms vesicles and crusts over. Potential complications include pneumonia, encephalitis, arthritis, and bacterial cellulitis. If the virus is contracted early in pregnancy, the damage is likely to be cutaneous, musculoskeletal, neurologic, and ocular. Infants can have intrauterine growth restriction, microcephaly, cerebellar and cortical atrophy, cataracts, limb malformations, and chorioretinitis (Gershon, 2005; Ehrbar et al, 2001; Mackowiak, 2002; van der Zwet et al, 2002). Viral infection in the last 3 weeks of pregnancy affects one in four newborns. The severity of neonatal disease is determined by the timing of the exposure. Infections are generally severe if contracted within 4 days before and 2 days after delivery. Severe viral respiratory distress with significantly depleted maternal passive antibody transmission puts the infant at an even greater risk for other complications. When maternal varicella infection occurs 5 to 21 days before delivery, the newborn has a much milder course of the disease and appears more capable of fighting the infection. This milder course is probably due to passive immunity transmitted to the infant via maternally derived antibodies (Gershon, 2005).

The diagnosis of varicella is made by isolation of HSV. Strict isolation of identified infants or of those whose symptoms are highly suspicious for infection is necessary. Vidarabine or acyclovir can be used for treatment of severe disease in newborns. Varicella-zoster immune globulin (VZIG) can be given to newborns to decrease the severity of infection in those exposed (Gershon, 2005).

Typically, if a mother has contracted varicella infection late in pregnancy, other persons, such as health care workers, family members, or other newborns, may have been exposed. Exposed susceptible persons should be protected with VZIG. A live attenuated varicella vaccine approved by the Food and Drug Administration is produced by Merck & Co. Inc., Whitehouse Station, NJ, (Gershon, 2005).

Gonorrhea

Neisseria gonorrhoeae is a species of small gram-negative diploid bacteria. They are diploid because they grow in pairs. Infection with this organism is seen most frequently in young adults aged 15 to 24 years. There are approximately 1 million new cases of gonorrhea each year. In females, infection is asymptomatic, which compromises detection of the disease. The organism is easily transmitted by infected tissue and secretions from the cervix, pharynx, urethra, or rectum. The incubation period is approximately 2 to 7 days. Pelvic inflammatory disease is often caused by the organism (Embree, 2005).

Clinical Manifestations

Gonorrhea infections are often mild but often cause blockage of the fallopian tubes. Perhaps 50% of women are asymptomatic with an infected cervix. In a pregnant woman, gonorrheal colonization of the cervix can cause inflammation and weakening of the fetal membranes and early rupture. Chorioamnionitis with *N. gonorrhoeae* as the causative organism can occur in the antepartum period and during labor and delivery; it is also related to increased risk of postpartum endometritis (Embree, 2005).

Disseminated gonococcal infection may present during pregnancy, causing arthritis, tendinitis, general aching, fever, and malaise. A previous history of gonorrhea presents a strong possibility that it may recur during pregnancy. Sexual partners should be screened and given treatment, because reinfection after treatment is common (Embree, 2005).

Gonococcal conjunctivitis in the newborn has historically been a risk from transmission via the birth canal. Prophylaxis has been mandated by law in the United States, and silver nitrate 1% solution or erythromycin is administered in both eyes of the neonate at birth. Fetal scalp electrodes have been identified as a potential method of organism transmission to the fetus. *N. gonorrhoeae* has been isolated from scalp abscesses, gastric and pharyngeal aspirates, conjunctival aspirates, and other blood and body fluids. Maternal and neonatal risks from exposure to the gonorrheal microorganism are significant and make it particularly important to screen for gonorrhea during pregnancy. Infected women have a higher incidence of premature labor, PROM, and infectious complications (Embree, 2005).

Prevention

Use of silver nitrate solution or erythromycin for prevention of gonococcal ophthalmia neonatorum is one of the early achievements in preventive medicine. Routine prophylaxis is mandated by law in the United States and has made a significant difference in the treatment of ocular disease. *Chlamydia* conjunctivitis has become far more common than gonococcal conjunctivitis in the neonate because of the continual screening for gonorrhea and the routine use of silver nitrate. Erythromycin ointment in both eyes is a more common prophylactic practice because it covers both gonococcal and chlamydial organisms (Embree, 2005).

Management: Mother

The appropriate treatment for a pregnant woman includes ceftriaxone, 250 mg intramuscularly once, plus erythromycin, 500 mg orally four times a day for 7 days. If gastrointestinal side effects are too severe, amoxicillin can be used. Follow-up, per the CDC, requires that cervical and rectal cultures for *N. gonorrhoeae* be obtained 4 to 7 days after treatment. Ideally, pregnant women should also receive treatment for chlamydia infection. In the nonpregnant woman, treatment with doxycycline, ofloxacin, and azithromycin is effective, but their use in pregnancy is not advised. Azithromycin has not been tested in pregnant women, but, if proven safe, only one dose would be required for effective treatment (Embree, 2005).

Management: Neonate

Infants who are delivered by an infected, untreated mother are usually given a complete infection workup, including a lumbar puncture, and placed on ampicillin and gentamicin therapy. If cultures confirm the presence of the microorganism and resistance is an issue, then infants should be treated with ceftriaxone, 25 to 50 mg/kg/day intravenously or intramuscularly in single doses, or cefotaxime, 25 mg/kg intravenously or intramuscularly every 12 hours (Embree, 2005). Education and support regarding the origin of the infectious agent are important in the treatment of gonorrhea. Sexual partners of infected persons should be encouraged to seek testing and appropriate antibiotic treatment for chlamydia as well as gonorrhea (Embree, 2005).

Hepatitis B Virus

The hepatitis B virus (HBV) is fairly large, approximately 42 nm in diameter. It is a double-stranded DNA–containing virus. Exposure to infected blood and body fluids, percutaneous introduction of blood, and administration of infected blood products are the principal routes of transmission. Contamination or infection of wounds can easily transmit the disease. The virus is fairly strong and is able to live on inanimate objects or fomites. Deactivation requires at least 1 minute in boiling water and extended autoclaving time.

In the adult, HBV infection produces systemic illness with general malaise, jaundice, anorexia, and nausea. Early stages of the disease may include fever, rash, and sore joints. Health care workers have historically been particularly vulnerable to this virus because of their repeated exposure to contaminated blood and body fluids and needle sticks. A carrier state of HBV can precipitate chronic liver disease (Lott & Kenner, 1994a, 1994b).

In certain areas of the world, such as Africa, Southeast Asia, and the Pacific Rim, the virus is considered endemic. In these areas, carrier rates are estimated to be 35%. Approximately 40% of these carriers have been identified as having been perinatally infected (Bradley, 2005).

Hepatitis B surface antigen (HBsAg) is an important test in assessing a woman's risk of transmitting HBV to her unborn child. The presence of HBsAg and hepatitis B e antigen (HBeAg) is the best indication of infectiousness. It is currently recommended that all pregnant women be screened at their first prenatal visit for HBsAg and HBeAg to prevent prenatal transmission (Bradley, 2005).

Infection early in pregnancy with HBV causes a 50% risk of neonatal HBV infection. Ninety percent of infants born to women who are positive for both HBsAg and HBeAg are at risk for development of HBV infection by their first birthday if they are not given treatment. Infants born to women who are positive for HBsAg but negative for HBeAg have lower rates of perinatal infection (20%) (Bradley, 2005). Infants who do not receive treatment are likely to become carriers, which may eventually lead to primary hepatocellular carcinoma. Treatment for these infants should be HBV vaccine along with hepatitis B immunoglobulin. For neonates whose mothers are HBsAg positive or exposed, HBV vaccine, 0.5 ml (10 mcg/ml), should be given intramuscularly in the anterolateral thigh at or within 24 hours of birth. Immunoglobulin (0.5 ml) should be given concurrently at a separate site. Vaccination should be repeated at 1 and 6 months: 0.5 ml; booster injections are suggested at 12 months and may need repeating at 5-year intervals. The vaccine can be used in infants who have been exposed to HIV. There is usually an immune response in these infants despite an altered CD4 count. The response does appear to be somewhat diminished (Bradley, 2005).

Vertical transmission of HBV may occur during vaginal delivery. The sharing of bodily secretions during sexual inter-

course can result in disease transmission also. HBV has a long incubation period—50 to 190 days, average 90 days. Current recommendations are for all pregnant women to be screened initially and again before delivery. Screening is essential to identify potential risk for perinatal transmission and for protection of those who are exposed to antigen-positive blood. Family clustering of HBV has been identified through spread via household contact (Bradley, 2005).

Clinical Manifestations

Prematurity, low birth weight and hyperbilirubinemia are clinical signs of HBV infection. Hepatosplenomegaly is also a common presenting symptom in an infant infected with a virus. An infant infected with HBV can be asymptomatic or present with a picture of fulminant infection (Bradley, 2005).

Risk Factors

Pregnant women in high-risk categories (i.e., they are known to have sexual contact with HBV-infected persons) should be screened so that appropriate follow-up can be provided. Persons in certain ethnic groups, such as Asians (Taiwanese especially) and Australian aborigines; intravenous drug users; and health professionals are at risk for the development of HBV. Individuals living in poor sanitary conditions are also at risk (Bradley, 2005).

Management and Prevention

Vaccination is recommended for individuals who are at risk for exposure to HBV, including health care workers, family members of chronic carriers, persons with large numbers of heterosexual partners, and intravenous drug users. HbsAg protein is administered to the deltoid muscle once and then again 1 month and 6 months later.

If the mother's antigen status is unknown at delivery, titers should be drawn and the woman should be vaccinated if the result is HbsAg positive. If the test results are unavailable or cannot be obtained, the neonate should be treated as if the mother were positive.

Proper and prompt identification of women in high-risk groups and knowledge of HBV status are important in the delivery room to determine whether the infant is at risk for infection. In accordance with universal infection control measures, appropriate barriers are used to protect health care workers from blood and body secretions. Delivery room and nursery personnel should always wear gloves when handling any new infant. The infant of a mother with confirmed HBV infection should be bathed with soap and water immediately, with special attention to removing all blood and secretions present on the skin and hair. The infant may be breastfed (unless the mother's nipples are cracked) and cared for routinely.

Chlamydia

Chlamydia is a genus of bacteria that grows between cells. Chlamydial infection is the most common sexually transmitted disease. Probably 50% of infected women of childbearing age are asymptomatic. Studies have shown that the infected population comprises sexually active women between 18 and 35 years of age having a high school education or less and three or more sexual partners in the previous 3 months (Darville, 2005; Miller, 2004). The infection can present as cervicitis, salpingitis, urethritis, or pelvic inflammatory disease.

Chlamydia trachomatis infection has been identified as causing a significant increase in the incidence of PROM, the number of low-birth-weight babies, and the rate of infant mortality (Darville, 2005; Miller, 2004). Thus, screening pregnant women for chlamydia is important (Hu et al, 2004). Treatment with erythromycin or clindamycin may prevent transmission to the newborn.

Clinical Manifestations

Chlamydia conjunctivitis can present in the newborn with a very watery discharge that may progress to purulent exudate. Application of erythromycin ointment at birth for ocular prophylaxis successfully treats both chlamydial and gonococcal conjunctivitis. Pneumonia can occur in newborns who have contracted chlamydia from their mother's genital tract. The incubation period is anywhere from 5 days to 3 to 4 months. Typical presentation is tachypnea, barrel chest, and an increased oxygen requirement. The infant may have interstitial infiltrations, hepatosplenomegaly, and increased eosinophils. In a prospective study of chlamydia, there was a 16% incidence of pneumonia in infants identified as being at risk for chlamydial infection (Darville, 2005; Miller, 2004).

Diagnosis of chlamydial infections is based on physical and laboratory examination; in cases of conjunctivitis, Giemsa-stained conjunctival scrapings provide a method of direct fluorescent antibody testing. The definitive diagnosis for chlamydial pneumonia is made by culture of the respiratory tract or identification of high levels of IgM antibodies to chlamydia.

Management and Prevention

Treatment of chlamydia infection in the newborn is usually with ampicillin and gentamicin if the infant's workup is for generic infection. Once the chlamydia organism is identified, more specific treatment is with erythromycin for 10 to 14 days.

If chlamydia is confirmed in a pregnant woman and treated, her sexual partners also require treatment. Rapid screening and diagnosis can be made using monoclonal antibodies.

Education and counseling regarding the method of transmission of chlamydia are important. This organism may be present for many years in the female genital tract and produce no symptoms. The organism does not respond to partial treatment; an infected woman and all her sexual partners must receive full treatment as soon as possible. Men should wear condoms during sexual relations to prevent transmission. Without treatment, the severe complications for the woman include pelvic inflammatory disease, ectopic pregnancy, and endometritis. The common newborn complication is pneumonia. Supportive ventilation in the newborn is usually necessary.

Viral Agents
Respiratory Syncytial Virus

Respiratory syncytial virus (RSV) is an infection usually found in older infants. It is thought that maternal antibodies protect infants for the first few weeks of life, but as passive immunity diminishes, these infants become more susceptible. Premature infants are more susceptible to the virus during their long-term hospitalizations. The most recent data available show that RSV was the leading cause of hospitalizations in infants annually from 1997 to 2000, according to a study by Leader and Kohlhase (2002).

Clinical Manifestations. An infant who is infected with RSV before 4 weeks of age may be asymptomatic or may have an upper respiratory infection with fever, bronchiolitis, apnea, or pneumonia. There may be a definite need for assisted ventilation, and deaths have occurred in rapidly fulminating disease, for which there is little available treatment. Small preterm infants who are already in significant pulmonary and cardiac jeopardy with respiratory distress syndrome or bronchopulmonary dysplasia are especially susceptible to development of severe infections. Nosocomial transmission of the virus between caretakers is possible; such transmission appears to result in less severe infection. The first clinical signs of transmission include a clear nasal discharge at approximately 10 to 52 days of life, followed by cough and wheezing. Radiologic changes compatible with pneumonia may also be found (Maldonado, 2005; Leader & Kohlhase, 2003; Wegner et al, 2004).

Treatment and Prevention. Good handwashing is extremely important in the prevention of transmission of RSV between critically ill patients. It has been shown that RSV-infected secretions can remain viable for up to 6 hours on countertops, 45 minutes on cloth gowns and paper tissues, and 20 minutes on skin. Thus, all infected infants should be cared for in cohort. Caretakers should be consistently assigned to decrease transmission rates. Gown and glove precautions can significantly reduce nosocomial transmission of RSV (Maldonado, 2005; Leader & Kohlhase, 2003; Wegner et al, 2004).

Any infant with a runny nose, nasal congestion, or unexplained apnea should be considered for isolation and investigated for RSV infection. Attention should be specific for those infants older than 4 weeks of corrected age. Specific cultures and screens should be performed because specific treatment is available if RSV is found.

Management. Treatment for identified RSV pneumonia is ribavirin. Ribavirin administration should be closely monitored by those who have been trained appropriately (Maldonado, 2005; Leader & Kohlhase, 2003; Wegner et al, 2004). Ribavirin can be administered safely to infants receiving mechanical ventilation and to infants in an oxygen hood. Specific safety precautions should be taken to protect the caretaker, because ribavirin has been identified as being potentially teratogenic. Protective measures include wearing a gown, gloves, and mask when in direct contact with the particles or mist containing ribavirin. Ideally, no pregnant woman would take care of an infant with RSV who is receiving ribavirin. Close monitoring of the pulmonary status, including the use of oxygen and mechanical ventilation, may be necessary. Isolation of the infected infant from other infants who could potentially be infected is important; the usual method for isolation is to minimize risk of the spread of the airborne virus and ribavirin particles.

Fungal Agents
Candida albicans

Candida species is a fungus that is frequently found in humans, and *C. albicans* is the most prevalent form in neonates. *Candida* organisms are oval, yeastlike cells that can bud to reproduce. *C. albicans* produces endotoxins, hemolysis, pyrogens, and proteolytic enzymes that are damaging to tissues (Maldonado et al, 2005; Triolo et al, 2002). Early recognition and treatment of fungal infection are imperative to prevent severe central nervous system complications and death.

Prolonged broad-spectrum antibiotic treatment for small premature infants may predispose infants to *Candida* overgrowth in the gastrointestinal tract. This overgrowth may predispose the infant to disseminated fungemia. Administration of hyperalimentation, frequent use of indwelling venous lines, and invasive procedures may also predispose the infant to *C. albicans* infection. One study has identified previous antibiotic therapy and assisted ventilation as the major factors that correlated to *Candida* infection (Maldonado et al, 2005; Triolo et al, 2002).

Clinical Manifestations

The newborn infected with *C. albicans* presents a picture similar to that of any septic infant. These newborns present with serious clinical signs of infection, often worsening with no presence of positive cultures. The infant is typically 20 to 30 days of age, has difficulties with oral feeds, depends on hyperalimentation, and has been given multiple courses of antibiotics. The infant may have respiratory distress, abdominal distention, guaiac-positive stools, carbohydrate intolerance, candiduria, temperature instability, and hypotension (Maldonado et al, 2005; Triolo et al, 2002).

Differential Diagnosis

A positive *Candida* culture should never be considered a contaminated specimen. Intermittently positive cultures may reflect transient candidemia, and, usually, removal of any indwelling catheters and lines and changing of antibiotic therapy may be indicated. In symptomatic low-birth-weight infants with positive systemic cultures, treatment should begin pending culture results.

Collaborative Management

The most effective drug for treatment of *C. albicans* infection is amphotericin B. This toxic, potent antifungal agent must be used cautiously. The initial dose is 0.1 to 0.3 mg/kg given intravenously over a period of 2 to 6 hours. The maintenance dosage is 0.5 to 1.0 mg/kg/day over 2 to 6 hours. Lower doses are started until higher doses can be tolerated. Increments of 0.1 mg/kg/day are used to increase the daily dose slowly. Many infants tolerate a total dose of 20 mg/kg if titrated over approximately 1 month. Often, if organ involvement is minimal, infants can be successfully given lower doses. If meningitis is suspected, 5-fluorouracil (5-FU) may be used. This antifungal agent acts to inhibit DNA synthesis so that *Candida* replication cannot occur.

Kidney toxicity is a major side effect of amphotericin B therapy because it causes renal vasoconstriction and decreases both renal blood flow and glomerular filtration rate. This damage can result in hyponatremia, hypokalemia, increased blood urea nitrogen, and increased creatinine, as well as acidosis. If the medication makes the patient oliguric, most physicians recommend stopping the drug until the next day. Thrombocytopenia, granulocytopenia, fever, nausea, and vomiting are the common side effects associated with amphotericin B. One major side effect of 5-FU is bone marrow depression, resulting in a decreased platelet count.

Because of the insidious onset of candidiasis, the septic infant who is not responding to traditional antibiotic treatment may have *Candida*. Catheter tips at intravenous sites and percutaneous lines should be changed and cultured. Urine can easily be cultured for the presence of *Candida*. Thrush and monilial rashes are indicative of candidiasis. These can easily be treated with oral and local antifungal agents (Maldonado et al, 2005).

Monitoring of infants receiving amphotericin B is challenging, because infants may have reactions to this medication. Blood pressure should be monitored every half hour, and urine output should be followed up closely. Vital signs and laboratory work, including liver enzyme tests, should be followed up daily to detect early signs of neonatal toxicity (Maldonado et al, 2005).

Nosocomial Infections

Both colonization and infection are nosocomial events, meaning "of or related to a hospital." The common meaning of the term *nosocomial* is "hospital acquired." Nursery-acquired infections are reported to the Centers for Disease Control and Prevention, which has a National Nosocomial Infections Surveillance System (Heath & Zerr, 2005).

The incidence of nosocomial infections in NICUs is 5% to 25% (Heath & Zerr, 2005). Critically ill infants who remain in a pathogen-filled environment are often in jeopardy because of their prolonged length of stay in the hospital. The mortality rate associated with these infections is between 5% and 20%, depending on the geographic area and specific birth-weight groups (Maldonado, 2005).

Coagulase-negative staphylococcus has been identified as a major cause of nosocomial infections. Low birth weight, multiple gestation, and prolonged hospitalization are significant factors for nosocomial infection. Yeast infections often occur if previous antibiotic therapy has been given. This infection is also associated with colonization of vascular catheters, assisted ventilation, and necrotizing enterocolitis (Maldonado, 2005).

Nursery epidemics can be caused by gram-negative and gram-positive or viral organisms because they have (1) the ability to colonize or infect human skin or the gastrointestinal tract, (2) the ability to be carried from person to person by hand contact, and (3) characteristics that allow existence on hands of personnel or in fluids or on inanimate objects, including intravenous fluids, respiratory support equipment, solutions used for medications, disinfectants, and banked breast milk (Maldonado, 2005).

Resistance to antibiotics is a serious problem in many NICUs, particularly with gram-negative enteric pathogens. Aminoglycoside resistance is a problem in many urban nurseries, as is colonization and infection with methicillin-resistant *S. aureus*. Respiratory infections with RSV, influenza virus, parainfluenza virus, rhinovirus, and echovirus occur in many nurseries. These are more difficult to identify and thus more difficult to report. CMV infection has been reported as a transfusion-related problem in low-birth-weight infants, thus prompting the current policy of using CMV-screened blood donors (Lamberson & Dock, 1992; Lamberson et al, 1988). Hepatitis A infection has also been reported as a transfusion-related problem that may develop in infants and staff in NICUs (Lin et al, 2001). Hepatitis C has been linked to use of immunoglobulins such as Gammagard by Baxter Laboratories, Deerfield, IL: (Lindenbach et al, 2005). Almost any organism given the right environment and support can become a nosocomially transmitted infection.

Infection Control Policies

Policies and procedures in nurseries should be set up by the hospital infection control committee based on the recommendations of the American Academy of Pediatrics and the CDC. The significance of these policies to newborns should be detailed in a hospital policy book. The following topics should be covered: (1) ocular prophylaxis, (2) skin and cord care, (3) nursery staff, (4) nursery design and environment, (5) handwashing, (6) staff apparel, (7) isolation, (8) visitors, (9) employee health, and (10) epidemic control (Maldonado, 2005). The simplest, most effective weapon for preventing infection is the liberal use of soap and water!

SUMMARY

Many factors place the neonate at high risk for infection. The nurse is in a unique role to implement methods for prevention of infection in nurseries, to detect early signs and symptoms of infection, and to participate in infection control. A better understanding of the neonatal immune system, methods of perinatal acquisition of organisms, common microorganisms, signs and symptoms of infections, and appropriate therapy provides the nurse with a sound basis for management of care as well as the development of hospital infection control policies for the NICU.

Case Study

IDENTIFICATION OF THE PROBLEM

Baby girl Smith is a 700-g, 27-week-gestation female born by emergency caesarean section secondary to significant fetal distress after a failed attempt to stop preterm labor. She was admitted to the NICU with respiratory distress.

ASSESSMENT: HISTORY AND PHYSICAL EXAMINATION

The pregnancy history was unremarkable until the development of preterm labor at $26\frac{1}{2}$ weeks. The mother had been hospitalized for 3 days with tocolytics and bed rest. Tocolytics were discontinued at 27 weeks due to maternal fever, leaking membranes, meconium-stained fluid, and decelerations of the fetal heart rate. Emergency caesarean section was performed due to the presence of fetal distress. Apgar scores were 4^1, 5^5, 8^{10}. Upon delivery, the neonate required positive-pressure ventilation, 100% FiO_2, and tactile stimulation.

DIFFERENTIAL DIAGNOSIS

Respiratory distress syndrome (RSD) secondary to surfactant deficiency

Respiratory distress secondary to meconium aspiration pneumonia

Respiratory distress secondary to sepsis

DIAGNOSTIC TESTS

Chest radiograph

CBC with differential and platelets

Blood cultures

WORKING DIAGNOSIS

The chest radiograph was consistent with RDS secondary to surfactant deficiency. The history of preterm labor, leaking membranes, and maternal fever suggests sepsis. The CBC revealed a low WBC with an increased number of immature to mature neutrophils, indicative of sepsis. The most likely cause of early-onset sepsis is group B beta-hemolytic streptococcus, although the history of leaking membranes could indicate a gram-negative organism.

DEVELOPMENT OF MANAGEMENT PLAN

The primary management for this baby was appropriate ventilatory support. She was placed on synchronous mechanical ventilation at 20/4, rate of 40 breaths/min, and 50% FiO_2. Exogenous surfactant replacement was implemented immediately. Umbilical artery and venous catheterization were performed; IV fluids of D_5W (100 ml/kg/day) were started to maintain fluid and electrolyte balance, provide nutrition, and allow blood-sampling. Ampicillin and gentamicin were started to provide coverage for most common gram-positive and gram-negative microorganisms. Continuing orders included serial CBCs; chemistry profiles, including electrolytes, calcium, and glucose; gentamicin levels; total parenteral nutrition; and trophic feedings of human milk at 24 hours of life.

IMPLEMENTATION AND EVALUATION OF EFFECTIVENESS

The baby's respiratory condition initially worsened, requiring increased ventilatory support to 24/4, rate of 60 breaths/min, and 80% FiO_2. After the second dose of exogenous surfactant, the baby's respiratory status improved and the ventilatory support was decreased in response to improved arterial blood gases, chest radiographs, and pulse-oximeter readings. By day 5 of life, the baby was extubated to nasal CPAP. The blood culture confirmed group B streptococcal infection and antibiotics were continued for 7 days.

REFERENCES

Adair CE et al (2003). Risk factors for early-onset group B streptococcal disease in neonates: a population-based case-control study. *Canadian Medical Association journal* 169:198.

Arvin AM et al (2005). Herpes simplex virus infections. In Remington JS, Klein JO, editors. *Infectious diseases of the fetus and newborn infant*, ed 6 (pp 845-866). Philadelphia: Saunders.

Baltimore RS (2003). Neonatal infection epidemiology and management. *Pediatric Drugs* 5(1):723-740.

Benedetto C et al (2004). Cervicovaginal infections during pregnancy: epidemiological and microbiological aspects. *Journal of maternal-fetal and neonatal medicine* 16:9-12.

Bortolussi R, Mailman TL (2005). Listeriosis. In Remington JS, Klein JO, editors. *Infectious diseases of the fetus and newborn infant*, ed 6 (pp 465-484). Philadelphia: Saunders.

Bradley JS (2005). Hepatitis. In Remington JS, Klein JO, editors. *Infectious diseases of the fetus and newborn infant*, ed 6 (pp 823-844). Philadelphia: Saunders.

Centers for Disease Control and Prevention (CDC) (2001). *Health information for international travel 2001-2002*. Atlanta, GA: Author.

Cooper LZ, Alford CA (2005). Rubella. In Remington JS, Klein JO, editors. *Infectious diseases of the fetus and newborn infant*, ed 6 (pp 893-926). Philadelphia: Saunders.

Darville T (2005). Chlamydia infections. In Remington JS, Klein JO, editors. *Infectious diseases of the fetus and newborn infant*, ed 6 (pp 385-392). Philadelphia: Saunders.

Dimpfl T, Gloning K (1995). Fever of undetermined origin in pregnancy—bear listeriosis in mind. *Journal of obstetrics and gynaecology* 15:184.

Edwards MS et al (2005). Group B streptococcal infections. In Remington JS, Klein JO, editors. *Infectious diseases of the fetus and newborn infant*, ed 6 (pp 406-464). Philadelphia: Saunders.

Ehrbar T et al (2001). A small for dates newborn girl with a mummified left arm. *European journal of pediatrics* 160:395-396.

Embree JE (2005). Gonococcal infections. In Remington JS, Klein JO, editors. *Infectious diseases of the fetus and newborn infant*, ed 6 (pp 393-402). Philadelphia: Saunders.

Gershon AA (2005). Chicken pox, measles, and mumps. In Remington JS, Klein JO, editors. *Infectious diseases of the fetus and newborn infant*, ed 6 (pp 693-738). Philadelphia: Saunders.

Gregg NM (1941). Congenital cataract following German measles in the mother. *Transactions of the Ophthalmological Society of Australia* 3:35.

Healy CM et al (2004). Features of invasive staphylococcal disease in neonates. *Pediatrics* 114:953-961.

Heath JA, Zerr DM (2005). Infections acquired in the nursery: epidemiology and control. In Remington JS, Klein JO, editors. *Infectious diseases of the fetus and newborn infant*, ed 6 (pp 1179-1206). Philadelphia: Saunders.

Hu D et al (2004). Screening for *Chlamydia trachomatis* in women 15 to 29 years of age: a cost-effectiveness analysis. *Annals of internal medicine* 141:501-513.

Ichiba H et al (2000). Neonatal listeriosis with severe respiratory failure responding to nitric oxide inhalation. *Pediatrics international* 42:696-698.

Ingall E et al (2005). Syphilis. In Remington JS, Klein JO, editors. *Infectious diseases of the fetus and newborn infant*, ed 6 (pp 545-580). Philadelphia: Saunders.

Kitajima H (2003). Prevention of methicillin-resistant *Staphylococcus aureus* infections in neonates. *Pediatrics international* 45:238-245.

Lamberson HV, Dock NL (1992). Prevention of transfusion-transmitted cytomegalovirus infection. *Transfusion* 32(3):196-198.

Lamberson HV et al (1988). Prevention of transfusion-associated cytomegalovirus (CMV) infection in neonates by screening blood donors for IgM to CMV. *Journal of infectious diseases* 157(4):820-823.

Langlet C et al (2003). An uncommon case of disseminated neonatal herpes simplex infection presenting with pneumonia and pleural effusions. *European journal of pediatrics* 162:532-533.

Leader S, Kohlhase K (2002). Respiratory syncytial virus-coded pediatric hospitalizations, 1997 to 1999. *Pediatric infectious diseases journal* 21:629-632.

Lim DV et al (1986). Reduction of morbidity and mortality rates for neonatal group B streptococcal disease through early diagnosis and chemoprophylaxis. *Journal of clinical microbiology* 23(3):489-492.

Lin FC et al (2001). Level of maternal antibody required to protect neonates against early-onset disease caused by group B streptococcus type Ia: a multicenter, seroepidemiology study. *Journal of infectious diseases* 184(8):1022.

Lindenbach BD et al (2005). Complete replication of hepatitis C virus in cell culture. *Science* 309(5734):623-626.

Lott JW, Kenner CA (1994a). Keeping up with neonatal infection: designer bugs, Part I. *American journal of maternal child nursing*. 19(4):207-213.

Lott JW, Kenner C (1994b). Keeping up with neonatal infection: designer bugs, Part II. *American journal of maternal child nursing*. 19(5):264-271.

Mackowiak PA (2002). A newborn with rash and chorioretinitis. *Clinical infectious diseases* 35:625-626.

Maldonado YA et al (2005). Less common viral infections. In Remington JS, Klein JO, editors. *Infectious diseases of the fetus and newborn infant*, ed 6 (pp 933-944). Philadelphia: Saunders.

Maldonado YA et al (2005). Pneumocystis and other less common fungal infections. In Remington JS, Klein JO, editors. *Infectious diseases of the fetus and newborn infant*, ed 6 (pp 1129-1176). Philadelphia: Saunders.

Miller KE (2004). *Chlamydia trachomatis* exposure in newborns. *American family physician* 69:727-730.

Neto EC et al (2004). Newborn screening for congenital infectious diseases. *Emerging infectious diseases* 10:1069-1073.

Ogunyemi D, Hernández-Loera GE (2004). The impact of antenatal cocaine use on maternal characteristics and neonatal outcomes. *Journal of maternal-fetal and neonatal medicine* 15:253-257.

Orschein RC et al (2005). Staphylococcal infections. In Remington JS, Klein JO, editors. *Infectious diseases of the fetus and newborn infant*, ed 6 (pp 513-544). Philadelphia: Saunders.

Palazzi D et al (2005). Bacterial sepsis and meningitis. In Remington JS, Klein JO, editors. *Infectious diseases of the fetus and newborn infant*, ed 6 (pp 247-296). Philadelphia: Saunders.

Peihong J et al (2001). Early congenital syphilis. *International journal of dermatology* 40:191-209.

Remington JS et al (2005). Toxoplasmosis. In Remington JS, Klein JO, editors. *Infectious diseases of the fetus and newborn infant*, ed 6 (pp 947-1092). Philadelphia: Saunders.

Stagno S, Britt W (2005). Cytomegalovirus infections. In Remington JS, Klein JO, editors. *Infectious diseases of the fetus and newborn infant*, ed 6 (pp 739-782). Philadelphia: Saunders.

Stoll BJ (2005). Neonatal infections: a global perspective. In Remington JS, Klein JO, editors. *Infectious diseases of the fetus and newborn infant*, ed 6 (pp 27-58). Philadelphia: Saunders.

Stoll BJ et al (2004). To tap or not to tap: high likelihood of meningitis without infection among very low birth weight infants. *Pediatrics* 113:1181-1186.

Triolo V et al (2002). Fluconazole therapy for *Candida albicans* urinary tract infections in children. *Pediatric nephrology* 17(7):550-553.

Uhl JR et al (2005). Use of the Roche LightCycler Strep B Assay for detection of group B streptococcus from vaginal and rectal swabs. *Journal of clinical microbiology* 43(8):4046-4051.

Van der Zwet WC et al (2002). Neonatal antibody titers against varicella-zoster virus in relation to gestational age, birth weight, and maternal titer. *Pediatrics* 109:79-87.

Visintine AM et al (1977). Infection in infants and children. *American journal of diseases of children* 131(4):393-397.

Wegner S et al (2004). Direct cost analyses of palivizumab treatment in a cohort of at-risk children: evidence from the North Carolina medicaid program. *Pediatrics* 114(6):1612-1619.

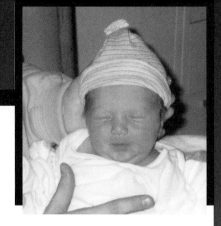

Chapter 10

Hematologic System

Gail A. Bagwell

The hematologic system is probably one of the least understood body systems of the neonate. But in order to provide the utmost care to the neonate, a thorough and complete understanding of the hematologic system and its components is necessary. The knowledge of how the blood cells develop and function as well as how the hemostatic system functions is essential in the understanding the diseases of the newborn that affect the hematologic system. Without this knowledge the nurse will miss many of the subtle signs and symptoms that indicate that a problem has arisen. This chapter discusses the hematologic and hemostatic systems, as well as the most common hematologic diseases of the newborn period.

OVERVIEW OF THE HEMATOLOGIC SYSTEM
Hematopoiesis
The hematopoietic system is characterized by the presence of pluripotent stem cells that differentiate into the three types of circulating blood cells: red blood cells (RBCs), white blood cells (WBCs), and thrombocytes (platelets). The formation, production, and maintenance of blood cells is referred to as hematopoiesis. Hematopoiesis is a continuous process that involves cell maturation and destruction concurrent with new cell production. Gestational age and postnatal age influence maturation and govern individual cell components, the level of activity, and the site of production.

The liver becomes the main site for hematopoiesis beginning at approximately 5 to 6 weeks' gestation. The production peaks at 4 to 5 months of age, then slowly regresses, with the bone marrow predominating from 22 weeks of gestation on. Also helping with hematopoiesis during the fetal period are extramedullary sites of the spleen, lymph nodes, thymus, and kidneys while the long bones are small.

Red Blood Cells
Erythropoiesis, the production of red blood cells, begins at approximately 3 to 4 weeks of gestation. The red blood cells (RBCs) are initially primitive megaloblasts, but when the liver becomes the primary site of hematopoiesis, a definitive line of RBCs is formed from the normoblasts, which progresses through several phases of refinement and accrue hemoglobin before reaching maturation. When the hemoglobin concentration of the normoblast reaches 34%, the nucleus is extruded and the cell becomes a reticulocyte. Approximately 1 to 2 days later, the reticulocyte becomes a mature RBC and is released into the bloodstream. The development of the RBC is identical in the bone marrow when it becomes the primary site of erythrocyte production.

The role of the red blood cell is to exchange oxygen and carbon dioxide between the lungs and tissues. Tissue oxygenation occurs by hemoglobin transport, whereas carbon dioxide removal is a reaction with carbonic anhydrase. Red blood cells also serve as a buffer to maintain acid-base balance.

The life span of fetal and newborn RBCs is much shorter than the adult RBC life span of 120 days. The term newborn's erythrocyte can last 60 to 70 days; that of a preterm infant, 35 to 50 days. One theoretic reason for this is the diminished deformability of the neonatal erythrocyte. Because of its larger size and cylindrical shape, the neonatal erythrocyte is more prone to destruction in the narrow sinusoids of the spleen.

The mean RBC count in the term newborn is in the range of 5.1 million to 5.3 million per milliliter, with an elevated reticulocyte count of 3% to 7% during the first 24 to 48 hours of life (Robertson & Shilkofski, 2005). Mean RBC counts in the premature infant range from 4.6 million to 5.3 million per milliliter, with a greater number of circulating immature RBCs reflected in a higher reticulocyte count (3% to 10%). In both groups of infants, the reticulocyte count falls abruptly to about 1% and the erythropoietin level drops to low, often undetectable, levels by the first week of life.

Hemoglobin
At 10 weeks' gestation, hemoglobin synthesis changes from the embryonic to the fetal form (hemoglobin F). The mechanism by which stem cells and progenitor cells perform this changeover remains unclear. Although low levels of a third form of hemoglobin, adult hemoglobin (hemoglobin A), are detectable at this time, hemoglobin F remains the predominant form during fetal development. At 30 weeks' gestation, 90% to 100% of hemoglobin is the fetal form; the remainder is hemoglobin A. Between 30 and 32 weeks, the percentage of hemoglobin F starts to decline. At 40 weeks, 50% to 75% of RBCs contain fetal hemoglobin; at 6 months of age, 5% to 8%; and at 1 year of age, 1%.

Each type of hemoglobin has properties that make it valuable at the time of its synthesis. Each has a different affinity for oxygen that varies its uptake and release to the tissue (Figure 10-1). Fetal hemoglobin has a high affinity for oxygen, binding it more readily at the intervillous spaces in the placenta when the fetal partial pressure of oxygen (PO_2) averages between 25 and 30 mm Hg. Adult hemoglobin has a decreased affinity for oxygen, which allows easier release of oxygen to the tissues when metabolic needs are high and the lungs are functional.

Erythropoietin
The factors that affect RBC production are still unclear, but erythropoietin appears to exert great control over erythro-

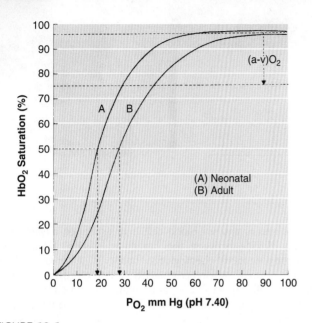

FIGURE **10-1**
The affinity for oxygen (i.e., the ability of the hemoglobin molecule to bind and hold the oxygen molecule) is markedly different between fetal and adult hemoglobin. Fetal hemoglobin has a greater affinity for oxygen. It is able to bind to oxygen more readily at the intervillous spaces of the placenta, a property that is useful in the low partial pressure of oxygen (PO_2) environment of the fetus. Adult hemoglobin has a diminished affinity for oxygen, which allows easier release of oxygen to the tissue when metabolic needs are higher than those that arise in the fetus. From Sacks L, Delivoria-Papadopoulos M (1984). Hemoglobin-oxygen interactions. *Seminars in perinatology* 8:168-183.

poiesis during late gestation. This circulating glycoprotein hormone, the gene of which is located on the seventh chromosome, is an obligate growth factor that stimulates stem cells to become committed progenitors of the erythrocyte (Figure 10-2). In adults the kidneys produce 90% to 95% of erythropoietin, but in the fetus the liver is considered the predominant site of production throughout most of gestation.

The major stimulus for erythropoietin release is diminished tissue oxygenation. In the absence of erythropoietin, hypoxia has no effect on the production of RBCs. However, if erythropoietin production is intact, hypoxia stimulates a rapid increase in erythropoietin levels, which remain elevated until hypoxia no longer exists. Although the liver is less responsive to hypoxia than the kidneys, production of erythropoietin in the fetus and newborn increases within minutes to hours after a precipitating event such as hypoxia. Erythropoietin acts by directly stimulating the RBC precursors, accelerating their passage through the various maturational stages. Although erythropoietin levels increase rapidly, no change in the number of erythrocytes is noted for approximately 5 days after a hypoxic stress. When erythropoietin stimulates production of excess RBCs, the red blood cells are released into the circulation before they have reached maturity (i.e., as reticulocytes); this is reflected in an elevated reticulocyte count.

Factors besides hypoxia that increase erythropoietin production in the newborn are maternal hypoxemia, smallness for gestational age, and poor placental function. Erythropoietin levels are also increased by testosterone, estrogen, thyroid hormone, prostaglandins, and lipoproteins. Cord blood levels normally are elevated compared with adult values but drop dramatically to almost undetectable levels in the newborn. The healthy newborn, therefore, produces few RBCs in the first few weeks of life because the hypoxic stimuli of low fetal PO_2 levels are no longer present. Erythropoietin levels do not increase in the term infant until 8 to 10 weeks of age, when tissue hypoxia caused by anemia is sensed by the kidneys.

The characteristics of the neonatal erythrocyte predispose both preterm and term infants to problems associated with hemolysis and immature hepatic response to erythrocyte destruction, as well as to the effects of shortened erythrocyte life span (as is seen in physiologic neonatal anemia and anemia of the premature infant). In addition to maturational influences, preexisting maternal diseases and intrauterine abnormalities can impair RBC function and production, resulting in increased oxygen and nutritional requirements for the growing fetus.

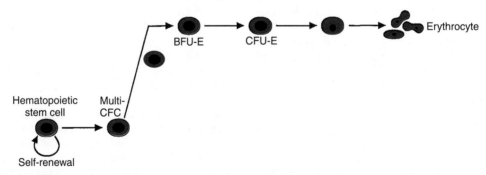

FIGURE **10-2**
Hematopoietic stem cells stimulated to become erythrocytes initially develop into multipotent colony-forming cells (*Multi-CFC*). A portion of the Multi-CFC become erythroid progenitor cells, the early and late erythroid burst-forming units (*BFU-E*), which eventually differentiate into erythroid colony-forming units (*CFU-E*). These progenitor cells progress to form the normoblast, the erythrocyte precursor. Multiple divisions and alterations of the normoblast lead to the development of the reticulocyte. When the reticulocyte extrudes its nucleus, it normally moves out of the predominant production sites (i.e., the liver or bone marrow) and into the blood. Modified from Luchtman-Jones L et al (2006). The blood and hematopoietic system. In Fanaroff A et al, editors. *Neonatal-perinatal medicine: diseases of the fetus and infant*, ed 8. Philadelphia: Mosby.

White Blood Cells

The formation of the white blood cells (WBCs) begins in the liver at approximately 5 to 7 weeks' gestation and then in the lymph nodes at 12 weeks' gestation, with the number of circulating WBCs increasing dramatically during the third trimester. The purpose of the white blood cell is to work against foreign proteins found in the body. The production and function of WBCs are also affected by gestational age; this subject is covered in more detail in Chapter 9.

Platelets

The production of platelets and clotting factors is also a function of gestational age. Although some factors are deficient at birth, several clotting factors and platelets are present in concentrations similar to adult levels. However, many of these components are functionally different from those of adults, possibly because of impaired activity or limited ability to respond to heightened needs. Coagulation dysfunction in the newborn may also be the result of genetic abnormalities (e.g., X-linked hemophilia), preexisting maternal illness (e.g., immune thrombocytopenic purpura), or infection (e.g., disseminated intravascular coagulation).

Platelet counts in the newborn do not vary much in relation to gestational age. Counts are similar from 27 to 40 weeks' gestation, with the range of normal falling between 215,000/mm^3 and 378,000/mm^3. At 32 weeks' gestation, platelet levels are comparable to those of an adult, but platelet function is not. Platelet counts under 150,000/mm^3 are considered thrombocytopenic.

Blood Volume

Normal blood values found shortly after birth reflect a time of maximum change. Blood values at birth depend on (1) the timing of cord clamping, (2) the infant's gestational age, (3) the blood sampling site, and (4) the technique used to obtain adequate blood flow.

The timing of cord clamping and the positional differences between the infant and the placenta can significantly influence newborn blood volume. Complete emptying of placental vessels before clamping can increase blood volume by 61%; one quarter of the placental transfusion occurs within the first 15 seconds, and half of the transfusion is complete by 1 minute.

The average blood volume is approximately 85 ml/kg of body weight in the term infant, though it can be as high as to 90 to 105 ml/kg in the preterm infant. The younger the infant's gestational age, the greater the blood volume will be per kilogram of body weight. The hemoglobin concentration and hematocrit are also functions of gestational age, especially in infants born before 32 weeks' gestation. The average mean hemoglobin concentration at 26 to 30 weeks is 13.4 g/dl, with an average mean hematocrit of 41.5% (Robertson & Shilkofski, 2005). In the term infant, mean hemoglobin values range from 16.5 to 18.5 g/dl, with mean hematocrit values between 51% and 56%. Mean hemoglobin values in postmature infants are higher than in the term infant, possibly as a result of progressive placental dysfunction and of oxygen deficit, which stimulates the release of erythropoietin. Table 10-1 summarizes the differences in hematologic values as a function of increasing gestational and postnatal age.

It is important to consider the sampling site and the quality of blood flow when interpreting laboratory values. The hemoglobin levels of capillary blood are 10% to 20% higher than those of venous and arterial blood. This discrepancy can be minimized by warming the extremity before drawing blood to enhance peripheral perfusion, allowing better spontaneous blood flow. Discarding the first few drops obtained on a capillary draw also improves the accuracy of the sample. Sampling by the venous route also requires care; poor blood flow through small-bore needles increases the chance of hemolysis, which can lead to sampling errors. Greater accuracy can be obtained by using the largest possible bore needle and removing the needle from the syringe before placing the sample in the specimen container. Gestational age also affects the discrepancy between reported capillary and venous results: the younger the gestational age, the larger the discrepancy. The key to accuracy in hematology laboratory values lies in the use of a consistent sampling site.

TABLE 10-1	Age-Specific Normal Blood Cell Values in Fetal Samples (26 to 30 Weeks' Gestation) and Neonatal Samples (28 to 44 Weeks' Gestation)						
Age	Hb (g%)[a]	HCT (%)[a]	MCV (fl)[a]	MCHC (g/% RBC)[a]	Reticulocytes	WBCs (×10^3/mm^3)[b]	Platelets (10^3/mm^3)[b]
26 to 30 weeks' gestation[c]	13.4	41.5	118.2	37.9	—	4.4	254
	(11)	(34.9)	(106.7)	(30.6)		(2.7)	(180 to 271)
28 weeks	14.5	45	120	31.0	(5-10)	—	275
32 weeks	15.0	47	118	32.0	(3-10)	—	290
Term[d] (cord)	16.5 (13.5)	51 (42)	108 (98)	33.0 (30.0)	(3-7)	18.1 (9 to 30)[d]	290
1 to 3 days	18.5 (14.5)	56 (45)	108 (95)	33.0 (29.0)	(1.8 to 4.6)	18.9 (9.4 to 34)	192
2 weeks	16.6 (13.4)	53 (41)	105 (88)	31.4 (28.1)		11.4 (5 to 20)	262
1 month	13.9 (10.7)	44 (33)	101 (91)	31.8 (28.1)	(0.1 to 1.7)	108 (4 to 19.5)	

Modified from Robertson J & Shilkofski N (2005). *Harriet Lane handbook*, ed 17. St Louis: Mosby

Hb, *Hemoglobin*; Hct, *hematocrit*; MCV, *mean corpuscular volume*; MCHC, *mean corpuscular hemoglobin concentration*; WBCs, *white blood cells*.

[a]*Data are mean (number in parenthesis is −2 standard deviations [SD]).*

[b]*Data are mean (number in parenthesis is −2 SD).*

[c]*In infants younger than 1 month, capillary Hb exceeds venous Hb: at 1 hour old, the difference is 3.6 g; at 5 days, 2.2 g; at 3 weeks, 1.1 g.*

[d]*Mean (95% confidence limits).*

TABLE 10-2	Blood Groups and Their Constituent Antigens (Agglutinogens) and Antibodies (Agglutinins)		
Genotype	**Blood Group**	**Agglutinogens**	**Agglutinins**
OO	O	–	Anti-A and anti-B
OA or AA	A	A	Anti-B
OB or BB	B	B	Anti-A
AB	AB	A and B	–

From Guyton AC, Hall JE (2006). Blood types, transfusion, tissue and organ transplantation. In Guyton AC, Hall JE, editors. Textbook of medical physiology, ed 11. Philadelphia: Saunders.

Blood Group Type

The RBCs have antigens located on the surface of the cell membranes that can cause antigen-antibody reactions. Blood is classified by group and types based on the antigens that are found on the RBC. The four major blood types are A, B, O, and AB. The most common blood types in the population are O at 47% and A at 41% (Guyton & Hall, 2006a). Antibodies to the antigens of different blood types occur naturally in the plasma (Table 10-2). For example, type A blood has A antigens on the cell surface but has circulating anti-B antibodies in the plasma. Type B blood has just the opposite, B antigens on the cell surface and anti-A antibodies in the plasma. Type AB blood has A and B antigens on the cell surface and neither antibody in the plasma, and type O blood has neither antigen on the cell surface and both anti-A and anti-B antibodies in the plasma. Antigens usually are polypeptides and complex proteins; antibodies are immunoglobulins (mostly IgG and IgM).

The other type of antigen is Rh antigens. Chromosome 1 stores the genetic material governing Rh antigens, but the number of genes involved in their synthesis has not been fully determined (Porter et al, 2003). There are three presumed Rh gene loci with the capability of producing five recognized antigens in the Rh complex: C, D, E, c, and e. The d antigen is considered an absence of antigen D because it cannot be isolated at present. Each individual has a paired set of these factors, having inherited a single set of C or c, D or d, and E or e from each parent. A predilection exists toward three particular combinations, two Rh positive (CDe and cDE) and one Rh negative (cde). Of these six factors, the two involved in Rh determination are D and d. The D antigen is most prevalent; its presence on the RBC indicates an Rh-positive cell, whereas its absence indicates an Rh-negative cell. Because of single-set inheritance from each parent, the potential exists for three different combinations of paired antigens: one pair being both d (Rh negative, homozygous), another pair being both D (Rh positive, homozygous), and the third pair being a combination of d and D (Rh positive, heterozygous). The end product is the production or absence of Rh antigen positioned on the surface of the RBC. The Rh antigen can be detected as early as 38 days' gestation on the fetal RBC and attains complete development during fetal life. This antigen is necessary for normal function of the RBC membrane and, unlike A and B antigens, which can be found in other tissues, it is confined exclusively to the RBC. Antibodies never occur naturally in the Rh system; exposure to the antigen is necessary to produce antibodies.

HEMOSTATIC SYSTEM

The components involved in blood coagulation and fibrinolysis (dissolution of a formed clot) are produced in the liver, vascular wall and tissue during early fetal life. Many of the clotting factors (procoagulants) and anticoagulants (inhibitors) can be identified during the 8th to 12th weeks of gestation. However, procoagulants, anticoagulants, and the substances responsible for dissolution of a clot, fibrinolytics, do not increase in number and function or reach adult levels simultaneously (Tables 10-3, 10-4, and 10-5). Some components increase with increasing gestational age, whereas others achieve normal adult levels several weeks to months before the fetus reaches term. Still other components do not achieve normal adult levels until several weeks to months after birth. Although the function of coagulation factors and anticoagulants in the fetus is not identical to that in an older child or adult, initial vascular response to injury by release of tissue thromboplastin is functional in the fetus as early as 8 weeks.

Hemostasis consists of a delicate and dynamic balance between factors that prevent exsanguination and those that keep the blood in a fluid form. The balanced interrelationship among four distinct components ensures orderly hemostasis and fibrinolysis when vascular integrity is destroyed or interrupted. The four constituents are vascular spasm, platelets and their activating substances, coagulation or plasma factors, and the fibrinolytic pathway.

Initial Steps in Hemostasis

Vascular Spasm

Initial hemostasis in a ruptured blood vessel consists of vascular spasm, which is a consequence of multiple mediator interactions, nervous reflexes, and localized muscle spasm. Although nervous reflexes are a response to pain, most of the vascular spasm is due to muscle contraction in the vessel wall secondary to direct injury. This vascular response to injury is present in an 8-week fetus and at term is the equivalent of adult norms in regard to capillary fragility and bleeding time. This component is gestational age dependent, as is evident in the increased capillary fragility shown by the preterm infant.

Platelet Plug Formation

The second mechanism of hemostasis after vascular injury is the formation of the platelet plug. Platelets coming into contact with an injured vascular wall adhere to the wall and form a platelet plug. This hemostatic plug is the primary means of closing small vascular holes at the capillary and small-vessel level. The platelets' ability to adhere on contact to a denuded vascular wall requires a glycoprotein, von Willebrand factor, which is synthesized by vascular endothelial cells and megakaryocytes. von Willebrand factor complexes with Factor VIII (antihemophilic factor) and both circulate jointly.

Platelets also have the ability to aggregate (stick to other platelets), forming large clumps. Aggregation is made possible by the platelet's ability to modify its shape and to secrete many biochemical substances (platelet release reaction) that enhance cohesion. When platelets and associated glycoproteins are activated by excess release of these biochemical substances during times of stress, fibrinogen receptors appear on the

TABLE 10-3   Normal Coagulation Test Results and Blood Levels of Coagulation Factors in the Fetus (19 to 27 Weeks' Gestation) and Newborn (28 Weeks' Gestation to Term)

Test/Factor	19 to 27 Weeks Mean ± SD	28 to 31 Weeks Mean (Boundary)	30 to 36 Weeks, Day 1 Mean (Boundary)	30 to 36 Weeks, Day 5 Mean (Boundary)	Full Term, Day 1 Mean (Boundary)	Full Term, Day 5 Mean (Boundary)
TEST						
Prothrombin time (PT) (seconds)	—	15.4 (14.6 to 16.9)	13 (10.6 to 16.2)	12.5 (10 to 15.3)	13 (10.1 to 15.9)	12.4 (10 to 15.3)
Activated partial thromboplastin time (AAPTT) (seconds)	—	108 (80 to 168)	53.6 (27.5 to 79.4)	50.5 (26.9 to 74.1)	42.9 (31.3 to 54.5)	42.6 (25.4 to 59.8)
Thrombin clotting time (TCT) (seconds)	—	—	24.8 (19.2 to 30.4)	24.1 (18.8 to 29.4)	23.5 (19 to 28.3)	23.1 (18 to 29.2)
FACTOR						
Fibrinogen (g/L)	1 ± 0.4	2.56 (1.6 to 5.5)	2.43 (1.5 to 3.73)	2.8 (1.6 to 4.18)	2.83 (1.67 to 3.99)	3.12 (1.62 to 4.62)
Factor II (units/ml)	0.12 ± 0.02	0.31 (0.19 to 0.54)	0.45 (0.2 to 0.77)	0.57 (0.29 to 0.85)	0.48 (0.26 to 0.7)	0.63 (0.33 to 0.93)
Factor V (units/ml)	0.41 ± 0.1	0.65 (0.43 to 0.8)	0.88 (0.41 to 1.44)	1 (0.46 to 1.54)	0.72 (0.34 to 1.08)	0.95 (0.45 to 1.45)
Factor VII (units/ml)	0.28 ± 0.04	0.37 (0.24 to 0.76)	0.67 (0.21 to 1.13)	0.84 (0.3 to 1.38)	0.66 (0.28 to 1.04)	0.89 (0.35 to 1.43)
Factor VIII (units/ml)	0.39 ± 0.14	0.79 (0.37 to 1.26)	1.11 (0.5 to 2.13)	1.15 (0.53 to 2.05)	1 (0.5 to 1.78)	0.88 (0.5 to 1.54)
von Willebrand factor (vWF) (units/ml)	0.64 ± 0.13	1.41 (0.83 to 2.23)	1.36 (0.78 to 2.1)	1.33 (0.72 to 2.19)	1.53 (0.5 to 2.87)	1.4 (0.5 to 2.54)
Factor IX (units/ml)	0.1 ± 0.01	0.18 (0.17 to 0.2)	0.35 (0.19 to 0.65)	0.42 (0.14 to 0.74)	0.53 (0.15 to 0.91)	0.53 (0.15 to 0.91)
Factor X (units/ml)	0.21 ± 0.03	0.36 (0.25 to 0.64)	0.41 (0.11 to 0.71)	0.51 (0.19 to 0.83)	0.4 (0.12 to 0.68)	0.49 (0.19 to 0.79)
Factor XI (units/ml)	—	0.23 (0.11 to 0.33)	0.3 (0.08 to 0.52)	0.41 (0.13 to 0.69)	0.55 (0.23 to 0.87)	0.55 (0.23 to 0.87)
Factor XII (units/ml)	0.22 ± 0.03	0.25 (0.05 to 0.35)	0.38 (0.1 to 0.66)	0.39 (0.09 to 0.69)	0.53 (0.13 to 0.93)	0.47 (0.11 to 0.83)
Prekallikrein (PK) (units/ml)	—	0.26 (0.15 to 0.32)	0.33 (0.09 to 0.57)	0.45 (0.26 to 0.75)	0.37 (0.18 to 0.69)	0.48 (0.2 to 0.76)
High-molecular-weight kininogen (HMWK) (units/ml)	—	0.32 (0.19 to 0.52)	0.49 (0.09 to 0.89)	0.62 (0.24 to 1)	0.54 (0.06 to 1.02)	0.74 (0.16 to 1.32)
Factor XIIIa (units/ml)	—	—	0.7 (0.32 to 1.08)	1.01 (0.57 to 1.45)	0.79 (0.27 to 1.31)	0.94 (0.44 to 1.44)
Factor XIIIb (units/ml)	—	—	0.81 (0.35 to 1.27)	1.1 (0.68 to 1.58)	0.76 (0.3 to 1.22)	1.06 (0.32 to 1.8)
Plasminogen (units/ml)	—	—	1.7 (1.12 to 2.48)	1.91 (1.21 to 2.61)	1.95 0.35 (44)	2.17 ± 0.38 (60)

Modified from Andrew M et al (1990). Development of the hemostatic system in the neonate and young infant. American journal of pediatric hematology/oncology 12:97-98; Andrew M et al (1987). Development of the human coagulation system in the full-term infant. Blood 70:166; and Andrew M et al (1988). Development of the human coagulation system in the healthy premature infant. Blood 72:1653.

TABLE 10-4	Normal Blood Levels of Coagulation Inhibitors in Newborns (30 Weeks' Gestation to Term)			
	30 to 36 Weeks' Gestation		**Full Term**	
Coagulation Inhibitors	**Day 1 Mean (Boundary)**	**Day 5 Mean (Boundary)**	**Day 1 Mean (Boundary)**	**Day 5 Mean (Boundary)**
Antithrombin III (ATIII) (units/ml)	0.38 (0.14 to 0.62)	0.56 (0.3 to 0.82)	0.63 (0.39 to 0.87)	0.67 (0.41 to 0.93)
Alpha$_2$-macroglobulin (α_2-M) (units/ml)	1.1 (0.56 to 1.82)	1.25 (0.71 to 1.77)	1.39 (0.95 to 1.83)	1.48 (0.98 to 1.98)
C1 esterase inhibitor (C1E-NH) (units/ml)	0.65 (0.31 to 0.99)	0.83 (0.45 to 1.21)	0.72 (0.36 to 1.08)	0.90 (0.6 to 1.2)
Alpha$_1$-antitrypsin (α_1-AT) (units/ml)	0.9 (0.36 to 1.44)	0.94 (0.42 to 1.46)	0.93 (0.49 to 1.37)	0.89 (0.49 to 1.29)
Heparin cofactor II (HCII) (units/ml)	0.32 (0.1 to 0.6)	0.34 (0.1 to 0.69)	0.43 (0.1 to 0.93)	0.48 (0.1 to 0.96)
Protein C (units/ml)	0.28 (0.12 to 0.44)	0.31 (0.11 to 0.51)	0.35 (0.17 to 0.53)	0.42 (0.2 to 0.64)
Protein S (units/ml)	0.26 (0.14 to 0.38)	0.37 (0.13 to 0.61)	0.36 (0.12 to 0.6)	0.5 (0.22 to 0.78)

Modified from Andrew M et al (1990). Development of the hemostatic system in the neonate and young infant. American journal of pediatric hematology/oncology 12:98-99; Andrew M et al (1987). Development of the human coagulation system in the full-term infant. Blood 70:167; and Andrew M et al (1988). Development of the human coagulation system in the healthy premature infant. Blood 72:1653.

TABLE 10-5	Normal Blood Levels of Fibrinolytic Components in Premature and Term Newborns			
	Premature Infants		**Full-Term Infants**	
Fibrinolytic Component	**Day 1 Mean (Boundary)**	**Day 5 Mean (Boundary)**	**Day 1 Mean (Boundary)**	**Day 5 Mean (Boundary)**
Plasminogen (units/ml)	1.7 (1.12 to 2.48)	1.91 (1.21 to 2.61)	1.95 (1.25 to 2.65)	2.17 (1.41 to 2.93)
Tissue plasminogen activator (TPA) (ng/ml)	8.48 (3 to 16.7)	3.97 (2 to 6.93)	9.6 (5 to 18.9)	5.6 (4 to 10)
Alpha$_2$-antiplasmin (α_2-AP) (units/ml)	0.78 (0.4 to 1.16)	0.81 (0.49 to 1.13)	0.85 (0.55 to 1.15)	1 (0.7 to 1.3)
Plasminogen activator inhibitor (PAI) (units/ml)	5.4 (0 to 12.2)	2.5 (0 to 7.1)	6.4 (2 to 15.1)	2.3 (0 to 8.1)

Modified from Andrew M et al (1990). Development of the hemostatic system in the neonate and young infant. American journal of pediatric hematology/oncology 12:102-103.

surface of the platelet. These receptors enhance the platelets' ability to bind fibrinogen, which in turn cross-links the platelets, allowing them to aggregate. This provides a tight mesh of clot around an injured vessel that controls bleeding (Figure 10-3). After 32 weeks' gestation, average platelet counts are comparable to those of term infants and adults, but the ability of platelets to aggregate is relatively diminished.

Coagulation

When bleeding cannot be controlled with merely a platelet plug, circulating plasma coagulation factors are triggered to form a network of fibrin that turns the existing plug into a hemostatic seal, which in turn completes hemostasis. Fibrin threads, necessary for clot formation, can develop within 15 to 20 seconds in the presence of normal coagulation factors. Within 3 to 6 minutes after vascular rupture, the entire opening is occluded by clot; within 30 to 60 minutes, the clot begins to retract, pulling the injured vascular portions together and further sealing the vascular end. This coagulation reaction involves several plasma proteins and three distinct phases. The first phase involves the formation of prothrombin activator,

followed by the activation of prothrombin to thrombin (formation of thrombin), and then concludes with the conversion of soluble fibrinogen to fibrin (fibrin clot formation) (Guyton & Hall, 2006b).

Phase I: Formation of Prothrombin Activator. According to the earliest theories on coagulation (cascade theory), prothrombin activator can be generated by two separate pathways, the intrinsic and extrinsic pathways. The intrinsic pathway is triggered by trauma or damage that occurs inside the vessel or to the blood itself and the extrinsic pathway is triggered by the production of tissue thromboplastin that is generated by vessel wall damage. This bimodal pathway can be interrupted or negated by a deficiency in platelets or any of the plasma coagulation factors or by the presence of inhibitors (anticoagulants) in the plasma. Selective activation of one of these pathways depends on the site and severity of injury.

Activation of the intrinsic pathway is slower because it lacks the major stimulus of the extrinsic pathway, tissue thromboplastin generated by vessel wall damage. The intrinsic pathway relies on blood trauma or injury within the vessel to

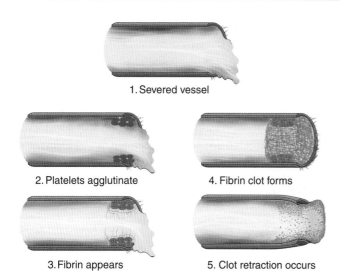

1. Severed vessel

2. Platelets agglutinate

3. Fibrin appears

4. Fibrin clot forms

5. Clot retraction occurs

FIGURE **10-3**
When vessel wall injury occurs, the initial clotting process begins with the formation of a platelet plug. Platelet activation stimulates fibrinogen receptors found on the surface of the platelets, which enhance their aggregation with other platelets and fibrinogen. The fibrin clot that forms retracts and occludes the damaged vascular wall. Redrawn from Guyton AC, Hall JE (2006). Hemostasis and blood coagulation. In Guyton AC, Hall JE, editors. *Textbook of medical physiology*, ed 11. Philadelphia: Saunders. From Seegers Witt (1948). *Hemostatic agents*. Courtesy Charles C Thomas Publishers, Ltd, Springfield, IL.)

alter platelets and plasma proteins and to convert dormant factors (zymogens), naturally found in circulating blood, into active proteolytic enzymes (Figure 10-4). Each activated enzyme subsequently reacts with the succeeding factor, changing it into its activated form. The steps of intrinsic activation of coagulation are as follows:

1. An activator (blood trauma, injury within the vessel, or contact with collagen) activates Factor XII, converting it to Factor XIIa, while simultaneously damaging platelets, which causes a release of platelet phospholipids.
2. Factor XIIa, in conjunction with prekallikrein and high-molar-weight kininogen, activates Factor XI, converting it to Factor XIa.
3. Factor XIa activates Factor IX, converting it to Factor IXa.
4. Factor IXa, platelet phospholipid, and Factor VIII combine to activate Factor X, converting it to Factor Xa.
5. Factor Xa combines with Factor V and platelet phospholipids to form prothrombin activator (prothrombinase), which releases thrombin from prothrombin. Calcium is required for this and the preceding two steps.

The extrinsic pathway can generate thrombin in a matter of seconds when injury occurs outside the vascular space (Figure 10-5). Tissue thromboplastin (tissue factor), composed of glycoproteins and phospholipids, is produced when tissue is injured. When plasma comes in contact with this substance, the initial intrinsic phases are bypassed and the following responses occur:

Intrinsic Pathway

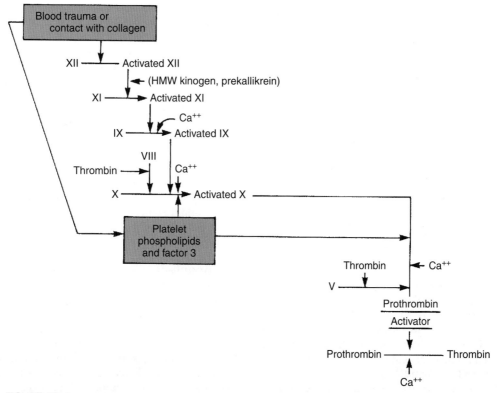

FIGURE **10-4**
The intrinsic pathway for initiating the clotting cascade is activated by trauma to the blood, injury within the vessel, or contact with collagen. *HMW*, High molecular weight. From Guyton AC, Hall JE (2006). Hemostasis and blood coagulation. In Guyton AC, Hall JE, editors. *Textbook of medical physiology*, ed 11. Philadelphia: Saunders.

Extrinsic Pathway

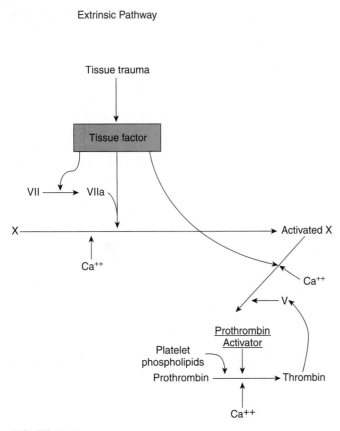

FIGURE **10-5**
The extrinsic pathway for initiating the clotting cascade can generate thrombin rapidly as a result of thromboplastin release from injured tissue. From Guyton AC, Hall JE (2006). Hemostasis and blood coagulation. In Guyton AC, Hall JE, editors. *Textbook of medical physiology*, ed 11. Philadelphia: Saunders.

1. Tissue thromboplastin or tissue factor (Factor III) activates Factor VII to Factor VIIa. These two factors form a complex with glycoprotein in the presence of ionized calcium (tissue factor–Factor VIIa complex) that activates Factor X, converting it to Factor Xa.
2. In the presence of calcium, Factor Xa forms complexes with phospholipids and Factor V to form prothrombin activator.

From this point on, the intrinsic and extrinsic pathways are identical, with both proceeding to phase II.

Phase II: Formation of Thrombin. Prothrombin activator from either of the two pathways continues the clotting cascade by further influencing the breakdown of the unstable plasma protein prothrombin. Prothrombin (Factor II) is synthesized by the liver under the influence of vitamin K, along with the other factors that form the prothrombin complex (Factors VII, IX, and X). When acted on by prothrombin activator, prothrombin forms the potent coagulant thrombin. The newly formed thrombin stimulates completion of the third and final phase of coagulation.

Phase III: Fibrin Clot Formation

Procoagulants. Thrombin promotes the conversion of fibrinogen (Factor I), a protein produced by the liver, into fibrin by splitting off two peptides from the soluble fibrinogen molecule. This exposes two sites, to which other split fibrin molecules can cross-link, forming an insoluble fibrin chain.

Fibrin stabilizing factor (Factor XIII) further strengthens the tight bond of this developing fibrin mesh. Fibrin stabilizing factor is naturally found in the plasma and is also secreted by entrapped platelets. The forming fibrin clot begins to contract and retract with the help of platelets that have actin-myosin action, the same action by which a muscle works. Extension of the clot into the surrounding circulating blood promotes further thrombosis. Thrombin from the clot has the ability to cleave prothrombin into more thrombin and enhances the production of prothrombin activator, thus acting as a potent biofeedback system for perpetuation of the clotting cascade.

Anticoagulants. Throughout the entire coagulation pathway, the action of the activated enzymes is modulated at each stage by multiple and specific inhibitors (anticoagulants). Consequently, coagulation is a process of balance between coagulation factors and naturally occurring inhibitors. Some of these anticoagulants are endothelial surface factors that prevent coagulation until the vessel's endothelial wall is damaged. One such factor is the smoothness of the wall, which prevents any adherence and subsequent activation; another is the monomolecular layer of protein covering the wall, which repels plasma clotting factors and platelets.

Two inhibitors, alpha$_1$-antitrypsin and C1 esterase inhibitor, interfere with the coagulation factors involved in the initial activation of the intrinsic pathway, as does Factor Xa despite its role in cleaving prothrombin into thrombin. Factor Xa rapidly binds with a tissue factor pathway inhibitor (TFPI) found in the plasma. This complex, TFPI–Factor Xa, joins with the tissue factor–Factor VIIa complex to form a quaternary complex that inhibits further activation of Factor X by tissue factor (Edstrom et al, 2000).

Thrombin also acts as its own inhibitor by stimulating activation of protein C, which inactivates Factors V and VIII in the presence of another vitamin K–dependent inhibitor, protein S. A deficiency of these two proteins has been implicated in cases of neonatal thrombosis.

Other inhibitors of thrombin formation are (1) fibrin threads created during clot formation, which absorb thrombin, thus removing it from circulation and eliminating its potential for further coagulation; (2) thrombomodulin, found on the endothelial surfaces of the body and in the plasma complexes with thrombin, which eliminates thrombin's ability to cleave fibrinogen; (3) alpha$_2$-macroglobulin, which inhibits proteases, including thrombin; (4) antithrombin III, which combines with thrombin, blocking the conversion of fibrinogen into fibrin; and (5) heparin cofactor II, which removes several activated procoagulants. Both antithrombin III and heparin are produced in the precapillary connective tissue of the lungs and liver.

Fibrinolysis. Once a clot develops, it can be invaded by fibroblasts that lay down connective tissue throughout the clot or it can be dissolved. The process of dissolution occurs by activation of naturally occurring factors that lyse the clot. Fibrinolysis is activated simultaneously with stimulation of the coagulation system, with powerful but inactivated anticoagulants built right into the clot (Figure 10-6). One of these anticoagulants, plasminogen, is manufactured by the liver, kidneys, and eosinophils. Under the influence of thrombin, activated Factor XII, tissue plasminogen activator (t-PA; located on the vascular endothelium) and urokinase plasminogen activator (u-PA; found in the urine), plasminogen is converted into plasmin, a proteolytic enzyme that

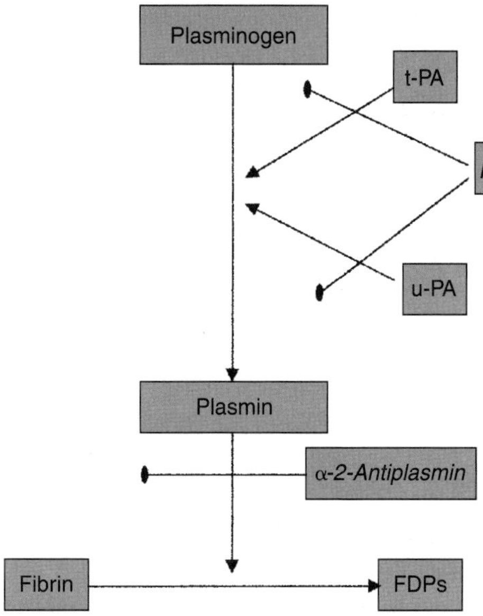

FIGURE **10-6**
The components of the fibrinolytic system involved in the lysis of a fibrin clot. *t-PA*, Tissue plasminogen activator; *PAI-1*, plasminogen activator inhibitor; *u-PA*, urokinase plasminogen activator; *FDPs*, fibrin degradation products. Modified from Edstrom C et al (2000). Developmental aspects of blood hemostasis and disorders of coagulation and fibrinolysis in the neonatal period. In Christensen R, editor. *Hematologic problems of the neonate*. Philadelphia: Saunders.

breaks down fibrin into fibrin split products. Plasmin not only digests the fibrin chains but also deactivates fibrinogen; Factors V, VII, and XII; and prothrombin. Plasmin can be inactivated by its inhibitor, alpha2-antiplasmin; tissue plasminogen activator can be inactivated by its inhibitor, plasminogen activator inhibitor-1.

In summary, both term and preterm newborns have the ability to create a balance between transitory deficiencies in the amount and function of a variety of clotting factors, platelets, and anticoagulant factors. The homeostasis between clotting factors and anticoagulants places the newborn in a mildly hypercoagulable state at birth. Compared with older children and adults, therefore, the newborn has no greater tendency to bleed but does have several differences in regard to coagulation components and reserves, including (1) gestational age-dependent variations in the concentrations of coagulation factors, anticoagulants, and fibrinolytics; (2) a faster turnover rate of components; (3) a slower rate of synthesis of components; and (4) limited ability to supply necessary components during times of increased need.

ASSESSMENT OF HEMATOLOGIC FUNCTION

Because infants respond to a variety of problems in a similar manner, many clinical findings (e.g., hypoglycemia, hypocalcemia, hypothermia, apnea, bradycardia, cyanosis, lethargy, poor feeding) warrant at least a complete blood count (CBC) to determine if a hematologic reason exists for these symptoms. With active bleeding, platelet counts, clotting studies, fibrinogen levels, and measurements of products of fibrinolysis (e.g., d-dimer, fibrin split products, or fibrin degradation products) can shed light on the type of blood dyscrasia present

BOX **10-1**
Physical Findings Helpful in Evaluating the Integrity of the Hematologic System
Obvious blood loss—hemorrhage Pallor Plethora Petechiae Ecchymosis Jaundice Hepatosplenomegaly Hematomas

and can direct the caregiver to the appropriate therapeutic response. These studies also provide a way to monitor and evaluate treatments. However, laboratory data are most helpful when they are used in conjunction with astute observation and physical assessment skills.

Several physical findings can help determine the well-being and homeostasis of the hematologic system (Box 10-1). Cutaneous abnormalities such as hematomas, abrasions, petechiae, and bleeding should alert the nurse to the possibility of a hematologic abnormality. Hepatosplenomegaly also can indicate abnormal breakdown of RBCs. Hepatosplenomegaly concurrent with hyperbilirubinemia and hemolysis can signal alloimmune problems (e.g., Rh and ABO incompatibilities) or acquired, congenital, or postnatal infection (e.g., cytomegalovirus infection, toxoplasmosis, herpes simplex infection, or hepatitis).

COMMON HEMATOLOGIC DISORDERS
Blood Group Incompatibilities

Blood group incompatibilities were first recognized in the 1940s with the discovery of the Rh grouping and the first test for detection of antibody-coated RBCs, devised by Coombs in 1946. Before the introduction of Rh immune globulin (RhIgG, RhIG, or RhoGAM) in 1964 and its release for general use in 1968, Rh incompatibility accounted for one third of all blood group incompatibilities. With the use of RhIgG, the frequency of Rh incompatibility has dropped significantly, and ABO has become the main blood group incompatibility, with sensitization occurring in 3% of all infants. Both incompatibilities involve maternal antibody response to fetal antigen, leading to RBC destruction by hemolysis. Rh antibody response is elicited on exposure to antigen and does not exist spontaneously, whereas anti-A and anti-B antibodies occur naturally. These entities also differ in the severity of the effect on the fetus and newborn and in the method of treatment.

Other minor blood groupings (e.g., Kell, C, E, Duffy, and Kidd) may also be involved in incompatibilities that result in hyperbilirubinemia, but Rh and ABO incompatibilities are the most common, accounting for 98% of all cases. There are 400 known RBC antigens that can induce antibody production. Some of these antibodies are induced after transfusion therapy with incompatible blood; others occur in response to the transfer of incompatible fetal blood cells into the maternal circulation during pregnancy. The Rh system alone has 40 discrete antigens, but only five (C, D, E, c, and e) are important.

ABO Incompatibility

Antigens or agglutinogens present on the RBC surface of each blood type, react with antibodies or agglutinins found in the plasma of opposing blood types. Of the 30 common antigens involved in antigen-antibody reactions, the ABO antigens are one of two groups most likely to be a problem, the other being the Rh group (Guyton & Hall, 2006a). As discussed earlier in this chapter, the four major blood types are A, B, O, and AB, with the antibodies to the antigens of different blood types occurring naturally in the plasma (Table 10-6).

With antigen and antibody in harmony, no RBC destruction occurs, but when a conflicting antibody is introduced into the circulation, RBC destruction may occur. RBCs have multiple binding sites to which opposing antibodies can attach. An antibody is capable of simultaneously attaching to several RBCs, thus creating a clump of cells. This clumping of cells, known as agglutination, can cause occlusion of small vessels and impair local circulation and tissue oxygenation. Fetal RBCs coated with antibodies attract phagocytes and macrophages that eventually destroy these agglutinated RBCs, usually through hemolysis by the reticuloendothelial cells in the spleen. Hemolysis can occur without preliminary agglutination, but it is a more delayed process because the body must first activate its complement system. High antibody titers (hemolysins) are required to stimulate this system, which causes the release of proteolytic enzymes that rupture the cell membrane.

In a transfusion reaction, when opposing blood types are mixed, the donor's RBCs are agglutinated, and the recipient's blood cells tend to be protected. The plasma portion of donor blood that contains antibodies becomes diluted by the recipient's blood volume, thus reducing donor antibody titers in the recipient's circulation. However, recipient antibody titers are adequate to destroy the donor RBCs by agglutination and hemolysis or by hemolysis alone. This is the situation in ABO incompatibility. In such cases, the maternal blood type usually is O, containing anti-A and anti-B antibodies in the serum, whereas the fetus or newborn is type A or B. Although incompatibility can occur between A and B types, it is not seen as frequently as AO or BO because of the globulin composition of the antibodies. In the O-type mother, the antibodies are usually IgG and can cross the placenta, whereas the antibodies of the type A or B mother frequently are IgM, which are too large to cross the placenta.

When transplacental hemorrhage (TPH) occurs between an ABO-incompatible mother and fetus, fetal blood entering the maternal circulation undergoes agglutination and hemolysis by maternal antibodies. This rapid response prevents the development of antibodies to other antigens present on fetal RBCs, because a time lapse is required for activation of the immune system. Consequently, fetal RBCs that are Rh positive in addition to being type A or type B are destroyed by naturally occurring anti-A or anti-B antibodies before any maternal antibodies to Rh factor (anti-D) can be produced.

TABLE 10-6	Comparison of Features Seen in Rh and ABO Incompatibility	
	Rh Incompatibility	**ABO Incompatibility**
BLOOD GROUP SETUP		
Mother	Negative	O
Infant	Positive	A or B
TYPE OF ANTIBODY	Incomplete (IgG)	Immune (IgG)
CLINICAL ASPECTS		
Occurrence in firstborn	5%	40% to 50%
Predictable severity in subsequent pregnancies	Usually	No
Stillbirth or hydrops	Frequent	Rare
Severe anemia	Frequent	Rare
Degree of jaundice	+ + +	+
Hepatosplenomegaly	+ + +	+
LABORATORY FINDINGS		
Direct Coombs' test (infant)	+	(+) or 0
Maternal antibodies	Always present	Not clear-cut
Spherocytes	0	+
TREATMENT		
Need for antenatal measures	Yes	No
Value of phototherapy	Limited	Considerable
Exchange transfusion		
Frequency	Approximately 67% of cases	Approximately 10% of cases
Donor blood type	Rh negative	Rh same as infant
	Group-specific when possible	Group O only
Incidence of late anemia	Common	Rare

From Ohls R (2001). Anemia in the newborn. In Polin R et al, editors. Workbook in practical neonatology, ed 3. Philadelphia: Saunders; modified from Naiman J (1982). Erythroblastosis fetalis. In Oski F, Naiman J, editors. Hematologic problems in the newborn, ed 3. Philadelphia: Saunders.

This naturally occurring phenomenon is the basis for the use of RhIgG, in which extrinsic anti-D destroys fetal cells before the maternal immune system can be activated to produce antibodies.

Despite this destruction of fetal RBCs, maternal anti-A or anti-B antibodies of the IgG form can freely cross the placenta and adhere to RBCs in the fetal circulation. For this reason, ABO incompatibility can occur in the first pregnancy (40% to 50% of total occurrences involve primigravidas) because TPH and inoculation of the mother with fetal blood are not necessary for the development of these naturally occurring antibodies. Since the A and B antigens on the fetal and neonatal RBCs are not well developed, only a small amount of maternal antibody actually attaches to the antigen. Other body tissues also have antigen sites to which some of the circulating antibodies can adhere, thereby decreasing the potential for RBC destruction. The resulting small amounts of IgG in the plasma do not stimulate activation of the complement system, therefore hemolysis is minimal. This lack of stimulation of the complement system and the above factors may explain why only 3% to 20% of infants of the 15% to 22% who are ABO incompatible with their mothers become symptomatic (Ozolek et al, 1994).

Erythrocyte antibodies are not usually present in the circulating blood until 2 to 8 months of postnatal age, which prevents maternal inoculation with fetal anti-A or anti-B antibodies. Antibody production then increases, reaching a maximum titer at 8 to 10 years of age (Guyton & Hall, 2006a). The newborn becomes inoculated with A and B antigens after birth through ingestion of food and the resulting bacterial colonization. This initiates production of anti-A or anti-B antibodies that circulate in the plasma, depending on the antigens present on the RBCs.

Clinical Manifestations. The chief symptom of ABO incompatibility is jaundice within the first 24 hours of life; 90% of all affected infants are female. Hemolysis and anemia are minimal, although signs of a mildly compensated hemolytic state are reflected in certain CBC values. The peripheral blood smear may show evidence of spherocytes, or RBCs lacking the normal central pallor and biconcave, disklike shape of the normal RBC. Because they are smaller than normal RBCs, spherocytes appear thicker. These physical characteristics result in abnormal fragility under osmotic stress. Spherocytes are not distensible or compressible because they lack the normal amount of loose cell membrane, making them more susceptible to destruction in the splenic sinusoids.

Additional laboratory findings include a positive direct Coombs' test result in 3% to 32% of cases (Ozolek et al, 1994) and positive results on both direct and indirect Coombs' tests in 80% of cases when micro techniques are used. The direct Coombs' test is a measurement of the presence of antibody on the RBC surface; the indirect Coombs' test is a measurement of antibody in the serum. ABO incompatibility can also be identified by the performance of an eluate test, which involves washing the RBCs of the newborn and testing the wash for anti-A or anti-B antibodies.

On physical examination, hepatosplenomegaly can be observed, a reflection of extramedullary erythropoiesis generated by the fetus in response to significant hemolysis. In an effort to compensate for increased cell destruction, the liver and spleen manufacture RBCs for a longer period than usually is seen in the fetus and newborn. Engorgement of the splenic sinusoids by hemolyzed RBCs contributes to splenomegaly.

Treatment. Since the antibodies involved in ABO incompatibility occur naturally, elimination of this type of incompatibility is virtually impossible. However, its effects on the fetus and newborn are much less dramatic and life-threatening than those of Rh incompatibility; therefore amniocentesis and monitoring of amniotic fluid bilirubin levels, intrauterine transfusions, and early delivery usually are not necessary. Nevertheless, problems associated with postnatal bilirubin clearance do arise, and phototherapy and possible exchange transfusion become part of the repertoire of care. These two treatment methods are discussed in further detail later in the chapter.

Rh Incompatibility

Incompatibilities involving the Rh system are the second most common alloimmune problem, but the severity of complications far surpasses that of ABO incompatibility. Antibodies never occur naturally in the Rh system; exposure to the antigen is necessary to produce antibodies. Such exposure is thought to occur through maternal inoculation with fetal RBCs by transplacental hemorrhage or through undetectable hemorrhage during labor, abortion, ectopic pregnancy, or amniocentesis.

Spontaneous TPH occurs in 50% to 75% of all pregnancies, with the greatest and most severe occurrence at the time of delivery. Fetal RBCs can be found in 6.7% of all pregnancies during the first trimester, 15% in the second trimester, and 28.9% in the third trimester (Porter et al, 2003). Spontaneous TPH allows fetal RBCs to pass into the maternal circulation, where antibodies develop in response to any foreign RBC antigen the mother does not possess. The risk of immunization depends on the ABO status of both mother and fetus and the size of the hemorrhage. On the basis of blood type, the risk for maternal Rh immunization in an ABO-compatible Rh-negative mother and Rh-positive fetus is 16%, whereas an ABO-incompatible pregnancy with an Rh-negative mother and Rh-positive fetus runs a 1.5% to 2% risk with each pregnancy. On the basis of the volume of TPH, if the hemorrhage is less than 0.1 ml RBCs, the overall risk for immunization is 3%; if the hemorrhage is greater than 5 ml, the risk increases to 50% to 65%.

The maternal Rh antibody is slow to develop and initially may consist exclusively of IgM, which cannot cross the placenta because of its molecular size. This is followed by the production of IgG, which can cross the placenta into the fetal circulation. The maximum concentration of the IgG form of antibody occurs within 2 to 4 months after termination of the first sensitizing pregnancy (Guyton & Hall, 2006a). If initial immunization occurs shortly before or at the time of delivery, the first Rh-positive infant born to such a mother may trigger the initial antibody response, but the infant will not be affected. However, subsequent exposure to RBCs of Rh-positive fetuses produces a rapid antibody response that consists mostly of IgG. This response results in antibody attachment to antigen sites on the fetal RBCs of these fetuses. The antibody coating of the RBCs forms the basis for a positive result on the direct Coombs' test. The affected RBCs undergo agglutination, phagocytosis, and eventually extravascular hemolysis in the spleen. The byproducts of hemolysis, especially bilirubin, pass through the placenta into the maternal circulation to be metabolized and conjugated by the maternal liver. The rate of destruction of fetal RBCs depends on the amount of anti-D antibodies on the cells, the effectiveness of anti-D antibodies in promoting phagocytosis, and the capability of the spleen's reticuloendothelial system to remove antibody-coated cells.

Erythroblastosis Fetalis

Hemolysis in the fetus caused by Rh incompatibility results in the disease known as erythroblastosis fetalis (EBF); the major consequences are anemia and hyperbilirubinemia. The name is derived from the presence of immature circulating RBCs (erythroblasts), which are forced into the circulation of affected fetuses to compensate for rapid destruction of fetal blood cells. The severity of the disease depends on the degree of hemolysis and the ability of the fetus's erythropoietic system to counteract the ensuing anemia. In an attempt to compensate for rapid destruction, the fetus continues to use extramedullary organs, such as the liver and spleen, which normally would have ceased RBC production after the seventh month of gestation.

Clinical Manifestations. The clinical manifestations of EBF are similar to those of ABO incompatibility but often are more intense (see Table 10-3). Jaundice results from an exaggerated rise in bilirubin, with the premature infant exhibiting an earlier rise and a more prolonged period of elevation. Hepatosplenomegaly may be found on physical examination, along with varying degrees of hydrops. Hydrops fetalis is a severe, total body edema often accompanied by ascites and pleural effusions. Although the pathogenesis is unclear, it is thought to be the result of congestive heart failure and intrauterine hypoxia from severe anemia, portal and umbilical venous hypertension caused by hepatic hematopoiesis, and low plasma colloid osmotic pressure induced by hypoalbuminemia. Low serum albumin levels are a consequence of altered hepatic synthesis, which may be due to local cellular necrosis and compromised intrahepatic circulation. All these factors can lead to portal and venous hypertension and edema. The severity of the anemia and hypoalbuminemia affects the degree of extravasation of fluid into the tissue.

Altered hepatic synthesis can impair production of vitamin K and vitamin K–dependent clotting factors, which can lead to hemorrhage in these infants. Petechiae and prolonged bleeding from cord and blood sampling sites may be initial signs of clotting abnormalities. Hypoglycemia that occurs secondary to hyperplasia of the pancreatic islet cells also is associated with EBF. Products of RBC hemolysis are thought to inactivate circulating insulin, promoting increased insulin release and subsequent pancreatic beta cell hyperplasia. Another theory suggests that potassium or amino acids released from hemolyzed cells may directly stimulate insulin production or indirectly produce this effect by increasing glucagon secretion. Approximately one third of surviving erythroblastotic infants have low blood glucose levels and elevated plasma insulin levels.

Antenatal Therapy. Adequate antenatal care is important in safeguarding the fetus that may be affected by EBF. Proper screening of any pregnant woman at her first prenatal visit is essential and should include blood type and Rh factor. If the mother is Rh negative, the father's blood type should also be ascertained. If the father is Rh positive, it is essential to determine Rh immunization of the mother by Coombs' testing, specifically the indirect Coombs' test. In addition to blood typing, a concise obstetrical history regarding any previous spontaneous or therapeutic abortions or delivery of an affected infant is important to ensure appropriate management of the current pregnancy. Women who are sensitized require more surveillance throughout the pregnancy than their unsensitized counterparts, and women who have previously given birth to affected infants require the greatest degree of care.

The unsensitized Rh-negative mothers can benefit from antenatal and postpartum administration of RhIgG. The Kleihauer-Betke test for fetal cells in the maternal circulation and the erythrocyte rosetting test that detects Rh-positive fetal cells may be useful screens for determining maternal candidates for RhIgG. Before the inception of RhIgG in 1964, when the first clinical trials were conducted, the frequency of Rh immunization was 7% to 8% in ABO-compatible pregnancies and 1% in ABO-incompatible pregnancies, with close to 50% of all perinatal deaths attributable to EBF. With the use of RhIgG after delivery, the incidence of Rh immunization was dramatically reduced to 1% to 1.8%. Because sensitization was known to occur without evidence of TPH at the time of delivery, the question was raised whether antenatal sensitization occurred in response to frequent, small, and undetectable hemorrhage before or during labor. For this reason, antenatal administration of RhIgG was initiated to eliminate such cases of alloimmunization. Antenatal administration has further reduced the incidence to as low as 0.1%. However, there will always be pregnancies in which RhIgG fails to suppress the formation of antibodies or in which administration is not feasible. Immunization is not effective if sensitization occurs before the initial antenatal screening or if the RhIgG dosage is inadequate to neutralize a massive TPH. For these reasons, it is estimated that the incidence cannot be reduced beyond 4 in 10,000 pregnancies even with the use of RhIgG.

RhIgG is assumed to adhere to any Rh-positive fetal RBCs that have invaded the maternal circulation. Agglutination, hemolysis, and removal of these foreign RBCs occur before the maternal immune system can recognize the invasion and develop antibodies that would transplacentally cross into the fetus.

Several obstetrical conditions, which may require RhIgG prophylaxis, because they can increase the risk of sensitization by increasing the chances of TPH are:
- Therapeutic or spontaneous abortion of any type; the incidence of TPH is higher with therapeutic abortion (three women in 30 may be sensitized)
- Amniocentesis, which has a 10% chance of causing TPH
- Ectopic pregnancies or hydatidiform moles
- Abdominal trauma
- Antepartum bleeding, as with placental abruption or placenta previa

Failure to administer RhIgG after such occurrences may leave these women at risk for sensitization. The American College of Obstetricians and Gynecologists recommends a dose of 50 mcg for high-risk situations that arise before 13 weeks' gestation and 300 mcg after 13 weeks' gestation, with the 300-mcg dose repeated at 28 weeks' gestation.

RhIgG has a half-life of 25 to 27 days and is effective for approximately 2 weeks after antigen exposure. The timing of the dose after delivery is important; administration within 72 hours of delivery is recommended. The dose after delivery allows a maximum estimated fetal transfusion of 30 ml of whole blood or 15 ml of packed RBCs, which leaves 1% of postpartum mothers without full coverage. If massive TPH is suspected, the dose of RhIgG may need to be increased to provide adequate amounts of anti-D antibodies. After administration of RhIgG, the Kleihauer-Betke test can be performed on the mother's blood to check for RBCs with fetal hemoglobin and to help determine the need for additional RhIgG.

By reducing the incidence of EBF, use of RhIgG has also reduced the number of available immunized donors that supply the polyclonal anti-D antibodies. The recent development of prophylaxis in the form of monoclonal antibodies against Rh D antigen has reached the stage of clinical trials and may afford an alternate source of RhIgG.

Other methods of monitoring the status and treating the fetus with EBF include ultrasonography, flow Doppler studies, amniocentesis, cordocentesis, intrauterine transfusions, and pharmacologic agent administration.

Treatment. On delivery of an infant with EBF, assessment of the newborn's cardiorespiratory status is of utmost importance. Because of ascites, pleural effusions, and circulatory collapse, these infants often require stabilization of the airway by intubation and mechanical ventilation. If peritoneal or pleural fluid prevents adequate chest excursion, paracentesis may be required to remove fluid from the abdominal cavity, or thoracentesis (chest tube insertion) may be needed to drain excess pleural fluid.

Delivery of an infant shortly after intraperitoneal transfusion may not allow adequate time for absorption of blood from the peritoneal cavity. The unabsorbed portion could lead to diminished lung expansion, resulting in respiratory failure or restricted mechanical ventilation. Such infants may require paracentesis for removal of blood from the peritoneal cavity.

After initiation of respiratory support, the infant should be assessed for adequacy of circulating blood volume. If the infant is severely hydropic, the inevitable anemia must be corrected with transfusions of packed RBCs, since an exchange transfusion may not be tolerated until the intravascular RBC volume is replenished. Transfusion is accomplished with O-negative or type-specific Rh-negative blood cross-matched against maternal blood. Initial use of a single-volume or partial exchange may offer a degree of cardiovascular stability before a double-volume exchange is attempted. Congestive heart failure, not present at the time of intravascular volume depletion, may become apparent as the infant is transfused. At times a severely affected infant may benefit from digitalization and diuretic therapy.

Prenatal damage to the liver can adversely affect the production of coagulation factors in such infants, making them prone to bleeding disorders. Hepatic damage can intensify any hyperbilirubinemia present, because the hepatic substances required for conjugation may also be impaired. Laboratory evaluation of the infant affected by EBF should consist of liver function studies, hematocrit determinations, and evaluation of coagulation status.

Nursing care of the infant affected by EBF involves scrupulous attention to the infant's cardiorespiratory status and vital signs. The infant needs to be positioned so as to reduce abdominal pressure on the diaphragm which will permit better chest expansion. Maintaining a normal PO_2 and avoiding overventilation may prevent barotrauma to lungs already compromised by pleural effusions. The lungs may be hypoplastic if

their growth has been sufficiently compromised by hydrops in utero, making ventilation difficult and predisposing the infant to extraventilatory air. Vital signs usually are assessed every hour until the infant's condition has stabilized. Hematocrit and bilirubin levels should be checked frequently during the first few hours and days of life to maintain adequate circulating blood volumes and to prevent toxic levels of bilirubin by timely initiation of therapy. If the cord bilirubin levels are significantly elevated, exchange transfusion may be necessary shortly after birth.

If bilirubin levels do not require immediate exchange, blood levels should be checked every 4 to 8 hours, depending on the initial cord blood levels and subsequent rate of rise. In Rh incompatibility, exchange is imminent if the rate of rise exceeds 1 mg/hr for the first 6 hours of life. The interval of blood sampling for bilirubin may be increased to 6 to 12 hours after the first 48 hours of life.

The major therapies used to control excessive unconjugated bilirubin levels are similar for all problems resulting in elevated unconjugated bilirubin levels. Phototherapy and exchange transfusion, the most frequently used therapies, are discussed later in the chapter.

Analysis of Laboratory Data. The following laboratory data can be helpful in the diagnosis and treatment of EBF:

- The mother's and infant's blood and Rh types.
- Coombs' reactivity: The infant's RBCs are coated with anti-D antibodies, resulting in a positive direct Coombs' test result; on occasion, the heavy coating of neonatal RBCs with antibody can lead to a false Rh typing (Rh negative); if the direct Coombs' test result is positive, the infant should be considered Rh positive.
- The infant's hematocrit, reticulocyte count, and RBC morphologic characteristics: The presence of immature cells or spherocytes helps distinguish Rh incompatibility from ABO incompatibility.
- Plasma bilirubin levels: The initial cord-blood bilirubin level and the rate of rise determine the appropriate timing of any exchange transfusion needed to control bilirubin levels. Cord bilirubin levels are closely associated with the severity of disease and the mortality rate.

Bilirubin Metabolism and Hyperbilirubinemia

Bilirubin production begins as early as 12 weeks' gestation. It is the primary degradation product of hemoglobin, although 20% to 30% is derived from nonerythroid sources such as tissue heme. Bilirubin is produced after completion of the natural life span of the RBC, but ineffective erythropoiesis or premature destruction of blood cells can increase its production. In RBC destruction, the aging or hemolyzed RBC membrane ruptures, releasing hemoglobin that is phagocytosed by macrophages. The hemoglobin molecule then splits into a heme portion and a globin portion. Bilirubin is derived from the degradation of the heme ring in the heme portion that binds to heme oxygenase. The ferric heme breaks down to the ferrous form and then is cleaved to form carbon monoxide and biliverdin. Biliverdin is further reduced to form bilirubin, and carbon monoxide joins with heme to form carboxyhemoglobin.

The four forms of circulating bilirubin are (1) conjugated bilirubin (which is excretable through the kidneys and intestines), (2) conjugated covalently bound bilirubin (which is attached to serum albumin and not found in neonates younger than 2 weeks of age), (3) unconjugated bilirubin (which is reversibly bound to albumin), and (4) free bilirubin (which is unconjugated and unbound). Measurement of conjugated (direct) bilirubin identifies the amount of bilirubin that reacts directly with van den Bergh's reagent. The portion of bilirubin reversibly bound to albumin is lipid soluble. It does not react with van den Bergh's reagent until it is combined with alcohol, hence the term unconjugated (indirect) bilirubin. Free bilirubin is not attached to albumin and can easily cross the blood-brain barrier, causing the damage seen in kernicterus. Measurements of conjugated and unconjugated bilirubin are important in the evaluation of the hyperbilirubinemic infant and provide valuable information for the diagnosis and method of treatment.

Although bilirubin is found in stool and amniotic fluid, the major route of elimination in the fetus is through the placenta. For this reason, bilirubin must be retained in the form that allows its passage into the maternal circulation. Consequently, the enzyme systems found in the fetus enhance the retention of bilirubin in the unconjugated form. Persistence of some of these fetal mechanisms during the newborn period can contribute to jaundice. Plasma concentrations of bilirubin usually are low in the fetus, except in cases of severe hemolytic disease. All bilirubin in the cord blood of the fetus is the unconjugated variety, which is effectively metabolized, conjugated, and excreted by the maternal liver and gallbladder. The mean cord blood bilirubin concentration in an infant unaffected by hemolytic disease is 1.8 mg/dl, regardless of the infant's gestational age or weight.

In the newborn, the major routes of bilirubin excretion are through the intestine and the kidneys. As the production of bilirubin exceeds the newborn liver's capacity to conjugate and eliminate it, plasma levels begin to rise rapidly. Jaundice becomes noticeable when the serum concentration reaches three times the amount normally present in the serum. The conjunctivae become visibly jaundiced at serum levels exceeding 2.5 mg/dl. In the full-term infant, jaundice usually becomes apparent within 2 to 4 days after birth and lasts until the sixth day, reaching a peak concentration of 6 to 7 mg/dl. Although infants born at 37 weeks' gestation or later are considered term, they are more likely to reach or exceed serum bilirubin levels of 13 mg/dl or higher than are infants born at 40 weeks' gestation. The preterm infant has cord-blood bilirubin levels similar to those of the term infant, but peak levels are higher, jaundice lasts longer, and levels peak later, at 5 to 7 days. Among preterm infants, 63% reach levels of 10 to 19 mg/dl, and 22% reach levels above 15 mg/dl.

Although the neonatal liver's conjugating mechanisms are reduced during the first few days of life, the liver is able to metabolize and excrete two thirds to three quarters of the bilirubin circulating throughout the body. Initially bilirubin is transported in the plasma, bound to albumin at two sites—a primary binding site that has a strong bond and a secondary site that has a weak bond. When available albumin binding sites are saturated, bilirubin circulates freely in the plasma. It is this portion of unconjugated bilirubin that can migrate into brain cells, causing damage known as kernicterus. The occurrence of kernicterus is related to the amount of diffusible, loosely bound bilirubin and the availability of albumin binding sites.

When bilirubin reaches the liver, it is transferred from plasma albumin, across the cell membrane of the liver, and into the liver cell. Two proteins, Y and Z, also called ligands, affect bilirubin transfer from plasma to liver. Here the bilirubin is either stored in the cell cytoplasm or removed from the ligands and conjugated in the hepatic endoplasmic reticulum. Conjugation is essential for the excretion of bilirubin into bile. Eighty percent of bilirubin is conjugated with glucuronic acid, becoming bilirubin glucuronide. Glucuronosyltransferase is the important hepatic enzyme required for the production of bilirubin glucuronide. Ninety-five percent of bilirubin glucuronide is excreted into bile and subsequently into the intestine.

Effective excretion of bilirubin from the intestine depends on the length of time needed for the passage of stool and on the presence of substances that break down conjugated bilirubin. The newborn may have diminished bowel motility and delayed meconium passage, which allow longer exposure of stool to bilirubin glucuronidase, the enzyme responsible for breaking down conjugated bilirubin. The action of this enzyme, in conjunction with the newborn's lack of the intestinal flora required to reduce bilirubin to urobilinogen, converts the conjugated form to the unconjugated form, which is then reabsorbed by the intestine.

Kernicterus

Kernicterus was rarely seen between the 1960s and the 1990s, but its incidence has risen since the mid-1990s with the advent of earlier home discharges. Kernicterus occurs when the albumin binding sites are filled which allows for increased amounts of free bilirubin to pass into the central nervous system (CNS). Free bilirubin easily crosses the blood-brain barrier and is transferred into the brain cells, causing obvious yellow staining of the brain tissue (kernicterus) that is similar to the effect on the skin. The areas of the brain usually affected by the staining are the hypothalamus, dentate nucleus, and cerebellum. Kernicterus is associated with varying degrees of neurologic damage, but a direct correlation cannot be drawn between serum bilirubin levels and the severity of involvement.

Many factors can influence the bilirubin binding capacity and increase the risk of kernicterus at lower bilirubin levels, including the following:

- *The total amount of available serum albumin:* Premature infants normally experience a relative hypoproteinemia and have fewer albumin binding sites available for free bilirubin.
- *The presence of other substances competing for available binding sites:* Certain drugs (e.g., sulfisoxazole, salicylates, sodium benzoate) compete with bilirubin for binding sites or replace bilirubin loosely attached to binding sites.
- *Acidosis and hypoxia:* Increased production of hydrogen ions and implementation of anaerobic metabolism can impede bilirubin binding. Albumin's ability to bind bilirubin drops to half its potential at a serum pH of 7.1, with free fatty acids produced during anaerobic metabolism competing for albumin binding sites. The simultaneous presence of acidosis and hypoxia, which can open the blood-brain barrier, can expose a sick infant to kernicterus at much lower serum bilirubin levels. Evidence also suggests that tests evaluating bilirubin binding capacity, rather than serum bilirubin concentrations, are better correlated with the appearance of subsequent CNS abnormalities.

Clinical Manifestations. Kernicterus usually becomes evident during the first 5 days of life. Its signs include lethargy or irritability, hypotonia, paralysis of upward gaze, high-pitched cry, poor eating, opisthotonic posturing, and spasticity. It is also associated with deafness, cerebral palsy, and tooth enamel abnormalities. The overall risk for kernicterus is 50% if serum bilirubin levels are 30 mg/dl or higher and 10% if levels are between 20 and 25 mg/dl. Preventing elevated levels of free bilirubin is the primary means of eliminating kernicterus. Prevention may require phototherapy for slowly rising levels but almost certainly demands exchange transfusion if the rise is rapid and marked.

Nonimmune Causes of Hyperbilirubinemia

Elevated bilirubin levels within the first 24 hours of life or levels exceeding 12 mg/dl are not considered physiologic and deserve investigation. Many conditions other than blood group incompatibilities can cause jaundice in the newborn. Most of the commonly seen disorders result in elevated levels of unconjugated rather than conjugated bilirubin. These pathologic conditions can be classified as (1) those that cause increased breakdown of RBCs (e.g., sepsis, drug reactions, and extravascular blood); (2) those that interfere with bilirubin conjugation (e.g., breast milk jaundice, drug interactions, hypothyroidism, acidosis, and hypoxia); and (3) those that cause abnormal bilirubin excretion (e.g., hypoxia or asphyxia, bowel obstruction, ileus, and congestive heart failure). The single factor most implicated in hyperbilirubinemia is prematurity, with the severity of jaundice directly correlated to declining gestational age. The premature infant is thought to be subject to a combination of increased RBC breakdown secondary to reduced RBC life span and impaired bilirubin conjugation as a result of liver immaturity.

Increased Red Blood Cell Breakdown

Several problems that arise in the perinatal period are associated with excessive and premature destruction of the RBCs by hemolysis. Neonatal bacterial and viral infections and intrauterine viral infections, especially those of the TORCH complex (toxoplasmosis, other agents, rubella, cytomegalovirus, and herpes simplex), have been implicated in the hemolytic destruction of RBCs. Certain medications, such as the synthetic analogues of vitamin K or large doses of natural vitamin K, also induce RBC destruction. Other conditions prevalent in the premature and term newborn can result in the extravasation of large amounts of blood (e.g., cephalhematoma and pulmonary or intracerebral hemorrhages). These extravascular collections of blood cells must undergo hemolysis to be reabsorbed by the body. Significant hemolysis, regardless of the cause, increases the bilirubin load on a metabolically immature neonatal liver. This increased load often results in hyperbilirubinemia in the newborn.

Interference with Bilirubin Conjugation

Breast Milk Jaundice. Breast milk jaundice affects approximately 2% to 4% of all breastfed babies and can be divided into two phases, early and late, each with a different time of onset and a different underlying cause. In early-onset breast milk jaundice, the infant is affected within the first few days of life. This condition is thought to be due to a combination of maternal and infant factors that lead to diminished fluid intake and dehydration. Predisposing maternal factors include limited maternal milk supply, engorgement, cracked nipples, poor feeding technique, and maternal illness or fatigue. Neonatal factors include poor suck, illness, lethargy that accompanies hyperbilirubinemia, and dehydration. Poor intake leads to poor stool output and increased enterohepatic resorption of bilirubin. The recommended treatment is phototherapy and alleviation of dehydration. Frequent breast feedings with avoidance of supplementation, in addition to lactation counseling, are advised.

Late-onset breast milk jaundice is a separate entity that is attributed to a change in the chemical or physical composition of breast milk; it usually occurs after the first 3 to 5 days of life (Wong et al, 2006). Bilirubin levels can reach 12 to 20 mg/dl between 8 and 15 days and may remain elevated for as long as 2 months. The infant appears healthy, and no evidence of RBC hemolysis is seen. This jaundice is believed to be caused by substances in breast milk that interfere with bilirubin conjugation or increase enterohepatic circulation, resulting in resorption of bilirubin from the intestine. Two substances found in breast milk, pregnanediol and nonesterified fatty acids, are thought to inhibit glucuronyl transferase, the enzyme necessary for bilirubin conjugation in the liver. However, the role of these two substances in the interference with glucuronyl transferase remains questionable.

Recent studies suggest the presence of an unknown substance in breast milk that enhances the breakdown of conjugated bilirubin deposited in the intestine before it can be eliminated in the stool. Conjugated bilirubin is broken down to the unconjugated form and reabsorbed by the small and large bowel. Unconjugated bilirubin diffuses easily into the blood supply of the bowel, where it is redistributed into the circulation.

When breastfeeding is discontinued, the bilirubin level falls within 24 to 48 hours, dropping to half its previous peak level by 48 hours. With resumption of breastfeeding, the bilirubin level starts to rise but at a much slower pace. Interruption of breastfeeding is not recommended; instead, continued and frequent breastfeeding is encouraged. However, the health care provider has the option to supplement nursing with formula or to interrupt breastfeeding and substitute formula, depending on the degree of bilirubin elevation. Supplementation of nursing with water or glucose water does not appear to have any effect on bilirubin levels in healthy term infants.

Drugs That Interfere with Bilirubin Conjugation. Certain medications ingested by the mother and passed transplacentally to the fetus (e.g., salicylates, sulfa preparations) can interfere with the ability of albumin to bind bilirubin. Administration of these drugs to the newborn can produce the same effect. Other medications, such as sodium benzoate, a commonly used preservative, compete with bilirubin for albumin binding sites.

Hypothyroidism. Hypothyroidism is one of the more common metabolic disorders associated with hyperbilirubinemia. Of all infants with hypothyroidism, 20% have elevated bilirubin levels lasting 3 to 4 weeks, with normalization of levels requiring up to 4 months. The suspected mechanism for jaundice is theorized to be a delay in glucuronosyltransferase synthesis or impairment of hepatic proteins that bind bilirubin and remove it from the plasma. The plasma membrane of liver cells may also be altered, resulting in decreased bilirubin influx into the hepatic cells.

Acidosis and Hypoxia. As previously stated in the discussion of kernicterus, a drop in serum pH alters albumin's ability to bind bilirubin. The accompanying increase in the production of free fatty acids promotes competition between fatty acids and bilirubin for binding sites. In animal models, respiratory acidosis but not metabolic acidosis increases movement of bilirubin across the blood-brain barrier.

Abnormal Bilirubin Excretion

Any disease state resulting in abnormal bilirubin excretion can raise serum bilirubin levels significantly. This is seen in hepatic dysfunction secondary to such entities as hypoxia or asphyxia, bowel obstruction, ileus, and congestive heart failure. However, these conditions have a tendency to elevate both the conjugated and unconjugated bilirubin levels. The diminished bowel motility associated with these conditions lengthens the time during which beta-glucuronidase, which is naturally present in the gut, can act on conjugated bilirubin in the stool. This enzymatic reaction converts conjugated bilirubin into the unconjugated form, which is reabsorbed into the intravascular compartment through the enterohepatic circulation. Direct hepatocellular damage associated with cholestasis and bacterial and viral infections can further impair the liver's ability to metabolize bilirubin.

Treatment of Hyperbilirubinemia

Phototherapy. The actual mechanisms by which phototherapy reduces unconjugated bilirubin and the exact mode of bilirubin excretion are not clearly understood. Photo-oxidation and photoisomerization are the two mechanisms thought to change bilirubin into water-soluble and excretable forms. Photo-oxidation involves the oxidation of bilirubin pigment deposited in the skin and its conversion into colorless products that can be excreted into the urine. Of the total body bilirubin concentration, 15% can undergo photodegradation through oxidation. Photoisomerization involves the conversion of bilirubin polymers present in the skin into excretable isomers. When the natural form of bilirubin is exposed to blue light at certain wavelengths, it undergoes photoisomerization. This changes it from a tetrapyrrole, a lipid-soluble substance, into five water-soluble isomers. Four of these isomers are excreted into bile without undergoing conjugation. Two are unstable isomers that are incorporated into bile and must be promptly eliminated from the gastrointestinal tract as a component of stool or they revert back to their natural forms, resulting in resorption of bilirubin from the gut and recirculation into the plasma. Two other isomers remain relatively stable and account for most of the bilirubin found in bile. The fifth isomer, lumibilirubin, is a stable, water-soluble form of bilirubin that is eliminated through urine and bile.

Phototherapy is also thought to enhance hepatic excretion of unconjugated bilirubin and to increase bowel transit time. When phototherapy is begun early, a 20% to 35% reduction in the serum bilirubin concentrations is noted by day 2 of life and a reduction of 41% to 55% by day 4. This reduction is more significant than the naturally occurring drop in the untreated infant.

Although no significant adverse effects are attributed to the use of phototherapy, it is not without associated side effects. Some of these problems include dermal rash, lethargy, abdominal distention, possible eye damage, dehydration caused by increased insensible water loss through the skin and digestive tract, thrombocytopenia, hypocalcemia, and secretory diarrhea possibly as a result of a temporary intestinal lactose deficiency. Another effect of phototherapy seen in infants with a significant direct bilirubin component is "bronze baby" syndrome. This syndrome is thought to be due to skin deposition of a photoproduct of bilirubin decomposition, possibly copper porphyrins, which cause bronzing of the skin and urine. Although no harmful effects can be attributed to the bronzing, it can last for several weeks to several months and is somewhat alarming to parents.

Phototherapy is not adequate therapy for a rapidly rising bilirubin level, but it is effective in the treatment of moderate hyperbilirubinemia that has not reached or exceeded levels known to be associated with kernicterus and in reducing the need for exchange transfusions after the first 12 hours of life. Intensive phototherapy can produce a decline of 1 to 2 mg/dl of total serum bilirubin within 4 to 6 hours (Bergman et al, 1994). This is a reflection of the length of exposure necessary for phototherapy to exhibit its effectiveness. The American Academy of Pediatrics (AAP) adopted a set of guidelines for the initiation of phototherapy and exchange transfusion in the term, healthy newborn (AAP, 2004) (Figure 10-7). Suggested bilirubin levels for initiation of therapy based on birth weight, including very low birth weight, are found on a chart devised by King and Jung (1990) (Figure 10-8). Recommended levels for the use of phototherapy or exchange transfusion must be adjusted downward for prematurity, acidosis, hypoxia, respiratory distress, asphyxia, and neurologic decompensation (Figure 10-9). Diminished bilirubin-binding capacity of albumin, decreased amounts of circulating albumin, and increased permeability of the CNS expose these infants to increased amounts of free bilirubin, which can easily cross the blood-brain barrier.

Although administration of intravenous immunoglobulin (IVIG) to the mother has produced contradictory results, its administration to infants with Rh hemolytic disease may be beneficial. Administration of IVIG to a group of infants with Rh incompatibility was associated with a reduction in the rate of exchange transfusion to 12.5%, compared with 69% in the control group. It is hypothesized that IVIG may interfere with receptors in the reticuloendothelium that are required to induce hemolysis. The optimum dosage has yet to be determined.

However, administration of albumin to an infant undergoing phototherapy may reduce the amount of bilirubin available in the skin for photoisomerization. In an attempt to saturate the increased available albumin binding sites, free bilirubin is drawn into the vascular compartment from the skin, where phototherapy exerts its effect. For this reason, use of albumin in the infant undergoing phototherapy should be carefully weighed.

Collaborative Management. Infants who require phototherapy benefit most from blue light in the wavelength range at which photoisomerization occurs most efficiently: that is, 420 to 460 nm. In addition to the appropriate wavelength, effective illumination must be maintained. Spectroradiometric readings of 4 to 6 mcW/cm²/nm are considered in the effective therapeutic range. For optimum therapy, phototherapy units should be checked for adequacy of light levels by nursing or bioengineering staff. Prolonged exposure to phototherapy lights may cause retinal damage, which can be minimized with adequate eye protection. Phototherapy units and eye

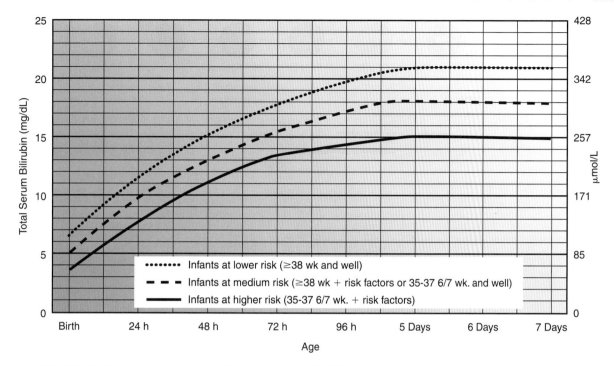

- Use total bilirubin. Do not subtract direct reacting or conjugated bilirubin.
- Risk factors = isoimmune hemolytic disease, G6PD deficiency, asphyxia, significant lethargy, temperature instability, sepsis, acidosis, or albumin <3.0 g/dL (if measured).
- For well infants 35-37 6/7 wk can adjust TSB levels for intervention around the medium risk line. It is an option to intervene at lower TSB levels for infants closer to 35 wks and at higher TSB levels for those closer to 37 6/7 wk.
- It is an option to provide conventional phototherapy in hospital or at home at TSB levels 2-3 mg/dL (35-50 mmol/L) below those shown but home phototherapy should not be used in any infant with risk factors.

FIGURE **10-7**

Guidelines for phototherapy in hospitalized infants of 35 or more weeks' gestation. From American Academy of Pediatrics, Subcommittee on Hyperbilirubinemia (2004). Management of hyperbilirubinemia in the newborn infant 35 or more weeks of gestation. *Pediatrics* 114(1):297-316. Copyright © 2004 American Academy of Pediatrics.

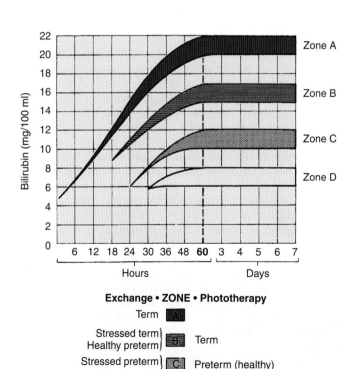

FIGURE **10-8**

The rate of increase in bilirubin levels, gestational age, and the newborn's general condition determine the type of treatment for hyperbilirubinemia and the rapidity of its initiation. This chart is a useful guideline for initiating phototherapy or exchange transfusion in hyperbilirubinemic infants. From Pernoll M et al (1986). Neonatal hyperbilirubinemia and prevention of kernicterus. In Pernoll M et al, editors. *Diagnosis and management of the fetus and neonate at risk*, ed 5. St Louis: Mosby.

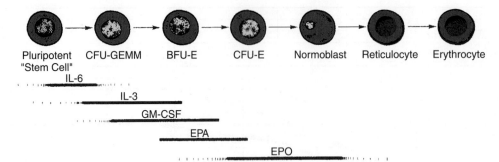

FIGURE **10-9**
The principal action of human recombinant erythropoietin is on the derivatives of the hematopoietic stem cells in the bone marrow that have been designated erythrocyte colony-forming units (*CFU-E*), the precursors of the red blood cell (RBC). *CFU-GEMM*, Colony-forming units—granulocytes, erythroid cells, macrophages, and megakaryocytes; *BFU-E*, erythrocyte burst-forming units; *IL-6*, interleukin-6; *IL-3*, interleukin-3; *GM-CSF*, granulocyte-macrophage colony-stimulating factor; *EPA*, erythroid potentiating activity; *EPO*, erythropoietin. From Christensen R (1989). Recombinant erythropoietic growth factors as an alternative to erythrocyte transfusion for patients with anemia of prematurity. *Pediatrics* 83:793-796.

protection should be removed for short periods throughout the day to provide the infant with visual stimulation and interaction with parents and caregivers. Nurses should also be aware that they may experience headaches from prolonged exposure to phototherapy lights.

Infants undergoing phototherapy require temperature stabilization appropriate for their size and overall condition. A larger infant who is basically well can be nursed in an open crib, but the sick term, premature, or low-birth-weight (LBW) infant requires temperature control through the use of open warmers or closed incubators. Adequate fluid intake and compensatory fluid adjustments for increased insensible water and stool loss may be required to prevent dehydration in these infants. While the infant is receiving phototherapy, bilirubin levels must be monitored frequently to assess the effectiveness of therapy and the need for exchange transfusion. Because phototherapy lights can alter blood bilirubin results, the lights should be turned off when drawing blood for serum bilirubin determinations.

Many hyperbilirubinemic infants who are healthy and not in need of thermoregulation or exchange transfusion can be cared for at home as long as the AAP guidelines are met. The parents of these infants must have access to home photo-therapy equipment and a medical supply company to service the equipment, as well as the support of their medical caregiver. If the infant can remain normothermic in an open crib without clothing, home phototherapy may be considered a cost-effective alternative to hospitalization. The same precautions regarding protective eye covering and adequate fluid intake must be observed in these infants. Frequent determination of bilirubin levels is required to ensure adequate treatment, and blood may be drawn daily for this purpose at the physician's office, the neighborhood hospital laboratory, or by a home health care worker.

Pharmacologic Agents. Phenobarbital is thought to accelerate bilirubin excretion by increasing its uptake and conjugation by the liver and by increasing its excretion by enhancing bile flow. However, no increased benefit is noted that cannot be achieved with phototherapy alone. No medications have been approved in the United States as therapy for inhibition of bilirubin synthesis, but clinical trials

have preliminarily shown that metalloporphyrins may be effective in controlling hyperbilirubinemia in the term and preterm infant. Metalloporphyrins are inhibitors of heme oxygenase, the enzyme involved in the degradation of heme to biliverdin, an intermediate in the synthesis of bilirubin. Tin-mesoporphyrin and tin-protoporphyrin are the two heme oxygenase inhibitors used in clinical trials as a prophylaxis and as treatment. Although these studies have shown beneficial effects, they are still in the initial stages of investigation.

Exchange Transfusion. Once done frequently in neonatal intensive care units, exchange transfusions are now rarely done. An exchange transfusion may be necessary, if bilirubin levels start to approach those associated with kernicterus despite phototherapy, to protect the CNS status of the jaundiced infant. The object of this procedure is to remove bilirubin and the antibody-coated RBCs from the newborn's circulation. In addition, exchange transfusion removes some of the circulating maternal antibodies and Rh-positive fetal RBCs while potentially normalizing the hematocrit. After a single-volume exchange, 75% of the newborn's RBC mass is removed; a double-volume exchange removes 85% to 90% of the cells. However, bilirubin removal is much less effective; only 25% of the infant's total body bilirubin is removed during a double-volume exchange. This probably occurs because the major portion of bilirubin is in the extravascular compartment, an area not affected by the exchange of blood volume. Rebound in bilirubin levels occurs within 1 hour of the exchange, with posttransfusion levels rising as high as 55% of pre-exchange values.

Although EBF remains the primary condition requiring exchange transfusion, the procedure also can be used to reduce levels of circulating metabolic toxins or exogenous drugs and to re-establish a normal hematocrit without further volume overload in anemia-induced congestive heart failure. The mortality rate for exchange transfusions is 1%. This rate includes death during the procedure or within 6 hours after its completion but excludes hydropic, kernicteric, or moribund infants.

The following criteria are used to determine the need for and timing of exchange transfusions, particularly in infants with EBF (Bergman et al, 1994):

TABLE **10-7**	Maximum Total Serum Bilirubin Concentration Allowed before Exchange Transfusion		
	Maximum Concentration (mg/dl)		
Birth Weight (g)	**Uncomplicated Course**	**Complicated Course**	
Under 1000	10	10	
1000 to 1249	13	10	
1250 to 1499	15	13	
1500 to 1999	17	15	
2000 to 2500	18	17	
2500 or over	25	20	

Adapted from Behrman R et al (2004). *The fetus and the neonatal infant.* In Behrman R et al, editors. *Nelson textbook of pediatrics,* ed 17. Philadelphia: Saunders.

- A cord blood bilirubin level over 4.5 mg/dl in term infants and 3.5 mg/dl in preterm infants
- A hemoglobin level under 8 g/dl and a bilirubin level over 6 mg/dl within 1 hour of delivery in a term infant
- A hemoglobin level under 11.5 g/dl and a bilirubin level over 3.5 mg/dl within 1 hour of delivery in a preterm infant
- An increase in bilirubin levels by 0.5 mg/dl/hr despite phototherapy
- A bilirubin level over 20 to 25 mg/dl in an uncompromised term infant (see Table 10-4), 18 mg/dl in the high-risk term newborn, and 10 to 18 mg/dl in the preterm infant, depending on gestational age and condition (Table 10-7)
- A bilirubin level over 10 to 17 mg/dl in a stressed or very immature preterm infant, over 10 to 12 mg/dl if hypoxia and acidosis are present

Identical criteria are used to determine the need for repeated exchange transfusion.

Side Effects of Exchange Transfusion. Exchange transfusion can have a marked effect on the cardiovascular status and the intravascular compartment, which is reflected in pressure changes, volume fluctuations, and biochemical balance. Significant morbidities such as anemia, air embolism, infection, bradycardia, necrotizing enterocolitis, thromboembolism and death can also occur as a result of an exchange transfusion. These are discussed more in depth on the website.

Collaborative Management of the Infant Undergoing an Exchange Transfusion. In addition to the general nursing care required by a sick infant, specific stabilization procedures are necessary for a successful exchange transfusion. A sample protocol for required care during an exchange is presented on the website.

Anemia
Pathophysiology
An infant is considered anemic if the hemoglobin or hematocrit value is more than two standard deviations below normal for their gestational age group (Luchtman-Jones et al, 2002). During the neonatal period, several abnormalities can evoke states of both acute and chronic anemia in the newborn.

These forms of anemia often precede and occur independently of the natural propensity for physiologic anemia that exists as a common entity among all infants, both term and preterm. The conditions that most commonly trigger these pathologic anemias are acute or chronic episodes of hemorrhage, acute or chronic RBC destruction and hemolysis, and blood sampling for laboratory analysis.

Acute Anemia. The physical presentation of acute anemia is more intense than that seen in the chronic form, because the causes of acute anemia are more emergent, life-threatening, and disruptive to the homeostasis of the infant (Box 10-2). The resulting cardiovascular collapse, followed closely by respiratory failure, can overwhelm the neonate with

---

BOX 10-2

Causes of Acute Anemia in the Newborn

Obstetric Accidents, Malformations of the Placenta and Cord
Rupture of a normal umbilical cord
- Precipitous delivery
- Entanglement

Hematoma of the cord or placenta
Rupture of an abnormal umbilical cord
- Varices
- Aneurysm

Rupture of anomalous vessels
- Aberrant vessel
- Velamentous insertion
- Communicating vessels in multilobed placenta

Incision of placenta during cesarean section
Placenta previa
Abruptio placentae

Occult Hemorrhage Before Birth
Fetoplacental
- Tight nuchal cord

Cesarean section
Placental hematoma
Fetomaternal
- Traumatic amniocentesis
- After external cephalic version, manual removal of placenta, use of oxytocin
- Spontaneous
- Chorioangioma of the placenta
- Choriocarcinoma

Twin to twin
- Chronic
- Acute

Internal Hemorrhage
Intracranial
Giant cephalhematoma, subgaleal, caput succedaneum
Adrenal
Retroperitoneal
Ruptured liver, ruptured spleen
Pulmonary

Iatrogenic Blood Loss

From Oski F, Naiman J (1982). Anemia in the neonatal period. In Oski F, Naiman J, editors. *Hematologic problems in the newborn.* Philadelphia: Saunders.

only marginal reserves. Immediate intervention and replacement of lost intravascular volume often are required to achieve stabilization. An infant experiencing an acute anemic episode (hemorrhage being the most common cause) has symptoms reflecting compromise of the cardiorespiratory system: shock, poor peripheral perfusion, poor respiratory effort or respiratory distress, tachycardia, pallor, lethargy, and hypotension. Before signs of acute anemia become apparent, the hemoglobin level must fall precipitously below 12 g/dl.

Acute blood loss results in a recognizable sequence of symptoms based on the volume loss:

- 7.5% to 15% volume loss: Little change is noted in heart rate and blood pressure, but stroke volume and subsequent cardiac output are reduced. Peripheral vasoconstriction occurs, resulting in diminished blood flow to the skeletal muscles, gut, and carcass.
- 20% to 25% volume loss: Hypotension and shock become apparent. Cardiac output is reduced, and peripheral vasoconstriction is present. Low tissue oxygen levels and acidosis become apparent.

Chronic Anemia. Prolonged, or chronic, anemia may not require rapid intravascular volume expansion, but it is by no means completely benign, as is seen with EBF or chronic twin-to-twin transfusion (Box 10-3). In both of these conditions, infants may require removal of intravascular volume and replacement with volume of a higher hematocrit before stabilization is achieved. Because these infants have had considerable time to adjust to chronic blood loss or hemolysis, the changes in vital signs may reflect poor oxygen-carrying capacity rather than hypovolemia. On physical examination, pallor usually is accompanied by hepatosplenomegaly, a reflection of the body's attempt to compensate for blood loss through extramedullary hematopoiesis. The blood smear may also reflect the long-standing nature of the problem; RBCs appear hypochromic and small, and a greater number of immature RBCs are seen.

Common Causes of Pathologic Anemia in the Newborn

Hemorrhage. Hemorrhage is one of the most common causes of pathologic anemia in the newborn. There are many different types of hemorrhage, but they can be classified into four distinct categories, each which will be discussed below.

Fetal-Maternal Transfusion Caused by Transplacental Hemorrhage. This phenomenon occurs in approximately 50% to 75% of all pregnancies and can be an acute or chronic process. An estimated 5.6% of pregnancies involve a fetal-maternal transfusion in the range of 11 to 30 ml of blood; another 1% involve an exchange of more than 30 ml. Fetal-maternal transfusions can be verified by the presence of fetal cells in the maternal circulation, which can be detected with the erythrocyte rosette test and the Kleihauer-Betke acid elution test for fetal hemoglobin in maternal blood. The erythrocyte rosette test specifically detects fetal RBCs. The Kleihauer-Betke test consists of an acid wash of a maternal blood smear followed by staining. Fetal hemoglobin resists elution from intact RBCs in an acid solution. Intact cells containing fetal hemoglobin can be distinguished microscopically, when stained, from adult erythrocytes. The presence of stained erythrocytes suggests contamination of maternal blood by fetal blood. This test is useful in identifying fetal RBCs in the mother's blood as long as no underlying

---

BOX 10-3

Causes of Chronic Anemia in the Newborn

Immunity disorders
- Rh incompatibility
- ABO incompatibility
- Minor blood group incompatibility
- Maternal autoimmune hemolytic anemia
- Drug-induced hemolytic anemia

Infection
- Bacterial sepsis
- Congenital infections
  - Syphilis
  - Malaria
  - Cytomegalovirus
  - Rubella
  - Toxoplasmosis
  - Disseminated herpes

Disseminated intravascular coagulation

Macroangiopathic and microangiopathic hemolytic anemias
- Cavernous hemangioma
- Large-vessel thrombi
- Renal artery stenosis
- Severe coarctation of aorta

Galactosemia

Prolonged or recurrent acidosis of a metabolic or respiratory nature

Hereditary disorders of the red cell membrane
- Hereditary spherocytosis
- Hereditary elliptocytosis
- Hereditary stomatocytosis
- Other rare membrane disorders

Pyknocytosis

Red cell enzyme deficiencies
- Most commonly glucose-6-phosphate dehydrogenase deficiency, pyruvate kinase deficiency, 5'-nucleotidase deficiency, and glucose-6-phosphate isomerase deficiency

Alpha-thalassemia syndrome

Alpha chain structural abnormalities

Gamma-thalassemia syndromes

Gamma chain structural abnormalities

From Oski F, Naiman J (1982). Anemia in the neonatal period. In Oski F, Naiman J, editors. *Hematologic problems in the newborn.* Philadelphia: Saunders.

---

condition increases the amount of fetal hemoglobin in the mother's blood.

Twin-to-Twin Transfusion. This phenomenon, which can be both acute and chronic, occurs in 15% to 33% of all monochorionic (monozygotic) twins, in which the placentas tend to be fused. The anastomosis usually is between an artery of one placenta and the vein of the other, although vascular connections may be artery to artery or vein to vein. In the chronic form of twin-to-twin transfusion, the size difference between twins can be helpful in determining the donor and the recipient. When the weight difference exceeds 20%, the smaller twin is always the donor. When the weight difference is less than 20%, either twin may be the donor. In such cases, hematocrit values prove useful in determining the donor and the recipient. The donor twin is anemic, and the blood count reflects increased hematopoiesis, as evidenced by an elevated reticulocyte count and increased numbers of immature RBCs. The recipient develops polycythemia but can exhibit signs of congestive heart failure and pulmonary or systemic hypertension. Laboratory data usually show a difference of 5 g/dl between donor and recipient hemoglobin values. Stillbirths are common in twin-to-twin transfusion, and both twins are at risk.

Obstetrical Accidents. Many obstetrical problems, especially those that occur before labor and delivery, can result in chronic as well as acute blood loss. Long-standing problems, such as placenta previa or partial abruption, usually result in anemia. However, acute hemorrhage rather than anemia is the case in problems that occur at the time of delivery. Examples are severe abruption, severing of the placenta during cesarean section, or umbilical cord rupture as a result of sudden tension on a short or tangled cord. A tight nuchal cord can reduce blood volume in a newborn by approximately 20%. Holding a newly delivered infant above the placenta can also reduce the hematocrit and blood volume because of the gravitational drainage of blood from the newborn into the placenta.

Internal Hemorrhage. A drop in the hematocrit during the first 24 to 72 hours that is not associated with hyperbilirubinemia usually is attributed to internal hemorrhage. Bleeding can occur in various parts of the body secondary to birth trauma or pre-existing anomalies. The areas of potential hemorrhage in the head include the subdural, subarachnoid, intraventricular, intracranial, and subperiosteal spaces. Infants can lose an estimated 10% to 15% of their blood during an intraventricular or intracranial hemorrhage. In cases of traumatic delivery or vacuum extraction, extensive scalp bleeding can result in significant blood loss, which can be estimated by measuring the increase in the head circumference. Each centimeter of increase represents an estimated 38 ml of blood lost from the intravascular compartment. Hemorrhage into the liver, kidneys, spleen, or retroperitoneal space can also occur in association with traumatic and breech deliveries.

Hepatic rupture occurs in approximately 1.2% to 5.6% of stillbirths and neonatal deaths; half of the hemorrhages are subcapsular. Infants with this disorder tend to be stable for 24 to 48 hours and then suddenly deteriorate. This deterioration seems to coincide with rupture of the capsule and hemoperitoneum. Hepatic rupture carries a poor prognosis, but rapid surgery preceded by multiple transfusions can save the infant. Splenic rupture is associated with severe EBF and should be suspected at the time of exchange transfusion if the central venous pressure is low rather than elevated. Signs of splenic rupture include scrotal swelling and peritoneal effusion without free air. Adrenal hemorrhage is seen more often in the infant of a diabetic or prediabetic mother and is characterized by a flank mass with bluish discoloration of the overlying skin.

Red Blood Cell Destruction and Hemolysis
Maternal-Fetal Blood Group Incompatibilities. Isoimmunization, as in ABO and Rh incompatibility, accounts for most cases of neonatal hemolysis. A reduced RBC life span caused by hemolysis usually is associated with a rise in the bilirubin level, 1 g of hemoglobin yielding 35 mg of bilirubin. Infants who have received intrauterine transfusions or exchange transfusions for blood group incompatibilities are predisposed to a hyporegenerative anemia that develops within the first few months of life. The pathophysiology is considered to be bone marrow suppression, possibly as a result of the increased amount of hemoglobin A received during the blood transfusions.

Acquired Defects of the Red Blood Cells. This hemolytic problem is seen in bacterial sepsis and viral infections, especially of the TORCH variety. Drug-induced RBC destruction, caused by either maternal ingestion or direct administration of the drug to the newborn, is another common cause of hemolysis. An example of this would be the hemolysis that could occur with administration of iron supplements to an infant with vitamin E deficiency.

Congenital Defects of the Red Blood Cells. Defects resulting in destruction of the RBCs can involve the cell membrane, enzymatic system, or hemoglobin component, as in glucose-6-phosphate dehydrogenase deficiency, thalassemia, and hereditary spherocytosis. Although these conditions can cause hemolysis in the newborn period, they are rare diseases.

Blood Sampling. Blood loss that occurs secondary to sampling is one of the two most frequent causes of chronic anemia in infants, the other being physiologic anemia of the newborn and premature infant. Among two groups of preterm infants admitted to neonatal intensive care units, the average blood loss from sampling during the first 4 to 6 weeks of life was 46 to 50 ml/kg; the severity of illness correlated with the amount of blood removed for sampling. Prudent blood sampling may eliminate unnecessary blood volume depletion and reduce the need for replacement transfusion therapy. Accurate recording of blood lost to sampling can prove beneficial in the assessment of a sick infant's circulatory status and volume needs. However, perfusion status and hematocrit values may be better determinants of the need for volume expansion or blood transfusions.

Differential Diagnosis
History. Acute and chronic anemia often can be distinguished from each other and from other problems by analyzing the family history for anemia or jaundice. The maternal history should be carefully examined for evidence of drug ingestion that may affect RBC life span or production, bleeding during the pregnancy or labor, or other incidents surrounding the delivery that may contribute to blood loss in the newborn.

Laboratory Findings. The type of anemia often can be identified on the basis of laboratory studies that evaluate RBC content and form.

- Hematocrit and hemoglobin levels can define the type as well as the degree of anemia. Blood loss during acute hemorrhage is rapid, with little evidence of the compensatory hematopoiesis seen in chronic anemia. RBCs are of normal size and have a normal hemoglobin mass, and no significant increase is seen in the number of immature RBCs. Hemoglobin values initially may not reflect hemorrhage because the intravascular volume contracts and masks volume loss. It may take several hours for intravascular equilibration to occur before the hemoglobin accurately reflects the extent of the hemorrhage. The site of hemoglobin or hematocrit sampling is important for obtaining accurate information, because capillary sticks on an infant in shock reflect venous stasis. A more accurate sample at this time would be from an arterial or venous source.
- Reticulocyte counts are useful in differentiating chronic and acute forms of anemia. Increased numbers of

immature RBCs reflect the degree of hematopoietic activity in response to anemia. Increased hematopoiesis requires a time lapse between the occurrence of anemia and stimulation of the hematopoietic centers.

- Peripheral blood smears are helpful in evaluating iron content and the size and shape of the RBC, which vary in different forms of anemia.
- Blood typing, Rh determination, and Coombs' testing can help identify blood group incompatibilities as causes of anemia.

Treatment

Collaborative Management of the Infant with Acute Anemia. The following measures are used to stabilize the condition of an infant with acute anemia:

- Basic resuscitation of the infant experiencing precipitous blood loss often includes stabilization of the airway by means of intubation and ventilation.
- Rapid line placement for fluid replacement, volume expansion, and blood sampling may require use of the umbilical vein or artery. Central venous pressure measurements can be helpful in assessing the degree of volume loss and the amount of replacement needed.
- If acute volume expansion is required, low-titer, type O-negative blood, plasma, albumin, or saline initially can be used in increments of 10 to 20 ml/kg until a type and cross-match replacement is available. Failure to respond may indicate continuing internal hemorrhage.
- After the infant's condition has been stabilized, laboratory tests and a physical examination should be performed to determine the cause of the anemia and to rectify the problem.
- Examination of the placenta and maternal blood sample testing for fetal hemoglobin may prove useful in determining the cause of the blood loss.

As with all newborns, the principles of care (provision of warmth, monitoring of vital signs, ongoing assessment, and accurate determination of intake and output) are essential to the well-being of the infant who has suffered acute blood loss. After initial stabilization, nursing care must include modifications that either eliminate recurrence of precipitous events or prevent further blood loss. Providing safe care to such infants requires adequate knowledge of the principles and procedures involved in volume expansion and the use of blood products. A review of the use of blood products can be found at the conclusion of this chapter.

Collaborative Management of the Infant with Chronic Anemia. The major focus of therapy for the infant with chronic anemia is control or elimination of the cause of the anemia. Several forms of chronic anemia in term and preterm infants are linked to dietary deficiencies that can be eradicated by replacement therapy. Chronic forms of anemia requiring symptomatic therapy can also be treated with transfusion therapy and erythropoietin.

Dietary Supplementation. The three major dietary factors that affect RBC production are iron, folate, and vitamin E. Because all three increase in amount with increasing gestational age, premature birth predisposes the immature infant to anemia as a result of insufficient stores.

Without benefit of iron supplementation, the hematopoiesis necessary to maintain a normal hemoglobin level depletes the infant's iron reserves by the time birth weight is doubled.

Various factors can further contribute to iron deficiency anemia, such as low birth weight, low initial hemoglobin levels, and blood loss through trauma, hemorrhage, or sampling. In the term infant, exhaustion of iron reserves normally occurs by 20 to 24 weeks' postnatal age, but this happens much earlier in the preterm infant. Iron stores needed for hemoglobin production are present in insufficient quantities at birth in the premature infant, making supplementation necessary during the first 2 to 4 months to prevent iron deficiency anemia.

In any gestational age group, iron depletion first becomes evident in reduced serum ferritin levels (serum ferritin being a measure of accumulated iron stores) and in the disappearance of stainable iron from the bone marrow. A subsequent reduction in the mean corpuscular volume (i.e., the size) of the RBC is followed by a drop in the hemoglobin level. Although prophylactic iron supplementation does not prevent the initial fall in hemoglobin, administration of 1 to 2 mg/kg/day of supplemental iron should supply term and preterm infants with adequate reserves; 3 to 6 mg/kg/day is recommended in iron-deficient infants or those receiving erythropoietin.

The relationship between serum ferritin levels and the administration of multiple transfusions to a population of newborn infants was evaluated to determine iron supplementation needs in this group. In a study by Arad and associates (1988), serum ferritin levels were measured in four groups of infants: (1) preterm infants transfused with more than 100 ml of packed cells, (2) preterm infants transfused with less than 100 ml, (3) nontransfused preterm infants, and (4) nontransfused term infants. At 4 to 5 months of age, the preterm infants receiving more than 100 ml of RBCs had the highest ferritin levels of all four groups. This would suggest that LBW infants receiving large volumes of RBCs could amass iron stores sufficient for new RBC production during the first 4 to 5 months without the need for additional iron supplementation.

Folate is the generic description for folic acid and its related compounds. Folate is a component of the B-complex vitamins involved in the maturation of RBCs, particularly the synthesis of DNA, which controls nuclear maturation and division. Because bone marrow is one of the body's faster growing and proliferative tissues, folic acid deficiency diminishes its ability to produce RBCs, resulting in a megaloblastic anemia.

High amounts of folate are present at birth in both term and preterm infants, but these levels drop rapidly, especially in LBW infants. It is estimated that approximately 68% of infants weighing less than 1700 g have subnormal levels of folate at 1 to 3 months of age. However, only a few infants actually develop anemia. Human milk and soy-based products contain an adequate amount of natural folate, but commonly used commercial products must be artificially enriched. Premature infant formulas are adequately enriched to satisfy a premature infant's folate needs provided that intake is sufficient. Because folate is absorbed in the duodenum and jejunum, any disease or medication that affects the absorptive surface of these areas can impair folate absorption.

Vitamin E, an antioxidant, is valuable in protecting the RBC membrane from destruction due to lipid peroxidation. Deficiency of this nutrient shortens the life span of the cell by exposing the unprotected, unsaturated membrane lipids to peroxidation and hemolysis. Infants are born in a state of relative vitamin E deficiency that is more intense in the smaller and more premature infants. Vitamin E is required in increasing amounts as the intake of polyunsaturated fatty acids increases. Deficiency becomes apparent in infants of birth weights less than 1500 g at approximately 4 to 6 weeks of age, resulting in decreased hemoglobin levels ranging from 7 to 10 g/dl. Administration of iron supplementation in the presence of this deficiency intensifies the hemolytic response. Signs and symptoms, as with many neonatal diseases, mimic those of other disease entities that occur in the neonatal period. One of the more obvious symptoms is edema of the feet, lower extremities, and scrotal area. The appearance of the RBC may vary, but abnormalities usually include fragmented or irregularly shaped cells, presence of spherocytes, and thrombocytopenia. Infant formulas are now enriched with adequate amounts of vitamin E, provided formula intake is sufficient.

Transfusion Therapy. Of all preterm infants admitted to an NICU, approximately 90% receive one transfusion in the first 6 weeks of life; 50% receive cumulative transfusions in excess of their total circulating RBC mass. In determining which infants may need subsequent transfusions after the first 2 weeks of life, gestational age of less than 30 weeks is the best predictor, regardless of severity of illness, number of transfusions during the first week, complications, or hematocrit level at birth. Only 14% of infants of more than 30 weeks' gestation require transfusions after 2 weeks of age.

Although a critically ill infant generally is maintained with a hematocrit above 40%, the benefits of transfusion therapy in the convalescent infant remain controversial. When the effects of transfusion therapy in the convalescent infant were studied, the elimination of symptoms attributed to anemia was not a consistent finding. In premature infants with hematocrits below 30%, apnea, bradycardia, dyspnea, feeding difficulties, poor weight gain despite good calorie intake, lethargy, tachypnea, tachycardia, and increased cardiac output and oxygen consumption appear to be relieved by transfusion therapy in some studies. There appears to be no overall relationship between hematocrit values and physiologic symptoms such as apnea, bradycardia, or changes in heart and respiratory rates, nor does abatement of these symptoms follow transfusion therapy.

In light of the controversy surrounding transfusions, evidence of impaired tissue oxygenation remains the ultimate criterion for the use of blood products. Measurement of lactic acid levels may prove helpful in determining which infants may benefit from transfusion therapy. When the oxygen-carrying capacity of hemoglobin is insufficient for tissue needs, anaerobic metabolism occurs, leading to excess production of lactic acid. Monitoring of lactic acid levels and transfusing only those infants with elevated levels may aid in establishing more sound criteria for transfusion therapy.

Several methods of blood preparation and use have been evaluated to minimize donor exposure and reduce the potential for transmitted disease. Studies suggest that packed RBCs with a shelf life of more than 5 days, and up to 42 days, are safe for use in neonatal transfusions (Gael, 2005; Basile & Southgate, 2004). This finding, combined with use of a sterile connection device that allows multiple aseptic entries into a unit of blood, would permit use of a designated unit for each infant at risk for multiple transfusions, thereby significantly reducing donor exposure (Gael, 2005). The desire to limit donor exposure must inevitably be balanced by the limited availability of banked blood. Multiple users on a blood unit

may reduce wastage but may possibly expose an infant to multiple donors.

Blood administered to the newborn is often irradiated, which causes cell membrane disruption and potassium leakage from the cell. The decision by the U.S. Food and Drug Administration to change its recommendations for the maximum storage time of irradiated blood from 42 to 28 days affects the length of use of a designated unit (Quinnan, 1993). Although older blood appears to be safe to administer, it is not recommended for rapid transfusions, administration of large aliquots, exchange transfusions, or treatment of coagulopathies.

The establishment of transfusion criteria can effectively minimize donor exposure. These guidelines help determine which infants would benefit from transfusion on the basis of symptoms, hematocrit value, and severity of illness.

Recombinant Human Erythropoietin Therapy. Cloning of the human erythropoietin (HuEPO) gene in 1985 resulted in the production of large amounts of HuEPO for use as an exogenous stimulant of erythroid progenitor cells in patients with anemia. HuEPO acts primarily on CFU-E, derivatives of the hematopoietic stem cells in the bone marrow and the precursors of the RBCs (Figure 10-10). Studies from the United States and England have shown the use of recombinant erythropoietin to be an effective replacement for transfusion therapy in raising the hemoglobin level in hyporegenerative anemia and end-stage renal disease. Further studies of preterm infants have demonstrated that HuEPO maintains the hematocrit level during the phase of normal anemia of the premature infant, with good proliferation of erythroid progenitor cells in response to HuEPO.

HuEPO has attained recognition as a standard of care for anemia of prematurity, because several clinical trials have established its effectiveness in reducing both the number of transfusions and the cumulative volume of transfused blood needed in treated patients (Messer et al, 1993; Ohls et al,

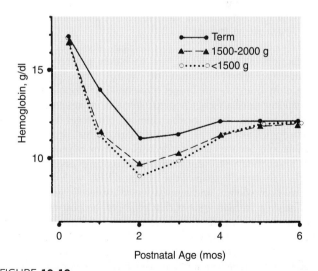

FIGURE **10-10**
Gestational age and birth weight are directly correlated with the timing of the postnatal drop in hemoglobin and with the nadir of the drop. Shown here are the differences between term infants and two groups of preterm infants, one weighing 1500 to 2000 g and the other less than 1500 g. From Brown M (1988). Physiologic anemia of infancy: normal red cell values and physiology of neonatal erythropoiesis. In Stockman J, Pochedly C, editors. *Developmental and neonatal hematology.* New York: Raven Press.

1993, 1995; Maier et al, 1994; Meyer et al, 1994). Donato and associates (2000) noted increased reticulocytosis in infants started early on erythropoietin but failed to see a reduction in transfusion requirements in those infants.

The usual response in preterm infants given HuEPO is an increase in blood levels of erythropoietin and reticulocytes, as well as RBC volume, 2 to 3 weeks after initiation of therapy. The accepted dosage of erythropoietin is 200 to 250 units/kg, given subcutaneously three times a week for 2 weeks, although a definitive therapeutic dosage has yet to be determined.

HuEPO has been evaluated for its effectiveness as an alternative to transfusion therapy for treatment of anemia in premature infants caused by (1) blood sampling, with administration beginning within the first 2 days of life (Maier et al, 1994; Ohls et al, 1995); (2) physiologic anemia of prematurity, with therapy starting at 1 to 4 weeks of age (Emmerson et al, 1993; Messer et al, 1993; Meyer et al, 1994; Shannon et al, 1995); and (3) anemia of bronchopulmonary dysplasia, with treatment starting at 3 months of age (Ohls et al, 1993).

Serum ferritin levels decline rapidly after initiation of HuEPO therapy in infants with normal pretreatment ferritin levels, despite prophylactic iron supplementation of 2 mg/kg/day. This predisposition to the development of iron deficiency anemia underlines the need for increased iron supplementation in infants treated with HuEPO. Also documented as a side effect of HuEPO therapy are transient thrombocytosis shortly after the initiation of therapy and transient neutropenia. The transient neutropenia can last as long as 2 months after discontinuation of therapy. It has been postulated that this phenomenon is due to a stimulant effect of HuEPO on megakaryocyte progenitors and a negative effect on granulocyte-monocyte progenitor cells. Before HuEPO was proven effective in raising hematocrit levels, its use was projected to eliminate the need for one third of all transfusions in premature infants.

Physiologic Anemia of the Newborn and Anemia of the Premature Infant

Shortly after birth, the physiologic regulator of RBC production, erythropoietin, falls to barely perceptible levels because the relative intrauterine hypoxia that stimulated its release in utero is no longer present. Erythropoietin levels remain low until another hypoxic stimulus occurs, one created by the normal drop in the hemoglobin level that marks physiologic anemia of the newborn. This drop in the hemoglobin level is due to decreased marrow production of RBCs secondary to diminished circulating erythropoietin levels, a shorter life span of the neonatal RBC with destruction of fetal hemoglobin, and hemodilution caused by growth.

The drop in hemoglobin that prompts the postnatal rise in erythropoietin directly correlates with the infant's gestational age and birth weight (Figure 10-11). The smaller and more immature infant reaches a lower nadir at an earlier postnatal age. The hemoglobin level in the term newborn reaches a nadir of 11.4 g/dl ± 0.9 in the first 2 to 3 months of life and plateaus at this level for approximately 2 more months before it gradually increases. Although there is no significant difference in cord blood hemoglobin levels between term infants and preterm infants born after 32 weeks' gestation, the drop in hemoglobin occurs earlier in the preterm infant, is more precipitous, and reaches a lower nadir. Starting at 2

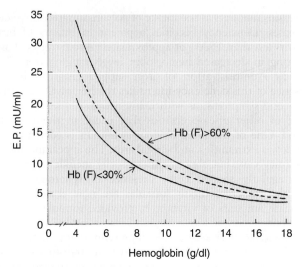

FIGURE 10-11
Because of the differences in oxygen affinity between adult and fetal hemoglobin, variations in the percentage of available fetal hemoglobin (hemoglobin F) affect erythropoietin levels. Improved oxygen uptake but decreased unloading at the tissue level is associated with hemoglobin F. Therefore the stimulus for erythropoietin production is diminished with lower concentrations of hemoglobin F (<30%). With higher concentrations (60%) of hemoglobin F, the stimulus response is an increase in erythropoietin production. At identical total hemoglobin levels, the stimulus for erythropoietin production is increased whenever the percentage of hemoglobin F exceeds the adult norm. From Stockman J et al (1977). The anemia of infancy and the anemia of prematurity: factors governing the erythropoietin response. *New England journal of medicine* 296:647. Copyright © 1977 Massachusetts Medical Society.

weeks of age, the preterm infant has a drop in hemoglobin of 1 g/dl/wk for the first several weeks; the nadir at 6 to 8 weeks of age is 2 to 3 g/dl lower than that of the term infant. An infant weighing 1000 to 1500 g at birth will have a mean hemoglobin nadir of 8 g/dl at 4 to 6 weeks of age.

Infants who have undergone exchange transfusion or multiple transfusions also have a greater fall in the hemoglobin level in the first 3 months of life. This phenomenon theoretically may be due to improved oxygen delivery to tissue associated with the replacement of fetal with adult hemoglobin. Adult hemoglobin has less affinity for oxygen because of the structural difference of the globin portion of the hemoglobin molecule. This, coupled with the increased amount of 2,3-disphosphoglycerate present in the blood, allows adult hemoglobin to release oxygen to the tissue more easily. Improved tissue oxygenation effectively lowers serum erythropoietin levels (Figure 10-12), resulting in decreased RBC production. Consequently, an infant undergoing intrauterine transfusion, exchange transfusion, or frequent postnatal transfusions has improved tissue oxygenation and a decreased erythropoietin level.

The switch in the predominant site of erythropoietin production during fetal life from the liver to the kidneys occurs concurrently with the change in hemoglobin to a more mature form. Hepatic production of erythropoietin in response to hypoxia is not as rapid as the kidneys' response, an adjustment that actually spares the fetus from polycythemia in utero. However, persistence of this hepatic pathway after premature birth may explain why the premature infant's hematocrit

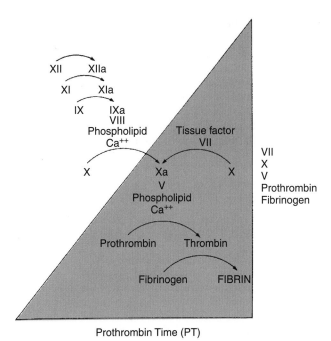

FIGURE **10-12**
Prothrombin time (PT) measures the prothrombin complex, which consists of Factors II (prothrombin), VII, IX, and X. These factors depend on vitamin K for synthesis. PT is also a measurement of the extrinsic pathway of coagulation. *Ca,* Calcium. From Lusher J (1987). Diseases of coagulation: the fluid phase. In Nathan D, Oski F, editors. *Hematology of infancy and childhood,* ed 3. Philadelphia: Saunders.

values reach a lower nadir that persists longer compared with the term infant. Although erythropoietin levels are reduced in the early newborn period, the erythroid progenitor cells in the bone marrow are exceedingly sensitive to erythropoietin and respond rapidly as blood levels increase. The normal erythropoietin level in infants beyond the newborn period is 10 to 20 munits/ml.

Physiologic anemia does not usually require any form of treatment. With good nutrition, the hemoglobin level in the term infant should start to rise by 3 months of age. With adequate nutrition and iron supplementation, the hemoglobin level in the preterm infant should start to increase by 5 months of age, eventually attaining hemoglobin values comparable to those of the term infant. It is the preterm infant with symptomatic anemia of prematurity who poses the question of transfusion vs HuEPO therapy, a question that has not yet been answered conclusively.

Polycythemia
Pathophysiology
Polycythemia, defined as a peripheral venous hematocrit over 65%, occurs in 4% to 5% of the total population of newborns, in 2% to 4% of term infants appropriate for gestational age, and in 10% to 15% of infants either small or large for gestational age. It has not been observed in infants of less than 34 weeks' gestation. Although the fetus lives in a low-PO_2 environment that should induce a polycythemic response, it protects itself by keeping hematocrit levels below 60%. This may be a function of slower fetal hepatic response to hypoxia compared with rapid renal response after birth. The average hematocrit on the first day of life is approximately 50% in the term infant and the preterm infant of more than 32 weeks'

gestation and 45% in the preterm infant of less than 32 weeks' gestation. During the first 4 to 12 hours of life, hemoglobin and hematocrit values tend to rise and then equilibrate, especially in infants receiving large placental transfusions.

The choice of sampling site can affect hematocrit values considerably, particularly during the early newborn period when peripheral circulation may be somewhat sluggish. Infants younger than 1 day of age either lack or have diminished cutaneous vasoregulatory mechanisms that reduce peripheral perfusion. Polycythemia further impairs peripheral circulation by increasing blood viscosity and reducing the flow rate. As blood viscosity increases, vascular resistance increases in the peripheral circulation and the microcirculation of the capillaries throughout the body. Compared with venous samples, the hematocrit levels of capillary samples are 5% to 15% higher, and those of umbilical vessel or arterial samples are 6% to 8% lower.

Three major factors determine blood viscosity: hematocrit, plasma viscosity (osmolality), and deformability of the RBCs. With hematocrit levels below 60% to 65%, blood viscosity increases in a linear fashion, but viscosity exponentially increases at higher hematocrit levels.

Variations in the components of plasma affect blood viscosity independent of the hematocrit. Abnormal composition of plasma protein, electrolytes, and other metabolites can either decrease or increase plasma viscosity. Such an increase in the presence of a high hematocrit further increases blood viscosity and reduces the blood flow rate. The ability of cells to modify their shape to successfully traverse the peripheral vascular bed and microcirculation also affects the blood flow rate. The degree of deformability of the cell determines its ability to pass through small vascular spaces; the greater the deformability of the cell, the quicker its passage. Less deformable cells can increase blood viscosity by occluding small vessels, causing sludging in the microcirculation that can lead to thrombosis and tissue ischemia.

The two major types of polycythemia are (1) the active form, which is caused by the production of an excess number of RBCs in response to hypoxia and other poorly defined stimuli; and (2) the passive form, which is caused by RBC transfusion to an infant secondary to maternal-fetal transfusion, twin-to-twin transfusion, or delayed cord clamping.

Active Polycythemia. Tissue hypoxia, regardless of the cause, elicits an increase in erythropoietin that stimulates RBC production. In the fetus, erythropoietin is produced initially by the liver and then by the kidneys, the adult production site. The kidneys' potential to release erythropoietin is active by 34 weeks' gestation. At this time, a renal erythropoietic factor reacts with a substance in the plasma to produce erythropoietin, the RBC stimulating factor. Hypoxia of the tissues adjacent to the renal tubules, where erythropoietin is thought to be produced, is the potent stimulator of this factor's release.

Many factors can lead to tissue hypoxia associated with the active form of polycythemia. These factors include the following:
1. Maternal factors that result in reduced placental blood flow
   - Pregnancy-induced hypertension
   - Older maternal age
   - Maternal renal or heart disease
   - Severe maternal diabetes (hematocrit values of 64% or higher are found in 42% of infants of a diabetic mother and 30% of gestational infants of a diabetic mother)

- Oligohydramnios
- Maternal smoking (the mechanism is thought to be production of carbon monoxide that crosses the placenta and induces a state of tissue hypoxia in the fetus)
2. Placental factors
   - Placental infarction
   - Placenta previa
   - Viral infections, especially TORCH
   - Postmaturity
   - Placental dysfunction that results in a small-for-gestational-age (SGA) infant
3. Fetal syndromes
   - Trisomies 13, 18, and 21
   - Beckwith-Wiedemann syndrome

Passive Polycythemia. Passive polycythemia is a result of increased fetal blood volume caused by maternal-fetal transfusion; twin-to-twin transfusion, with one twin being polycythemic and the other anemic; or delayed cord clamping. A diagnosis of maternal-fetal transfusion can be considered when (1) the infant's blood is found to contain larger amounts than expected of adult hemoglobin, IgA, or IgM; (2) RBCs in the infant's blood have maternal blood group antigens, if the mother's and the infant's blood groups are different; or (3) XX cells are found in an XY infant. In twin-to-twin transfusion, morbidity and mortality are comparable in both groups of affected infants, with one twin being anemic and the other polycythemic. By far, however, the most common cause of fetal transfusion is delayed cord clamping with positioning of the newborn below the level of the placenta. Delayed cord clamping can increase the circulating volume by as much as 60% and can raise the hematocrit value by 10%.

Clinical Manifestations

Symptoms of polycythemic hyperviscosity, which usually are evident within the first few days after birth, reflect compromise of various organ systems. The most commonly seen findings include the following:

1. Neurologic symptoms
   - Lethargy
   - Hypotonia
   - Tremulousness
   - Exaggerated startle
   - Poor suck
   - Vomiting
   - Seizures
   - Apnea
2. Cardiovascular symptoms
   - Plethora
   - Cardiomegaly
   - Electrocardiographic changes (right and left atrial hypertrophy, right ventricular hypertrophy)
3. Respiratory symptoms
   - Respiratory distress
   - Central cyanosis
   - Pleural effusions
   - Pulmonary congestion and edema
4. Hematologic symptoms
   - Thrombocytopenia
   - Elevated reticulocyte level
   - Hepatosplenomegaly
5. Metabolic symptoms
   - Hypocalcemia

- Hyperbilirubinemia
- Hypoglycemia

Hypoglycemia found in conjunction with polycythemia can be a reflection of (1) increased glucose consumption by an overabundant number of RBCs; (2) increased cerebral extraction of glucose secondary to hypoxia; (3) a state of hyperinsulinemia caused by increased erythropoietin levels; or (4) decreased hepatic glucose production as a result of sluggish hepatic circulation. Hyperbilirubinemia associated with polycythemia is a reflection of increased byproducts of RBC destruction.

The complications of polycythemia center around the increased resistance to blood flow related to hyperviscosity; blood flow to all organ systems is impaired by sluggish circulation. Pulmonary blood flow can be dramatically compromised, resulting in pulmonary hypertension, retained lung fluid, and respiratory distress syndrome. Taxation of the heart by an increased vascular load can lead to congestive heart failure and left to right shunting across the foramen ovale or ductus arteriosus. Sludging of blood in the microcirculation of the kidneys can lead to renal vein thrombosis and renal failure. Impairment of blood flow to the bowel can lead to necrotizing enterocolitis.

Treatment

Although most infants with polycythemia are asymptomatic or minimally symptomatic, the hematocrit level and the presence of symptoms, even if minimal, should form the basis of treatment. Because hematocrit levels of 65% can lead to neurologic abnormalities and levels of 75% or higher are always associated with neurologic changes, an infant with a venous hematocrit of 65% or higher should be considered for partial exchange transfusion.

Partial exchange results in dramatic improvement in symptomatic infants, relieving congestive failure and improving CNS function. It also corrects hypoglycemia, relieves respiratory distress and cyanosis, and improves renal function.

Partial exchange transfusion should be done as the venous hematocrit (Hct) approaches 65% and as symptoms appear; 5% albumin or crystalloid is suggested as replacement for the removed aliquot of blood. With the advent of stricter precautions for prevention of viral transmission by blood products, use of fresh-frozen plasma would not seem advisable. The formula for calculating the partial replacement of blood volume is

$$\text{Replacement volume} = \frac{\text{Observed Hct} - \text{Desired Hct}}{\text{Observed Hct}} \times \text{Blood volume}$$

Collaborative Management of the Infant with Polycythemia

The care of any newborn infant should include a screening hematocrit determination for polycythemia by 12 hours of age. This allows both detection of any infant with polycythemia and adequate observation before symptoms become apparent. Because the initial sample usually is obtained by heel stick or finger stick, detection of a high value should be followed by venipuncture confirmation. The infant should be kept adequately hydrated and closely monitored for hypoglycemia and hypocalcemia. A hematocrit value over 65% should prompt careful observation of the infant for any symptoms associated with hyperviscosity. If symptoms appear, the infant should undergo partial exchange transfusion. During the partial exchange, the same care should be provided as that given during a single-volume or double-volume exchange transfusion.

COMMON COAGULATION DISORDERS IN THE NEWBORN

Hemorrhagic Disease of the Newborn

The liver produces most of the clotting factors, including those of the prothrombin complex. Adequate function of this complex requires the specific action of vitamin K, which is continuously synthesized by bacteria in the bowel. Vitamin K is not directly involved in the synthesis of these factors but is required for the conversion of precursor proteins produced by the liver into active factors having coagulant capabilities. Vitamin K is especially necessary for conversion of prothrombin binding sites into forms that can bind calcium, which is required for the completion of many steps in the clotting cascade.

Vitamin K–dependent factors reach approximately 30% to 70% of adult levels in the cord blood of term infants but quickly drop to half that amount if the infant is not given vitamin K. Because these factors are gestational age dependent, the more premature the infant, the lower the levels at birth. The exaggerated drop after birth may be due to poor placental transfer of maternal vitamin K, immature liver function, and delayed synthesis of vitamin K by the bowel. Vitamin K–dependent factors slowly rise but do not reach normal adult levels until approximately 9 months of age. Administration of approximately 25 mcg (0.025 mg) of vitamin K can prevent this decline and normalize the prothrombin time.

Hemorrhage during the early neonatal period that can be attributed to a deficiency of vitamin K–dependent factors is classified as hemorrhagic disease of the newborn, of which there are three identified forms. The early form, the least common type, is characterized by bleeding within the first 24 hours of life, usually associated with maternal anticonvulsant therapy. It is theorized that anticonvulsants may induce fetal hepatic enzymes involved in the degradation of already low levels of fetal vitamin K. Early neonatal bleeding cannot be prevented by postnatal administration of vitamin K. Daily antenatal administration of large doses of oral vitamin K (10 mg) to mothers receiving anticonvulsant therapy for at least 10 days before delivery was found to be beneficial to the newborn. Vitamin K crosses the placenta, elevating newborn levels of vitamin K for 10 days after birth, with the increase in levels correlating with the timing of the last prenatal dose.

The classic form of hemorrhagic disease usually occurs during the first 2 to 5 days of life and manifests as generalized and, occasionally, dramatic bleeding. The most common sites are the gastrointestinal tract, umbilicus, circumcision site, skin, and internal organs. The usual cause is inadequate intake of breast milk in an infant who has not received prophylactic vitamin K. Breast milk provides adequate vitamin K to prevent this disorder if it is taken in sufficient quantities.

The late form of hemorrhagic disease, which occurs after the first week of life, is more devastating than the early form because of the higher incidence of intracranial hemorrhage (the risk approaches 63%). Permanent neurologic sequelae are seen in 24% of affected infants, and the mortality rate can be as high as 14%. This form of hemorrhagic disease is associated with chronic disease states that interfere with fat absorption or the performance of intestinal flora. Both early and late hemorrhagic disease of the newborn are intensified in breastfed infants. Definitive diagnosis rests on a history of lack of vitamin K prophylaxis at birth and a prolonged prothrombin time (Figure 10-12), which measures the prothrombin complex clotting factors (Factors II, VII, IX, and X). One test, the protein induced by vitamin K absence or antagonist-II (PIVKA-II) test, is useful in identifying proteins induced by vitamin K deficiency that appear in the plasma of vitamin K–deficient infants. These proteins consist of the inert and functionally defective precursors of prothrombin that are produced when vitamin K levels are deficient.

Several factors can predispose an infant to hemorrhagic disease of the newborn. Almost all these factors involve some form of hepatic dysfunction. The most obvious predisposing factor is failure of an infant to receive prophylactic vitamin K postnatally. Other risk factors include maternal ingestion of anticonvulsants and coumarin anticoagulants (which interfere with the action of the prothrombin complex factors), birth asphyxia, prolonged labor, and breastfeeding.

Human milk has a lower vitamin K content than cow's milk. Infants receiving a commercial formula for 24 hours have prothrombin times similar to those of infants receiving vitamin K after birth. Infants with hepatic dysfunction or bowel malabsorption, although not found strictly in the early neonatal period, can develop vitamin K deficiency despite having received prophylaxis at birth. Such disorders as chronic diarrhea, biliary atresia, hepatitis, cystic fibrosis, and prolonged parenteral nutrition do not allow adequate vitamin K production and can result in low prothrombin complex factors. These infants benefit from weekly vitamin K supplementation (1 mg given intramuscularly), the dose recommended by the AAP (2002) for postnatal newborn prophylaxis. The suggested preparation for administration to the newborn is the natural aqueous solution of vitamin K rather than the synthetic preparation, which can cause hemolysis. Because of preterm infants' hepatic immaturity and inability to effectively synthesize clotting factors, these infants' response to vitamin K is not as predictable as that of term infants.

Controversy continues over whether intramuscular or oral prophylaxis should be used. At one time, intramuscular administration of vitamin K was linked to the occurrence of childhood cancers; however, this charge has not been substantiated by research. The use of one or two oral doses of vitamin K as an effective treatment is also disputed, and research is needed to determine its efficacy. Research continues in an effort to determine the appropriate timing and number of oral doses of vitamin K and to develop a better oral preparation. Alternative therapies are also being investigated, including antenatal maternal dosing to prevent antenatal intraventricular hemorrhage and postnatal maternal dosing as prophylaxis in the breastfed infant.

Kumar and colleagues (2001) reported that premature infants have high plasma vitamin K levels in the first 2 weeks of life as a result of intramuscular and parenteral supplementation. These researchers measured vitamin K levels in infants who were given 1 mg of vitamin K intramuscularly at birth and who then were given vitamin K parenterally at a dosage of 60 mcg/day for those less than 1000 g and 130 mcg/day for those weighing more than 1000 g. This research suggests that further studies need to focus on vitamin K levels in the premature infant and attempts need to be made to determine the adequate dose.

Active bleeding caused by hemorrhagic disease of the newborn may require blood replacement or the use of fresh-frozen plasma for immediate clotting factor replacement.

Hemophilia
Pathophysiology
Hemophilia A and B are the most common inherited bleeding disorders. Classic hemophilia (hemophilia A) is the most frequently inherited coagulation abnormality, accounting for 90% of all genetically linked coagulopathies and 80% to 85% of all hemophilias, whereas hemophilia B occurs in 10% to 15%. Both diseases are passed from mother to son as an X-linked trait. Hemophilia A is caused by factor VIII deficiency and hemophilia B is caused by a factor IX deficiency. Both factors are essential in normal thrombin production. They are needed for the activation of pathway of factor X, which converts prothrombin to thrombin. The absence of either factor severely impairs the body's ability to generate both thrombin and fibrin. A hemophiliac's problem is not that of bleeding more rapidly, but of abnormal clot formation. This results in hemorrhage with a potential for significant blood loss. When the clot does form it is often fragile, and rebleeding can occur if proper treatment did not occur.

The severity of the disease is dependent on the baseline level of factor VIII or factor IX. Levels of 1% to 2% are associated with severe disease, 2% to 5% with moderate disease, and over 5% with mild disease, a level at which active bleeding rarely occurs. In a retrospective study of hemophiliacs, approximately 44% of a group of severe hemophiliacs were symptomatic during the first week of life, whereas only 14% of a mildly affected group displayed any bleeding during the first 7 days of life.

Diagnosis
Infants affected with hemophilia have a prolonged partial thromboplastin time and decreased factor, but the prothrombin time, thrombin time, and platelet count are relatively normal. The major symptom of hemophilia is bleeding, most often from the circumcision site, scalp, umbilicus, and brain. Not all severe hemophiliacs bleed after circumcision in the early newborn period. The reason for this is unknown, but it has been suggested that tissue thromboplastin release, caused by the circumcision clamp on the foreskin, may initiate the extrinsic pathway and clotting cascade, preventing excessive bleeding.

Prenatal diagnosis is possible, but the results are not always accurate. Diagnosis involves measurement of the ratio of factor antigen to coagulant antigen on blood samples of fetuses of more than 20 weeks' gestation. If diagnosed with Factor VIII deficiency, the infant should also be evaluated for von Willebrand disease.

Treatment
The ultimate goal of treatment for hemophilia is to raise the defective or deficient factor to a level that will prevent bleeding. In order to have replacement products be as free as possible of transfusion-transmissible diseases, it is recommended that recombinant products be used rather than plasma-derived products. Recombinant factor VIII concentrates are preferred

for hemophilia A, whereas either plasma-purified factor IX or a monoclonal immunoaffinity is preferred for hemophilia B.

Desmopressin (DDAVP, 1-desamino-8-D-arginine vaso-pressin) is now the treatment of choice for mild to moderate hemophilia A, in patients who have shown a response to the drug in trials. This medication is not effective in the treatment of hemophilia B. The effectiveness and applicability of this therapy in the newborn is still unknown, but currently it is not recommended if the infant is younger than 3 months of age. Amicar, an antifibrinolytic agent, is also showing some benefit in the treatment of hemophilia.

Thrombocytopenia
The normal range of platelets is 150,000 to 450,000/mm^3; the average count in the newborn is approximately 250,000/mm^3. Platelet counts below 150,000/mm^3 are considered abnormal and should be subject to investigation for a possible pathologic process. Platelet function in the neonate reaches normal adult levels between the fifth and ninth postnatal days. Although 14% of all preterm infants and 4% of all term infants are thrombocytopenic, with platelet counts below 150,000/mm^3, not all of these infants are ill.

Thrombocytopenia is the most common bleeding disorder in the newborn; 20% of all NICU admissions have platelet counts below 50,000/mm^3, and 80% of sick infants have counts below 100,000/mm^3. However, the pathogenesis of the thrombocytopenia can be determined in only 60% of these infants. Abnormalities of the platelet count are due to increased destruction or decreased production, and the underlying cause is mediated by maternal, placental, neonatal, or iatrogenic factors. In most thrombocytopenic newborns, platelet counts are low as a result of increased destruction rather than bone marrow depression. The overall mortality rate for infants with thrombocytopenia is 34%; 22% of these infants exhibit a bleeding diathesis. Infants with a platelet count below 20,000/mm^3 are at particularly high risk for bleeding.

Maternal Factors
Thrombocytopenia is the most common form of hemostatic problem present during pregnancy; 5% to 7% of healthy mothers have platelet counts below 150,000/mm^3. Some of the maternal factors associated with thrombocytopenia are maternal drug ingestion (e.g., chloramphenicol, hydralazine, tolbutamide, and thiazides), maternal eclampsia and hypertension, placental infarction, and immune-mediated maternal platelet antibodies.
Immune-Mediated Maternal Platelet Antibodies
Idiopathic Thrombocytopenia. With immune-mediated thrombocytopenia, in which maternal antibodies destroy platelets, 80% of cases are caused by the autoimmune form, or maternal idiopathic thrombocytopenic purpura (ITP), which strikes women during the second to third decade of life. ITP, now also referred to as autoimmune thrombocytopenia, is a pre-existing condition in which maternal lymphocytes produce IgG antiplatelet antibodies (PAIgG) that attack maternal platelets, usually reducing the platelet count to below 150,000/mm^3. These antibodies are specifically directed at platelet antigen and bind to platelets, which are then phagocytosed by cells carrying a specific receptor, the Fc receptor. The greatest number of cells with this receptor are found in the reticuloendothelial system of the spleen, which is

also the major site of PAIgG production. ITP is often confused with HELLP syndrome, which, in addition to a low platelet count, involves hemolysis and elevated liver enzymes.

Because IgG can cross the placenta, fetal platelets can also be destroyed by the transplacental passage of platelet antibodies, resulting in thrombocytopenia in the fetus and newborn. The mortality rate is 1% to 10% in these affected infants, and the condition can persist postnatally for as long as 4 months.

Neonatal Alloimmune Thrombocytopenia. The remaining 20% of immune-mediated thrombocytopenias are caused by an alloimmune (isoimmune) reaction in which maternal antibodies are produced against foreign fetal platelets (paternally inherited), whereas maternal platelet levels remain normal. This reaction occurs when fetal platelets, which have an antigen not found on maternal platelets, pass into the maternal circulation. The resultant generation of maternal antibodies in response to the fetal platelets is similar to the mechanism behind Rh incompatibility. Unlike Rh incompatibility, alloimmune thrombocytopenia affects 33% to 50% of first pregnancies. The mother develops IgG antibodies that eventually cross into the fetal circulation, resulting in platelet destruction. The PlA1 alloantibodies are responsible for 50% to 80% of neonates with alloimmune thrombocytopenia. This phenomenon occurs in approximately 1 in 2000 to 1 in 5000 live births. The mortality rate of 10% to 15% in alloimmune thrombocytopenia is higher than that in ITP, because bleeding tends to be more severe. The incidence of intracranial hemorrhage in utero is reported to be as high as 10% to 15%, with most cases occurring between 30 and 35 weeks' gestation. Treatment consists of transfusion of maternal platelets, exchange transfusion, and use of IVIG. Platelets usually normalize in the newborn by 4 weeks of age.

Antenatal Treatment. Antenatal treatment is not universally agreed on, but several sources suggest administration of corticosteroids 1 to 2 weeks before delivery and administration of multiple aliquots of IVIG within 7 to 9 days of delivery. Steroids and IVIG are theorized to work in similar fashion by (1) diminishing the production of antiplatelet antibodies, (2) interfering with antibody attachment to the surface of the platelets, and (3) reducing platelet destruction by interfering with phagocytic receptors in the reticuloendothelial system. Suggested steroid therapy consists of prednisone (1 to 2 mg/kg/day, orally) for 2 to 3 weeks. When the desired increase in platelet count occurs, usually within 3 weeks, the dose is tapered to a level that will maintain a platelet count over 50,000/mm³. IVIG can be administered in several different doses and for different lengths of time, but the regimen most often used is 400 mg/kg/day given intravenously for 5 days, with an increase in the platelet count expected within 7 to 9 days. In patients who are unresponsive to these two therapies, splenectomy may be necessary to remove the major site of antibody production and platelet destruction.

Serious bleeding during labor and delivery occurs only in infants with platelet counts below 50,000/mm³. Scalp sampling in fetuses of mothers with ITP and delivery by cesarean section of infants with platelet levels below 50,000/mm³ are recommended.

Postnatal Treatment. Postnatal treatment consists of platelet transfusion, exchange transfusion with blood less than 2 days old, steroid therapy (prednisone, 1 to 5 mg/kg/day), and IVIG. The major difference in therapy between ITP

and alloimmune thrombocytopenia is the use of washed, irradiated, maternal platelets in infants with alloimmune thrombocytopenia.

Neonatal Factors

Neonatal factors associated with thrombocytopenia include asphyxia, an Apgar score of less than 7, disseminated intravascular coagulation, exchange transfusion, infection, smallness for gestational age, necrotizing enterocolitis, hyperbilirubinemia and phototherapy, meconium aspiration, cold injury, polycythemia, pulmonary hypertension, and cardiopulmonary bypass procedure. Treatment of thrombocytopenia caused by neonatal factors consists initially of amelioration of the underlying problem, followed by symptomatic treatment with platelet transfusion. Transfusion therapy should be considered if platelet counts are in the range of 50,000/mm³ to 100,000/mm³ and active bleeding is present. Platelet transfusion should be considered when the level is below 50,000/mm³ even if active bleeding is not present.

A helpful formula for estimating the rise in platelets after transfusion is as follows: one tenth the volume (in milliliters) of a unit of platelets per kilogram of weight raises the platelet count by 50,000/mm³.

Disseminated Intravascular Coagulopathy

Disseminated intravascular coagulation (DIC) is marked by a generalized deficiency of coagulation factors and platelets, which leaves the infant predisposed to hemorrhage. Because this condition is triggered by a pre-existing illness and does not occur independently, treatment consists of identification and resolution of the underlying problem. Releases of tissue factor and substantial injury to endothelial cells are the two major mechanisms that precipitate DIC (Mitchell & Cotran, 1999). The factors most often associated with bleeding that occurs secondary to DIC are obstetrical complications, respiratory distress syndrome, hypoxia, hypotension, necrotizing enterocolitis, and sepsis. Occasionally thrombosis of large vessels can trap platelets and consume an amount of clotting factors sufficient to cause DIC. Mortality rates reach 60% to 80% in infants with DIC who experience severe bleeding.

The hematologic picture of DIC (Table 10-8) reflects a depletion of platelets, prothrombin, fibrinogen, angiotensin III (AT III), protein C, and Factors V, VIII, and XIII. The prothrombin time and partial thromboplastin time are prolonged and are not corrected by the addition of fresh-frozen plasma to the blood sample. The fibrinolytic system is also stimulated, as evidenced by the presence of degradation products of fibrinolysis (i.e., fibrin degradation products or fibrinolytic split products). A commonly used test, measurement of d-dimer, serves as an evaluation of the activation of the fibrinolytic system in that it measures degradation of cross-linked fibrin. However, the d-dimer test may not be very helpful in the newborn because the result commonly is positive in infants who do not have a consumptive coagulopathy.

Successful treatment of DIC depends on alleviation of the underlying cause. Palliative treatment consists of replacement of deficient clotting factors with fresh-frozen plasma and cryoprecipitate, platelet transfusions, and exchange transfusion. Heparin is used infrequently because it carries a higher risk of hemorrhage; it is used only when large-vessel thrombosis occurs.

TABLE 10-8	Hematologic Findings in Disseminated Intravascular Coagulation
Hematologic Feature	**Finding**
Uniformity of clotting defect	Variable
Capillary fragility	Usually abnormal
Bleeding time	Often prolonged
Clotting time	Variable
One-stage prothrombin time	Moderately prolonged
Partial thromboplastin time	Prolonged
Fibrin degradation products	Present
Factor V	Diminished
Fibrinogen	Often diminished
Platelets	Often diminished
Red cell fragmentation	Usually present
Response to vitamin K	Diminished or absent
Associated disease	Severe; may include sepsis, hypoxia, acidosis, or obstetric accident
Previous history	Associated diseases; administration of vitamin K

From Oski F (1976). Hematological problems. In Avery G, editor. Neonatology. Philadelphia: Lippincott.

Differential Diagnosis of Newborn Coagulopathies

Analysis of a number of factors often can aid in the identification of the specific coagulopathy affecting an infant. Careful evaluation of the following factors can pinpoint the correct diagnosis and influence the choice of therapy or intervention:

- A familial history of a bleeding disorder, such as hemophilia
- A maternal history of a bleeding disorder, as in auto-immune thrombocytopenia
- An obstetrical history that suggests a possible abnormality, as in maternal alloimmunization or hypofibrinogenemia
- An adverse neonatal history, such as with hypoxia or asphyxia
- Failure to administer prophylactic vitamin K at birth
- Physical manifestations of a bleeding disorder (e.g., obvious bleeding, the presence or absence of petechiae or ecchymosis) and the infant's overall condition
- Laboratory data that identify specific abnormalities, such as specific coagulation factor deficiencies, thrombocytopenia, and prolonged prothrombin time, partial thromboplastin time, and clotting times

Collaborative Management of a Coagulopathy

Care of an infant with a bleeding diathesis should be aimed at prevention of further injury or bleeding. Supportive care of fragile tissue and limiting the number of blood draws from sites other than central catheters are of great importance in the infant who lacks adequate clotting factors to control bleeding. Appropriate administration of platelets, clotting factors, or blood products requires the correct equipment, the correct method of administration, and conscientious monitoring of vital signs to ensure effective therapy without causing further harm to the infant. Wise decisions regarding replacement blood products are now important in light of the severe and potentially lethal sequelae of acquired infection. Adopting guidelines for transfusion therapy may safeguard infants and eliminate unnecessary exposure to blood products (Table 10-9). Monitoring of laboratory tests to determine continuing needs and the efficacy of therapy is important throughout the infant's course of therapy.

When blood or blood products are administered, the infant must be evaluated continuously for signs of fluid overload and untoward reaction. Although blood reactions are rare in the newborn, they tend to occur within the first 15 minutes of blood or blood product administration. Signs of such reactions include rashes, tachycardia, hypertension, hematuria, cyanosis, and hyperthermia. Throughout the acute course of illness, the hematocrit values and the state of perfusion, rather than the percentage of the infant's blood volume removed, should govern the decision on whether to transfuse. Symptoms of hypovolemia include metabolic acidosis, hypotension, poor perfusion, tachycardia, cyanosis, and shock.

BLOOD COMPONENT REPLACEMENT THERAPY

Whole Blood

This product is not used for routine volume expansion because of the hematocrit dilution that occurs. It is used in surgical procedures that require large volumes of blood for replacement, for exchange transfusions, and for priming heart-lung oxygenators for extracorporeal membrane oxygenation.

Packed Red Blood Cells

Blood is "hard spun" to concentrate cells and allow the supernatant to be removed. Because of this form of preparation, less volume can be administered. Packed RBCs can be reconstituted with normal saline, 5% albumin, or fresh-frozen plasma. Packed RBCs can be used in exchange transfusions or in the treatment of anemia in the acutely ill or symptomatic convalescent infant.

Washed Red Blood Cells

For additional protection, RBCs can be washed to remove as much of the plasma, nonviable RBCs, WBCs, and metabolic wastes as possible. To further eliminate the possibility of a graft-versus-host reaction, cells can be irradiated with 5000 rad; this prevents T-lymphocyte proliferation and, when done in conjunction with washing, can remove up to 95% of T lymphocytes.

Frozen Deglycerolized Red Cells

Frozen storage of deglycerolized RBCs allows preservation of rare units of blood, but the cost of preparation increases considerably. In addition, this product tends to have a higher potassium content and hemoglobin concentration. Centrifuging it, removing the supernatant, and diluting it to the desired hematocrit tend to control these problems.

Fresh-Frozen Plasma

A whole unit of fresh-frozen plasma can be thawed, but once entered, it is good for only 6 hours. If, however, it is packaged in aliquots, such as a quad pack, before freezing and then thawed, the quad pack unit is good for 24 hours once it has thawed. Fresh-frozen plasma provides a rich source of coagulation factors; 10 to 15 ml/kg, which contains 1

TABLE 10-9	Example of Transfusion Guidelines for Preterm Infants	
Hematocrit (%)/ Hemoglobin (g/dl)	**Ventilator Requirements or Symptoms**	**Transfusion Volume**
Hct ≤ 35/Hb ≤ 11	Infants requiring moderate or significant mechanical ventilation (mean airway pressure over 8 cm; H_2O and fractional concentration of oxygen in inspired gas [FiO_2] over 40%)	15 ml/kg of packed red blood cells (PRBCs) over 2 to 4 hours
Hct ≤ 30/Hb ≤ 10	Infants requiring minimal mechanical ventilation (any mechanical ventilation or continuous positive airway pressure [CPAP] >6 cm; H_2O and FiO_2 ≤ 40%)	15 ml/kg PRBCs over 2 to 4 hours
Hct ≤ 25/Hb ≤ 8	Infants receiving supplemental oxygen who do not require mechanical ventilation, but for whom one or more of the following is a factor: • Tachycardia (heart rate over 180) or tachypnea (respiratory rate over 80) for 24 hours or longer • Increased oxygen requirement from the previous 48 hours; specifically, a fourfold or greater increase in nasal cannula flow (e.g., 0.25 to 1 L/min) or an increase in nasal CPAP of 20% or more from the previous 48 hours (e.g., 10 to 12 cm H_2O) • Elevated lactate concentration (2.5 mEq/L or higher) • Weight gain of less than 10 g/kg/day over the previous 4 days while receiving at least 100 kcal/kg/day • Increase in episodes of apnea and bradycardia (more than nine episodes in a 24-hour period or two or more episodes in 24 hours requiring bag and mask ventilation) while receiving therapeutic doses of methylxanthines • Surgery	20 ml/kg PRBCs over 2 to 4 hours (if infant is fluid sensitive, divide into two 10 ml/kg volumes)
Hct ≤ 20/Hb ≤ 7	Infants without any symptoms who have an absolute reticulocyte count under 100,000 mcl*	20 ml/kg PRBCs over 2 to 4 hours (if infant is fluid sensitive, divide into two 10 ml/kg volumes)

Modified from Ohls R (2001). Anemia in the newborn. In Polin R et al, editors. Workbook in practical neonatology, ed 3. Philadelphia: Saunders.
The absolute reticulocyte count is determined by multiplying the number of red blood cells by the percentage of uncorrected reticulocytes

international units/ml of all clotting factors, raises the overall level of clotting factor activity by 20% to 30%. Fresh-frozen plasma often can normalize prolonged prothrombin and partial thromboplastin times in the newborn who has a generalized deficiency in quantity and activity of available clotting factors.

Platelets

The number of platelets available for circulation after transfusion depends on the storage time. In transfusions using platelet bags less than 7 days old, the rise in platelet levels is comparable to the rise seen with the use of fresh platelets. Use of packs older than 7 days achieves only 70% of the rise seen with the use of fresh platelets. Platelets also can be concentrated by centrifuge if smaller volumes are required. An important caveat: platelets require a special administration set for proper infusion.

Granulocytes

Granulocytes, which are used for infusion in septic infants with severe neutropenia, are prepared from fresh donor blood through the process of plasmapheresis. WBCs are removed from the unit of blood, but a large number of RBCs remain. For this reason, the donor unit must be typed and cross-matched to the infant for blood type and Rh compatibility. WBCs usually are irradiated to eliminate donor T cells in an effort to prevent graft-versus-host responses. The use of granulocyte transfusions remains controversial.

Cryoprecipitate

This form of plasma preparation is rich in Factors VIII and XIII and fibrinogen and is useful in the treatment of hemophilia. Because it is a single-donor collection, the risk for infection is lower than with pooled substances. Each unit of cryoprecipitate transfused raises fibrinogen levels by 200 mg/dl per 100 ml of the infant's blood volume.

Factor Concentrates

Factor concentrates are used as specific therapy for identified factor deficiencies. They are obtained from pooled plasma and expose the recipient to multiple donors, thereby increasing the potential for infection, especially with hepatitis B, CMV, and AIDS. Eighty percent of cases of hepatitis B-infected blood can be identified by the third-generation screening tests, and blood screening is also available for CMV. Because the risk for transmission of HIV is increased by pooled concentrates, it is now recommended that concentrates be treated with heat, solvent, steam, detergent, or ultraviolet light to kill any virus that may be present. Currently it is unclear whether such treatment alters or inactivates the clotting activity of factor concentrates.

Case Study

IDENTIFICATION OF THE PROBLEM

A 6-day-old infant is admitted to the neonatal intensive care unit (NICU) with a history of jaundice and lethargy from her local pediatrician's office. A total serum bilirubin (TSB) test drawn at the pediatrician's office had a result of 42 mg%.

ASSESSMENT: HISTORY AND PHYSICAL EXAMINATION

The baby girl was born at 36 weeks' gestation at 3.16 kg to a 24-year-old gravida 1, para 1 mother of Macedonian descent. The pregnancy was complicated by positive maternal group B bacterial streptococcal cultures, and the mother was treated with penicillin chemoprophylaxis. The baby was born by a spontaneous vaginal delivery without complications. The baby was vigorous at birth with Apgar scores of 8 and 9. The mother's blood type was O Rh positive, and the infant's type was A Rh positive. The Coombs' test was positive. The breastfed infant had an unremarkable course but was noted to be jaundiced at 30 hours of age. A TSB test was done with a result of 12.9 mg%. She was discharged home at 40 hours of age.

On admission to the NICU, the infant was noted to be severely jaundiced but pink. Her vital signs were within normal limits (NL), with an axillary temperature of 98.4° F, heart rate of 130 beats/min, respiratory rate of 62 breaths/min, and blood pressure of 58/35 mm Hg with a mean of 45 mm Hg. Her weight on admission was noted to be 2.78 kg, a 12% loss. Her examination was nonremarkable, except for her decreased response to stimuli, poor muscle tone, poor suck, and a decreased Moro reflex. Her glucose screen was 55.

DIFFERENTIAL DIAGNOSIS

Many conditions are known to cause jaundice and lethargy in the newborn. The most common are hyperbilirubinemia, ABO incompatibility, G6PD, hypothyroidism, dehydration secondary to inadequate breast feeding, sepsis, and kernicterus.

DIAGNOSTIC TESTS

To determine the cause of the jaundice and lethargy, a CBC with differential, repeat TSB, electrolytes, calcium, glucose, liver function tests, and T4/TSH, G6PD screen, a hemoglobin electrophoresis, and blood culture all need to be ordered.

WORKING DIAGNOSIS

The baby's repeat bilirubin was 43%; her CBC showed a WBC of 12.1/mm^3, with 35% segs and 4% bands; her hemoglobin was 10.1 g%; her hematocrit was 28.5%; and her reticulocyte count was 2%. The G6PD screen was adequate. Electrolytes, liver function tests, calcium, and glucose were within normal limits, and free T4 was 1.3 ng/dl (NL: 0.9 to 2.1), but TSH was 24.98 milli–international units (NL: 1.7 to 9.1). The hemoglobin electrophoresis was "A, F." These test results suggest a working diagnosis of hyperbilirubinemia secondary to ABO incompatibility and hypothyroidism.

DEVELOPMENT OF MANAGEMENT PLAN

The main goal for an infant with a bilirubin of 43% is to reduce the bilirubin level as quickly as possible to prevent kernicterus. While the blood is being typed and cross-matched, the infant needs to be placed in a neutral thermal environment, made NPO, have a peripheral IV placed, begin D10 with 0.2 normal saline with 20 mEq KCl/L at 120 ml/kg/hr, and started on antibiotics. An attempt should be made to do a cutdown of the umbilical cord to place an umbilical vein and arterial catheter for the exchange transfusion. Double phototherapy lights need to be started as well.

IMPLEMENTATION AND EVALUATION OF EFFECTIVENESS

A double volume exchange transfusion was done over several hours. The infant received a calcium and glucose boluses during the transfusion for low calcium and glucose. Phototherapy lights were continued after the transfusion. Her laboratory tests of TSB, electrolytes, CBC with differential, glucose, and calcium were repeated after the exchange transfusion was completed. Her postprocedure TSB level was 24.6%.

During the exchange the baby became apneic, which required her to be intubated and ventilated for 2 days. She received antibiotics for 3 days and phototherapy for 5 days and was started on Synthroid for her abnormal TSH.

On day of life 12, the TSB was 10.1 mg%. On examination, the infant was slightly hypertonic. A BAER was normal, but an MRI was consistent with kernicterus. She was discharged home with a referral made to the neonatal developmental clinic and early intervention to follow her developmental status.

REFERENCES

American Academy of Pediatrics (AAP) and the American College of Obstetrics and Gynecology (ACOG) (2002). *Guidelines for perinatal care*, ed 5. Elk Grove Village, IL: AAP.

American Academy of Pediatrics, Provisional Committee for Quality Improvement and Subcommittee on Hyperbilirubinemia (2004). Management of hyperbilirubinemia in the newborn infant 35 or more weeks of gestation. *Pediatrics* 114:297-316.

Arad I et al (1988). Serum ferritin levels in preterm infants after multiple blood transfusions. *American journal of perinatology* 5(1):40-43.

Basile LA, Southgate WM (2004). Transfusion therapy. *Neonatal and infant nursing reviews* 4(4):223-230.

Bergman D et al (1994). American Academy of Pediatrics: practice parameter: management of hyperbilirubinemia in the healthy term newborn. *Pediatrics* 94:558-561.

Donato H et al (2000). Effect of early versus late administration of human recombinant erythropoietin on transfusion requirements in premature infants: results of randomized, placebo-controlled, multicenter trial. *Pediatrics* 105:1066.

Edstrom C et al (2000). Developmental aspects of blood hemostasis and disorders of coagulation and fibrinolysis in the neonatal period. In Christensen R, editor. *Hematologic problems of the neonate*. Philadelphia: Saunders.

Emmerson AJ et al (1993). Double-blind trial of recombinant human erythropoietin in preterm infants. *Archives of disease in childhood* 68:291-296.

Gael S (2005). Selection of blood components for neonatal transfusion. *Neonatal reviews* 6(7):e351-355.

Guyton AC, Hall JE (2006a). Blood types, transfusion, tissue and organ transplantation. In Guyton AC, Hall JE, editors. *Textbook of medical physiology*, ed 11. Philadelphia: Saunders.

Guyton A, Hall JE (2006b). Hemostasis and blood coagulation. In Guyton AC, Hall JE, editors. *Textbook of medical physiology*, ed 11. Philadelphia: Saunders.

King J, Jung A (1990). Phototherapy. In Nelson N, editor. *Current therapy in neonatal-perinatal medicine*. Philadelphia: BC Decker.

Kumar D et al (2001). Vitamin K status of premature infants: implications for current recommendations. *Pediatrics* 108:117-122.

Luchtman-Jones L et al (2002). The blood and hematopoietic system. In Fanaroff A, Martin R, editors. *Neonatal-perinatal medicine*, ed 7. St Louis: Mosby.

Maier RF et al (1994). The effect of epoetin-beta (recombinant human erythropoietin) on the need for transfusion in very-low-birth-weight infants. *New England journal of medicine* 330:1173-1178.

Messer J et al (1993). Early treatment of premature infants with recombinant human erythropoietin. *Pediatrics* 92:519-523.

Meyer MP et al (1994). Recombinant human erythropoietin in the treatment of anemia of prematurity: results of a double-blind, placebo-controlled study. *Pediatrics* 93:918-923.

Mitchell R, Cotran R (1999). Hemodynamic disorders, thrombosis and shock. In Cotran R et al, editors. *Robbins pathologic basis of disease*, ed 9. Philadelphia: Saunders.

Ohls RK et al (1993). A randomized, double-blind, placebo-controlled trial of recombinant erythropoietin in treatment of the anemia of bronchopulmonary dysplasia. *Journal of pediatrics* 23:996-1000.

Ohls RK et al (1995). Efficacy and cost analysis of treating very-low-birth-weight infants with erythropoietin during their first 2 weeks of life: a randomized, placebo-controlled trial. *Journal of pediatrics* 126:421-426.

Ozolek JA et al (1994). Prevalence and lack of clinical significance of blood group incompatibility in mothers with blood type A or B. *Journal of pediatrics* 125:87-91.

Porter TF et al (2003). Immunologic disorders in pregnancy. In Scott J et al, editors. *Danforth's obstetrics and gynecology*, ed 9. Philadelphia: Lippincott.

Quinnan G (1993). *Recommendations regarding license amendments and procedures for gamma irradiation of blood products*. Washington, DC: U.S. Department of Health and Human Services, Center for Biologics Evaluation and Research, Food and Drug Administration.

Robertson J, Shilkofski N (2005). *Harriet Lane handbook*, ed 17. St Louis: Mosby.

Shannon KM et al (1995). Recombinant human erythropoietin stimulates erythropoiesis and reduces erythrocyte transfusions in very-low-birth-weight preterm infants. *Pediatrics* 95:1-8.

Wong RJ et al (2006). Neonatal jaundice and liver disease. In Martin R, Fanaroff A, Walsh M, editors. *Neonatal-perinatal medicine*, ed 8, St Louis: Mosby.

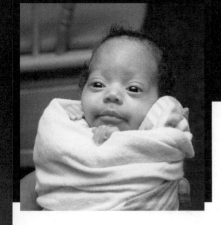

Chapter 11

Musculoskeletal System

Joyce M. Butler

Abnormalities of the neonatal musculoskeletal system range from a subtle brachydactyly to a fatal form of osteogenesis imperfecta congenita. Causes range from uterine malpositioning of the fetus to autosomal dominant disorders. Regardless of the clinical significance, an overt structural defect can become the focus of parental attention. Assessment of the musculoskeletal system—which can have multiple normal variants—and knowledge of pathogenesis, sequelae, treatment, and prognoses for deformities of this system is imperative to the clinician. Delay in diagnosis and treatment may contribute to a less than optimal outcome of the musculoskeletal deformity. Appropriate education of the family by the health care professional is often paramount to a beneficial outcome because many musculoskeletal disorders require compliance with long-term therapy.

Deformities of the musculoskeletal system create not only functional problems, but, in some cases, visible defects as well. The appearance of the deformity and type of dysfunction may greatly affect how the parent views the neonate, affecting the infant's potential for positive growth and development. Proper assessment and description of the musculoskeletal system requires the clinician to be familiar with the associated terminology. Box 11-1 identifies some of the more common terms used when describing the musculoskeletal system.

This chapter identifies some of the most common musculoskeletal defects identified in the newborn period. In addition, it describes the management as well as the long-term implications of the functional and aesthetic problems encountered with musculoskeletal defects and dysfunction.

ASSESSMENT

Astute systematic observation is the key tool for assessing the neonatal musculoskeletal system. Visual inspection should begin in one body region—cephalic or caudal—and progress along the body in an organized fashion. For the initial examination, view the infant in a quiet resting state to assess posture, positioning, and identification of any overt anomalies. Active movement by the infant allows the clinician to view muscle tone and active ranges of motion. Manipulation is used to assess passive range of motion, including joint mobility. Radiologic studies as well as simple body measurements aid the clinician in identifying covert musculoskeletal deformities.

Maternal history is reviewed for uterine anomalies such as the bifid uterus, amniotic fluid volume, and fetal movement during gestation, as well as the birthing process. Family history is also important to obtain, as mild forms of defects, such as osteogenesis imperfecta, may be misdiagnosed in a family as simply short stature. In developing a differential diagnoses, the

clinician must be aware that a combination of deformities present in a neonate may be a small part of a larger syndrome. Conversely, congenital anomalies that present in combination may be coincidental findings.

SKELETAL DYSPLASIAS/CONNECTIVE TISSUE DISORDERS

The most dramatic birth defects involving the musculoskeletal system include skeletal dysplasias and connective tissue disorders such as achondroplasia, hypochondroplasia, thanatophoric dysplasia, and osteogenesis imperfecta. These defects can be mild, even diagnosed later in life, or fatal, presenting immediately in the newborn period. These types of defects involve an abnormality in endochondral ossification (long bone formation) or involving the development of the connective tissue.

Osteogenesis Imperfecta
Anatomy and Pathophysiology

Osteogenesis imperfecta (OI) is a connective tissue disorder with genetic origins. The primary pathophysiologic defect involves the collagen structure. A genetic mutation occurs either in the COL1A1 or COL1A2 gene responsible for collagen formation (Lashley, 2005). Collagen (the major extracellular protein) formation fails to progress beyond the reticulin fiber stage. Further significant disruption in the collagen formation in OI includes a defect in cross-linking that results in decreased collagen stability. Although osteoblastic activity appears normal, typically no collagen is produced. Any tissue containing collagen, such as sclerae, bones, ligaments, and teeth, may be affected. Through various clinical, genetic, and biochemical studies, OI has been determined to be heterogeneous; it may result from autosomal recessive or autosomal dominant disorders as well as from spontaneous mutations (Spitz, 1996). Clinical presentations of OI range from mild affectations to individuals with fatal prognoses. The overall incidence in Western countries is reported as 1:20,000 live births (Lashley, 2005).

Based on a classification system by Sillence and Danks (1978), OI is divided into four major groups; two are autosomal recessive, and two are autosomal dominant. Two of the groups (OI types I and IV) are further subdivided according to the absence or presence of dentin (involving the teeth) abnormalities (dentinogenesis imperfecta). Dentinogenesis imperfecta occurs when the dentin layer is affected concomitant with constriction of the pulp space. The clinical appearance of dentinogenesis imperfecta involves teeth that are grayish blue to brown in color. The teeth are typically worn

BOX 11-1

Common Musculoskeletal Terms

Valgus: positioning an anatomical part away from the body's midline; a part that is in **abduction**

Varus: positioning an anatomical part inward, or toward the body's midline; a part that is in **adduction**

Equinus: flexion of the midfoot/sole

Talipes: foot, generally used to describe various foot deformities

Clinodactyly: deviation of fingertips resulting in a bent or curved appearance

Camptodactyly: Permanent flexion of one or more finger joints

Reduction: restoration to a normal position

Plagiocephaly: misshapen skull/head

down because of decreased resistance to pressure. The deciduous teeth are more often affected than the permanent teeth. It is important to explain to the parents that the aesthetic appearance of the child may improve with the emergence of permanent teeth.

Continuing on the Sillence and Danks categories, additional groups of OI have been defined. Types V and VI, which are considered to be extensions of the type IV group of OI, do not appear to have defects in the type I collagen genes (Glorieux et al 2000, 2002).

Clinical Presentation

OI type I is an autosomal dominant disorder with variable penetrance. Simply stated, the clinical appearance of affected individuals in the same family may range from mild to severe.

The clinical presentation of this disorder is evident in the neonatal period in 10% of affected individuals. Fractures are the primary sign in neonates. Affected neonates typically have normal height and weight for their gestational age. Other clinical features include severe hearing impairment, with an incidence of 40:1, and preponderance for bruising. The sclerae are often bluish as well; however, this is difficult to define in the neonatal period.

OI types I and IV are subdivided into types 1/IVA and 1/IVB depending on the presence of dentinogenesis imperfecta. Dentin abnormalities are found in OI type 1/IVB. These are identified as the child matures.

Prenatal diagnosis of type I is difficult, as most cases do not exhibit fractures in utero as do the more severe forms of OI, which exhibit repeated fractures and bowing of the fetal extremities. In one recent study, the percentage of OI type I diagnosed prenatally was 3.4% vs 49% of OI type II diagnosed in the prenatal period (Cubert et al, 2001). If a family history is significant for osteogenesis, prenatal testing evaluating the collagen through a chorionic villus sample can determine abnormal collagen formation indicating a mutation in either the COL1A1 or COL1A2 genes, although this is not 100% effective. Ultrasonography may detect more severe forms with early fractures and bowing of extremities.

OI type II is also referred to as the perinatal-lethal type. It is an autosomal recessive disorder that results in death either in utero or in the perinatal/neonatal period. Prenatal diagnosis is possible with this condition because of the multiple in utero

fractures and bowing of extremities. Death can occur through damage to vital organs—brain, liver, and lungs—which are not protected by the fragile bony structures. The ribcage tends to be narrow and shortened with severe distress noted with spontaneous breathing. Affected infants are small for gestational age with shortened body and legs, but the head appears large for body size. Both upper and lower extremities tend to be shortened and deformed with multiple fractures. Radiographic films demonstrate both old and new multiple fractures and crumbled long bones. Ribs and bones may also appear thin and difficult to discern. Trauma of birth exacts a further toll on the appearance of these infants and contributes to the maceration of the head and limbs.

OI type III is a rare, severe disorder with autosomal recessive inheritance pattern. This is the most severe type for those surviving the neonatal period. Fractures may be present at birth, and the clinical course may simulate OI type II. Variations between types II and III are identified on physical examination. Neonates with OI type III have normal height and weight for gestational age at birth. Although multiple rib fractures may appear on chest radiographs, the beaded rib appearance is absent. The long bones in OI type II are crumbled, whereas the bones in type III have multiple fractures and calcifications. The extremities do not usually appear deformed, as in type II; however, individuals affected with OI type III have the shortest stature for all survivors of OI disorders. Mortality rates for children and young adults with OI type III are high because of the development of severe kyphoscoliosis and pulmonary complications.

OI type IV is similar to type I in that it is an autosomal dominant disorder with variable penetrance. OI type IV resembles type I in terms of presentation. Newborns rarely have identified fractures, but a number of fractures occur as the child begins to ambulate, with increased weight bearing. These infants also present with growth that is average for gestational age. The growth pattern can change, however, as the child matures, because of increased bowing and kyphoscoliosis, with a short stature compared to a normal height at maturity in milder forms of type I. OI type IV can also progress to a more severe form depending on the degree of kyphoscoliosis and vertebral compression fractures, often resembling type III. Unlike type III, life span in type IV is not affected.

Differential Diagnosis

Milder forms can be difficult to diagnose in the neonatal period. Only 10% of mild OI cases will present in the neonatal period. In these milder cases, fractures in the neonatal period may result from birth trauma. Fractures are most abundant in the arms, legs, clavicles, and ribs. A comprehensive connective tissue workup is not indicated in isolated neonatal fractures; however, this should prompt a more in-depth history of the family in terms of number of broken bones and so forth, as mild OI cases can be easily overlooked.

Multiple rib fractures in a neonate may prompt respiratory compromise because the pain from the fractures thwarts the infant's breathing attempts. OI may be suspected when it is difficult to wean an infant from ventilatory support and other pathologic causes have been ruled out. In such cases, chest radiographs should be closely inspected for rib fractures and callus formation. Case reports have also identified newborns who sustained fractures of the femurs during routine examination of the hip for dysplasia.

In contrast, the severe forms of OI may imitate skeletal dysplasias with a dwarf/short-limbed appearance. These can be distinguished by radiographs, as the skeletal dysplasias may have a short-limbed dwarf appearance without fractures, whereas the bowing and short-limbed appearance of an infant with OI is due to multiple fractures and crumbling long bones.

Diagnosis

Accurate diagnosis of OI disorders is of primary concern for the affected individual and family. Recurrence rates and inheritance patterns vary among the recessive and dominant forms as well as spontaneous mutations.

Radiographic studies as well as tissue and blood sampling for genetic evaluation lead to the actual diagnosis of osteogenesis imperfecta. Diagnosis is often made on clinical presentation with genetic/collagen studies used to confirm the diagnosis.

As many as 10% to 15% of affected individuals may test negative for OI based on collagen studies, and up to 5% of those with clinical evidence of OI may have normal genetic/DNA assays. In addition, there is a delay of several weeks before collagen and genetic/DNA assays can be completed, on average.

Diagnoses of child abuse have been incorrectly reported in mild OI cases with the onset of fractures and more obvious bruising occurring as the infant begins to mature toward the end of the first year of life. The delay between presentation and confirmation of OI is extremely disruptive and upsetting to the family suspected of child abuse.

Treatment

No treatment for the underlying pathologic cause of OI disorders exists. Therefore management of OI centers on support and promotion of independence in terms of mobility, function, and social integration. Rehabilitation techniques include active range of motion, strengthening exercises, stretching, and coordination exercises. Water activities are well tolerated, even in severely affected patients. Outcome appears to be enhanced when physical and occupational therapies are instituted promptly after birth, condition allowing. Independent living is improved in the population when the affected individual is mobile. One study evaluated the ability of children with OI to walk and reported that the type of OI was the most important clinical indicator for the ability to walk (Engelbert et al, 2000). Children with type III and IV had a lower chance of walking than those with type I. Positive clinical signs associated with the development of the ability to walk included rolling over before 8 months, supported sitting before 9 months, sitting without support by 12 months, and pulling to a standing position without support before 12 months (Engelbert et al, 2000).

Rodding surgery is a surgical technique used as an aid to improve the chances of ambulation or to improve a bone with frequent or poorly healing fractures. Children older than 1 year can be considered for this surgery. A long bone—typically the femur or tibia, but the arm or spine can also be involved—is threaded onto a stainless steel or titanium rod. This rod acts like an internal splint to stabilize the bone. Fractures may still occur with the splinted bone, but the rod will assist in maintaining the bone in alignment.

Ongoing research continues to evaluate the use of biophosphonates. This group of medications is aimed at reducing the activity of the osteoclasts in bone (the cells that break down and resorb bone) and increasing the life and activity of the osteoblasts (the cells which make new bone). The individual with OI will still have abnormal bone formation, but the volume of bone (density) would theoretically increase.

One study involving a treatment period of 5 years demonstrated increased bone density, reduced bone pain, increased mobility, and decreased fractures in 30 children diagnosed with moderate to severe OI. (Glorieux et al, 1998). Among the limitations of this study is the fact that it was a nonblinded, small study for which no control (placebo) group was included. Further studies involving biophosphonates are ongoing.

In addition, bone marrow transplants are also receiving attention after a report that three children demonstrated improvement in bone mineral density, better growth, and fewer fractures following bone marrow transplants from their respective siblings (Horwitz, 1999). Further investigation continues in an effort to identify benefits of this therapy for individuals with OI.

Management

In the neonatal period, infants with OI are managed according to clinical presentation and maturity for a particular gestational age. Health care professionals as well as family are reminded to handle the infant carefully. Padded splints for the extremities may help reduce the incidence of accidental fractures, and signs should be posted on the infant's bed as a reminder of handling techniques. As the infant grows, padded orthotic devices support the trunk and extremities to reduce the incidence of skeletal deformities such as kyphoscoliosis.

Vascular checks of casted or splinted extremities are required. Pallor would be indicative of decreased or poor arterial flow with cyanosis a sign of venous stasis. Although pulse checks may be helpful, the clinician should realize that by the time a pulse is absent, irreparable harm may have occurred. For this reason, parents should be taught to assess color and capillary refill rather than pulse palpation.

An infant with OI necessitates skin care in terms of positioning. Bedding should be of the type to discourage decubitus formation as the infant may have minimal spontaneous movement secondary to pain from fractures. Splints (e.g., rolled blankets or sandbags) placed beside the infant's chest stabilize the thoracic wall and potentiate effective ventilation. These splints appear to be most effective in cases of multiple rib fractures.

Pain relief through medication and supportive measures is a necessity. The infant may react to pain caused by multiple fractures through facial grimacing and crying on movement. Alterations in vital signs (e.g., tachycardia, tachypnea, and hypertension), irritability, and restlessness have also been attributed to pain in the neonate.

Proper handling is a key to avoiding additional fractures. Never pick up an infant or child from under the arms, as this places excessive pressure on the shoulders and ribs. Diapering should be accomplished by gently lifting the lower body with a hand placed under the buttocks, never by pulling up at the ankles.

Because of the limited movement of infants and children with more severe forms of OI and increased fractures, many children experience a developmental delay. Physical therapy and occupational therapy working with the family and child are necessary to augment continuing development.

Acutely, respiratory complications are evident immediately following delivery in severe OI. These infants typically have a critical course and, because of the severity of their disease, are often the ones with greatest mortality in the newborn period. Intubation is necessary after delivery, and the majority rarely wean off this support. Infants affected with milder forms of OI presenting in the newborn period may experience periods of tachypnea and oxygen needs with increased activity and PO feedings. This may be due to multiple rib fractures resulting in pain and decreased tidal volume with inspiration. As the child ages, respiratory complications may become more apparent when the complication of kyphoscoliosis is present, as the thorax is compromised and compressed. In these situations, shortness of breath, fatigue, and sleep apnea may occur.

Skeletal Dysplasia

Skeletal dysplasia identifies a group of clinical disorders that involve abnormal endochondral ossification. It includes achondroplasia, hypochondroplasia, and thanatophoric dysplasia, all of which present with a short-limbed skeletal dysplasia at varying ages of development.

Achondroplasia

Although the word *achondroplasia* was once used to describe any form of dwarfism, it is now recognized as one distinct type of dwarfism having characteristic features. Achondroplasia has an autosomal dominant pattern of inheritance and is the most common nonlethal skeletal dysplasia. Most cases occur by spontaneous mutation. The incidence of achondroplasia has varied in the past as a result of multiple forms of skeletal dysplasia diagnosed as achondroplasia. The incidence if 2.5 per 100,000 live births. One risk factor for spontaneous mutation that involves achondroplasia appears to be advanced paternal age.

Achondroplastic infants can be identified at birth with a rhizomelic shortening of the extremities. In other words, when the arms are viewed, the upper arm (humerus bone) will appear more severely shortened when compared to the lower arm (radius and ulnar bones). The same holds for the lower extremities, where the thigh (femur) will appear more severely shortened than the lower leg (tibia and fibular bones). The infant who is affected with achondroplasia also presents with a disproportionately large head with frontal bossing and depressed nasal bridge. The hands are small with a trident configuration that describes the appearance of the fingers and an increased spacing between the long and ring fingers. Identification of mild hypotonia and limitation of elbow extension with laxity in most other joints is also noted in the achondroplastic child. These neuromuscular and skeletal anomalies—including the mild hypotonia, rhizomelia, joint laxity, and reduced elbow extension—can produce a delay in gross motor milestones but generally improve to normal over the first few years of life. Central intelligence is normal in most cases.

Hypochondroplasia

Hypochondroplasia is rarely noted at birth, as the length of the infant is often normal. The short stature becomes clinically apparent around 24 months of age. This condition is rarely diagnosed in the neonatal period but may present with macrocephaly. Hypochondroplastic children and adults experience some of the similar orthopedic complications as the achondroplastic individual. Some of these include joint and lower back pain.

Thanatophoric Dysplasia

Thanatophoric dysplasia is the third in this series of common skeletal dysplasias. It is a lethal defect and is often compared to osteogenesis imperfecta, type II in terms of its clinical scenario after birth, with death usually in several hours or days. Mortality is high secondary to pulmonary hypoplasia. The clinical presentation of thanatophoric dysplasia describes a fetal environment of reduced fetal movements and polyhydramnios. Hypotonia in the neonate with macrocephaly, often presenting as a clover leaf–shaped skull, is believed secondary to early fusion of the coronal and lambdoidal sutures. The limbs are short and bowed (Figure 11-1) with severe brachydactyly or short digits. The thorax is very narrow and short (Figure 11-2), reminding the clinician of the abnormal pulmonary development and severe pulmonary hypoplasia. The abdomen has a protuberant appearance. Almost all cases of thanatophoric dysplasia result from a new genetic mutation.

Differential Diagnosis. The differential diagnosis of a neonate with dwarflike appearance includes achondroplasia, OI type II, thanatophoric dwarfism, asphyxiating thoracic dysplasia, lethal short limb–polydactyly syndromes, and achondrogenesis. In achondroplasia, the patient has markedly shortened limbs and often bowing of the lower limbs, but

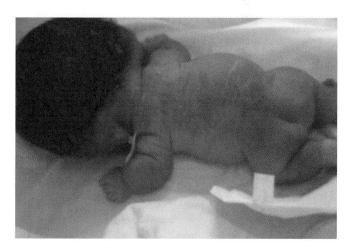

FIGURE **11-1**
Thanatophoric dysplasia: shortened, bowed extremities.

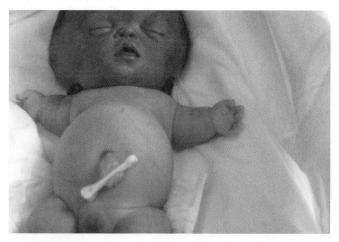

FIGURE **11-2**
Thanatophoric dysplasia: narrow thorax and protuberant abdomen.

radiographic studies do not show evidence of multiple fractures and long-bone crumbling as seen in OI type II. Thanatophoric dwarfism and achondrogenesis, both typically fatal in the neonatal period, are characterized by an extremely narrow chest and marked defective ossification, respectively.

Management. Management of skeletal dysplasias depends on the long-term outcome for the specific type of dysplasia. As noted in the previous section, many of these skeletal dysplasias presenting in the newborn period are lethal during the newborn period. With nonlethal varieties, the complications are primarily neurologic and involve the spinal nerves. Anatomic configuration of the intraspinal canal results in pressure on the cord and spinal nerves. This pressure produces chronic backache and, in the most severe scenario, paraplegia. Referrals to physical and occupational therapists, along with long-term orthopedic follow-up, can reduce some of the complications. If these changes in the spinal column do occur, the child is at greatest risk for development of increased respiratory difficulties, mobility problems, self-concept and self-esteem concerns, physical pain, and central or peripheral nervous system neuropathies.

Sisk and colleagues (1999) described a 38% incidence of obstructive sleep apnea in children with achondroplasia. Apnea usually presented in early childhood. Adenotonsillectomy was more successful than adenoidectomy; follow-up surgery in the two groups was reported as 18% and 90%, respectively.

Because children with achondroplasia have a different appearance than their peers, any exaggeration of the condition can add to a faulty self-concept. As the child grows, continual assessment by health care professionals and the parents concerning the personal image that the child is developing is prelude to a positive self-esteem. Positive support of parents during the neonatal period through comments about what the infant is doing and how the infant looks may provide a role model of positive behavior that the parents can emulate with the child.

ARTHROGRYPOSIS

Historically, the term *arthrogryposis* (curved, hooked joint) has been used not only to provide a description of a clinical appearance but also as a diagnosis for various conditions. The one common denominator for conditions termed arthrogryposis is the presence of multiple congenital joint contractures. More than 150 known conditions feature multiple congenital contractures as the dominant feature; many of these conditions are syndromes unrelated to a chromosomal or genetic problem.

The most common forms of arthrogryposis multiplex congenital are autosomal dominant distal arthrogryposis, amyoplasia, multiple pterygium syndrome, and cerebro-oculo-facio-skeletal syndrome. Pena-Shokeir syndrome is a rare presentation of arthrogryposis associated with severe pulmonary hypoplasia. Most affected infants die in the neonatal period or in the first 12 months of life (Hall, 1981).

Genetic counseling varies depending on whether arthrogryposis is the primary diagnosis or whether it is a part of a more complex syndrome or genetic defect. Genetic variations have included spontaneous mutation, X-linked, as well as autosomal dominant and recessive.

Pathology

Arthrogryposis involves congenital, nonprogressive limitation of movement in two or more joints in different body areas. The deformity primarily results from fibrous and fatty changes in muscles secondary to decreased fetal movement. Although muscles undergo normal embryologic development, they are replaced by fibrous and fatty tissue after a reduction of normal fetal movement. The physiologic muscle changes subsequently produce contracted joints. Animal studies have produced congenital joint contractures by decreasing fetal movement through various processes. Ultimately, any process that result in limited intrauterine movement by the fetus can lead to multiple congenital contractures. The severity of such contractures increases with a longer duration of limited movement. If movement is limited early in fetal development, the severity of contractures will be more severe. The causes of decreased fetal movement can be classified into three categories, which are listed in Table 11-1.

Diagnosis

Classification of the affected body parts is necessary prior to further diagnosis. Amyoplasia, classic arthrogryposis, is of a sporadic nature. It has a typical appearance with symmetrical joint involvement, usually of all four limbs, and decreased muscle mass. Frequency of joint involvement increases from proximal to distal joints. Therefore, severe equinovarus deformities are almost universal and the wrists are typically flexed. The elbows and knees can be in a flexed or extended position; however, in most cases, both upper and lower extremities are in extension. Dimpling may be noted at the elbows and knees. Shoulders are internally rotated. Normal skin creases overlying the joints are absent, and the skin is tense and glossy.

Facial features are characterized by mild micrognathia. A midline hemangioma of the eyes, nasal bridge, and forehead may be present and usually fades with time. A less severe form, distal arthrogryposis, features limb involvement primarily of the hands and feet. Fingers tend to be overlapping with clenched fists, thumbs flexed into palms, and fingers with ulnar deviation (clinodactyly). Camptodactyly can also be identified

TABLE **11-1**	Etiology of Decreased Fetal Movement
Category	**Examples**
MYOPATHIC Abnormal muscle function secondary to failure of muscle formation or degeneration	Congenital muscular dystrophy Absence of muscles
NEUROPATHIC Abnormal nerve function or innervation that involves either CNS or peripheral nervous system Abnormal connective tissue	Drugs or toxins CNS malformations: decreased number of anterior horn cells
MECHANICAL LIMITATION Produces compression within uterus	Multiple gestation Amniotic rupture Oligohydramnios Uterine myomas or bifid uterus

CNS, *Central nervous system.*

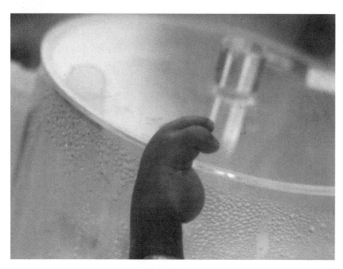

FIGURE **11-3**
Arthrogryposis: severe ankle extension (talipes equinus) and midfoot flexion.

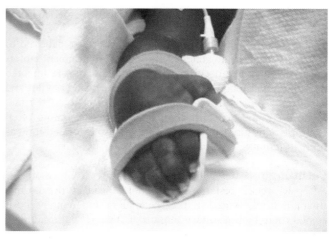

FIGURE **11-4**
Arthrogryposis: hand splint.

as well as positional foot abnormalities; individuals generally have normal intelligence. Figure 11-3 illustrates the severe contracture involving the ankle with talipes equinus (midfoot flexion).

Genetic evaluation is required to identify a possible abnormality. If a specific genetic etiology or specific syndrome is located, an attempt at characterizing the long-term prognosis is improved. Otherwise the family is counseled as to the uncertainty of neurologic development. It is recognized that congenital contractures are not resolved or healed, but remain a limitation during one's lifetime.

In addition to genetic evaluation, diagnosis may be achieved with the use of muscle biopsy and nerve conduction tests, as well as imaging of the brain and spinal cord.

Collaborative Management

Excluding infants with concurrent central nervous system (CNS) dysfunction, infants with multiple congenital contractures have excellent prognoses. The goal of collaborative management is to achieve and maintain an acceptable range of motion in the affected joints. With appropriate management, independent living is attainable for many individuals.

During the newborn period, it is often a challenge to hold, feed, and care for these infants because of the extended upper and lower extremities and reduced inability to easily position these limbs due to the contractures. Physical therapy should be initiated early in the neonatal period. In the past, infants with multiple congenital contractures were casted; however, this therapy was found to produce additional muscle atrophy secondary to the immobilization. Currently, physical therapy is used in conjunction with splinting when necessary. Splints are molded and shaped specifically for each limb dependent on severity of contractures and positioning (Figure 11-4).

Physical therapy is a lifetime process, and parents are taught the techniques to use with their children. Parental or family involvement is a key factor in the success of the therapy for these infants. Creativity on the part of the health care professional as well as on the part of the parents complements efforts to manipulate the rather rigid infant during feedings,

sleeping, holding, and daily care activities. Parents may need referrals to agencies providing respite care or assistance from volunteers to maintain daily care needs.

Theoretically, the development of congenital contractures is a result of decreased fetal movement. Therefore, researchers continue to examine ways to stimulate fetal movement for those considered at high risk for the development of multiple congenital contractures. High-risk individuals include those with a positive family history of arthrogryposis, maternal complaints of decreased fetal movement, oligohydramnios, and positive family history of muscle, nerve, CNS, or connective tissue abnormalities that might lead to decreased ability to move fetal body parts during development.

If in utero contractures develop secondary to fetal akinesia, the theory is that any stimulation of movement has the potential for preventing contractures. Stimulation could be in the form of intrauterine physical therapy and drugs such as caffeine for fetal stimulation.

Prognosis

The long-term prognosis for multiple congenital contractures depends on the extent of involvement. Mortality rates are low for those without CNS involvement (1% to 7%). For those with CNS involvement, mortality rates rise to almost 50%.

DEVELOPMENTAL DYSPLASIA OF THE HIP (DDH)

Developmental dysplasia of the hip refers to any manifestation of hip instability, ranging from subluxation to complete dislocation. DDH remains a common problem despite almost universal neonatal screening. Reports indicate success rates as high as 100% for the diagnosis of DDH in the neonatal period, yet these same reports also suggest that neonatal screening programs are ineffective. Although controversy surrounds the usefulness of neonatal screening programs for the diagnosis of DDH, these programs have led to earlier diagnosis and treatment for many infants. Because some infants possess normal hip movement, some examinations may initially be normal, yet later exhibit abnormal hip development. Dysplastic hip screenings should be performed at routine health visits at 2 weeks and again at 2, 4, 6, 9, and 12 months of age.

Reports of the incidence of DDH vary. The incidence in the United States is approximately 1.5 per 1000 live births. Differences in DDH vary between ethnic groups, believed to be multifactorial, with genetic, ethnic, and environment factors all involved in the occurrence rates. Caucasians are affected more often, although the incidence rises in Scandinavian and Mediterranean countries. Females are affected 6 to 8 times more often, and generally the left hip is affected more often than the right hip. Incidence of DDH is also increased in first-born children.

Pathology

After 40 weeks' gestation, the femoral head in the normal infant is firmly seated in the acetabulum and remains positioned there by the surface tension of the synovial fluid. The hips of a normal infant are difficult to dislocate. Conversely, the infant with a dysplastic hip has a loosely fitting femoral head and acetabulum. Because of this pathophysiologic phenomenon, the femoral head can assume several abnormal positions in an infant with DDH. One such position is termed subluxation. Subluxation occurs when the femoral head can be moved to the edge of the acetabulum but not completely out of it. Another position is termed dislocatable hip. A dislocatable hip exists when the femoral head can be displaced from the acetabulum by manipulation but returns to the acetabulum afterward. The femoral head can also be found in a completely dislocated position at birth. Dislocated hips may or may not be reduced by manipulation.

DDH is a dynamic disorder that may improve or deteriorate with or without treatment. Thus, the joint may spontaneously dislocate and reduce (return to normal position) with normal neonatal movement. At the initial phase of the disorder, seen during the neonatal period, no other significant pathologic concerns exist. With time, this simple mechanism progresses in complexity because of adaptive changes. DDH can eventually progress to permanent reduction, complete dislocation, or dysplasia (abnormal development). More than 60% of infants with hip instability stabilize within the first week of life, and 88% stabilize postnatally within the second month. Only 12% of infants with initial hip instability are considered to have DDH with potential for progression.

When complete dislocation occurs, pathologic changes occur to the femoral head, acetabulum, and ilium. This complete dislocation is due to the adaptive changes that occur in the adjacent tissue and bone. The long-term complication of dislocation, when adequate treatment has not occurred, is degenerative changes of both the femoral head and the acetabulum. Once adaptive changes occur, risk for progressive degeneration despite treatment increases. The subluxated hip, when not diagnosed in the neonatal period, is generally diagnosed at adolescence, when the stress of puberty and rapid growth spurts occur. With subluxation, the femoral head is laterally displaced and pushed upward into the joint, although not completely out of the acetabulum. As the child grows and increased weight bearing occurs, the femoral head slides around and moves to the joint's edge. Degenerative changes result from this continual sliding. Sclerosis of the underlying bone, loss of cartilage, and formation of degenerative cysts are the most common degenerative changes (Cooperman & Thompson, 2002).

The pathology associated with an increase of DDH in primigravidas may be due to the unstretched uterine and abdominal muscles, oligohydramnios, and the high association of fetal breech positioning in primigravidas. In addition, the increased incidence of DDH in females appears secondary to the fact that twice as many females as males present in the breech position, and females appear to have heightened laxity in response to maternal relaxin hormones. The breech position remains a major contributory factor in the development of DDH. Increased incidence of left hip involvement appears secondary to the tendency of the fetus to lie with its left thigh against the maternal sacrum. This position forces the left hip into a posture of flexion and adduction. Thus the femoral head is covered more by the joint capsule than by the acetabulum.

Diagnosis

In the neonatal period, the Ortolani and Barlow maneuvers are useful in making the diagnosis of DDH. The Ortolani test is used to identify a dislocated hip of a newborn, and the Barlow test is used to determine whether the hip is dislocatable (Barlow, 1962; Ortolani, 1976). In practice, both procedures are done in sequence. For examination the infant is placed on a firm surface in the supine position, in a relaxed and quiet state. Only one hip is examined at a time. To perform the Ortolani test, the clinician stabilizes the infant's pelvis with one hand and with the other hand grasps the infant's thigh on the side to be tested. The examiner's middle finger is located over the greater trochanter (lateral aspect of upper thigh), and the thumb is around the base of the knee wrapping around to the inner thigh. The hip and knee are in flexion. The infant's leg is then gently abducted (legs pulled away from midline) with an anterior lift. In a positive Ortolani test, a "clunk" is heard with abduction. This clunk occurs as the dislocated femoral head slides over the posterior rim of the acetabulum and into the hip socket. False positive diagnoses of DDH have occurred when the examiner misinterprets a normal "click" for a clunk. A click is not a sign of DDH, but may be heard as a result of snapping of ligaments or tendons, and most clicks are normal. If a click is noted, it is important to follow up within a period of weeks for re-evaluation.

Barlow's test attempts to manipulate the femoral head out and posteriorly out of the socket. If there is little to no movement of the hip during these exams, the hip may be dislocated and is not able to be reduced, thereby providing a false negative test for hip dislocation. Family and case history may be more significant, as the risk of DDH in an infant is increased if either of the parents were diagnosed with this developmental disorder.

When the femoral head is subluxated, the examiner may observe a sliding motion in the hip joint during physical examination. This sliding motion can be characteristic of an unstable hip joint. Most cases of unstable hips spontaneously resolve without treatment. As there is no way to determine which hips will reduce and stabilize without treatment, treating all unstable hips is the best approach. The use of ultrasonography is not universally recommended as a screening tool for DDH (Woolacott, 2005). The use of periodic physical exams for the confirmation/diagnosis and treatment of hip dysplasia is deemed the most acceptable in terms of screening guidelines.

After 6 months of age, the Ortolani and Barlow maneuvers are inappropriate and the examiner at that time will monitor leg length, walking gait, and skin creases over the legs and hips for asymmetry. Radiographic studies of the hip after 6 months of age can identify a poorly formed acetabulum.

It is important to note that the American Academy of Pediatrics (AAP) recommends that if a newborn is discharged before 48 hours of age, he or she should be reexamined with a repeat hip exam 2 to 4 days after discharge (Morey, 2001).

Collaborative Management

The goal of management is to achieve and maintain reduction of the unstable hip. The sooner treatment is implemented, the greater the chance for successful outcome. Various splint devices are used to treat DDH in infants. Examples of splints include the Pavlik harness, von Rosen splint, Denis Browne hip adduction splint, and Frejka pillow splint. The most commonly used splint for neonates is the Pavlik harness. Once commonly used, the triple diaper method (to maintain legs in abduction) is not recommended by the AAP for use in stabilizing a hip.

The Pavlik harness allows for spontaneous hip and lower extremity movement while maintaining reduction of the hip joint. It can be worn comfortably during all aspects of normal newborn care, including diaper changes. The Pavlik harness can be adjusted for growth. It is indicated for use in newborns and infants up to 6 to 8 months of age. Use of this harness is contraindicated for infants able to stand and for those in whom the hip joint is not reducible by manipulation, specifically the Ortolani procedure, because the infant may attempt to bear weight while wearing the harness, thus potentially pushing the hip out of alignment. This movement counteracts reduction of the hip joint. The greatest danger is of the child become entangled in the parachute-like straps while attempting to push up to a standing position. A major factor influencing the success of the Pavlik harness is parental compliance with the treatment. With this condition, extensive parental education is imperative. The use of the harness is typically around 3 months.

Long-Term Consequences and Complications

As with most therapeutic treatments, the potential for iatrogenic complications exists. Complications observed following DDH treatment include avascular necrosis, redislocation, and acetabular dysplasia. Complications can result from either inadequate or overly aggressive treatment.

An additional complication that has been reported with the use of the Pavlik harness is the development of brachial plexus palsy (Mostert et al, 2000). The tension of the shoulder harness appears related to this complication. The harness may be applied too tightly or may not be modified with the infant's growth, resulting in downward pressure on the brachial plexus nerves and subsequent neuropathy.

Alternatives include closed reduction with traction or open reduction with casting. A hip spica cast is most often used with infants. Care then includes observance for poor pedal pulses, decreased peripheral circulation, pain, skin excoriation or abrasions, and possible development of respiratory infections resulting from decreased mobility. Parents are taught to evaluate for these complications and care needs prior to discharge.

CLUBFOOT

The classic clubfoot, talipes equinovarus, refers to a dysmorphic foot with hindfoot equinus, forefoot adduction, and midfoot supination. The term *clubfoot* may also be used to describe milder talipes conditions, including talipes calcaneus and talipes varus.

Foot deformities are among the most common birth defects. Clubfoot has an incidence of 1 in 1000 live births. Males are affected nearly twice as often as females, and, in infants with unilateral presentation, most defects appear on the right.

Pathology

The precise mechanism of development of clubfoot has not been irrefutably established. Some researchers allude to the theory of intrauterine malposition, whereas others, noting a high incidence in families with a positive history of the disorder, ascribe it to a genetic cause.

Gaining popularity is the theory that clubfoot is a multifactorial disorder involving a genetic predisposition coupled with environmental forces such as oligohydramnios, primiparity, macrosomia, and multiple fetuses.

This disorder is apparent at birth. The skin overlying the lateral aspect of the foot may be taut, whereas the medial aspect may have increased skin folds and creasing. The affected foot is typically smaller than a normal foot. In older children, the calf muscle may be noticeably decreased in size. Milder talipes conditions may be returned to the neutral position by manipulation.

Collaborative Management

Early diagnosis and treatment of clubfoot are essential. In the early newborn period, joints, muscles, and ligaments may be more compliant to corrective manipulation without surgical intervention. This may involve serial casting as frequently as 2- to 4-day intervals. Surgery may be required in as many as 50% of clubfoot deformities. Difficulty with skin closure has been reported as a complication following correction of severe clubfoot. This is especially true if the affected foot has received prior surgery. Special shoe splints or braces may be used toward the end of any successful treatment.

Difficulty for the parents and caretakers is with handling, bathing, and dressing the infant with casting. Reinforcing the use of serial casting as a means of avoiding surgery is necessary.

SYNDACTYLY

Fusion, or webbing, between two digits is referred to as syndactyly. This condition is the most common anomaly of the hand, with an incidence of 1 in 2250 live births. Males are affected slightly more than females. In 50%, both hands are involved in a symmetric presentation. Syndactyly of the fingers may be accompanied by syndactyly of the toes.

Pathology

Although most occurrences of syndactyly appear secondary to spontaneous mutation, familial predisposition has been reported, thus indicating an autosomal dominant pattern. Syndactyly may also be associated with a specific syndrome such as Apert's syndrome.

There are four classifications of syndactyly. Complete syndactyly occurs when the fusion is from the base to the tip of the digit. Fusion that does not extend to the tip of the digit is termed incomplete. Simple syndactyly refers to digits connected by skin and soft tissue. Fused digits involving an osseous connection are considered complex syndactyly. Abnormal nerve and vessel configurations may accompany complex syndactyly.

Diagnosis and Management

Diagnosis is by appearance, although radiographic films may identify the involvement with complex syndactyly, especially when more than two digits are involved.

Management, including the type and timing or treatment, is dependent on its classification. Surgery is directed toward promoting normal function and appearance. Fingers of unequal length should be separated by 6 to 12 months of age to prevent curvature of the longer finger from deviating toward the shorter finger. If more than two adjacent digits are involved, surgery is often performed in stages to prevent vascular compromise of the middle digit(s).

Prognosis is favorable for normal function and appearance, except in cases of complex syndactyly involving not only bone but also vascular and nervous tissue. These cases may be associated with some postoperative loss of function.

Parents of infants with syndactyly are instructed in physical therapy, specifically in massage of the interconnecting skin. Massage of the webbed or interconnecting skin provides stretching, allowing for easier skin repair when needed.

POLYDACTYLY

Polydactyly is any duplication of digits beyond the normal five. It is the second most common hand anomaly. Polydactyly is believed to be caused by duplication of a single embryonic bud. African Americans are affected 10 times more often than Caucasians. African Americans more often have postaxial polydactyly (duplication of the fifth digit), whereas preaxial polydactyly (duplication of the thumb) occurs primarily in Caucasians. Central axial polydactyly is the duplication of the ring, long, or index finger. Central axial polydactyly is often associated with complex syndactyly. Polydactyly may be further classified into three types. Type I is merely a rudimentary soft tissue mass connected by a pedicle. Treatment of this type involves simple excision, which is often performed in the newborn prior to discharge. Type II is a partial duplication with involvement of the phalanges. Type III, a rare occurrence, involves complete duplication of the metacarpal and phalanges.

Collaborative Management

Treatment of polydactyly, types II and III, centers around functional capacity first and appearance second. The infant is observed for the function of the dominant digit, and efforts are made to remove the least functional counterpart. If both duplicated digits appear to be equally functional, surgery is then used to promote an aesthetic appearance. Reparative surgery is generally completed by 3 years of age.

AMNIOTIC BAND SYNDROME

Amniotic band syndrome, with an incidence ranging from 1 in 2250 to 1 in 15,000 live births, is characterized by uncommon, asymmetric fetal deformities. Deformities that have been attributed to amniotic banding include congenital limb amputation, syndactyly, constriction bands, clubfoot, craniofacial defects such as cleft lip and palate, and visceral defects such as gastroschisis and omphalocele (Baraitser & Winter, 1996).

Pathology

Two theories—endogenous and exogenous—serve to explain the cause of amniotic band syndrome. The endogenous theory postulates that the deformities are caused by an innate derangement of the primary embryonic cell layers from which the tissues and organs develop. The presence of amniotic bands, according to this theory, is a late development with no clinical significance.

The exogenous, and seemingly more popular, theory contends that early amniotic rupture allows the fetus to move into close approximation to the chorion by entering the chorionic cavity. The ruptured amnion then forms fibrous strings or bands. These bands can adhere to the skin, thus altering normal morphogenesis (e.g., cleft lip or palate, omphalocele), or disrupt the vascular integrity, resulting in gastroschisis. Amniotic bands have been found encircling normally developed structures, thus resulting in congenital amputations, construction rings with lymphedema distal to the ring, and facial clefts in nonanatomic distribution. Postural deformities such as clubfoot are believed to be caused by the fetus' close approximation to the chorion.

Diagnosis

Many clinicians believe amniotic bands must be present for the diagnosis of amniotic band syndrome. However, others believe the presence of fetal deformities in a nonanatomic pattern, without obvious bands, is sufficient to establish the diagnosis. Congenital deformations, such as the visceral and craniofacial aspects, in the absence of amniotic bands may go undiagnosed as amniotic band syndrome. Figure 11-5 is an example of an amniotic band constriction ring noted on the arm of an infant with unilateral cleft lip or palate. Evidence of this constriction ring indicates that development of the lip and palate were at one time normal, but development altered with the present of amniotic bands.

Collaborative Management

Notwithstanding the inherent problems associated with omphaloceles, gastroschisis, encephaloceles, clubfoot, syndactyly, and facial clefts, the clinician must be attuned to the unique complications of constricting bands. Constricting bands are usually associated with edema distal to the band. The resulting edema and vascular compromise contribute to complications such as skin breakdown, necrosis, and thromboembolus formation that result from venostasis and infection. Care should include frequent vascular checks to assess perfusion. Trauma and tissue breakdown are discouraged through positioning and skin care. Observation for localized areas of necrosis is stressed.

As with other aesthetically disappointing musculoskeletal disorders, the family requires emotional and psychologic

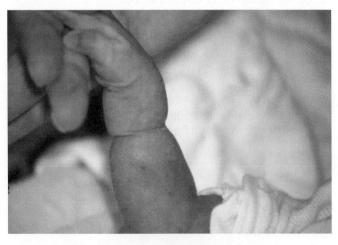

FIGURE **11-5**
Amniotic band syndrome: constriction rings.

support as adjustment to and acceptance of the infant are allowed to occur. Parents may be fearful that an extremity will be lost due to necrotic tissue formation or infection. These fears may be justified, and the parents should be prepared for this possibility. Complete surgical repair may not be possible during the infant's initial hospitalization, thus necessitating frequent hospitalizations during the early developing years.

CONGENITAL MUSCULAR TORTICOLLIS

Torticollis, with an incidence of 0.4% of all live births, is another musculoskeletal deformity with unknown pathogenesis. It is a disorder of the sternocleidomastoid muscle.

Pathology

Several theories exist as to the cause of congenital torticollis, including genetics, abnormal uterine positioning, and neurogenic and ischemic injury to the sternocleidomastoid muscle. Whatever the cause, this pathologic disorder consists of a fibrous contraction of the sternocleidomastoid muscle. Typically, the ipsilateral trapezius muscle is atrophic.

Diagnosis

Torticollis can present during the neonatal period. Presentation includes a 1- to 3-cm hard palpable mass in the neck on the affected side accompanied by abnormal positioning of the head. Infants with congenital torticollis tilt the head to the affected side, and the chin is pointed upward and in the opposite direction. Facial asymmetry may be a later sign. The face and skull on the affected side appear smaller.

Vertebral radiographs are necessary to evaluate for any vertebral anomalies that may also mimic abnormal head and neck posturing.

Collaborative Management

Physical therapy and positioning are instituted with diagnosis. Congenital torticollis generally resolves within the first year of life. Persistent torticollis past 12 months may require surgery to release and lengthen the tight muscle. For children with untreated torticollis or with torticollis unresponsive to therapy, the shoulder on the affected side is raised to compensate for the abnormal head positioning. This form of compensation may lead to cervical and lumbar scoliosis as well as chronic back pain.

BIRTH TRAUMA

Birth trauma includes both mechanical and asphyxial events occurring during delivery. This trauma may be secondary to pressure and distortion. This can occur despite exemplary obstetrical care. Birth trauma occurs in approximately 2 to 7 per 1000 live births. A positive association exists between birth trauma and macrosomia, prematurity, breech presentation, dystocia, and cephalopelvic disproportion.

Clinical Presentation and Pathology

Birth trauma includes abrasions, ecchymoses, erythema, cephalohematomas, caput succedaneum, fractures, brachial plexus damage, and nerve palsies. Clavicular fractures are the most common fractures diagnosed as birth trauma. Clavicles are at an increased risk for fractures during shoulder dystocia in a vertex presentation or with arms extended during a breech delivery (Cooperman & Thompson, 2002).

Physical examination findings related to birth trauma may appear only as bruising, abrasions, and petechiae that overlie the affected part. Further diagnostic methods should be used when the infant exhibits pain on movement, limited motion, and abnormal passive positioning of an extremity or head movement.

Skull fractures may present as cephalohematomas. Skull fractures are most often linear and typically involve the parietal bones. Symptomatic evidence of a nondepressed skull fracture may resemble signs of increased intracranial pressure secondary to epidural hemorrhage. Clinical presentation may include changes in tone, hypertonicity or hypotonicity, arching of the back with the head in hyperextension, and respiratory compromise. Usually, no treatment is indicated for asymptomatic skull fractures. Depressed skull fractures, however, may require elevation of the depressed area.

Vertebral fractures are incurred in difficult breech deliveries in which longitudinal traction in combination with a twisting motion may occur. Fractures commonly involve the seventh cervical and first thoracic vertebrae. Treatment depends on the extent of resultant nerve damage but often requires some form of traction.

The most common nerve injury attributed to birth trauma is brachial plexus damage and resulting nerve palsy. This injury involves damage to the network of nerve fibers in the neck and shoulder, referred to as the brachial plexus. Involvement may occur in the upper portion (Erb-Duchenne palsy), lower portion (Klumpke's palsy), or both portions (complete brachial plexus palsy). Erb-Duchenne palsy is the most common form. The affected arm is limp and in a position of elbow extension with internal rotation. Moro reflex is diminished but the grasp reflex is intact. Klumpke's palsy involves paralysis of the hand and wrist. Complete brachial plexus palsy results in paralysis of the entire arm.

Diagnosis

Diagnosis of birth trauma is based on physical assessment findings. These are usually visible at birth or in the immediate postnatal period. Physical findings should be confirmed by radiologic evaluation as well as to rule out additional findings such as an unsuspected fracture with Erb's palsy.

Collaborative Management

Treatment of birth trauma depends on the type and severity of the trauma. Often, supportive measures may be the only intervention required. For instance, brachial plexus injuries require immobilization in a neutral position using braces or slings. Passive range-of-motion exercises should be instituted at 7 to 10 days of age.

Clavicular fractures also respond to supportive management. Typically, the arm is maintained against the body with the elbow flexed and arm across the chest. This position limits movement, thereby decreasing pain and possible trauma to the site. Callus formation stabilizes the fracture by 10 days of age. A hard, palpable knot can often be felt with this callus formation.

CRANIOSYNOSTOSIS

The bones that constitute the skull are joined with fibrous joints. These joints are lined with a thin layer of fibrous tissue. Separation of these joints allows for remodeling of the skull at the time of delivery and for rapid growth of the head during the early developmental years. The skull consists of five main sutures: coronal, lambdoidal, squamosal, sagittal, and metopic.

The signal for normal closure of these sutures is not very clear, but is believed secondary to multiple factors—including vascular, hormonal, genetic, mechanical, and local factors. Complete fusion of these sutures is anticipated in the second or third decade of life.

Premature closure of any suture in the skull results in a clinical condition called craniosynostosis. The early closure of a cranial suture typically starts at one point and progresses along the suture line. Premature closure may occur prenatally or postnatally. Simple craniosynostosis defines the premature fusion of one suture; complex craniosynostosis indicates that two or more sutures are fused. Primary craniosynostosis, the most common form, is not associated with a known disorder. Secondary craniosynostosis is associated with an underlying pathology, such as hyperthyroidism, thalassemia, Apert's syndrome, Crouzon's syndrome, and Cole-Carpenter syndrome.

Pathology and Clinical Characteristics

Clinical characteristics depend on which suture is affected. The closure of one suture does not allow growth in that area, but generally increases growth in the other areas of the skull. When the sagittal suture is involved, the head presents as dolichocephalic, with a long and narrow-appearing skull and increased length from front to back. Bossing of the frontal and occipital regions accompanies this long and narrow appearance. The coronal suture is the second most common (sagittal closure is first) suture involved in premature closure. The clinical appearance is a skull that is wide from side to side, but short from front to back, also termed brachydactyly. Bilateral lambdoidal craniosynostosis could be identified with a flattened occipital region, whereas unilateral lambdoidal craniosynostosis has a flattened area on one side of the occiput and appears asymmetrical when compared to the other side. Long-term supine positioning of the infant can also produce this appearance.

Positional asymmetric skull appearance, not related to abnormal suture closure, is generally seen in those infants with a neuromusculoskeletal defect that will not allow the child to move its head from side to side spontaneously. Congenital torticollis can result in an asymmetrically flat occipital region as the infant tilts the head toward the affected side.

Isolated metopic craniosynostosis will produce a deformity with a narrow, protruding forehead. Facial development of the skull is also affected, and orbital hypotelorism is also noted with this defect.

Diagnosis and Management

Diagnosis is preceded by suspicion of the abnormal physical appearance of the skull. There is persistent or progressive abnormal skull growth—often with the head circumference intact for age. Craniosynostosis is usually confirmed with a CT scan of the skull.

Surgical therapy is required for the treatment of this disorder. The complexity of the procedure increases with the number of sutures involved and the cranial remodeling at the time of surgery. Often serial craniotomies are required for full correction. The fused suture is removed, and to prevent repeat early closure and reduce osteoblastic activity, a material is used to line the sutures. Often a helmet is required for the child to wear for a period of time to improve cranial remodeling.

There is an increased incidence of mental dysfunction when more than one suture is involved. This does not appear related to the early suture closing, but rather, from early brain development/formation and growth. This is also observed with more complex syndromes.

TAR SYNDROME: THROMBOCYTOPENIA–ABSENT RADIUS

TAR is classified by the bilateral absence of radii and hypomegakaryocytic thrombocytopenia, typically less than 150,000 mm^3. This anomaly is associated with some degree of ulnar hypoplasia. The ulna may be either hypoplastic or absent.

There is also an increase in eosinophils. Multiple other defects can be noted, including congenital heart disease (33%) and mental deficiency (7%).

Pathology

There is an autosomal recessive inheritance pattern, although most cases are spontaneous. The greatest pathology can occur in the neonatal period and correlates to the severity of thrombocytopenia, which can induce intracranial hemorrhages. An increased incidence of hemorrhagic death has been reported with some viral illness, especially involving the GI system. This increased incidence of mortality has been reported at 40% (Jones, 2005). Hematologic complications improve with age—hence the reduced mortality and morbidity associated with this syndrome after the first year of life.

A complication encountered as the child matures is the gross motor developmental delay experienced by the abnormal hands and arms. Most children who are affected with this syndrome might require some type of adaptive device but rarely perform well with prostheses, as they learn to compensate with their existing limbs (McLaurin et al, 1999).

Collaborative Management

The primary management in the newborn period centers on the platelet levels. Because of increased risk of bleeding, platelet transfusions may be required. In addition, handling and phlebotomy via heel sticks should be kept to a minimum to reduce bruising.

SUMMARY

Although the majority of musculoskeletal defects in the newborn are nonlethal and often not long-term functional problems, they may become the focus of the parents' attention. This can be attributed to the perception that the infant does not meet their preconceived idea of the "perfect child." An understanding of the development of the musculoskeletal system and pathology for various defects can assist the clinician in teaching and supporting the family and infant. In addition, recognizing the subtle abnormalities can prompt the clinician to evaluate for additional, often subtle, associated defects that could have serious genetic implications.

Case Study

IDENTIFICATION OF THE PROBLEM

A term newborn was delivered at 37 weeks' gestation after a pregnancy complicated by lack of routine prenatal care, early rupture of membranes, early loss of amniotic fluid volume, and reduced fetal movements later in gestation.

At the time of delivery, the infant was noted to have multiple contractures involving the hips, knees, ankles, wrists, fingers, elbows, and shoulders. She was admitted to the NICU after delivery for further evaluation and care, including diagnostic workup.

ASSESSMENT: HISTORY AND PHYSICAL EXAMINATION

A female infant was delivered at 37 weeks' gestation. This was the first pregnancy for the 19-year-old mother. Maternal history consisted of limited prenatal care with initial prenatal visit at 18 weeks, at which time she was admitted with leaking membranes. This early complication did not progress to early delivery or maternal chorioamnionitis. There was apparent resolution of amniotic fluid leakage with maternal bed rest during this period. An ultrasound demonstrated borderline low amniotic fluid levels but normal fetal movement and development.

After discharge, the mother did not return for further prenatal visits; she presented at the local hospital with complaints of rupture of membranes at 37 weeks' gestation. On further questioning, the mother described reduced fetal movement over the previous several weeks.

The mother was not compliant with the prescribed prenatal vitamins or iron with only random dosing habits. Maternal laboratory test results were benign: negative for *Chlamydia* and gonorrhea, nonreactive rapid plasma reagin (RPR), negative for human immunodeficiency virus (HIV) serology, and negative hepatitis studies.

Upon admission to the hospital, fetal monitoring demonstrated variable fetal heart rate (FHR) decelerations; ultrasound noted transverse lie with reduced fetal movements and abnormal posturing of fetal extremities.

Delivery was by urgent cesarean section with general anesthesia. Apgar scores were 7 and 8 at 1 and 5 minutes, respectively.

At the time of delivery, the infant exhibited a weak cry and mild depression that improved easily with tactile stimulation and drying. No ventilatory support was required.

On examination she had contractures involving extension of the elbows, knees, and ankles, with severe talipes equinovarus present. Flexion of hip, wrists, and fingers, which overlapped into palms, pronated forearms. The shoulder girdle was tight with inability to move the upper arms toward midline. Facies with flat affect and compressed/flattened nares were observed, as well as plagiocephaly involving flattened frontal bone.

Hemodynamics and respiratory effort and oxygenation were unaffected. No murmur was noted on examination, with benign GI examination and three-vessel cord noted as well. Spinal examination was performed without dimpling or masses noted. Cranial sutures were slightly separated with small/open anterior and posterior fontanelles. The infant had periods of quiet/alert behavior, sucked vigorously with intact swallowing ability, and reacted easily to sound and light touch.

DIFFERENTIAL DIAGNOSIS

The appearance of multiple congenital contractures may be secondary to a number of specific medical conditions. Chromosomal anomalies, neuropathic abnormalities, and abnormal muscle development and/or innervation are key concerns for development of fetal/neonatal contractures. In addition, reduced space for fetal movement secondary to abnormal uterine space (bifid uterus or presence of uterine tumors) as well as oligohydramnios may all limit the movement of the fetus.

Arthrogryposis (multiple congenital contractures), regardless of exact cause, appears to result from reduced fetal movement over time. Therefore, any condition, whether intrinsic such as abnormal karyotype or extrinsic with the lack of amniotic fluid, can result in the development of multiple congenital contractures.

DIAGNOSTIC TESTS

Systematic evaluation is needed with the appearance of multiple contractures in an effort to isolate the cause of the reduced movement during gestation.

Genetics evaluation including karyotype with high-resolution banding is needed. Radiographic imaging (CT or MRI) of brain parenchyma and ventricular system should be ordered; echocardiogram and renal sonogram are needed to evaluate for other anomalies.

Electromyography can evaluate the innervation of the muscular system, and a muscular biopsy can identify absence or abnormalities of muscle formation. Basic radiographs of the spine and bony structures can also be useful to evaluate for old fractures that might be noted with types of osteogenesis imperfecta. Viral cultures and/or immunoglobulin M levels may identify an infectious process. Ophthalmology evaluation is needed to assess for retinal degeneration and opacities.

WORKING DIAGNOSIS

The chromosome analysis was normal, 46XX. CT scan of the brain and spine was also normal. Further examinations, including echocardiogram, renal sonogram, and ophthalmology examination, were normal.

Electromyography was normal, indicating normal innervation and nerve conduction ability.

Muscle biopsy in some areas demonstrated change of muscle tissue to a fibrous, fatty tissue, which is a classic finding in arthrogryposis. The muscle changes to a fatty tissue with fibrous bands secondary to absent movement. This is a permanent change, and muscle tissue does not return to these areas.

Continued

Case Study—cont'd

With the absence of a specific neuromuscular or genetic etiology, the development of arthrogryposis appears related to early loss of amniotic fluid volume limiting uterine space. Without serial prenatal visits, repeated evaluation of further fluid loss and fetal movement was not assessed, placing this fetus at risk for complications.

DEVELOPMENT OF MANAGEMENT PLAN

There is no cure for this disorder; the long-term outcome depends on the presence or absence of associated airway or pulmonary pathology.

This infant was able to breathe easily on room air and did not demonstrate contractures of the jaw, which can limit oral feeding success. Without life-threatening complications, a normal life span is expected. Difficulties with daily living will be a lifelong problem.

The goal of management is to improve daily functioning in all stages of life and development, including feeding, sitting, and ambulation, as well as gaining use of arms and fingers.

Early physical therapy to stretch contractures and improve movement is a key factor and requires family participation and access to health care facilities.

Splinting augments physical therapy efforts by placing the affected joints and limbs in a normal posture or position. Earlier use of serial casting was of little value, as it hampered the usefulness of physical therapy and need for stretching and movement to the areas.

Brief serial casting for the severe clubfeet was completed, followed by further physical therapy and later surgery to restructure the foot and ankle. Postsurgical splints for the ankles and feet improved her later efforts at ambulation.

IMPLEMENTATION AND EVALUATION OF EFFECTIVENESS

Discharge was accomplished with redundant teaching of the mother and family members regarding how to pick up and hold the infant as well as how to change diapers and bathe the infant. Handling of this infant could be difficult because of her stiff extremities and joints. With improper handling, broken bones or dislocated joints could occur. In addition, with the inability to cuddle the infant as a result of her stiff posture, the mother appeared to have difficulties bonding with and holding the infant.

Social work services and home health nursing visits were arranged to assess, teach, and encourage the mother and other family members in the care of this infant.

Despite multiple home and transportation services and assistance, the mother became noncompliant with this infant's return visits to physical therapy and other follow-up with overall poor outcome of this infant's progress. The outlook for achieving the long-term goal of an independent and functional lifestyle for this infant is poor due to dysfunctional family dynamics and compliance.

REFERENCES

Baraitser M, Winter RM (1996). *Color atlas of congenital malformation syndromes.* St Louis: Mosby.

Barlow TG (1962). Early diagnosis and treatment of congenital dislocation of the hip. *Journal of bone and joint surgery* 44B:292-301.

Cooperman DR, Thompson GH (2002). Neonatal orthopedics. In Fanaroff AA, Martin RJ, editors. *Neonatal-perinatal medicine: diseases of the fetus and infant,* ed 7. St Louis: Mosby.

Cubert RR et al (2001). Osteogenesis imperfecta: mode of delivery. *Obstetrics & gynecology* 97:66-69.

Engelbert RH et al (2000). Osteogenesis imperfecta in childhood prognosis for walking. *Journal of pediatrics* 137:397-402.

Glorieux FH et al (1998). Cyclic administration of pamidronate in children with severe osteogenesis imperfecta. *New England journal of medicine* 339(14):947-952.

Glorieux FH et al (2000). Type V osteogenesis imperfecta: a new form of brittle bone disease. *Journal of bone and mineral research* 15(9):1650-1658.

Glorieux FH et al (2002). Osteogenesis imperfecta type VI: a form of brittle bone disease with a mineralization defect. *Journal of bone and mineral research* 17(1):30-38.

Hall JG (1981). An approach to congenital contractures (arthrogryposis) [review]. *Pediatric annals* 10(7):15-26.

Horwitz EM (1999). Transplantability and therapeutic effects of bone marrow derived mesenchymal cells in children with osteogenesis imperfecta. *Nature medicine* 5(3):309-313.

Jones KL (2005). *Smith's recognizable patterns of human malformation,* ed 6. Philadelphia: Saunders.

Lashley FC (2005). *Clinical genetics in nursing practice,* ed 3. New York: Springer.

McLaurin RM et al (1999). Management of thrombocytopenia–absent radius (TAR) syndrome. *Journal of pediatric orthopedics* 19:289-296.

Morey SS (2001). The American Academy of Pediatrics. AAP develops guidelines for early detection of dislocated hips. *American family physician* 63:565-566.

Mostert AK et al (2000). Results of Pavlik harness treatment for neonatal hip dislocation to Graf's sonographic classification. *Journal of pediatric orthopedics* 19:289-296.

Ortolani M (1976). Congenital hip dysplasia in the light of early and very early diagnosis. *Clinical orthopedics and related research* 119:6-10.

Sillence D, Danks D (1978). The differentiation of genetically distinct varieties of osteogenesis imperfecta in the newborn period. *Clinical research* 26:178A.

Sisk EA et al (1999). Obstructive sleep apnea in children with achondroplasia: surgical and anesthetic considerations. *Otolaryngology–head and neck surgery* 120:248-254.

Spitz JL (1996). *Genodermatosis: a full color clinical guide to genetic skin disorders.* Baltimore: Williams & Wilkins.

Woolacott NF (2005). Ultrasonography in screening for developmental dysplasia of the hip in newborns: systematic review. *British medical journal* 330:1413.

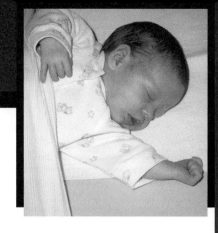

Chapter 12

Neurologic System

Susan Tucker Blackburn • Georgia R. Ditzenberger

The central nervous system (CNS) is one of the extraordinarily complex systems of the human body. Normal function of the CNS is critical to the function of every organ in the body and for the integration of organ systems that coordinate physiologic and neurobehavioral processes. Neurologic dysfunction during the neonatal period can arise from insults that occur before, during, or after birth. Such insults can affect the infant's ability to survive the perinatal and neonatal periods and can have implications for later developmental and cognitive outcome. Thus, alterations in neurologic function in the neonate have significant immediate and long-term consequences for the infant and family. Early recognition of infants at risk for neurologic dysfunction and prompt implementation of appropriate interventions are crucial for the survival and for the reduction of long-term morbidity.

This chapter examines the structural and functional development of the CNS in the embryo, fetus, and neonate and the basis for common congenital and developmental anomalies. Neurologic assessment of the neonate and related diagnostic techniques are also presented, as are selected pathophysiologic problems that affect the central and peripheral nervous systems. The neurologic problems examined include neonatal seizures, intracranial hemorrhage, white-matter injuries, hypoxic-ischemic encephalopathy (HIE), structural alterations, and birth injuries. Figure 12-1 shows the general structure of the central nervous system.

CENTRAL NERVOUS SYSTEM DEVELOPMENT AND STRUCTURAL ABNORMALITIES

Many disorders of the neurologic system are related to defects in the development of the organs of the CNS. The development of the CNS can be divided into six stages: (1) neurulation, (2) prosencephalic development, (3) neuronal proliferation, (4) neuronal migration, (5) organization, and (6) myelinization. These stages overlap, and development progresses at different rates in various sections of the CNS. Embryologic development of the CNS begins shortly after fertilization, and maturation continues after birth until adulthood. The CNS therefore is one of the earliest systems to begin development and one of the last to reach maturity. The stages of CNS development are summarized in Table 12-1. CNS development is controlled by developmental genes in a complex cascade of gene expression along the anterior-posterior axis of the embryo (Murphy et al, 2005).

Neurulation

Primary neurulation, or dorsal induction, during the first 3 to 4 weeks of gestation involves formation of the primitive brain and spinal cord. The CNS arises as a thickening of the ectoderm on the dorsal portion of the embryo at about 18 days' gestation. The brain and spinal cord develop from this thickening, which is called the neural plate. The neural plate invaginates, forming the midline neural groove along the dorsal surface of the embryo. The parallel folds of tissue on either side of this groove are called the neural folds. The neural folds eventually form the forebrain, midbrain, hindbrain, and spinal cord. By the end of the third postconceptional week, the neural folds fuse to form the neural tube. The cranial portion of the lumen of the neural tube forms the ventricles; the caudal portion forms the central canal of the spinal cord. The tissues of the neural tube interact with surrounding mesoderm tissue (somites) to stimulate development of the bony structures of the CNS (i.e., the skull and vertebrae).

In the fusion of the neural folds, some of the neuroectodermal cells on the upper margins are not incorporated into the neural tube. These cells form the neural crest, which lies between the neural tube and the surface ectodermal layer. The neural crest tissue forms the peripheral nervous system, which includes the cranial, spinal, and autonomic system ganglia and nerves, Schwann cells, melanocyte (pigment) cells, meninges, and skeletal and muscular components of the head (Moore & Persaud, 2003).

Closure of the neural tube begins in the occipitocervical region at about 22 days' gestation. The neural folds do not fuse simultaneously; fusion proceeds in cephalic and caudal directions from this site. For several days the neural tube is fused toward the central area but is open at both ends. The end areas are known as the rostral (anterior) and the caudal (posterior) neuropores. The cranial end of the neural tube closes at approximately 24 days' gestation. Fusion of the cranial portion forms the forebrain. Failure of closure leads to anencephaly. The caudal neuropore, which is in the future lumbosacral area, closes in a rostrocaudal direction at approximately 26 days' gestation (Volpe, 2001b). Once both neuropores are closed, the neural tube is a closed, fluid-filled system that has no further connection to the amniotic cavity unless a defect is present. Failure of the neuropores to close gives rise to neural tube defects (NTDs). Because differentiation of the surrounding mesodermal tissue (somites) into vertebrae, cranium, and dura depends on interaction with the neural tube, NTDs involve not only the neural elements but also the bony structures and meninges.

Secondary neurulation consists of two phases: canalization and regressive differentiation. These processes form the spinal cord caudal to the upper lumbar area. Development of the lower lumbar, sacral, and coccygeal areas begins at 28 to

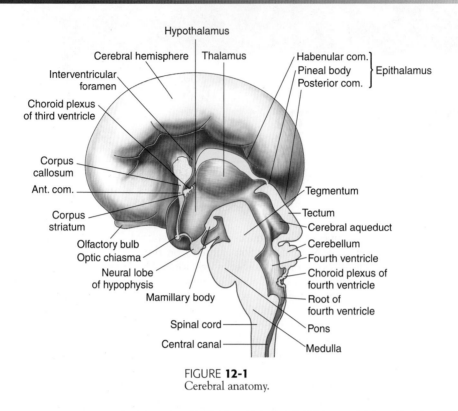

FIGURE **12-1**
Cerebral anatomy.

TABLE **12-1**	Stages in the Development of the Central Nervous System and Related Developmental Defects	
Stage	**Peak Period of Occurrence**	**Developmental Defects**
Neurulation	3 to 4 weeks' gestation	Neural tube defects, anencephaly, encephalocele, spina bifida cystica (meningocele, meningomyelocele, myeloschisis), dermal sinus
Prosencephalic development	2 to 3 months' gestation	Holoprosencephaly, holotelencephaly
Neuronal proliferation	3 to 4 months' gestation	Microcephaly vera, macrencephaly, neurofibromatosis, other neurocutaneous disorders
Neuronal migration	3 to 5 months' gestation	Hypoplasia or agenesis of the corpus callosum, schizencephaly, lissencephaly, pachygyria, polymicrogyria
Organization	6 months' gestation to 1 year of age	Alterations in brain development secondary to the effects of Down syndrome and trisomies 13, 14, and 15; behavioral alterations; mental retardation
Myelinization	8 months' gestation to 1 year of age	Brain hypoplasia, neurologic deficits

Compiled from Scher MS (2001). Brain disorders of the fetus and neonate. In Klaus MH, Fanaroff AA, editors. Care of the high-risk neonate, ed 5 *(pp 481-527). Philadelphia: Saunders; Hill A, Volpe JJ (1989).* Fetal neurology. *New York: Raven Press; and Volpe JJ (2001).* Neurology of the newborn, ed 4. *Philadelphia: Saunders.*

32 days' gestation from an undifferentiated cell mass at the caudal end of the neural tube. Vacuoles develop that gradually coalesce, enlarge, and contact the caudal end of the neural tube. This period of canalization is followed by a period of regressive differentiation, which lasts until after birth and is characterized by regression of much of the caudal cell mass (Volpe, 2001b).

Disorders of Neurulation

Congenital anomalies that arise during the period of neurulation result from failure of neural tube closure. NTDs include anencephaly, encephalocele, and spina bifida. Of NTDs, 80% result from failure of neural tube closure at either the cranial or the caudal end (Moore & Persaud, 2003).

NTDs usually are accompanied by alterations in vertebral, meningeal, vascular, and dermal structures; these anomalies include anencephaly, encephalocele, spina bifida occulta, and myelomeningocele. NTDs arise from genetic and environmental influences. They have a familial incidence and an increased genetic susceptibility. With one affected family member, the overall risk for defects in subsequent offspring in the United States is 2% to 3%, which doubles with two or more affected family members; the risk is greater if the previously affected offspring had a lesion at T11 or higher (Volpe, 2001b). The incidence is higher with younger and older mothers, maternal diabetes, a history of miscarriages, maternal folate deficiency, and maternal exposure to drugs such as valproic acid (Kaufman, 2004).

Folic acid supplementation at conception reduces the rate of NTDs (Klusmann et al, 2005). Folate is a cofactor for enzymes needed in DNA and RNA synthesis and is important to a cell's ability to methylate proteins, lipids, and myelin and to the actions of other B vitamins. The American Academy of Pediatrics (AAP) recommends that women of childbearing age consume 0.4 mg of folate daily; for women who previously have had an infant with a neural tube defect, the recommendation is 4 mg daily (AAP, 1999). A neural tube defect can be identified prenatally through maternal serum screening, ultrasound examination, and measurement of the alpha-fetoprotein level of the amniotic fluid. Antenatal screening for NTDs involves analysis of maternal serum alpha-fetoprotein (AFP), which is done as part of the maternal screening at 16 to 18 weeks' gestation. Elevated AFP levels (greater than 2.5 multiples of the median) are followed up with an ultrasonographic examination and, if that is not definitive, by analysis of amniotic fluid AFP levels (Murphy et al, 2005). AFP is a major fetal glycoprotein, similar to the albumin produced in the fetal liver from 6 weeks' gestation. Concentrations of AFP peak at 13 to 15 weeks' gestation. Normally the AFP concentration of the cerebrospinal fluid is significantly higher than that of the amniotic fluid; therefore when CSF leaks into the amniotic fluid, as occurs with an open neural tube defect, the AFP level of the amniotic fluid is elevated (Mizejewski, 2003).

Anencephaly. Anencephaly is caused by failure of the anterior neural tube to fuse in the cranial area. Since the advent of perinatal diagnosis and folic acid therapy, the incidence of anencephaly has declined to 0.2 per 1000 live births (Murphy et al, 2005). Because fusion of the anterior neural tube forms the forebrain, anencephalic infants have minimal development of brain tissue. The brain tissue that does develop is poorly differentiated and becomes necrotic with exposure to amniotic fluid; this results in a mass of vascular tissue with neuronal and glial elements and a choroid plexus marked by partial absence of the skull bones (Volpe, 2001b). Because anencephaly is caused by failure of the neural tube to close cranially, this defect occurs before 24 to 26 days' gestation (around the period of rostral neuropore closure).

Anencephalic infants often have other anomalies. Three fourths are stillborn; the remainder die during the neonatal period, and few are still alive at 1 week (Murphy et al, 2004; Volpe, 2001b). Management of infants with anencephaly is supportive, involving provision of warmth and comfort until the infant dies. Families require emotional support and assistance in coping with their grief over the birth of an infant with a defect and the death of their infant.

Encephalocele. The incidence of encephalocele is 1 to 2 per 10,000 live births (Murphy et al, 2005). Encephaloceles arise from failure of closure of a portion of the neural tube in the anterior region. Although this defect can occur in any region, approximately three fourths occur in the occipital region. The sac protrudes from the back of the head or the base of the neck. The next most common area is the frontal region, with involvement of the orbit, nose, and/or nasopharynx (Back, 2005; Volpe, 2001b). Hydrocephalus, which may be present at birth or develop after surgical repair, occurs with 50% of occipital encephaloceles because of alterations in the posterior fossa (Weindling & Rennie, 2005). Encephaloceles may occur in association with meningomyelocele.

The protruding sac varies considerably in size, and the size of the external sac does not correlate with the presence of neural elements. For example, a large occipital sac may contain minimal neural tissue, whereas a small sac may contain parts of the cerebellum or accessory lobes; some occipital lesions have no neural elements in the sac (Volpe, 2001b). If the sac is leaking CSF at birth, immediate repair is necessary. If the defect is covered by skin, surgery may be delayed until a complete workup, including skull radiography, computed tomography (CT) or cranial ultrasonography, magnetic resonance imaging (MRI) and electroencephalography (EEG) can be performed. Surgical closure helps prevent infection and helps facilitate feeding and other care. A ventriculoperitoneal shunt is inserted if hydrocephaly is present. The prognosis is poor if significant brain tissue is contained within the sac. The mortality rate and later outcome are significantly better for infants with anterior defects than for those with posterior defects (Back, 2005). Other management includes prevention of infection and trauma and positioning to avoid pressure on the defect. Promotion of normothermia is essential, especially in infants with CSF leakage, because these infants are at risk for thermoregulatory problems caused by evaporative losses. Postoperative management includes assessment of ventilation and perfusion, comfort measures, monitoring of neurologic and motor function, promotion of normothermia, prevention of infection, positioning to prevent pressure on the operative site, and monitoring of the site for CSF leakage.

Families of infants with an encephalocele need initial and continuing support and counseling. Initial parental care involves assisting parents with the shock of the defect and its appearance and with their grief over having an infant with an anomaly, as well as helping the parents deal with the outcome implications of this defect. Nursing care also involves enhancing parent-infant interaction and involving the parents in the infant's care when they are ready. Teaching before discharge includes skin care, positioning, exercises, handling and feeding techniques, and activities to promote growth and development.

Spina Bifida. Spina bifida is a general term used to describe defects in closure of the neural tube that are associated with malformations of the spinal cord and vertebrae. Spina bifida arises from defects in closure of the caudal neuropore (open defects) or during secondary neurulation (closed defects). Defects range from minor malformations of minimal clinical significance to major disorders that result in paraplegia or quadriplegia and loss of bladder and bowel control. The two major forms of spina bifida are spina bifida occulta and spina bifida cystica.

Spina bifida occulta occurs in 5% to 10% of the normal population (Weindling & Rennie, 2005). This disorder is a vertebral defect at L5 or S1 that arises from failure of the vertebral arch to grow and fuse between 5 weeks' gestation and the early fetal period (Moore & Persaud, 2003). Spina bifida occulta is a defect in the formation of the caudal portion of the spinal cord (secondary neurulation). Most of those with condition have no problems, and the defect may go unrecognized. A few individuals have underlying abnormalities of the spinal cord or the nerve roots, or both; diastematomyelia (division of the spinal cord or nerve roots in an anteroposterior direction by a bony spicule or cartilaginous band); or dermoids or dermal sinuses (Weindling & Rennie, 2005). These abnormalities usually are manifested externally by a hemangioma, dimple, tuft of hair, or lipoma in the lower lumbar or sacral area. A dermal sinus is a tract of squamous epithelium that connects to the dura mater; this defect is found in the midline, usually in the lumbosacral area corresponding to the location of the caudal neuropore. A dermal sinus occasionally is recognized at birth, but more often it is diagnosed later, after repeated episodes of meningitis.

Spina bifida cystica is a generic term for NTDs characterized by a cystic sac containing meninges or spinal cord elements, or both, along with vertebral defects. Epithelium or a thin membrane covers the sac. This defect occurs in approximately 1 in 1000 live births, and, as with anencephaly, the incidence has declined in recent years (Moore & Persaud, 2003; Murphy et al, 2005). The three main forms of spina bifida cystica are meningocele, myelomeningocele, and myeloschisis. Spina bifida cystica can occur anywhere along the spinal column but is seen most often in the lumbar or lumbosacral area. A meningocele involves a sac that contains meninges and CSF, but the spinal cord and nerve roots are in their normal position.

Myelomeningocele accounts for 80% of spina bifida cystica. The sac contains spinal cord or nerve roots, or both, in addition to meninges and CSF. During development the nerve tissues become incorporated into the wall of the sac, impairing differentiation of nerve fibers (Moore & Persaud, 2003). Infants with myelomeningocele have neurologic deficit below the level of the sac. Approximately 80% of these malformations occur in the lumbar area, which is the final area of neural tube fusion. This defect occurs at 26 to 30 days' gestation, around the time of caudal neuropore closure. Myeloschisis is a severe defect in which no cystic covering exists, leaving the spinal cord open and exposed. Myeloschisis is thought to arise from a local overgrowth of the neural plate, which prevents neural tube closure. This defect probably occurs between 18 and 23 days' gestation. The spinal cord in affected patients is a flattened mass of neural tissue. These infants have significant neurologic deficits and are at great risk for infection. This defect can involve the entire length of the spinal cord and can occur in association with anencephaly (Moore & Persaud, 2003).

With myelomeningocele or myeloschisis, the spinal cord or nerve roots, or both, are displaced dorsally; defects of the muscle and bony structures exist lateral to the defect. The lesions are covered with skin or meninges or both. If the sac is covered with meninges, there is a risk of rupture during delivery, along with leakage of CSF and the risk of infection and dehydration. Many infants also have an associated Arnold-Chiari malformation, often with secondary aqueductal stenosis that results in a noncommunicating form of hydrocephalus. An Arnold-Chiari malformation is also a defect in neural tube closure. This malformation involves a group of anomalies, including displacement of the medulla, fourth ventricle, and lower cerebellum into the cervical canal; bony defects of the occiput, foramen magnum, and cervical vertebrae; and obstruction of the foramen magnum, leading to hydrocephalus (Weindling & Rennie, 2005). Infants with NTDs may also have cardiac, intestinal, orthopedic, and other neurologic anomalies.

The defect may vary greatly in size but is apparent on examination of the infant. The protruding sac usually is in the lumbosacral area and is covered with skin or meninges. Fluid may be leaking from a partly or completely ruptured sac.

Infants with this defect have altered tone and activity of the lower extremities and may assume a froglike posture. With bowel and bladder involvement, dribbling of urine and feces may be noted. The neurologic deficit varies with the level of the defect. The sensory level generally tends to approximate the motor level but may be several segments lower because of differences in the pattern of innervation between sensory and motor fibers (Kaufman, 2004). Infants with NTDs may have evidence of hydrocephalus at birth. Ultrasonography, CT, or MRI can be used to determine the size of the ventricular system, to rule out aqueductal stenosis and an Arnold-Chiari malformation, and to monitor ventricular status and the development of hydrocephalus. Renal dysfunction may develop as a result of recurring urinary tract infections.

Immediate management includes stabilization and prevention of trauma to or infection of the sac and its contents. The infant is monitored for signs of infection, including signs of sepsis or meningitis and localized infection, including redness or discharge from the sac. Warmth and hydration are provided, and fluid and electrolyte status is monitored. These infants are at greater risk of hypothermia and dehydration because of the open lesion, which lacks the normal protective skin covering.

The infant is positioned prone or on the side to reduce tension on the sac. A roll between the legs at hip level assists in maintaining abduction of the legs; a foot roll is used to maintain the feet in a neutral position. Change of position from prone to side lying or side to side, as well as range-of-motion exercises, helps prevent skin breakdown and contractures. Low Trendelenburg position may be used to reduce CSF pressure on the sac. If the infant must be temporarily placed in a supine position for a procedure, a donut roll can be used to prevent pressure on the sac. Postoperative positioning also involves use of the prone or side-lying position, maintenance of body alignment, prevention of hip abduction, and prevention of pressure on the operative site with holding. The sac must be kept free of fecal or urine contamination. Meticulous skin care, consisting of keeping the skin clean and dry and removing urine and stool, helps prevent skin breakdown and infection. The timing and characteristics of urination and stool excretion are observed to help determine the degree of deficit.

For many infants with NTDs, immediate closure and aggressive care constitute the appropriate management. Unless the defect is severe or is associated with multiple life-threatening anomalies, more than 90% of infants with myelomeningocele survive the neonatal period. If the defect goes untreated, 15% to 30% survive and are left with increased deficit. Immediate closure, therefore, is the treatment of choice for most infants (Hirose, 2001; Volpe, 2001b). Immediate closure reduces the risk of infection and improves the prognosis by reducing further deterioration of the spinal cord and nerve tracts. Early closure also facilitates caregiving. A large defect may require several surgical procedures for complete closure. If the defect is completely covered by epithelium, surgery may be delayed for a short period so that function can be evaluated further. All infants with NTDs are evaluated and monitored for hydrocephalus. Urologic function and renal function also are assessed continually. All infants with involvement of the spinal cord or nerve roots, or both, require multidisciplinary follow-up and continuing care to deal with neurologic, urologic, orthopedic, and psychologic problems.

Families of infants with NTDs need initial and continuing support and counseling. Initial parental care involves assisting parents with the shock of the defect and its appearance and with their grief over having an infant with an anomaly. Nursing care also involves enhancing parent-infant interaction and involving the parents in the infant's care when they are ready. Teaching before discharge includes skin care, positioning, exercises, handling and feeding techniques, and provision of activities to promote development. Many areas have spina bifida associations and parent-to-parent support programs to which parents can be referred for peer support.

In utero repair of neural tube defects at 19 to 25 weeks' gestation has been reported to reduce postnatal complications such as hindbrain herniation and hydrocephalus (Lee & Harrison, 2005; Walsh & Adzick, 2003). Significant improvement in sensorimotor function has generally not been reported and an increase in obstetrical complications, such as preterm labor, oligohydramnios, and premature rupture of the membranes, has been reported (Hirose et al, 2003; Murphy et al, 2005). Clinical trials are ongoing.

The prognosis varies with the level and severity of the defect. Most infants with lesions lower than S1 will walk unaided; those with lesions higher than L2 generally will have some wheelchair dependency; bowel and bladder function are controlled at the level of S2 to S4 (Hirose et al, 2003; Volpe, 2001b). However, these limitations are changing as a result of improved perinatal management and new technologies, and more children are ambulatory now than previously. Infants with a myelomeningocele involving a small lumbosacral lesion, without accompanying hydrocephalus or other anomalies, have some degree of neurologic deficit. These infants may be paraplegic but have a good prognosis for eventual independent function. Infants with myeloschisis have a poor prognosis. Many of these infants die of sepsis in the neonatal period. Those who survive have severe neurologic impairments. The prognosis has also improved with the current early and aggressive treatment of infants without major cerebral lesions, hemorrhage, infection, high spinal cord lesions, or advanced hydrocephalus (Volpe, 2001b).

Prosencephalic Development

Prosencephalic development, or ventral induction, involves early development of the brain and ventricular system, which occurs during the second to third month of gestation (peaking at 5 to 6 weeks). The brain develops from the cranial end of the neural tube beginning at the end of the fourth week. During this period, the three primary brain bulges (or vesicles) and cavities are formed, after fusion of the neural folds in the cranial area. Development of the face is associated with prosencephalic development of the CNS; consequently, alterations in brain development often result in facial malformations (Back, 2005; Moore & Persaud, 2003).

The primary brain bulges are the forebrain (prosencephalon), the midbrain (mesencephalon), and the hindbrain (rhombencephalon). During the fifth week, the forebrain divides into two secondary vesicles, the telencephalon and the diencephalon, and the hindbrain divides into the metencephalon and the myelencephalon. The derivatives of each of these structures form the structures of the definitive brain. The third and fourth ventricles are formed from cavities within the rhombencephalon and diencephalon; the aqueduct of Sylvius links these two ventricles. The lateral ventricles arise from cavities in the cerebral hemispheres and are connected to the third ventricle by the foramen of Monro (see Figure 12-1). Early growth of the neural tube is most rapid in the forebrain region. To give these structures space to grow, the neural tube bends at several points, forming the mesencephalic (midbrain area), cervical (junction of the hindbrain and spinal cord), and pontine flexures.

Disorders of Prosencephalic Development

Malformations that occur during this period generally are thought to arise around the fifth to sixth weeks of gestation. Infants with these anomalies have a poor prognosis, and many are lost in early pregnancy or are stillborn. Malformations of the forebrain include holoprosencephaly and holotelencephaly. Holoprosencephaly is an abnormality in cleavage of the hemispheres that arises from genetic or possibly environmental alterations. Failure of horizontal, transverse, and sagittal cleavage of the prosencephalon disrupts formation of the telencephalon and the diencephalon and their derivatives. The resultant brain has a single monoventricular cerebral mass enclosed by a membrane; aplasia of the optic tract, with absence of the olfactory tracts and bulbs, corpus callosum, and supralimbic cortex, also is characteristic. Microcephaly, hydrocephaly, and facial anomalies also may be seen (Volpe, 2001b). With holotelencephaly, the parts of the brain that develop from the telencephalon form a single spheroid structure; the diencephalon and its derivatives are less affected.

Congenital hydrocephalus can also arise during this period. At about 6 weeks' gestation, three critical events occur that are related to the formation and circulation of CSF: (1) development of secretory epithelium in the choroid plexus, (2) perforation of the roof of the fourth ventricle, and (3) formation of the subarachnoid space. Alterations in the second and third events give rise to a communicating form of hydrocephalus (Volpe, 2001b).

Neuronal Proliferation

The development of neurons and glial cells involves proliferation in the germinal matrix; migration (to their final destination) in the next stage of CNS development; differentiation of glial cells (during the period of organization) into specific cell types; alignment of neurons; and the development of interneuron and glial-neuron relationships. The peak period of neuronal proliferation lasts from 2 to 4 months' gestation. During this stage, further development occurs in the subventricular and ventricular zones, where neurons and glial cells are derived from stem cells in the germinal matrix. Initial proliferation involves primarily neurons and radial glia, which are needed for neuron migration. Proliferation of other glia and their derivatives (astrocytes and oligodendrocytes) occurs intensively during the stage of organization, at 5 to 8 months' gestation. During the most intense period of proliferation, before 32 to 34 weeks' gestation, the periventricular area receives a large proportion of the cerebral blood flow. This area is vulnerable to hemorrhage in preterm infants.

Disorders of Neuronal Proliferation

Disorders of proliferation arise from inadequate or excessive proliferation of neuronal derivatives, glial derivatives, or glial cell derivatives. Because mature neurons cannot divide, the eventual number of neurons is determined early in gestation. Insults may alter the neuronal-glial stem cells (reducing the number of neurons or glial cells) or may alter cell growth (resulting in smaller cells) (Volpe, 2001b). The resulting disorders include micrencephaly, macrencephaly, and neurofibromatosis. Micrencephaly may be due to a reduction in either the size (micrencephaly vera) or number (radial microbrain) of stem cells.

Micrencephaly vera is associated with a small brain size (caused by a decrease in the size of the proliferating units) that occurs at 2 to 4 months' gestation. These infants often do not have marked neurologic deficits or seizures during the neonatal period, but later they are severely retarded. Micrencephaly vera may be caused by genetic factors (autosomal recessive or dominant trait, X-linked recessive trait, or translocation) or by environmental factors (irradiation, metabolic alteration, or infection). Micrencephaly vera is found with maternal rubella, fetal alcohol syndrome, maternal cocaine use, and maternal phenylketonuria with elevated phenylalanine levels during pregnancy (Murphy et al, 2005; Volpe, 2001b).

Macrencephaly results in a large brain size because of excessive proliferation of neuronal elements or nonneuronal elements, or both. Macrencephaly is associated with genetic disorders (including Beckwith-Wiedemann syndrome, Sturge-Weber syndrome, and achondroplasia), chromosomal disorders (e.g., Klinefelter and fragile X syndromes), and neurocutaneous disorders, such as neurofibromatosis. Neurofibromatosis involves excessive proliferation of nonneuronal elements in the CNS and mesodermal structures of the body, with cutaneous stigmata (Volpe, 2001b). The onset occurs after neuronal proliferation, at the time of glial cell proliferation during organization. Infants with more than five café au lait spots larger than 5 mm in diameter at birth should be further evaluated for neurofibromatosis (Tappero & Honeyfield, 2003).

Neuronal Migration

The peak period for the neuronal migration stage is 3 to 5 months' gestation. This stage is characterized by the movement of millions of cells from their point of origin in the subependymal germinal matrix of the periventricular region (see Figure 12-1) to their eventual loci in the cerebral cortex and cerebellum. The process of neuronal migration is critical to the formation of the cortex, gyri, and deep nuclear structures. Development of the gyri and sulci follows a predictable pattern that is linked to gestational age. At 21 to 25 weeks' gestation, the central ventricles are large and the brain agyric; gyral development begins by the end of this period.

The mechanisms that guide neuronal migration are not completely understood, but they are mediated by signaling proteins, surface molecules, and receptors on both the neurons and the radial glia (Ikonomidou et al, 2001). Radial glia act as guides for migrating cells. These glia later transform into astrocytes (Volpe, 2001b). The cerebral cortex has essentially achieved its full complement of neurons by 20 weeks' gestation. Later, migration predominantly involves glial cells. The migration of the neurons to both the cortex and the cerebellum is assisted by the radial glia.

Disorders of Neuronal Migration

Errors or exogenous insults before or after birth can alter migration of neurons and glial cells. Alterations in migration can result in hypoplasia or agenesis of the corpus callosum, agenesis of a part of the cerebral wall (schizencephaly), or gyral anomalies (pachygyria, lissencephaly, and polymicrogyria).

The preterm infant may be especially vulnerable to gyral alterations. Rapid development of the gyri begins at 26 to 28 weeks' gestation and continues through the third trimester into the postbirth period. Development of gyri results in a marked increase in cerebral surface area (Back, 2005; Volpe, 2001b).

Organization

The peak period for organization is about the fifth month of gestation to 1 year after birth. However, organizational processes continue for many years after birth, especially in the cerebellum. Some processes, such as synaptogenesis, continue until death. Organizational processes allow the nervous system to act as an integrated whole. These processes include (1) establishment of subplate neurons, which serve as transient "way stations" by providing a place of synaptic contact for axons that ascend from the thalamus and other areas in which connecting cortical neurons are not yet in place; (2) attainment of the proper alignment, orientation, and layering of cortical neurons; (3) arborization or differentiation and branching of axons and dendrites; (4) differentiation of the glial cells; (5) development of synaptic connections ("wiring" of the brain); (6) balancing of excitatory and inhibitory synapses; and (7) cell death and selective elimination of neuronal processes (Volpe, 2001b).

The process of cell death and selective elimination of neuronal processes is important in adjusting the size of individual neurons to their anticipated need and also is an important component of brain plasticity in infants. In the developing brain, neuronal processes targeted for elimination can be saved if they are needed because of damage to other processes; by this means, functional ability is preserved. Excitatory neurotransmitters, such as glutamate, mediate neural development and organization by acting on N-methyl-D-aspartate (NMDA) receptors (Ikonomidou et al, 2001; Sanchez & Jensen, 2001).

Disorders of Organization

Organization of the brain is susceptible to insults from errors of metabolism, abnormal chromosomes, and perinatal insults. Organizational processes are particularly vulnerable in the preterm infant being cared for in an intensive care unit during this period. Alterations in arborization and wiring of the brain can lead to hypersensitivity, poorly modulated behavior, and all-or-nothing responses. Alterations in organization are seen in infants with Down syndrome, who have abnormal development of the axons and dendrites and altered synaptic formation, fragile X syndrome (the most common cause of inherited mental retardation in males), Angelman syndrome (microdeletion on the long arm of maternal chromosome 15), phenylketonuria, congenital rubella, and trisomies 13, 14, and 15 (Ikonomidou et al, 2001; Sanchez & Jensen, 2001).

Myelinization

The myelinization stage involves development of myelin sheaths around nerve fibers in the nervous system. Oligodendrocytes (central nervous system) or Schwann cells (peripheral nerves) form sheaths. The lipoprotein plasma membranes of these cells wrap themselves around the nerve fibers for several layers. Myelinization of fiber tracts tends to occur before maturation of functional ability (Moore & Persaud, 2003).

Myelinization begins early in pregnancy and continues to adulthood. The peak time for myelinization is 8 months' gestation to 2 years of age (Kinney, 2005). This process begins before birth in the peripheral areas, first in the peripheral motor nerves and then in the peripheral sensory nerves. Myelinization also begins before birth in the CNS, moving upward from the brainstem. In the CNS, myelinization occurs first in the sensory areas and then in the motor areas. Myelinization of ascending pathways in the spinal cord, brainstem, and thalamus is completed by about 30 weeks' gestation, and myelinization from the thalamus to the cortex is completed by 37 weeks (Volpe, 2001b). This has implications for neonatal pain management. From birth to adulthood, myelinization proceeds within the cerebral hemispheres in conjunction with development of higher associative and sensory functions. Myelinization is important in most nerve tracts in the CNS because it insulates individual fibers to enhance specificity of connections, increases the number of alternative pathways, and markedly increases the speed of transmission (Volpe, 2001b).

Disorders of Myelinization

Myelinization is susceptible to damage from exogenous influences, particularly malnutrition, which can lead to a range of neurologic deficits in which hypoplasia of the cerebral white matter occurs. Primary hypoplasia of the white matter with vacuolization of the myelin occurs in postnatal malnutrition, congenital hypothyroidism, and amino and organic acidopathies such as maple syrup urine disease, homocystinuria, and phenylketonuria. This defect in myelinization can lead to severe neurologic deficits in these infants (Volpe, 2001b).

NEUROLOGIC ASSESSMENT

Assessment of neurologic function is an initial step in evaluating an infant's response to the transition to extrauterine life and the impact of perinatal events and pathophysiologic problems on the central and peripheral nervous systems. Assessment of neurologic function and identification of dysfunction encompass several components, including the history, physical examination, neurologic examination, laboratory tests, and other diagnostic techniques.

History

Risk factors noted in the maternal, obstetrical, and neonatal histories can be useful in identifying infants at risk for neurologic dysfunction and specific pathophysiologic factors. Specific risk factors for each problem discussed here are identified later in individual sections. General maternal or family historical factors that must be examined include a family history of NTDs; chromosomal or genetic abnormalities or other malformations; maternal substance abuse; chronic maternal health problems; maternal age, nutritional status, and exposure to teratogens; and the outcome of previous pregnancies.

Obstetrical risk factors include prematurity, postmaturity, placental problems (e.g., abruptio placentae and placenta previa), use of analgesia or anesthesia, and maternal problems (e.g., infection, hypertension, and substance abuse). A large-for-gestational-age (LGA) infant, prolonged or precipitate labor, forceps delivery, and abnormal presentation increase the risk of birth trauma and hemorrhage. Alterations in intrauterine growth and polyhydramnios may be present with an infant who has a CNS malformation. Fetal distress, hypoxia, ischemia and low Apgar scores are associated with intracranial hemorrhage and HIE.

Because neurologic dysfunction also can arise from postnatal problems, the infant's postbirth history is evaluated for status at birth and resuscitation required, ischemic or hypoxic episodes, shock, hypoperfusion, hemorrhage, infection, and metabolic or electrolyte aberrations. The infant's record is also reviewed for clinical signs, such as seizures or alterations in activity, tone, and state, which are associated with neurologic dysfunction.

Physical Examination

A comprehensive physical examination is an important component of the assessment of any infant at risk for or showing evidence of neurologic dysfunction. Infants are examined especially for evidence of infection and birth trauma, such as ecchymosis, edema, lacerations, and fractures. Temperature, blood pressure, color, and respiratory pattern also are assessed. The infant is examined for signs of vascular alterations, such as a port wine stain along trigeminal nerve branches, which may indicate Sturge-Weber syndrome. The characteristics of the infant's cry (e.g., robustness, presence in response to aversive stimuli, and pitch) may also be useful. Funduscopic examination may be performed to assess for chorioretinitis (associated with intrauterine viral infection), papilledema (seen with cerebral edema, although less reliably in neonates), and congenital anomalies (Amiel-Tison, 2001).

Specific parameters that are particularly important for the nurse to assess in infants with neurologic problems are (1) the head size, shape, and rate of growth; (2) the sutures and fontanelles; (3) whether major and minor anomalies are present; and (4) the vertebral column. Because CNS anomalies often are associated with other anomalies and syndromes, the infant also is examined for major anomalies of body systems and for isolated or clustered minor malformations, such as low-set or abnormally shaped ears, micrognathia, and hypertelorism of the eyes. The vertebral column is inspected and palpated for evidence of NTDs. Signs that may indicate an underlying defect include hair tufts, dimples, and fistulae.

Head Size, Shape, and Rate of Growth

The monitoring and plotting of head circumference are basic components of health care for all infants, regardless of gestation or health status. The largest circumference is measured, which usually is the occipitofrontal circumference (OFC), about 1 cm above the eyes. The measurement is plotted on the appropriate growth grid for the infant's gender and gestation. The most accurate measurements are made with a metal or plastic tape marked in centimeters. Paper tapes tend to stretch and are less accurate but can be used for initial screening and for infants whose head size raises no concern. The occipitofrontal circumference generally ranges from 32.6 to 37.2 cm in term infants. Infants with caput succedaneum or overriding sutures may need to be remeasured after 3 days to obtain a more accurate measurement (Amiel-Tison, 2001). The head usually grows a maximum of 0.5 cm per week in term infants. Head growth in preterm infants usually is 0.5 cm in the first and second weeks, 0.75 cm during the third week, and 1 cm per week thereafter (Scher, 2001).

Serial measurements must be made to identify changes in the rate of growth as well as in size. Changes in the growth rate are important because an infant may have a significant increase or decrease in head growth but remain within the 10th to 90th percentiles on standard head growth grids. The occipitofrontal circumference should be measured several times over the first days after birth to obtain an accurate baseline after molding and edema from birth have resolved. Head circumference is measured weekly on preterm or ill infants. More frequent measurements may be made if the infant is at risk of developing progressive ventricular dilation.

Head shape can also reflect perinatal events and specific anomalies. The forces of labor and delivery may deform the head, but these changes are transient and disappear within a few days. Infants with craniosynostosis (premature closure of one or more sutures) and hydrocephalus have abnormal head configurations.

Sutures and Fontanelles

The entire head is inspected and palpated, and each suture and fontanelle is assessed. The anterior fontanelle is assessed while the infant is in a quiet state and in a semiupright or sitting position. The fontanelle should be open, soft, and flat. Pulsation may be felt normally in a newborn but can be associated with elevated blood pressure. A sunken or depressed fontanelle is seen with dehydration, and a bulging fontanelle is noted with increased intracranial pressure (ICP). The anterior fontanelle usually is diamond shaped and may be small at birth if molding and overriding of the sutures are present; the size increases within a few days to the usual dimensions seen in term infants (i.e., 3 to 4 cm long by 1 to 3 cm wide). The anterior fontanelle closes at 8 to 16 months of age. The anterior fontanelle may bulge slightly with increased tension when the infant cries and may be slightly depressed when the infant is placed in an upright position. The posterior fontanelle closes any time from 8 months' gestation to 2 months after birth. If open at birth, it is 1 to 3 cm wide and has a triangular shape. In rare cases a "third fontanelle" may be palpated along the sagittal suture between the anterior and posterior fontanelles; this is not a true fontanelle but a defect in the parietal bone. It can be palpated in normal infants, but it is also seen in infants with Down syndrome or hypothyroidism (Tappero & Honeyfield, 2003).

A 4- to 5-mm separation (up to 1 cm) of all the sutures except the squamosal (temporoparietal) suture is normal in the newborn. The squamosal suture should not be separated more than 2 to 3 mm, especially in the term or near-term (late preterm) infant. Overriding of the bones and molding from delivery may modify this finding in the first few days after birth. Abnormal findings include persistence of suture separation over time, increased separation of the sutures, and separation of the squamosal suture by more than 2 to 3 mm. With increased ICP, separation of the sutures occurs in a specific order: sagittal, coronal, metopic and lambdoidal, and squamosal; therefore separation of the squamosal suture is the most clinically significant (Amiel-Tison, 2001). The cranial bones are inspected and palpated so that fractures, extradural hemorrhage, edema, and areas of uneven ossification of the cranial bones or craniotabes can be identified.

Neurologic Examination

The neurologic examination is useful for evaluating for the presence and determining the extent of neurologic dysfunction in the neonate, for monitoring recovery, and as a prognostic indicator. Factors such as gestational age, health status, the infant's state, medications, and timing of feedings must be considered in the interpretation of neurologic findings. Parameters examined in the assessment of neurologic status include level of consciousness, activity, tone, posture, reflexes, and evaluation of selected cranial nerves (Amiel-Tison, 2001; Brown, 2005; Rennie, 2005a; Volpe, 2001a). The optimum state of the infant during a neurologic examination is quiet and alert.

Level of Consciousness

Neurologic insults frequently alter the infant's level of consciousness. The level of consciousness may range from normal states of consciousness for gestation to hyperexcitability, irritability, lethargy, hyperalertness, and stupor or coma. The three clinical levels of consciousness that best correlate with outcome are hyperalertness, lethargy, and stupor or coma. In the hyperalert state, the infant has an increased sensitivity to sensory stimulation, with wide-open eyes but with a diminished blink response and ability to fixate and follow (Amiel-Tison, 2001). A lethargic infant responds to tactile and noxious stimuli, but the responses are delayed. A stuporous or obtunded infant's response is limited to noxious stimuli, and a comatose infant shows no response to tactile or noxious stimuli (Volpe, 2001a). Hyperexcitability and irritability can be assessed by noting an infant's response to caregiving actions and medical procedures, as well as the baby's state during intercaregiving intervals and ability to use self-consoling maneuvers or to be soothed by others.

Activity, Tone, and Posture

Infant activity, tone, and general position are assessed, along with spontaneous positioning of the extremities and hands. The infant first is assessed while lying in a resting position. A frog-leg position while supine is seen in immature infants, after breech delivery, and in infants who have experienced severe asphyxia or who have major health problems or neuromuscular disorders (Amiel-Tison, 2001). The quality and symmetry of activity with spontaneous and elicited movement are assessed. Alterations in symmetry of the trunk, face, and extremities at rest or with spontaneous movement suggest congenital anomalies, birth injury, or neurologic insult. Tight fisting is an abnormal sign. A cortical thumb (inside thumb on closure of the hand) may be normal, but it is abnormal if persistent. Opisthotonos and decerebrate or decorticate posturing may also occur.

Abnormal movements include seizure activity, jitteriness, and tremors, although the last two findings often are normal. The characteristic movements seen with tremors in the neonate vary with the underlying disorder. Tremors associated with metabolic problems usually are low-amplitude, high-frequency movements, whereas tremors associated with CNS problems usually are high-amplitude, low-frequency movements. Jitteriness is a common finding in infants because of the lack of myelinization of the pyramidal tracts. A major function of these tracts is to inhibit spinal reflexes. In the neonate, these unmyelinated tracts respond in a mass way to central arousal with peripheral hyperexcitability. Spontaneous or elicited movement can set off tremors. Tremors can also be associated with metabolic abnormalities, asphyxia, or drug withdrawal. Tremors and jitteriness must be differentiated from seizures. Jitteriness is stimulus sensitive and is not marked by gaze or eye deviations. The predominant movement in jitteriness is tremulousness (rather than the clonic movement seen in seizures), which ceases with passive flexion (Rennie, 2005a).

Resting, passive, and active tone is assessed. Resting tone is evaluated by observing the infant at rest in a supine position. Passive tone is evaluated by examining extensibility, which involves maneuvers used in the neuromuscular component of gestational age assessment. Assessment of active tone involves altering the infant's posture to obtain directed motor responses (Amiel-Tison, 2001). Common maneuvers are righting reactions of the legs and trunk and examination of neck flexors and extensors. Righting reactions are elicited by holding the infant upright with the feet on a firm surface. The infant's ability to straighten the legs and trunk is assessed. Neck flexors and extensors are assessed using the pull-to-sit maneuver. Infants with peripheral nerve injuries, neuromuscular disorders, alterations at the neuromuscular junction, and spinal cord injuries tend to be hypotonic and have muscle weakness. Infants with CNS disturbances secondary to asphyxia, intracranial hemorrhage, Down syndrome, or metabolic disturbances tend to be hypotonic without muscle weakness (Amiel-Tison, 2001; Scher, 2001). Hypertonia is seen less often than hypotonia in neonates with neurologic problems. Marked extensor hypotonia may be seen in association with severe hypoxic-ischemic injury, bacterial meningitis, or massive intraventricular hemorrhage (Scher, 2001; Volpe, 2001a).

Reflexes

Primary and tendon reflexes are assessed. In infants with neurologic dysfunction, these reflexes may be diminished, absent, or accentuated. The primary reflexes include sucking, grasping, crossed extension, automatic walking (stepping), and the Moro reflex. They should be present, symmetric, and reproducible in the neonatal period and should gradually disappear during infancy (Volpe, 1998). The primary reflexes are affected by gestational age, but all are present to some degree by 28 to 32 weeks' gestation. The tendon reflexes assessed in the neonate are the biceps, knee, and ankle jerk. All should be present after about 33 weeks' gestation, but can be difficult to interpret (Brion et al, 2003; Rennie, 2005a). Ankle clonus generally is not a significant finding in the neonate.

Examination of Selected Cranial Nerves

Full cranial nerve assessment generally is not performed on the neonate. However, function of these nerves can be evaluated using several relatively simple maneuvers: fixation and following, pupillary responses, doll's eye response, hearing, vestibular response, and suck and swallow (Table 12-2).

TABLE **12-2**	Nursing Assessment of Selected Cranial Nerves in the Newborn	
Nerve	**Assessment**	**Implications**
Optic (II)	Blink in response to light (consistent by 28 weeks' gestation)	Visual system intact to the level of the superior colliculi (does not indicate visual cortex function)
	Fixation on object placed approximately 19 cm in front of infant's face (consistent by 32 weeks' gestation)	Presence of vision
	Follows object with eyes and by turning head (consistent by 37 weeks' gestation)	
	Examination of external eye	Evaluation of abnormalities (e.g., cataracts, irregularities of size or shape, microphthalmos, or scleral hemangiomas)
	Funduscopic examination (ophthalmoscope set at 2 to 4 diopters)	Normal newborn optic disc is pale or grayish-white; observe for abnormalities (e.g., retinal hemorrhage or lesion)
Oculomotor (III), trochlear (IV), and abducens (VI)	Pupillary reactivity (equal and responsive to light; appears by 28 weeks' gestation and consistent by 32 weeks)	Intact cranial nerve III; unequal or nonresponsive pupils in infants over 32 weeks' gestation are associated with increased intracranial pressure or hemorrhage
	Doll's eye maneuver (vestibular response; present by 25 weeks' gestation): hold infant in an upright position at arm's length and rotate in both directions	Stimulation of semicircular canals with impulses sent to the brainstem via nerves III, VI, and VII. Normal response is isotonic deviation of the eyes away from the direction of movement; lack of response is associated with brainstem dysfunction or excessive administration of sedatives such as phenobarbital; disconjugate eye movements and some nystagmoid movements occasionally are seen normally during the first 3 weeks
Trigeminal (V)	Elicit the corneal reflex (may not be reliable in newborn) or observe for a grimace on pinprick	Facial sensation (not usually done routinely but may be useful with an infant with facial paralysis)
	Elicit sucking and ability of infant to bite down on examiner's finger	Masticatory power
Facial (VII)	Observe appearance and symmetry of face at rest and during spontaneous and elicited movement	Abnormalities associated with birth injury and cerebral insults

Continued

TABLE 12-2	Nursing Assessment of Selected Cranial Nerves in the Newborn—cont'd	
Nerve	**Assessment**	**Implications**
Acoustic (VIII)	Evaluate auditory function by noting response (blink or startle) to sudden loud noise (seen by 28 weeks' gestation) or (in more mature infants) by cessation of movement and turning to sound while in a quiet, alert state	A gross assessment of auditory function; failure of the infant to respond while in a quiet, alert state in a quiet environment on repeated examinations indicates the need for examination of auditory function
Trigeminal (V), facial (VII), glossopharyngeal (IX), vagus (X), and hypoglossal (XII)	Evaluate sucking (V, VII, XII), swallowing (IX and X), and gag reflex (IX and X)	Impairment interferes with feeding and may indicate or be associated with cerebral insult

Compiled from Amiel-Tison C (2001). *Clinical assessment of the infant nervous system.* In Levene MI et al, editors. Fetal and neonatal neurology and neurosurgery, ed 3 (pp 99-120). Edinburgh: Churchill Livingstone; Scher MS (2001). *Brain disorders of the fetus and neonate.* In Klaus MH, Fanaroff AA, editors. Care of the high-risk neonate, ed 5 (pp 481-527). Philadelphia: Saunders; Rennie JM (2005a). *Neurological problems of the neonate: assessment of the neonatal neurological system.* In Rennie JM, editor. Roberton's textbook of neonatology, ed 4 (pp 1093-1105). Edinburgh: Churchill Livingstone; and Volpe JJ (2001b). *Neurology of the newborn, ed 4.* Philadelphia: Saunders.

Clinical Signs Associated with Neurologic Dysfunction

Clinical manifestations of neurologic dysfunction can be specific, nonspecific, or subtle. Five types of clinical signs are commonly seen in infants with neurologic problems: (1) CNS depression, (2) hyperirritability, (3) increased ICP, (4) seizures, and (5) movement alterations. Seizures are discussed later. Signs and symptoms of CNS depression, hyperirritability, increased ICP, and movement alterations are listed in Table 12-3.

Diagnostic Techniques

Diagnostic techniques that may be used with infants suspected of neurologic problems include neurophysiologic studies, radiographic assessment, structural brain imaging, and measurement of cerebral blood flow, measurement of ICP, cerebral blood flow determination, radionucleotide assessment, cerebral angiography, brainstem-evoked responses, EEG, and lumbar puncture. The three types of brain structural imaging most often used are ultrasonography, CT, and MRI. Head ultrasound (HUS) examination is used most often to evaluate intracranial structures. HUS is portable, fast, and done at the bedside and involves nonionizing radiation. Cranial and sagittal images can be evaluated by means of the anterior fontanelle and periventricular leukomalacia by means of the posterior fontanelle. Scans can be real time and multiplanar. Doppler sonography can be used to evaluate cerebral blood flow. HUS is limited in evaluating the posterior fossa and is not useful for interparenchymal and meningeal areas (Papile, 2002; Rennie, 2005a; Scher, 2001).

CT, which uses ionizing radiation, and MRI, which uses nonionizing radiation, are useful for examinations in the axial or coronal plane; they also can be helpful if HUS is unsatisfactory. MRI, although not always available, generally is preferable to CT except in cases involving calcifications or acute hemorrhage and is useful in predicting outcome in infants with hypoxic-ischemic encephalopathy (du Plessis, 2005; Scher, 2001). MRI is slower and usually requires sedation or anesthesia. CT may also require sedation but has greater

sensitivity and specificity, especially in infants with unexplained neurologic signs (Barnes & Taylor, 1998).

Laboratory tests are performed to assist in the diagnosis of specific neurologic disorders and to identify underlying causes. The CSF is examined for signs of hemorrhage (increased red blood cells, increased protein, decreased glucose, and xanthochromia) and to rule out infection. Xanthochromia often is a late sign and may reflect an elevated protein level rather than the presence of blood. If the ICP is increased, the pressure of the CSF on needle insertion may reflect this. Other laboratory evaluations include the hematocrit value, serum glucose level, electrolyte levels, blood gases, and acid-base status. A sepsis workup or screening for toxoplasmosis, rubella, cytomegalovirus, and herpes simplex (TORCH) is performed if intrauterine infection or neonatal sepsis and meningitis are suspected. A genetic workup and other metabolic studies are performed if errors of metabolism or other inherited disorders are thought to be present.

GENERAL MANAGEMENT

Management specific to each type of neurologic dysfunction is described in later sections. However, in the nursing care of infants with neurologic dysfunction, common nursing diagnoses and management techniques that must be considered with all infants and their families are listed below. Those marked with an asterisk (*) are discussed in other chapters.

1. Alteration in level of consciousness
   - Monitor infant's state, activity level, responsiveness, eye movements, head circumference, and vital signs; also monitor for seizure activity and signs of increased ICP.
   - Position infant so as to promote skin integrity, prevent contractures, and reduce ICP (i.e., head in midline and slightly elevated).
   - Monitor fluid and electrolyte status.
   - Maintain adequate ventilation and perfusion.
   - Implement comfort measures.

TABLE 12-3	Clinical Manifestations of Central Nervous System Dysfunction
Alteration	**Clinical Manifestations**
Central nervous system depression	Altered level of consciousness
	Weak, absent cry
	Weak, absent primary reflexes
	Poor feeding
	Decreased activity
	Decreased passive tone
	Decreased active tone
	Altered respirations
Hyperirritability	Sharp, excessive crying
	Hyperactivity
	Exaggerated passive tone
	Hypertonia
	Difficult to console
	Low sensory threshold
Increased intracranial pressure	Irritability
	Lethargy
	Increased head circumference
	Palpable sutures, especially squamous
	Bulging, tense fontanelle
	Increased extensor tone of neck
	Downward deviation of eyes
	Vomiting (late)
	Dilated head veins (late)
Seizures	See Table 12-5
Movement alterations	Jitteriness, tremors
	Decerebrate posturing
	Decorticate posturing
	Opisthotonos

Data from Amiel-Tison C (2001). Clinical assessment of the infant nervous system. In Levene MI et al, editors. Fetal and neonatal neurology and neurosurgery, ed 3 (pp 99-120). Edinburgh: Churchill Livingstone; Brown LW (2005). Neurologic examination. In Spitzer AR, editor. Intensive care of the fetus and neonate, ed 2 (pp 767-774). St Louis: Mosby; Rennie JM (2005a) Neurological problems of the neonate: assessment of the neonatal neurological system. In Rennie JM, editor. Roberton's textbook of neonatology, ed 4 (pp 1093-1105). Edinburgh: Churchill Livingstone.

- Maintain an appropriate thermal environment.
- Reduce environmental stressors.
- Promote neurobehavioral stability.

2. Potential for injury related to trauma or infection
   - Use aseptic technique.
   - Use sterile technique when appropriate.
   - Position infant to prevent contamination of defects or operative sites.
   - Monitor for signs of localized infection or neonatal sepsis.
   - Handle infant gently.
   - Position infant to reduce potential of trauma or contamination.

3. Impairment of skin integrity
   - Position infant in alignment and change position regularly.
   - Use foam, sheepskin, lambskin, or waterbeds.
   - Massage skin gently to stimulate circulation.
   - Use appropriate skin care measures.

4. Alteration in comfort*

5. Impaired mobility
   - Position infant in alignment and change position regularly.
   - Promote skin integrity.
   - Use gentle range-of-motion exercises.

6. Alteration in thermoregulation*

7. Alteration in nutrition*

8. Promote neurobehavioral organization and development*

9. Altered family processes*

10. Grieving (family)*

NEONATAL SEIZURES

Seizures are the most common neurologic sign during the neonatal period. They are not a disease in themselves but a sign of underlying disease processes that have resulted in an acute disturbance within the brain (Volpe, 2001b). If left untreated, these disorders can lead to permanent damage of the CNS or other tissues. Disease processes associated with seizures in the neonate include primary CNS disorders, hypoxic-ischemic events, systemic diseases, and metabolic insults. The reported incidence of neonatal seizures ranges from 2 to 3 per 1000 live births (Rennie & Boylan, 2003). Seizures are seen more often in preterm infants (10 to 15 per 1000 live births) than in term infants (1 per 1000 live births) (Rennie, 2005b; Rennie & Boylan, 2003). Perinatal hypoxia-ischemia accounts for 50% to 60% of all neonatal seizures (Zupanc, 2004). Seizure activity may be an acute, recurrent, or chronic phenomenon. Neonatal seizures usually are acute and disappear within the first few weeks after birth. Recurrent or continuous seizures increase the risk of neurologic damage from the seizure activity itself (Mizrahi, 2001).

Pathophysiology

Seizures are the result of excessive, synchronous electrical discharge or depolarization in the brain that produces stereotypic, repetitive behaviors. Depolarization and repolarization of the nerves are caused by the movement of sodium and potassium across the cell membrane. The inward migration of sodium ions (Na^+) results in depolarization; repolarization is produced by the outward migration of potassium ions (K^+). These processes require an energy-dependent pump and energy in the form of adenosine triphosphate (ATP).

The specific mechanism that causes neonatal seizures is unknown. Such seizures might be the result of one or more of these mechanisms: (1) disturbances in energy production and the Na^+-K^+ pump, (2) altered neuronal membrane permeability to sodium, and (3) imbalances in excitatory and inhibitory neurotransmitters (Volpe, 2001a; Zupanc, 2004).

A disturbance in energy production, with changes in the movement of Na^+ and K^+ across the neuronal membrane, can lead to an imbalance between depolarization and repolarization. The movement of K^+ (repolarization) unbalances the movement of Na^+ (depolarization). Changes in energy production occur secondary to hypoxemia, ischemia, and hypoglycemia. Alterations in the permeability of the neuronal membrane to sodium can occur with hypocalcemia. Calcium normally binds with proteins in the cell membrane to inhibit Na^+ movement. A decrease in the availability of calcium would increase inward movement of Na^+ and lead to depolarization. Hypomagnesemia also increases membrane permeability to Na^+, and alkalosis or hyponatremia, as well, can lead to seizures through this mechanism.

Imbalances in neurotransmitters lead to a relative excess of excitatory neurotransmitter (glutamate or acetylcholine) over inhibitory neurotransmitter (gamma-aminobutyric acid or GABA) and increase the rate of depolarization. This can occur as a result of an excess of excitatory substance (associated with hypoxemia, ischemia, and hypoglycemia) or a deficiency of inhibitory substance. Pyridoxine deficiency leads to an inhibitory neurotransmitter deficiency by depressing activity of the enzyme responsible for synthesis of gamma-aminobutyric acid. Elevated levels of excitatory inhibitors derived from ammonia are seen in preterm infants who have an excessive protein intake or in infants who have liver dysfunction after severe hypoxic-ischemic events (Volpe, 2001a; Zupanc, 2004).

Biochemical Effects of Seizures

Seizures result in increased energy expenditure by the organism, which leads to the following sequence of biochemical events: (1) breakdown of ATP to adenosine diphosphate with release of energy; (2) increased glycolysis, stimulated by adenosine diphosphate, with conversion of glycogen to glucose; (3) increased production of pyruvate, which is used by the mitochondria in ATP production; (4) increased oxygen and glucose consumption; (5) increased production of lactate from pyruvate, stimulated by increased adenosine diphosphate; and (6) lactate/H^+-stimulated local vasodilation, which increases local blood flow and substrate availability (Volpe, 2001a; Zupanc, 2004). The rise in blood pressure associated with seizures also increases cerebral blood flow and substrate availability. Seizures result in a marked decrease in brain glucose concentrations because the cells to replenish ATP supplies use much of the available glucose.

Repetitive seizures in the neonate eventually alter brain lipid and protein metabolism and energy metabolism, resulting in a reduction in total brain DNA, RNA, protein, and cholesterol. In animal models these deficiencies lead to impairment of cellular proliferation, differentiation, and myelinization (Volpe, 2001a, b). The effects in the human neonate are unclear but of concern. Brain damage caused by seizure activity could be the result of alterations in protein metabolism or the energy supply, or it could be the result of damage from asphyxia or edema.

Seizures in Neonates Compared with Those in Older Children and Adults

Seizures are more common and expressed differently in the neonate than in older individuals because of structural and functional differences in the neonatal brain. The peak time for organizational processes in the brain is from the sixth month of gestation to 1 year after birth; therefore term and especially preterm infants have relatively immature brain organization at birth. This lack of organization results in an inability to propagate and sustain generalized seizures. For example, the neonate's brain lacks the arborization and synaptic connections (wiring) necessary for a firing neuron to recruit adjacent neurons to fire synchronously. Inadequate organization also leads to a slower response to stimuli (Volpe, 2001b). The lower rate of nerve conduction, limited myelinization, and smaller number of connections between neurons alter the threshold for neuron firing and ability to propagate seizures (Holmes et al, 2002; Volpe, 2001b; Zupanc, 2004).

The neonate has more inhibitory than excitatory synapses; this is actually a protective mechanism because it reduces the chance that a generalized seizure will be propagated in the cerebral cortex. As a result, cortical seizures are rare in neonates (Volpe, 2001b). The newborn has more excitatory (glutamate) than inhibitory neurotransmitters. In addition, GABA, the main inhibitory neurotransmitter in adults, is excitatory in the newborn (Rennie, 2005b). The glutamate level is increased (it is needed by the brain for neuronal development and organization); maturation of the inhibitory system is delayed; and the number of NMDA receptors that respond to glutamate is increased (Holmes et al, 2002; Rennie, 2005b; Zupanc, 2004). Seizure activity in these infants is more likely to be generated in areas of the brain that are more mature, such as the temporal lobe and subcortical structures, especially in the limbic area. The limbic area, located above the corpus callosum, is one of the oldest parts of the brain in terms of embryologic development. This area is involved with behaviors such as sucking, drooling, chewing, swallowing, oculomotor deviations, and apneic episodes, behaviors typical of those seen with subtle seizures in the neonate (Volpe, 2001b).

Assessment

Seizures are a clinical manifestation associated with various underlying pathologic processes (Table 12-4) including hypoxia, ischemia, hypoglycemia, hypocalcemia, intracranial hemorrhage, infection (meningitis, congenital viral infections, viral encephalopathy), congenital anomalies of the CNS, and other metabolic disturbances, such as alkalosis, hypomagnesemia, hypernatremia, and hyponatremia. Less common causes of seizures are drug withdrawal from opiates or barbiturates, genetic disorders of amino and organic acid metabolism, kernicterus, hyperviscosity, and local anesthetic intoxication.

Seizures can be difficult to recognize in neonates because the clinical manifestations often are subtle and can be associated with other disorders or can involve individual behaviors such as grimacing, startle, sucking, and twitching. Seizures also can occur with minimal or no outward signs. Recognition of seizures in the neonatal period requires careful, continuous assessment by the nurse of all infants at risk. Clinical manifestations may include abnormal movements or alterations in tone of the trunk or extremities; abnormal facial, oral, tongue, or ocular movements; and respiratory problems (Mizrahi, 2001). Specific examples of each of these are listed in Table 12-5.

Types of Seizures

Various classifications of neonatal seizures are used, some focusing primarily on clinical and behavioral manifestations, others on the presence or absence of electroencephalographic correlates (Granelli & McGrath, 2004; Rennie, 2005b). Volpe's (2001b) classification identifies, in order of decreasing frequency, the following seizure types: subtle, tonic, clonic (multifocal and focal), and myoclonic.

Subtle seizures are the most common type of seizure seen in neonates, particularly among preterm infants. This type of seizure often is missed because the clinical manifestations may be difficult to recognize and distinguish from other events. The

TABLE 12-4	Major Causes of Neonatal Seizures	
Cause and Frequency (% of Total)	**Usual Age at Onset (Days)**	**Predominant Type of Seizure**
Hypoxic-ischemic injury (50% to 60%)	After 1 (often 6 to 18 hours after birth); 90% in first 72 hours	Subtle (all), generalized tonic, multifocal clonic
Intracranial hemorrhage (10%)		
IVH	1 to 4	Subtle progressing to tonic
SAH	2 to 3	Any type
SDH	1 to 2	May be focal
Hypocalcemia (15%)		
Early	1 to 3	Usually focal or multifocal
Late	4 to 7	Usually focal or multifocal
Hypoglycemia (10%)	1 to 2	Usually focal or multifocal
Infections (5% to 10%)		
Bacterial meningitis	4 to 7	Any type; may be tonic
Viral encephalopathy	2 to 15	Any type
Congenital viral infection	3 to 7	Tonic, myoclonic
CNS malformations (<5% to 10%)	2 to 10 (often not until several months of age)	Tonic, myoclonic
Drug withdrawal (rare)	3 to 34	Tonic or myoclonic
Local anesthetic intoxication* (uncommon)	Before 1 (1 to 6 hours after birth)	Tonic

Compiled from Scher M (2001). Brain disorders of the fetus and neonate. In Klaus MH, Fanaroff AA, editors. Care of the high-risk neonate, ed 5. Philadelphia: Saunders; Scher MS (2005). Neonatal seizures. In MacDonald MG et al, editors. Avery's neonatology: pathophysiology and management of the newborn, ed 5 (pp 1005-1025). Philadelphia: Lippincott Williams & Wilkins; Stevenson DK, Sunshine P (1989). Neonatal seizures. Fetal and neonatal brain injury. Toronto: Decker; Torrence C (1985). Neonatal seizures. Neonatal network 4:9-16, 21-22; Volpe JJ (2001). Neurology of the newborn, ed 4. Philadelphia: Saunders; and Zupanc ML (2004). Neonatal seizures. Clinics in perinatology 51:961-978. IVH, Intraventricular hemorrhage; SAH, subarachnoid hemorrhage; SDH, subdural hemorrhage; CNS, central nervous system. *Caused by accidental injection of local anesthetic into the scalp during placement of paracervical, pudendal, or epidural blocks or during injection of local anesthetics at delivery.

TABLE 12-5	Clinical Manifestations of Seizures in the Neonate
Type of Manifestation	**Specific Alterations**
Abnormal movement or alterations of tone in the trunk and extremities	Clonic (generalized or multifocal, migratory) Altering hemiclonic tonic (single extremity), extension of arms and legs ("decerebrate-like"), extension of legs and flexion of arms ("decorticate-like"), or generalized Myoclonic (isolated or general) Bicycling movements of legs Swimming or rowing arm movements Loss of tone with general flaccidity
Facial, oral, and tongue movements	Sucking Grimacing Twitching Chewing, swallowing, yawning
Ocular movements	Tonic horizontal eye deviation Staring, blinking Nystagmoid jerks
Respiratory manifestations	Apnea (usually preceded or accompanied by one or more subtle manifestations) Hyperpneic or stertorous breathing

Modified from Clancy RR (1983). Neonatal seizures. In Polin RA, Berg F, editors. Workbook in practical neonatology. Philadelphia: Saunders; Gale E (1981). Neonatal seizures. In Perez R, editor. Protocols for perinatal nursing practice. St Louis: Mosby; Mizrahi EM (2001). Neonatal seizures and neonatal epileptic syndromes. Neurology clinics 19:427-463.

behaviors most commonly seen with subtle seizures are (1) tonic, horizontal deviations of the eyes with or without nystagmoid jerking; (2) repetitive blinking or fluttering of the eyelids; (3) drooling, sucking, or tongue thrusting; and (4) swimming or rowing movements of the arms with occasional bicycling movements of the legs (Rennie, 2005b; Scher, 2005; Volpe, 2001b). Apnea may occur but usually is the result of the underlying cause of the seizure in the preterm, rather than of the seizure per se, and rarely occurs as an isolated seizure event (Zupanc, 2004).

The most common form of tonic seizure is the generalized tonic seizure, which usually involves tonic extension of all the extremities but sometimes is limited to one extremity or is manifested by tonic flexion of all limbs. Generalized tonic seizures can be confused with decorticate or decerebrate posturing. Other signs may include eye deviations, apnea, and occasional clonic movements. This type of seizure is the one seen most frequently in preterm infants, especially those with intraventricular hemorrhage and hypoxic-ischemic insults. Generalized tonic seizures often are accompanied by apnea or decerebrate-type postures or both. Occasionally, focal tonic seizures may occur, which are characterized by sustained asymmetric posturing of the limbs, trunk, or neck. Focal tonic seizure activity may be difficult to differentiate from voluntary movement (Scher, 2005; Volpe, 2001b).

Clonic seizures may be multifocal or focal. Because multifocal clonic (migratory) seizures involve the cortex, they are more characteristic of term infants but occasionally may be seen in older preterm infants. This type of seizure involves rhythmic, jerky clonic movements of one or more limbs that migrate to other parts of the body in a random fashion. Multifocal clonic seizures can be confused with jitteriness. These seizures are associated with diffuse hyperexcitability of the cortex, such as occurs with metabolic derangements (Mizrahi, 2001).

Focal clonic seizures also are seen more frequently in term than in preterm infants. This form of seizure is characterized by localized clonic jerking that usually is confined to one limb or the face. Focal clonic seizures may be associated with focal traumatic CNS injuries, such as cerebral contusions and infarcts, or may be a response to a severe metabolic disturbance or asphyxia and occur in combination with other seizure types (Mizrahi, 2001).

Myoclonic seizures are uncommon in term infants and are rarely seen in preterm infants. These seizures are characterized by single or multiple sudden jerks with flexion of the upper (most common) or lower extremities and occasionally the trunk and neck. Myoclonic seizures are most often seen with inborn errors of metabolism or other metabolic problems.

Management

Management of neonatal seizures has two goals: (1) to determine and treat the underlying cause of the seizures and (2) to protect the infant from injury during and after the seizure. Determining the cause involves assessment of the perinatal and neonatal history, a physical examination, laboratory evaluation, and other diagnostic studies. Previous events that may indicate the underlying cause include the delivery history, bleeding, birth trauma, hypoxic-ischemic events, exposure to infectious agents and other teratogens, maternal substance abuse, and postbirth illnesses.

The physical examination includes evaluation of the infant's general health and neurologic status. Routine laboratory studies include electrolyte levels; glucose, calcium, magnesium, and blood urea nitrogen levels; hematocrit value; blood gases; and pH. A blood culture and lumbar puncture also are often performed. A lumbar puncture helps to rule out both infection and CNS bleeding. Other laboratory and diagnostic studies may include CT, ultrasonography, MRI, skull radiography, TORCH screening, amino acid screening (for inborn errors of metabolism), or EEG. The results of an interictal EEG can provide information for the prognosis, more so in a term than a preterm infant.

Seizures must be recognized, seizure activity documented, and the infant protected and supported during and after the seizure. Observing and documenting seizure activity involves noting and recording (1) the time the seizure begins and ends; (2) the body parts involved (e.g., extremities, eyes, head); (3) a description of motor movement, eye deviations, and pupillary reactions; and (4) the infant's respiratory status, color, state, level of consciousness, and postictal status.

During the seizure, the infant's airway must be maintained, vital signs monitored, and the infant assessed for adequacy of respiration and heart rate to maintain ventilation and perfusion. To protect the infant from injury during the seizure, the nurse should not force anything into the infant's mouth or try to restrain the infant's extremities. The nurse should try to turn the infant's head to the side, if possible. After the seizure, the infant's condition should be monitored, and supportive care should be provided so that ventilation, oxygenation, adequate fluids, glucose, and warmth are maintained. The nurse also should assess the infant for signs related to the events that can cause seizure activity in the neonate to help determine the cause of the seizure and prevent additional seizures.

Treatment of the underlying cause of the seizure is a priority for preventing more seizures and neurologic damage. Management of intracranial hemorrhage and CNS anomalies is discussed later in this chapter. Management of other conditions, such as hypoxic-ischemic events, metabolic and electrolyte disorders, infections, and drug withdrawal, are discussed in detail in other chapters. Continual monitoring of blood gases, acid-base status, serum glucose, and fluid and electrolyte status is important for any infant with seizures. Infants who have seizures, regardless of the cause, require intravenous administration of glucose because seizure activity depletes brain glucose and energy supplies (Scher, 2005). Alterations in oxygenation and acid-base status can occur as a complication of the apnea associated with a seizure or the physiologic consequences of seizure activity. Fluid and electrolyte management should be appropriate to the underlying cause of the seizures. For example, fluids are restricted initially in infants with cerebral edema and perinatal hypoxic-ischemic injury.

The issues of when to treat with anticonvulsant drugs and for how long are controversial (Granelli & McGrath, 2004; Wirrell, 2005; Zupanc, 2004). Some clinicians favor early, aggressive therapy, whereas others do not because neonatal seizures often abate spontaneously. Recurrent or prolonged seizures require treatment with anticonvulsants to reduce the risk of brain injury. The first-line anticonvulsant in the neonate is phenobarbital. Other drugs used include phenytoin (Dilantin) or fosphenytoin (generally recommended for IV use over phenytoin) and benzodiazepines such as lorazepam and midazolam (Granelli & McGrath, 2004; Mizrahi, 2001; Zupanc, 2004). Blood levels of these drugs must be monitored carefully to ensure therapeutic levels and prevent toxicity. Cardiovascular status and respiratory function must also be monitored. Refractory seizure may require alternative agents such as clonazepam, lidocaine, carbamazepine, diazepam, valproate, or primidone (Mizrahi, 2001; Zupanc, 2004).

Because anticonvulsants can be respiratory, myocardial, and CNS depressants or can compete with bilirubin for albumin binding, the infant's cardiorespiratory status, color, and neurologic status are monitored in addition to drug effectiveness. Parent teaching includes helping the family to understand the cause and significance of the seizure or seizures and any diagnostic tests that are planned. Discharge teaching of parents includes recognition of seizure manifestations, care of the infant during and after a seizure, and administration of anticonvulsants (dosage and side effects) if administration of these drugs is to be continued after discharge.

Outcomes

The mortality rate for infants with seizures has declined in recent years, from approximately 40% before 1969 to less than 15% currently. Benign seizures in otherwise healthy infants during the first week have a good prognosis (Mizrahi, 2001). Among infants who have repeated seizures, the percentage that show later developmental problems is 25% to 35% or higher (Holmes & Ben-Ari, 2001; Volpe, 2001b). Preterm infants tend to recover more rapidly from a seizure than do term infants; however, mortality and later morbidity are higher in preterm infants. The prognosis for infants who have seizures during the neonatal period is influenced by (1) the time of onset, (2) the cause of the seizure, (3) the interictal EEG results, (4) responsivity to treatment, and (5) the frequency and duration of the seizures (Granelli & McGrath, 2004; Mizrahi, 2001; Scher, 2001; Zupanc, 2004). Seizure onset less than 48 hours after birth has a poor prognosis, whereas onset after 4 days generally has a good prognosis. Clonic seizures have a better prognosis than the other types (Mizrahi, 2001). The EEG results are a better prognostic sign in term than in preterm infants.

The poorest prognosis is seen with seizures associated with severe hypoxic-ischemic injury, grade III or grade IV intraventricular hemorrhage, herpes infection, some bacterial meningitis, and CNS malformations. The best prognosis is seen in infants with seizures that occur secondary to late hypocalcemia, hyponatremia, and uncomplicated subarachnoid hemorrhage. Other causes have a mixed prognosis (Volpe, 2001b). Repeated or prolonged seizures can lead to brain injury by altering cerebral blood flow and delivery of oxygen and nutrients, by depleting brain glucose and energy stores, and by interfering with ventilation (Volpe, 2001b).

HYPOXIC-ISCHEMIC ENCEPHALOPATHY

Hypoxic-ischemic encephalopathy (HIE) occurs as a result of injury to the brain from a combination of systemic hypoxemia and diminished cerebral perfusion that leads to ischemia. The hypoxemia and ischemia may occur simultaneously or sequentially. HIE may occur secondary to prenatal, intrapartal, or postnatal insults. Hypoxic-ischemic damage to the brain occurs in both preterm and term infants. The site of injury varies with maturational changes in the vascular anatomy and metabolic activity of the brain. In the preterm infant younger than 32 to 34 weeks' gestation, hypoxic-ischemic damage usually is associated with germinal matrix hemorrhage/intraventricular hemorrhage (GMH/IVH). The incidence of severe forms of HIE has declined markedly as a result of advances in perinatal care. Most perinatal hypoxic-ischemic events are mild with minimal effects. The insult is significant enough to cause transient organ dysfunction in 4 to 6 per 1000 live births and result in death or significant neurologic sequelae in 1 per 1000 live births (du Plessis, 2005; Madan et al, 2005).

Pathophysiology

After 33 to 34 weeks' gestation, blood flow and brain metabolic activity become less prominent in the germinal matrix and periventricular area and shift to the cortical area. Hypoxia and ischemia in older preterm and term infants, therefore, are more likely to damage areas of the peripheral and dorsal cerebral cortex. Five types of lesions have been identified in infants with HIE: (1) selective neuronal necrosis; (2) status marmoratus of the neurons of the basal ganglia and thalamus, with loss of neurons in these areas; (3) parasagittal cerebral injury; (4) periventricular leukomalacia (primarily in preterm infants); and (5) focal or multifocal ischemic brain necrosis (Hill, 2005; Levene & Evans, 2005; Volpe, 2001b).

The primary lesion for the hypoxic injury is neuronal necrosis in the cortices of the cerebrum and cerebellum, with damage to the gray matter at the depths of the sulci. Neurons of the brainstem may also be injured. Areas of necrosis may extend into the white matter and into the gray matter of the basal ganglia (du Plessis, 2005). The primary ischemic injury occurs in the posterior portion of the parasagittal region secondary to watershed or border zone infarcts. The border zone is at the junctions of the anterior, middle, and posterior cerebral arteries and the superior and inferior cerebellar arteries. This area is farthest from the original source of the brain blood supply of the major cerebral vessels. Thus, with localized ischemia, such as occurs when the infant has systemic hypotension or hypoperfusion, this area receives the least amount of blood.

With hypoxia and systemic hypotension, cerebral perfusion is maintained at first by cerebral vasodilation and redistribution of blood flow to the brain from other organs. If the hypoxia and ischemia continues, brain fluid balance and cerebral blood flow are altered; energy is depleted; ischemia and edema develop; and neurophysiologic activity is disrupted.

At the cellular level, neurologic injury is caused by energy depletion, accumulation of extracellular glutamate, and activation of glutamate NMDA receptors (du Plessis, 2005). This process occurs in two phases. The initial insult and effects of hypoxia lead to hyperpolarization with an influx of sodium, potassium, and water into the cell. This interferes with the cell's ability to produce an action potential, with failure of the sodium-potassium pump and cell edema. Calcium moves into the cell via voltage-dependent ion channels opened by the changes in the sodium-potassium pump. This reduces calcium currents and release of neurotransmitters. These events may be protective mechanisms to reduce neuronal excitability and conserve oxygen. However, reperfusion and reoxygenation may lead to buildup of free oxygen radicals and primary neuronal death. If the hypoxia and ischemia persist, NMDA receptors are activated, which further increases intracellular calcium (entering the cell via glutamate-controlled ion channels). More glutamate is released and accumulates to toxic levels. Nitric oxide (NO) is also released and accumulates. NO, which at normal levels promotes vasodilation and increased blood flow, reaches toxic levels, leading to production of excess free oxygen radicals and further activation of NMDA receptors. NO combines with superoxide free radicals to produce the toxic peroxynitrates, causing further cell damage. This late reperfusion phase (usually beginning 6 to 12 or more hours after the initial insult) is characterized by hyperexcitability and cytotoxic edema and damage caused by the release of free oxygen radicals and NO, inflammatory changes, and imbalances in inhibitory and excitatory neurotransmitters with secondary neuronal death due to necrosis or apoptosis (Bloch, 2005; Buonocore & Perrone, 2004; du Plessis, 2005; Ferriero, 2004; Levene & Evans, 2005; Saugstad, 2001). After a hypoxic-ischemic insult, the entire cortex initially may be edematous, and further ischemic damage may occur as a result of compression of the cortex against the skull.

Assessment

HIE in term or late preterm infants usually is found in infants following asphyxial events. Nonneurologic signs and symptoms related to the underlying hypoxia and ischemia are discussed elsewhere. Most term infants with HIE demonstrate a characteristic pattern of neurologic findings over the first 72 hours of life, including seizures, altered level of consciousness, altered tone, altered activity, irregular respirations, apnea, poor or absent Moro reflex, abnormal cry, poor suck, and altered pupillary responses and eye movements.

Clinical signs can be graded, ranging from mild to severe. Mild HIE is characterized by mild depression or hyperalertness, irritability, and sympathetic nervous system excitation (tachycardia, dilated pupils). These infants have a good Moro reflex and deep tendon reflexes and generally are symptomatic for less than 24 hours or so. Infants with moderate insults demonstrate lethargy interspersed with brief arousal, decreased tone, altered primary reflexes, and increased parasympathetic tone (bradycardia, decreased pupil size and blood pressure) and may develop seizures. Infants with severe insults have varying levels of consciousness initially but then become stuporous or comatose. These infants have depressed deep tendon and Moro reflexes, hypotonia, and most develop seizures (du Plessis, 2005; Levene & Evans, 2005). Seizures occur in up to 60% of infants with HIE with a usual onset at 12 to 14 hours of age (Zupanc, 2004). The types of seizures most often seen are multifocal clonic seizures in term infants, although myoclonic clonic and subtle seizures may also be seen (du Plessis, 2005).

Management

Infants with HIE have multiorgan and multisystem problems that arise from the original hypoxic-ischemic insult. As a result, management of these infants is complex and requires a coordinated team effort. Acute management of infants with HIE focuses on delivery room resuscitation and stabilization and management of the primary problem and related alterations in the cardiovascular, pulmonary, gastrointestinal, and renal systems. Management of these systems is discussed elsewhere. Prompt identification and treatment of seizures is needed to prevent further alterations in ICP and cerebral blood flow. Management of these infants in relation to neurologic problems focuses on elimination of the original hypoxia, alleviation of tissue hypoxia, and promotion of adequate cerebral perfusion and brain oxygenation and maintenance of an adequate glucose supply (du Plessis, 2005; Shankaran, 2002; Volpe, 2001b).

Interventions are directed toward establishing ventilation and adequate perfusion and preventing or minimizing hypotension, hypoxia, acidosis, rapid alterations in cerebral blood flow and systemic blood pressure, and severe apneic and bradycardic episodes. Hyperoxia is also avoided because this state can result in cerebral vasoconstriction and diminished perfusion. The infant's neurologic status is continually

monitored and documented, as are oxygenation, temperature, and blood pressure. HIE must be differentiated from other neurologic dysfunctions caused by trauma, infection, or CNS anomalies. An extensive workup to define the type, extent, and location of the injury may include cranial ultrasonography, brainstem auditory evoked potentials, MRI, EEG, and measurements of cerebral blood flow, ICP, and the creatinine kinase level.

Other parameters that are monitored are the serum and urinary electrolyte levels and osmolality; blood urea nitrogen, serum creatinine, and glucose levels; and fluid and electrolyte balance. These infants are at risk for hypocalcemia secondary to release of excessive phosphorus from the breakdown of ATP that occurred to produce energy; the need for energy arises in response to the stress induced by perinatal hypoxic-ischemic injury. The excess phosphorus is also related to use of bicarbonate to correct acidosis induced by these events. After hypoxic-ischemic events, an infant is at risk for hypoglycemia as a result of depletion of stores from high energy; therefore, provision of adequate glucose for energy and interventions to reduce energy expenditure are important. Fluid status and intake and output are monitored to prevent fluid overload and to reduce localized increases in pressure; fluids are restricted although effectiveness of this intervention has not been evaluated with clinical trials (Kecskes et al, 2005). Fluid management is critical not only for treating the cerebral edema but also for managing the alterations in renal function and problems such as acute tubular necrosis that frequently accompany moderate to severe forms of HIE.

Research continues into newer therapeutic and neuroprotective strategies, such as mild induced hypothermia, calcium channel blockers, and antioxidant agents (Calvert & Zhang, 2005; du Plessis, 2005; Hamrick & Ferriero, 2003; Jensen et al, 2003). Induced mild hypothermia has been used to reduce secondary reperfusion injuries (Perlman, 2004). Techniques studied include both selective cooling of head with mild systemic hypothermia (34° to 35° C) or whole-body cooling (Gluckman et al, 2005; Jacobs et al, 2003; Shankaran et al, 2002). Cooling is generally for 24 to 72 hours and is begun by 6 hours postbirth (6 hours is a therapeutic window demonstrated in sheep between insult and further cell death (du Plessis & Volpe, 2002) for neuroprotective interventions. Most human studies report beneficial effects in terms of improved survival and outcome with no significant adverse effects (Gunn et al, 2005; Wyatt & Robertson, 2005). However, even with cooling, mortality and morbidity remain high. Gluckman et al (2005) in the CoolCap Study reported that cooling may be less effective if cooling started after onset of seizures or in infants with most severe EEG changes prior to therapy.

Fluctuations in systemic blood pressure with increased ICP and altered cerebral hemodynamics can occur as a result of caregiving or environmental stress; therefore developmentally supportive care of these infants to reduce stress is essential. As the infant recovers, opportunities for sensory experiences are an important part of care. These experiences can be introduced slowly, as the infant can tolerate them without becoming stressed and overloaded. Physiologic and neurologic status is monitored and documented at regular intervals. The infant is observed for changes in level of consciousness, tone, and activity and for evidence of seizures. Seizures are recognized and treated promptly to prevent further injury. Positioning and skin care are important, especially for hypoactive, obtunded, or comatose infants. The interventions listed in Table 12-6 to alter ICP and promote oxygenation in infants at risk for GMH/IVH can also be used for infants with HIE.

Parents need initial and continuing support in dealing with their infant's critical illness; the lack of infant responsiveness if the infant is hypoactive, stuporous, or comatose; the possibility of death; and the implications for later neurologic deficits. Parent teaching focuses on promoting an understanding of the

infant's health status and care and providing anticipatory guidance regarding changes in the infant's state, as well as the outcome. The parents need to be shown how to interact with and care for their infant in a developmentally appropriate manner, with the goal of promoting opportunities for interaction while minimizing stressful events. The nurse can model this type of care for the parents and provide anticipatory guidance in the ways the infant's needs and care will change as

TABLE 12-6	Nursing Care to Reduce the Risk of Germinal Matrix Hemorrhage/Intraventricular Hemorrhage (GMH/IVH)*
Intervention	**Rationale**
1. Position the infant with the head in the midline and the head of the bed slightly elevated.	Intracranial pressure (ICP) is lowest with the head in the midline and the head of the bed elevated 30 degrees. Turning the head sharply to the side causes obstruction of the ipsilateral jugular vein and can increase ICP.
2. Avoid tight, encircling phototherapy masks.	Pressure on the occiput can increase ICP by impeding venous drainage.
3. Avoid rapid fluid infusions for volume expansion. • Know the normal blood pressure (BP) for the infant's weight and age. • If the infant is not hypovolemic, suggest dopamine therapy to maintain BP.	Rapid increases in intravascular volume can rupture the capillaries in the germinal matrix, and this risk may be even greater if the infant has a history of hypoxia and hypotension. Even modest, abrupt increases in BP may cause GMH/IVH.
4. If sodium bicarbonate (NaHCO$_3$) therapy is necessary to correct a documented metabolic acidosis, give a dilute solution slowly.	The role of NaHCO$_3$ is unclear, but rapid infusions may cause elevations in carbon dioxide, possibly dilating cerebral vessels and contributing to a pressure-passive cerebral circulation.
5. Monitor BP diligently. Inform physician if a fluctuating pattern in the arterial pressure tracing is noted in high-risk infants receiving ventilation.	The blood flow velocity in the anterior cerebral artery is reflected by the pattern of the simultaneously recorded arterial BP.
6. Monitor closely for signs of pneumothorax, including: (a) Increase in mean BP, especially increases in diastolic BP (early) (b) Increased heart rate (c) Changes in breath sounds, which may or may not be appreciated (d) Diminished arterial oxygen pressure (PaO$_2$) (e) Increased arterial carbon dioxide pressure (PaCO$_2$) (f) Shift in cardiac point of maximum impulse (g) Hypotension and bradycardia (late)	Pneumothorax may precede GMH/IVH. The sum of hemodynamic changes caused by pneumothorax is flow under increased pressure in the germinal matrix capillaries. Changes in vital signs can be early indicators of pneumothorax.
7. Maintain temperature in neutral thermal range.	Hypothermia has been associated with GMH/IVH.
8. Suction only as needed.	Even brief suctioning episodes (20 sec) can increase cerebral blood flow velocity, BP, and ICP and reduce oxygenation.
9. Avoid interventions that cause crying. • Consider long-term methods of achieving venous access to avoid frequent venipunctures. • Critically evaluate all manipulations and handling. • Use analgesics for stressful procedures.	Crying can impede venous return, increase cerebral blood volume, and compromise cerebral oxygenation in sick infants.
10. Maintain blood gas values within a normal range. • Use continuous noninvasive monitoring of oxygenation. • Adjust the fractional concentration of oxygen in inspired gas (FiO$_2$) as needed to maintain the transcutaneous oxygen pressure (TcPO$_2$) or pulse oximeter values within desired range. • Avoid interventions that cause hypoxia.	Hypoxia and hypercapnia are associated with the development of GMH/IVH. These events increase cerebral blood flow and may impair the neonate's already limited ability to autoregulate the cerebral blood flow. Hypoxia can injure the germinal matrix capillary endothelium.

Modified from Kling P (1989). Nursing interventions to decrease the risk of periventricular-intraventricular hemorrhage. *Journal of obstetric, gynecologic, and neonatal nursing 8*:462.
*Premature neonates are most vulnerable to GMH/IVH during the first 4 days of life; approximately 50% of hemorrhages occur in the first 24 hours. Attempts to minimize the risk of GMH/IVH should begin immediately after birth, even before the infant has reached the special care nursery.

the baby matures. Parents can also be involved in devising and implementing a developmental plan of care for their infant.

Outcomes

The prognosis, which varies with the extent and severity of the insult and the resulting brain injury, ranges from death before or shortly after birth to severe neurologic impairment to minimal or no sequelae. Specific sequelae may not be apparent for several months or longer. Some infants make a significant recovery, although the rate and degree of recovery vary. MRI or CT can be used to assess the location, degree, and extent of the injury (Levene & Evans, 2005). Sequelae of HIE in term infants are related to the site of injury (e.g., the cortex); they include mental retardation, microcephaly, cortical blindness, hearing deficits, and epilepsy. Generally, infants with mild HIE do well, as do most infants with moderate HIE of less than 5 days' duration. Infants with moderate HIE of longer duration or severe HIE have a higher mortality rate and later cognitive and motor problems (du Plessis, 2005).

GERMINAL MATRIX AND INTRAVENTRICULAR HEMORRHAGE

Germinal matrix hemorrhage/intraventricular hemorrhage (GMH/IVH) is the most common type of intracranial hemorrhage seen in the neonatal period. GMH/IVH is seen almost exclusively in preterm infants, particularly those weighing less than 1500 g. The incidence in this group of infants has declined and currently ranges from 15% to 20% (Madan et al, 2005). The risk of GMH/IVH increases with decreasing gestational age. GMH/IVH occurs but is rare after 35 to 36 weeks' gestation because of the involution of the subependymal germinal matrix and alterations in cerebral blood flow patterns that occur after this time (Levene, 2001a). The major risk factors for GMH/IVH in the neonate are prematurity and hypoxic events interrelated with the anatomic and physiologic processes that make the periventricular site particularly vulnerable. Any perinatal or neonatal event that results in hypoxia or alters cerebral blood flow or intravascular pressure increases the risk of GMH/IVH.

GMH/IVH is classified by the location and severity of the hemorrhage. A grade I or slight hemorrhage is characterized by isolated germinal matrix hemorrhage; a grade II or small hemorrhage by intraventricular hemorrhage with normal ventricular size; and a grade III or moderate hemorrhage by intraventricular hemorrhage with acute ventricular dilation. A grade IV or severe hemorrhage involves both intraventricular and brain parenchyma hemorrhage (Madan, et al, 2005; Papile, 2002).

Pathophysiology

The neuropathophysiology of GMH/IVH involves a complex interaction of intravascular, vascular, and extravascular factors. In infants of less than 28 to 32 weeks' gestation, the hemorrhage generally arises from the subependymal germinal matrix at the head of the caudate nucleus near the foramen of Monro. On those rare occasions when GMH/IVH occurs in term infants, bleeding usually arises from the choroid plexus rather than from the germinal matrix (Volpe, 2001b).

The germinal matrix includes the tissue underlying the ependymal wall of the lateral ventricles. In many preterm infants, the hemorrhage begins as a microvascular event in the germinal matrix and is confined to the subependymal area.

In the rest, the original hemorrhage ruptures into the lateral ventricles and then into the third and fourth ventricles. The blood eventually collects in the subarachnoid space of the posterior fossa, often extending into the basal cistern (see Figure 12-1) (Levene & de Vries, 2001). Rupture of the hemorrhage from the germinal matrix into the ventricles may serve a protective function by decompressing the hemorrhagic area and reducing further tissue destruction. Progressive ventricular dilation may occur as the result of obstruction of CSF flow by an obliterative arachnoiditis or as the result of blood clots at the level of the aqueduct of Sylvius or the foramen of Monro (Scher, 2001; Cherian et al, 2004). With severe hemorrhages, blood may also be found in the periventricular white matter. This usually is due not to extravasation of blood from the ventricles but to an associated insult in the white matter that increases the risk of CP (Madan et al, 2005; Cherian et al, 2004).

The neuropathologic consequences of GMH/IVH include (1) destruction of the germinal matrix and its glial precursor cells, (2) infarction and necrosis of periventricular white matter, and (3) posthemorrhagic hydrocephalus (Volpe, 2001b). As the IVH moves from the germinal matrix area into the surrounding white matter, periventricular hemorrhagic infarction associated with intraparenchymal echodensities develops. The appearance of this parenchymal lesion is associated with increased mortality and neurodevelopmental sequelae (Volpe, 2001b). Infants with GMH/IVH may also have periventricular leukomalacia (PVL). However, PVL is thought to arise as a consequence of hypoxic-ischemic injury and is not caused by the GMH/IVH per se (Madan et al, 2005; Volpe, 2001b).

Intravascular Factors

Intravascular hemodynamic factors play a prominent role in the pathogenesis of GMH/IVH. These factors include distribution of blood to the periventricular region, pressure-passive cerebral blood flow, and venous hemodynamics. The stages of CNS development characteristic of preterm infants born at less than 32 to 33 weeks' gestation increase the risk of hemorrhage in the periventricular area.

Periventricular Blood Flow

The subependymal germinal matrix is a transient structure that begins to thin after 14 weeks and has almost completely involuted by 36 weeks' gestation (Levene, 2005; Volpe, 2001b). This is the site where neuroectodermal cells that serve as precursors for neurons (before about 24 weeks' gestation) and glial cells develop. These cells subsequently migrate to their eventual locus in the cerebral cortex. Processes involved in the proliferation, differentiation, and migration of these cells result in an area that is highly vascularized and metabolically active. Before 32 weeks' gestation, a significant portion of the total cerebral blood flow goes to the periventricular germinal matrix, primarily to support neuroblast and glioblast mitotic activity and migration. Any factor that increases cerebral blood flow can result in overperfusion of the periventricular region. After 32 to 34 weeks' gestation, cell proliferation and migration decline. The germinal matrix becomes less prominent and receives a smaller proportion of the cerebral blood supply. At this point, the greater proportion of blood flow is to the rapidly differentiating cerebral cortex (Madan, et al, 2005; Papile, 2002; Volpe, 2001b).

Cerebral Autoregulation

The blood vessels of the brain normally are protected from marked alterations in flow by autoregulatory processes. If cerebral autoregulation is intact, the arterioles constrict or dilate to maintain a constant cerebral blood flow despite fluctuations in systemic blood pressure. Hypoxia and hypoxemia in the neonate alter cerebral autoregulation. This alteration can lead to a pressure-passive system in which cerebral blood flow varies directly with arterial pressure. Subsequent alterations in systemic blood pressure or cerebral blood flow, or both, are transmitted directly to the brain and, in particular, to the area receiving the greatest proportion of cerebral blood flow; that is, the fragile, thin-walled vessels of the germinal matrix. Thus rapid fluctuations in systemic blood pressure or cerebral blood flow (i.e., moving from increased to decreased flow and vice versa) also increase the risk of vessel rupture (de Vries & Rennie, 2005; Volpe, 2001b). Altered hemodynamics with fluctuations in blood flow can occur with positive pressure ventilation, rapid volume expansion, hypercapnia, and possibly reduced hematocrit and blood glucose values. Increased systemic blood pressure and, potentially, cerebral blood flow also can occur with caregiving events, such as handling, suctioning, and chest physical therapy (Volpe, 2001b).

Venous Hemodynamics

Increased venous pressure, arising from events such as myocardial failure or positive-pressure ventilation, can also be transmitted directly to the capillaries of the germinal matrix. These events can impede cerebral venous return, leading to stasis and venous congestion, which then lead to increased venous pressure and vessel rupture. The point of vulnerability in the venous drainage system of the brain is at the level of the foramen of Monro and the caudate nucleus (the usual site of GMH/IVH). At this location there is a U-shaped turn in the venous drainage system where the confluence of the thalamostriate, terminal, and choroidal veins forms the internal cerebral vein, which empties into the great vein of Galen. This results in a sharp change in the direction of blood flow and predisposes to turbulent venous flow with stasis and thrombus formation and an area vulnerable to increased intravascular pressure (Volpe, 2001b). In addition, the pliable skull of the preterm infant can easily be deformed, obstructing the major venous sinuses and increasing venous pressure.

Vascular Factors

The capillary bed of the germinal matrix is immature and has large, irregular, thin-walled vessels, a feature that increases its vulnerability to rupture. The capillary walls thicken with increasing gestational age. The fragility of these vessels is due partly to the lack of thickness and strength of the basement membrane and the lack of collagen and smooth muscle. With migration of the neuronal and glial cells and their derivatives, the germinal matrix undergoes involution. The immature capillary bed is remodeled into the definitive, mature capillary bed (Madan et al, 2005; Volpe, 2001b). The epithelial cells of these capillaries are dependent on oxidative metabolism and thus are easily injured by hypoxic events. This characteristic increases the likelihood of leakage or rupture if transmural pressure increases. Because these vessels require an adequate supply of oxygen to maintain their functional integrity, decreased cerebral blood flow can lead to hypoxic-ischemic injury. These vessels are also susceptible to ischemia because they tend to lie in the vascular border zone, or "watershed" area (see the section on HIE). Both increased and decreased cerebral blood flow, therefore, can be involved in the pathogenesis of GMH/IVH.

Extravascular Factors

The capillary bed of the highly vascularized germinal matrix is embedded in gelatinous material that is deficient in supportive mesenchymal elements, thus providing poor support for the fragile blood vessels. In addition, excessive fibrinolytic activity occurs in the periventricular area. As a result, a small initial bleed may not clot off and be localized, but rather may continue to enlarge and rupture into the ventricles, or the cerebral parenchyma, or both (Volpe, 2001b).

Assessment

Perinatal events that can lead to fetal and neonatal hypoxia include maternal bleeding, fetal distress, perinatal hypoxic-ischemic injury, prolonged labor, preterm labor, and abnormal presentation. Neonatal hypoxic events, such as respiratory distress, apnea, and hypotension, further increase the risk of intraventricular hemorrhage (Hill, 2005). Events associated with impeded venous return, increased venous pressure, or both include assisted ventilation, high positive inspiratory pressure, prolonged inspiratory duration, continuous positive airway pressure, and air leak. Venous pressure can also be increased by compression of the infant's skull during vaginal delivery, application of forceps, and use of constricting head bands. Rapid administration of hypertonic solutions (e.g., sodium bicarbonate and glucose), rapid volume expansion, hypernatremia, hypercarbia, caregiving interventions, and environmental stress can increase cerebral blood flow. Hypercarbia causes cerebral vasodilation, thus increasing blood flow. Hypertonic solutions given rapidly or in a large bolus alter osmotic gradients between the brain and the blood. Repeated or prolonged seizures raise the blood pressure and can lead to hypoxia (Volpe, 2001b).

The clinical manifestations of this disorder often are nonspecific and are not well correlated with later sonographic evidence of bleeding. Therefore a high index of suspicion, along with careful monitoring, is important for infants at risk. The diagnosis usually is made by cranial ultrasonography to determine the presence and severity of GMH/IVH and the progression of the hemorrhage, as well as to monitor later complications such as PVL and progressive ventricular dilation. However, ultrasonography is limited in its ability to identify small amounts of blood in normal size ventricles (Papile, 2002).

More than 90% of infants with GMH/IVH bleed within the first 72 hours after birth; 50% of the bleeding occurs in the first 24 hours after birth (de Vries & Rennie, 2005). Approximately 10% to 20% of infants observed serially with cranial ultrasonography after bleeding demonstrate progressive increases in the size of the hemorrhage over a 24- to 48-hour period (de Vries & Rennie, 2005). Late hemorrhages are seen after a few days or weeks in about 10% of infants. Late hemorrhages are seen primarily in preterm infants with severe, prolonged respiratory problems. A new hemorrhage or an extension of a previous one may develop in these infants. A GMH/IVH may also develop before birth in some infants.

The signs and symptoms of GMH/IVH are often nonspecific and subtle. The clinical signs that correlate most closely with

CT evidence of hemorrhage are (1) a decreasing hematocrit value or failure of the hematocrit value to increase after a transfusion; (2) a full anterior fontanelle; (3) changes in activity level; and (4) decreased tone (Volpe, 2001b). Other clinical signs associated with GMH/IVH are impaired visual tracking, increased tone of the lower limbs, neck flexor hypotonia, and brisk tendon reflexes (Levene & de Vries, 2001).

Besides a declining hematocrit value, laboratory evidence suggestive of GMH/IVH involves CSF findings indicative of hemorrhage: increased red blood cell levels, increased protein levels, decreased glucose levels, and xanthochromia (often a later finding and caused by increased protein). Extremely low CSF glucose levels, or hypoglycorrhachia, can be found several days to a week (usually 5 to 15 days) after the hemorrhage in some infants.

The patterns of clinical manifestations seen in individual infants vary widely and range from silent or subtle to catastrophic. At one end of the continuum are the 25% to 50% of infants with GMH/IVH who have only silent, subependymal bleeding with no or minimal clinical signs (de Vries & Rennie, 2005). The hemorrhage is discovered during routine ultrasonographic screening. Other infants may show an unexplained fall in hematocrit (by 10% or more) or failure of the hematocrit to rise after a transfusion (Volpe, 2001b). Other clinical manifestations, if present, include alterations in level of consciousness or stupor, hypotonia, abnormal eye movements or positions, and altered mobility. These infants generally survive. Later developmental outcome varies, depending on the severity of the hemorrhage.

Catastrophic deterioration usually involves major hemorrhages that evolve rapidly over several minutes or hours. Clinical findings include stupor progressing to coma, respiratory distress progressing to apnea, generalized tonic seizures, decerebrate posturing, fixation of pupils to light, and flaccid quadriparesis. This clinical presentation is associated with a declining hematocrit value, bulging fontanelle, hypotension, bradycardia, temperature alterations, hypoglycemia, and syndrome of inappropriate antidiuretic hormone. Infants with catastrophic hemorrhages have a high mortality rate and, if they survive, a poor prognosis for later development (Volpe, 2001b).

Management

Management of GMH/IVH involves prevention of hemorrhage in infants at risk, acute care of infants with current bleeding, pharmacologic therapies, and management of posthemorrhagic ventricular dilation. Routine ultrasonographic screening of infants at risk for GMH/IVH can identify infants with silent bleeding or bleeding associated with nonspecific, subtle symptoms. Prevention or risk reduction begins in the perinatal period, with the prevention of preterm birth, perinatal hypoxic-ischemic injury, and birth trauma. Administration of antenatal steroids is associated with a decreased incidence of GMH/IVH (Hill, 2005; Linder et al, 2003).

Postbirth prevention and risk-reduction activities include resuscitation by trained NICU team and interventions to prevent or reduce hypoxic or ischemic events; to prevent rapid changes in cerebral blood flow, fluctuations in systemic blood pressure, and hyperosmolarity; and to prevent or minimize fluctuations in ICP. By identifying these vulnerable infants, interventions can be instituted to prevent new bleeding or extensions of existing hemorrhage. Continual assessment of fetal and neonatal oxygenation and perfusion is important so that subtle alterations can be recognized and clinicians can intervene early to prevent cerebral hyperperfusion and stabilize cerebral blood flow and pressures. Prompt resuscitation at birth minimizes hypoxemia and hypercarbia, which can alter cerebral autoregulation. Hypertonic solutions and volume expanders are administered slowly, with careful monitoring of vital signs and color. Activities that can increase ICP or cause wide swings in arterial or venous pressure are avoided or minimized when possible, especially during the first 72 hours of life. Because seizures can alter cerebral blood flow and ICP, they must be recognized promptly and treated.

Acute treatment of infants with GMH/IVH involves providing physiologic support by maintaining oxygenation, perfusion, normothermia, and normoglycemia. Physical manipulations and handling are minimized, as are environmental stressors, to reduce the risk of hypoxia and of fluctuations in arterial blood pressure and cerebral blood flow. The infant's position is also important. The infant can be placed prone or side lying. The head is positioned in the midline or to the side, but without flexing the neck. The head of the bed can be elevated slightly. The Trendelenburg position is avoided. Vital signs, blood pressure, tone, activity, and level of consciousness are monitored frequently. The care of infants with progressive ventricular dilation is discussed in the section on hydrocephalus. Developmental interventions, such as containment or swaddling during aversive procedures such as endotracheal suctioning, may promote greater physiologic stability during these procedures and a more rapid return to baseline (McLendon et al, 2003). Specific interventions are listed in Table 12-6.

Pharmacologic therapies, including administration of phenobarbital, indomethacin, vitamin E, and fibrinolytic agents, have been tried prophylactically to reduce the incidence of hemorrhage or to prevent more severe bleeding or neurologic damage, or both. Research findings have been inconsistent for all of these therapies, and some infants have done worse with these therapies (Brion et al, 2003; Crowther & Henderson-Smart, 2003; Fowlie & Davis, 2003; Hill, 2005).

Parent care involves recognition and discussion of parental concerns about their infant's immediate and long-term prognosis and teaching regarding GMH/IVH, its implications and management. The parents need to be shown how to interact with and care for the infant at risk for GMH/IVH in a developmentally appropriate manner, with the goal of promoting opportunities for interaction while minimizing stressful events. The nurse can model this type of care for parents and provide anticipatory guidance in the ways in which the infant's needs and care will change as the baby matures. Parents can also be involved in devising and implementing a developmental plan of care for their infant to reduce environmental stressors.

Management of Progressive Ventricular Dilation

Because progressive posthemorrhagic ventricular dilation is seen in 25% to 35% of GMH/IVH, infants with a history of GMH/IVH are followed with serial cranial ultrasonography. Posthemorrhagic hydrocephalus develops after birth at varying times after the initial insult. Head size can increase without increases in ICP (normopressive hydrocephalus) because of the neonate's soft, malleable skull and open sutures and fontanelles. A tense fontanelle may be noted when the infant is placed in an upright position. Progressive ventricular dilation initially may cause compression and damage to the cortex without causing any change in head size and may be apparent only on ultrasound. Signs of increased ICP (e.g., bulging anterior fontanelle, setting-sun sign, dilated scalp veins, and widely separated sutures) tend to be later findings. In most infants, the ventricular dilation occurs slowly, without increased ICP. Ventricular growth spontaneously arrests in approximately half of these infants within about 30 days. The remaining infants continue to demonstrate ventricular dilation and increased ICP (de Vries & Rennie, 2005; Volpe, 2001a; Whitelaw, 2001).

The initial treatment for normopressive hydrocephalus is observation, because in many of these infants, ventricular growth arrests spontaneously without therapy. Progressive ventricular dilation with increasing ICP is managed with a ventriculoperitoneal shunt or, if the infant is too ill or too small for surgery, with temporary ventricular drainage. A ventriculoperitoneal shunt is the shunt of choice in infants and children because this type is easier to insert, revise, and lengthen and has a lower risk of infection than a ventriculoatrial shunt. One end of a radiopaque catheter is placed in the lateral ventricle, usually on the right side, and the other end is placed in the peritoneal cavity. The catheter contains a one-way valve that is palpable on the side of the head near the ear. The shunt needs multiple revisions during childhood for growth and for malfunctioning. Major complications of ventriculoperitoneal shunts are infection and obstruction. Too-rapid drainage of CSF immediately after insertion of the shunt can lead to herniation of the brain or subdural hematoma.

After surgery, these infants are positioned on the side opposite the shunt, with the head of the bed flat or slightly elevated to prevent rapid loss of CSF and decompression. The valve should not be pumped unless this action is specifically ordered. The position can be rotated to supine every few hours to prevent skin breakdown. The skin should be kept clean and dry. The infant can also be placed on sheepskin or lambskin to prevent skin breakdown.

Infants with a shunt are observed for signs of localized or systemic infection, ileus, and shunt obstruction. Obstruction of the shunt leads to accumulation of CSF, enlargement of the head, and signs of increased ICP. Infection of the shunt may appear as localized redness or drainage around the incision, temperature instability, altered activity, or poor feeding. Fluid status and intake and output are monitored, and the infant is observed for signs of dehydration from too rapid loss of CSF. Signs of too-rapid decompression include a sunken fontanelle, agitation or restlessness, increased urine output, and electrolyte abnormalities. Parent teaching before discharge includes care of the infant and shunt, including positioning and skin care. Parents must be comfortable in handling and caring for their infant before discharge. They should know the signs of shunt malfunction, increased ICP, infection, and dehydration. Continuing follow-up care of the infant and parental support are important. Parents may be referred to parent groups for peer support. The long-term outcome generally has not been improved by the use of serial lumbar puncture, administration of drugs to reduce CSF production, or use of fibrinolytic agents to dissolve clots (de Vries & Rennie, 2005).

Outcomes

The severity and extent of the hemorrhage and the presence of associated problems (e.g., respiratory distress syndrome, perinatal hypoxic-ischemic injury, and sepsis) influence mortality and morbidity. Infants with a history of GMH/IVH are also at risk for developing posthemorrhagic ventricular dilation, which may be normopressive or associated with increased ICP. Infants with small or mild hemorrhages survive and generally have a good outcome, with a low incidence of major neurologic sequelae and posthemorrhagic ventricular dilation. Infants with moderate hemorrhage have a 5% to 20% mortality rate, and ventricular dilation develops in 15% to 25% of survivors. Mortality in infants with severe hemorrhage averages 50%, with development of progressive ventricular dilation in 55% to 80%. Although infants with severe hemorrhages tend to have significant motor and cognitive deficits, some seem to escape significant long-term sequelae. The incidence of neurologic sequelae ranges from 15% in infants with moderate hemorrhage to 35% to 90% in infants with severe hemorrhages. Sequelae include cerebral palsy (CP), developmental retardation, sensory and attention problems, learning disorders, and hydrocephalus (de Vries & Rennie, 2005; Levene & de Vries, 2001; Madan et al, 2005; Volpe, 2001b).

WHITE-MATTER INJURY IN PRETERM INFANTS

White-matter injury (WMI) is the most common severe neurologic insult seen in preterm infants (de Vries & Rennie, 2005). White-matter hypoxic-ischemic injury includes both focal cystic necrotic lesions, referred to as periventricular leukomalacia (PVL), seen in 3% to 15% of surviving very-low-birth-weight (VLBW) infants, and the more common diffuse noncystic lesions associated with disturbances in myelinization seen in at least 26% of survivors (Back & Rivkees, 2004; de Vries & Rennie, 2005; Wiswell & Graziani, 2005). Leukomalacia refers to change in the brain's white matter reflective of softening. WMI often is associated with GMH/IVH, but it is a separate lesion that may also occur in the absence of GMH/IVH. PVL is a symmetric, nonhemorrhagic, usually bilateral lesion caused by ischemia from alterations in arterial circulation (Wiswell & Graziani, 2005). Time of onset is variable.

Risk factors include any event during the prenatal, intrapartal, or postbirth periods that results in cerebral ischemia; this includes asphyxia, GMH/IVH, hypoxia, hypercarbia, hypotension, cardiac arrest, and infection (in which blood flow is diminished by the action of endotoxins). The major risk factors are GMH/IVH, asphyxia, and chorioamnionitis (Wiswell & Graziani, 2005).

Pathophysiology

PVL begins with ischemic necrosis of the white matter dorsal and lateral to the external angles of the lateral ventricles, especially in the border zone area. The border zone is the area farthest from the original source of the cerebral blood supply and thus is most susceptible to ischemic damage from diminished cerebral blood flow. PVL often extends into the cortical white matter (Volpe, 2001b). Pathologic changes begin with patchy areas of focal ischemic coagulation that may occur as early as 5 to 8 hours after the initial hypoxic-ischemic insult. This is followed within a few days by proliferation of macrophages and astrocytes, along with endothelial and glial infiltration. Later changes include thinning of the white matter and liquefaction in the central portion of the necrotic area, as well as cavitation, cystic changes, and decreased myelinization (de Vries & Levene, 2001). Cerebral atrophy leads to expansion of the lateral ventricles and hydrocephalus.

The pathogenesis of WMI is due to the interaction of three maturation-dependent factors: (1) immature vascular supply to the white matter that reduces oxygen delivery to vulnerable areas of the brain; (2) impairments in cerebral autoregulation; and (3) vulnerabilities of the premyelinating oligodendrites, which are especially vulnerable to damage from reactive oxygen and nitrogen species (free radicals), glutamate, adenosine, and cytokines (Kinney, 2005; Volpe, 2001a). Damage to the premyelin-producing oligodendrites leads to release of cytokines (indicating an inflammatory process), glutamate, and free radicals (Back & Rivkees, 2004; Wiswell & Graziani, 2005). Oligodendrocyte development and survival are impaired, leading to altered myelinization with subsequent motor, cognitive, and behavioral neurodevelopmental problems. Axonal damage and disruption also occur (Kinney, 2005). Perinatal infection and an immune-mediated inflammatory response with release of proinflammatory cytokines are increasingly thought to play a prominent role in PVL pathogenesis (Kadhim et al, 2001).

Assessment

PVL is a compilation of prenatal or postnatal insults or both. Often no clinical findings are specific to PVL during the first weeks of life unless the damage is severe. Cranial ultrasonography can identify infants at risk for or who have early signs of PVL, although HUS is not as sensitive in the diagnosis of PVL as it is with GMH/IVH; MRI can identify changes early and is especially useful with diffuse WMI (Wiswell & Graziani, 2005). Infants at risk for WMI should undergo serial cranial ultrasonographic examinations and again at discharge and with later follow-up. With severe damage, neuromotor abnormalities and signs of ventricular enlargement develop. As the infant matures, neurologic and motor deficits become apparent.

Management

Initial management focuses on treating the primary insult and its attendant complications and preventing further hypoxic-ischemic damage. This involves preventing or minimizing hypotension, hypoxia, acidosis, and severe apneic and bradycardic episodes. HUS and MRI are used serially to diagnose PVL and to follow its progression in infants at risk. Later management involves care related to residual problems, such as spastic diplegia and hydrocephalus. Nursing interventions focus on acute management of the primary problem and supportive care for the infant and parents. Nurses have a major role in identifying signs of hypoxia and ischemia and instituting interventions to prevent further ischemic damage. These interventions are similar to those described earlier and in Table 12-6. Environmental stressors may increase the risk for development of GMH/IVH and subsequent PVL or may cause associated developmental problems. Developmental and environmental interventions, therefore, are important aspects of nursing care.

Parents need initial and continuing support in dealing with their infant's illness and the risk of later neurologic problems. Parent teaching should focus on promoting an understanding of the infant's health status and care and providing anticipatory guidance and follow-up care. The parents can be shown how to interact with and care for their infant in a developmentally appropriate manner to foster parent-infant interaction and to promote infant organization and development. The nurse can model this type of care for the parents and can provide anticipatory guidance as the infant's needs and care change.

Outcomes

Infants with PVL may die in the neonatal period, usually from the original hypoxic, hemorrhagic, or infectious insult rather than from PVL per se. Infants with WMI are at higher risk for later developmental problems that affect motor, cognitive, and visual function (Wiswell & Graziani, 2005). The most prominent sequelae in survivors, especially those with multifocal cystic lesions around the lateral ventricles, is spastic diplegia with or without hydrocephalus (Calvert & Zhang, 2005). In infants with spastic diplegia, descending fibers from the motor cortex cross the affected area around the ventricles. Because the leg motor fibers are closest to the ventricles, spastic diplegia of the leg is the most common sequela. With extension of the damage, arm involvement with spastic quadriplegia may occur. Damage to the optic radiations in this area leads to visual deficits (Wiswell & Graziani, 2005). Infants with diffuse WMI are more likely to develop cognitive and neurobehavioral impairments (Calvert & Zhang, 2005).

BIRTH INJURIES

Traumatic injury to the central or peripheral nervous system can occur during the perinatal or postnatal period. Most of these injuries happen during the intrapartum period and may occur with perinatal hypoxic-ischemic events. Perinatal events most frequently associated with birth injury include midforceps delivery, shoulder dystocia, low forceps delivery, birth weight exceeding 3500 g, and second stage of labor lasting longer than 60 minutes. The incidence of injury has declined markedly in recent years as a result of improvement in obstetrical care and increased use of cesarean sections for abnormal presentations. However, birth injuries can also arise from trauma during a cesarean section or resuscitation.

Injuries that occur before the intrapartum period usually are caused by compression or pressure injuries from an unusual fetal position. The risk of injury to the central or peripheral nervous system is greater with malpresentation (especially breech), malposition, prolonged or precipitate labor, prematurity, multiple gestation, shoulder dystocia, macrosomia, and instrumental delivery. The most prevalent types of injury to the nervous system are extracranial hemorrhage, intracranial hemorrhage, skull fractures, spinal cord injury, and peripheral nerve injury.

Extracranial Hemorrhage

Caput succedaneum and cephalohematoma are the most common types of birth injury, as well as the most benign. Caput succedaneum is characterized by soft, pitting, superficial edema that is several millimeters thick and overlies the presenting part in a vertex delivery. This edematous area lies above the periosteum and thus crosses suture lines. The edema consists of serum or blood, or both. Infants with caput succedaneum may also have ecchymosis, petechiae, or purpura over the presenting part. Caput succedaneum occurs in infants after a spontaneous vertex delivery or after the use of a vacuum extractor. This type of extracranial hemorrhage requires no care other than parent teaching regarding its cause and significance. It resolves within a few days after birth with no sequelae.

Cephalohematoma occurs in 1.5% to 2.5% of newborns (Madan et al, 2005). It involves subperiosteal bleeding, usually over the parietal bone but possibly over other cranial bones. Cephalohematoma usually is unilateral but can be bilateral. This type of hemorrhage is seen most often in males, after the use of forceps, after a prolonged, difficult delivery, and in infants born to primiparas. The characteristic finding is a firm, fluctuant mass that does not cross the suture lines. The mass often enlarges slightly by 2 to 3 days of age. Approximately 5% of infants with unilateral and 18% with bilateral cephalohematomas have a linear skull fracture underlying the mass (Madan et al, 2005). In rare cases an infant may have a subdural or subarachnoid hemorrhage.

A cephalohematoma is limited to the periosteal area and does not cross suture lines; it can take weeks to months to resolve completely. Conversely, caput succedaneum crosses suture lines, may be accompanied by ecchymosis, and resolves within a few days after birth. Caput succedaneum and cephalohematoma over the occipital bone must be differentiated from encephalocele. In contrast to extracranial hemorrhage, an encephalocele is characterized by pulsations, increased pressure (tenseness) with crying, and the appearance of a bony defect on radiographic studies.

Infants with a cephalohematoma generally have no symptoms. Management includes parent teaching and monitoring for the development of hyperbilirubinemia. Occasionally an infant with a large cephalohematoma becomes anemic. These infants should also be monitored for symptoms of intracranial hemorrhage or skull fracture. Generally, cephalohematomas resolve between 2 weeks and 6 months of age, and most resolve by 8 weeks. Calcium deposits occasionally develop, and the swelling may remain for the first year.

Subgaleal Hemorrhage

Subgaleal or subaponeurotic hemorrhage is the most serious form of extracranial hemorrhage in newborns (Rennie, 2005a). Blood collects in a large potential space between the galea aponeurotica and the periosteum of the skull through which large emissary veins pass (Uchil & Arulkumaran, 2003). The area is called a potential space because it can greatly expand, with accumulations of up to 260 ml (more than the entire blood volume of some newborns) (Furdon & Clark, 2001). Traction or application of intense shearing forces to the scalp pull the aponeurosis from the vault and rupture these veins

Subgaleal hemorrhage occurs in 4 per 10,000 spontaneous vaginal deliveries and 59 per 10,000 vacuum-assisted deliveries (Uchil & Arulkumaran, 2003). The incidence is also increased with precipitous deliveries, macrosomia, and severe dystocia, and with failed vacuum deliveries requiring forceps (Uchil & Arulkumaran, 2003). Use of soft silastic cups (rather than the rigid hard cup) with vacuum extractors is associated with fewer scalp injuries, although the soft cups are more likely to fail (Johanson & Menon, 2000). Mortality is 17% to 25%; however, if the infant survives the hemorrhage and does not develop HIE, the hemorrhage usually resolves in 2 to 3 weeks and outcomes are good (Rennie, 2005a).

Subgaleal hemorrhage is a clinical emergency. These infants usually present at birth or within a few hours (occasionally at a few days) (Uchil & Arulkumaran, 2003). Clinical findings include a firm, ballotable head mass that crosses sutures and fontanelles (often extending from the orbital ridge, around the ears to the neck) and increases in size after birth. Each centimeter of enlargement is estimated to be equivalent to 40 ml of blood loss (Rennie, 2005a). The mass mimics edema and shifts with head repositioning. Infants usually show signs of pain on manipulation of the scalp or head (Furdon & Clark, 2001; Uchil & Arulkumaran, 2003). Infants may present with a rapidly falling hematocrit, anemia, hypovolemia, pallor, hypotension, tachycardia, tachypnea, hypotonia, and other signs of shock (Rennie, 2005a; Uchil & Arulkumaran, 2003). Management includes rapid recognition, cardiovascular and respiratory monitoring, administration of blood and volume expanders, and control of bleeding (Furdon & Clark, 2001; Rennie, 2005a; Steinbach, 1999).

Case Study

IDENTIFICATION OF THE PROBLEM

A term female infant was delivered vaginally, assisted with a Malmström (metal) vacuum apparatus. The infant was limp and pale upon delivery with Apgar scores of 5^1, 4^5. The infant was successfully resuscitated by 10 minutes of age, with spontaneous respirations resumed, and heart rate was greater than 100 beats/min. She remained pale with thready pulses and poor peripheral perfusion. The infant was brought to the neonatal intensive care unit.

ASSESSMENT: HISTORY AND PHYSICAL EXAMINATION

The term female infant was delivered vaginally to a 24-year-old G2 P1 woman following prolonged labor at term after an uncomplicated pregnancy. The vaginal delivery was assisted with a Malmström (metal) vacuum apparatus. Upon delivery, the infant was limp and pale; Apgar scores were 5^1, 4^5. The infant was pale with thready pulses, poor peripheral perfusion, and heart rate of 180 beats/min on admission. Umbilical catheters were placed and 20 ml/kg Plasmanate was given for volume expansion; dopamine was initiated because of low blood pressure and ongoing poor perfusion. A rapidly enlarging scalp hematoma was noted during this time. The infant was given an emergency blood transfusion of 15 ml/kg, and a disseminated intravascular coagulation (DIC) panel was sent to the laboratory.

Gestational age was term with a birth weight of 3.3 kg; OFC and length were not available. She had a boggy, enlarging scalp hematoma; eyes were equal and reactive to light, positive red reflex and normal facies. Her lungs were clear and equal to bases with a gasping respiratory effort. Heart rate was regular with no murmur noted. Poor peripheral perfusion, capillary blood refill time greater than 5 seconds, and thready pulses were noted. The abdomen was soft and nontender with no hepatosplenomegaly or masses palpable and a three-vessel cord. Genitourinary examination revealed normal female infant genitalia. The anus appeared patent. On neurologic examination she was noted to have decreased responses, with eyes open and unblinking. Extremities were well formed; muscle tone was very decreased. Skin was pale with slightly cyanotic undertones; extremities were cool and mottled.

Continued

Case Study—cont'd

DIFFERENTIAL DIAGNOSES

The differential diagnoses were (1) subgaleal hemorrhage; (2) perinatal hypoxic-ischemic injury; (3) shock; (4) DIC; (5) intracranial hemorrhage; (6) rule out sepsis; and (7) rule out congenital cardiac defects.

DIAGNOSTIC TESTS

To start differentiating between the most likely diagnoses a variety of tests were needed. Laboratory tests obtained were a complete blood tests with differential and coagulation panel. Imaging tests ordered were a head CT scan, transcutaneous Doppler and nuclear medicine flow scan, and electroencephalogram (EEG).

WORKING DIAGNOSIS

Laboratory results on admission were WBC/differential benign, hematocrit (Hct) 21%, platelet count 168,000/mm³, prothrombin time (PT) greater than 100 seconds, partial thromboplastin time (PTT) greater than 100 seconds, fibrinogen 54 mg/dl, and D-dimers 2 to 4 mg/ml. Other diagnostic tests results were (1) head CT scan (performed within 4 hours of age): extensive blood within the extracranial soft tissues, mild intraventricular and subarachnoid hemorrhage; (2) transcranial Doppler and nuclear medicine flow scan (performed at 24 hours of age): no cerebral blood flow; and (3) EEG (performed on day of life 3): absence of cortical activity. These findings along with the data from the history and physical assessment suggested a working diagnosis of extensive subgaleal hemorrhage with hematoma.

DEVELOPMENT OF MANAGEMENT PLAN

The treatment plan was (1) colloids to treat DIC, Hct changes; (2) monitoring; (3) mechanical ventilation as needed; (4) fluid support; (5) blood, tracheal, surface cultures for bacterial and/or viral infections; (6) antibiotics; (7) sodium bicarbonate boluses to correct metabolic acidosis; and (8) vasopressors to maintain adequate blood pressure and cerebral blood flow.

IMPLEMENTATION AND EVALUATION OF EFFECTIVENESS

The treatment plan was implemented immediately after birth and admission to the neonatal intensive care unit. The infant was intubated within the first half hour of life because of her ongoing gasping respirations and given multiple blood transfusions, fresh-frozen plasma with cryoprecipitate transfusions, and multiple sodium bicarbonate and normal saline boluses. Respiratory status and blood pressure were normalized within the first hour of life, and metabolic acidosis and coagulation panel results were normalized within the first 24 hours of life. Severe brain involvement was suspected on day of life 2, with the dismal results of the Doppler and flow scan; brain death was determined on day of life 3, with the flat EEG results. All bacterial and viral cultures were negative, and liver function tests were normal. The infant received a total of 476 ml neonatal red blood cells, 8 units of cryoprecipitate, and 140 ml of fresh-frozen plasma to normalize the coagulation studies by 24 hours of age. Life support was terminated on day of life 4; the autopsy was remarkable for an extensive subgaleal hematoma and moderate subarachnoid and subdural hemorrhage.

Other Types of Intracranial Hemorrhage

In addition to GMH/IVH, several other clinically important types of intracranial bleeding can occur in the neonate, including primary subarachnoid hemorrhage, subdural hemorrhage, and intracerebellar hemorrhage. These types of hemorrhage arise from trauma or hypoxia during the perinatal period.

Primary Subarachnoid Hemorrhage

Primary subarachnoid hemorrhage (SAH) is the most prevalent form of intracranial hemorrhage in neonates and the least clinically significant for most infants. SAH occurs in both preterm and term infants but is more common in preterm infants. SAH may occur alone (primary SAH) or as a secondary event with other forms of intracranial hemorrhage. For example, with GMH/IVH, blood moves into the subarachnoid space via the fourth ventricle.

Pathophysiology. Primary SAH consists of bleeding into the subarachnoid space that is not secondary to subdural or intraventricular bleeding. In neonates, the source of the bleeding is venous blood; in older children and adults, SAH usually involves arterial blood. With primary SAH, blood leaks from the leptomeningeal plexus, bridging veins, or ruptured vessels in the subarachnoid space (Levene, 2005). This type of

hemorrhage is associated with trauma or asphyxia. Trauma that causes increased intravascular pressure and capillary rupture is the underlying causal event in most term infants with SAH. In preterm infants, SAH usually is the result of asphyxial events. Factors that place an infant at risk for SAH include birth trauma, prolonged labor, difficult delivery, fetal distress, and perinatal hypoxic-ischemic events.

Assessment. Three clinical presentations have been described for infants with SAH (Volpe, 2001b). The most common is a preterm infant with a minor SAH. These infants are asymptomatic. The hemorrhage is discovered accidentally, for example, during a lumbar puncture as part of a sepsis workup. With the second type of clinical presentation, term or preterm infants may show isolated seizure activity at 2 to 3 days of age or preterm infants occasionally may present with apnea. Between seizures, the infant appears and acts healthy ("well baby with seizures"). Infants in both of these groups survive and usually do well developmentally. The third type of clinical presentation involves infants with a massive SAH that has a rapid and fatal course. This presentation is rare and often is associated with both a severe asphyxial event and birth trauma. Blood in the CSF on lumbar puncture indicates the possibility of SAH, but true hemorrhage must be distinguished from a bloody tap. MRI and CT also can help confirm the diagnosis; ultrasonography is unreliable with SAH (Levene, 2005).

Management. Management of these infants begins with efforts to prevent or reduce the risk of trauma and hypoxia during the perinatal period, so as to reduce the risk of development of SAH. Infants with SAH are observed for seizures and other neurologic signs during the early neonatal period. Nursing care is primarily supportive and includes maintenance of oxygenation and perfusion and provision of warmth, fluids, and nutrients. Nursing management also involves helping the parents to understand the basis for and cause and prognosis of SAH, as well as the care of their infant. Occasionally, infants with massive, acute SAH may require a craniotomy.

Outcomes. Generally, infants with SAH survive, and asymptomatic infants do well. Up to half of symptomatic infants with severe, sustained traumatic or hypoxic injury with further damage to the CNS have neurologic sequelae (Hill, 2005; Volpe, 2001b). Hydrocephalus occasionally develops in infants with a history of SAH as a result of obstruction of CSF flow by adhesions. These infants should undergo repeat ultrasonographic examinations to monitor ventricular dilation.

Subdural Hemorrhage

Subdural hemorrhage (SDH) is more common in term than preterm infants. The incidence of SDH has declined markedly as a result of improvements in obstetrical care. This decrease has been particularly notable in term infants (Hill, 2005; Levene, 2005). Risk factors include precipitous, prolonged, or difficult delivery, use of midforceps or high forceps, prematurity, cephalopelvic disproportion, and macrosomia. SDH is seen more often in infants born to primiparas, possibly because of the more rigid birth canal. Infants with abnormal presentations (e.g., breech, foot, brow, or face) are also at higher risk for SDH. Early recognition of SDH is critical for infants with severe bleeding who require surgical intervention.

Pathophysiology. SDH in newborns is almost always caused by trauma during the perinatal period. Bleeding occurs between the dura and the arachnoid and may be unilateral or bilateral. The bleeding occurs over the cerebral hemispheres or posterior fossa with or without tentorium or falx cerebri lacerations (see Figure 12-1). The cerebral hemispheres are the most common site for SDH. Bleeding usually occurs over the temporal convexity, with rupture of superficial cerebral veins or of "bridging" veins between the superomedial aspect of the cerebrum and the superior sagittal sinus. Because the superficial veins over the cerebrum are poorly developed in the preterm infant, this type of hemorrhage is seen less often in these infants. Bleeding over the posterior fossa involves bleeding below the tentorium and compression of the brainstem. Dural tears at the junction of the falx and tentorium near the attachment of the great vein of Galen are also associated with compression of the brainstem and midbrain (Levene, 2005; Volpe, 2001b).

Assessment. SDH must be distinguished from other types of intracranial hemorrhage and neurologic problems. This differentiation often can be accomplished by evaluating the infant's history and presentation and, if the infant is having seizure activity, by ruling out other causes of seizures. SDH over the cerebral hemispheres often is associated with SAH. SDH also occurs with extracranial hemorrhages, such as cephalohematoma and subgaleal, subconjunctival, and retinal

hemorrhages; skull fractures; and brachial plexus or facial palsies (Levene & de Vries, 2001; Volpe, 2001b). MRI or CT can assist in confirming the diagnosis; HUS is less reliable (Madon et al, 2005).

Clinical signs of SDH relate to the site of the bleeding and the severity of the hemorrhage. Three patterns are seen in infants with bleeding over the cerebral hemispheres (Volpe, 2001b). The first pattern is seen in most neonates with SDH; these infants have a minor hemorrhage and are asymptomatic or have signs such as irritability and hyperalertness. With the second pattern, seizures develop during the first 2 to 3 days of life and usually are focal. Other neurologic signs, which may be absent or present, include hemiparesis; pupils that are unequal and respond sluggishly to light; full or tense fontanelle; bradycardia; and irregular respirations. The third pattern is seen in a few infants who have no or nonspecific signs in the neonatal period but in whom signs appear at 4 weeks to 6 months of age. These infants generally show increasing head size as a result of continued hematoma formation, poor feeding, failure to thrive, altered level of consciousness and, occasionally, seizures caused by the chronic subdural effusion.

Infants with abnormal neurologic signs from birth often have had bleeding over the posterior fossa with tentorial lacerations. Signs include stupor or coma, eye deviation, asymmetric pupil size, altered pupillary response to light, tachypnea, bradycardia, and opisthotonos. As the clot enlarges, these infants rapidly deteriorate, with signs of shock appearing over minutes to hours. The infant becomes comatose and has fixed, dilated pupils and altered respirations and heart rate, which culminate in respiratory arrest. Infants with small tears in the posterior fossa may have no clinical manifestations for the first 3 to 4 days of life. During this time, the clot gradually enlarges until signs of increased ICP appear. As the brainstem becomes compressed, the infant's condition deteriorates, and oculomotor abnormalities, altered respiration, bradycardia, and seizures occur (Volpe, 2001b).

Management. SDH often can be prevented or its severity diminished by reducing trauma during the perinatal period. Treatment of infants who have bleeding over the cerebral hemispheres is supportive. Infants with a history of perinatal trauma or other risk factors are observed for seizures and other neurologic signs. Care is primarily supportive and includes maintenance of oxygenation and perfusion and provision of warmth, fluids, and nutrients. Nursing management also involves helping the parents to understand the basis for and the cause and prognosis of this type of hemorrhage, as well as the care of their infant.

Symptomatic infants with bleeding over the temporal convexity and increased ICP may require surgical evacuation if the infant's condition cannot be stabilized neurologically. Massive posterior fossa hemorrhage requires craniotomy and surgical aspiration of the clot (Levene & de Vries, 2001). Infants at risk for SDH should be monitored carefully over the first 4 to 6 months after birth for late signs of bleeding and hematoma formation. Monitoring of these infants includes observation of head size, growth, feeding, activity, and level of consciousness, as well as monitoring for seizure activity.

Outcomes. The prognosis varies with the location and severity of the hemorrhage. Infants with bleeding over the cerebral hemispheres who are asymptomatic do well, as do most infants who have transient seizures in the neonatal period if no associated cerebral injury is present. Early diagnosis with CT or MRI has improved the outcome for infants with posterior fossa hemorrhage (Volpe, 2001b). Most infants with bleeding over the tentorium or falx cerebri die; severe hydrocephalus and neurologic sequelae usually develop in those that survive (Hill, 2005).

Intracerebellar Hemorrhage

Intracerebellar hemorrhage is rare and is thought to be the result of hypoxia. These hemorrhages occur in both term and preterm infants but are more common in preterm infants. Intracerebellar hemorrhage is seen during autopsy in infants with a history of perinatal hypoxic-ischemic events or severe respiratory distress syndrome (or both) and GMH/IVH. Intracerebellar hemorrhage also occurs secondary to trauma, especially in very-low-birth-weight (VLBW) infants. Mechanical deformation of the occiput during forceps or breech delivery and compression of the compliant skull during fixation of the head for caregiving procedures or with use of constrictive head bands may also be predisposing factors (Volpe, 2001b).

Two presentations have been described. Many infants are critically ill from birth, with rapidly progressive apnea, a declining hematocrit value, and death within 24 to 36 hours. Other infants are less ill initially, and symptoms develop up to 2 to 3 weeks of age. Clinical manifestations include apnea, bradycardia, hoarse or high-pitched cry, eye deviations, opisthotonos, seizures, vomiting, hypotonia, and diminished or absent Moro reflex. Hydrocephalus often develops in these infants as early as the end of the first week after birth. The prognosis is poor in survivors, especially those born prematurely or with severe hemorrhage (Levene & de Vries, 2001).

Skull Fracture

Two types of skull fractures, linear and depressed, are seen in newborns. Skull fractures occur in utero, during labor, with forceps delivery, or during a prolonged, difficult labor with compression and battering of the fetal skull against the maternal ischial spines, sacral promontory, or symphysis pubis (Levene, 2001b). The fetal skull often is able to tolerate mechanical stressors relatively well, because it is flexible, malleable, poorly ossified, and less mineralized than the adult skull. Depressed fractures occur after forceps delivery but occasionally are seen after a vaginal or cesarean birth. Compression of the skull causes buckling of the inner table without a break in the continuity of the skull.

Linear fractures usually occur over the frontal or parietal bones. These fractures often are associated with extracranial hemorrhage and may underlie a cephalohematoma; they usually are asymptomatic. Skull radiographs are required for the diagnosis. Intracranial hemorrhage rarely complicates linear fractures. Some infants may have underlying cerebral injury or may have a "growing fracture," which is a rare complication in which a dural tear allows the leptomeninges to extrude into the fracture site (Paige & Carney, 2002). A depressed skull fracture manifests as a visible, palpable depression, or dent in the skull, usually over the parietal area. These fractures often are described as resembling a Ping-Pong ball because the depression does not involve any loss of bone continuity. Unless underlying cerebral contusion or hemorrhage is present, no other signs or symptoms are seen.

The diagnosis is confirmed with skull radiographs or CT scans. CT is performed to identify cerebral contusions or hemorrhage. Nursing assessment includes monitoring these infants for signs of neurologic dysfunction, intracranial hemorrhage, meningitis, and seizures, although these findings are rare. Parents usually are concerned about their infant's appearance (with a depressed fracture) and the possibility of brain damage. They need support and teaching. Infants with uncomplicated linear fractures require no special management. Follow-up monitoring usually is recommended so that a growing fracture and development of a leptomeningeal cyst can be ruled out. Infants with basal fractures are treated for shock and hemorrhage. If the infant has leakage of CSF, antibiotics usually are given prophylactically to prevent meningitis.

In some infants with a depressed fracture, the fracture elevates spontaneously within the first week. Most clinicians recommend manually elevating an uncomplicated depressed fracture that does not elevate spontaneously within a few days (Paige & Carney, 2002). After this time, manual elevation is more difficult or impossible. Several techniques have been used for manual elevation, including gentle pressure and use of a breast pump or vacuum extractor, with varying results (Paige & Carney, 2002). Surgical intervention usually is necessary if manual elevation fails, if the fracture is more severe and bone fragments are in the cerebrum, if neurologic deficits exist, or if ICP is increased.

Linear fractures heal spontaneously with no sequelae unless underlying cerebral damage or a growing fracture is present. Basal fractures are associated with high mortality and poor developmental outcome. Infants with depressed fractures that are small or treated early (or both) have a good prognosis. Infants with large fractures, especially if treatment is delayed, have a greater risk of sequelae. Unless a depressed fracture has lacerated the dura (a rare occurrence), neurologic deficits in these infants usually are caused by cerebral injury from the original trauma or a hypoxic event, or both, rather than by the fracture per se (Paige & Carney, 2002). Infants with skull fractures should undergo regular evaluation of growth and development during infancy and early childhood.

Spinal Cord Injury

Spinal cord injuries are uncommon and usually occur in the midcervical to lower cervical and upper thoracic areas. Injury can occur at any point along the cord. Spinal cord injuries are caused by excessive traction, rotation, and torsion of the vertebral column and neck. Injury usually does not result from compression, but rather from stretching of the spinal cord, which is less flexible than the bony vertebral column. Damage to the spinal cord ranges from complete transection to laceration, edema, hemorrhage, and hematoma formation. Hemorrhage into the lining of the arteries may result in thrombosis, infarction, and ischemic cord damage. Risk factors are breech delivery (major factor), dystocia, macrosomia, and cephalopelvic disproportion (Levene, 2001b; Madan et al, 2005).

Infants with partial spinal cord injury have subtle neurologic signs and variable degrees of spasticity. Infants with high cervical or brainstem injuries are stillborn or die shortly after birth from respiratory depression, shock, and hypothermia. Infants with midcervical or upper cervical injury may be stillborn, born with marked respiratory depression, or have respiratory depression, with the neurologic injury going unrecognized until flaccidity, immobility of the legs, urine retention, or all three are noted. If born alive, these infants usually die within the first week, after development of progressive central respiratory depression that often is complicated by pneumonia. Other findings in this group of infants include relaxation of the abdominal wall, absent sensation in the lower half of the body, absent deep tendon and spontaneous reflexes, brachial plexus injury, and constipation. This group also includes infants with injuries at the C8 to T1 level who usually survive, and may have a transient paraplegic paralysis at birth. Infants with mild injury may recover most or all of their function. Infants with moderate to severe damage are paraplegic or quadriplegic and have permanent neurologic damage (Levene, 2001b; Madan et al, 2005).

Initially, clinical manifestations are those of spinal cord shock, with hypotonia, weakness, flaccid extremities, sensory deficits, relaxed abdominal muscles, diaphragmatic breathing, Horner syndrome (ipsilateral ptosis, anhidrosis, and miosis), and a distended bladder. Infants with low cervical lesions have shallow, paradoxical respirations; these infants do not sweat. The skin over the affected area is dry and warm. Pinprick and deep tendon reflexes are absent. Areflexia may be noted over the upper and lower extremities in some infants. The degree of neurologic insult often cannot be accurately evaluated until the infant has recovered from the initial period of spinal shock and any edema or hemorrhage has been reabsorbed (Paige & Carney, 2002). After several weeks or months, a paraplegic autonomic hyperreflexia develops that is characterized by periodic mass reflex response. This results in tonic spasms of extremities, spontaneous micturition, and profuse sweating over the paralyzed area.

Initial management focuses on stabilization, treatment of associated problems (e.g., asphyxia, hemorrhage, shock), and management of respiratory depression. Infants with mid-cervical to upper cervical or brainstem lesions require assisted ventilation. Parents are in shock initially and need time to grieve. They need continuing support and teaching regarding the care of the infant. Ongoing management of these infants and their families requires a multidisciplinary team that includes the disciplines of nursing, medicine, neurology, neurosurgery, physical therapy, orthopedics, urology, social work, and psychology. Ultrasonography, CT, or MRI may be performed to determine the level and the extent of injury.

Skin integrity over the paralyzed area must be maintained to prevent pressure areas and skin breakdown. Thermoregulation may be a problem, because evaporative loss through the skin is reduced over the affected body parts in the initial period of the recovery process. The infant is positioned and repositioned regularly to promote normal alignment of body parts and prevent development of contractures and decubiti. The affected areas should be kept clean and dry and massaged with gentle, passive range-of-motion exercises. These infants need meticulous bowel and bladder care to prevent urinary tract infection and skin excoriation. Glycerin suppositories at regular intervals can help normalize bowel function. Infants are also monitored for signs of respiratory infection and pneumonia. Parental teaching before discharge focuses on normal baby care issues and concerns, as well as the special needs of a paralyzed infant.

The prognosis depends on the level and severity of the injury, but it generally is poor. Many infants with spinal cord injury are stillborn or die shortly after birth, particularly those with midcervical to high cervical or brainstem injuries. Those who survive have varying degrees of residual paralysis, respiratory problems, and bowel and bladder dysfunction, depending on the level of the injury. Most surviving infants

have a spastic quadriplegia. Infants with involvement of the intercostal muscles and diaphragm often are ventilator dependent.

Peripheral Nerve Injuries

Peripheral nerve injuries result from stretching, compression, twisting, hyperextension, or separation of nerve tissue (Madan, et al, 2005; Paige & Carney, 2002). Injury can occur before, during, or after birth. Damage can range from swelling of the nerve to complete peripheral degeneration (with later total recovery) to complete division of all structures. The more common sites affected are the brachial plexus and the facial, phrenic, radial, median, and sciatic nerves. This type of injury is seen predominantly in term or LGA infants.

Injury to the radial nerve usually results from compression of the nerve caused by fracture of the humerus during a breech delivery or by intrauterine compression of the arm. The infant has wrist drop with a normal grasp reflex. Recovery usually occurs over the first few weeks to months. Median and sciatic nerve injuries are generally postnatal iatrogenic events. Median nerve injury can be a complication of brachial or radial arterial punctures. These infants have diminished pincer grasp and thumb strength and a flexed fourth finger. Recovery is variable. Sciatic nerve injuries are often permanent. They arise from trauma from a misplaced intramuscular injection or from ischemia from an injection of hypertonic solutions into the gluteal muscle. Infants with this type of injury have diminished abduction and distal joint movement. Hip adduction, rotation, and flexion are unaffected (Madan et al, 2005; Paige & Carney, 2002).

Facial Nerve Palsy

Facial nerve palsy has an incidence of 0.23% (Levene, 2001b). Injury to the peripheral nerve is caused by trauma from oblique application of forceps, prolonged pressure on the nerve during labor from the maternal sacral promontory, or pressure from an abnormal fetal posture. Although some investigators have not found any differences in incidence between forceps and spontaneous vaginal deliveries, others have noted a correlation between the type of forceps and the incidence of injury. The facial nerve of the newborn is superficial after it emerges from the stylomastoid foramen. As a result, the nerve is vulnerable to compression injury at this site or as it traverses the ramus of the mandible. The temporofacial and cervicofacial nerve branches are most often involved. The injury is most common on the left. Because the prognosis is favorable, the injury appears to be caused by hemorrhage or edema into the nerve sheath rather than by disruption of the nerve fibers (Volpe, 2001b).

Facial nerve paralysis must be distinguished from asymmetric crying facies and nuclear agenesis. Asymmetric crying facies results from absence of the depressor muscle of the angle of the mouth. These infants close their eyes normally when crying, but the mouth does not move down and out. They suck without dribbling. This disorder generally is benign. Nuclear agenesis (Möbius syndrome) is a more severe disorder characterized by congenital paralysis of the facial muscles.

Clinical manifestations vary, depending on whether the injury is to the central nerve, the peripheral nerve, or the peripheral nerve branch. The complete peripheral nerve injury results in a unilateral inability to close the eye or open the mouth. The lower lip on the affected side does not depress during crying, nor does the forehead wrinkle. The affected side appears full and smooth, with obliteration of the nasolabial fold. These infants dribble milk while feeding. The infant may be unable to close the eye on the affected side. Central injury usually results in a spastic paralysis of the lower portion of the face contralateral to the side of CNS injury without involvement of the eyes or forehead. Peripheral nerve branch injury results in varying degrees of paralysis of the forehead, eye, or lower face, depending on the branch involved. The paralysis is apparent at birth or within 1 to 2 days after birth.

Almost all infants recover completely. Improvement usually is apparent by 1 to 4 weeks, and complete recovery occurs after several months in most infants (Levene, 2001b). Infants with severe nerve regeneration have a longer recovery period and may occasionally require later cosmetic surgery.

Nursing management involves parent counseling and teaching and prevention of complications. The eye on the affected side is patched, and 1% methylcellulose eye drops are instilled every 3 to 4 hours to prevent corneal damage. Dribbling with sucking can be a transient problem. If no improvement is noted by 7 to 10 days or if further loss of function occurs, a neurosurgical consultation usually is recommended. With partial degeneration, physical therapy, massage, or electrical stimulation may be used, although the efficacy of these therapies is controversial and not well documented. Electromyography, nerve excitability, or nerve conduction latency examinations may be performed to evaluate the extent of the damage.

Brachial Plexus Injury

Brachial plexus palsy involves injury of the C5 to T1 nerve roots and is seen almost exclusively in term infants. The incidence ranges from 0.6% to 2.6% (Pondaag et al, 2004). Injury to the brachial plexus results from excessive lateral flexion, rotation, or traction on the neck (McNeely & Drake, 2003). The degree of injury varies, ranging from edema and hemorrhage of the nerve sheath to avulsion of the nerve root from the spinal cord. With mild to moderate injury the axons are shattered, but the nerve sheaths remain intact. This degree of intactness of the nerve sheaths promotes regeneration of the nerve by 3 to 4 months, with full recovery by 3 to 15 months in most infants (McNeely & Drake, 2003; Noetzel et al, 2001). Severe injuries result in radicular rupture or intraspinal tearing of the nerve and division of the nerve into radicles. If radicular rupture occurs, the root loses contact with the spinal cord. These injuries do not recover spontaneously (Levene, 2001b).

Brachial plexus injuries usually are unilateral and on the left side. Fracture of the clavicle may occur in conjunction with this type of injury. Brachial plexus injury can be seen in uncomplicated deliveries and after cesarean birth, but is usually associated with vaginal delivery of LGA infants, shoulder dystocia, breech and other abnormal presentations, and prolonged labor or difficult delivery. Spontaneous injuries may occur from compression of the shoulder as it passes over the sacral prominence (Levene, 2001b).

Clinical manifestations vary with the location and severity of the injury. Signs of injury usually are apparent from birth but may be delayed for several days to a few weeks in some infants. The major types of injury are Erb's palsy, or upper plexus injury involving C5 to C7, and Klumpke's palsy, or lower plexus injury at C5 to T1 (Levene, 2001b). With Erb's palsy, the shoulder and upper arm are involved, and denervation of the deltoid, supraspinous, biceps, and brachioradialis muscles occurs. The arm lies passively at the infant's side, abducted and

internally rotated, and the forearm is pronated. The wrist and fingers are flexed. This posture is referred to as the "waiter's tip" position. The Moro reflex is absent, and the biceps and radial reflexes are diminished or absent on the affected side; the grasp reflex is normal. Klumpke's palsy is seen primarily in breech infants whose arm has been hyperabducted and delivered with the head affecting the flexors of the wrist and hand. Cervical sympathetic fibers may also be affected; sweating and sensation are absent in the affected hand and arm. The infant holds the affected arm at the side of the thorax with the hand in a claw hand posture. The Moro and grasp reflexes are absent, and the triceps reflex is diminished or absent on the affected side; biceps and radial reflexes are present. If the T1 root is affected, the infant manifests Horner syndrome (ipsilateral ptosis, anhidrosis, and miosis) (Levene, 2001b).

With total (Erb-Klumpke) palsy, the entire arm and hand are involved as a result of injury to the nerve roots of the brachial plexus from C5 to T1. Complete paralysis of the upper and lower arm and hand, flaccidity, and accompanying sensory, trophic, and circulatory changes are noted. Deep tendon and Moro reflexes are absent. If the C4 roots are also affected, an associated phrenic nerve (diaphragmatic) paralysis occurs. Involvement of the T1 root leads to Horner syndrome in about one third of these infants (Levene, 2001b).

Initial management focuses on protecting the arm until localized edema and pain have subsided. MRI or CT are used to visualize the degree of injury. The affected arm is immobilized with shoulder and elbow splints to prevent contractures and further stretching of the plexus. After edema subsides, at about 7 to 10 days, physical therapy gradually is instituted as the infant can tolerate it. Initially the regimen may involve gentle, passive range-of-motion exercises. These infants have continued physical therapy consisting of massage and exercise over the first months until total or partial recovery occurs. Infants with a brachial plexus injury should be evaluated for associated problems, including fractures and respiratory difficulty secondary to phrenic nerve paralysis.

If improvement is not noted within the first few months, electromyography and nerve conduction studies are performed to determine the extent of the damage, to follow recovery, and to determine whether surgical intervention is needed, although surgery is controversial (Levene, 2001b). Infants with brachial plexus injuries often experience considerable pain during movement of the affected arm in the first few weeks after birth. Nursing management is directed at reducing passive and active movement of the arm and providing comfort measures to reduce pain. Splints are removed intermittently to reduce the risk of abduction contractures. The paralyzed arm is supported in a position of relaxation. Parent teaching regarding positioning, prevention of contractures, and exercise is essential.

The prognosis depends on the level and severity of the injury. Approximately 65% to 95% of infants have full recovery with supportive care (McNeely & Drake, 2003; Noetzel et al, 2001). Many recover by 3 to 4 months of age and more than 90% by 2 to 3 years (Pondaag et al, 2004). Erb's palsy, the most common type of injury, has the best prognosis for full recovery. Infants with total paralysis are most likely to have residual paralysis. Residual functional deficits include alteration in abduction and external rotation of the shoulder; restricted movement of the elbow, forearm, and hand; and hand weakness (Noetzel et al, 2001). These functional impairments can lead to abnormal muscle development and arm growth.

Phrenic Nerve Palsy

Phrenic nerve palsy is caused by injury of the cervical nerve roots at C3 to C5. The injury results from tearing of the nerve sheath, which is accompanied by edema and hemorrhage. Phrenic nerve palsy is frequently associated with Erb-Klumpke paralysis. Risk factors, especially breech delivery, are similar to those for brachial plexus injury. Paralysis of the diaphragm is a result of damage to the phrenic nerve. The injury usually is unilateral and on the right side. Because the diaphragm is paralyzed, infants with phrenic nerve injury have respiratory difficulty. This phenomenon must be differentiated from CNS, cardiac, and pulmonary problems (Paige & Carney, 2002).

Infants with mild to moderate phrenic nerve injury may have early respiratory difficulty, suggestive of hypoventilation that stabilizes or improves. The infant may have recurrent episodes of cyanosis and dyspnea. The breathing pattern is altered. In these infants, breathing involves primarily thoracic movement with minimal or no abdominal excursions. Infants with complete avulsion or bilateral injuries have severe respiratory distress from birth, with tachypnea, apnea, and a weak cry (Paige & Carney, 2002).

Management focuses on promoting ventilation and oxygenation. Infants may be placed on nothing by mouth status (NPO) initially, and feeding may be instituted as the infant's respiratory status improves. Infants with severe distress require positive pressure ventilation or constant positive airway pressure for support until recovery occurs. Electrical pacing of the diaphragm and rocking beds have also been used (Paige & Carney, 2002). Surgical plication of the diaphragm is performed if no improvement is noted or if the infant is still ventilator dependent at 4 to 6 weeks of age. The infant is positioned on the affected side. If the infant cannot be fed, adequate fluid and calories must be provided. Feeding is instituted gradually. Initially, the infant may need to be gavage fed. When oral feeding is started, the infant is fed slowly and given ample opportunity for rest and monitoring of respiratory status. Because recovery takes several months, parents must be taught feeding, positioning, and comfort techniques. The developmental needs of infants requiring prolonged hospitalization must be met; sensory input and play activities appropriate to their maturity and health status must be provided. Most infants recover by 6 to 12 months of age. Other infants recover clinically but have residual abnormalities of diaphragmatic movement on radiography (Paige & Carney, 2002).

SUMMARY

Infants with neurologic dysfunction present a significant challenge to the neonatal nurse. The nurse must respond to infants with life-threatening conditions, such as perinatal hypoxic-ischemic injury and intracranial hemorrhage; to those with transient problems, such as an isolated seizure; and to those with chronic problems, such as NTDs. Nurses must also deal with their own responses and those of the families of infants who may die during the neonatal or early infancy periods or whose short-term and long-term outcome may be altered by the extent of neurologic insult. To optimally care for these infants and their families, nurses must understand the basis for and the implications of specific types of neurologic dysfunction; they must recognize the clinical manifestations of these types of dysfunction; and they must respond appropriately in concert with other health care professionals.

The nursing care of infants who have or who are at risk for neurologic dysfunction involves assessment and monitoring of the infant's neurologic status and responses to the extrauterine environment, as well as of subtle signs that may indicate a change in status. Nursing management of the infant involves activities to address alteration in level of consciousness, potential for injury related to trauma or infection, impairment of skin integrity, alterations in comfort, impaired mobility, alterations in thermoregulation, alterations in nutrition and fluid and electrolyte status, and promotion of neurobehavioral organization and development. The nurse must also assess family coping, interactive processes, knowledge, and grieving to assist the family in coping with the birth of an ill infant and, for many families, with the uncertainty or certainty of long-term neurologic deficits in their infant.

Case Study

IDENTIFICATION OF THE PROBLEM

A 6-day-old former term infant turned blue at home on day 4 of life and was admitted to the local hospital. While there, the infant was screened for sepsis (normal complete blood count [CBC] and differential, negative cultures for viral and bacterial sepsis). On day 2, at the local hospital, the infant had a seizure consisting of lip smacking, apnea, cyanosis, and bicycling of lower extremities; was given 10 mg/kg phenobarbital; and was taken to CT, which showed a right intraventricular hemorrhage. The infant was transferred to the NICU of the tertiary care hospital. Social maternal history is significant because a cousin died of "fits" at 3 months of age; other relatives suffered frequent bone fractures or sundown eye sign. Father is reportedly short-statured with short-statured children.

ASSESSMENT: HISTORY AND PHYSICAL EXAMINATION

A 6-day-old former term neonate was delivered vaginally following an uncomplicated pregnancy with a birth weight of 2990 g. Prenatal laboratory results were remarkable for positive group B streptococcus (GBS) vaginal culture, for which the mother received prophylactic perinatal antibiotics. The infant did well after delivery, breast-fed vigorously, and was discharged home with his mother on day 2 of life. At the time of admission, his weight was 2950 g, occipitofrontal circumference (OFC) was 33 cm, and length was 49.5 cm. On examination, the infant was somewhat sleepy and irritable with handling.

His anterior fontanelle was large and soft, with sutures split to just above eyebrows, and his lateral sutures were proximate. His pupils were equal and reacting to light, with

Continued

Case Study—cont'd

bilateral red reflex and sunset eyes when crying. His nares were patent bilaterally, and palate and clavicles were intact. His lungs were clear and bilaterally equal with easy work of breathing with spontaneous respirations. His heart had regular rhythm and rate, and no murmur was noted with peripheral pulses 2+ in all extremities, good peripheral perfusion, and capillary blood refill time was about 3 seconds. His abdomen was soft and nontender with his liver at right costal margin (RCM) and no hepatosplenomegaly or masses palpable; his umbilical stump was dry. He appeared to be a normal male infant with testes bilaterally descended into a well-developed scrotum. He arched with handling, moved all extremities with increased tone, and exhibited an occasional tongue thrust. Examination showed positive sunset eyes, positive gag reflex, positive blink response, and no clonus. His extremities were well formed with good muscle mass, and his skin was pale pink with good turgor and healing areas from previous lab draws and intravenous access attempts. No petechiae or rashes were noted.

DIFFERENTIAL DIAGNOSES

The differential diagnoses were (1) seizures of unknown etiology; (2) rule out herpes simplex infection and other viral or bacterial meningitis; (3) rule out brain structure abnormalities; (4) rule out nonaccidental trauma (NAT); (5) rule out intracranial and intraventricular hemorrhage (ICH, IVH); and (6) hypoventilation.

DIAGNOSTIC TESTS

To begin to differentiate between the diagnoses, a variety of tests were needed. Laboratory tests obtained were a complete blood count with differential, electrolytes, blood urea nitrogen (BUN), ionized calcium, alkaline phosphorus, ammonia level, lactate, serum glutamic-oxaloacetic transaminase (SGOT), blood and central spinal fluid (CSF) bacteria and viral cultures, and urine drug screen. Imaging tests ordered were serial EEGs, MRI of the brain, and head CT. Pediatric specialists consulted were the NAT team, and neurology, metabolic, and endocrine services.

WORKING DIAGNOSIS

Laboratory results were as follows: WBC 10.6, segmented cells 27, bands 0, lymphocytes 39, monocytes 27, eosinophils 4, hematocrit (Hct) 60.2%, platelet count 254,000; sodium 132, potassium 4.7, chloride 96, bicarbonate 29, calcium 11.9, ionized calcium 1.42, phosphorus 2.9, alkaline phosphorus less than 5, ammonia 45, lactate 2.2, blood urea nitrogen (BUN) less than 1, and serum glutamic-oxaloacetic transaminase (SGOT) 33. The blood and CSF cultures were negative for bacteria and viral growth. The urine drug screen was negative. These laboratory results effectively ruled out sepsis, meningitis, electrolyte imbalances, and metabolic disease as etiologies for seizure activity. The extremely low alkaline phosphorus, low phosphorus, and high calcium and ionized calcium levels were indicators for endocrine disease.

The EEG was moderately abnormal due to excessive background discontinuity and prominent high-amplitude spikes and polyspikes, but no seizures were noted. The ophthalmic examination was normal without ocular hemorrhages. The MRI revealed hemorrhage located either in subependymal location or cavum velum interpositum not consistent with shear injury, and the subsequent head CT determined the placement of the hemorrhage in the right thalamic area with extension into the lateral ventricles and stable ventricle size. A repeat EEG on hospital day 7 was significantly improved but still mildly abnormal due to focal moderate amplitude, midline vertex, and negative spikes without seizure activity. A skeletal radiographic study showed no fractures; however, there was evidence of metaphyseal fraying in the lower extremities consistent with developing rickets. The imaging results ruled out NAT and other structural causes for the clinical presentation of seizure-like activity. The results gave further support for endocrine disease due to the early radiographic indication for rickets.

The NAT team, consisting of a pediatric developmental specialist, neurologist, ophthalmologist, and patient advocate, concluded that the seizures were not caused by brain injury due to nonaccidental trauma. After assessing the infant, examining the laboratory tests, and reviewing the scans, the neurology service concluded that the etiology of the seizures was not structural or related to brain injury but most likely due to pyridoxine deficiency or some endocrine or metabolic syndrome. After evaluation of all diagnostic results, endocrinologists considered the seizures to be related to hypophosphatasia. The working diagnosis was a 6-day-old infant with seizures due to probable hypophosphatemia.

DEVELOPMENT OF MANAGEMENT PLAN

The management plan was to monitor the infant; provide respiratory, fluid, and nutritional support with a low-calcium formula; initiate vitamin D supplements to delay bone decalcification and rickets; provide teaching for the parents; and arrange follow-up with the primary care provider and the pediatric neurology, orthopedic, and endocrinology services.

IMPLEMENTATION AND EVALUATION OF EFFECTIVENESS

During the examination phase, pyridoxine was given for a seizure-like event on hospital day 2 that included bicycling, sneezing, clonic-tonic movements with Cheyne-Stokes–like respiratory pattern. Maintenance pyridoxine was given until hospital day 10, when it was determined the seizures were caused by hypophosphatemia. The infant was NPO with peripheral intravenous fluids until a special low-calcium formula could be delivered, and vitamin D supplements were started to delay bone decalcification and rickets. At time of discharge, the infant was taking good amounts of the formula by nipple and gaining weight slowly. His mother was learning what little there is to know about this rare congenital disease and learning to prevent fractures as much as possible. The prognosis for symptomatic congenital hypophosphatasia is poor, with death usually occurring within the first year of life. Follow-up care was arranged with neurology, orthopedics, and endocrinology.

Case Study

IDENTIFICATION OF THE PROBLEM

A term infant male was limp and not breathing well after birth. The certified nurse midwife (CNM) performed mask-delivered positive pressure ventilation with room air with improvement in respiratory effort. Apgar scores were 1^1, 2^5, 4^{10}, 5^{15}. The infant was brought to the neonatal intensive care center. On admission, the infant continued to manifest poor respiratory effort, and nasal continuous positive pressure (NCPAP) of 6 cm H_2O was initiated with 0.50 FiO_2.

ASSESSMENT: HISTORY AND PHYSICAL EXAMINATION

The infant boy was born at 40 6/7 weeks by vaginal delivery to a 24-year-old, G1 P0 >1 woman at home with a CNM present. Prenatal laboratory results and history were unremarkable with negative GBS status. The pregnancy was uncomplicated. Membranes were spontaneously ruptured with clear fluid approximately 11 hours prior to delivery, and no maternal fever was documented; the mother received antibiotics about 4 hours prior to delivery. Active pushing in second stage was 4 hours, followed by shoulder dystocia after the infant's head was delivered.

The infant's birth weight was 3765 g, OFC was 37 cm, and length was 54 cm. His anterior fontanelle was soft, flat, sutures opposed, proximate with a right cephalohematoma; eyes were equal and reactive to light with a positive red reflex; nares were bilaterally patent, and palate and clavicles were intact. His breath sounds were coarse bilaterally, slightly decreased over lower the right lung field. Increased work of breathing was manifested with increased subcostal and substernal retractions, slight tracheal tug, and flared nares. He was mildly tachycardic, but no murmur was noted. Peripheral pulses were 1+ in all extremities with poor peripheral perfusion and capillary blood refill time of more than 4 seconds. His abdomen was soft and nontender with no hepatosplenomegaly or masses palpable and a three-vessel cord. He was responsive and alert on admission, with well-formed extremities and slightly decreased muscle tone. His skin was pale pink and slightly mottled, with acrocyanosis and circumoral cyanosis.

Nasal CPAP was initiated to support respiratory effort. The infant was noted to be slightly shocklike; peripheral intravenous fluids were initiated at 80 ml/kg/day maintenance and a fluid bolus was given; umbilical arterial and venous catheters were attempted but unsuccessful. After the chest radiograph confirmed right pneumothorax, needle aspiration was performed for small amount of air. Subsequent radiographs showed pneumothorax resolved. Infant initially improved but on day 2 of life developed apnea, tonguing, lip smacking, and rhythmic extremity movement.

DIFFERENTIAL DIAGNOSES

The differential diagnoses for an infant following a difficult delivery with positive pressure ventilation include (1) respiratory distress vs transient tachypnea of the newborn (TTN); (2) rule out pneumothorax; (3) rule out hypoxic ischemic encephalopathy; (4) rule out intracranial hemorrhage; (5) rule out sepsis; (6) shock; and (7) rule out seizures. Other diagnoses that should be ruled out include congenital cardiac defects and metabolic or endocrine defects.

DIAGNOSTIC TESTS

The initial differentiation between diagnoses in this case required evaluation of blood cultures for bacteria and viral growth, CBC with differential, electrolytes, lactic acid, and ammonia levels, amino acid assays and urine organic acids, and liver function tests. Imaging tests were chest radiography, head CT, MRI, and serial EEGs. A consult was obtained from pediatric neurology.

WORKING DIAGNOSIS

The CBC/differential results were unremarkable for sepsis, and the cultures were negative. The chest radiograph obtained soon after admission revealed a small right pneumothorax. The head CT at 24 hours of age was normal with no evidence of hydrocephalus, ischemia, or intracranial hemorrhage. The first EEG at 48 hours of age revealed moderate to severely abnormal EEG due to discontinuous low-amplitude background with asynchrony and frequent, subclinical, electrographic seizures from midline vertex and left central region. The second EEG at 72 hours of age showed improvement from initial EEG with no electrographic seizures. There were positive sharp transient waves that were of concern for underlying structural abnormalities and can be consistent with anoxic and hypoxic events as reflected with clinical presentation. The third EEG at 5 days of age was abnormal due to predominately right temporal sharp waves and possibly two brief electrographic seizures. An MRI at 11 days of age showed abnormalities on T2 and DWI consistent with perinatal HIE.

The working diagnosis was seizures due to hypoxic-ischemic encephalopathy, with secondary diagnoses of respiratory distress and pneumothorax.

DEVELOPMENT OF MANAGEMENT PLAN

The management plan included (1) monitoring; (2) respiratory support with mechanical ventilation as needed; (3) fluid support; (4) sepsis screen; (5) antibiotics; and (6) needle aspiration with chest tube insertion if indicated.

IMPLEMENTATION AND EVALUATION OF EFFECTIVENESS

The management plan was implemented soon after admission to the NICU. Antibiotics were given for 48 hours for the sepsis screen. The right pneumothorax was reduced with needling and resolved without further intervention. The infant exhibited seizure activity, confirmed with EEG, and was loaded with phenobarbital 15 mg/kg × 1, with resolution of the seizure. Infant was subsequently intubated at approximately 36 hours of age for a prolonged apnea event requiring positive pressure ventilation and given

Continued

Case Study—cont'd

another 15 mg/kg phenobarbital loading dose and initial lorazepam (Ativan) dose to control seizures.

Metabolic etiology was ruled out with normal lactic acid and ammonia levels and normal amino acid assays and urine organic acids results. State metabolic screening results were expedited and were normal. Infant's neurologic examination deteriorated over the first 4 days, with the infant presenting with no gag, no corneal reflex, passive hypertonicity, active hypotonia, consistent and rhythmic hyperventilation, and periodic apnea, clonic-tonic movements of predominately the left extremities by the end of day 3 of life, and persisting through day 5 of life. Maintenance phenobarbital was initiated on day 3 of life, and lorazepam was given periodically for seizure activity during days 4 to 5 of life. Seizures were no longer observed after day 5 of life; infant gradually improved clinically with improved passive and active tone, improved gag, and positive corneal reflex. Infant was extubated on day 6 of life to high-flow nasal cannula of 2 L/min flow of room air; weaned quickly to room air without nasal cannula flow. Feeds of expressed mother's milk had been initiated per gavage tube on day 3 of life; infant was tolerating full volume by day 7 by gavage every 3 hours. Breast-feeding and nipple feeds were initiated on day 8, but infant needed most of his feeds by gavage at time of discharge on day 18. Infant was discharged with phenobarbital; follow-up care was arranged for neurology clinic and EEG 1 month after discharge. The infant was breast-feeding well, gaining weight, and thriving at the neurology follow-up appointment.

REFERENCES

American Academy of Pediatrics, Committee on Genetics (1999). Folic acid for the prevention of neural tube defects. *Pediatrics* 104:325.

Amiel-Tison C (2001). Clinical assessment of the infant nervous system. In Levene MI et al, editors. *Fetal and neonatal neurology and neurosurgery*, ed 3 (pp 99-120). Edinburgh: Churchill Livingstone.

Back SA (2005). Congenital malformations of the central nervous system. In Taeusch HW et al, editors. *Avery's diseases of the newborn*, ed 8 (pp 938-964). Philadelphia: Saunders.

Back SA, Rivkees SA (2004). Emerging concepts in periventricular white matter injury. *Seminars in perinatology* 28:405-414.

Barnes PD, Taylor GA (1998). Imaging of the neonatal central nervous system. *Neurosurgery clinics of North America* 9:17-47.

Bloch JR (2005). Antenatal events causing neonatal brain injury in preterm infants. *Journal of obstetric, gynecologic, and neonatal nursing* 34:358-366.

Brion LP et al (2003). Vitamin E supplementation for prevention of morbidity and mortality in preterm infants. *Cochrane database of systematic reviews* 4:CD003665.

Brown LW (2005). Neurologic examination. In Spitzer AR, editor. *Intensive care of the fetus and neonate*, ed 2 (pp 767-774). St Louis: Mosby.

Buonocore G, Perrone S (2004). Biomarkers of hypoxic brain injury in the neonate. *Clinics in perinatology* 31:107-116.

Calvert JW, Zhang JH (2005). Pathophysiology of an hypoxic-ischemic insult during the perinatal period. *Neurological research* 27:246-260.

Cherian S et al (2004). The pathogenesis of neonatal post-hemorrhagic hydrocephalus. *Brain pathology* 14:305-311.

Crowther CA, Henderson-Smart DJ (2003). Phenobarbital prior to preterm birth for preventing neonatal periventricular hemorrhage. *Cochrane database of systematic reviews* 2:CD00164.

de Vries LS, Levene MI (2001). Cerebral ischemic lesions. In Levene MI et al, editors. *Fetal and neonatal neurology and neurosurgery*, ed 3 (pp 373-406). Edinburgh: Churchill Livingstone.

de Vries LS, Rennie JM (2005). Neurological problems of the neonate: preterm brain injury: preterm cerebral hemorrhage. In Rennie JM, editor. *Roberton's textbook of neonatology*, ed 4 (pp 1148-1169). Edinburgh: Churchill Livingstone.

du Plessis AJ (2005). Perinatal asphyxia and hypoxic-ischemic brain injury in the full term infants. In Spitzer AR, editor. *Intensive care of the fetus and neonate*, ed 2 (pp 775-802). St Louis: Mosby.

du Plessis AJ, Volpe JJ (2002). Perinatal brain injury in the preterm and term newborn. *Current opinion in neurology* 15:151-157.

Ferriero D (2004). Neonatal brain injury. *New England journal of medicine* 35:1984-1995.

Fowlie PW, Davis PG (2003). Prophylactic indomethacin for preterm infants: a systematic review and meta-analysis. *Archives of disease in childhood child fetal and neonatal edition* 88:F464-F466.

Furdon A, Clark D (2001). Differentiating scalp swelling in the newborn. *Advances in neonatal care* 1:22-27.

Gluckman PD et al (2005). Selective head cooling with mild systemic hypothermia after neonatal encephalopathy: multicentre randomized trial. *Lancet* 365:663-670.

Granelli SLP, McGrath J (2004). Neonatal seizures: diagnosis, pharmacologic interventions and outcomes. *Journal of perinatal and neonatal nursing* 18:275-287.

Gunn AJ et al (2005). Therapeutic hypothermia: from lab to NICU. *Journal of perinatal medicine* 33:340-346.

Hamrick SEG, Ferriero D (2003). The injury response in the term newborn brain: can we neuroprotect? *Current opinion in neurology* 16:147-154.

Hill A (2005). Neurological and neuromuscular disorders. In MacDonald MG et al, editors. *Avery's neonatology: pathophysiology and management of the newborn*, ed 5 (pp 1384-1409). Philadelphia: Lippincott Williams & Wilkins.

Hirose S et al (2001). Fetal surgery for myelomeningocele. *Current opinion in obstetrics and gynecology* 13:215-222.

Hirose S et al (2003). Fetal surgery for myelomeningocele: panacea or peril? *World journal of surgery* 27:87-94.

Holmes GL, Ben-Ari Y (2001). The neurobiology and consequences of epilepsy in the developing brain. *Pediatric research* 49:320-325.

Holmes GL et al (2002). New concepts in neonatal seizures. *NeuroReport* 13:A3-A8.

Ikonomidou C et al (2001). Neurotransmitters and apoptosis in the developing brain. *Biochemistry and pharmacology* 62:401-405.

Jacobs S et al (2003). Cooling for newborns with hypoxic ischaemic encephalopathy. *Cochrane database of systematic reviews* 4:CD003311.

Jensen A et al (2003). Perinatal brain damage—from pathophysiology to prevention. *European journal of obstetrics, gynecology and reproductive biology* 22(110, Suppl 1):S70-S79.

Johanson R, Menon V (2000). Soft versus rigid vacuum extractor cups for assisted vaginal delivery. *Cochrane database of systematic reviews* 2:CD000446.

Kadhim H et al (2001). Inflammatory cytokines in the pathogenesis of periventricular leukomalacia. *Neurology* 56:1278-1284.

Kaufman BA (2004). Neural tube defects. *Clinics in perinatology* 51:389-419.

Kecskes Z et al (2005). Fluid restriction for term infants with hypoxic-ischaemic encephalopathy following perinatal asphyxia. *Cochrane database of systematic reviews* 3:CD004337.

Kinney HC (2005). Human myelinization and perinatal white matter disorders. *Journal of neurological sciences* 228:190-192.

Klusmann A et al (2005). A decreasing rate of neural tube defects following the recommendations for periconceptional folic acid supplementation. *Acta paediatrica* 94:1538-1542.

Lee H, Harrison MR (2005). Surgery for fetal malformations. In Spitzer AR, editor. *Intensive care of the fetus and neonate*, ed 2 (pp 203-212). St Louis: Mosby.

Levene MI (2001a). The asphyxiated newborn infant. In Levene MI et al, editors. *Fetal and neonatal neurology and neurosurgery*, ed 3 (pp 471-504). Edinburgh: Churchill Livingstone.

Levene MI (2001b). Disorders of the spinal cord, cranial and peripheral nerves. In Levene MI et al, editors. *Fetal and neonatal neurology and neurosurgery*, ed 3 (pp 695-708). Edinburgh: Churchill Livingstone.

Levene M (2005). Neurological problems of the neonate: intracranial hemorrhage at term. In Rennie JM, editor. *Roberton's textbook of neonatology*, ed 4 (pp 1120-1128). Edinburgh: Churchill Livingstone.

Levene MI, de Vries LS (2001). Neonatal intracranial hemorrhage. In Levene MI et al, editors. *Fetal and neonatal neurology and neurosurgery*, ed 3 (pp 372-399). Edinburgh: Churchill Livingstone.

Levene M, Evans DJ (2005). Neurological problems of the neonate: hypoxic-ischemic brain injury. In Rennie JM, editor. *Roberton's textbook of neonatology*, ed 4 (pp 1128-1148). Edinburgh: Churchill Livingstone.

Linder N et al (2003). Risk factors for intraventricular hemorrhage in very low birth weight premature infants: a retrospective case-control study. *Pediatrics* 111(5 Pt 1):e590-595.

Madan A et al (2005). Central nervous system injury and neuroprotection. In Taeusch HW et al, editors. *Avery's diseases of the newborn*, ed 8 (pp 965-992). Philadelphia: Saunders.

McLendon D et al (2003). Implementation of potentially better practices for the prevention of brain hemorrhage and ischemic brain injury in very low birth weight infants. *Pediatrics* 111(4 Pt 2):e497-e503.

McNeely PD, Drake JM (2003). A systematic review of brachial plexus surgery for birth-related brachial plexus injury. *Pediatric neurosurgery* 38:57-62.

Mizejewski GJ (2003). Levels of alpha-fetoprotein during pregnancy and early infancy in normal and disease states. *Obstetrical and gynecological survey* 58:804-826.

Mizrahi EM (2001). Neonatal seizures and neonatal epileptic syndromes. *Neurology clinics* 19:427-463.

Moore KL, Persaud TVN (2003). *The developing human: clinically oriented embryology*, ed 7. Philadelphia: Saunders.

Murphy AA et al (2005). Malformations of the central nervous system. In Spitzer AR, editor. *Intensive care of the fetus and neonate*, ed 2 (pp 867-894). St Louis: Mosby.

Noetzel MJ et al (2001). Prospective study of recovery following neonatal brachial plexus injury. *Journal of child neurology* 16:488-492.

Paige PL, Carney B (2002). Neurologic disorders. In Merenstein G, Gardner S, editors. *Handbook of neonatal intensive care*, ed 5 (pp 665-676). St Louis: Mosby.

Papile L (2002). Intracranial hemorrhage. In Fanaroff AA, Martin RJ, editors. *Neonatal-perinatal medicine*, ed 7 (pp 879-886). St Louis: Mosby.

Perlman JM (2004). Brain injury in the term infant. *Seminars in perinatology* 28:415-424.

Pondaag W et al (2004). Natural history of brachial plexus palsy; a systematic review. *Developmental medicine and child neurology* 48:138-144.

Rennie JM (2005a). Neurological problems of the neonate: assessment of the neonatal neurological system. In Rennie JM, editor. *Roberton's textbook of neonatology*, ed 4 (pp 1093-1105). Edinburgh: Churchill Livingstone.

Rennie JM (2005b). Neurological problems of the neonate: seizures. In Rennie JM, editor. *Roberton's textbook of neonatology*, ed 4 (pp 1105-1119). Edinburgh: Churchill Livingstone.

Rennie JM, Boylan GB (2003). Neonatal seizures and their treatment. *Current opinions in neurology* 16:177-181.

Sanchez RM, Jensen FE (2001). Maturational aspects of epilepsy mechanisms and consequences for the immature brain. *Epilepsia* 42:577-585.

Saugstad OD (2001). Resuscitation of the asphyxic newborn infant: new insight leads to new therapeutic possibilities. *Biology of the neonate* 79:258-260.

Scher MS (2001). Brain disorders of the fetus and neonate. In Klaus MH, Fanaroff AA, editors. *Care of the high-risk neonate*, ed 5. Philadelphia: Saunders.

Scher MS (2005). Neonatal seizures. In MacDonald MG et al, editors. *Avery's neonatology: pathophysiology and management of the newborn*, ed 5 (pp 1005-1025). Philadelphia: Lippincott Williams & Wilkins.

Shankaran S (2002). The postnatal management of the asphyxiated term infant. *Clinics in perinatology* 29:675-692.

Shankaran S et al (2002). Whole-body hypothermia for neonatal encephalopathy: animal observations as a basis for a randomized, controlled pilot study in term infants. *Pediatrics* 110:377-385.

Steinbach MT (1999). Traumatic birth injury: intracranial injury. *Mother baby journal* 4:513-519.

Tappero EP, Honeyfield ME (2003). *Physical assessment of the newborn*, ed 3. Santa Rosa, CA: NICU Ink.

Uchil D, Arulkumaran S (2003). Neonatal subgaleal hemorrhage and its relationship to delivery by vacuum extraction. *Obstetrical and gynecological survey* 58:687-693.

Volpe JJ (1998). Neonatal neurologic evaluation by the neurosurgeon. *Neurosurgery clinics of North America* 9:1-16.

Volpe JJ (2001a). Perinatal brain injury: from pathogenesis to neuroprotection. *Mental retardation and developmental disabilities research review* 7:56-64.

Volpe JJ (2001b). *Neurology of the newborn*, ed 4. Philadelphia: Saunders.

Walsh DS, Adzick NS (2003). Fetal surgery for spina bifida. *Seminars in neonatology* 8:197-205.

Weindling AM, Rennie JM (2005). Neurological problems of the neonate: central nervous system malformations. In Rennie JM, editor. *Roberton's textbook of neonatology*, ed 4 (pp 1180-1203). Edinburgh: Churchill Livingstone.

Whitelaw A (2001). Neonatal hydrocephalus—clinical assessment and nonsurgical treatment. In Levene MI et al, editors. *Fetal and neonatal neurology and neurosurgery*, ed 3 (pp 739-752). Edinburgh: Churchill Livingstone.

Wirrell EC (2005). Neonatal seizures: to treat or not to treat? *Seminars in pediatric neurology* 12:97-105.

Wiswell TE, Graziani LJ (2005). Intracranial hemorrhage and white matter injury in preterm infants. In Spitzer AR, editor. *Intensive care of the fetus and neonate*, ed 2 (pp 803-816). St Louis: Mosby.

Wyatt JS, Robertson NJ (2005). Time for a cool head—neuroprotection becomes a reality. *Early human development* 81:5-11.

Zupanc ML (2004). Neonatal seizures. *Clinics in perinatology* 51:961-978.

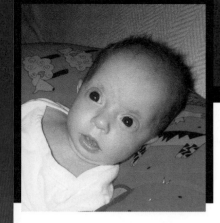

Chapter 13

Auditory System

Kathleen Haubrich

Hearing is a prerequisite to typical cognitive, social, and emotional development. Any impairment of hearing, either temporary or permanent, from birth to 18 months can have a profound effect on the auditory stimulation necessary for language development. Sensory deprivation affects the acquisition of communication skills, even though the hearing loss may be corrected.

The importance of early identification of hearing impairment in the neonate has been well documented in the literature (Kennedy et al, 2000). A study of childhood language development and academic achievement reported that hearing impairment has a significant impact on the development of a child as evidenced by limited speech production skills (Gallaudet University, Center for Assessment and Demographic Study, 1998). Karchmer and Allen (1999) looked at another aspect of childhood development, receptive and expressive language skills, and found that children with a hearing impairment demonstrated a significant delay in the development of these skills and slower academic achievement.

To prevent or minimize the detrimental effects on social, cognitive, and educational development, hearing impairment must be identified as early as possible. Statistics indicate that the incidence of significant bilateral hearing loss is about 1 to 2 per 1000 newborn infants in a well-baby nursery and about 2 to 4 per 100 infants in the neonatal intensive care unit (White et al, 2000). Moderate to profound hearing impairment is reported in fewer than 2% of infants at risk, and approximately 1 in 100 infants are born deaf.

Despite the sequelae of auditory impairment in infants and young children, the average age at which hearing impairment is identified, in settings without a screening program, is 12 to 40 months of age, beyond the critical stage for speech and language development (Russ et al, 2002).

The Joint Committee on Infant Hearing (2000) of the American Academy of Pediatrics (AAP), in a report on early identification of hearing impairment in infants and young children, concluded that all infants should be screened for hearing impairment. The task force based its conclusion on two premises: first, advances in technology have led to better screening methods, and second, using limited, risk-based criteria fails to identify 50% to 70% of children born with impairment.

This chapter reviews the assessment of the auditory system and discusses the collaborative management of the conditions presented.

ANATOMY OF THE EAR

The ear is the anatomic unit involved in hearing and equilibrium. It consists of three parts: the external ear, the middle ear, and the inner ear. The external ear is composed of the auricle (pinna) and the external ear canal (Figure 13-1). A complex cartilage framework gives structure to the auricle. Because of this anatomic position, the auricle is susceptible to trauma from external forces. The external ear canal is curved posterosuperiorly and anteromedially. The canal is oval in shape, and the long axis is positioned superoinferiorly. Normally, the outer portion of the canal is cartilaginous, and the medial portion is bony. Before 34 weeks' gestation, the pinna is a slightly formed, cartilage-free double thickness of skin. In the newborn, however, most of the canal is cartilaginous and collapsed. But as ear development ensues, the cartilage becomes firmer, making the outer two thirds of the canal more patent (Figure 13-2). Cerumen glands and tiny hairs are present in the outer portion of the cartilaginous canal. The medial two thirds of the canal lies immediately over a bony area and is referred to as the osseous region. The auditory meatus assumes an irregular path from the concha to the tympanic membrane.

At the termination of the external canal is the eardrum, or tympanic membrane, which forms the boundary between the outer and the middle ear (Figure 13-3). The tympanic membrane has a complicated shape that loosely resembles a flat cone, and it moves with changes in air pressure. Because the tympanic membrane is oval and translucent, the middle ear structure often can be visualized through it. The short and long processes of the malleus are attached to the fibrous layer of the tympanic membrane and are visible on the lateral surface. The middle ear cavity is an air-filled space connected by an air cell system posterior to the mastoid and by the eustachian tube anterior to the nasopharynx. Neither of these communications is in a dependent position for drainage of fluids. Ciliated columnar cells cover the walls of the tympanic cavity and mastoid air cells. Secretory cells are distributed throughout the middle ear, with the greatest number in the eustachian tube. In the middle ear, the malleus, incus, and stapes occupy the region between the tympanic membrane and the oval window of the middle ear. During otoscopic examination, the long process of the incus often can be seen through the tympanic membrane.

The stapedius and the tensor muscles of the tympanic membrane attach in the middle ear to the malleus and the stapes by tendons. The chorda tympani nerve passes across the

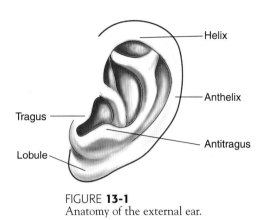

FIGURE **13-1**
Anatomy of the external ear.

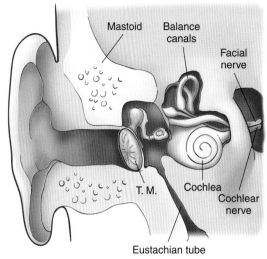

FIGURE **13-3**
General framework of the outer, middle, and inner ear. *T.M.*, Tympanic membrane. Redrawn from Pappas D (1985). *Diagnosis and treatment of hearing impairment in children.* San Diego, CA: College-Hill Press.

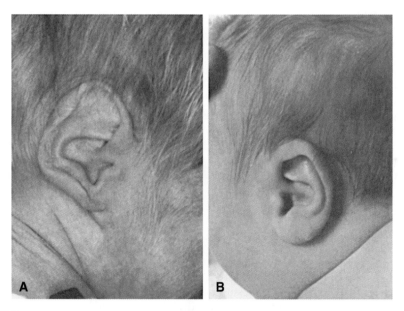

FIGURE **13-2**
Premature (**A**) and full-term (**B**) ear. From Schreiner RL, Bradburn NC (1987). *Care of the newborn,* ed 2. New York: Raven Press.

posterior surface. The medial wall of the middle ear cavity contains the oval and round windows. Between these two windows, the lower portion of the cochlea forms a prominence known as the promontorium tympani on the medial wall of the middle ear.

The inner ear consists of a bony labyrinth composed of three parts: the semicircular canals, the vestibule, and the cochlea. A dense, bony capsule in the petrous protein of the temporal bone surrounds these hollow spaces; this capsule contains perilymph and endolymph. Each of the semicircular canals has a dilated portion at the end, referred to as ampullae,

which contain the crista ampullaris, a vestibular sense organ. In the vestibule, the utricle and saccules are formed; these structures saccules contain sensory endings important for maintaining equilibrium.

The cochlea is a tubular structure with 212 spirals; it closely resembles a snail shell, having a base and an apex. The cochlea is divided into the scala vestibuli and the scala tympani. The two tracts connect at the apex. The scala vestibuli begins at the oval window, and the scala tympani terminates at the round window. The basilar membrane side of the duct gives rise to the organ of Corti, the organ of hearing. The organ of

Corti includes hair cells and supporting cells; attached to the hair cells is a gelatinous membrane called the tectorial membrane.

The membranous labyrinth of the inner ear is composed of connective tissue filled with endolymph that forms in the bony labyrinth. Hair cells of the cochlea and the vestibular labyrinth are attached by afferent nerve fibers to the neurons of the auditory system, the spiral ganglion, and Scarpa's ganglion in the temporal bone. Efferent nerve fibers from ganglia form the auditory and vestibular division of the eighth cranial nerve and exit the temporal bone on its posterior surface to enter the brainstem.

PHYSIOLOGY OF AUDIOLOGIC FUNCTION
External Ear

The external ear consists of the auricle (pinna) and the external auditory meatus (external canal). The primary function of the external ear is to funnel sound to the tympanic membrane. Absence of the auricle contributes to difficulty in sound localization.

Middle Ear

Advancing sound entering the auditory canal directly strikes the tympanic membrane. This membrane and the ossicles serve as transmitters from the outer ear to the inner ear. The malleus, which is continuous with the tympanic membrane and is connected with the incus and stapes, moves the ossicles. Ossicles transfer sound energy into the inner ear through the oval window, which holds the stapes by means of an angular ligament.

The middle ear is lined with respiratory mucosa composed of ciliated columnar epithelial cells, supporting cells, and secretory cells. Secretory cells secrete mucus that forms a complex mucous layer. The cilia of the middle ear interact with the mucus by transporting mastoid and middle ear secretions through the eustachian tube to the nasopharynx, where they are swallowed. This mechanism is known as the mucociliary transport system. Glycoproteins in the mucus determine the viscosity and elasticity of the middle ear mucus. Mucus that is too thick or too thin impedes effective transport of bacteria and cellular debris from the mastoid and middle ear cleft: this transport has a protective effect against ear infections. In addition to serving as an exit for secretions into the nasopharynx, the eustachian tube equalizes the pressure between the middle ear and the ambient atmosphere.

Inner Ear

Before this point in the hearing mechanism, all of the sound energy is contained in the air-filled spaces of the external and middle ear. From the stapes onward, the pathway for sound moves through fluid-filled spaces. When sound is transferred from the tympanic membrane to the inner ear, the stapes creates a fluid wave that is transmitted to the round window. This transmission creates fluid waves that travel from the basal aspect of the cochlea to the apex. As the fluid wave moves, it displaces the basilar membrane. Maximum movement of the basilar membrane occurs at the point specific to the frequency of sound entering the ear; that is, high-frequency sounds cause minimal disturbance at the basal end of the cochlea, and low-frequency sounds cause minimal disturbance at the apex.

Vibrations in the basilar membrane cause movement of the organ of Corti. This organ contains receptor hair cells that are on the basilar membrane. Vibrations of the hair on the hair cells cause either polarization or depolarization, depending on the direction of the bend. When sufficient depolarization occurs, action potentials are produced that are propagated along the auditory pathway to the auditory cortex. The cochlea provides input by coding information about loudness and frequency in the action potentials sent to the cortex, giving meaning to the sound. Hair cells of the spiral organ of Corti are stimulated as they touch the tectorial membrane. Hair cells act as transducers that convert mechanical energy into electrical impulses; this action occurs in the fibers of the spiral ganglion. Axons of these cells become the auditory nerve (vestibulocochlear nerve). Nerve fibers pass to the medulla, the pons, and the midbrain, and finally to the temporal lobes of the cortex, where the impulses are interpreted as sound.

The vestibular system is similar to the auditory system. Fluid moves within the vestibular labyrinth when the head moves. The semicircular canals respond to angular acceleration (rotation), and the utricle and saccule respond to linear acceleration (position). Movement of endolymph exerts force on the hairs of the sensory cells of the cristae and the maculae. Depolarization of the sensory cells produces action potentials, which are transmitted to the vestibular cortex. The vestibular apparatus functions in conjunction with proprioception and visual orientation to maintain balance.

HEARING IMPAIRMENT

The American Speech-Language-Hearing Association (ASHA) defines hearing impairment as "a loss of auditory sensitivity that can be measured at birth and for which intervention strategies are known and available." Hearing impairment represents a spectrum of hearing loss classified as mild, moderate, severe, or prolonged (Spivak, 1998). The criterion for measuring bilateral conductive and sensorineural hearing deficit in children is 1000 to 4000 Hz, the frequency range that is important for speech recognition.

Types of Hearing Impairment

The types of hearing impairment have been classified according to the location of the problem. Impairment may be one of three types: conductive, sensorineural, or a combination of these. Conductive losses arise from conditions that affect the outer and middle ear; sensorineural loss results from inner ear disorders; and combination losses result from disruptions in both areas of the ear.

Conductive Hearing Loss

Conductive hearing loss exists when dysfunction in the outer or middle ear disrupts the normal sequence of sound localization and vibration. Frequently the external auditory meatus becomes occluded by cerumen (wax), which impedes the transmission of sound. Otitis media, an infection of the middle ear, is the most common cause of conductive hearing loss. In this instance, fluid accumulates in the middle ear, preventing the tympanic membrane and ossicular chain from vibrating normally. The infection also can occur secondary to newborn diseases such as bronchopulmonary dysplasia (Gray et al, 2001). Often related to hearing loss are congenital syndromes, such as CHARGE (posterior coloboma, hearing defect, choanal atresia, retardation, and genital and ear anomalies) (Acham & Walch, 2001).

Congenital deformities of the outer ear also can affect the neonate's ability to hear. Because the function of the external ear is to funnel sound, variations in the structure and protrusion of the pinna may contribute to conductive hearing loss.

A missing or deformed pinna can result from a malformation of the auricular folds. Atresia of the auditory meatus or abnormal development of the ossicular chain may arise from defective development of the branchial chain.

Individuals with conductive hearing loss have difficulty hearing low-frequency sounds (i.e., those in the 125- to 500-Hz range). Management of the neonate with conductive hearing loss is directed toward early observation, detection, and intervention to eliminate the source of infection, to remove the blockage, and to provide amplification, resulting in the restoration of normal hearing.

Sensorineural Hearing Impairment

Sensorineural hearing impairment results from damage to the sensory nerve endings of the cochlea or dysfunction of the auditory nerve (eighth cranial nerve). A typical characteristic of inner ear dysfunction is the inability of the inner ear to interpret fluid changes in the cochlea. With sensorineural loss, hearing is normal at low frequencies; sound deficits are evident at frequencies above 1000 Hz.

Sensorineural hearing loss may manifest as a congenital inner ear abnormality, resulting in congenital deafness. Other conditions that may cause sensorineural hearing loss are trauma to the inner ear, the effects of certain drugs, prolonged exposure to loud noise, infections, infectious conditions such as measles, and the effects of aging.

IDENTIFICATION OF THE HEARING-IMPAIRED INFANT

Physical Examination

The physical examination of the infant should be performed in a quiet, warm, draft-free area appropriate for observation and inspection of auditory structures and function. Observing the infant's behavior before examining the ear yields baseline assessments. The alert, normal full-term newborn reacts by turning toward the sound of human speech or ring of a bell; this infant also startles to the stimulus of a loud noise. Observation of the preterm infant is deferred to a later time, prior to discharge when the behavioral response has matured. Observation of infant response alone provides only a crude estimate of neonatal hearing ability.

Inspection of the Ear

Inspection of the ear begins with the medial and lateral surfaces of the pinna and the surface of the scalp, face, and neck. Development of the pinna correlates with the infant's gestational age. At term, the pinna of the newborn is well shaped and has sufficient cartilage to maintain normal shape and resistance (see Figure 13-2). Before 34 weeks' gestation, the pinna is a slightly formed double thickness of cartilage. The relationship of the pinna to the other structures of the head and face is important in the initial assessment. With normal placement, the helix is located at the level of the outer canthus and the tragus is roughly level with the intraorbital rim. Low-set auricles frequently are associated with abnormalities of the urinary system. Unilateral conductive hearing loss may be present in children with normal-size pinnae and unilateral absence of the superior crus or in patients with

a fused anthelix-helix; thickened, hypertrophied ear lobes; a "cup" ear; and a protruding pinna. The pinna may be abnormally small (microtia) or absent (anotia). Atresia (closure of the external auditory canal) may be observed. The condition is classified as mild, indicating a small ear canal; medium, indicating that a bony atretic plate has replaced the canal with ossicular malformation; or severe, indicating a small or absent ear canal and middle ear space.

Several combinations of atresia and microtia may be seen; therefore all children with these abnormalities should be suspected of having middle ear abnormalities. These infants may also have sensorineural hearing loss. Atresia often is observed with cranial, facial, mandibular, or acrofacial dysostoses. Abnormalities of the skeletal system or chromo-somal aberration may also be accompanied by atresia. Aural atresia may be associated with facial, labial, or palatal clefts. Infants with atresia often have conductive hearing loss related to the inability of the ear canal to transmit sound.

Preauricular abnormalities, including pits or tags (Figure 13-4) and branchial fistulas, often are accompanied by external or middle ear malformations. These appendages may be present with an otherwise normal-appearing pinna. Preauricular tags or pits usually require only cosmetic surgery or excision if they are draining.

The pinna should be inspected for location and for its relationship to other facial structures. Normal attachment is to the side, level with the middle third of the face, and fixed in position to the lateral aspect of the external auditory canal. The major convolutions of the pinna are the helix, anthelix, tragus, antitragus, and lobule. The lobule of the external ear has no cartilage. The angle of placement of the pinna is almost vertical, and if the angle is more than 10 degrees off normal, it is considered abnormal. The superior helix is located at the outer canthus of the eye, and the tragus is roughly level with the infraorbital rim.

Low-set auricles frequently are associated with other abnormalities of the first and second branchial cleft and with abnormalities of the urinary system. Other abnormalities that may be noted are skin tags, sinuses, or pits, which often

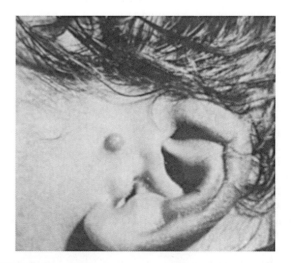

FIGURE **13-4**
Preauricular tag. From Schreiner RL, Bradburn NC (1987). *Care of the newborn*, ed 2. New York: Raven Press.

are associated with other auditory or renal malformations. The pinna often may be observed to have bruising from a forceps delivery. Depending on the degree of bruising, the discoloration should subside within the first week of life.

The external auditory meatus should then be observed for patency. Atresia or stenosis of the external meatus may be seen. This abnormality results in a conductive hearing loss because sound transmissions are blocked; the condition should be noted as part of the physical findings.

Inspection of the Middle Ear and Tympanic Membrane

The depths of the external meatus can be examined with a brightly illuminated pneumatic otoscope. Vernix caseosa frequently is encountered in the ear canal of the neonate. The otoscope is introduced into the ear canal by exerting gentle traction posterosuperiorly on the auricle. In the neonate, the tympanic membrane lies in a nearly horizontal plane. The tympanic membrane is visualized through the collapsed neonatal ear by gently dilating the ear canal with the speculum as the cartilaginous canal is traversed. The tympanic membrane should be examined for thickness, vascularity, and contour. All areas, including the area above the short process of the malleus (pars flaccida), should be visualized for completeness. Normally the tympanic membrane appears translucent. White shadows of the ossicles usually can be seen through the membrane. The mobility of the tympanic membrane can be assessed by applying intermittent pressure through a bulb or by blowing through a polyethylene tube connected to an otoscope.

Otitis media can occur in the first days of life and can be diagnosed by otoscopic examination. Otitis media often manifests as a poorly mobile, bulging, yellow, opacified tympanic membrane. Complications of otitis media are common. Otitis media with middle ear effusion may cause hearing loss, perforation of the tympanic membrane, and possibly intracranial complications, including meningitis, encephalitis, and brain abscess (Vartiainen, 2000). Middle ear effusion occurs in both outpatient and inpatient groups of neonates.

Inspection of the Head and Neck

The anatomy of the head and neck should be assessed for deficits as part of the screening process for all neonates. Ear anomalies associated with head and neck anomalies may occur as a result of a primary regional defect; secondary to a primary defect in an area contiguous to the temporal bone; as part of an inherited defect involving the skeletal system; or as part of a chromosomal disorder. Malformations of the head and neck may be relatively simple or complex. Any neonate with a defect, even a minor one, should be closely examined for hidden major malformations.

Nose

Examination of the nose should be directed toward identification of suspicious defects, such as unusual broadness with a flat base and a short length (saddle nose), small nostrils, and notched alae. Deformities of the nose often appear with other craniofacial abnormalities.

Mouth

Defects in the oral cavity are the most common defect associated with hearing impairment. A child with cleft lip or palate has a deficiency in the palate musculature that is primarily related to the inability of the tensor muscle of the velum palatinum to dilate the eustachian tube actively during swallowing. Hearing problems may be observed in patients with cleft palate, depending on the patient's age on examination and the means of the exploration.

Cleft lip or palate leaves the child vulnerable to the effusion of fluid and, as a result, to varying degrees of hearing loss. The consequences of effusion raise the rate of otitis media, for which 50% to 90% incidences have been reported. The hearing loss associated with cleft lip or palate generally is conductive; however, sensorineural and combination losses have been reported. Infants younger than 12 months of age who had cleft palate that was surgically repaired often have a detectable degree of hearing loss. The degree of loss is directly related to the severity of the palatal defect.

Eyes

Deformities of the eyelids are the most common abnormality involving the eyes. A variation in eyelid configuration has been noted in which the upper eyelid forms an almost vertical curve at the level of the medial limit of the cornea and fuses with the lower eyelid. The distance of the two medial angles is increased. These findings typically are noted in Waardenburg's syndrome, an autosomal dominant disorder that results in mild to severe sensorineural hearing loss in 50% of patients. The hearing loss may be unilateral or bilateral and progressive.

Epicanthal folds, which are true vertical folds extending from the nasal fold into the upper eyelid, are commonly noted in infants with Down syndrome, or trisomy 21. Other physical features seen in Down syndrome are low-set ears, small pinnae, and a narrow external ear canal. Infants with this syndrome tend to have recurrent otitis media and anomalies of the middle ear ossicles. The incidence of hearing loss is high, and the condition may be the sensorineural, conductive, or combination type.

Hair

An unusual hair texture or hairline should raise suspicion in the assessment for abnormalities associated with hearing loss. Twisted hair (pili torti) has been associated with sensorineural hearing loss. The hair may be twisted, dry, brittle, or easily broken. Aberrant scalp hair patterns may also be significant.

Neck

Defects of the neck that may be associated with hearing impairment are branchial cleft fistulas and mildly webbed or shortened neck. Not all infants with defects of the head or neck also have hearing impairments; many variations may be observed in the normal neonate (Jones, 1988). The presence of such defects does increase the risk of hearing impairment, however, and should be followed up in the long-term interest of the child.

HISTORY

The importance of a comprehensive history for identifying the infant at risk cannot be overemphasized. The newborn carries a history extending back to the time of conception and is influenced by both perinatal events and parental genetic composition. Gathering of data on the infant's history is the first step in identifying infants at risk for hearing impairment. A thorough history of familial hearing loss, either presenting at birth or childhood through adolescence, is significant.

Family History

More than 50 types of hereditary hearing loss have been described. A significant number of hearing impairments may be classified as genetically based. Hereditary hearing loss must be identified on the basis of a thorough medical and family history, which should include the following components:

1. Determination of the cause and circumstances under which the hearing impairment was first noticed: Many different circumstances surrounding the onset of the hearing loss may cause it to be labeled as congenital or hereditary or both. An example of hearing loss that is hereditary and not congenital is Alport's syndrome, an autosomal dominant trait resulting in deafness that appears at 8 years of age.
2. A complete family history: This should include a history of previous and current pregnancies.
3. An extended family history of data relating to hearing impairments of both immediate and extended family members.
4. A thorough physical examination: The head and neck region, particularly, should be examined for abnormalities.
5. Selective testing procedures for assessing possible causes of sensorineural hearing loss.

A form can be used to obtain information on familial hearing loss from the mother. Although the questions easily may be asked orally, the form provides a structure that can ensure consistency and is the preferred method of data gathering in most settings. The questionnaire should be given to all new mothers and should be completed prior to discharge. The questionnaire provides an excellent opportunity for educating the mother on normal speech and language development.

HEREDITARY HEARING LOSS

Autosomal Dominant Inheritance

Autosomal dominant inheritance accounts for 10% to 25% of cases of hereditary hearing impairment. The hearing loss may be unilateral or bilateral, and males and females are affected equally. Autosomal dominant hearing disorders vary in severity ("variable expressivity") and in progression of hearing loss. A typical example of an autosomal dominant hearing disorder occurs in Waardenburg's syndrome, which is characterized by hypertelorism, a high nasal bridge, synophrys, and hypoplastic alae nasi. Pigmentation abnormalities include a white forelock, partial albinism, hypopigmentation of the fundi, blue irises, and premature graying. In this syndrome, severe to profound bilateral sensorineural hearing loss is present with integumentary system involvement. The histopathologic characteristics are absence of the organ of Corti and atrophy of the spiral ganglion.

Another example of an autosomal dominant hearing loss with incomplete penetrance and variable expression occurs in Treacher Collins syndrome. Major features of the syndrome include facial anomalies; small, displaced, or absent external ears; external auditory canal atresia; and poorly developed or malformed tympanic ossicles. Deafness generally is complete and conductive.

Klippel-Feil syndrome, if familial, is another example of autosomal dominance with variable expression. The characteristics of this syndrome are craniofacial disorders, fusion of some or all of the cervical vertebrae, cleft palate (occasionally), and severe sensorineural hearing loss. Crouzon's disease is another disorder in which hearing loss is attributed to autosomal dominance with variable expression. An abnormally shaped head, a beaked nose, and marked bilateral exophthalmos caused by premature closure of the cranial sutures characterize this disease. Hearing loss may be conductive or sensorineural because of middle ear deformities.

Autosomal Recessive Inheritance

Autosomal recessive inheritance accounts for about 40% of childhood deafness. An estimated one in eight individuals is a carrier for a recessive form of hearing impairment. The incidence of recessive inheritance is higher in marriages of recent common ancestry. This type of union increases the possibility that each parent will be the carrier of an identical defective gene that may express itself as an abnormal trait. Hearing loss in people with an autosomal recessive gene tends to be more severe than in those with autosomal dominant inheritance, because most cases of recessive hearing loss are associated with Scheibe's deformity of the cochlea. With Scheibe's dysplasia, the entire organ of Corti is rudimentary; hair cells are missing, and the supporting cells are distorted or collapsed. The vestibular membrane usually is collapsed. Pendred's syndrome, a condition marked by hearing loss and goiter detected in the first 2 years of life, is an example of an autosomal recessive disorder.

X-Linked Disorders

Approximately 3% of hereditary deafness is due to the X-linked mode of transmission (Northern & Downs, 1984). The mutant gene is on the X chromosome, and males transmit only Y chromosomes to their male offspring; therefore only males are affected. The female is the carrier and has the chance to transmit the gene to 50% of her sons, who manifest the disease, and 50% of her daughters, who carry the abnormality. The hearing loss characteristically is not present at birth but develops in infancy to varying degrees. X-linked hearing losses, with exceptions, are sensorineural, and some retention of hearing in all frequencies often occurs. Recessive, or X-linked, Duchenne's muscular dystrophy is an example of this type of disorder. Characterized by muscle wasting, the severe infantile form of muscular dystrophy also is associated with mild to moderate sensorineural hearing loss.

Cytogenetic Disorders

Cytogenetic disorders are caused by structural changes in one or more of the chromosomes or by errors in the distribution of the chromosomes. Down syndrome, which is caused by an extra chromosome 21, is the most common chromosomal aberration syndrome, with an incidence of 1 in 600 to 800 births. Approximately 5% of cases of Down syndrome are due to translocation and fusion of part of chromosome 21 to chromosome 14. Children with trisomy 21 have a high incidence of hearing loss.

Characteristic otologic findings that have an impact on the hearing performance of these children during the early years are (1) a high incidence of stenosis of the external auditory canal, (2) a high incidence of serous otitis media, and

(3) a high incidence of cholesteatoma-persistent growth of squamous epithelium from the ear canal into the middle ear or mastoid through a tear in the tympanic membrane.

The narrowed segment is located at the junction of the cartilaginous and bony portions of the canal. With increasing age, the canal has been noted to assume a more typical appearance as the thickened tissue recedes.

The degree of hearing loss in these infants varies but is rarely ever profound. On examination of the aperture, some of these children are found to have congenital ossicular malformations and destruction caused by inflammations arising from chronic infection.

Mental retardation is a clinical condition frequently seen with Down syndrome. The impact of the otologic handicap on the developmental potential of these children is uncertain. Because of the high incidence of hearing loss in this group, early and frequent monitoring is imperative. Collaborative research studies must be done to identify factors affecting the otologic problems of infants with Down syndrome and to devise early strategies to optimize these infants' potential.

OTHER PERINATAL AND POSTNATAL FACTORS ASSOCIATED WITH HEARING LOSS

Elevated Bilirubin Level

Hyperbilirubinemia, also referred to as neonatal jaundice, occurs when an excess of bilirubin is present in the blood. The condition can be neurotoxic to the infant at high concentrations. Jaundice is observed in approximately 60% of term infants and in 80% of preterm infants. Any number of factors that interfere with the transport of bilirubin to the liver or that reduce or prevent the metabolization of bilirubin in the liver can lead to toxic levels of the unconjugated bilirubin. Unconjugated bilirubin can cross the blood-brain barrier. Kernicterus, a neurologic syndrome, results from the deposit of unconjugated bilirubin in the basal ganglia of the brain, causing motor and sensory deficits, mental deficits, or death. Exchange transfusions are performed to lower the bilirubin level in infants at risk of developing kernicterus. For neonatal problems, hyperbilirubinemia is the most common sequela that results in deafness. The Joint Committee on Infant Hearing (2000) of the AAP has suggested that infants with a bilirubin level that exceeds the indications for an exchange transfusion are at risk for hearing impairment.

Low Birth Weight

Low birth weight (under 1500 g), especially when associated with such complications as hyperbilirubinemia and perinatal asphyxia, is widely accepted as a risk factor for congenitally acquired hearing impairment. Reports of hearing loss in low birth weight (LBW) infants put the incidence in the range of 4% to 16%. Other conditions that have been reported to enhance the risk of neurologic sequelae, including hearing impairment, are acidosis, sepsis, ototoxic drug therapy, sound trauma, and hypoglycemia. Determining the exact cause of hearing loss in neonates with multiple risk factors remains difficult. Any of these factors alone may cause hearing impairment, but when they are associated with immature physiologic status, the risk of hearing impairment increases. The hearing loss most often demonstrated in LBW infants is the sensorineural type, particularly in the high-frequency range. Prolonged intubation and otitis media have been correlated with hearing loss in LBW infants.

The higher incidence of hearing loss in LBW infants has been attributed to several factors, including (1) the infant's premature physiologic status; (2) perinatal complications (e.g., hyperbilirubinemia, hypoxia, acidosis, and apneic spells), which are likely to cause brain damage in LBW infants; (3) the constraints of intensive care; and (4) the combined effects of the preceding factors.

The "constraints of intensive care" refers to the iatrogenic factors common in the care of newborns admitted to the neonatal intensive care unit (NICU) that have an impact on the incidence of hearing impairment. These factors include ambient noise and exposure to ototoxic drugs.

Galambos and colleagues (1994) presented a retrospective study of hearing loss in level two (n = 1527) and level three (n = 4374) graduates. Their findings indicated that 1.4% of level two and 2.1% of level three infants failed two rounds of auditory brainstem response (ABR) testing and subsequently required hearing aid devices within the first year of life.

Ototoxic Drugs

The effects of ototoxic drugs commonly used in the care of LBW infants, which potentiate damage to the cochlea or to the vestibular portion of the inner ear, have been well documented. Drugs that have been reported to be potentially ototoxic include antibiotics, diuretics, and antimalarial pharmaceuticals. There appears to be considerable individual susceptibility to these ototoxic drugs, which usually cause bilateral symmetric hearing loss of varying degrees. Numerous factors may enhance the risk of ototoxicity, including elevated serum drug levels; decreased renal function; use of more than one ototoxic drug simultaneously or in increased doses or for an extended period; the infant's age, health, and heredity; and concurrent noise.

Specific aminoglycosides reported for more than a decade to have ototoxic potential include amikacin, clindamycin, gentamicin, kanamycin, tobramycin, and vancomycin. The ASHA (Joint Committee on Infant Hearing, 1994) guidelines suggested that aminoglycoside therapy administered for longer than 5 days in combination with loop diuretics be added to the risk criteria for potential sensorineural hearing loss.

Caution is indicated to monitor peak and trough serum concentrations of antibiotics, as well as creatinine clearance, to avoid high systemic levels in infants with impaired renal function.

Sound Trauma

The potential for noise-induced hearing loss in the neonate has been the subject of numerous reports in the literature. In the NICU, numerous sources constantly generate background and alarm noise.

The noise level in the NICU has been reported to be 20 dB higher than that in the well-baby nursery. The noise level of incubators per se does not cause sensorineural hearing loss in otherwise healthy preterm infants. Sudden noises in the NICU have been reported to cause hypoxemia in preterm infants, which leads to a decrease in transcutaneous oxygen tension and an increase in intracranial pressure, heart rate, and respiratory rate.

Nearly all the reported sound pressure levels of incubators (60 to 80 dB) are consistently lower than the risk level for adults. However, the damage risk level for adults, 90 dB, is based on intermittent exposure to noise; neonates are subject to continuous exposure for weeks and months at a time.

In recent years more research has focused on sound levels in the NICU and ways to reduce them (Walsh-Sukys et al, 2001). Graven (2000) performed a systematic review of NICU noise levels to determine the adverse reactions that were found, such as hearing loss. Philbin and associates (1999) recommended that the overall continuous sound level in any bed space or patient care area not exceed 55 dB. When background noise exceeds 50 dB, sleep is disturbed (Robertson & Philbin, 1996). Operating an NICU at sound levels below 50 dB requires careful attention to design and the cooperation of all those working on the unit.

Newborns at risk for hearing impairment may be exposed to hazardous sound levels during transport. For example, in a helicopter the noise level can reach 90 to 110 dB. Use of ear protectors during air transport has been suggested. These earmuffs also are used worldwide in many units to reduce noise for infants transported by ground or air.

Adding recorded voice and music to the environment of the preterm infant is a practice widely used to enhance the auditory environment. Sound sources should be kept a reasonable distance from infants' ears, and the sound level should be kept below 55 dB (Philbin & Klass, 2000). White and associates (2000) have developed NICU design standards that include recommendations both for safe lighting and for sound levels.

DIFFERENTIAL DIAGNOSIS

No differential diagnosis exists for deafness, although generally a differential diagnosis to determine the etiology of the hearing impairment is listed. The emphasis is not on the deafness but on what neonatal or infant issues might incorporate deafness as one of the symptoms.

DIAGNOSTIC TESTS

Laboratory testing is not of benefit in the diagnosis of deafness; however, if a genetic syndrome is suspected, biochemical evidence may be of benefit in determining the etiology. Connexin 26 is a genetic marker for deafness. Laboratory testing for perinatal infections such as cytomegalovirus (CMV), syphilis, and other TORCH infections may be indicated.

For bilateral hearing loss, markers for general inflammatory disease, such as sedimentation rate, rheumatoid factor, or 68-kDa protein a marker specially for autoimmune ear disease may be evaluated.

IMAGING STUDIES

Computed tomographic (CT) scanning and magnetic resonance imaging (MRI) may be used to establish a malformation of the cochlea or cochlear nerve. MRI scanning may be used to identify an enlarged vestibular aqueduct, in the case of a sensitive ear in a child with a minor head trauma who presents with deteriorating hearing.

SCREENING METHODS FOR IDENTIFICATION OF HEARING LOSS

Factors are presented to facilitate identification of infants at risk for hearing impairment (American Speech-Language-Hearing Association, Joint Committee on Infant Hearing, 1994, 2000). Universal screening for hearing loss (UNHS) is required by law in more than 30 states and is performed routinely in some health care systems in other states. Selective

---

BOX 13-1
Risk Identification Criteria: Neonates (Birth to 28 Days)
The risk factors that identify those neonates at risk for sensorineural hearing impairment include:
1. An illness or condition requiring admission of 48 hours or greater to a NICU.
2. Stigmata or other findings associated with a syndrome known to include a sensorineural or conductive hearing loss.
3. Family history of permanent childhood sensorineural hearing loss.
4. Craniofacial anomalies, including those with morphologic abnormalities of the pinna and ear canal.
5. In utero infection such as cytomegalovirus, herpes, toxoplasmosis, or rubella.

From Joint Committee on Infant Hearing (2000). Year 2000 position statement: Principles and guidelines for early hearing detection and intervention program. *American journal of audiology* 9:9-29.

---

screening of high-risk neonatal indicators is used as the basis for selection in the absence of universal screening. Institutions are advised to use the ASHA Joint Committee's high-risk neonatal indicators associated with sensorineural and/or conductive hearing loss (Box 13-1) as a guide to identifying infants in need of hearing screening. These factors are also used to determine which infants need follow-up despite a normal initial screening result. If only infants who are identified as having one or more high-risk factors are screened, 50% to 70% of children with impairment remain unidentified (Thompson et al, 2001).

Hearing screening is a method of detecting hearing impairment before the deficit becomes obvious in the infant. In the past 15 years, programs and procedures for screening newborns have been developed, modified, and improved. The goal of any screening program is to accomplish the task rapidly, accurately, and economically.

The AAP Task Force on Newborn and Infant Hearing (1999) has endorsed universal screening of all newborns. Audiologic follow-up is required for infants whose history indicates that degenerative disease or intrauterine infection may cause progressive, fluctuating, or late-onset hearing loss. In all cases, before discharge the parents should be informed about speech and hearing milestones (Figure 13-5) and should be provided with information about community agencies available for long-term follow-up if needed. Because the intent of all screening programs is to identify hearing impairment before 3 months of age and to habilitate hearing-impaired children no later than 6 months of age, program development is essential (Joint Committee on Infant Hearing, 2000).

Peripheral Measurements of Hearing Function

Assessment of hearing function in the neonate has focused on a two-tiered approach in which the evoked otoacoustic emissions (EOAE) test is used initially, and the automated ABR test is used as follow-up for infants who show hearing impairment on the initial screening. Otoacoustic emissions are low-intensity

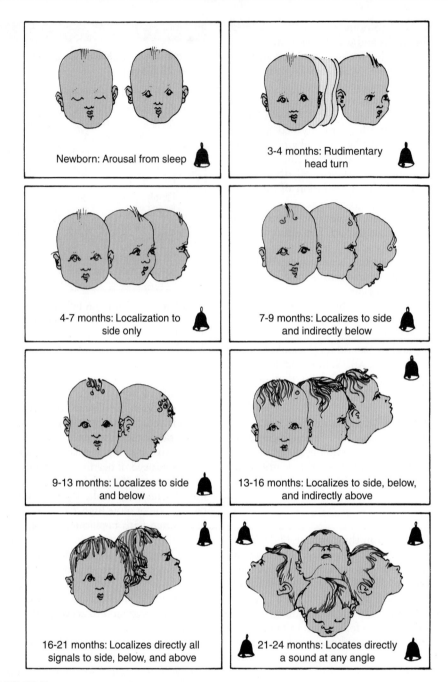

FIGURE **13-5**
Maturation of auditory response. From Northern J, Downs M (1984). *Hearing in children*. Baltimore: Williams & Wilkins.

sounds that can be measured by placing a sensitive microphone in the ear canal. Hearing screening using otoacoustic emissions is quick, inexpensive, and relatively accurate.

If hearing impairment is detected on the EOAE test, the ABR test can confirm the validity of that result. The ABR test records the electrical potentials that arise from the auditory nerve system. During this test, disk electrodes are attached to the vertex and mastoid areas, and repetitive sounds are presented to the ear in the form of clicks caused by a direct current pulse. The recorded response is a sequence of waves that represents the action potential of the auditory nerve. The

wave latencies in infants at risk tend to show smaller and more prolonged responses. The absolute latency of the ABR waves depends on the intensity of the click stimulus. Reducing the click stimuli from 60 dB to 30 to 40 dB identifies thresholds of hearing. Absence of all waves indicates the presence of a peripheral lesion.

An abnormal ABR result may be defined as one that shows an absence of response at 40 dB or a wave V latency that exceeds the norm by two standard deviations. Wave V responses are used to determine abnormality because they are highly repeatable in infants and show little variability in normal-hearing subjects. The ABR test appears to be a sensitive method in that no false-negative results have been reported. Considering that any screening method should be quick, inexpensive, and easily administered and should allow easy interpretation of results on a large number of infants, the drawback to the ABR test is that it is more costly than the EOAE test. Nevertheless, the ABR test can be justified as the initial neonatal hearing test, especially in preterm or high-risk infants. The Joint Committee on Infant Hearing (1994, 2000) specifies that an audiologist should supervise the infant hearing screening program.

In some infants whose initial ABR test results meet risk criteria, continuing audiologic follow-up and management may be appropriate. These infants include those with risk factors associated with possible progressive or fluctuant loss, such as a family history of progressive hearing loss, CMV infection, and persistent fetal circulation.

Infants who do not demonstrate a repeatable ABR wave V to the signal presented at 40 dB in at least one ear should have a comprehensive hearing evaluation at no later than 6 months of age. This follow-up includes a general physical examination, including examination of the head and neck; otoscopy and otomicroscopy; identification of relevant physical abnormalities; and laboratory tests for perinatal infections. A comprehensive audiologic evaluation may include additional evoked potential evaluation and acoustic emittance measurements. Although precise data on hearing sensitivity cannot be obtained until the infant can respond to operant conditioning test procedures at approximately 6 months of age, habilitation should not be delayed. The treatment protocols can be modified as additional hearing evaluation data become available. Many institutions are now using the ABR and EOAE tests as early as 24 hours of age. The rationale is that the earlier a problem is identified, the sooner treatment can be started (Ronge, 1997).

Infants can be fitted with hearing aids before 3 months of age. Attention to early identification, amplification, and education does not necessarily ensure speech and language acquisition but certainly facilitates it, even in the most profoundly hearing-impaired child.

DEVELOPMENT OF A TREATMENT PLAN FOR THE HEARING-IMPAIRED NEONATE

Two of the recommendations of the Joint Committee on Infant Hearing (1994, 2000) are that hearing screening of all infants be completed before discharge or no later than 3 months of age, and that whenever possible, the diagnostic process be completed and habilitation begun by 6 months of age. An infant with a positive hearing test result should be retested within 6 weeks of the initial screening procedure. Infants whose history indicates that they are at risk for late-onset hearing loss should be observed by periodic audiologic testing.

For the infant with a confirmed hearing loss, efforts are directed at treatment. In accordance with Public Law 99, early intervention services are (1) evaluation and assessment and (2) development of an individualized family service plan. The full evaluation plan is to be completed within 45 days of referral. This plan may include various methods directed at treatment of serous otitis media, which is a major cause of temporary conductive hearing loss. For the infant with a permanent conductive hearing loss, amplification with a

hearing aid may facilitate stimulation in the early critical period. Infants can be fitted with a hearing aid device as soon as the impairment is diagnosed. In addition to amplification, the family should be taught total communication skills that will enhance interaction between the sender and the receiver. The basic premise is to use every means to communicate, such as gesturing, touching, and attending to stimuli.

Hearing screening is a task for a team of professionals that includes pediatricians, otolaryngologists, audiologists, neurologists, and nurse practitioners. Local public health agencies may provide services such as data collection and referral. Many large metropolitan medical centers have speech and hearing centers as part of a broad base of services ranging from diagnosis to rehabilitation. At the national level, the following organizations provide health professionals and consumers with information on the diagnosis and treatment of hearing impairments: American Speech-Language-Hearing Association (ASHA), 10801 Rockville Pike, Rockville, MD 20852, www.professional.asha.org; National Institute on Deafness and other Communication Disorders, Wise Ears, www.nih.gov/nidcd/health/wise.

IMPLEMENTATION AND EVALUATION

The overall goal of any treatment program for the hearing impaired is to optimize the infant's potential communication skills and abilities. To achieve this goal, a comprehensive evaluation, follow-up, and management system must be implemented. The multidisciplinary, multiservices approach should be instituted only when all components are available to the infant and the family (American Speech-Language-Hearing Association, 1994).

In addition to qualified professionals and services, other factors influence the management and habilitation of the hearing-impaired infant. These factors can facilitate or hamper entry into the system and compliance with the treatment regimen (Box 13-2).

Outcome measures of the treatment program are early identification and implementation of a comprehensive habilitation plan to maximize communication potential and parental acceptance of the infant's disability.

The infant with severe to profound hearing impairment who is not at risk for recurrent otitis media and who does not get satisfactory results with a hearing aid is a candidate for cochlear implants (discussed next). For the hearing-impaired infant, multiple referral sources exist in which a multidisciplinary approach optimizes the infant's potential for growth and development.

BOX 13-2

Factors Influencing the Management and Habilitation of the Hearing-Impaired Infant

Factors That Facilitate Management
Parental involvement
Expeditious arrangements for referral

Factors That Hamper Management
Long waiting list
Poor communication between speech and hearing departments

Cochlear Implants

Cochlear implants are not new, but they increasingly are being used to treat infants with sensorineural hearing loss. The implants are electronic devices that are more sensitive to sound than traditional hearing aids. The external part of the device is surgically placed in the skin behind the ear, and the internal electrodes are placed in the inner ear at the cochlea. Rather than amplifying sound, the implant replaces the nonfunctional transmission of sound in the inner ear; it allows the brain to understand sound signals. In the United States about 7000 children have received cochlear implants (www.nidcd.nih.gov, 2001). Implants work only if some spiral ganglion cells are present to transmit the auditory signal. The implants take sound signals and convert them to electrical stimuli. The sound is conveyed by electrodes, which can be placed in several arrangements, and then transmitted to an external processor. A single-channel or multiple-channel (as many as 22) unit can be used to process the sound.

An issue for patients of any age with any type of cochlear implant is the comfortable level of sound (Donaldson et al, 2001). This sometimes is difficult to determine in infants, who are easily stimulated. The impact of implants on speech and language development is also an area of research (Sarant et al, 2001). The implant consists of a microphone, speech processor, transmitter, receiver, and electrodes. Ongoing studies are needed to determine if implants have a positive effect on language acquisition and speech perception and at what age should they be done. To date, the outcome has been promising; children who received implants before language acquisition are in some cases developing close to the normal range. The later the child receives the implants, the more likely it is that speech patterns will remain disturbed. (More information on cochlear implants is available online at http://www.nidcd.nih.gov/health/pubs hb/coch.htm.)

Parental Support

Support for the parents of a hearing-impaired child is based on the foundation of trust and acceptance between the practitioner and the family. Notification of a hearing impairment is an extremely traumatic and deeply disturbing situation for the parents, one that often provokes denial. Often, identification of the problem is delayed because the parents cannot admit that something is wrong. Some practices in the diagnostic workup for hearing impairment seem to favor separation of the parents from the diagnostic process. EOAE and ABR testing

may foster denial because the findings are abstract, and parents need to have visible, tangible evidence of the impairment. The practitioner plays a major role in reiterating, interpreting, and reinforcing the information conveyed by the audiologist. Sensitivity to the parents' need to grieve the loss of the "perfect child" is important. Acceptance of the handicap can be aided by enlisting the parents as co-diagnosticians. Asking the parents what they think the problem is and making them part of the decision-making process objectifies the diagnoses and aids future compliance with the habilitative regimen. By listening to the parents' feelings of inadequacy and by indirect teaching, practitioners can help the parents acquire more fruitful coping strategies.

The mother-infant relationship is potentially damaged when the infant is hearing impaired. Reciprocal communication that normally occurs between the mother and the infant on an affective and a verbal level has been reported to be diminished with infants who are hearing impaired. The handicapped infant may miss intended signals from parents and may emit signals that are not understood. The parents must capture their infant's visual attention so that their efforts are effectively stimulating. An asynchrony may develop that can retard the infant's ability to acquire language even beyond the limits of the hearing loss itself. The family can be taught total communication skills (gesturing, touching, and attending) to support interaction with the infant.

SUMMARY

Hearing is a prerequisite speech acquisition and lays the foundation for future social and intellectual growth. There is a preponderance of evidence that supports the vital role of auditory stimulation for language acquisition in the first 18 months of life. Early infant hearing screening has been mandated by national organizations and put into law in most states. History of perinatal events, family history, and physical examination of the newborn are important components of early screening, but do not identify all infants with hearing loss. The most accurate measurement of hearing in the newborn is the auditory brainstem response (ABR) test measuring the latent potential of wave 5 of the auditory nerve. Testing should ideally be performed in the hospital soon after birth or before 3 months of age. Abnormal test results identifying a hearing impairment indicate the need to habilitate hearing-impaired children no later than 6 months of age. Support and cooperation of the parents of a hearing-impaired child is essential.

Case Study

IDENTIFICATION OF THE PROBLEM

The infant in this case study is currently a 50-day-old Caucasian male ready for discharge from the neonatal intensive care unit. On admission, the infant's weight was 1498 g. The infant required bubble CPAP for the first 12 hours, but was easily weaned to room air. Temperature regulation was initially accomplished via a warmed isolette, and the infant was weaned to an open crib. The infant was initially started on an IV of D10W at 100 mL/kg/day. Initial attempts to maintain suck reflex were fraught with difficulty

and an occupational therapy consult for feeding was secured. A number of nipple adaptations were tried and an indwelling feeding tube proved to be the best vehicle for nutrition. The infant demonstrated slow but steady weight gain to 2403 g.

ASSESSMENT: HISTORY AND PHYSICAL EXAMINATION

A male Caucasian infant was born via spontaneous vaginal delivery. Membranes ruptured spontaneously 8 hours prior

Case Study—cont'd

to delivery. Amniotic fluid was noted to be scant and clear at the time of rupture. Group B streptococcus (GBS) culture was negative at the last prenatal visit, 2 weeks prior to delivery. A neonatal nurse practitioner attended the delivery. Apgar scores of 6 and 8 were assigned, and the infant was transferred to the NICU via a warmed isolette. The infant's weight on admission was 1498 g, and admitting vital signs were temperature 36.8° C, heart rate 162 beats/min, respiratory rate 66 breaths/min, and blood pressure 58/36 mm Hg (mean arterial pressure 41 mm Hg).

Physical examination revealed microcephaly and a soft, flat anterior fontanelle. A dysplastic pinna with microtia was noted in the right ear. The left ear displayed a hypoplastic pinna with patent ear canal. The ears were normally placed on the head. The eyes displayed a palpebral fissure with downward slanting and absent eyelashes on the lower lids. Bilateral breath sounds were clear; HRR without murmur. The abdomen was soft and round, with a three-vessel cord and positive bowel sounds. The patient had normal male genitalia, patent anus, and intact spine. Neonatal reflexes were intact. The gestational assessment was 34-week small-for-gestational-age (SGA) male.

DIFFERENTIAL DIAGNOSIS

A variety of differential diagnoses are possible for this 34-week SGA male infant:

- Cleft palate
- Microcephaly
- Dysplastic right pinna with microtia
- Hypoplastic left ear
- Micrognathia
- Mild RDS

DIAGNOSTIC TESTS

To begin differentiating between the syndromes that have facial abnormalities, a complete physical examination of other body systems can assist in differentiating the diagnosis of Treacher-Collins syndrome (TCS). TCS can be distinguished from Nager syndrome and Miller syndrome if no abnormalities are present in the hands or arms. TCS can be distinguished from oculoauriculovertebral conditions such as Goldenhar syndrome because facial involvement is bilateral and the spinal column is intact.

Testing includes CT scan, genetic testing for TCOF1 (Treacher-Collins syndrome), TORCH studies, ABR testing, genetic workup, and head ultrasound.

WORKING DIAGNOSIS

The CT scan revealed marked micrognathia, microcephaly, and cleft palate, with a normally developed brain. TORCH studies were negative. ABR testing revealed abnormal results bilaterally. Genetic testing revealed a normal male chromosomal composition. Genetic testing for TCOF1 was positive. Head ultrasound was normal.

DEVELOPMENT OF MANAGEMENT PLAN

The management plan for this patient includes the following:

- Parent education for TCS
- Referral to TCS website: www.treachercollinsfnd.org
- Follow-up appointment for ABR testing and evaluation for amplification measures
- Referral to plastic surgery diagnostic center
- Referral to genetic counseling center
- Follow-up appointment at digestive clinic
- Social service consult for community resources
- Parental teaching of habilitation communication techniques and care of the infant's feeding tube

IMPLEMENTATION AND EVALUATION OF EFFECTIVENESS

The mother was consistently involved with the care of the infant; however, her visits were limited due to dependence on public transportation. Weekly care conferences that included the mother were held to update and seek input from the care team members. The infant was referred for further auditory testing and fitted for amplification in the left ear. The infant was evaluated by the plastic surgery center, and a management plan was developed that included repair of the cleft palate and surgical reconstruction of the jaw area with the ultimate goal of removal of the feeding tube. Genetic testing of the familial linkages revealed that the mother tested positive for the marker on chromosome 5 called TCOF1 and was advised that future pregnancies carry a 50% chance of inheriting the disorder.

REFERENCES

Acham A, Walch C (2001). Mondini dysplasia without functional impairment in the framework of a CHARGE association. *Laryngorhinootologie* 80(7):381-384.

American Academy of Pediatrics (AAP) (2000). Joint Committee on Infant Hearing 2000 position statement. *Pediatrics* 106(4):798-817.

Donaldson GS et al (2001). Effects of the clarion electrode positioning system on auditory thresholds and comfortable loudness levels in pediatric patients with cochlear implants. *Archives of otolaryngology, head neck surgery* 127(8):956-960.

Galambos R et al (1994). Identifying hearing loss in the intensive care nursery: a 20-year summary. *Journal of the American Academy of Audiology* 5(3):151-162.

Gallaudet University, Center for Assessment and Demographic Study (1998). Thirty years of the annual survey of deaf and hard of hearing children and youth: a glance over the decades. *American annals of the deaf* 142(2):72-76.

Graven SN (2000). Sound and the developing infant in the NICU: conclusions and recommendations for care. *Journal of perinatology* 20(8 Pt 2):S88-S93.

Gray PH et al (2001). Conductive hearing loss in preterm infants with bronchopulmonary dysplasia. *Journal of paediatric child health* 37(3):278-282.

Joint Committee on Infant Hearing (1994). *Joint Committee on Infant Hearing Year 1994 position statement*. Available at: http://professional/asha.org/resources/legislative/joint_statement.cfm.

Joint Committee on Infant Hearing (2000). *Joint Committee on Infant Hearing year 2000 position statement: principles and guidelines for early hearing detection and intervention programs*. Available at: http://www.infanthearing.org/jcih/.

Jones KL, editor (1988). *Smith's recognizable patterns of human malformation,* ed 4. Philadelphia: Saunders.

Karchmer MA, Allen TE (1999). The functional assessment of deaf and hard of hearing students. *American annals of the deaf* 144(2):68-77.

Kennedy CR et al (2000). Current topic: neonatal screening for hearing impairment. *Archives of disease in childhood* 83:377-383.

Northern JL, Downs MP (1984). *Hearing in children.* Baltimore: Williams & Wilkins.

Philbin MK, Klass P (2000). Behavior effects of auditory experience on the term newborn. *Journal of perinatology* 20(8):68-76.

Philbin MK et al (1999). Recommended permissible noise criteria for occupied, newly constructed, or renovated hospital nurseries. *Journal of perinatology* 19(8 Pt 1):559-563.

Robertson A, Philbin MK (1996). Studies of sound and auditory development. Paper presented at the conference on the Physical and Developmental Environment of the High Risk Neonate, January 31, 1996. Clearwater Beach, FL: University of South Florida College of Medicine.

Ronge LJ (1997). Making a sound decision. *AAP news* 13(4):10-11.

Russ SA et al (2002). Six year effectiveness of a population based two tier infant hearing screening programme. *Archives of disease in childhood* 86:245.

Sarant JZ et al (2001). Variation in speech perception scores among children with cochlear implants. *Early hearing* 1:18-28.

Spivak LG, editor (1998). *Universal newborn hearing screening.* New York: Thieme.

Task Force on Newborn and Infant Hearing (1999). *Early identification of hearing impairment in infants and young children.* Elk Grove Village, IL: American Academy of Pediatrics.

Thompson DC et al (2001). Universal hearing screening: summary of evidence. *Journal of the American Medical Association* 286(16):2000-2010.

Vartiainen E (2000). Otitis media with effusion in children with congenital or early onset hearing impairment. *Journal of otolaryngology* 29(4):221-223.

Walsh-Sukys M et al (2001). Reducing light and sound in the neonatal intensive care unit: an evaluation of patient safety, staff satisfaction, and costs. *Journal of perinatology* 21(4):230-235.

White R et al (2000). *Neonatal intensive care unit structure and design: recommended standards.* Tampa, FL: University of South Florida.

Chapter 14

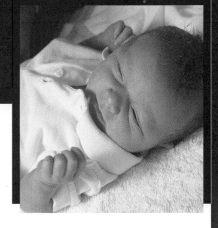

Ophthalmic System

Frances Strodtbeck

The eye begins to develop early in gestation, making this body system vulnerable to insults during the growth process. Neonatal visual problems occur as a result of transplacental, congenital, or neonatal infections; congenital or genetic malformation; exposure to drugs; or abnormal adaptation of the developing eye and its vascularity to stimuli such as oxygen. Visual disturbances in the newborn can range from minor refractory problems to complete blindness. Early detection and treatment are essential if the best possible outcome is to be achieved.

This chapter briefly outlines the embryologic development of the eye, reviews the key points of assessment of the newborn's eyes, and describes specific ophthalmic dysfunctions. Collaborative management and appropriate nursing care are also discussed.

EMBRYOLOGY

Our understanding of the forces that control and govern the development of the eye is growing but limited. About 2 weeks after fertilization, the embryonic plate elongates, and the primitive streak develops along the dorsal surface. The brain and eye develop from the neuroectoderm anterior to the primitive streak. The optic pits (optic sulci) are formed by the indentation of neuroectoderm. Closing of the neural tube leads to movement of the optic pits laterally and outward, toward the surface ectoderm. This movement results in the formation of the optic vesicles (Moore et al, 2003).

As the optic vesicle approaches the outer wall of the embryo, it stimulates a focal thickening of cells called the lens placode. At the fourth week of gestation, this tissue invaginates, forming the optic cup. The inferior portion of the cup is the last to close. The two layers of the optic cup oppose one another to form the retina. At the same time, the lens placode sinks beneath the ectoderm and later becomes the crystalline lens. Mesoderm surrounding the optic cup differentiates to form the sclera, choroid, and part of the cornea (Moore et al, 2003).

Mesoderm anterior to the lens develops into the pupillary membrane; the periphery of the pupillary membrane becomes the iris. The center degenerates to form the pupil. Ectoderm that covers the mesodermal folds appears above and below the lens placode to form the eyelids. The eyelids are fused until about 26 weeks' gestation. The lacrimal gland, the lacrimal drainage system, and the eyelashes form from the ectoderm that covers these folds. Tear production does not begin until 2 to 4 months after birth, when the lacrimal system process is complete (Moore et al, 2003).

ASSESSMENT OF THE EYES

History

A thorough history is imperative to determine whether risk factors for eye problems are present. A complete family, medical, pregnancy, and psychosocial history, along with a maternal review of systems, should be obtained. The interviewer should ask questions related to the family history of vision problems (e.g., strabismus, glaucoma, retinoblastoma) and refractive errors (e.g., myopia). The maternal history should include questions about exposure to infectious diseases such as gonorrhea, chlamydiosis, rubella, and cytomegalovirus (CMV) infection, which are known to cause significant eye problems in newborns. The perinatal history should include questions about any difficulties that might have resulted in hypoxia or anoxia, conditions associated with adverse optical changes. Previous pregnancies that resulted in preterm births can provide important information about prior experience with retinopathy of prematurity (ROP).

Examination

Examining the eyes of a newborn can be a challenge. Care must be taken during the examination process to protect the newborn from injury and cold stress. The infant's state is also important for a successful examination. Newborns in the quiet, alert state are more responsive to visual stimuli.

Most important information about the eyes of the newborn can be obtained from inspection and observation. An examination with an ophthalmoscope usually is not indicated, except when the inspection and observation findings suggest serious problems, such as cataracts or glaucoma.

It is easier to examine the newborn's eyes when they are spontaneously open. Dimming the lights, talking to the infant, and holding the baby upright may facilitate natural opening of the eyes. Newborn eyes should be assessed for their shape, symmetry, and size and for the presence of obvious features, such as eyebrows and eyelashes. The eyes should appear clear, unswollen, and without discharge. Occasionally, irritation may result from the prophylactic drops or ointment used to prevent ophthalmia neonatorum. The eyelids should be evaluated for redness or swelling and for evidence of colobomas and abnormal tumor masses. Inability to elevate the eyelids or ptosis (drooping) of one or both eyelids may lead to amblyopia or poor visual development. The presence of unusual folds and the slant of the eye should be noted. The pupils should be checked for size, equality, reaction to light, and accommodation. The color and clarity of the red reflex should be checked. In African American infants, the reflex may be pale orange rather than red (Fletcher, 1998).

The cornea should be evaluated for clarity and size. A cloudy cornea may be caused by congenital glaucoma, errors of metabolism, or congenital corneal dystrophy. Trauma at birth can result in injury to the cornea, giving the cornea a hazy appearance.

Directly behind the iris is the lens. Cloudiness or opacity in the lens is by definition a cataract. An ophthalmologist should evaluate any cataract found in a newborn as soon as possible to determine if it is visually significant. Surgery should be performed to remove vision-threatening cataracts as soon as the infant is able to tolerate the procedure. Early surgery is critical to the prevention of amblyopia (lazy eye), which develops in these eyes when the condition is ignored for a few months.

Leukocoria is the descriptive term for a whitish-appearing pupil. This condition is almost always indicative of a serious eye problem. The differential diagnosis of leukocoria includes cataract, retinoblastoma, persistent hyperplastic primary vitreous, retrolental fibroplasia, toxocariasis, and Coats' disease.

Because infants with fetal alcohol syndrome can have coloboma, cataract, and microphthalmos, the presence of these findings should alert the examiner to look for other features of the syndrome (Hug et al, 2000). The maternal history should also be re-evaluated for alcohol use during the pregnancy.

The posterior pole of the eye (optic nerve, macula, and blood vessels) is examined with an ophthalmoscope after the pupil is dilated (Figure 14-1). Because a newborn often squirms and moves the head to avoid the light of the ophthalmoscope, an assistant should stabilize the infant's head and body. Giving the infant a bottle or pacifier as a calming measure often is helpful. A topical anesthetic, such as 0.5% proparacaine HCl ophthalmic solution, should be instilled to dull the corneal and conjunctival sensitivity and decrease the newborn's pain. The assistant may separate the eyelids, or a small pediatric eyelid speculum can be used. Care should be taken to avoid causing a corneal abrasion while the speculum is inserted. Normal saline should be used to prevent corneal drying, especially under the heat of a radiant warmer.

For more involved eye examinations, such as those for screening preterm infants for retinopathy of prematurity (ROP), an eyelid speculum and sclera depressor are used (Figure 14-2). Topical anesthetics and comfort measures to minimize or prevent pain are required (Marsh et al, 2005). Insertion of the eyelid speculum and manipulation of the newborn's eye with the sclera depressor, regardless of gestational age, causes the newborn distress leading to pain (Rush et al, 2004; Gal et al, 2005). Comfort measures such as nesting and use of sucrose pacifiers are appropriate nursing interventions to use prior to insertion of the speculum and during eye examination (Gal et al, 2005; Marsh et al, 2005).

About 34% of newborns show retinal hemorrhage, most often in the posterior pole. The risk of retinal hemorrhage is greater with vacuum-assisted delivery and diminished with delivery by cesarean section. More than 90% of the hemorrhages resolve within 2 weeks; however, resolution of retinal hemorrhage in the newborns of women who have had induced labor may take up to 5 weeks.

The infant's ability to see can be assessed by getting the newborn to fix on and follow brightly colored objects. The examiner should hold the object steady about 7 to 9 inches from the infant's eye until the newborn fixes on it (the examiner notes the reflection of the object in the middle of the

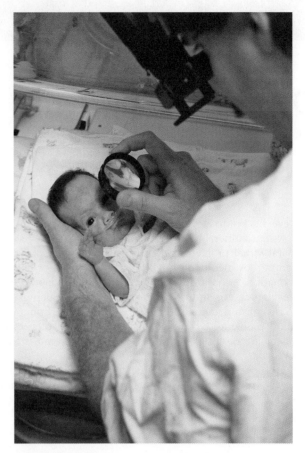

FIGURE **14-1**

A preterm infant undergoing indirect ophthalmoscopy for ROP screening. Used with permission of National Eye Institute, National Institutes of Health (http://www.nei.nih.gov/photo/inst.asp).

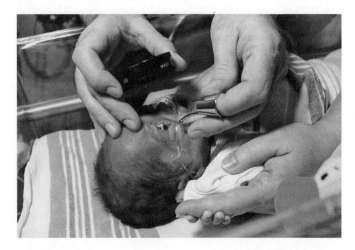

FIGURE **14-2**

ROP eye examination using an eyelid speculum and sclera depressor. Used with permission of National Eye Institute, National Institutes of Health (http://www.nei.nih.gov/photo/inst.asp).

newborn's pupil). Newborns should be able to follow an object about 90 inches either left or right from a midline or central position. Care should be taken to eliminate distractions and to avoid talking because infants respond best to the presentation of one stimulus at a time.

Several important measurements should be obtained. The interpupillary distance and the width of the palpebral fissure should be determined; abnormal values may indicate an underlying syndrome, such as fetal alcohol syndrome. The interpupillary distance (the distance from midpupil to midpupil when the eyes are looking forward) determines whether the eyes are spaced appropriately. Abnormal findings are hypotelorism (eyes too close together) or hypertelorism (eyes too far apart). The width of the palpebral fissure is the distance from the medial canthus to the lateral canthus of each eye; this measurement determines the appropriateness of the opening for the eye. The measurements obtained should be compared with published norms to determine if the value is normal or abnormal. Infants of diabetic mothers (except those born to women with gestational diabetes) should be carefully examined for displaced inner canthi, lens opacity, microphthalmos, tear duct obstruction, and ocular lipoma.

Determining visual acuity in a newborn is difficult. Several methods can be used, including visual preference charts and visual evoked potentials. At term, newborn visual acuity ranges from 20/100 to 20/400, depending on the testing method used. This improves to 20/80 to 20/200 by 4 months of age, 20/40 to 20/80 by 12 months of age, and 20/20 by 2 years of age. According to a recent study described by the authors as the "largest study in the world literature looking at refractive errors at birth against gestational age," all newborns are born with some degree of myopia (Varughese et al, 2005). The authors examined 1200 newborns with gestational ages ranging from 24 to 43 weeks in the first week of life. The degree of myopia was inversely proportional to the gestational age, with the most significant myopia seen in very low birth weight newborns. Approximately 68% of the newborns also had astigmatism.

Attention should also be given to an eye motility examination. In the neonate, the position of the eyes varies greatly. Most infants display intermittent outward deviation (exotropia), which usually disappears within the first few months of life. Any constant inward (esotropia) or outward deviation should be evaluated for a possible nerve or muscle palsy. Intermittent nystagmus (rapid movements of the eye) is a common finding in the newborn. Persistent nystagmus is abnormal; patients with this disorder should be referred for further evaluation (Fletcher, 1998).

Eye Drops

Great care must be taken in the selection of dilating drops for use in newborns. Systemic absorption of the eye drops, although unavoidable to some extent, can cause severe reactions, including death. Cardiovascular consequences, including arterial hypertension, a predisposing factor for intracranial hemorrhage, have been reported in premature infants. Necrotizing enterocolitis (NEC) and feeding intolerance have also been reported in premature infants after eye examinations.

Excess medication that flows out of the eyelids is easily absorbed through the porous skin of the newborn and should be wiped off to prevent systemic absorption. Medication can also be absorbed from the nasolacrimal system; this can be minimized by applying pressure with a fingertip over the nasolacrimal duct for approximately 1 minute after instillation of the drops.

The mydriatics most often used are cyclopentolate, phenylephrine, and tropicamide. For maximum dilation and minimum risk of side effects, a combination of drugs routinely is used in most clinical settings. According to Chew and colleagues (2005), the combination of cyclopentolate 0.2% and phenylephrine 1% produced better mydriasis with few systemic side effects in infants with dark irises. This randomized, double-blinded clinical trial compared cyclopentolate 1% and phenylephrine 2.5%, tropicamide 1% and phenylephrine 2.5%, and cyclopentolate 0.2% and phenylephrine 1% in preterm infants undergoing screening for ROP. Although all three regimens resulted in papillary dilation, the cyclopentolate 1% + phenylephrine 2.5% and tropicamide 1% + phenylephrine 2.5% treatments were associated with significant increases in blood pressure. One half of the subjects in the cyclopentolate 1% + phenylephrine 2.5% group developed feeding intolerance. In another prospective, randomized study, eight different regimens were studied in a population of full-term infants (Ogut et al, 1996). The drug associated with maximum side effects was phenylephrine 2.5%. The safest drug was tropicamide 1%, whereas cyclopentolate 0.5% in combination with tropicamide 0.5% and phenylephrine 2.5% produced the best mydriasis. According to Bolt et al (1992), phenylephrine 2.5% and tropicamide 9.5% produced mydriasis in preterm infants without systemic adverse effects. A complete list of ophthalmic medications commonly used in the newborn is presented in Table 14-1.

After the examination, the infant's eyes should be shielded from light until the pupils return to normal size. The eyes can be covered with occlusive eye shields, such as phototherapy shields, or a cover can be placed over the baby's incubator. Unshielded, dilated eyes are very sensitive to light. Excessive light entering a dilated pupil may cause intense pain. In premature infants or those with underlying health problems, the reaction to the pain may involve systemic responses, such as apnea, bradycardia, cyanosis, and agitation.

DIAGNOSTIC TESTS

A variety of diagnostic tests can be used to further evaluate the newborn for eye abnormalities. These tests are not routinely performed and require the expertise of specially trained ophthalmologists.

Electroretinography

An electroretinogram (ERG) may be obtained when retinal disease is suspected. The ERG provides information about retinal and photoreceptor function. Before an ERG is done, the infant should be sedated and the pupils pharmacologically dilated. Black, opaque patches are placed over each eye for a minimum of 30 minutes before testing, which is done in a special darkroom. The examiner wears a red light similar to that used in photographic darkrooms; this allows the examiner to operate the equipment and visualize the patient. For the test, the examiner removes one patch, instills another drop of dilating drug, and places a special contact lens electrode on the eye's surface. A photic stimulator then generates white flashes of varying intensities. The eye's response to these stimuli is recorded continuously in a manner similar to that used to obtain an electroencephalogram (EEG).

Visual Evoked Potentials

Visual evoked potentials (VEPs) provide information about the functioning of the visual system by measuring activity evoked by neurons in different afferent pathways. Unlike ERGs, VEP testing does not require any medication. The

TABLE 14-1	Commonly Used Eye Medications
Generic Name	**Brand Name**
TOPICAL ANESTHETICS	
Proparacaine hydrochloride	Alcaine, Ophthaine, Ophthetic
Tetracaine hydrochloride	Anacel, Pontocaine
MYDRIATICS (DILATING DROPS)	
Atropine sulfate	Atropisol, BufOpto Atropine, Isopto-Atropine
Cyclopentolate hydrochloride	Cyclogyl
Homatropine hydrobromide	Isopto Homatropine
Phenylephrine hydrochloride	Mydfrin, Neo-Synephrine
Scopolamine hydrobromide	Isopto Hyoscine
Tropicamide	Mydriacyl
ANTI-INFLAMMATORY AGENTS	
Dexamethasone	Maxidex Ophthalmic Suspension
Dexamethasone sodium phosphate	Decadron Phosphate
Fluorometholone	FML Liquifilm Ophthalmic
Prednisolone acetate	Econopred, Pred Forte, Pred Mild
Prednisolone sodium phosphate	AK-Pred, Inflamase Forte, Inflamase, Metreton
ANTI-INFECTIVES	
ANTIBACTERIALS	
Bacitracin	
Chloramphenicol	Chloromycetin, Chloroptic, Econochlor
Erythromycin	Ilotycin
Gentamicin sulfate	Garamycin
Polymyxin B sulfate	
Silver nitrate 1%	
Sulfacetamide sodium	Bleph-10, Cetamide, Sodium Sulamyd
Tetracycline hydrochloride	Achromycin
Tobramycin	Tobrex
ANTIVIRALS	
Idoxuridine	IDU
Trifluridine	Viroptic
Vidarabine	Vira-A
MISCELLANEOUS	
Fluorescein sodium	Diagnostic drops for corneal abnormalities
Timolol maleate	Timoptic (antiglaucoma medication)

testing is done in a darkened room with the infant held on an assistant's lap. EEG electrodes are placed on the infant's head, and a light flash stimulating lamp is directed toward the baby's eyes. Responses to light stimuli, called flash evoked responses, are then recorded. VEP testing can be used to estimate function and maturation of the primary cortex and the geniculo-cortical visual system. This may provide useful information in the management of infants with delayed visual maturation and other neurologic problems, including hydrocephalus and intraventricular hemorrhage (Kraemer et al, 1999).

Digital Image Analysis

Digital image analysis (DIA) is used in conjunction with optic fundal photographs to evaluate the morphology of the optic nerve. Because the retina develops from the brain, studying the eye can provide clues to central nervous system (CNS) problems. With DIA, a computer-assisted digital mapping system is used to analyze photographs of the fundus. This technology may provide information helpful to an understanding of the relationship between pathologic conditions of the CNS and retinal problems (Hellström, 1999).

A new digital camera, the RetCam 120 (Massie Research Laboratories, Inc., Dublin, CA), is gaining popularity in neonatal and pediatric units. The RetCam 120 is a portable digital camera designed for wide-field, real-time images of the retina. The camera has a hand-held unit that enables it to be used at the bedside. The camera can be operated by specially trained individuals rather than retinal specialty ophthalmologists. The technology has been used on infants with retinopathy of prematurity (ROP), shaken baby syndrome, and retinoblastoma. Although the RetCam 120 is 100% specific for retinopathy of prematurity, its sensitivity ranges from 46% to 76% (Yen et al, 2002), making it an unacceptable substitute for indirect ophthalmoscopy. In addition, the device causes distress to the neonate (Mehta et al, 2005).

NEONATAL CONJUNCTIVITIS

Any conjunctivitis that occurs in the first 28 days of life is classified as neonatal conjunctivitis, according to the World Health Organization (WHO). Neonatal conjunctivitis can be classified as aseptic or septic. Aseptic conjunctivitis is often a chemical reaction to prophylactic medication administered shortly after birth to prevent gonorrheal disease of the newborn's eyes. The Center for Disease Control's National Nosocomial Infections Surveillance (NNIS) program defines conjunctivitis as the isolation of culture positive pathogens from purulent discharge obtained from the conjunctiva or contiguous tissues such as eyelids or cornea, or redness and/or pain in the conjunctiva or eye and the presence of one of the following: purulent discharge, organisms and/or white blood cells present in the gram stain of the exudate, positive antigen test, positive viral culture, positive single antibody titer, or the presence of multinucleated giant cells visible under microscopy (Horan & Gaynes, 2004). This definition is used for infections in neonatal intensive care units; although, it has recently been shown to miss 38% of the cases of neonatal conjunctivitis in two large neonatal intensive care units (Haas et al, 2005).

Septic conjunctivitis in the newborn is an infection of the conjunctiva (the thin, translucent mucous membrane covering the cornea) caused by a variety of bacteria, viruses, and other organisms. The incidence of septic neonatal conjunctivitis in the United States is 1% to 2%. Chlamydial infection has replaced gonorrhea as the most common cause of septic eye infection. Septic neonatal conjunctivitis usually manifests with a discharge that develops shortly after birth. Because the origins of newborn conjunctivitis can vary, laboratory investigations are important in determining the exact cause. In some cases of conjunctivitis, rapid treatment is important to prevent vision loss.

The presentation of neonatal conjunctivitis varies with the cause of the inflammation or infection. Some findings, such as purulent eye discharge and erythema and edema of the eyelids and conjunctivae, are present in most cases. Transient tearing or watery discharge may be noticed early in the infection process.

Aseptic Neonatal Conjunctivitis

Most U.S. states require prophylaxis against neonatal gonorrheal conjunctivitis. According to the American Academy of Pediatrics (AAP), topical 1% silver nitrate solution, 0.5% erythromycin ointment, and 1% tetracycline ointment are equally effective (AAP, 2000). Although not available commercially as single-dose vials or tubes, 2.5% povidone-iodine solution is gaining recognition as another treatment option.

Although silver nitrate has largely been replaced by erythromycin as the drug of choice for neonatal ocular prophylaxis, the older drug is still used in some units. Silver nitrate drops typically cause an irritant reaction that leads to conjunctival edema, redness, and watery discharge. The reaction starts within a few hours of instillation of the drops, usually resolves within 48 hours, and is self-limiting. Labo-

ratory cultures and smears should be obtained to rule out an infectious cause for the conjunctivitis. Parents should be informed of the benign nature of the inflammation once the proper diagnosis has been made. The eyes should be cleansed frequently of any secretions to prevent skin irritation.

Silver nitrate is effective against *Neisseria gonorrhoeae* and most bacteria; however, it is not effective against *Chlamydia* organisms. For this reason, some states substitute tetracycline ointment or erythromycin ointment for routine prophylaxis. In areas with a high incidence of penicillinase-producing *N. gonorrhoeae*, silver nitrate is the drug of choice (Laga et al, 1989).

Erythromycin and tetracycline ointments are effective against a variety of microorganisms, including chlamydia. These ointments rarely cause irritation to the newborn's eyes. Because erythromycin is only about 80% effective, a second dose may be needed.

Chlamydial Conjunctivitis (Inclusion Conjunctivitis)

In recent years *Chlamydia trachomatis* has been recognized as the most common cause of conjunctivitis in the newborn. The bacteria are transmitted from the infected mother to the infant at birth, and conjunctivitis usually appears 4 to 14 days later. The condition may be mild or moderate, and with proper treatment it resolves within 6 weeks. Clinical symptoms include swelling of one or both eyelids and mucopurulent discharge. Chronic infection can lead to more serious consequences, such as conjunctival scarring, adhesions of the eyelid, and deposits of connective tissue under the cornea.

The diagnosis is made from laboratory tests. The conjunctiva is scraped with a spatula, and a smear is made for Giemsa staining; classically this reveals a dark-staining cytoplasmic inclusion body. Direct immunofluorescent antibody staining or enzyme immunoassay should be done to confirm the diagnosis.

Topical eye treatment should consist of application of sulfacetamide or tetracycline drops or ointment for 3 weeks. Although the eye infection generally is not serious, a chlamydial pneumonitis develops in 11% to 20% of infected neonates. Systemic therapy with oral erythromycin estolate or erythromycin ethylsuccinate for 3 weeks often is necessary to eradicate the organism from the respiratory tract.

Gonorrheal Conjunctivitis

Routine prophylaxis of neonates has greatly reduced the incidence of gonorrheal conjunctivitis. Because of the potential for blindness from this infection, early detection and prompt treatment are critical. Gonorrheal conjunctivitis typically manifests as an acute, purulent, bilateral conjunctivitis with eyelid edema. If not treated appropriately, the infection may progress rapidly to corneal ulceration and endophthalmitis. Gram stains and cultures should be performed routinely in all cases of neonatal conjunctivitis. The presence of *N. gonorrhoeae* confirms the diagnosis. Treatment consists of administration of intravenous or intramuscular antibiotics and application of topical ointment to the eye. Irrigation of the eye with sterile saline may be necessary to remove drainage.

Staphylococcal Conjunctivitis

Staphylococcal conjunctivitis is a bacterial infection usually acquired during vaginal delivery or by contact with an infected mother or nursery personnel. Symptoms normally appear

2 to 4 weeks after birth. In most cases the conjunctivitis is mild and produces a purulent discharge. It may progress to corneal ulceration, endophthalmitis, or generalized skin infection. The diagnosis is made with cultures and Gram stain. Because staphylococci can be found in the conjunctivae of healthy neonates, laboratory results should be interpreted cautiously. Treatment includes application of topical bacitracin or erythromycin ointment and cleansing of exudate from the eyelids.

Herpes Simplex Conjunctivitis

Herpes simplex infection at birth may be a feature of either localized or systemic disease. The neonate usually is infected during passage through the birth canal. The conjunctivitis manifests with eyelid swelling, conjunctival inflammation, corneal opacity, and epithelial dendrites. The dendrites can best be seen if the cornea is stained with a fluorescein dye and then examined under the blue light of a portable slitlamp. The onset of the conjunctivitis usually is 2 to 14 days after birth. The disseminated form of the disease may also lead to cataracts and optic neuritis.

Diagnosis through laboratory findings is based on conjunctival epithelia scrapings for Giemsa staining and tissue cultures. The Giemsa stain should reveal multinucleated giant cells and intranuclear inclusion. Fluorescent antibody techniques are also helpful for making the diagnosis. This disease should always be kept in mind when the mother or father has a history of genital herpes. Treatment should be instituted with application of the topical antiviral trifluridine. Systemic treatment may be helpful in disseminated cases.

Infectious Conjunctivitis Caused by Other Microorganisms

Case reports describing neonatal infectious conjunctivitis caused by unusual microorganisms are increasing in the professional literature. Although most of the case reports describe infections in hospitalized premature infants, two reports concerned full-term infants who were readmitted with conjunctivitis caused by *Neisseria meningitidis* (Dinakaran & Desai, 1999; Lehman, 1999). Both infants required local and systemic treatment and were discharged home. Because *N. meningitidis* can cause a serious infection resulting in significant morbidity and mortality, it is important to differentiate this organism from other gram-negative diplococci, such as *N. gonorrhoeae* (Lehman, 1999). Individuals exposed to *N. meningitidis* are considered high-risk contacts and should be treated with chemoprophylaxis (Lehman, 1999).

Two cases of serious eye infection in preterm infants caused by *Pseudomonas aeruginosa* have been reported (Shah et al, 1999; Wasserman et al, 1999). A 910-g boy born at 27 weeks' gestation developed meningitis and multiple brain abscesses subsequent to the conjunctivitis. This infant was discharged at 2 months of age with no apparent visual impairment. The other infant, a 736-g boy born at 24 weeks' gestation, was found to have *P. aeruginosa* sepsis. Several days later a purulent discharge from the eyes was noted. Examination of the eyes revealed bilateral endophthalmitis, perforated cornea, and possible total retinal detachment in one eye. A detailed eye examination was not possible because of the infant's unstable condition. The baby subsequently died of overwhelming sepsis, and no autopsy was performed (Wasserman et al, 1999).

Premature infants in the neonatal intensive care units (NICU) frequently are colonized with a variety of *Candida* species. Despite the increased incidence of *Candida* sepsis in premature infants, ocular involvement usually is limited to a retinochoroiditis that resolves with systemic antifungal therapy. Several reports have been published describing severe candidal eye disease that required surgical intervention (Shah et al, 2000; Johnston & Cogen, 2000). Two of the reports described the development of a cataract, one in an infant born at 29 weeks' gestation and the other in an infant born at 32 weeks' gestation. Both infants required a lensectomy and vitrectomy (Shah et al, 2000; Johnston & Cogen, 2000; Drohan et al, 2002). The third report concerned an infant born at 28 weeks' gestation who developed recurrent *Candida* lens abscess and endophthalmitis, which required lensectomy and vitrectomy for treatment (Drohan et al, 2002).

The conjunctiva can also be the portal of entry of nosocomial pathogens. A case report from Italy describes the horizontal transmission of *Candida parapsilosis*, a pathogen normally associated with indwelling catheters (e.g., percutaneously inserted central lines), from the nursing staff to a preterm infant (Lupetti et al, 2002). The preterm infant developed candidemia. Molecular typing determined the organism was transferred from the hands of two nurses to the infant's conjunctiva, and then to the bloodstream.

Adenovirus type 8 was the cause of two outbreaks of keratoconjunctivitis in neonatal intensive care units in Europe (Percivalle et al 2003; Chaberny et al, 2003). The virus was identified with polymerase chain reaction, and antibody technologies were used to document the presence of the virus in patients and nursery staff.

Lacrimal Dysfunction
Obstructed Nasolacrimal Duct

Blockage of the nasolacrimal duct occurs when the duct fails to canalize at the entrance to the nose. This blockage occurs in 2% of all newborns and is the most common cause of chronic conjunctivitis in infants. After 1 month of age, the infant shows excessive tearing and pooling in the medial canthal region and signs of infection. Pressure on the lacrimal sac area usually causes pus or mucus to exude from the puncta. Because the problem resolves spontaneously in 50% of affected neonates by 6 months of age, conservative treatment involving lacrimal massage and application of topical antibiotics is recommended. Obstruction that lasts beyond this point may require lacrimal probing. Nasolacrimal duct blockage must be differentiated from congenital glaucoma, a foreign body on the eye, or corneal injury or inflammation.

Mucocele

Mucoceles occur because of the one-way valve effect at the end of the nasolacrimal duct. Mucus accumulates or amniotic fluid is trapped in the nasolacrimal sac, and the infant develops a bluish mass in the inferomedial region of the eyelid. This swelling most often is confused with a hemangioma. If simple massage does not decompress the mucocele, probing of the nasolacrimal duct may be necessary.

RETINOPATHY OF PREMATURITY

Retinopathy of prematurity (ROP), a disease arising from proliferation of abnormal blood vessels in the newborn retina, was first reported by Terry in 1942. His description of a fibrous growth behind the lens and retinal detachment in premature infants gave birth to the name retrolental fibroplasia (RLF).

CLASSIFYING RETINOPATHY OF PREMATURITY

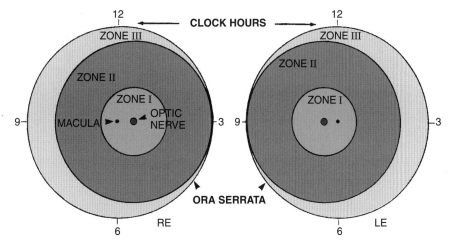

FIGURE **14-3**

International classification of retinopathy of prematurity. Zones and clock hours are used to describe the location and extent of ROP in the retinas of the right eye *(RE)* and the left eye *(LE)*. From Anonymous (1984). An international classification of retinopathy of prematurity. *Pediatrics* 74(1):127-133.

The name was changed to retinopathy of prematurity in 1984 by an international committee charged with providing a uniform classification system for the disease. The classification system uses a standard description of the location of retinopathy (using zones and clock hours), the severity of the disease (stage), the presence of special risk factors (plus disease), and the features of regression (International Committee on Retinopathy of Prematurity, 1984) (Figure 14-3). The International Committee for the Classification of ROP (2005) recently published several revisions to its original recommendations. The three changes introduced are (1) recognition of a more virulent form of ROP, aggressive posterior ROP, or AP-ROP; (2) an intermediate grade of plus disease (pre-plus) that occurs between normal posterior pole vessels and frank plus disease; and (3) a clinical tool for estimating the extent of zone I involvement.

AP-ROP is defined as a rapid, progressive form of ROP that quickly progresses to stage 5 disease if left untreated. Characteristics of AP-ROP include posterior location and prominence of plus disease, usually in zone I or posterior zone II. Because of the aggressive nature of this disease, the diagnosis of AP-ROP is normally made during a single examination. The definition of plus disease was modified from four quadrants to two quadrants. The new recommendations also call for using a plus (+) symbol after the stage number to designate the presence of plus disease (e.g., stage 3+).

ROP was responsible for an epidemic of blindness in young children in the 1940s and early 1950s until the link to supplemental oxygen therapy was made in 1952. Subsequently, the practice of limiting oxygen administration in the care of premature infants led to the near disappearance of the disorder. Improvements in neonatal health care in the past 30 years have increased the survival of preterm infants, yet ROP remains the leading cause of blindness in premature infants. With the advent of surfactant replacement therapy, there was initial elation that the incidence and severity of ROP was decreasing (Hussain et al, 1999); however, reports since then are conflicting. Recent data from Denmark suggest that progress toward eradicating ROP has halted (Fledelius & Kjer,

2004, Fledelius et al, 2004). These investigators have seen an increase in the incidence of ROP (from 10% to 31%) and in the number of cases needing ablation therapy.

This problem is further complicated by differences in study methodology, years studied, and the introduction of new definitions such as threshold and prethreshold ROP. Despite the differences, most authors are in agreement that ROP is a significant disease in very-low-birth-weight and gestational-age preterm infants. Detailed information on the incidence and severity of ROP is summarized in Table 14-2.

Pathophysiology

ROP is a disease caused by an abnormal adaptation of normal maturational processes in the face of physiologic stress. The disease develops gradually and is divided into six stages of increasing clinical severity (see Table 14-3). Definitions of terminology used in conjunction with the stages of ROP are provided in Box 14-1.

The key factor in the development of ROP, especially in premature infants, is the developing retinal blood vessels. The pathophysiology of ROP occurs in two phases. Phase I is delayed growth of the retinal vascularity following preterm birth. Phase II occurs when the hypoxia created during phase I stimulates the growth of new blood vessels (Smith, 2003). Retinal vascularization begins at the optic nerve at about 16 weeks' gestation. Retinal vascular development proceeds slowly and reaches the retinal periphery (ora serrata retinae) during the ninth month of gestation (Vander, 1994). The incompletely vascularized retina has a peripheral avascular zone that varies in size with the degree of immaturity of the retina (Smith, 2003). The in utero growth of retinal blood vessels is stimulated by the release of vascular endothelial growth factor (VEGF) and insulin-like growth factor-1 (IGF-1). VEGF is found at the front line of the growing retinal blood vessels, whereas IGF-1 is maintained at a constant level in the retinal microenvironment. VEGF is a cytokine regulated by the amount of oxygen (hypoxia). IGF-1 is a non–oxygen-regulated cytokine involved in the regulation of endothelial cell survival and proliferation (Smith, 2004).

TABLE 14-2	Summary of Recent Studies on Incidence and Severity of ROP				
First Author	**Location of Study**	**Years Included**	**Gestational Age of Subjects**	**Birth Weight of Subjects**	**Type of Study**	**Significant Findings**
Good	USA (Early Treatment for ROP Cooperative Group)	2000–2002		<1250 g	Prospective	Incidence of ROP 68% with more Zone I and prethreshold disease than in the CRYO-ROP study of 1986–1987. Incidence unchanged by race; however, more prethreshold disease seen in white infants
Markestad	Sweden	1999–2000	22 to 27 weeks	500 to 999 g	Prospective, observational	33% of 23-week preterms needed ROP treatment compared to 0% at >25 weeks
Chiang	New York State, USA	1996–2000	All newborns hospitalized for >28 days		Population-based cohort	ROP incidence by BW: <600 g, 32%; 600 to 799 g, 38%; 800 to 999 g, 30%; 1000 to 1199 g, 17%; 1200 to 1499 g, 8%; 1500 to 1999 g, 4%; 2000 to 2499 g, 2%
Hussain	Connecticut, USA	1989–1997	22 to 36 weeks	600 to 1832 g	Retrospective	21% all ROP; ≥Stage 3, 5%; None in >32 weeks
Gilbert	International ROP Group	1996–2002	25.3 to 33.5 weeks	410 to 2700 g	Observational	Mean GA/BW for severe ROP for: Highly developed countries: Canada, 25.6/759; USA, 25.4/763; UK, 25.3/737. Moderately developed countries: Argentina, 30.2/1263; Brazil, 27.7/952; Chile, 26.8/903; Colombia, 29.2/1122; Cuba, 30.7/1285; Ecuador, 33.5/1259; Peru, 29.1/1051. Poorly developed countries: India, 29.3/1243; Vietnam, 29.9/1284
Lee	Canada	1996–1997	All admissions to level 3 units		Population-based cohort	Incidence of ROP: <1500 g, 43%; ≥ Stage 3, 11%

Larsson	Sweden	1988–1990 and 1998–2000	<1500 g	Prospective comparison to 1988–1990 data in same geographic region	Total ROP stayed the same (36.4% 2000 vs 40% in 1990) Change in distribution noted: Incidence by GA: ≤26 weeks, 23% vs 14% 27 to 29 weeks, 42% vs 48% 30 to 32 weeks, 32% vs 30% ≥33 weeks, 4% vs 9% Incidence by BW: ≤750 g, 9% vs 5% 751 to 1000 g, 27% vs 24% >1000 g, 64% vs 72%
Hameed	UK	1990–1994 and 1995–1999	≤1250 g	Observational comparison in same geographic region	Survival, 76% (1995–1999) Survival, 62% (1990–1994) ≥Stage 3, 12% (1995–1999) ≥Stage 3, 4% (1990–1994)
O'Connor	Rhode Island, USA	1994–2000	<1250 g	Retrospective review	Incidence of ROP increased from 40% to 54% Incidence of threshold ROP increased from 2% to 5% Highest incidence and severity seen in BW <750 g
Fledelius	Denmark	1993–1997	<1750 g	Retrospective	Incidence of ROP, 10%

TABLE **14-3**	Stages of Retinopathy of Prematurity

I	Mildly abnormal blood vessel growth. Many children who develop stage I improve with no treatment and eventually develop normal vision. The disease resolves on its own without further progression.
II	Moderately abnormal blood vessel growth. Many children who develop stage II improve with no treatment and eventually develop normal vision. The disease resolves on its own without further progression.
III	Severely abnormal blood vessel growth. The abnormal blood vessels grow toward the center of the eye instead of following their normal growth pattern along the surface of the retina. Some infants who develop stage III improve with no treatment and eventually develop normal vision. However, when infants have a certain degree of Stage III and "plus disease" develops, treatment is considered. "Plus disease" means that the blood vessels of the retina have become enlarged and twisted, indicating a worsening of the disease. Treatment at this point has a good chance of preventing retinal detachment.
IV	Partially detached retina. Traction from the scar produced by bleeding, abnormal vessels pulls the retina away from the wall of the eye.
V	Completely detached retina and the end stage of the disease. If the eye is left alone at this stage, the baby can have severe visual impairment and even blindness.

From National Eye Institute (2006): Retinopathy of prematurity (ROP) resource guide. Bethesda, Maryland: National Eye Institute. Available at: http://www.nei.nih.gov/health/rop/index.asp#5. Accessed September 13, 2006.

BOX **14-1**

Terminology Used in Describing ROP

Term	Definition
Plus disease	≥2 quadrants of vessel tortuosity and fullness at the optic nerve
Popcorn	Scarring resulting from isolated tufts of regressed neovascularization
Hot dog	"Red hot" active ridge of abnormal vessel growth that is increasing in size; may become the site of retinal detachment
Prethreshold disease	Zone 1: Any number of clock hours of stage 1 or 2 without plus disease
	Zone 2: Any number of clock hours of stage 3 without plus disease, any number of clock hours of stage 2 with plus disease, and plus disease with <5 contiguous and <8 composite clock hours of stage 3 disease
Threshold disease	Zone 1: Any stage 1 plus or 2 plus or any stage 3, with or without plus disease
	Zone 2: Presence of ≥5 contiguous or ≥8 composite clock hours of stage 3 with plus disease

The STOP-ROP Multicenter Study Group (2000). Supplemental therapeutic oxygen for prethreshold retinopathy of prematurity (STOP-ROP), a randomized, controlled trial. I: primary outcomes. *Pediatrics* 105:295-310.

Following preterm birth, the normal growth of the retina vascularity stops and some of the already developed vessels are lost. The retina, however, remains metabolically active and becomes hypoxic because of the lack of blood vessels. This hypoxia becomes a potent inducer of new vessel growth (neovascularization) by stimulating the expression of VEGF at 32 to 34 weeks' postmenstrual age. As the new blood vessels proliferate, they tend to grow into the vitreous and can cause bleeding and the formation of fibrous tissue (Smith, 2003).

Many preterm infants in the NICU receive supplemental oxygen to treat their respiratory distress. The hyperoxia caused by oxygen use suppresses VEGF and IGF-1 resulting in programmed cell death, or apoptosis, of vascular endothelial cells, which in turn causes hyperoxia-induced vaso-obliteration and scarring of the retinal vessels (Smith, 2004).

As the preterm infant matures, the growing retina triggers a release of VEGF, and IGF-1 levels also rise. This creates an environment for new vessel growth (neovascular proliferation) that leads to progression of the retinopathy (Smith, 2003). Mild degrees of ROP are often transient and regress once the abnormal stimuli are removed or corrected. Moderate retinopathy can lead to excessive fibrous tissue formation or scarring in the peripheral retina, which may lead to traction on the macula and reduced vision. In severe cases of ROP, fibrous tissue development may lead to retinal detachment and blindness. Severely affected neonates may also have leukocoria, glaucoma, or both.

Risk Factors

ROP is a multifactorial disease that occurs primarily in premature infants. Although many risk factors have been identified, prematurity and low birth weight remain the most important factors leading to the development of ROP (Markestad et al, 2005; Allegaert et al, 2004b; Chiang et al, 2004). Other risk factors include use of supplemental oxygen, intraventricular hemorrhage, sepsis, multiple births, acidosis, and blood transfusions. Risk factors identified in the postsurfactant era from the management of extremely preterm infants (23 to 25 weeks' gestation) include birth weight less than 1000 g, glucocorticoid steroid use, maternal preeclampsia, ventilator days, continuous positive pressure ventilation, intrauterine growth restriction (IUGR), male gender, fluctuating oxygen saturations and/or PaO_2, and renal insufficiency defined as creatinine greater than 1.5 mg/dl (York, 2004; Anderson, 2004; Allegaert et al, 2004a; Darlow et al, 2005; Todd et al, 1994). A relationship between glucocorticoid steroid use and ROP is questioned by other investigators (Wright & Wright, 1994). Although dopamine use has been suggested by Liu et al (2005) and Mizoguchi et al (1999), others dispute this, stating that dopamine use is reflective of cardiovascular instability in the critically ill preterm infant, rather than being an independent risk factor for ROP (Allegaert et al, 2004a). Factors associated with the development of threshold ROP include maternal preeclampsia, occurrence of pulmonary hemorrhage, continuous positive airway pressure (CPAP), and duration of mechanical ventilation (Shah et al, 2005).

Unusual risk factors have also been reported. These most likely represent factors specific to the individual reporting unit. Lang et al (2005) found an increase in threshold ROP in native Alaskan males, despite similar or better prenatal and NICU variables when compared to non-native Alaskan infants in a

Washington State unit. British investigators describe a case of severe ROP in a 26-week gestation, IUGR preterm infant with a birth weight of 525 g who was undergoing treatment with sildenafil acetate (Viagra, Pfizer, Inc., New York, NY) (Marsh et al, 2004). At 5 weeks of age, the infant's condition worsened secondary to sepsis from coagulase-negative *Staphylococcus* and *Candida* and he was started on nitric oxide. After 3 days with no improvement in oxygenation, the infant was started on sildenafil and began improving. The infant was noted to have no ROP at examinations performed during 31 to 33 weeks of postmenstrual age (PMA). During the examination at 34 weeks PMA, "bilateral iris neovascularization, hazy media, and dilated and tortuous fundal vessels," 7 clock hours of stage 3 ROP zone II on the right, and 5 clock hours on the left were noted. The authors also mentioned that they have seen an increase in treatable ROP that coincides with the use of sildenafil in their unit. They concluded that this case "may link its use (sildenafil) to the development of aggressive ROP" (Marsh et al, 2004).

Fluctuating and higher oxygen levels in preterm infant blood have also been implicated as a risk factor for ROP (Askie, 2004; York et al, 2004; Anderson et al, 2004; Saugstad, 2005). Fluctuating PaO_2 in preterm infants weighing less than 1500 g increased the risk for threshold ROP in York et al's study (2004). In a national survey of the relationship between pulse oximeter practices in the first 2 weeks of life and ROP, the authors found that 58% of the surveyed units maintained different criteria for acceptable saturation ranges in the first 2 weeks of life as compared to the acceptable ranges for preterm infants greater than 2 weeks of age (Anderson et al, 2004). Although the average rate of stage 3 or higher ROP was not significantly different in the centers with higher saturation ranges compared to those with lower saturation ranges, the rate of retinal ablation surgery was significantly higher in centers that maintain maximum saturations above 98% in the first 2 weeks of life. They also noted that rates of surgery and greater than stage 3 ROP were higher in units that maintained maximum saturations above 92% after the first 2 weeks of life. This study suggests that preterm infants should be kept in oxygen saturations less than or equal to 92%.

For some variables linked to the development of ROP, the evidence is less conclusive, and no direct link to the treatment or management of medically unstable premature infants has been established. Often these factors are interlinked; they include antioxidant deficiencies; administration of beta-adrenergic blockers late in pregnancy for preterm labor; maternal bleeding; apnea of prematurity; use of xanthines, such as caffeine and theophylline; abnormal blood gas findings; the number of days on mechanical ventilation; early intubation; ambient lighting; hypotension; NEC; and patent ductus arteriosus treated with indomethacin (Arroe & Peitersen, 1994).

Other factors such as breast milk feedings and the use of nitric oxide in the treatment of respiratory distress in preterm infants may provide some protection against the development of ROP. Hylander et al (2001) found that preterm infants weighing less than 1500 g at birth who received human milk feedings had a lower incidence of ROP when compared to preterm infants who were formula fed. The positive benefit of human milk feeding remained after adjusting for confounding variables such as birth weight, race, and duration of oxygen therapy. Mestan et al (2005) reported that treatment with nitric oxide improved the neurodevelopmental outcomes of preterm infants at 2 years of age. The incidence of severe ROP was 24% in the nitric oxide group and 46% in the placebo group of preterm infants.

Although most ROP occurs in premature infants, rare cases of the disease have been reported in full-term infants, stillborn infants, and infants who were not given supplemental oxygen. In a large cohort study of all newborns hospitalized in New York State, 17 infants with birth weights greater than 2000 g had a discharge diagnosis of ROP (Chiang et al, 2004). None of the infants required treatment for their ROP. A recent case report describes severe retinopathy with bilateral retinal detachment almost identical to ROP in a full-term infant with hypoplastic left heart syndrome (Ahmad & Hirose, 2004). This infant had "areas of avascular retina, significant retinal neovascularization, fibrous proliferation, and tractional detachment" (Ahmad & Hirose, 2004). The authors concluded that cyanotic heart disease "can cause a retinopathy with chronic retinal vascularization and retinal detachments" (Ahmad & Hirose, 2004). These reports, along with the striking similarity of disease presentation from infant to infant, have led some to conclude that ROP may have a genetic component. Further research is needed to increase our understanding of the cause and the pathophysiology of this disease.

Treatment

Treatment of ROP can be divided into three categories: preventive, interdictive, and corrective. Until premature birth can be abolished, the major focus of ROP treatment is early detection and appropriate follow-up of significant disease. Javitt and colleagues (1993) estimated that properly timed screening and treatment for ROP is not only cost saving but also may save approximately 320 infants per year from a lifetime of blindness. Despite the international effort to standardize ROP and the efforts of the several multicenter, randomized clinical trials, no universally accepted guidelines exist for the screening of premature infants. Screening protocols vary from institution to institution, among different countries, and even with the level of development of the countries. Several widely used, published guidelines are summarized in Table 14-4.

Preventive Treatment

Other preventive strategies in use or under consideration are antioxidant therapy, oxygen monitoring, and modification of environmental light. High doses of the antioxidant vitamin E gained popularity in the 1980s as a prophylactic therapy for ROP; however, clinical studies failed to document a protective effect. Significant side effects, such as sepsis, NEC, intraventricular hemorrhage, and death, were noted, prompting most nurseries to avoid the use of high-dose vitamin E (Pierce & Mukai, 1994). Preliminary evidence suggests that penicillamine, an antioxidant used in the treatment of hyperbilirubinemia in Hungary, may lower the incidence of ROP; however, the substance has not been tested for this purpose outside of Hungary. Inositol, an antioxidant found in breast milk and other dietary sources, is also under investigation. Preliminary data reveal an unexpected reduction in the incidence of ROP in treated infants (Phelps, 1992). Other investigators are exploring whether bilirubin is protective against ROP. Multicenter, randomized, controlled studies are needed to determine the true value of these antioxidants.

TABLE 14-4	Guidelines for Retinopathy of Prematurity Screening Examinations	
Recommending Group	**Infant Criteria**	**First Examination Due**
American Academy of Pediatrics, American Academy Ophthalmology, American Association of Pediatric Ophthalmology & Strabismus	Birth weight <1500 g *or* gestational age <28 weeks; selected infants between 1500 and 2000 g with an unstable clinical course who are believed to be at high risk	4 to 6 weeks of chronological age *or* within 31 to 33 weeks' postmenstrual age, whichever is later
Canadian Pediatric Society, Canadian Association of Pediatric Ophthalmologists	Birth weight ≤1500 g *or* gestational age ≤30 weeks	4 to 6 weeks' postmenstrual age
British College of Ophthalmologists	Birth weight ≤1500 g ***and/or*** gestational age ≤31 weeks	6 to 7 weeks' postmenstrual age

Oxygen monitoring has been the major emphasis in the prevention of ROP. Elaborate policies and practices for continuous monitoring of oxygenation have evolved over the years, including invasive methods (fiberoptic umbilical catheters) and noninvasive techniques (transcutaneous oxygen monitoring, pulse oximetry). Despite these efforts, few data indicate a safe level of oxygenation in infants at risk for ROP. Early efforts at restricting oxygen delivery in the 1950s and 1960s traded visual problems for neurologic sequelae. The current practice of minimizing oxygen exposure while preserving optimum functioning of vital organs must continue until research determines the appropriate strategies. As previously discussed in risk factors, fluctuating oxygen level can increase the risk for ROP.

Environmental lighting in nurseries has been implicated as a contributing factor in the development of ROP. Although the clinical studies that claim to show this relationship have many limitations, some authorities believe the data are sufficient to warrant concern. It was hoped that multicenter clinical trials would shed some light on the subject (Seiberth et al, 1994); however, no data are available to answer the question. Many nurseries instituted reduced environmental lighting and shielding of incubators as part of a developmental approach to care.

Interdictive Treatment

The second strategy for treating ROP focuses on therapies aimed at minimizing or preventing blindness once the disease has developed. Interdictive therapies include cryotherapy and laser photocoagulation.

Cryotherapy was developed in the 1970s in Japan. It gained popularity in the United States in the 1980s after the release of data from the Cryotherapy for Retinopathy of Prematurity Study. The study was terminated early, when preliminary analysis revealed a significant benefit in eyes treated with cryotherapy (Phelps, 1992). The improvements noted in study subjects persisted in follow-up studies (Cryotherapy for Retinopathy of Prematurity Cooperative Group, 1988; Good et al, 2005).

Cryotherapy is a surgical procedure involving insertion of a probe cooled with liquid nitrogen on the medial aspect of the eye. Confluent spots on the avascular retina are ablated (destroyed by freezing), reducing the release of an angiogenic factor that appears to induce retinal vasoproliferation. Although the exact way in which cryotherapy works remains unknown, substantial evidence indicates that the therapy

works and improves the outcome of ROP (Cryotherapy for Retinopathy of Prematurity Cooperative Group, 1988; Trese, 1994; Coats, 2005; Palmer et al, 2005).

Despite its proven benefits, cryotherapy is not a benign procedure. Ocular and other complications can occur. Ocular complications include edema of one or both eyelids, laceration of the conjunctiva, intraocular hemorrhage, and late retinal detachment (Vander, 1994). Other complications reported include apnea, bradycardia, arrhythmias, increased oxygen requirement, seizures, and in rare cases, cardiorespiratory arrest.

Neonatal nurses and other health care professionals should work closely with the ophthalmologist performing the cryotherapy. Infants undergoing the procedure must have their pupils dilated because of the need for indirect ophthalmoscopy. Although the procedure usually is performed using local anesthesia, it can severely stress the infant. The oculocardiac reflex, a vagal nerve-mediated reflex, may be set off during the procedure, causing bradycardia. Triggering of this reflex can be prevented by preoperative administration of atropine. It is imperative that the infant's cardiorespiratory status be closely monitored throughout the procedure and the immediate postoperative period. It is also recommended to have analgesia during and after the procedure. Premature infants, especially those with bronchopulmonary dysplasia, often have increased oxygen requirements and apnea episodes after cryotherapy. Nasal stuffiness, another common side effect of cryotherapy, may be partly responsible for the increase in apnea or oxygen requirements or both (Phelps, 1992).

Laser photocoagulation, the newest technique, has virtually replaced cryotherapy as the treatment of choice for ROP. Argon and infrared diode lasers have been used successfully to ablate the avascular retina in a manner similar to that used in cryotherapy. Advantages of laser photocoagulation therapy include technical ease of performance; usefulness in posterior ROP that is difficult to treat with cryotherapy; less stress to the infant; fewer side effects; and fewer delayed consequences of myopia and retinal detachment. Using cost-utility analysis, health care economists have also determined that laser ablation surgery for threshold ROP is cost effective (Brown et al, 2004; Brown & Brown, 2005). Laser ablation therapy can result in angle-closure glaucoma in infants with severe ROP (Trigler et al, 2005).

Recent evidence suggests that earlier treatment of ROP is more important than the type of treatment. The Early Treatment for ROP randomized, clinical trial found that unfavorable outcomes at 9 months' follow-up were significantly reduced the early treatment eyes (Early Treatment for ROP Cooperative Group, 2003). Both cryotherapy and laser photocoagulation therapy were used in the clinical trial, and the study group recommended retinal ablation therapy "for any eye with Type I ROP" and serial examinations for those with Type 2 ROP. Other researchers noted that retinal detachment developed in 14% of eyes treated with ablation therapy (Coats, 2005). In another study comparing early versus conventional treatment of prethreshold disease, no significant differences were noted in the prevalence of myopia or high myopia (Davitt et al, 2005). Thus, it appears that early treatment of ROP may be beneficial to the infant and is not associated with increased risks of adverse outcomes such as myopia.

Corrective Treatment

The focus of corrective treatment is surgery for the repair of detached retinas. Scleral buckling, vitrectomy, or both, with or without lensectomy, are the techniques most often used. Scleral buckling involves the placement of a silicone or plastic band around the globe of the eye. The band is constricted, which brings the sclera closer to the retina, facilitating retinal reattachment. This procedure often is performed in conjunction with cryotherapy or laser therapy to salvage any remaining vision (Gupta et al, 2002).

When retinal detachment progresses beyond the point of scleral buckling, the ophthalmologist must consider anatomic reattachment of the retina. Vitrectomy involves surgically opening the eye, removing the lens, and gently excising the proliferative scar tissue; this allows the retina to lie against the pigmented epithelium and reattach (Trese, 1994).

Despite the skill required for these procedures, most infants who undergo corrective therapy do not have significant improvement in their vision. According to a recent systematic review of the literature on scleral buckling and vitrectomy, retinal reattachment rates varied from 0.8% to 90% (Ertzbischoff, 2004). The best surgical reattachments rates (>50%) occurred when the surgery was performed on infants between 2 and 9 months of age. In addition, the level of visual function did not correlate with the degree of retinal reattachment. Poor visual outcomes occurred regardless of the timeliness or delay in surgical reattachment (Ertzbischoff, 2004).

Outcomes

Outcome studies suggest that the incidence of long-term problems has been underestimated. Although studies on the natural history of ROP in the postsurfactant era consistently support an increased rate of mild ROP which usually regresses, the consequences of severe ROP, especially stage 3 or greater disease, remain less than desirable. At 18 months of age, 34.5% of preterm infants with threshold ROP had complications consisting of strabismus, nystagmus, myopia, and late retinal detachment (O'Connor et al, 2003). Fifteen percent of the infants were legally blind. In a 15-year outcome study of premature infants with threshold disease enrolled in the multicenter trial of cryotherapy for ROP (CRYO-ROP), 30% to 45% of treated eyes had unfavorable outcomes, and blindness occurred in 36% of treated eyes (Palmer et al, 2005). Despite the high rate of poor outcomes in treated eyes, the rate was significantly lower than that observed in control eyes. Of concern was the finding that new retinal detachments were noted at the 10-year examination. On a positive note, the authors also reported that 30 eyes had 20/20 or better vision at the 15-year examination (Palmer et al, 2005). Jandeck et al (2004) describe using pars plana vitrectomy in a group of preterm infants who developed late-onset retinal detachment from vitreoretinal changes caused by ROP. Retinal reattachment was achieved in 90% at follow-up ranging from 7 months to 7 years of age. Tufail et al (2004) reported on the clinical findings, management, and outcomes in a group of older children and adults with regressed ROP that progressed into rhegmatogenous retinal detachment (RRD). RRD occurs when vitreous humor enters the potential space beneath the retina through a break in the retina. The influx of fluids causes the retina to separate from the underlying retinal pigment epithelium. The mean age at presentation of RRD was 22 years and 90% of the eyes were myopic. The neonatal histories included prematurity (mean gestational age 29 weeks), low birth weight (mean birth weight 1110 g), and a mean length of stay in the NICU of 12 days. Three individuals developed intraventricular hemorrhage and two had necrotizing enterocolitis. This group of former preterm infants also had a variety of nonretinal problems including cataracts, strabismus, nystagmus, esotropia, amblyopia, lattice peripheral retinal degeneration, and peripheral retinal pigmentary changes. The authors noted that "RRD can also occur in eyes with previously treated ROP and the late vitreoretinal sequelae of treated acute ROP may come to replace spontaneously regressed ROP as a vitreoretinal surgical challenge in the future" (Tufail et al, 2004).

Prematurity without ROP is also associated with poor visual outcomes. According to Cooke et al (2004), preterm infants are three times more likely to wear glasses, three to four times more likely to have poor visual acuity or stereopsis (3D vision or depth perception), and 10 times more likely to have strabismus. None of the subjects in this study required treatment for ROP and only 7% had stage 3 ROP. Poor school performance in this population of preterm infants was also attributed to the visual impairments. Because none of the infants with poor visual outcomes had intraventricular hemorrhages or periventricular leukomalacia, poor school performance could not be explained by neurologic problems. Larssen et al (2005) showed that preterm infants have decreased distance and near vision acuities when compared to full-term infants. Despite reports that prematurity may interfere with color vision, a prospective case controlled study of preterm infants born before 33 weeks compared to full-term controls showed that both groups had similar chromatic contrast thresholds (measurement of red-green color differences) and achromatic contrast sensitivity (measurement of ability to detect shades of gray and other neutral colors) (Jackson et al, 2003).

Collaborative Care

Health professionals have to be concerned about care of the individual infant with ROP and the families of those infants. Oftentimes, the nursery nurse may be caring for a convalescing infant who is transported back to a community hospital, or an infant who is discharged prior to the first ROP screening examination. Attar et al (2005) found that infants back transported to a community hospital often missed their follow-up eye examinations when compared to those discharged directly from the regional perinatal-neonatal unit. The same authors also found that infants discharged prior to the first ROP exam were more likely to miss follow-up eye care than those infants who had their first examination while in the NICU.

The development of ROP is concerning to parents of premature infants. Open communication between the neonatal health care team and the parents is crucial for helping the parents successfully cope with the stress of a hospitalized premature infant. It is important to determine the amount of information a parent can handle. At first, general information about the relationship of ROP and prematurity can be shared with the parents. After the first eye examination has been performed, the information can be specific to their baby. The neonatal health care team must work closely with the ophthalmologist to provide a consistent message to the family. Information shared should take into account known cultural differences, such as that the occurrence of severe ROP is higher in white infants than in those of other racial groups (Gupta et al, 2002). Parent teaching should focus on providing a basic understanding of ROP, the purpose of the screening examinations, and the importance of regular vision testing for their infant after discharge. Explanations of eye examination results may need reinforcing as parents try to assimilate an overwhelming amount of information. Misconceptions about the disease and the use of oxygen need to be corrected.

Once ROP is diagnosed in an infant, parents may need more support than usual. Some parents may exhibit denial because they cannot see any physical evidence of a problem. Families of infants who need surgical intervention may feel greater stress from their concern for their infant's vision and the added communication with an ophthalmologist or retinal surgeon. Nursery staff members can help parents cope by providing support during decision-making sessions with the eye specialists, by asking questions to clarify information, and by reinforcing information provided. It is also important to determine if parents are obtaining information from outside sources such as the World Wide Web. An analysis of 114 Internet sites on ROP found that 62.5% of the sites evaluated contained fair to poor information (Martins & Morse, 2005). Of the websites analyzed, 25% were academic, 20% were organizational, and 55% were commercial.

Information given to the parents about the prognosis of ROP in their infant must be included in any discharge planning. Parents need to understand that eye problems are more common in premature infants and may develop in infants with regressed ROP. Myopia (nearsightedness), strabismus (crossed eye), astigmatism, and amblyopia (lazy eye) are common sequelae. Glaucoma and late retinal detachment are common sequelae in infants with severe ROP.

Clearly, early detection and referral to programs for visual impairment are essential. Parents need to understand the importance of regular eye examinations by a pediatric ophthalmologist or by an ophthalmologist knowledgeable about ROP and its complications. Many families may benefit from referral to community resources, support groups, and special programs for children with visual problems.

Last, the nursing staff and unit managers have to maintain vigilance about infection control practices during eye examinations or ablation treatment conducted in the NICU. Major risk factors for nosocomial infection are unwashed or poorly washed hands and the sterility of instruments such as eyelid speculums. In a recent survey of NICU nurse managers representing 290 units, 72% reported that they provide the instruments for eye examinations and 17% reported instruments are provided by the ophthalmologist (Hered, 2004). Nineteen percent of units reported that they reuse instruments. Eye infections due to ROP screening exams were acknowledged by 9% of the units. This study provides evidence that there is no consistency in practice regarding the sterility of ophthalmic instrumentation. Standards for best practice in this arena need to be developed to minimize the risk of nosocomial infections in this group of high-risk preterm infants.

CONGENITAL DEFECTS

Aniridia

Aniridia is a severe ocular abnormality that manifests as a bilateral absence of the iris. Cataracts, corneal pannus, macular dysfunction, and glaucoma usually accompany the defect. Most of these infants have significantly diminished visual acuity, to a level of 20/200 or worse. About 20% to 30% of children with the noninherited form of aniridia eventually develop Wilms' tumor of the kidney.

Persistent Hyperplastic Primary Vitreous

Persistent hyperplastic primary vitreous is a unilateral disorder that affects both genders equally. It results from persistence of the hyoid vessels that connect the optic nerve and the posterior surface of the lens. It should be considered in the differential diagnosis of leukocoria. The involved eye invariably is small, and a mature cataract often is present. Surgery may improve the integrity of the eye, but useful vision usually is not restored.

Capillary Hemangioma of the Eyelid

Capillary hemangioma of the eyelid, a blood vessel tumor, usually appears before 6 months of age. It tends to enlarge, stabilize, and then regress by the time the child is 5 years old. The tumor usually is elevated and reddish purple. Capillary hemangiomas often are referred to as strawberry nevi because of their appearance.

Superficial tumors of the eyelid cause cosmetic and visual problems. Pressure on the globe from the tumor may result in significant astigmatism and subsequently amblyopia. If the tumor is large, it may cover the pupil and prevent normal visual development. Deep tumors in the orbit may manifest with proptosis. These tumors may be treated with surgical removal, radiation, or steroid injection. Tumors that are exclusively cosmetic should be allowed to regress without intervention.

Ptosis

Ptosis is a drooping of one or both eyelids as a result of neurologic, muscular, or mechanical factors. If the ptosis is significant enough to cover the pupil, a dense amblyopia may result. If bilateral ptosis is present, the infant may have slowed motor development and delayed ambulation later in life. These problems are caused by the awkward, chin-up position the child must maintain in order to see. Mild ptosis that causes a problem with appearance generally is not repaired until the child is 4 or 5 years old because the results usually are better at this age.

A thorough family history should be obtained. Several familial syndromes are associated with ptosis, including blepharophimosis syndrome and double-elevator palsy.

Significant birth trauma may result in damage to the cervical ganglion and in an infantile Horner's syndrome, in which the infant has different-colored pupils, miosis, anhidrosis (lack of sweating), and mild ptosis. Direct trauma to the eyelid or a tumor in the eyelid may also cause ptosis. Surgical repair corrects this defect easily.

Congenital Glaucoma

Congenital glaucoma occurs in approximately 1 in 25,000 births. Glaucoma is a disease in which the intraocular pressure is elevated to a level sufficient to damage the optic nerve. Because of the blinding potential of this disease, it must be detected early in the infant's life and treated properly. The affected neonate shows tearing, light sensitivity, eyelid spasm, and a large, cloudy cornea. The disease is slightly more common in males than in females. The diagnosis often is missed until the child is about 2 to 3 months of age. Conditions associated with glaucoma include trisomy 21, congenital rubella, Marfan syndrome, neurofibromatosis, oculodentodigital syndrome, Rieger's syndrome, Sturge-Weber syndrome, Rubinstein-Taybi syndrome, and Weill-Marchesani syndrome (Gupta et al, 2002).

It is critical that congenital glaucoma be differentiated from other diseases that have similar symptoms. Nasolacrimal duct obstruction involves tearing but does not cause light sensitivity or a cloudy cornea. Difficult labor or forceps injury may damage the cornea and cause temporary clouding, but the intraocular pressure is not elevated, a hallmark feature of glaucoma. The large eyes of the infant with congenital glaucoma may appear beautiful to the parents, but health professionals should be alert to the possibility of this disease.

The abnormality in congenital glaucoma is a deformity of the filtering system that controls the level of intraocular pressure in the eye. Congenital glaucoma is treated surgically. The results usually are good, but parents must be educated about the need for continued monitoring of this condition throughout the child's life.

Congenital Cataracts

The causes of significant lens opacity in the newborn are numerous. Cataracts are an important cause of blindness because they may interfere with the process of visual development early in the infant's life. For this reason, visually significant cataracts must be detected and treated before they cause amblyopia, which may be unresponsive to the most persistent treatment.

Heredity is an important cause of congenital cataracts. A thorough family history is critical in determining the cause of the lens opacity. The inheritance pattern may be autosomal dominant, autosomal recessive, or sex linked. A maternal history of diabetes, x-ray exposure, or malnutrition may be an important factor in cataract formation. In premature infants, transient cataracts or insignificant opacities are commonly seen as a result of remnants of developmental tissues. ROP can also lead to cataracts in premature infants. Several inborn errors of metabolism cause cataracts, including galactosemia, Alport's syndrome, Fabry's disease, and Lowe syndrome. Intrauterine rubella infection is also associated with cataracts in the neonate.

Cataract surgery early in life is critical to the infant's visual rehabilitation. Useful vision is especially difficult to achieve in eyes with monocular cataracts. It is important for nurses to work closely with the infant's parents. The parents' persistence in handling contact lenses and in amblyopia therapy often determines the outcome for their child's vision.

Retinoblastoma

Retinoblastoma is the most common intraocular neoplasm in childhood. The tumor occurs in approximately 1 in 20,000 live births. Most cases appear sporadically and occur in infants with no family history of the disease. An autosomal dominant pattern usually is responsible for the 5% to 10% of inherited retinoblastomas, most of which are bilateral. Autosomal dominant transmission occurs with an estimated 85% penetrance (Brantley & Harbour, 2001). A somatic mutation accounts for 80% of unilateral tumors.

The most common presenting symptom is leukocoria. Most of the tumors are not detected in the neonatal period, except in infants with a positive family history. The tumor is highly malignant and may spread to the bone marrow, CNS, or other organs. Untreated patients rarely survive. The standard treatment for advanced cases of retinoblastoma is enucleation. Less severe cases are treated with radiation, laser photocoagulation, or cryotherapy. Children with this tumor require close follow-up for possible recurrence after treatment. Parents must be educated about the disease so that they are aware of the need for constant monitoring of their child.

CONGENITAL INFECTIONS
Cytomegalovirus Infection

Congenital cytomegalovirus (CMV) infection occurs in most infants with symptomatic disease and infrequently in asymptomatic infants. Ocular lesions include chorioretinitis, optic nerve atrophy, strabismus, cataract, macular scarring, and visual impairment. In a recent report from the Congenital CMV Longitudinal Study Group, 22% of the infants with symptomatic CMV disease had moderate to severe vision impairment, compared with 1% of the asymptomatic infants with CMV disease (Coats et al, 2000). The two common causes of severe visual impairment were optic atrophy and cortical visual impairment. Strabismus was also present in many of the symptomatic infants (Coats et al, 2000). Because of the risk for later development of strabismus and amblyopia, the authors recommend lifelong eye examinations for symptomatic infants (Coats et al, 2000).

Like many of the herpes family viruses, CMV can become active after periods of dormancy. Parents should be advised of this so that they can seek appropriate eye care if their child develops vision problems later in life.

Rubella

Congenital rubella is responsible for a wide variety of ocular complications, including pigmentary retinopathy, glaucoma, cataract, and microphthalmos. Although the clinical presentations range across a wide spectrum, newborns classically have hearing, eye, and cardiac defects.

Currently the incidence of congenital rubella syndrome is low; however, new information from long-term follow-up studies suggests that the prevalence of ocular problems is nearly twice the previously thought rate (78% instead of 43%). Several trends have also been noted, including an increase in cases of delayed disease and new associations of combination problems. Microphthalmia, cataracts, and glaucoma are more likely to occur in combination than independently. Pigmentary retinopathy produces a characteristic salt-and-pepper appearance and can result in sudden vision loss during adulthood. Poor visual acuity and diabetic retinopathy are also of concern in individuals with congenital rubella syndrome. The parents of an infant with congenital rubella need to understand that vision problems may occur at any time and that they must have their child screened regularly.

Herpes Simplex Virus

Herpes simplex virus causes a wide variety of eye disorders in newborns. Corey and Flynn (2000) recently reported a case of congenital herpes simplex infection that resulted in bilateral persistent fetal vasculature of the eye. Persistent fetal vasculature occurs when intraocular vessels fail to involute in utero. This involution is a normal part of eye development.

Varicella

Although rare, congenital infection caused by varicella, commonly known as chickenpox, produces eye anomalies in more than 50% of affected infants. These defects include microphthalmia, chorioretinitis, enophthalmia, cataract, optic nerve atrophy, nystagmus, and anisocoria (Choong et al, 2000).

Toxoplasmosis

Toxoplasma gondii is a parasitic organism with an affinity for brain and eye tissue. As with many other congenital infections, ocular anomalies vary depending on fetal age at the time of infection. The most common clinical presentation is a focal necrotizing retinochoroiditis. Other ocular manifestations include microphthalmia, traction retinal detachment, nystagmus, strabismus, cataracts, disruption of the retinal pigment epithelium, retinal dysplasia, and vitreitis (Berk et al, 2000; Roberts et al, 2001). A recent study of congenital toxoplasmosis suggests that the inflammatory response mounted by the fetus and newborn contributes to irreversible retinal damage (Roberts et al, 2001).

Lymphocytic Choriomeningitis Virus

A new congenital viral infection, lymphocytic choriomeningitis virus (LCV), must be added to the list of viruses that cause ocular defects (Barton et al, 2002). Congenital LCV infection was first reported in the United States in 1993. LCV is a single-strand RNA virus found in rodents, including house mice and hamsters. Outbreaks of LCV infection associated with mice tend to occur in trailer parks, inner-city dwellings, and substandard housing. Laboratory mice and hamsters can also cause outbreaks among laboratory personnel. The virus probably is transmitted by airborne droplets and by food contaminated by rodent urine or feces. It also may be transmitted by the bite of an infected animal (Barton et al, 2002; Mets et al, 2000).

Neonates with congenital infection usually have microcephaly, hydrocephaly, and chorioretinitis. In a recent report, a 3-day-old boy who had microcephaly at birth was found to have chorioretinitis, conjunctivitis, congenital glaucoma, and a serious cardiac defect (single ventricle and pulmonary atresia). Further testing revealed positive antibody titers for LCV (Mets et al, 2000). Mets and colleagues concluded that "congenital lymphocytic choriomeningitis virus infection may be more common than previously appreciated" and that "serologic testing . . . should be part of the standard workup for

congenital chorioretinitis" (Mets et al, 2000). It also might be prudent to counsel women to avoid handling pet mice and hamsters during pregnancy.

OTHER DISORDERS THAT AFFECT THE EYES
Fetal Alcohol Syndrome

Ocular abnormalities often are overlooked in infants with fetal alcohol syndrome (FAS) because of the CNS damage, facial dysmorphia, and severe intrauterine growth restriction present in these infants. Abnormalities of the eyes common in infants with FAS include microphthalmos, coloboma, nystagmus, cataracts, glaucoma, microcornea, amblyopia, phthisis, persistent hyperplastic primary vitreous, and refractive errors. Most affected infants have diminished visual acuity. A recent study found ocular evidence of FAS in previously undiagnosed children evaluated for developmental delay or hyperactivity disorders or both (Hug et al, 2000). This study suggests that FAS should be included in the differential diagnosis of infants undergoing eye examination for developmental delay or hyperactivity disorders.

Maternal Diabetes

Although maternal diabetes is recognized for its teratogenic effects, craniofacial anomalies are rarely reported. The presence of oculoauriculovertebral (OAV) complex in 14 infants of diabetic mothers who were insulin dependent or who were treated with oral hyperglycemic medications throughout their pregnancies has been reported (Ewart-Toland et al, 2000). Women with gestational diabetes were excluded from the study. The specific ocular anomalies noted in these infants were lens opacity, microphthalmia, optic nerve hypoplasia, laterally displaced inner canthi, tear duct obstruction, and ocular lipomas. Wang et al (2002) suggest that OAV occurs as a result of faulty neural crest cell migration in diabetic women with poor control during pregnancy.

Periventricular Leukomalacia

Periventricular leukomalacia (PVL) has replaced ROP as the major cause of visual impairment in premature infants (Jacobson et al, 1998). Impairments found in infants with PVL included diminished visual acuity, eye movement disorders, and visual field restriction. Other eye problems included optic disc anomalies, nystagmus, strabismus, delayed visual maturation, and visual perceptual-cognitive problems (Jacobson & Dutton, 2000). These visual problems persist into childhood, according to a recent report from France (Porton-Deterne et al, 2000).

Intraventricular Hemorrhage

Intraventricular hemorrhage (IVH) without PVL is also associated with ocular morbidity (O'Keefe et al, 2001). Strabismus was present in 47% of infants with grade I and grade II IVH and in 42% of infants with grade III and grade IV IVH. Optical atrophy was present in 25% of infants with IVH. The incidence of ROP was also higher in this population of infants; no significant relationship to the grade of IVH was noted. Visual impairments were also common in infants with IVH, including smaller than average visual field, poor grating acuity, and poor recognition acuity (O'Keefe et al, 2001).

SUMMARY

Visual disturbances, although sometimes difficult to detect, have a dramatic impact on a newborn's behavioral and psychosocial development. PVL has replaced ROP as the most common cause of serious eye disease in premature infants. Despite significant advances in the diagnosis, treatment, and follow-up of infants with very low birth weight and prematurity, visual morbidity continues to be a concern as smaller neonates survive neonatal intensive care.

Treatment of vision problems requires collaborative efforts among the neonatal health care team, the ophthalmologist, and the families of affected children. Clear, consistent communication between health care providers and parents, parental education, and good follow-up are important to the quality of care.

Case Study

IDENTIFICATION OF THE PROBLEM

Premature infants are at risk for complications from immature function of organ systems, effects of environmental conditions, and as consequences of therapies for support and treatment of conditions related to their immature organ system functions. This case study presents some of the challenges faced by these patients and their care providers. The infant in the following case study is currently 70 days old (36 weeks' corrected gestational age). He is on ad libitum feedings and in an open crib. His medications are aldactazide, sodium chloride (NaCl) supplements, and pediatric multivitamins with iron. He is also on nasal cannula oxygen for chronic lung disease.

ASSESSMENT: HISTORY AND PHYSICAL EXAMINATION

JR was born October 27, 2005, at 26 weeks' gestation to a 30-year-old, gravida 2 para 1 mother whose pregnancy was uncomplicated until the onset of preterm labor. She received prenatal care and is O negative, RPR nonreactive, rubella immune, GC negative, *Chlamydia* positive (treated during pregnancy), hepatitis B negative, and HIV negative. The urine drug screen was also negative. JR was born by repeat cesarean section when it was determined that preterm labor could not be stopped. Apgar scores were 7 and 9 (1 and 5 minutes, respectively). Birth weight was 771 g. He was intubated, given one dose of Survanta, and placed on SIMV with the following settings: 34% oxygen, PIP 16, PEEP 5, and rate 30 in the delivery room. Umbilical lines were placed.

Physical Assessment December 28, 2005

General	Pink, warm, prompt elastic recoil
HEENT	Slight dolichocephaly, anterior fontanelle soft, full; sutures not split; eyes clear, no drainage or redness; fixes and follows on objects; nasal cannula in place and secure; nares and septum without lesions or deviations; palates intact, strong suck
Chest	Bilateral breath sounds equal and clear; S1 and S2 regular, no murmurs; precordium quiet; pulses strong, regular and equal; capillary refill <3 seconds
Abdomen	Soft, protuberant with active sounds in all quadrants, no organomegaly, small umbilical hernia
GU	Preterm male genitalia, testes partially descended; right inguinal hernia reducible
Extremities	Symmetrical, no dislocated hips
Neuro	Alert, responsive to interaction; tone appropriate for gestational age

Summary Problem List (In order of appearance)

1. **Health maintenance**—26-week, AGA preterm
   At risk for IVH—Head ultrasounds were normal × 3
   At risk for NEC—Did not have any problems with feedings
   Thermoregulation—Weaned to open crib at 6 weeks of age (32 weeks' corrected gestational age)
   At risk for RSV—Received Synagis on November 11 and December 10, 2005
   Immunizations—Hepatitis B vaccine on December 12, 2005
   Hearing screen—Left ear did not pass × 2
2. **Respiratory distress**
   Electively extubated on day of life (DOL) 2 and placed on nasal cannula oxygen at 1 L/min.
3. **Possible sepsis**
   Received a 48-hour course of ampicillin and gentamicin. Serial CBCs and cultures were negative.
4. **Fluid, electrolytes, and nutrition**
   NPO for 3 days and started on total parenteral nutrition. Trophic feedings started on DOL 4. Advanced to full enteral feedings of 150 ml/kg/day of preterm formula 24 cal/oz on DOL 15 and started on pediatric multivitamins with iron. TPN was restarted when he was made NPO for indomethacin therapy and surgery. He was back on full feedings on November 27, 2005, and his weight was 1506 g. He weighed 1875 g on December 15, 2005, and 2164 g on December 28, 2005.
5. **Apnea of prematurity**
   Started on Cafcit 2 days prior to extubation on DOL 4 and was discontinued on December 6, 2005 (DOL 46). No apnea noted afterwards.
6. **Anemia of prematurity**
   Placed on erythropoietin during first week of life and followed with weekly hematocrits (Hct). His lowest Hct was 30.5%. Erythropoietin discontinued on December 12, 2005. No blood transfusions were required.
7. **Patent ductus arteriosus**
   On DOL 17, he developed pulmonary edema and a murmur and was given a dose of furosemide. Cardiac ECHO revealed a large patent ductus arteriosus (PDA) with left-to-right shunting. He was started on indomethacin and aldactazide. The PDA closed with treatment; however, clinical symptoms reappeared 3 days later, and a second course of indomethacin was given. On November 18, 2005 (DOL 27), JR underwent a PDA ligation with an uncomplicated postoperative course.

Continued

Case Study—cont'd

8. **Chronic lung disease**

   On DOL 34, he was started on aldactazide for pulmonary edema and chronic lung changes on chest radiograph. Supplemental NaCl was started 1 week later. He was switched from nasal cannula oxygen to high-flow nasal cannula (Vapotherm) at 4 L/min for increased work of breathing. He was weaned to regular nasal cannula on December 17, 2005. Currently, JR remains on nasal cannula oxygen at $1/4$ L/min, aldactazide, and sodium supplements.

9. **Pneumonia**

   On November 25, 2005, he presented with increasing respiratory distress. A workup for sepsis was done, and he was started on ampicillin and tobramycin. The chest radiograph showed patchy infiltrates and chronic changes. His CBC was slightly left shifted. All cultures were negative. He received a 7-day course of antibiotics for presumed pneumonia.

10. **Retinopathy of prematurity (ROP)**

    First eye examination, December 5, 2005, on DOL 45—Immature vascularity in both eyes (stage 0, zones 2-3 bilaterally). Follow-up examination was scheduled for 2 weeks later.

    Second eye examination, December 12, 2005—Stage 1-2, zone 2 with questionable plus disease. Follow-up examination was scheduled for 1 week.

    Third examination, December 26, 2005—Stage 2-3+, zone 2 on right; stage 2+, zone 2 on left. Patient was referred for laser treatment.

    December 28, 2005; eye examination by retinal specialist—Stage 3+, zone 2 bilaterally. Laser photocoagulation was performed.

11. **Social**—JR's parents are married with one older child who is 4 years old. His father works full-time, and his mother plans to work part-time when JR comes home

(she is currently working full-time). They rent a house and live about 15 miles from the hospital. Both parents visit almost daily and perform JR's care during the visits. They are comfortable feeding, bathing, and dressing him; changing his leads; and taking him in and out of the crib. There is family in the area for support, and both parents are actively involved in their church.

DIAGNOSTIC TESTS

Indirect ophthalmoscopy by pediatric retinal specialist:

October 27, 2005	At risk for ROP
December 5, 2005	Immature retinal vascularity (stage 0, zone 2-3 ROP)
December 19, 2005	Prethreshold ROP (stage 1-2, zone 2, ? plus disease)
December 26, 2005	Severe ROP with plus disease (stage 2-3+, zone 2 in right eye, stage 2+, zone 2 in left)
December 28, 2005	Threshold ROP (stage 3+, zone 2 bilaterally)

WORKING DIAGNOSIS

Progressive retinopathy of prematurity

DEVELOPMENT OF MANAGEMENT PLAN

Laser photocoagulation to both eyes on December 28, 2005

IMPLEMENTATION AND EVALUATION OF EFFECTIVENESS

The retinal specialist determined that JR needed laser treatment immediately and scheduled the procedure for the same day as his examination. JR was placed on prednisolone acetate 1% ophthalmic solution TID for 5 days following surgery. A follow-up eye examination is scheduled for 1 week after surgery.

REFERENCES

Ahmad OF, Hirose T (2004). Severe retinopathy in a child with hypoplastic left heart syndrome. *American journal of ophthalmology* 137(3):566-567.

Allegaert K et al (2004a). Dopamine is an indicator but not an independent risk factor for grade 3 retinopathy of prematurity in extreme low birthweight infants. *British journal of ophthalmology* 88:309-310.

Allegaert K et al, on behalf of the EpiBel Study Group (2004b). Threshold retinopathy at threshold of viability: the EpiBel study. *British journal of ophthalmology* 88:239-242.

American Academy of Pediatrics (AAP) Committee on Infectious Disease (2000). *Red book 2000.* Elk Grove Village, IL: AAP.

Anderson CG et al (2004). Retinopathy of prematurity and pulse oximetry: a national survey of recent practices. *Journal of perinatology* 24:164-168.

Arroe M, Peitersen B (1994). Retinopathy of prematurity: review of a seven-year period in a Danish neonatal intensive care unit. *Acta paediatrica* 83(5):501-505.

Askie L (2004). Appropriate levels of oxygen saturation for preterm infants. *Acta paediatrica supplement* 93(444):26-28.

Attar MA (2005). Barriers to screening infants for retinopathy of prematurity after discharge or transfer from a neonatal intensive care unit. *Journal of perinatology* 25(1):36-40.

Barton LL et al (2002). Lymphocytic choriomeningitis virus: emerging fetal teratogen. *American journal of obstetrics and gynecology* 187(6):1715-1716.

Berk TA et al (2000). Underlying pathologies in secondary strabismus. *Strabismus* 8(2):69-75.

Bolt B et al (1992). A mydriatic eye drop combination without systemic effects for premature infants: a prospective double-blind study. *Journal of pediatric ophthalmology and strabismus* 29(3):157-162.

Brantley MA Jr, Harbour JW (2001). The molecular biology of retinoblastoma [review]. *Ocular immunology inflammation* 9(1):1-8.

Brown MM, Brown GC (2005). How to interpret a healthcare economic analysis. *Current opinion in ophthalmology* 16(3):191-194.

Brown MM et al (2004). Value-based medicine and vitreoretinal diseases. *Current opinion in ophthalmology* 15(3):167-172.

Chaberny IE et al (2003). An outbreak of epidemic keratoconjunctivitis in a pediatric unit due to adenovirus type 8. *Infection control and hospital epidemiology* 24(7):514-519.

Chew C et al (2005). Comparison of mydriatic regimens used in screening for retinopathy of prematurity in preterm infants with dark irides. *Journal of pediatric ophthalmology and strabismus* 42(3):166-173.

Chiang MF et al (2004). Incidence of retinopathy of prematurity from 1996 to 2000: analysis of a comprehensive New York State patient database. *Ophthalmology* 111:1317-1325.

Choong CS et al (2000). Congenital varicella syndrome in the absence of cutaneous lesions. *Journal of paediatrics and child health* 36(2):184-185.

Coats DK (2005). Retinopathy of prematurity: involution, factors predisposing to retinal detachment, and expected utility of preemptive surgical reintervention. *Transactions of the American Ophthalmological Society* 103:281-312.

Coats DK et al (2000). Ophthalmologic findings in children with congenital cytomegalovirus infection. *Journal of AAPOS* 4(2):110-116.

Coats DK et al (2005). Involution of retinopathy of prematurity after laser treatment: factors associated with development of retinal detachment. *American journal of ophthalmology* 140(2):214-222.

Cooke RWI et al (2004). Ophthalmic impairment at 7 years of age in children born very preterm. *Archives of diseases in childhood fetal and neonatal edition* 89:F249-F253.

Corey RP, Flynn JT (2000). Maternal intrauterine herpes simplex virus infection leading to persistent fetal vasculature. *Archives of ophthalmology* 18(6):837-840.

Cryotherapy for Retinopathy of Prematurity Cooperative Group (CRPCG) (1988). Multicenter trial of cryotherapy for retinopathy of prematurity: preliminary results. *Archives of ophthalmology* 106(4):471-499.

Darlow BA et al, Australian and New Zealand Neonatal Network (2005). Prenatal risk factors for severe retinopathy of prematurity among very preterm infants of the Australian and New Zealand Neonatal Network. *Pediatrics* 115(4):990-996.

Davitt BV et al, for the Early Treatment for ROP Cooperative Group (2005). Prevalence of myopia at 9 months in infants with high-risk prethreshold retinopathy of prematurity. *Ophthalmology* 112:1564-1568.

Dinakaran S, Desai SP (1999). Central serous retinopathy associated with Weber-Christian disease. *European journal of ophthalmology* 9(2):139-141.

Drohan L et al (2002). *Candida* (amphotericin-sensitive) lens abscess associated with decreasing arterial blood flow in a very low birth weight preterm infant. *Pediatrics* 110(5):65-68.

Early Treatment for Retinopathy of Prematurity Cooperative Group (2003). Revised indications for the treatment of retinopathy of prematurity: results of the early treatment for retinopathy of prematurity randomized trial. *Archives of ophthalmology* 121(12):1684-1694.

Ertzbischoff LM (2004). A systematic review of anatomical and visual function outcomes in preterm infants after scleral buckle and vitrectomy for retinal detachment. *Advances in neonatal care* 4(1):10-19.

Ewart-Toland A et al (2000). Oculoauriculovertebral abnormalities in children of diabetic mothers. *American journal of medical genetics* 90(4):303-309.

Fledelius HC, Kjer B (2004). Surveillance for retinopathy of prematurity in a Danish county. Epidemiological experience over 20 years. *Acta ophthalmololologica Scandinavica* 82:38-41.

Fledelius HC et al (2004). Surveillance for retinopathy of prematurity in a Copenhagen high-risk sample 1999–2001. Has progress reached a plateau? *Acta ophthalmololologica Scandinavica* 82:32-37.

Fletcher MA (1998). *Physical diagnosis in neonatology.* Baltimore: Lippincott Williams & Wilkins.

Gal P et al (2005). Efficacy of sucrose to reduce pain in premature infants during eye examinations for retinopathy of prematurity. *Annals of pharmacotherapy* 39(6):1029-1033.

Gilbert C et al (2005). Characteristics of infants with severe retinopathy of prematurity in countries with low, moderate, and high levels of development: implications for screening programs. *Pediatrics* 115(5):518-525.

Good WV et al, Early Treatment for Retinopathy of Prematurity Cooperative Group (2005). The incidence and course of retinopathy of prematurity: findings from the early treatment for retinopathy of prematurity study. *Pediatrics* 116(1):15-23.

Gupta BK et al (2002). The eye. In Fanaroff AA, Martin RJ, editors. *Neonatal-perinatal medicine: diseases of the fetus and newborn,* ed 7. St Louis: Mosby.

Haas J et al (2005). Epidemiology and diagnosis of hospital-acquired conjunctivitis among neonatal intensive care unit patients. *Pediatric infectious disease journal* 24(7):586-589.

Hameed B et al (2004). Trends in the incidence of severe retinopathy of prematurity in a geographically defined population over a 10-year period. *Pediatrics* 113(6):1653-1657.

Hellström A (1999). Optic nerve morphology may reveal adverse events during prenatal and perinatal life: digital image analysis. *Survey of ophthalmology* 44(Suppl 1):S63-S73.

Hered RW (2004). Use of non-sterile instruments for examination for retinopathy of prematurity in the neonatal intensive care unit. *Journal of pediatrics* 145(3):308-311.

Horan TC, Gaynes RP (2004). Surveillance of nosocomial infections. In Mayhall CG, editor. *Hospital epidemiology and infection control,* ed 3 (pp 1659-1702). Philadelphia: Lippincott Williams & Wilkins.

Hug TE et al (2000). Clinical and electroretinographic findings in fetal alcohol syndrome. *Journal of AAPOS* 4(4):200-204.

Hussain N et al (1999). Current incidence of retinopathy of prematurity, 1989–1997. *Pediatrics* 104(3):26-34.

Hylander MA et al (2001). Association of human milk feedings with a reduction in retinopathy of prematurity among very low birth weight infants. *Journal of perinatology* 21(6):356-362.

International Committee for the Classification of Retinopathy of Prematurity (2005). The international classification of retinopathy of prematurity revisited. *Archives of ophthalmology* 123(7):991-999.

International Committee on Retinopathy of Prematurity (ICROP) (1984). An international classification of retinopathy of prematurity. *Pediatrics* 74(1):127-133.

Jackson TL et al (2003). Monocular chromatic contrast threshold and achromatic contrast sensitivity in children born prematurely. *American journal of ophthalmology* 136(4):710-719.

Jacobson LK, Dutton GN (2000). Periventricular leukomalacia: an important cause of visual and ocular motility dysfunction in children [review]. *Survey of ophthalmology* 45(1):1-13.

Jacobson L et al (1998). Periventricular leukomalacia causes visual impairment in preterm children: a study on the aetiologies of visual impairment in a population-based group of preterm children born 1989–95 in the county of Varmland, Sweden. *Acta ophthalmologica Scandinavica* 76(5):593-598.

Jandeck C et al (2004). Late retinal detachment in patients born prematurely: outcome of primary pars plana vitrectomy. *Archives of ophthalmology* 122(1):61-64.

Javitt J et al (1993). Cost-effectiveness of screening and cryotherapy for threshold retinopathy of prematurity. *Pediatrics* 91(5):859-866.

Johnston WT, Cogen MS (2000). Systemic candidiasis with cataract formation in a premature infant. *Journal of AAPOS* 4(6):386-388.

Kraemer M et al (1999). The neonatal development of the light flash visual evoked potential. *Documenta ophthalmologica* 99(1):21-39.

Laga M, Meheus Piot P (1989). Epidemiology and control of gonococcal ophthalmia neonatorum. *Bulletin World Health Organization* 67(5):471-477.

Lang DM et al (2005). Is Pacific race a retinopathy of prematurity risk factor? *Archives of pediatric and adolescent medicine* 159(8):771-773.

Larsson E et al (2002). Incidence of ROP in two consecutive Swedish population based studies. *British journal of ophthalmology* 86:1122-1126.

Larsson EK et al (2005). A population-based study on the visual outcome in 10-year-old preterm and full-term children. *Archives of ophthalmology* 123(6):825-832.

Lee SK et al, and Canadian NICU Network (2000). Variations in practice and outcomes in the Canadian NICU network: 1996–1997. *Pediatrics* 106(5):1070-1079.

Lehman SS (1999). An uncommon cause of ophthalmia neonatorum: *Neisseria meningitidis. Journal of AAPOS* 3(5):316.

Liu PM et al (2005). Risk factors of retinopathy of prematurity in premature infants weighting less than 1600 g. *American journal of perinatology* 22(2):115-120.

Lupetti A et al (2002). Horizontal transmission of *Candida parapsilosis* candidemia in a neonatal intensive care unit. *Journal of clinical microbiology* 40(7):2363-2369.

Markestad T et al (2005). Early death, morbidity, and need of treatment among extremely premature infants. *Pediatrics* 115(5):1289-1298.

Marsh CS et al (2004). Severe retinopathy of prematurity (ROP) in a premature baby treated with sildenafil acetate (Viagra) for pulmonary hypertension. *British journal of ophthalmology* 88:306-307.

Marsh VA et al (2005). Efficacy of topical anesthetics to reduce pain in premature infants during eye examinations for retinopathy of prematurity. *Annals of pharmacotherapy* 39(5):829-833.

Martins EN, Morse LS (2005). Evaluation of internet websites about retinopathy of prematurity patient education. *British journal of ophthalmology* 89(5):565-568.

Mehta M et al (2005). Pilot study of the systemic effects of three different screening methods used for retinopathy of prematurity. *Early human development* 81(4):355-360.

Mestan KK et al (2005). Neurodevelopmental outcomes of premature infants treated with inhaled nitric oxide. *New England journal of medicine* 353(1):23-32.

Mets MB et al (2000). Lymphocytic choriomeningitis virus: an underdiagnosed cause of congenital chorioretinitis. *American journal of ophthalmology* 130(2):209-215.

Mizoguchi MB et al (1999). Dopamine use is an indicator for the development of threshold retinopathy of prematurity. *British journal of ophthalmology* 83(4):425-428.

Moore K et al (2003). *Before we are born: essentials of embryology and birth defects*. Philadelphia: Saunders.

O'Connor MT et al (2003). Is retinopathy of prematurity increasing among infants less than 1250 g birth weight? *Journal of perinatology* 23:673-678.

Ogut MS et al (1996). Effects and side effects of mydriatic eyedrops in neonates. *European journal of ophthalmology* 6(2):192-196.

O'Keefe M (2001). Ocular significance of intraventricular haemorrhage in premature infants. *British journal of ophthalmology* 85(3):357-359.

Palmer EA et al, and the Cryotherapy for ROP Cooperative Group (2005). 15-year outcomes following threshold retinopathy of prematurity: final results from the multicenter trial of cryotherapy for retinopathy of prematurity. *Archives of ophthalmology* 123(3):311-318.

Percivalle E et al (2003). A comparison of methods for detecting adenovirus type 8 keratoconjunctivitis during a nosocomial outbreak in a neonatal intensive care unit. *Journal of clinical virology* 28(3):257-264.

Phelps DL (1992). Retinopathy of prematurity. *Current problems in pediatrics* 22(8):349-371.

Pierce EA, Mukai S (1994). Controversies in the management of retinopathy of prematurity. *International ophthalmology clinics* 34(3):121-148.

Porton-Deterne IF et al (2000). Ocular motility and visuo-spatial attention in children with periventricular leukomalacia. *Brain and cognition* 43(1-3):362-364.

Roberts F et al (2001). Histopathological features of ocular toxoplasmosis in the fetus and infant. *Archives of ophthalmology* 119(1):51-58.

Rush R et al (2004). Systemic manifestations in response to mydriasis and physical examination during screening for retinopathy of prematurity. *Retina* 24(2):242-245.

Saugstad OD (2005). Oxygen for newborns: how much is too much? *Journal of perinatology* 25(Suppl 2):S45-S49.

Seiberth V et al (1994). A controlled clinical trial of light and retinopathy of prematurity. *American journal of ophthalmology* 118(4):492-495.

Shah GK et al (2000). Intralenticular *Candida* species abscess in a premature infant. *American journal of ophthalmology* 129(3):390-391.

Shah S et al (1999). Bacteremia, meningitis and brain abscesses in a hospitalized infant: complications of *Pseudomonas aeruginosa* conjunctivitis. *Journal of perinatology* 19(6 Pt 1):462-465.

Shah VA et al (2005). Incidence, risk factors of retinopathy of prematurity among very low birth weight infants in Singapore. *Annals of the Academy of Medicine of Singapore* 34(2):169-178.

Smith LE (2003). Pathogenesis of retinopathy of prematurity. *Seminars in neonatology* 8:469-473.

Smith LE (2004). Pathogenesis of retinopathy of prematurity. *Growth hormone & IGF research* 14(Suppl A):S140-S144.

Todd DA et al (1994). Retinopathy of prematurity in infants less than 29 weeks' gestation at birth. *Australian and New Zealand journal of ophthalmology* 22(1):19-23.

Trese MT (1994). Surgery for retinopathy of prematurity. *International ophthalmology clinics* 34(3):105-111.

Trigler L et al (2005). Case series of angle-closure glaucoma after laser treatment for retinopathy of prematurity. *Journal of AAPOS* 9(1):17-21.

Tufail A et al (2004). Late onset vitreoretinal complications of regressed retinopathy of prematurity. *British journal of ophthalmology* 88:243-246.

Vander JF (1994). Retinopathy of prematurity: diagnosis and management. *Journal of ophthalmic nursing and technology* 13(5):207-212.

Varughese S et al (2005). Refractive error at birth and its relation to gestational age. *Current eye research* 30(6):423-428.

Wang R et al (2002). Infants of diabetic mother are at increased risk for the oculo-auriculo-vertebral sequence: a case-based and case-control approach. *Journal of pediatrics* 141(50):611-617.

Wasserman BN et al (1999). *Pseudomonas*-induced bilateral endophthalmitis with corneal perforation in a neonate. *Journal of AAPOS* 3(3):183-184.

Wright K, Wright P (1994). Lack of association of glucocorticoid therapy and retinopathy of prematurity. *Archives of pediatric and adolescent medicine* 148(8):848-852.

Yen KG et al (2002). Telephotoscreening to detect retinopathy of prematurity: preliminary study of the optimum time to employ digital fundus camera imaging to detect ROP. *Journal of AAPOS* 6(2):64-70.

York JR et al (2004). Arterial oxygen fluctuation and retinopathy of prematurity in very-low-birth-weight infants. *Journal of perinatology* 24(2):82-87.

Chapter **15**

Fluids, Electrolytes, Vitamins, and Minerals

Sergio DeMarini • Linda L. Rath

Water and electrolytes are vital components of the body at any age. The laws that regulate fluid and electrolyte balance in the newborn are the same as those that control this process in children and adults. However, the newborn's body water distribution is both quantitatively and qualitatively different. Furthermore, rapid changes occur at the time of birth, and sick newborns pose additional challenges. Consequently, water and electrolyte homeostasis is of vital importance and special care is required to maintain an appropriate balance, especially in very-low-birth-weight (VLBW) infants.

In this chapter the recommendations of the American Academy of Pediatrics (AAP) have been followed whenever possible. In all other instances the conclusions drawn are based on current medical evidence in the field.

WATER AND ELECTROLYTES
Water
Water is the main component of the human body. It is distributed both inside and outside the cells; therefore, a practical simplification is to classify total body water (TBW) as intracellular water (ICW) and extracellular water (ECW). ICW is the total amount of water in all the body's cells. ECW is the total amount of water outside the cells; it comprises the water in the interstitial space and in the intravascular space (plasma).

Physiology
The distribution of TBW between intracellular and extracellular spaces depends on the water's relative content of solutes (electrolytes, proteins): that is, on its relative osmolality. The total number of solute particles in solution determines the osmolality of a solution. Osmolality values are expressed in osmoles or milliosmoles per kilogram of water (Osm/kg or mOsm/kg). Because cell membranes are completely permeable to water but not to most solutes, water shifts from one compartment to the other until equilibrium is established between the osmolalities on both sides of the membrane. The osmolality of intracellular and extracellular spaces, therefore, is equal,

although the composition of ICW is different from that of ECW; sodium (Na) is the main extracellular ion, whereas potassium (K) is the main intracellular ion. The size of a compartment depends on the number of osmoles in it, which in turn determines the water content.

In each compartment, a main solute acts to keep water in the compartment:
- The volume of the intracellular compartment is maintained mainly by K salts and is regulated by the Na-K cellular pump.
- The volume of the extracellular compartment is maintained mainly by Na salts and is regulated by the kidneys.
- In the extracellular space, the volume of the intravascular compartment is maintained mainly by the colloidal osmotic pressure of plasma proteins.

Changes in Water Distribution
TBW declines with growth (Figure 15-1). It constitutes more than 90% of the total body weight in the first trimester of gestation, about 80% at 32 weeks' gestation, about 78% at 40 weeks' gestation, and approximately 60% to 65% at the end of the first year of life. The ratio of ECW to ICW also changes with growth. ECW declines from approximately 60% of body weight in the second trimester to about 45% at term. Correspondingly, ICW increases from about 25% of body weight in the second trimester to approximately 33% at term.

At birth an acute expansion of ECW is superimposed on the gradual changes that took place during fetal life. This is due to (1) placental transfusion, (2) reabsorption of lung fluid, and (3) water and electrolytes shift from the intracellular to the extracellular space (Baumgart & Costarino, 2000). The newborn at birth, therefore, is in a state of excess extracellular fluid, a condition that is particularly prominent in preterm infants (TBW and ECW are greater at lower gestational ages). Because the excess ECW is lost through diuresis, some weight loss (5% to 10% in term infants) usually occurs as a consequence of these physiologic changes in body water distribution. Postnatal loss and regaining of weight reflect changes

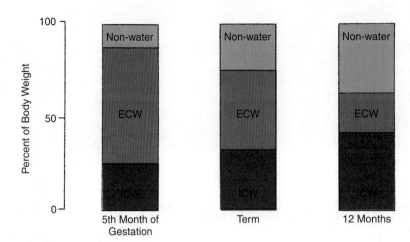

ECW: Extracellular water
ICW: Intracellular water

FIGURE **15-1**
Changes in body water distribution. *ECW*, Extracellular water; *ICW*, intracellular water.

in the interstitial water component of ECW, whereas plasma volume remains essentially unchanged. In preterm infants, the postnatal weight loss is greater (usually 10% to 20%) and occurs more frequently in the smallest infants. As long as the intravascular volume is adequate and serum electrolytes are normal, it appears inappropriate to replace all fluid losses during the first days of life. Administration of large amounts of fluids increases the risk of symptomatic patent ductus arteriosus (PDA) and bronchopulmonary dysplasia (BPD).

Water Balance and Body Metabolism

The human body loses a variable amount of water and electrolytes daily. To maintain body fluid balance, fluid losses must be replaced periodically. Maintenance fluid requirements are calculated to replace water and electrolytes normally lost through urine, stool, skin, and the respiratory tract. Water turnover is part of cellular metabolism and usually is related precisely to the basal metabolic rate. The basal metabolic rate is the amount of energy the body must produce to maintain homeostasis at rest and in a thermally neutral environment. Carbohydrates, lipids, and proteins are the substances used to produce energy. Waste products are heat, nitrogen, carbon dioxide, and water. To excrete waste products, the body normally loses water through the kidneys (to eliminate nitrogen), the skin (to eliminate excess heat), and the respiratory tract (to eliminate carbon dioxide). Therefore a high body energy expenditure means a large amount of waste products and, consequently, large water losses.

The cells generate some water as a byproduct of cell metabolism (i.e., water of oxidation). This amount of water, which must be subtracted from fluid requirements, is approximately equal to water losses in stools; therefore the latter can be omitted from the usual calculations of required water intake.

Water Requirements

Maintaining the overall body water and salt composition requires replacement of renal water and electrolyte losses and insensible water losses from the respiratory tract and skin evaporation. An approximate estimate of maintenance fluids is as follows: 100 ml of water is needed for each 100 kilocalories (kcal) of energy expended.

Although this relationship between metabolic rate and water loss holds true in full-term infants, it is not valid in preterm infants. Immature renal function, very high insensible water losses as a result of skin immaturity and a higher body surface area to body mass ratio, and neonatal illnesses significantly affect fluid balance (Baumgart & Costarino, 2000). Although values for fluid requirements are available (Table 15-1), they provide only an approximate guideline for the individual infant.

Fluid requirements may be determined more accurately if factors that influence insensible water loss (IWL) are taken into account (Table 15-2). For example, radiant warmers and phototherapy increase insensible water loss, whereas use of a plastic blanket under a radiant warmer or adequate humidification in an incubator reduces IWL.

Effects of Postnatal Adaptation on Water Requirements

Fluid management is easier if one remembers a few simple principles: (1) to separate water from sodium requirements; (2) to keep maintenance fluids separate from fluids given to correct electrolyte abnormalities; and (3) to recognize the pattern of neonatal diuresis. Monitoring a newborn's urine output can help to individualize fluid requirements. According to Lorenz and colleagues (1995), most preterm infants show a definite postnatal pattern of diuresis, which has three phases: the prediuretic phase, the diuretic phase, and the homeostatic phase (Table 15-3). The prediuretic phase occurs in the first 48 to 72 hours of life. In this phase, the glomerular filtration rate, urine output, and sodium and potassium excretion are all very low. Water is lost mainly by IWL. Because only water is lost through the skin, the appropriate steps in calculating fluid intake during this phase are the following:

TABLE 15-1	Approximate Water Requirements of Newborns in the First Week of Life			
	Birth Weight			
Time Period	**Under 1000 g**	**1000 to 1500 g**	**1501 to 2000 g**	**Full Term**
First 48 hours	80 to 140	60 to 100	60 to 80	40 to 60
End of first week	150 to 200	140 to 160	110 to 150	100 to 150

Amounts are given as ml/kg/d.

TABLE 15-2	Factors Affecting Water Loss in Neonates
Increases Water Loss	**Reduces Water Loss**
WATER LOSS FROM THE SKIN	
Low gestational age	High humidity in incubator
Forced convection in incubator	Double-walled incubator
Radiant warmer	Plastic heat shield
Hyperthermia	Plastic blanket
Activity	Semipermeable skin patches
Phototherapy	
WATER LOSS FROM THE RESPIRATORY TRACT	
Tachypnea	Continuous distending pressure with humidified gas
Inadequate humidification	Artificial ventilation with humidification
RENAL WATER LOSS	
Diuretics	Renal failure
Osmotic diuresis (hyperglycemia, mannitol)	Inappropriate secretion of antidiuretic hormone
Congenital adrenal hyperplasia	Congestive heart failure

- Intake is limited to insensible water losses.
- No sodium, chloride, or potassium is given.
- The standard intravenous solution should provide glucose at a rate of 4 to 6 mg/kg/min (with increasing amounts of amino acids).

As only skin water losses occur during this phase, preterm infants appear to be predisposed to hypernatremia. Early sodium supplementation offers no advantage and increases the risk of hypernatremia.

The diuretic phase usually begins on day 2 to 5 of life. Urine output and sodium and potassium excretion all increase abruptly. This phase seems to be triggered by atrial natriuretic peptide (ANP), which is released by myocardial cells in response to atrial stretching. The proposed mechanism is as follows: falling pulmonary vascular resistance leads to increased venous return to the left atrium and to release of ANP. ANP in turn causes increased natriuresis (Modi, 2003). In this phase, fluid intake is adjusted as follows:

- Water intake is increased to maintain a normal serum sodium concentration and to obtain a total weight loss of about 10% in term newborns and between 10% and 20% in preterm infants.
- Sodium (to keep the serum Na level normal) and potassium (when the serum K level declines) should be added to the intravenous solution.

In the homeostatic phase, which follows the diuretic phase, diuresis stabilizes. The goal of fluid and electrolyte intake in this phase is to allow an adequate caloric intake and growth, without causing fluid overload.

Appropriate administration of fluid is important, because both excessive fluid restriction and fluid overload lead to clinical consequences (Figure 15-2). Excessive fluid restriction may lead to dehydration, hyperosmolality, hypoglycemia, and hyperbilirubinemia. In preterm infants, high volumes of parenteral fluids have been associated with a higher incidence of PDA, BPD, and necrotizing enterocolitis (NEC). It is important to realize that the occurrence of BPD has been correlated with fluid volume administered during the first 4 days of life. Maintaining the fluid and electrolyte balance,

TABLE 15-3	Pattern of Postnatal Diuresis in Preterm Infants During the First Week of Life		
	Phases of Postnatal Diuresis		
Factors	**Prediuretic**	**Diuretic**	**Homeostatic**
Age	First 2 days	2 to 5 days	After 2 to 5 days
Diuresis	Very low	Sudden increase	Varies with intake
Urine	Very low	Sudden increase	Varies with intake
	Interventions		
Water	Fluid restriction	Allow physiologic weight loss	Provide calories for growth
Sodium	None	Provide enough to maintain normal serum sodium level	Provide growth allowance

From Lorenz JM et al (1995). Phases of fluid and electrolyte homeostasis in the extremely low birth weight infant. Pediatrics 196:484-489.

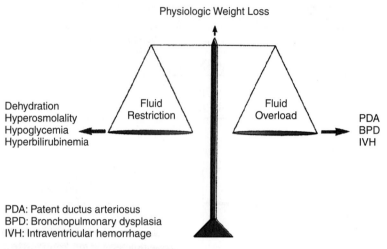

FIGURE **15-2**
Risks of fluid administration.

therefore, is extremely important in preterm infants. Close monitoring of clinical hydration, body weight, urine output, and the serum Na concentration should allow the best possible decisions on fluid administration.

Sodium

Sodium is the main extracellular ion, constituting, with its salts, more than 90% of the total amount of solutes in the extracellular space. Sodium is absorbed in both the small intestine and the colon; the largest amount is absorbed in the jejunum. Sodium absorption involves several mechanisms:

- Passive absorption, after glucose absorption, secondary to the flow of water
- Active absorption, stimulated by glucose and amino acids
- Active absorption, uncoupled with glucose, involving the Na-K pump
- Active absorption in exchange with hydrogen ions

The overall process is very efficient. Adults normally absorb 98% of ingested sodium. The kidneys excrete sodium, which is filtered by glomeruli and reabsorbed throughout the tubules and the collecting ducts. Most of the sodium is absorbed with chloride (Cl), but small amounts are absorbed in exchange with potassium ions (K^+) or hydrogen ions (H^+). Under normal circumstances, 96% to 99% of filtered sodium is reabsorbed. The main factors involved in the regulation of sodium resorption are the oncotic and hydrostatic pressures in the peritubular capillaries and the action of aldosterone, which increases the absorption of sodium in exchange with K^+ or H^+. Although antidiuretic hormone does not affect the excretion of sodium directly, it can influence the serum Na concentration indirectly because it regulates the excretion or resorption of free water.

The Na concentration in human milk is 12 to 20 mEq/L (12 to 20 mmol/L). The current recommendation for standard formulas is 20 to 60 mg/100 kcal (6 to 17 mEq/419 kJ [kilojoules]) (AAP, 1998). The recommendation for growing preterm infants is 3 to 5 mEq/kg/day (Tsang et al, 2005). Because of their high urinary loss of sodium, very low birth weight (VLBW) infants (those weighing less than 1500 g) may require temporarily up to 8 mEq/kg/day by the end of the first week of

life. Thereafter, urinary losses in these infants are gradually reduced. The normal serum Na concentration ranges from 130 to 150 mEq/L. Disorders of sodium balance are listed in Box 15-1.

Hyponatremia. Hyponatremia (a serum Na level below 130 mEq/L) is caused by retention of water relative to sodium. When the serum Na concentration and, therefore, serum osmolality decline, water moves into cells. The increased water content in the brain causes the signs and symptoms of hyponatremia. Vomiting, lethargy, and apnea may occur with

---

BOX **15-1**

Disorders of Sodium Balance

Hyponatremia

Early
Perinatal asphyxia
Respiratory distress syndrome
Diuretics
Nebulization associated with nasal continuous positive airway pressure
Hypotonic fluid administered to mother during labor

Late
Very low birth weight infant fed human milk or standard formula
With overhydration: congestive heart failure, renal failure
With dehydration: adrenal insufficiency, vomiting, diarrhea, peritonitis

Hypernatremia

With Dehydration
Vomiting, diarrhea with inadequate fluid replacement
Osmotic diuresis (hyperglycemia, mannitol)
Radiant warmers
"Hyperosmolar state" in infants weighing less than 800 g

With Overhydration
Excessive administration of sodium bicarbonate ($NaHCO_3$)
Errors in administration of sodium chloride (NaCl)

various degrees of hyponatremia, but seizures and coma usually are not seen unless the serum Na concentration falls below 115 mEq/L. Neonatal hyponatremia usually is classified as early or late, depending on the timing of the occurrence.

Early Hyponatremia. Early hyponatremia, which often occurs in the first 2 days of life, is caused by extrinsic perinatal factors. It is not influenced by parenteral administration of additional sodium and water. Early hyponatremia most often is caused by perinatal asphyxia. The mechanism is diminished excretion of free water, which is caused by increased secretion of antidiuretic hormone (syndrome of inappropriate secretion of antidiuretic hormone, or SIADH) and impairment of renal function by hypoxia. Severe respiratory distress syndrome (RDS) also predisposes newborns to hyponatremia, probably for the same reasons.

Early hyponatremia can be iatrogenic in origin. Possible causes include administration of large volumes of hypotonic fluid to the mother during labor; nebulization with nasal continuous positive airway pressure (CPAP), resulting in water overload; and use of diuretics with excessive free water replacement. Infants with early hyponatremia usually are in a state of excess water, and fluid restriction is the appropriate treatment.

Late Hyponatremia. The most common form of late hyponatremia typically is seen after the first week of life in growing VLBW infants fed either human milk or standard formulas. These infants have a negative sodium balance in the first weeks of life because of a combination of factors, including an inadequate sodium intake and temporary unresponsiveness of the renal tubules to aldosterone (Baumgart & Costarino, 2000). VLBW infants initially may require amounts as high as 8 mEq/kg/day to obtain a positive sodium balance. Spontaneous improvement in sodium balance within weeks is the rule.

At any time, neonatal hyponatremia may occur in association with overhydration (dilutional hyponatremia) or dehydration (true hyponatremia).

Hyponatremia with overhydration may occur in newborns with congestive heart failure (congenital heart disease, PDA), renal failure, or SIADH. Because total body sodium is increased but TBW is even more increased, administration of sodium would only cause additional expansion of the extracellular space, which can aggravate the infant's condition. Fluid restriction is the treatment.

Either renal or extrarenal sodium and water losses can cause hyponatremia with dehydration. Renal losses usually result from adrenal insufficiency (salt-losing type of congenital adrenal hyperplasia, adrenal hemorrhage), although infants with a urinary tract obstruction occasionally may have similar electrolyte disorders. Extrarenal losses may result from disorders such as vomiting, diarrhea, and peritonitis. Treatment is directed both at the underlying disorder and at volume replacement with sodium chloride (NaCl)–containing solutions. The amount of sodium needed to correct a low serum Na level can be calculated according to the standard formula:

Na to be given = 0.6 × Weight (kg) × (Desired serum Na –
(mEq/mmol)   Actual serum Na)

The correction usually is made over several hours, and the target is a serum Na concentration of about 135 mEq/L. However, this general rule has two important exceptions:

- If shock is present or impending, normal saline should be given intravenously (IV) and rapidly at 10 to 20 ml/kg

over 20 to 30 minutes; this treatment is repeated until arterial blood pressure is normal.
- With symptomatic hyponatremia, which almost always occurs only when the serum Na level is below 115 mEq/L, hypertonic saline should be infused. However, because either an abrupt or a large increase in osmolality carries the risk of intracranial hemorrhage and congestive heart failure (CHF), the aim of the initial correction in this case should be a lower than normal serum Na concentration, such as 120 to 125 mEq/L. Even if hyponatremia is asymptomatic, hypertonic saline is used if serum Na is below 120 mEq/L, to prevent symptoms.

Hypernatremia. Hypernatremia (a serum Na level over 150 mEq/L) is an increase in the serum Na concentration. It may be accompanied by dehydration or, in rare cases, by overhydration. Hypernatremia with dehydration is caused by an insufficient water intake, by increased renal or extrarenal water losses, or by a combination of these two factors. Hypernatremia with overhydration usually is iatrogenic in origin.

When hypernatremia and, therefore, hyperosmolality develop, water moves out of the cells into the extracellular space to achieve an osmotic equilibrium between intracellular and extracellular fluid. This attempt to equilibrate intracellular and extracellular fluids, results in volume depletion of the intracellular space. Brain cells can protect themselves, maintaining their intracellular volume by generating new solutes, called idiogenic osmoles. Idiogenic osmoles are substances (amino acids, polyols, trimethylamines) synthesized by the brain as a protective response to serum hyperosmolality. Idiogenic osmoles are neither produced nor catabolized rapidly; therefore this mechanism is effective within certain limits and only if hyperosmolality does not develop too rapidly. Similarly, correction of hypernatremia with hypotonic solutions should not be performed rapidly, because idiogenic osmoles cannot be metabolized quickly and cerebral edema can occur as a result of movement of water into brain cells.

In VLBW infants, sodium restriction during the first 3 to 5 days of life (i.e., no sodium other than with transfusions) may prevent hypernatremia and reduce the need for parenteral fluid.

Hypernatremia with Dehydration. Hypernatremia with dehydration results from water losses for which fluid replacement is inadequate. Water loss may occur from the gastrointestinal tract (vomiting, diarrhea). Inadequate replacement of fluids may include failure to provide the appropriate water intake, especially when this shortcoming is compounded by administration of high-solute fluids. Renal water loss may occur when an increased amount of solute, such as glucose or mannitol, must be excreted (osmotic diuresis). Significant IWL through the skin occurs when infants are placed under radiant warmers, and the magnitude of these losses is inversely related to gestational age.

Hypernatremia with dehydration must be corrected slowly, because cerebral edema can easily develop. Intravascular volume should be restored quickly with isotonic fluids, but water deficits should be corrected slowly and with great caution by administration of hypotonic fluids.

A hyperosmolar state can occur in the first days of life in infants of less than 26 weeks' gestation who weigh less than 800 g. These infants' immature skin and large surface allow massive evaporative losses of free water, which results in significant dehydration (weight loss of 20% or more in the first

48 hours) accompanied by hypernatremia, hyperkalemia, and hyperglycemia, without oliguria (Baumgart & Costarino, 2000). Once this hyperosmolar state is fully established, correction involves the risk of volume overload. The suggested strategy for preventing this syndrome is as follows:

- IWL through the skin is reduced by using an incubator with a high relative humidity (instead of an overhead warmer), with or without a plastic shield or Saran wrap blanket or semipermeable membranes such as Tegaderm (3M, St. Paul, MN).
- The infant's weight, urine output, serum Na level, and glucose concentration are monitored frequently.
- Sodium is restricted, and the smallest volume of fluids is given that allows the serum Na concentration to be maintained within normal limits (the initial rate is 80 to 100 ml/kg/day with subsequent increases, usually without exceeding 150 ml/kg/day).

Hypernatremia with Overhydration. Hypernatremia with overhydration is almost always iatrogenic in origin. It may occur after administration of sodium bicarbonate during cardiopulmonary resuscitation or for acidosis or RDS, or it may arise from errors in the administration of NaCl with fluids. Because administration of sodium increases serum osmolality, it results in a shift of water into the intravascular space. An acute expansion of plasma volume may result in intracranial bleeding and heart failure with pulmonary edema. Treatment of hypernatremia with overhydration involves restricting sodium intake and providing diuretic therapy.

Potassium

Potassium is the main intracellular cation. Its concentration in cells is maintained by the membrane sodium-potassium adenosine triphosphatase (Na$^+$,K$^+$-ATPase) pump. Because potassium is involved in the regulation of cell membrane potential, variations in the serum K concentration have important effects. Although every cell is susceptible to fluctuations in the serum K concentration, the effects on myocardial cells are the most prominent and severe. Dietary potassium is mainly absorbed in the small intestine by passive absorption, and it is actively secreted in the colon. The kidneys excrete potassium. Probably all filtered potassium is reabsorbed in the proximal tubule. Potassium is then secreted by the distal tubules in exchange with sodium in a process regulated by aldosterone. The amount of potassium secreted normally is proportional to intake, so that balance is maintained. Stable, growing preterm infants have a K retention rate similar to that of the fetus (about 1.0 to 1.5 mEq/kg/day).

The potassium requirement for both preterm and full-term infants is 2 to 3 mEq/kg/day. The current recommendation for standard infant formulas is 80 to 200 mg/100 kcal (14 to 34 mEq/419 kJ) (AAP, 1998). The recommendation for growing preterm infants is 1.5 to 2.7 mEq/419 kJ (Tsang et al, 2005).

The normal serum concentrations are 3.5 to 5 mEq/L. Disorders of potassium balance are listed in Box 15-2.

Hypokalemia. Hypokalemia (a serum potassium level below 3.5 mEq/L) can be caused by inadequate intake, gastrointestinal losses (diarrhea, vomiting, continuous aspiration, and removal of gastrointestinal contents), and renal losses (diuretics, steroid therapy, renal tubular acidosis, and Bartter's syndrome).

The consequences of hypokalemia are related to the effects on muscle cells. Although abdominal distention and

---

BOX 15-2

Disorders of Potassium Balance

Hypokalemia
Inadequate intake
Gastrointestinal losses: vomiting, diarrhea, continuous gastric aspiration
Renal losses: diuretics, steroids, renal tubular acidosis

Hyperkalemia
Excessive intake
Impaired excretion: renal failure, congenital adrenal hyperplasia
Movement of potassium out of cells: catabolic states, acidosis

---

diminished bowel motility may occur, the cardiac effects are of much greater concern, and an electrocardiogram (ECG) may be a better measure of serious toxicity than the serum K concentration. ECG changes include a depressed ST segment, a flattened T wave, and a higher U wave. A prolonged P-R interval, a widening QRS complex, and various arrhythmias may follow, particularly in newborns treated with digoxin.

Treatment involves potassium replacement. Potassium chloride should be given very slowly (less than 0.3 mEq/kg/hr), and the serum K concentration or ECG, or both, should be checked frequently. Rapid IV administration of potassium may cause fatal arrhythmias.

Hyperkalemia. Hyperkalemia (usually defined as a serum K level over 6.5 mEq/L) can be caused by an excessive intake of potassium, impaired excretion (renal failure, salt-losing congenital adrenal hyperplasia), or increased movement of potassium from intracellular to extracellular space (catabolic states, acidosis of any origin). Spurious hyperkalemia must be ruled out. This condition can be caused by venipuncture (injury to red blood cells), which must be ruled out. Hyperkalemia occurs in approximately 50% of infants whose birth weight is less than 1000 g, and it is especially common in infants with low urine output in the first hours of life. The proposed mechanism is an increased potassium flow from the intracellular to the extracellular compartment, caused by a decline in the activity of Na$^+$,K$^+$-ATPase. Increased catabolism does not seem to play a significant role. Cardiac toxicity is the main issue and is better reflected by ECG changes than by the serum K concentration. The typical ECG sequence is peaked T waves, disappearance of P waves, and a widening QRS complex, which fuses with the T wave to form a sine wave. Ventricular fibrillation may follow.

Treatment is directed at the underlying disorder, but several temporary measures can be taken, including administration of the following:

- 10% calcium gluconate (1 ml/kg, IV), to antagonize the effect of hyperkalemia on the myocardium
- Sodium bicarbonate (1 to 2 mEq/kg, IV), to raise the blood pH and, consequently, increase potassium influx into cells.
- Salbutamol, by aerosol, to try to increase cellular uptake of potassium
- Infusion of glucose and insulin, at a ratio of 4 g of glucose to 1 unit of insulin, to increase cellular uptake of potassium

- Furosemide (1 mg/kg, IV), to increase renal excretion
- A potassium-binding resin, Kayexalate (1 g/kg, by rectum or by mouth), to increase intestinal excretion

All these measures are temporary. If the serum K concentration continues to rise and exceeds 8 mEq/L, peritoneal dialysis or exchange blood transfusions, using a mixture of washed red blood cells (RBCs) and fresh-frozen plasma (to avoid a high blood K level), should be instituted.

Chloride

Chloride is the main inorganic anion in the extracellular fluid, and together with sodium, it is essential for maintenance of plasma volume. Chloride is administered as NaCl in the diet. Intestinal absorption is passive in the jejunum. It occurs secondary to sodium absorption. In the ileum and colon, chloride is actively absorbed in exchange with bicarbonate. Normally only minimal amounts of chloride are lost in the feces. Chloride is excreted by the kidneys: like sodium, it is filtered by the glomeruli and reabsorbed throughout the tubules and collecting ducts. Normally 99% of the filtered chloride is reabsorbed.

Chloride resorption is inversely related to bicarbonate resorption. The serum concentrations of chloride and bicarbonate are also inversely correlated, which keeps the total anion concentration (Cl^- and HCO_3^-) constant. For this reason, although chloride has no buffer effect, it plays an important part in acid-base regulation. When chloride is retained in the body, the serum bicarbonate level declines and metabolic acidosis follows. When chloride is lost from the body, the serum bicarbonate level rises and metabolic alkalosis ensues.

The current chloride recommendation for infant formulas is 55 to 150 mg/100 kcal [10 to 28 mEq/419 kJ]] (AAP, 1998). The recommendation for growing preterm infants is 2.3 to 6.4 mEq/419 kJ (Tsang et al, 2005). Normal serum Cl concentrations are 90 to 112 mEq/L in full-term infants and 100 to 115 mEq/L in preterm infants. Disorders of chloride balance are listed in Box 15-3.

Hypochloremia. Hypochloremia (a serum Cl level below 90 mEq/L) may be caused by diminished intake or by increased loss of chloride (gastrointestinal or renal). Clinical manifestations include metabolic alkalosis, hypokalemia and, in the case of a chronic disturbance, failure to thrive.

Insufficient intake has occurred with some old soy formulas that had very low chloride content. The diagnosis of insufficient chloride intake is based on the dietary history and on the absence of urinary chloride, which indicates a normal ability to retain chloride to compensate for the low intake. Prolonged vomiting (pyloric stenosis) or continuous aspiration and removal of gastric contents (e.g., necrotizing enterocolitis, abdominal surgery) can increase gastrointestinal losses of chloride as hydrochloric acid (HCl).

Congenital chloridorrhea is a rare disorder of severe diarrhea, beginning at birth, caused by impairment of the active Cl transport system in the ileum and colon. Analysis of feces shows an acid pH and a greatly increased Cl concentration. Diarrhea is caused by the osmotic effect of excess chloride, and hypokalemia ensues as a secondary consequence of diarrhea. Treatment involves a diet low in NaCl and potassium supplementation. The most common cause of increased renal loss of chloride is diuretic therapy. Frequent indications for this treatment in infancy are congestive heart failure and, especially, BPD.

Chronic administration of furosemide, which often is part of the treatment for BPD, may cause chloride deficiency with secondary metabolic alkalosis. Alkalosis, in turn, causes hypoventilation and an increase in the arterial carbon dioxide pressure ($PaCO_2$). This clinical picture can simulate pulmonary edema, but in this case the treatment should not be additional diuretic therapy (as in pulmonary edema), but rather correction of the hypochloremia.

Metabolic alkalosis with hypochloremia and hypokalemia caused by increased renal loss of chloride is the characteristic feature of Bartter's syndrome, in which the underlying mechanism is a defect in tubular resorption of chloride. Elevated urinary Cl and prostaglandin concentrations are diagnostic. Replacement with NaCl and potassium chloride (KCl) or treatment with indomethacin (a prostaglandin antagonist), or both, is usually effective.

Hyperchloremia. Hyperchloremia (a serum Cl level over 115 mEq/L) usually is associated with metabolic acidosis and can be caused either by bicarbonate depletion or by an excessive chloride intake. Diarrhea is the most common cause of hyperchloremic metabolic acidosis, because in the intestine chloride is absorbed with sodium, and bicarbonate is excreted with potassium. Increased loss of bicarbonate occurs with renal tubular acidosis. Usually only the proximal type is diagnosed in the neonatal period, and it occurs mainly in male infants. The renal threshold for bicarbonate drops below normal and the acidity of the urine is not diminished in this condition, and the result is a hyperchloremic metabolic acidosis. The condition is self-limited, and the diagnosis is based on the demonstration that the renal bicarbonate threshold is lower than normal. When the serum bicarbonate concentration is lower than the normal threshold, bicarbonate is retained and acid urine is produced.

Hyperchloremia may follow excessive administration of NaCl. Overtreatment with NaCl may be absolute, as in accidental errors in administration, or relative, as in renal failure. In the latter case, excretion is impaired and can be exceeded by an otherwise "normal" intake; NaCl administration, therefore, must be reduced accordingly. Finally, apparent hyperchloremia, together with increased serum concentrations of other electrolytes, can occur with dehydration when there is a water deficit in relation to solute.

BOX 15-3

Disorders of Chloride Balance

Hypochloremia

Decreased intake: some soy formulas
Increased gastrointestinal losses: vomiting (pyloric stenosis), continuous gastric aspiration, congenital chloridorrhea
Increased renal losses: diuretics, Bartter's syndrome

Hyperchloremia

Increased bicarbonate losses: renal tubular acidosis
Excessive administration of NaCl: absolute or relative (renal failure)
Hypertonic dehydration (apparent hyperchloremia)

Calcium and Phosphorus

Calcium (Ca) is the most abundant mineral in the human body. It is an essential component of the skeleton and plays an important role in muscle contraction, neural transmission, and blood coagulation. Phosphorus (P) is essential for bone mineralization, erythrocyte function, cell metabolism, and generation and storage of energy.

The calcium content of human milk is about 39 mg/100 kcal (0.97 mmol/419 kJ), and the phosphorus content is about 19 mg/100 kcal (0.61 mmol/419 kJ). The current recommendations for standard formulas are 60 mg/100 kcal (1.5 mmol/419 kJ) for calcium and 30 mg/100 kcal (0.97 mmol/419 kJ) for phosphorus (AAP, 1998). The recommendations for growing preterm infants are 1.9 to 5.0 mmol/419 kJ for calcium and 1.5 to 4.1 mmol/419 kJ for phosphorus (Tsang et al, 2005). With parenteral nutrition, a calcium intake of 60 to 80 mg/kg/day (1.5 to 2.0 mmol/kg/day) and a phosphorus intake of 45 to 60 mg/kg/day (1.5 to 1.9 mmol/kg/day) is recommended (Tsang et al, 2005). To avoid precipitation in the parenteral solution, the Ca concentration should be maintained between 500 and 600 mg/L (12.5 to 15 mmol/L), and the P concentration should be maintained between 390 and 470 mg/L (12.5 to 15 mmol/L).

Calcium. Calcium transport in the intestine occurs by both passive and active processes. Active intestinal transport involves carriers called calcium-binding proteins. Vitamin D in its active form, 1,25-dihydroxyvitamin D, is essential for the active process. Parathyroid hormone (PTH) is involved only through stimulation of production of 1,25-dihydroxyvitamin D. Vitamin D deficiency and almost any form of intestinal malabsorption can impair calcium transport. Corticosteroids diminish calcium absorption by inhibiting its transfer in the intestinal mucosa. Anticonvulsants can directly inhibit intestinal transfer of calcium (phenytoin) or can interfere with vitamin D metabolism (phenobarbital and phenytoin).

The serum Ca concentration is maintained within narrow limits by the action of parathyroid hormone, 1,25-dihydroxyvitamin D, and calcitonin. PTH and 1,25-dihydroxyvitamin D increase the serum Ca level, and calcitonin reduces it.

The kidneys excrete calcium, and filtered calcium is reabsorbed in most segments of the tubules. Parathyroid hormone increases tubular resorption of calcium, whereas calcitonin is thought to increase calcium excretion. Disorders of calcium balance are listed in Box 15-4.

Hypocalcemia. Neonatal hypocalcemia is defined as an ionized serum Ca concentration below 4.4 mg/dl (1.1 mmol/L) in full-term infants. For preterm infants, for whom insufficient normative data on ionized calcium are available, a total serum Ca concentration below 7 mg/dl (1.75 mmol/L) continues to be a reasonable definition. Hypocalcemia conventionally is divided into early hypocalcemia, which occurs in the first 2 days of life, and late hypocalcemia, which occurs after the first 2 days, usually at about 1 week of age. Neonatal hypocalcemia may be asymptomatic or can cause symptoms such as irritability, tremors, poor feeding, muscle twitching, and seizures.

Early hypocalcemia is relatively common and sometimes is caused by perinatal factors. Approximately 30% of preterm infants (those less than 37 weeks' gestation), 35% of birth-asphyxiated infants, 17% to 32% of infants of insulin-dependent diabetic mothers, and up to 90% of VLBW infants (those weighing less than 1500 g) develop hypocalcemia in the first days of life (DeMarini & Tsang, 2001). Several factors appear to be involved, including abrupt termination of maternal calcium supply, temporary functional hypoparathyroidism (in

---

BOX 15-4

Disorders of Calcium Balance

Hypocalcemia

Early
Preterm infant
Infant of insulin-dependent diabetic mother
Perinatal asphyxia

Late
Cow milk–based formula
Hypomagnesemia
Hypoparathyroidism
Maternal vitamin D deficiency
Osteopetrosis

Hypercalcemia
Excessive administration of calcium or vitamin D (or both)
Subcutaneous fat necrosis
Williams' syndrome
Idiopathic hypercalcemia
Hyperparathyroidism
Hypophosphatasia
Bartter's syndrome
Congenital carbohydrate malabsorptions
Familial hypocalciuric hypercalcemia

---

infants of diabetic mothers), an increased calcitonin concentration (in asphyxiated and preterm infants), and 1,25-dihydroxyvitamin D resistance (in VLBW infants).

Late hypocalcemia typically occurs by the end of the first week of life and is caused by an increase in the dietary phosphate load. It was relatively common with the use of evaporated cow milk formulas, the phosphate content of which greatly exceeded that of human milk. Current formulas have a phosphorus content closer to that of human milk, and late neonatal hypocalcemia is much less common, although it has not disappeared. Maternal vitamin D deficiency may be a predisposing factor. Phototherapy appears to be a cofactor associated with neonatal hypocalcemia, especially in preterm infants. The mechanism is not completely understood.

In rare cases late hypocalcemia can occur as a consequence of subclinical maternal hyperparathyroidism: maternal hypercalcemia leads to fetal hypercalcemia, which suppresses the fetal parathyroid glands. After birth, when the maternal source of calcium is no longer available, the suppressed parathyroid glands are unable to maintain a normal serum Ca concentration. Because the maternal hyperparathyroidism often is asymptomatic, neonatal hypocalcemia may provide the initial clue to the maternal disease. Another uncommon but serious condition that can cause symptomatic hypocalcemia is severe hypomagnesemia (see the section on Magnesium later in the chapter).

Several factors complicate the choice of treatment for neonatal hypocalcemia: (1) It may coexist with other perinatal complications, such as asphyxia and hypoglycemia, which can cause similar clinical signs; (2) it may be associated with seizures without being the cause of the seizures; and (3) in most cases, the condition is asymptomatic and self-limited.

If the hypocalcemia is asymptomatic, 10% calcium gluconate (9.4 mg of elemental calcium per milliliter) may be given orally (PO) at a rate of 75 mg/kg/day divided into six equal doses. If hypocalcemia is symptomatic (e.g., seizures), 10% calcium gluconate must be given intravenously at a rate of 2 ml/kg over 10 minutes; the heart rate should be closely monitored and the infusion stopped immediately at the first sign of bradycardia.

Hypercalcemia. Hypercalcemic disorders (a serum Ca level over 11 mg/dl [2.75 mmol/L]), such as subcutaneous fat necrosis, Williams' syndrome, congenital hyperparathyroidism, Bartter's syndrome, and familial hypocalciuric hypercalcemia, are exceedingly rare among newborns. Hypercalcemia usually is of iatrogenic origin and results from excessive administration of calcium or vitamin D.

The clinical signs, which are nonspecific, include constipation, polyuria, and bradycardia. Nephrocalcinosis and nephrolithiasis caused by hypercalcemia can be aggravated by dehydration and administration of furosemide.

Treatment of hypercalcemia is as follows:

- Calcium and vitamin D supplementation is suspended, and dietary intake of Ca and vitamin D is restricted (human milk or vitamin D—free formula is given).
- Urinary excretion of calcium is promoted by fluid administration (about twice the maintenance requirement).
- In the case of vitamin D excess, glucocorticoids are given to reduce intestinal absorption and bone resorption of calcium.
- With failure of other interventions, pamidronate can be given, although experience with biphosphonates in newborns is limited. Pamidronate is generally given at a dose of 1 mg/kg, as a single 4-hour infusion. In case an additional dose is needed, it should not be given prior to 6 to 7 days, as serum Ca nadir usually occurs by day 6.

Phosphorus. Phosphorus is absorbed mainly in the jejunum by both active and passive diffusion. Absorption depends mainly on the absolute amount of phosphorus in the diet, the relative concentrations of calcium and phosphorus (an excessive amount of either can diminish absorption of the other), and whether substances are present that bind to phosphorus and make it unavailable for absorption (e.g., phytates in soy-based formulas).

The kidneys excrete phosphorus; normally about 10% to 15% of the filtered phosphorus is excreted. Parathyroid hormone directly influences phosphorus excretion through its phosphaturic effect. Disorders of phosphorus balance are listed in Box 15-5.

BOX 15-5

Disorders of Phosphorus Balance

Hypophosphatemia
Rickets/osteopenia of prematurity
Inadequate parenteral phosphorus administration
Malabsorption
Familial hypophosphatemias: vitamin D-resistant rickets, X-linked hypophosphatemia, Fanconi syndrome

Hyperphosphatemia
Impaired excretion of phosphorus: renal failure
Hypoparathyroidism
Excessive parenteral or enteral administration of phosphorus

Hypophosphatemia. Hypophosphatemia (a serum P level below 4 mg/dl [1.29 mmol/L]) is a common feature in preterm infants with rickets of prematurity, which is caused by insufficient intake of calcium and phosphorus. Rickets of prematurity is common in VLBW infants fed regular formulas, especially human milk with low phosphorus content. Preterm formulas provide a higher concentration of calcium and phosphorus and can produce bone mineralization similar to intrauterine bone mineralization. In very rare cases, hypophosphatemia is caused by neonatal hyperparathyroidism.

In infancy, hypophosphatemia can be caused by diseases of vitamin D metabolism (vitamin D–dependent rickets) or by disorders of renal phosphorus transport (familial hypophosphatemic rickets).

Severe hypophosphatemia (a serum P level below 1 mg/dl [0.32 mmol/L]) is uncommon and may occur only in newborns receiving parenteral alimentation with an inadequate amount of phosphorus. Respiratory failure and decreased myocardial performance have been described as possible consequences of severe hypophosphatemia.

Hyperphosphatemia. Neonatal hyperphosphatemia (a serum P level over 7 mg/dl [2.26 mmol/L]) can be caused by ingestion of milk formulas containing high amounts of phosphorus, by excessive parenteral administration of phosphorus, by impaired phosphorus excretion (renal failure), or by defects in hormonal regulation (hypoparathyroidism). Severe hyperphosphatemia may cause metastatic calcifications and hypocalcemia. Management includes alimentation with human milk or with a low-phosphorus formula (e.g., Similac PM 60/40, Columbus, OH, Ross Laboratories) and calcium supplementation to increase binding to phosphorus and its fecal excretion. Reducing the parenteral phosphorus intake usually resolves parenteral hyperphosphatemia. In renal failure, 1,25-dihydroxyvitamin D, which exerts its effects independent of functioning renal tissue, can be given to counteract hypocalcemia secondary to hyperphosphatemia.

Supplementation with 1,25-dihydroxyvitamin D and calcium may be used to treat hypoparathyroidism that arises from maternal hyperparathyroidism (transient hypoparathyroidism) or from DiGeorge syndrome (permanent hypoparathyroidism, which includes some or all of the following features: aplasia of the thymus and parathyroid glands, T-cell immunodeficiency, defects of the aortic arch, and peculiar facies).

Magnesium

Magnesium (Mg) is distributed primarily in the skeleton and the intracellular space. It is involved in energy production, cell membrane function, mitochondrial function, and protein synthesis.

Magnesium is absorbed by passive diffusion throughout the small intestine. Absorption is related to intake, and approximately 50% to 70% of dietary magnesium is absorbed. The kidneys primarily regulate the serum Mg concentration; under normal circumstances, less than 5% of the filtered magnesium is excreted. Parathyroid hormone increases the serum Mg concentration, possibly through mobilization from bone. An acute decline in the serum Mg concentration increases secretion of parathyroid hormone, but chronic magnesium deficiency reduces PTH secretion and therefore may cause hypocalcemia.

The magnesium content of human milk is about 5 mg/ 100 kcal (0.21 mmol/419 kJ). The recommendation for standard

---

BOX 15-6

Disorders of Magnesium Balance

Hypomagnesemia
Infant of diabetic mother
Infant small for gestational age
Malabsorption syndromes
Isolated intestinal magnesium malabsorption

Hypermagnesemia
Maternal treatment with magnesium sulfate (e.g., for tocolysis, pre-eclampsia)
Excessive magnesium administration with parenteral nutrition

---

formulas is 6 mg/100 kcal (0.25 mmol/419 kJ) (AAP, 1998). The recommendation for growing preterm infants is 0.3 to 0.6 mmol/419 kJ (Tsang et al, 2005).

In parenteral nutrition, an intake of 4.3 to 7.2 mg/kg/day (0.2 to 0.3 mmol/kg/day) is recommended. The Mg concentration in the parenteral solution should be maintained between 36 and 48 mg/L (1.5 to 2 mmol/L) to avoid precipitation. Disorders of magnesium balance are listed in Box 15-6.

Hypomagnesemia. Theoretically, magnesium transfer from mother to fetus might be impaired with placental malfunction, and placental insufficiency appears to predispose the infant to neonatal hypomagnesemia (a serum Mg level below 1.6 mg/dl [0.66 mmol/L]). In infants of diabetic mothers, hypomagnesemia appears to be a consequence of maternal magnesium depletion. Any severe malabsorption syndrome can cause magnesium deficiency, and an isolated defect in intestinal absorption of magnesium has been described.

Hypomagnesemia in the neonatal period usually is transient (except in malabsorption cases) and asymptomatic, but it can cause hyperexcitability and, occasionally, severe intractable hypocalcemic seizures that are unresponsive to calcium infusion and anticonvulsants. The mechanism of the resultant hypocalcemia is diminished secretion of PTH caused by magnesium depletion. The treatment is 0.2 ml/kg of 50% magnesium sulfate given intramuscularly (IM) or intravenously. This dose can be repeated, with monitoring of the serum Mg concentration every 12 hours, until normomagnesemia is achieved.

Hypermagnesemia. Neonatal hypermagnesemia (a serum Mg level over 2.8 mg/dl [1.15 mmol/L]) is an iatrogenic event caused either by parenteral nutrition or, more commonly, by maternal treatment with magnesium sulfate (MgSO$_4$) for tocolysis or preeclampsia. Other causes are administration of magnesium-containing antacid for treatment of stress ulcers and treatment of persistent pulmonary hypertension of the newborn with MgSO$_4$. Reported clinical signs of hypermagnesemia include hyporeflexia, lethargy, and respiratory depression. Neonatal serum Mg concentrations rarely rise to potentially dangerous levels and often gradually return to normal after several days. Hypermagnesemia does not cause hypocalcemia in the neonatal period and appears to be associated only with hypotonia. Usually no treatment is necessary. In severe cases, exchange blood transfusion has been used to lower the elevated serum concentrations.

WATER-SOLUBLE VITAMINS
Thiamine (Vitamin B$_1$)
Thiamine is a necessary coenzyme in carbohydrate and amino acid metabolism. Intestinal absorption is both active and passive; transport is active at physiologic concentrations and passive at pharmacologic concentrations. Thiamine is absorbed throughout the small intestine, but mainly in the duodenum. The kidneys excrete thiamine, and urinary excretion varies according to dietary intake.

The thiamine content of human milk is about 210 mcg/L. For standard formulas, the AAP (1998) recommends a minimum content of 40 mcg/100 kcal (0.12 mcmol/419 kJ). The recommendation for growing preterm infants is 0.5 to 0.7 mcmol/kg/day (Tsang et al, 2005). The recommended parenteral intake for stable preterm infants is 0.6 to 1.0 mcmol/kg/day.

Deficiency
Thiamine deficiency results in beriberi, but it is almost never seen in the neonatal period. Infantile beriberi occurs only in breastfed infants of thiamine-deficient mothers. The clinical signs, which become apparent after 1 to 4 months, include aphonia, cardiac signs (dyspnea and cyanosis), and neurologic signs (bulging fontanelle and seizures). Thiamine deficiency can be determined from reduced activity of the erythrocyte enzyme transketolase or by measuring the whole blood thiamine concentration.

Toxicity
Thiamine toxicity has not been reported with oral administration and is very rare in parenteral administration. Very large IV doses of thiamine have caused anaphylaxis and respiratory depression in adults.

Riboflavin (Vitamin B$_2$)
As part of the coenzymes flavin adenine dinucleotide (FAD) and flavin mononucleotide (FMN), riboflavin is involved in electron transport and is essential to glucose, amino acid, and lipid metabolism. Riboflavin is absorbed in the proximal part of the small intestine, and amounts in excess of needs are excreted unchanged in the urine. The average riboflavin content of human milk is approximately 350 mcg/L (Tsang et al, 2005). The AAP (1998) recommends a concentration of 60 mcg/100 kcal (0.16 mcmol/419 kJ) for standard formulas and 200 to 300 mcg/100 kcal (0.53 to 0.80 mcmol/419 kJ) for stable preterm infants. Riboflavin is degraded by light (both sunlight and phototherapy) but is resistant to pasteurization.

Deficiency
Riboflavin deficiency results in epithelial abnormalities (stomatitis, cheilosis, glossitis, seborrheic dermatitis), normocytic anemia, and vascularization of the cornea. Riboflavin intake does not seem to be sufficient in preterm infants fed human milk, especially if the infant undergoes phototherapy. The significance of this deficiency is unclear, but supplementation may be reasonable. However, although the vitamin is inactivated by light, clinical riboflavin deficiency caused by phototherapy has never been reported.

Toxicity
There are no toxic effects of riboflavin. However, grossly abnormal parenteral intakes have been associated to obstructive uropathy in a preterm infant.

Vitamin B₆

Vitamin B_6 is the generic term used to describe three substances: pyridoxine, pyridoxal, and pyridoxamine. The metabolic functions of these vitamins include synthesis of neurotransmitters, heme, and prostaglandins and inter-conversion of amino acids. Absorption occurs in the proximal small intestine by passive diffusion and phosphorylation takes place in the liver. Vitamin B_6 needs are related to protein intake, the mean vitamin/protein ratio being 15 mcg/g.

The vitamin B_6 content of human milk ranges from 130 to 310 mcg/L, depending on maternal intake of the vitamin (Tsang et al, 2005). The AAP (1998) recommends a concentration of 60 mcg/100 kcal (0.29 mcmol/419 kJ) for standard formulas and 125 to 175 mcg/100 kcal (0.61 to 0.85 mcmol/419 kJ) for preterm infants. Vitamin B_6 is inactivated by light. Pyridoxal and pyridoxamine are heat labile, whereas pyridoxine is heat stable and is used for milk fortification.

Deficiency

Vitamin B_6 deficiency can develop with any severe mal-absorption and with dietary deprivation (human milk low in vitamin B_6, improperly sterilized milk, goat milk). Clinical signs include hypochromic microcytic anemia, failure to thrive, irritability, and seizures. Isoniazid binds to and inactivates vitamin B_6; therefore infants receiving this drug may need vitamin B_6 supplementation. Neonatal pyridoxine-dependent seizures are caused by a congenital abnormality of vitamin B_6 metabolism, and pharmacologic doses of vitamin B_6 are needed.

Toxicity

There are no reports of vitamin B_6 toxicity in newborns. However, seizures and sensory neuropathy have been reported in adults taking large doses of pyridoxine.

Cyanocobalamin (Vitamin B₁₂)

Vitamin B_{12} is essential to the synthesis of DNA nucleotides and to carbohydrate and lipid metabolism. Vitamin B_{12} is also necessary in cell folate metabolism. It can be synthesized only by microorganisms and is absent in plants. Absorption of vitamin B_{12} takes place in the distal third of the ileum and requires the presence of intrinsic factor, a glycoprotein secreted by the stomach. The vitamin is transported in plasma by a specific protein (transcobalamin II). Vitamin B_{12} is stored in the liver and preterm infants have much lower stores than term newborns.

The average cobalamin concentration in mature human milk is about 0.7 mcg/L (0.51 nmol/L). The AAP (1998) recommends a cobalamin content of 0.15 mcg/100 kcal (0.11 nmol/419 kJ) in standard formulas and 0.25 mcg/100 kcal (0.18 nmol/419 kJ) for preterm ones. The current recommended intake for growing preterm infants is 0.3 mcg/kg/d (0.22 nmol/kg/day) (Tsang et al, 2005).

Deficiency

Vitamin B_{12} deficiency causes hematologic changes (megalo-blastic anemia, thrombocytopenia, leukopenia with hyper-segmentation of neutrophils) and neurologic changes (demyelination of the spinal cord and mental retardation). Neurologic manifestations may precede anemia. Because liver stores at birth are very large and usually sufficient for most of the first year of life, vitamin B_{12} deficiency rarely develops in infancy.

Since body stores significantly exceed needs, nutritional deficiency occurs exclusively in infants fed breast milk from strictly vegetarian (vegan) mothers. Deficiency in such infants has been described at as early as 4 months of age: signs include developmental delay and anemia. Both vegan mothers and their infants have high urinary concentrations of methyl-malonic acid, as a biochemical marker. Vitamin B_{12} deficiency can develop in infants with short-bowel syndrome if the terminal ileum (the site of absorption) is resected. The onset of vitamin B_{12} deficiency from intrinsic factor deficiency occurs at about 6 months of age. Congenital transcobalamin II deficiency is a rare but important cause of vitamin B_{12} deficiency; signs can occur after only 6 weeks of life, and mental retardation is invariably present. Because both folic acid and vitamin B_{12} deficiency can cause megaloblastic anemia and because folic acid can interfere with vitamin B_{12} metabolism, the differential diagnosis becomes important. A large folate intake may mask the hematologic signs of vitamin B_{12} deficiency and can aggravate the neurologic damage.

Toxicity

Toxicity from vitamin B_{12} has not been reported.

Folic Acid

Folic acid is essential to the synthesis of nucleic acids and to the metabolism of some amino acids. Maximum absorption of folic acid takes place in the proximal jejunum. Absorption is active with physiologic doses of folic acid and mainly passive with pharmacologic doses. Folic acid is stored in the liver in small amounts, but its half-life is prolonged by enterohepatic recirculation. Folic acid can be synthesized by intestinal bacteria.

The average folate concentration in mature human milk is approximately 85 mcg/L (191 nmol/L), although heat treatment reduces the concentration in milk. The current recommendation for standard formulas is 4 mcg/100 kcal (9 nmol/419 kJ) (AAP, 1998). For preterm infants, the current recommended intake is 25 to 50 mcg/kg/day (56 to 113 nmol/kg/day) (Tsang et al, 2005).

Deficiency

Signs of deficiency include hypersegmentation of neutrophils, megaloblastic anemia, poor growth, irritability, and hypotonia. Neurologic disorders, such as seizures and mental retardation, are seen only with the congenital, isolated defect of folic acid absorption. Folic acid deficiency may be associated with prematurity (rapid growth and diminished hepatic stores), hemolytic disease of the newborn (increased erythropoiesis), anticonvulsant therapy (interference with absorption), prolonged antibiotic therapy (diminished production from intestinal bacterial flora), and any malabsorption syndrome.

Toxicity

There are no reports on toxic effects of folic acid in infancy. However, at least theoretically, very large doses of folic acid may reduce the serum concentration of phenytoin. In preterm infants, folic acid may diminish zinc absorption.

Ascorbic Acid (Vitamin C)

Vitamin C is required for collagen synthesis, for normal function of osteoblasts and fibroblasts, for metabolism of some amino acids, and for synthesis of neurotransmitters. It also acts as an antioxidant. Ascorbic acid is actively absorbed in the small intestine, and a feedback mechanism apparently regulates absorption of the vitamin. Very large doses of vitamin C appear to diminish the efficiency of intestinal absorption and to leave affected individuals prone to rebound deficiency once intake declines. Vitamin C is excreted by the kidneys either unchanged or as oxalic acid.

The vitamin C concentration in human milk is about 50 mg/L (284 mcmol/L). The AAP (1998) recommends a concentration of 8 mg/100 kcal (45 mcmol/419 kJ) for standard formulas. The recommendations for stable preterm infants are 18 to 24 mg/kg/day (102 to 136 mcmol/kg/day) (Tsang et al, 2005). Heat treatment (e.g., pasteurization) significantly reduces vitamin C content in milk.

Deficiency

Vitamin C deficiency is very rare but can occur in infants fed pasteurized, unsupplemented cow milk or vitamin C–deficient breast milk. Vitamin C deficiency is associated with transient tyrosinemia and neonatal scurvy.

Transient tyrosinemia arises from a partial enzymatic deficiency that causes an elevation in the serum concentration of the amino acid tyrosine. The tyrosine concentration declines with administration of vitamin C. Transient tyrosinemia is common, occurring in as many as 10% of full-term infants and 30% of preterm infants during the first week of life. The amount of dietary tyrosine also plays a role, because a high protein intake and casein-predominant formulas can increase the serum tyrosine concentration. With the current whey-based formula, this appears to be less of a problem. Additionally, since these transiently elevated concentrations are so common, it seems unlikely that they could be regarded as abnormal.

Neonatal scurvy is very rare. It is characterized by hemorrhages in the skin, subperiosteal spaces, and costochondral cartilage; by anemia resulting from diminished iron absorption; and by failure to thrive. Rebound scurvy, or scurvy that develops after abrupt discontinuation of a large vitamin C intake, has been reported in infants of mothers who took large amounts of vitamin C during their pregnancy (Schanler, 1997).

Toxicity

Large doses of vitamin C may diminish vitamin B_{12} absorption, increase iron absorption, and increase the incidence of nephrolithiasis in congenital disorders such as oxalosis and cystinuria.

Niacin

Niacin includes nicotinic acid and its amide, nicotinamide. As components of the coenzymes nicotinamide adenine dinucleotide (NAD) and nicotinamide adenine dinucleotide phosphate (NADP), niacin is involved in mitochondrial electron transport, lipid synthesis, and glycolysis.

Niacin can also derive from the amino acid tryptophan: consequently, dietary intake of both niacin and tryptophan is evaluated to calculate niacin requirements. For this reason, it is customary to use niacin equivalents (1 mg of niacin = 1 niacin equivalent = 60 mg of tryptophan).

The average concentration of niacin in human milk is 0.8 niacin equivalents/100 kcal, which also is the recommended concentration for standard formulas (AAP, 1998). The

recommendation for growing preterm infants is 3.6 to 4.8 mg/kg/day (30 to 40 mcmol/kg/day) (Tsang et al, 2005). Heating and storage do not significantly affect the niacin content in milk.

Deficiency

Pellagra (rough skin) is the consequence of niacin deficiency. In adults, signs include dermatitis and inflammation of the mucous membranes, diarrhea, and dementia.

Toxicity

Toxicity is related to the proportion of nicotinic acid and may manifest in adults as cutaneous vasodilation, arrhythmias, and increases in intestinal motility and gastric acid secretion.

FAT-SOLUBLE VITAMINS
Vitamin A

Vitamin A exists in many isomeric forms; the basic and most active component is all-trans retinol. Vitamin A can be administered in different forms (retinol itself, palmitate esters of retinol, provitamins) and in different units (micrograms, international units). Vitamin A activity usually is defined as the equivalent weight of retinol (retinol equivalent [RE]). One RE is equal to 1 mcg or 3.33 international units of retinol and to 6 mcg or 10 international units of the provitamin beta carotene. Dietary retinol is absorbed in the proximal intestine, and under normal circumstances, about 50% is absorbed. Retinol is incorporated into chylomicrons and transported to the liver, where it is stored as retinyl esters, mainly in the stellate cells. From the liver, retinol is released into the circulation according to needs. It is transported in plasma, bound to retinol-binding protein, and delivered to tissues. Although liver stores are the main body reserve, vitamin A is stored also in eyes and lungs. Retinol facilitates the visual process in the rod cells of the retina and plays a role in regulating and differentiating epithelial cells. Retinol appears to be necessary for normal lung growth.

With parenteral nutrition, a considerable amount of retinol is lost during delivery, due to both photodegradation and adherence to tubing. Loss during infusion can be corrected by adding vitamin A to IV lipids (Werkman et al, 1994). The average vitamin A concentration in mature human milk is approximately 600 to 2000 international units/L. The AAP (1998) recommends a concentration of 250 to 750 international units (75 to 225 RE/100 kcal) for standard formulas. The recommendation for growing preterm infants is 700 to 1500 international units/kg/day (Tsang et al, 2005). Higher intakes (2000 to 3000 international units/kg/day) may be needed in infants with chronic lung disease (Greer, 2005).

Deficiency

The classic signs of vitamin A deficiency (night blindness, dryness of the cornea progressing to ulceration, perifollicular dermatitis) are of no value in the neonatal period. In clinical practice, a serum retinol concentration below 10 mcg/dl (0.35 mcmol/L) is accepted as indicative of unequivocal vitamin A deficiency. In preterm infants, deficiency is commonly defined by a serum retinol concentration below 20 mcg/dl (0.7 mcmol/L).

Vitamin A deficiency may occur with any form of fat malabsorption (diminished absorption), in preterm infants (low hepatic stores and diminish intake), in infants given parenteral nutrition (adherence of retinol to plastic tubing), and in infants with bronchopulmonary dysplasia. In infants with BPD, vitamin A deficiency may not absolute but relative, possibly owing to an increased requirement for vitamin A. Based on this hypothesis, several trials have been conducted to prevent BPD with large parenteral doses of vitamin A. The results have been analyzed in a Cochrane Review (Darlow & Graham, 2001). At dosages of 2000 to 5000 international units given intramuscularly three times a week, there was no overall difference in oxygen use at one month of age. Vitamin A supplementation was associated with a significant but small reduction in oxygen use at 36 weeks' postconceptional age from 62% to 55% (RR: 0.85). There was no difference in length of stay. As BPD is typically a multifactorial disease and shows marked variations among units, there is no uniform consensus on such therapy.

Toxicity

Vitamin A toxicity occurs from significant overdosage. The clinical signs are those of increased intracranial pressure: bulging anterior fontanelle, vomiting, and other neurologic symptoms. Doses of up to 8500 international units/kg/day have been given to preterm infants without recognizable side effects (Mactier &Weaver, 2005).

Vitamin D

Vitamin D is essential for normal metabolism of calcium and phosphorus. Through the effects of its active form, 1,25-dihydroxyvitamin D, it is necessary for parathyroid hormone action in mobilizing calcium and phosphorus from bone; for intestinal absorption of calcium and phosphorus; and, indirectly, for bone formation.

Vitamin D can be obtained through the diet or can be synthesized by the skin after exposure to sunlight. Regardless of its origin, vitamin D is transported to the liver, where it is converted into 25-hydroxyvitamin D (25-OHD), and subsequently to the kidneys, where it is converted into the final, active metabolite, 1,25-dihydroxyvitamin D. 25-OHD is the major circulating vitamin D metabolite, and it is regarded as an indicator of vitamin D status. It is transferred from mother to fetus, and maternal vitamin D deficiency may be a predisposing factor for late neonatal hypocalcemia.

The serum concentration of 1,25-dihydroxyvitamin D appears to be tightly regulated. The synthesis of 1,25-dihydroxyvitamin D is facilitated by PTH, hypocalcemia, and hypophosphatemia. Placental transfer of 1,25-dihydroxyvitamin D has been demonstrated only after pharmacologic maternal doses. It is not clear if maternal-fetal transfer occurs, at least in significant amounts, under normal circumstances.

The current recommendation is a daily intake of 400 international units for both full-term and preterm infants (AAP, 1998). Breastfed full-term infants receiving adequate exposure to sunlight ($\frac{1}{2}$ to 2 hours per week average with face and hands exposed) do not appear to require vitamin D supplementation. However, as adequate sunlight exposure is difficult to assess, AAP recommends a supplement of 200 international units/day for all breastfed infants, until they are weaned to at least 500 ml/day of vitamin D–fortified milk (Gartner & Greer, 2003).

Deficiency

Vitamin D deficiency results in bone demineralization or rickets. Clinical signs are craniotabes, frontal bossing, widened ribs with enlargement of the costochondral junctions, and muscle weakness.

Laboratory findings include a low serum 25-OHD concentration (as a result of diminished intake); an increased serum PTH level, stimulated by a transiently low blood calcium level (to maintain a normal serum Ca level); normal or increased 1,25-dihydroxyvitamin D level (as a result of PTH stimulation); and restored serum Ca and low serum P concentrations (as a result of the effects of PTH).

Rickets can be caused by inadequate vitamin D intake, by inadequate exposure to sunlight, and by any form of fat malabsorption. Rickets or osteopenia of prematurity, a common disorder in VLBW infants, is caused neither by dietary vitamin D deficiency nor by abnormality of vitamin D metabolism, but by insufficient intake of calcium and phosphorus. A vitamin D dose of 200 international units/kg/day, up to a maximum of 400 international units/day, maintains a normal vitamin D status in preterm infants (Backström et al, 1999).

Toxicity

Excessive doses of vitamin D can cause hypercalcemia, restlessness, polyuria, and failure to thrive. Calcinosis occurs mainly in the kidneys but may also occur in the cardiovascular system, lungs, and intestine.

Vitamin E

Vitamin E is made up of several compounds, named tocopherols, which are important biologic antioxidants; among these, α-tocopherol is believed to be most active. Vitamin E acts as a free radical scavenger and protects the polyunsaturated fatty acid of biologic membranes from peroxidation.

Oral administration of either α-tocopherol or α-tocopherol acetate results in satisfactory absorption. However, fixed oral daily doses of vitamin E can produce variable serum concentrations. Moreover, absorption may be diminished in sick infants. Tocopherols are absorbed in the jejunum and transported by either chylomicrons or low-density lipoproteins to body tissues. The serum tocopherol concentration may not reflect the tissue concentration, because tocopherol is carried by plasma lipoproteins, which are diminished in the newborn. Vitamin E is stored mainly in adipose tissue and in the liver.

Vitamin E is excreted mainly in feces. Biliary excretion is small, and urine excretion is almost negligible. The half-life of tocopherol is approximately 2 days. Because excretion is minimal, vitamin E is cleared from serum by tissue uptake or metabolic degradation, or both.

The average vitamin E concentration in mature human milk is about 2 to 3 international units/L. The recommendation of the American Academy of Pediatrics (1998) for standard formulas is based on both caloric intake and dietary content of polyunsaturated fatty acids: 0.7 international units of vitamin E/100 kcal or at least 0.71 international units of vitamin E per gram of linoleic acid. During the first 2 to 3 weeks of life of enterally fed preterm infants, intake usually is too low to achieve vitamin E sufficiency; therefore the vitamin should be supplemented at a dosage of 6 to 12 international units/kg/day (Tsang et al, 2005).

Pharmacologic doses of vitamin E have shown no benefit for physiologic anemia of prematurity or BPD. The effects on retinopathy of prematurity (ROP) and on intraventricular hemorrhage (IVH) remain controversial. Vitamin E may reduce the overall risk of IVH, but has no effect on severe IVH (grade 3 and 4). With regard to ROP, the overall risk is unchanged, but the risk of developing severe ROP seems to be reduced. Vitamin E supplementation is associated with an increased risk of neonatal sepsis (Brion et al, 2003). Doses exceeding 25 international units/kg/day may result in tissue concentrations greater than those needed for maximum antioxidant effect.

Deficiency

Vitamin E deficiency can occur in two categories of patients: (1) Infants with severe forms of fat malabsorption can develop vitamin E deficiency and neurologic and myopathic abnormalities over several years, and (2) preterm infants fed milk formulas both low in vitamin E and high in polyunsaturated fatty acids may develop, at about 2 months of age, a syndrome consisting of anemia, thrombocytosis, and peripheral edema. Anemia was aggravated by iron supplementation. This syndrome does not seem to occur with current preterm formulas.

Toxicity

Very large doses of vitamin E can cause calcification at injection sites, creatinuria, inhibition of wound healing, and fibrinolysis. An increased incidence of necrotizing enterocolitis has been associated with high oral doses of a hyperosmolar preparation. An intravenous preparation, tocopherol acetate in polysorbate, has been associated with a fatal syndrome consisting of renal failure, thrombocytopenia, hepatomegaly, cholestasis, and ascites.

Vitamin K

Two forms of vitamin K are naturally available: vitamin K_1, or phylloquinone, which is synthesized by plants, and vitamin K_2, or menaquinone, which is synthesized by animals.

Vitamin K is required for the synthesis of coagulation factors II, VII, IX, and X and for conversion of inactive precursors into active clotting factors. Other vitamin K–dependent proteins include plasma protein C and S, osteocalcin, and renal Gla protein. Dietary vitamin K is absorbed in the small intestine and transported with chylomicrons through the lymphatic system. Intestinal bacteria synthesize vitamin K, and this form probably is absorbed in the colon. In adults, about 50% of the total amount of vitamin K in the body comes from intestinal bacteria. The intestine is sterile at birth, and no significant synthesis of vitamin K by the intestinal flora occurs in the first few days of life. The usual intestinal bacteria of breastfed infants do not appear to synthesize vitamin K. The vitamin is stored in the liver, but storage capacity appears to be limited. Excretion occurs mainly with bile in the feces; urinary excretion is quantitatively less important.

The concentration of phylloquinone in human milk is about 2.1 mcg/ml (4.6 mcmol/L); it is about 4.9 mcg/ml (10.9 mcmol/L) in cow milk and 55 to 58 mcg/ml (122 to 129 mcmol/L) in formulas (Greer, 1997). Dietary intake of vitamin K, therefore, depends on both the quality and quantity of ingested milk. A deficiency state is seen almost exclusively in breastfed infants who do not receive vitamin K.

The following recommendations have been made for vitamin K supplementation:

- At birth: 0.5 to 1 mg (1.1 to 2.2 mcmol) given IM
- Infants receiving total parenteral nutrition: Daily supplementation at a dosage of 10 mcg/kg (22 nmol/kg)

or a weekly bolus injection of 0.3 to 1 mg (0.66 to 2.2 mcmol)
- Standard formulas: A minimum concentration of 4 mcg/100 kcal (9 nmol/419 kJ) (AAP, 1998)
- Preterm infants: An intake of 6.66 to 8.33 mcg/100 kcal (15 to 18.5 nmol/419 kJ)

Deficiency

Vitamin K deficiency may result in vitamin K deficiency bleeding (VKDB). Bleeding usually occurs from the umbilical stump or after minor procedures (e.g., circumcision, blood sampling), but serious events such as gastrointestinal and cerebral hemorrhages are also possible.

Three clinical forms of VKDB, early, classic, and late, have been recognized.

- The early type occurs on the first day of life in infants born to mothers receiving anticonvulsant therapy (phenytoin, phenobarbital). These infants should be given an injection of vitamin K intramuscularly immediately after birth. This form of the disease may be prevented by antepartum maternal vitamin K supplementation.
- The classic type occurs between 2 and 10 days of life in breastfed infants who were not given vitamin K at birth. This form can be prevented by both IM and oral vitamin K supplementation.
- The late type, the most common form of the disease, occurs at 2 to 12 weeks of age, in breastfed infants with inadequate or no prophylaxis and in infants with fat malabsorption. This type is frequently complicated by intracranial bleeding, and it has a high mortality rate.

According to the AAP, vitamin K should be given to all newborns as a single intramuscular dose of 0.5 to 1 mg (AAP, 2003). Such a prophylaxis prevents the late form of VKDB, with the rare exception of severe malabsorption syndromes (Von Kries, 1999). Multiple daily or weekly oral doses, during the first 12 weeks of life, may be as effective as a single dose given intramuscularly (Wariyara et al, 2000).

Toxicity

There is no evidence of vitamin K toxicity, except for RBC hemolysis and hyperbilirubinemia after administration of large doses of the synthetic vitamin K_3 (menadione).

TRACE MINERALS
Zinc

Zinc, as a cofactor, is necessary for the synthesis of nucleic acids and for the metabolism of proteins, lipids, and carbohydrates; it therefore is essential to normal growth and development.

Zinc accumulation in the fetus mainly occurs during the third trimester. Consequently, preterm infants have lower body stores than full-term infants. However, stores are limited in both full-term and preterm infants, and dietary intake is essential for maintaining optimum zinc status in the newborn. Zinc is absorbed in the duodenum and proximal jejunum. Although cases of zinc deficiency in breastfed infants have been reported, zinc absorption is greater from human milk than from formulas. Excretion occurs mainly through feces; urinary excretion is far less important.

The zinc concentration in human milk ranges from 60 to 22 mcmol/L (Atkinson & Zlotkin, 1997) and declines over time. Healthy preterm infants given 23 mcmol/kg/day show a retention rate similar to the intrauterine accretion rate (Wastney et al, 1999).

The recommended concentration of zinc for standard formulas is 500 mcg/100 kcal (7.5 mcmol/419 kJ) (AAP, 1998). The current recommendation for enteral feedings in growing preterm infants is 1000 to 3000 mcg/kg/day (15.3 to 45.9 mcmol/kg/day) (Tsang et al, 2005). With parenteral nutrition, a zinc intake of 400 mcg/kg/day (6.1 mcmol/kg/day) is recommended for stable preterm infants.

Deficiency

Zinc deficiency can arise from inadequate intake, diminished absorption (preterm infant), or increased loss (malabsorption syndromes, ostomies). A serum zinc concentration below 40 mcg/dl (6.1 mcmol/L) is generally accepted as an indication of deficiency. However, in mild, subclinical zinc deficiency, serum zinc concentration can be in the low normal range.

Dietary zinc deficiency has been reported only in breastfed preterm infants, owing to the large variations in the zinc concentration of human milk. Signs of deficiency include reduced growth velocity, acro-orificial rash, hypoproteinemia, and generalized edema. In preterm infants, postnatal zinc supplementation seems to have a positive effect on linear growth (Diaz-Gomez et al, 2003). Acrodermatitis enteropathica is an autosomal recessive disease that involves a defect in the intestinal absorption of zinc. The disease is characterized by a dermatitis that affects the extremities and perioral/perigenital areas; diarrhea; and failure to thrive, which progresses to thymic atrophy and immunodeficiency.

Toxicity

Zinc toxicity has not been reported in newborns. Overdosage may result in copper deficiency and an increase in the serum cholesterol concentration.

Copper

Copper is necessary for normal functioning of oxidative enzymes (e.g., cytochrome oxidase) and for synthesis of collagen, melanin, and catecholamines. Both full-term and preterm infants are born with significant liver stores (Atkinson & Zlotkin, 1997). Active absorption takes place mainly in the duodenum. Copper absorption appears to be greater with human milk than with formulas. In plasma, approximately two thirds of copper is bound to ceruloplasmin. In newborns, limited ceruloplasmin synthesis results in low plasma ceruloplasmin and, consequently, a low serum copper concentration. Neither the serum copper level nor the ceruloplasmin concentration is an adequate index of copper status in the first weeks of life. Preterm infants show lower copper and ceruloplasmin levels than term infants for many months. Copper excretion occurs almost exclusively through the bile.

Despite wide variation in copper content, human milk appears adequate for both full-term and preterm infants. The recommended copper concentration for standard formulas is 60 mcg/100 kcal (0.93 mcmol/419 kJ) (AAP, 1998). The recommendation for stable, growing preterm infants is 120 to 150 mcg/kg/day (1.9 to 2.4 mcmol/kg/day). With parenteral nutrition, a copper intake of 20 mcg/kg/day (0.31 mcmol/kg/day) is recommended for stable preterm infants (Tsang et al, 2005).

Deficiency

Copper deficiency can result from inadequate intake (cow milk, total parenteral nutrition) or increased loss (malabsorption syndromes, ostomies).

Clinical signs of copper deficiency include pallor (as a result of anemia and hypopigmentation), hypotonia, psychomotor retardation, hypochromic anemia unresponsive to iron therapy, neutropenia, osteoporosis, pseudoscurvy, and failure to thrive (Atkinson & Zlotkin, 1997; Hoyle et al, 1999). Signs are usually identified after the first month of life.

Toxicity

Copper toxicity has not been reported in newborns. However, IV administration of normal amounts to infants with cholestasis results in liver damage, because excess copper cannot be excreted. Exogenous copper intoxication may be one of the causes of infantile cirrhosis (Dieter et al, 1999).

MANAGEMENT

Obtaining vascular access in a sick newborn has become as routine a part of the admission procedure as obtaining vital signs and weighing the patient. Nurses and physicians are responsible for providing peripheral or central vascular access and ensuring safe delivery of IV fluids. They also must be able to recognize the signs and symptoms of disorders in hydration and prevent complications that may be associated with fluid administration.

Assessment and Evaluation in Fluid and Electrolyte Therapy

The estimation of a patient's fluid and nutritional needs depends on the infant's age and weight and the disease process involved. The fluid and electrolyte needs of a 4-kg infant with perinatal asphyxia and seizures are different from those of a 32-week, 1750-g infant with RDS or a 23-week, 460-g infant with multiple complex needs. These infants represent varying points on the continuum of fetal growth and development; each represents a different disease process; and each also requires careful management of fluid and electrolytes to maintain homeostasis.

Fluid needs can be calculated using body weight, body surface area, or caloric expenditure (Behrman et al, 2004). Caloric expenditure is an easy method in which the infant's caloric needs are calculated, and fluid and electrolyte requirements are related to it. To begin these calculations, it must be remembered that 1 kcal is the amount of heat needed to raise the temperature of 1 L of water by 1° C. Caloric expenditures up to 10 kg = 100 calories/kg/24 hours. For example, a 1700-g infant would expend 170 calories in 24 hours, whereas a 460-g infant would expend 46 calories in 24 hours. This can be expressed as Energy intake = Energy stored + Energy expended + Energy excreted (Ambalavanan, 2002).

Caloric expenditures can be modified by an increase or decrease in body temperature and by specific disease states. Caloric expenditure can be used to determine water needs, because for every 100 calories metabolized, 100 ml of fluid is needed (Behrman et al, 2004). Water needs are determined by calculating IWL from the skin and pulmonary system and actual losses from the urine, stool, and sweat (Table 15-4).

Insensible water loss (IWL) can be affected by a variety of factors, including skin integrity and the degree of that integrity. An example of this is the newborn infant with a large

TABLE 15-4	Fluid Intake and Output in Neonates	
	Range (ml/100 cal/24 hr)	Average* (ml/100 cal/24 hr)
OUTPUT		
Insensible water losses		
Pulmonary	10 to 20	15
Skin	25 to 35	30
Urine	50 to 70	60
Stool	5 to 10	7
Sweat	0 to 20	0
INTAKE		
All fluids consumed		112
Water of oxidation		−12

Average maintenance requirement is 100 ml/100 cal/day.

TABLE 15-5	Electrolyte Components of Intravenous Fluids	
Solution	mEq Na/1000 ml	mEq Na/100 ml
D_5W ½ NS (dextrose 5%, ½ strength, normal saline)	77	7.7
D_5W ¼ NS	38.5	

Na, Sodium.

gastroschisis. This midline abdominal wall defect predisposes the infant to large insensible water losses because of the exposed abdominal organs and absent omentum or peritoneum. Another example is a 23-week, 400-g infant with the typical "translucent" skin that has not yet formed a protective keratin layer; this condition predisposes the infant to dehydration secondary to large insensible water loss through the skin. Environmental factors also affect IWL; these factors include the presence or absence of humidity and increased or decreased ambient temperature. The use of radiant warmers has long been understood to affect an infant's fluid status by increasing insensible losses in a relatively open, unprotected environment. Phototherapy has similar effects, with the additional problem of thermoregulation. Increases in the metabolic rate, body temperature, and activity all must be included in the calculation of fluid needs.

Fluids usually are calculated on a daily basis, taking into consideration past losses, projected losses, and maintenance requirements. However, depending on the disease process, fluids may need to be calculated more often, even as often as every 4 hours, to keep up with losses and to make appropriate adjustments in fluid therapy. A general estimate of fluid requirements can be calculated on the basis of the guidelines presented in Table 15-1. Again, these are just guidelines; requirements differ according to gestational age and disease process. The fluid requirement for a premature, low-birth-weight infant may be as high as 150 to 200 ml/kg/day in some cases during the first 24 hours of life; on the other hand, for a full-term, asphyxiated infant, fluids may be restricted to no more than 40 to 50 ml/kg/day for the first 72 hours of life.

Electrolyte requirements usually are calculated on the basis of 100 calories metabolized:

- Sodium: 2 to 3 mEq/100 cal/24 hours (2 to 3 mEq/kg/day)
- Potassium: 1 to 2 mEq/100 cal/24 hours (1 to 2 mEq/kg/day)

Standard IV solutions containing a predetermined amount of sodium are routinely used in neonatal intensive care units (e.g., 5% dextrose in 0.45% NaCl) with potassium chloride and other electrolytes or minerals added as indicated (Table 15-5).

Caloric requirements cannot be met solely by the IV solutions commonly used in NICUs (i.e., 5% or 10% dextrose). These solutions are relatively low in calories; there are only 4 calories per gram of glucose (carbohydrate). The number of

calories in intravenous solutions is calculated on a percent solution and based on grams per 100 ml. Therefore 5% dextrose in water (D_5W) contains 5 g of dextrose per 100 ml of fluid, 10% dextrose in water ($D_{10}W$) contains 10 g/100 ml, and so on. To carry this calculation further, D_5W and $D_{10}W$ IV solutions contain 20 and 40 calories, respectively (D_5W = 5 g/100 ml at 4 cal/g = 20 cal).

The dextrose concentration used also depends on the infant's gestational age and renal function. The premature kidneys, unable to concentrate urine and conserve electrolytes and glucose, may alter glucose excretion, "spilling sugar" into the urine. An essential test of the infant's response to IV glucose therapy can easily be done at the bedside with a urine dipstick and a few drops of urine. This test can detect glucose, protein, ketones, and blood in the urine and can determine the pH level, an important indicator of acid-base balance.

Determination of the specific gravity is another essential bedside test that requires only a few drops of urine. The specific gravity, which normally is between 1.008 and 1.012, is an early indicator of hydration status. The urine dipstick and specific gravity tests should be performed at least every shift while the infant is receiving IV fluids and more often as the infant's condition warrants.

Fluid intake and output should be strictly monitored to ensure adequate hydration. Giving too much or too little fluid affects urine output (UOP), as do disease processes such as acute renal failure and drug administration (e.g., indomethacin or aminoglycoside antibiotics). UOP is monitored and calculated hourly over a 24-hour period. It should be no less than 1 ml/kg/hour/day. For example, for a 2-kg infant:

$$UOP = 240 \text{ ml/24 hours} = 10 \text{ ml/2 kg} = 5 \text{ ml/kg/hour}$$

This is an adequate UOP for an infant of this weight and gestation.

For infants requiring long-term IV therapy, total parenteral nutrition (TPN) is used to improve nutritional status, and it may be started within the first 24 to 72 hours of life. TPN spares protein, increases calories and, when used in conjunction with Intralipid (Abbott Labs, Abbott Park, IL), an IV fat emulsion preparation, further maximizes caloric intake. If the TPN solution is infused through a peripheral vein, the glucose concentration is limited to no more than 12.5% because of the risks of tissue irritation and sloughing with infiltration; however, if the solution is infused through central lines, a higher glucose concentration may be used. With this route, in addition to the increased glucose concentration (which increases calories), higher concentrations of protein, fat, and other essential minerals and trace elements may be infused.

Caloric supplementation with TPN is as follows:
- Glucose: (4 cal/g): 2.5 to 12.5 g/100 ml (e.g., 2.5% to 12.5% solutions)
- Protein (4 cal/g): 1 to 3 g/kg/day; 4 to 12 cal/kg/day
- Fat (9 cal/g): Up to 4 g/kg/day (20% emulsion, 2 cal/ml)

The nurse is responsible for monitoring hourly fluid intake and should always double-check fluid orders to ensure that the ordered rate and solution are appropriate for that infant.

Weight is an important indicator of overall fluid status. Infants are usually weighed daily; extremely-low-birth-weight (ELBW) infants and infants with excessive fluid losses and needs may be weighed more often (i.e., every 12 hours or even every 6 hours) with fluid needs recalculated on the basis of weight changes. It is important to weigh infants carefully, because inaccuracies that show extreme weight fluctuations can have a detrimental impact on therapy. For example, an inaccurate weight measurement showing an increase of 100 g in a 12-hour period for an infant with severe RDS may result in giving that infant an unnecessary dose of furosemide. The infant should be weighed nude, with as much equipment removed as possible (e.g., ECG leads, probes), at the same time each day, and on the same scale. In-bed scales that give constant weight readouts simplify the weighing process and cause the infant minimal stress.

The physical examination can reveal changes in the infant's fluid status and should be used in conjunction with laboratory data to plan interventions in fluid and electrolyte therapy. A general assessment for hydration status includes the infant's color, skin turgor, activity, mucous membranes, fontanelles, vital signs, and UOP, as follows:

- Color: Pink and well perfused rather than pale and mottled (indicates dehydration)
- Skin turgor: Good turgor, rather than "tenting" (indicates dehydration) or edematous and shiny (indicates fluid overload)
- Activity: Active with good tone, rather than lethargic and hypotonic (indicates dehydration or overhydration)
- Mucous membranes: Pink and moist, rather than dry and gray (indicates dehydration)
- Fontanelles: Soft and flat, rather than depressed (indicates dehydration) or tense and full (may indicate overhydration)
- Vital signs: Heart rate, rhythm, blood pressure and temperature within normal range for gestational age
- UOP: Normal (e.g., approximately 1 ml/kg/hr), rather than excessive (indicates overhydration), diminished, or absent (indicating dehydration)

SUMMARY

The care of infants with alterations in fluid and electrolyte balance presents a management challenge for both physicians and nurses. A thorough understanding of the underlying pathophysiology and the rationale for therapy enables the health care team to provide more informed care for these infants and to anticipate and prevent problems.

REFERENCES

Ambalavanan N (2002). Fluid, electrolyte, and nutrition management of the newborn. Available at: http://www.emedicine.com. Retrieved October 1, 2005.

American Academy of Pediatrics, Committee on Nutrition (1998). *Pediatric nutrition handbook.* Elk Grove Village, IL: American Academy of Pediatrics.

American Academy of Pediatrics, Committee on Fetus and Newborn (2003). Controversies concerning vitamin K and the newborn. *Pediatrics* 112: 191-192.

Atkinson SA, Zlotkin SH (1997). Recognizing deficiencies and excesses of zinc, copper, and other trace elements. In Tsang RC et al, editors. *Nutrition during infancy.* Cincinnati, OH: Digital Educational Publishing.

Backström MC et al (1999). Randomised controlled trial of vitamin D supplementation on bone density and biochemical indices in preterm infants. *Archives of disease in childhood: fetal and neonatal edition* 80: F161-F166.

Baumgart S, Costarino AT (2000). Water and electrolyte metabolism in the micropremie. *Clinics in perinatology* 27:131-146.

Behrman RE et al (2004). *Nelson textbook of pediatrics.* Philadelphia: Saunders.

Brion LP et al (2003). Vitamin E supplementation for prevention of morbidity and mortality in preterm infants. *Cochrane database of systematic reviews,* CD003665.

Darlow BA, Graham PJ (2001). Vitamin A supplementation for preventing morbidity and mortality in very low birth weight infants (Cochrane Review). In *The Cochrane library,* Issue 2, Oxford.

DeMarini S, Tsang RC (2001). Disorders of calcium, phosphorus, and magnesium metabolism. In Fanaroff AA, Martin RJ, editors. *Neonatal perinatal medicine.* St Louis: Mosby.

Diaz-Gomez NM et al (2003). The effect of zinc supplementation on linear growth, body composition, and growth factors in preterm infants. *Pediatrics* 111:1002-1009.

Dieter HH et al (1999). Early childhood cirrhosis in Germany between 1982 and 1994 with special consideration of copper etiology. *European journal of medical research* 4:233-242.

Gartner LM, Greer FR (2003). American Academy of Pediatrics, Section on Breastfeeding and Committee on Nutrition. Prevention of rickets and vitamin D deficiency: new guidelines for vitamin D intake. *Pediatrics* 111:908-910.

Greer FR (1997). Special needs and dangers of fat-soluble vitamins A, E, and K. In Tsang RC et al, editors. *Nutrition during infancy.* Cincinnati, OH: Digital Educational Publishing.

Greer FR (2005). Vitamin A, E and K. In Tsang RC et al, editors. *Nutritional needs of the preterm infant: scientific basis and practical guidelines.* Cincinnati, OH: Digital Educational Publishing.

Hoyle GS et al (1999). Pseudoscurvy caused by copper deficiency. *Journal of pediatrics* 134:379.

Lorenz JM et al (1995). Phases of fluid and electrolyte homeostasis in the extremely low birth weight infant. *Pediatrics* 196:484-489.

Mactier H, Weaver LT (2005). Vitamin A and preterm infants: what we know, what we don't know and what we need to know. *Archives of diseases of childhood: fetal and neonatal edition* 90:F103-F108.

Modi N (2003). Clinical implications of postnatal alterations in body water distribution. *Seminars in neonatology* 8:301-306.

Schanler RJ (1997). Who needs water-soluble vitamins? In Tsang RC et al, editors. *Nutrition during infancy.* Cincinnati, OH: Digital Educational Publishing.

Tsang RC et al (2005). *Nutritional needs of the preterm infant: scientific basis and practical guidelines.* Cincinnati, OH: Digital Educational Publishing.

Von Kries R (1999). Oral versus intramuscular phytomenadione: safety and efficacy compared. *Drug safety* 21:1-6.

Wariyara U et al (2000). Six years' experience of prophylactic oral vitamin K. *Archives of disease in childhood: fetal and neonatal edition* 82:F64-F68.

Wastney ME et al (1999). Zinc absorption, distribution, excretion, and retention by healthy preterm infants. *Pediatric research* 45:191-196.

Werkman SH et al (1994). Effect of vitamin A supplementation of intravenous lipids on early vitamin A intake and status of premature infants. *American journal of clinical nutrition* 59:586-592.

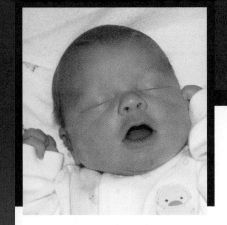

Chapter 16

Neonatal and Infant Pharmacology

Beth Shields

Neonatal and infant pharmacology requires an understanding of the impact of immature organ systems on pharmacologic drug response. Research in pharmacology has lagged behind the enhanced survival rates for sick newborn infants of all birth-weight subgroups. Optimal understanding of infant pharmacology is of vital importance, as the average number of drugs administered to premature infants weighing less than 1000 g ranges from 15 to 20 (Soldin et al, 2002; Raj, 2005). This chapter will review the basic principles of neonatal and infant drug therapy. Discussion of the nursing implications is included.

GENERAL PRINCIPLES OF DRUG THERAPY

The individualization of drug therapy in premature and term infants is essential because of rapid and variable maturation of all physiologic and pharmacologic processes. The phrase *therapeutic orphans*, coined more than 25 years ago, stresses the relative lack of drug safety and efficacy information in the pediatric population (Shirkey, 1968). Thirty years later, published literature on the use of medications in the pediatric population remains sparse. Three-fourths of prescription drugs marketed in the United States lack pediatric use information (Committee on Drugs, 2002). Conducting well-controlled trials is difficult, and therapeutic regimens are often supported by case reports, small studies, or past experiences of a particular clinician.

PEDIATRIC OFF-LABEL USE

The Food and Drug Administration (FDA) approves the initial labeling of a medication. However, once a drug is FDA approved, it may be prescribed by a licensed provider for any indication deemed appropriate. Over the past several years, legislation has been passed to encourage that safety, pharmacogenomic, pharmacokinetic, and pharmacodynamic data be collected to aid in pediatric-specific labeling for medications. The Food and Drug Modernization Act is one important piece of legislation. The strongest incentive of this act is a 6-month patent exclusivity awarded to a product if pediatric labeling is obtained (Brummel, 2001; Spielberg, 2001; Yaffe, 2003; Woo, 2004). A list of drugs with such current exclusivity are outlined in the Pediatric Exclusivity Provision (Best Pharmaceuticals Act for Children, 2001, http://www.fda.gov/cder/pediatric).

PEDIATRIC DOSING METHODS

Infants are not small adults and, as such, cannot simply be given a portion of an adult dose. Drug dosages must be prescribed for each infant on an individual basis. Their unique pharmacotherapeutic requirements predispose this population to errors in individual dosage calculations. Guidelines have been developed in an attempt to prevent dosing errors in this diverse patient population (American Academy of Pediatrics, 2003; Levine et al, 2001).

Several dosing methods have been used to calculate the optimal drug dose for both preterm and full-term infants. Pediatric dosage handbooks employ dosing methods based on age, body weight, and body surface area (BSA) as well as pharmacokinetic dosing (Taketomo et al, 2004; Young & Mangum, 2004). Each method provides only an estimate, and dosages must constantly be reevaluated and adjusted according to clinical efficacy and toxicity.

To calculate a drug dosage based on age or body weight, it is important to understand the meaning of terms commonly used in the pediatric population (Table 16-1). Because of ease of calculation, dosing based on weight (mg/kg/dose or mg/kg/day) is the most common method. Weight-based dosing is expressed as a dosage range vs an absolute dose. Dosing based on BSA (mg/m^2/dose) requires both a weight and height to accurately assess an infant's BSA. Lack of appropriate pediatric dosing information makes this method impractical except with steroids and chemotherapeutic agents. Pharmacokinetic dosing is discussed in detail in the following sections.

ADVERSE DRUG EFFECTS

Like the elderly, infants are prone to adverse drug events (ADEs). An ADE is an injury (both preventable and not preventable) that results from the use of a drug (Holdsworth, 2003; Woods, 2005). Unique drug delivery factors including individual dosage calculations, preparation of small doses from concentrated commercial solutions, and slow IV rates make neonates more prone to ADEs.

Neonates are particularly predisposed to ADEs because of immature metabolic and excretion pathways as well as potential drug exposures during pregnancy, delivery, and lactation. A study that included 800 infants exposed to medications through breast milk revealed that 11% of infants experienced ADEs. The rate of adverse events rose to approximately 16% when multiple medications were used during breastfeeding (Howard & Lawrence, 2001).

Several classic neonatal ADEs have occurred because of lack of knowledge or forethought regarding developmental differences between neonates and older infants and children.

TABLE 16-1	Pediatric Drug Dosing: Age/Weight Terminology	
Term	**Definition**	
Gestational age (GA)	By dates: number of weeks from the onset of mother's last menstrual period until birth	
	By examination: assessment of gestation (time from conception until birth) by a physical and neuromuscular examination	
Low-birth-weight (LBW)	Birth weight of <2500 g	
Very-low-birth-weight (VLBW)	Birth weight of <1500 g	
Small-for-gestational-age (SGA)	Birth weight <10th percentile for GA	
Appropriate for gestational age	Birth weight between age (AGA) 10th and 90th percentile for GA	
Large for gestational age (LGA)	Birth weight >90th percentile for GA	
Postnatal age (PNA)	Chronologic age (in days) after birth	
Postconceptional age (PCA)	GA at birth plus PNA	
Preterm infant	<37 completed weeks GA at birth	
Full-term infant	38 to 42 weeks GA at birth	
Neonate	0 to 28 days PNA	
Infant	1 month to 1 year of age	
Child	1 to 12 years of age	

Data adapted from El-Chaar G (2003). Pharmaceutical care in premature infants. US pharmacist HS13-HS31; and Committee on Fetus and Newborn, American Academy of Pediatrics (AAP) (2004). Age terminology during the perinatal period. Pediatrics 114(5):1326-1364.

Examples of such ADEs include chloramphenicol-associated gray baby syndrome, neonatal gasping syndrome, and numerous case reports of ADEs caused by absorption of drugs through the skin of newborn infants (Robertson, 2003a, 2003b; Kaushal et al, 2001).

The enhanced survival of extremely premature infants must raise awareness concerning increased risk of serious short- and long-term adverse effects of neonatal drug therapy. Recent data support an increased incidence of neurodevelopmental delay and cerebral palsy in infants treated with systemic dexamethasone in the prevention of chronic lung disease. Furthermore, studies have demonstrated conflicting short- and

long-term neurologic outcomes in infants treated with inhaled nitric oxide therapy (Committee on Fetus and Newborn, 2002; Mestan et al, 2005; Van Meurs et al, 2005).

DEVELOPMENTAL PHARMACOKINETICS

Pharmacokinetics is the study of a drug concentration vs time and encompasses the absorption, distribution, metabolism, and elimination (ADME) of a drug and its metabolites in the body. Developmental pharmacokinetics—or the change in the ADME of drugs with organ maturation—is a well-known phenomenon (Table 16-2). To fully comprehend the ADME of drugs, pharmacokinetic terminology must be applied. Standard

TABLE 16-2	Developmental Pharmacokinetics in the Neonate		
Route of Administration	**ADME**	**Alteration in Kinetics**	**Therapeutic Implication**
Oral	Absorption	Prolonged gastric emptying time	Delayed oral absorption; decrease serum peak concentrations
Oral	Absorption	Relative achlorhydria	Increased absorption of basic drugs; decreased absorption of acidic drugs
Intramuscular	Absorption	Decreased muscle mass, decreased muscle blood flow, decreased muscle activity	Decreased/erratic drug absorption
Percutaneous	Absorption	Decreased thickness of stratum corneum; increased skin hydration, increased BSA/weight ratio	Increased percutaneous absorption, increased systemic toxicity
All*	Distribution	Increased ECF and TBW	Increased doses (mg/kg) for water-soluble drugs
All*	Distribution	Decreased plasma protein binding (PPB)	Increased volume of distribution, increased free fraction
All*	Metabolism	Immature hepatic enzyme activity	Decreased drug clearance
All*	Excretion	Immature glomerular and tubular function	Decreased drug clearance

Data from Soldin OP et al (2002). Review: therapeutic drug monitoring in pediatrics. Therapeutic drug monitoring 24(1):1-8; El-Chaar G (2003). Pharmaceutical care in premature infants. US pharmacist HS13- HS31; Woo TM (2004). Pediatric pharmacology update: essential concepts for prescribing. Advance nursing practice 12(6):22-27; and Kearns GL et al (2003). Developmental pharmacology—drug disposition, action, and therapy in infants and children. New England journal of medicine 349(12):115-1167.
BSA, Body surface area; ECF, extracellular fluid; TBW, total body water.
*All routes of administration include oral, parenteral, percutaneous, and rectal.

TABLE **16-3**		Pharmacokinetic Terminology
Pharmacokinetic Term	**Abbreviation**	**Definition**
Bioavailability	F	The extent to which a drug enters the systemic circulation
Volume of	Vd	The relation between the distribution amount of drug in the body and the measured plasma concentration
Clearance	Cl	The ability of eliminating organs to remove a drug from the blood or plasma
Elimination half-life	$t^{1/2s}$	The time required for half the amount of drug present in the blood to disappear
Steady-state concentration	Cpss	A concentration at which the rate of drug administration is equal to the rate of drug elimination

Data adapted from Soldin OP et al (2002). Review: therapeutic drug monitoring in pediatrics. Therapeutic drug monitoring 24(1):1-8.

pharmacokinetic terminology is used when describing the ADME of medications (Table 16-3).

In addition to the pharmacokinetics of a drug, the pharmacodynamics of a particular medication is also important. Pharmacodynamics is the relationship between the pharmacokinetics of a drug and its therapeutic or toxic effects in a specific patient. Pediatric drug dosing regimens are influenced by both the effect of the body on a drug (pharmacokinetics) as well as the effect of a drug on the body (pharmacodynamics) (Figure 16-1). Recent data support age-dependent differences in the interaction of a drug and its receptors, ultimately resulting in an altered pharmacodynamic response. (Kearns et al 2003).

Absorption

Absorption refers to the translocation of a drug from the site of administration into the systemic circulation. With the exception of the intravenous route, all other routes of administration require a drug to cross membranes in order to reach the systemic circulation and exert its pharmacologic effects. Bioavailability is the pharmacokinetic term that has been used to describe the extent to which a drug enters the systemic circulation (Soldin et al, 2002). Drugs administered via the intravenous route are 100% bioavailable.

Drug absorption depends on the physiochemical properties of the drug—including molecular weight, degree of ionization, lipid solubility, and drug formulation characteristics. In addition, patient-dependent factors, many of which are age-related, affect drug absorption (Kearns et al, 2003; Woo, 2004; El-Chaar, 2003; Soldin et al, 2002).

Medications are administered to infants via many routes including oral (PO), intravenous (IV), intramuscular (IM), percutaneous, and rectal administration. Parenteral administration (IV) of drugs is important when a rapid response is desired or clinical status precludes oral absorption. Muscle tone, muscle mass, and regional blood flow to the area influence absorption of medications from an IM injection. Neonates, particularly premature neonates, may have significantly decreased muscle mass, as muscle mass is directly proportional to an infant's gestational age (Kearns et al, 2003; El-Chaar, 2003). The IM injection of a medication may result in a delay in peak serum concentrations due to poor or erratic absorption. Medications commonly administered to neonates via the IM route include vitamin K, ampicillin, and gentamicin.

Absorption from the gastrointestinal tract depends on factors including gastric acidity, gastric emptying time, bacterial colonization of the gastrointestinal tract, intestinal transit time and permeability, and biliary and pancreatic function (Kearns et al, 2003; El-Chaar, 2003; Woo, 2004). The maturation of gastric pH differs in preterm vs. term infants and seems to correlate with postnatal age rather than postconceptional age. The gastric pH at birth approaches 6 to 8 because of the presence of residual amniotic fluid, falls to approximately 1.5 to 3 several hours after birth, and then slowly increases over the next 10 days in term infants. The lack of gastric acid output early in postnatal life is called *relative achlorhydria.*

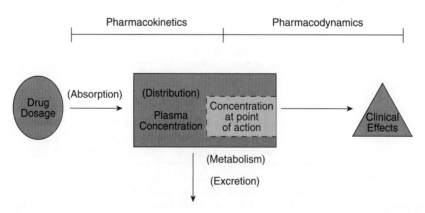

FIGURE **16-1**
Relationship between pharmacokinetics and pharmacodynamics. From McLeod HL, Evans WE (1992). Pediatric pharmacokinetics and therapeutic drug monitoring. *Pediatrics in review* 13(11):420.

Gastric pH will reach adult values by 2 years of age (Woo, 2004; El-Chaar, 2003). Gastric pH affects drug ionization and drug absorption. A more basic environment (higher gastric pH) will decrease the absorption of acidic drugs (i.e., phenytoin, phenobarbital) and favor the oral absorption of more basic or acid-labile drugs (i.e., ampicillin, penicillin, and erythromycin).

Most drugs are absorbed in the small intestine. Therefore gastric emptying time will play an important role in both the rate and extent of oral drug absorption. Gastric emptying time is delayed in the neonatal patient, especially in the premature infant. Gastric emptying may be prolonged up to 6 to 8 hours and may not attain adult values until 6 to 8 months of age. Oral absorption may also be delayed in the neonate because of decreased intestinal transit time and activity of pancreatic enzymes as well as low concentrations of intraluminal bile acids (Kearns et al, 2003; Woo, 2004; El-Chaar, 2003).

Percutaneous absorption or absorption through the skin depends on skin integrity, blood flow to the skin, thickness of the epidermal layer (i.e., stratum corneum), skin hydration, and the ratio of surface area per kilogram of body weight (BSA to weight ratio) (El-Chaar, 2003). Percutaneous absorption may be increased substantially in newborn infants because of an underdeveloped stratum corneum, smaller amounts of subcutaneous fat, and increased skin hydration. Maturation of premature skin is related to postnatal age, and the attainment of an epidermal layer similar to that of a full-term neonate occurs within 3 weeks of postnatal life. The greater the BSA to weight ratio, the greater the absorption of a drug is on a per-kilogram basis with topical medications. The ratio of a newborn's skin to body surface area is approximately three times that of an adult. Systemic toxicity has been described in neonates after the administration of topical iodine, hexachlorophene, salicylic acid, epinephrine, and corticosteroids (Woo, 2004). The rectal mucosa may serve as a site of drug absorption in neonates who are unable to take medications by mouth, and in whom rapid IV access cannot be achieved. Rectal absorption is dependent on regional blood flow, retention of the drug in the rectum, and chemical properties of the drug. The rectal route of administration results in less efficient absorption when compared to the oral route, and in many instances higher mg/kg doses may be required (El-Chaar, 2003). Medications commonly administered via the rectal route in infants include acetaminophen, diazepam, chloral hydrate, and sodium polystyrene sulfonate.

Distribution

Once a medication has reached the blood stream, it will distribute among various organs, fluids, and tissues. The distribution of drugs within the body is influenced by many factors including total body water, total body fat, plasma and tissue binding, membrane permeability, and the infant's hemodynamic status. The pharmacokinetic term used to describe the relation between the amount of drug in the body and the measured plasma concentration is the apparent volume of distribution (Vd) (El-Chaar, 2003).

Total body water can be divided into intracellular and extracellular spaces. At birth, a full-term neonate is approximately 80% water, with 45% as extracellular and 35% as intracellular fluid. By 1 year of age a child is approximately 60% water, with 20% extracellular and 40% intracellular fluid (Kearns et al, 2003) (Figure 16-2). Body fat is approximately

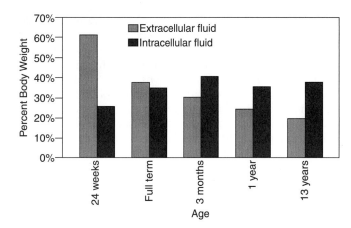

FIGURE **16-2**
Changes in total body water distribution with age. From Massanari MA. Age-based competency assessment of pharmacists in pediatrics, part II: application of developmental pharmacokinetics to pediatric pharmacy practice. *Journal of pediatric pharmacy practice* 2(3):143.

1% of the total body composition of a premature infant at 29 weeks' gestational age, increases to approximately 15% at term, and is 25% of total body composition between 1 and 2 years of age. Water-soluble medications have a much higher volume of distribution in neonates than in adults; therefore neonatal dosing is higher on a per-kilogram basis (i.e., gentamicin, vancomycin). Fat-soluble medications have a much smaller distribution volume in a neonate than in an adult. Neonatal dosing of medications that are fat-soluble is lower on a per-kilogram basis (Kearns et al, 2003; El-Chaar, 2003; Woo, 2004).

Several physiologic variables can produce both quantitative and qualitative differences in plasma and tissue binding of drugs. In general, neonatal plasma protein binding of drugs is decreased in comparison to adults. The decrease in plasma protein binding in neonates is a result of several factors, including the decreased formation of plasma proteins by the immature neonatal liver. Albumin is the major drug-binding protein in plasma and binds primarily to acidic drugs (i.e., phenobarbital, phenytoin). A lower plasma pH may decrease protein binding of acidic drugs, and the presence of endogenous substances may compete for protein binding sites. Endogenous substances in the neonate include free fatty acids and bilirubin, as well as transplacentally acquired interfering substances such as hormones and pharmacologic agents. Reduction in protein binding of drugs leads to an increase in the unbound or active component of the drug (Jew et al, 2002; Kearns et al, 2003).

Metabolism

Drug metabolism is influenced by genetic factors (pharmacogenomics), age, and the activity of drug-metabolizing enzymes. Most drugs are fat-soluble and require biotransformation into more water-soluble substances before elimination from the body. This process of biotransformation occurs mainly in the liver, and produces active as well as inactive metabolites.

The two main types of drug metabolism are phase I (nonsynthetic) and phase II (synthetic) reactions. Phase I reactions include oxidation, reduction, methylation, hydrolysis, and hydroxylation. The cytochrome P450 mixed-function oxidase system is responsible for most phase I reactions. Phase II reactions include conjugation with glycine, glucuronic acid, and sulfate. Phase I reactions appear to mature more rapidly, meeting or exceeding adult capacity by 6 months of age. Phase II reactions reach adult levels in children by 3 to 4 years of age. Maturation of these enzymatic pathways will affect neonatal metabolism of medications and thereby affect the clinical response to medications. Examples of drug toxicity in neonates with immature metabolic pathways include the gray baby syndrome, caused by decreased capacity to glucuronidate chloramphenicol, and neonatal gasping syndrome in neonates decreased capacity for glycination of the benzyl alcohol found in flush solutions (Robertson, 2003a).

Neonates may use different pathways to metabolize drugs than older infants and children use. These pathways may result in a modified pharmacologic response to medications. For example, neonates are not able to metabolize morphine adequately to its 6-glucuronide metabolite, a metabolite that is 20 times more active than morphine as an analgesic. Theophylline, a drug commonly used for the treatment of apnea of prematurity, presents another example of altered metabolic pathways. Theophylline is oxidized to inactive components in adults but is N-methylated to caffeine, a pharmacologically active agent in the neonate (El-Chaar, 2003).

Maturation of hepatic enzymes may also be influenced by prenatal or postnatal exposure to enzyme-inducing (i.e., phenobarbital, phenytoin, rifampin) or enzyme-inhibiting (i.e., cimetidine, erythromycin) agents. One drug may alter the metabolism of another medication, thereby increasing or decreasing effectiveness, creating toxicity, or producing subtherapeutic levels. Drug activity may also be interfered with by concurrent disease states. Interferences such as these are referred to as drug–disease state interactions (El-Chaar, 2003).

Elimination

Systemic clearance (Cl) is the ability of the eliminating organs, (kidney, liver, lung, skin) to remove a drug from the blood or plasma. Drugs and their metabolites are primarily eliminated by the kidneys. The principle renal mechanisms responsible for drug excretion include glomerular filtration, tubular secretion, and tubular reabsorption, all of which are immature at birth. Overall renal function increases with age, although as with hepatic metabolism, the maturation rate of individual physiologic functions varies (Figure 16-3). Glomerular filtration matures several months before tubular secretion; tubular reabsorption is the last to mature. The glomerular filtration is directly proportional to gestational age after 34 weeks' gestation. The increase in glomerular filtration after birth depends on postconceptional age and is influenced by increased cardiac output, decreased peripheral vascular resistance, increased mean arterial pressure, and increased surface area for filtration. The clinical importance of increases in glomerular filtration become apparent when one examines drugs excreted primarily by filtration such as gentamicin and vancomycin. Tubular reabsorption and secretion are also decreased in the neonate. Ampicillin, a drug commonly used in the neonatal population, undergoes tubular secretion (El-Chaar, 2003; Woo, 2004).

The elimination half-life ($t^{1}/_{2}$) of a drug refers to the time it takes for half the amount of drug in the blood to be eliminated. The volume of distribution and clearance of a medication are determinants of a drug's half-life. Half-life is an important factor in determining the appropriate interval between drug doses. Drugs with a long half-life are given at less frequent

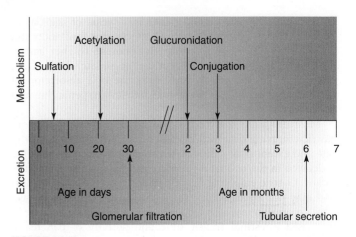

FIGURE **16-3**
The time line of expected maturation of metabolic pathways in the neonate to 6-month-old infant. From Massanari MA. Age-based competency assessment of pharmacists in pediatrics, part II: application of developmental pharmacokinetics to pediatric pharmacy practice. *Journal of pediatric pharmacy practice* 2(3):145.

dosing intervals, whereas those with shorter half-lives may need to be given via a continuous infusion (Jew et al, 2002; Soldin et al, 2003).

With constant drug dosing, the elimination half-life will determine the time to reach the so-called steady-state serum concentration. Steady state refers to the time at which the rate of drug administration equals the rate of drug elimination. When drug concentrations are monitored in clinical practice, steady-state concentrations should be obtained. Steady-state concentrations are reached in approximately five half-lives. This factor explains the rationale for administering a loading dose for medications with long half-lives. A loading dose is a single dose of a medication that is used to rapidly attain a serum concentration and therefore the desired clinical effect. A loading dose produces a higher circulating concentration earlier in the therapeutic course as opposed to waiting five half-lives. In neonates, loading doses are commonly administered for theophylline, caffeine, phenobarbital, phenytoin, and digoxin (Jew et al, 2002; Soldin et al, 2003).

THERAPEUTIC DRUG MONITORING

Therapeutic drug monitoring (TDM) is the use of serum drug concentrations and pharmacokinetic and pharmacodynamic principles to regulate drug dosages. TDM is of particular importance in the neonatal population, which may under- or over-respond to the usual dosing regimens. Additional unique considerations in the neonate include the precise delivery of very small doses and volumes of medications, the availability of blood for measurement of drug concentrations, interference of endogenous substances with drug assays, frequent changes in neonatal pharmacokinetic parameters, and the extrapolation of therapeutic serum concentrations from adult data to the neonatal population (Soldin et al, 2003; Jew et al, 2002).

TDM is used for drugs in which a correlation between the measured plasma concentration and drug efficacy or toxicity exists. Drugs with narrow therapeutic indexes are ideal candidates for TDM. A drug exhibits a narrow therapeutic index if the plasma concentration required for therapeutic effects is relatively close to the concentration known to produce toxicity. Drugs for which TDM is used in the neonatal population

TABLE 16-4	Neonatal Therapeutic Drug Monitoring	
Drug	**Trough Serum Concentration**	**Peak Serum Concentration**
Theophylline (AOP)	6 to 12 mcg/ml	
Caffeine	5 to 20 mcg/ml	
Phenobarbital	20 to 40 mcg/ml	
Phenytoin	8 to 15 mcg/ml	
Gentamicin	<2 mcg/ml	4 to 12 mcg/ml
Vancomycin	5 to 10 mcg/ml	25 to 40 mcg/ml
Digoxin	0.9 to 2 mcg/ml	

Data adapted from Jew R et al (2002). Therapeutic drug monitoring in neonates. Philadelphia College of Pharmacy reports on neonatal pharmacotherapy 2(2):1-25; *and El-Chaar G (2003). Pharmaceutical care in premature infants.* US pharmacist HS13-HS31.

include theophylline, caffeine, phenobarbital, phenytoin, gentamicin, vancomycin, and digoxin (Soldin et al, 2003; El-Chaar, 2003). TDM allows the clinician to aim for a therapeutic range, which is usually safe and effective, with minimal drug toxicity.

With the exception of drugs administered via a continuous infusion, drug concentrations in the plasma are not static. The time of blood sampling relative to the time of drug administration is of utmost importance. For some medications both trough and peak concentrations are monitored, whereas with other medications it is routine to monitor trough concentrations (Table 16-4). Obtaining levels once a patient achieves steady-state concentrations provides the most accurate information with regard to drug efficacy or toxicity. Patients with altered organ function or rapidly changing clinical status may require closer monitoring of serum concentrations than do other patients.

Certain medications such as phenytoin are highly plasma protein-bound. For these medications, two types of assays are available, including total and free serum concentrations. Free levels indicate the amount of free, unbound drug that is available to exert its effects on target tissues. When free phenytoin serum assays are not available, caution must be used in the interpretation of total serum concentrations. Levels may be falsely interpreted as low when the actual amount of active drug is adequate or toxic (Soldin et al, 2003).

FETAL AND INFANT EXPOSURE TO MATERNAL MEDICATIONS

Fetal Exposure

Virtually any medication or substance given to the mother, either intentionally or inadvertently can cross the placental membrane. The amount of drug that passes into the fetal circulation depends on several factors—including the molecular weight, protein binding, lipid solubility, and ionization of the drug; maternal drug serum concentrations; and integrity of the placental barrier. Physiologic changes during pregnancy can affect absorption, distribution, metabolism, and excretion of medications in the mother. Fetal exposure to a medication may lead to deleterious effects on the exposed fetus or may result in minimal or no adverse outcomes.

Labeling a drug as a teratogen indicates the potential of a medication to produce congenital malformations in an infant. A medication may not be a teratogen but may produce other

---

BOX 16-1

Pregnancy Risk Categories

Category	Description
A	Adequate and well-controlled studies in pregnant women have not shown an increased risk of fetal abnormalities.
B	Animal studies have revealed no evidence of harm to the fetus; however, there are no adequate and well-controlled studies in pregnant women. **or** Animal studies have shown an adverse effect, but adequate and well-controlled studies in pregnant women have failed to demonstrate a risk to the fetus.
C	Animal studies have shown an adverse effect, and there are no adequate and well-controlled studies in pregnant women. **or** No animal studies have been conducted, and there are no adequate and well-controlled studies in pregnant women.
D	Studies, adequate and well-controlled or observational, in pregnant women have demonstrated a risk to the fetus. However, the benefits of therapy may outweigh the potential risk.
X	Studies, adequate and well-controlled or observational, in animals or pregnant women have demonstrated positive evidence of fetal abnormalities. The use of the product is contraindicated in women who are or may become pregnant.

From Meadows M (2001). Pregnancy and the drug dilemma. *FDA consumer magazine*, May-June, US Food and Drug Administration.

untoward effects on the infant, such as respiratory depression or sedation seen with maternal narcotic administration just prior to delivery. Drug companies have been required since 1983 to assign each medication a pregnancy risk category (Box 16-1) (Brent, 2001; St Onge et al, 2004).

Lactation Exposure

An often-overlooked source of exposure to medications is transfer from the maternal circulation into breast milk. The safety and potential risks to the nursing infant must be considered during maternal drug use. Maternal drug use includes over-the-counter drugs, prescription drugs, illicit drugs, and, more recently, herbal products. A recent survey of 14,000 breastfeeding women revealed that 79% took at least one medication, and each woman averaged 3.3 different medications during the course of breastfeeding her infant (Howard & Lawrence, 2001).

The pH and size of a drug molecule, protein-binding properties, lipid and water solubility, and diffusion rate will all influence the quantity of drug that passes from maternal serum into breast milk. Additional considerations include the time the medication is taken in relation to the period of nursing, the amount or dose of medication, the pharmacokinetics of the drug, the length of nursing, and the amount of milk ingested.

TABLE 16-5	American Academy of Pediatrics: Drugs Contraindicated During Breastfeeding
Drug	**Reported or Possible Effect**
Amphetamines	Irritability, poor sleeping
Anticancer drugs	Possible immunosuppression, questionable effects on growth
Cocaine	Cocaine intoxication
Heroin	Tremors, restlessness, vomiting, poor feeding
Marijuana	Structural changes in nursing brain in laboratory animals
Phencyclidine (PCP)	Potent hallucinogen
Radioactive compounds	Radioactivity in breast milk

Adapted from American Academy of Pediatrics Committee on Drugs (2001). The transfer of drugs and other chemicals into human milk. Pediatrics 108(3):776-789.

The American Academy of Pediatrics Committee on Drugs periodically publishes guidelines regarding the transfer of drugs and chemicals into human milk. Specific medications are considered contraindicated in the breastfeeding infant (American Academy of Pediatrics, 2001) (Table 16-5). In addition, websites are available that provide the most recent information on newer drugs and breastfeeding (Dr Hale's pharmacology website, 2005; http://www.ibreastfeeding.com).

MEDICATION ADMINISTRATION

Once an appropriate drug dosage is established, the optimal route and method of drug administration is also of utmost importance. Many commercially available dosage forms are not suitable for use in the pediatric patient population. Developmental considerations with regard to medication administration must also be considered.

Oral Administration

Many drugs prescribed for infants and children are not available in suitable oral dosage forms. Oral medications are administered to an infant via a nipple, dropper, syringe, or feeding tube. The preferred dosage form for infants is an alcohol-free, sugar-free, dye-free, and low-osmolality liquid preparation. However, orally administered medications may only be commercially available as tablets or capsules or as concentrated oral solutions or suspensions. High-osmolality substances administered to the neonate have been associated with many adverse effects, including the development of necrotizing enterocolitis and decreased intestinal transit time.

Preparation and delivery of small therapeutic doses from concentrated commercial oral solutions may be difficult. Alteration (dilution or compounding) of an adult dosage form raises issues regarding compatibility and stability. Commonly prescribed oral medications that are not commercially available in a liquid formulation include rifampin, captopril, and spironolactone. Oral medications may also contain silent or inactive ingredients that supply the "delivery system" of the drug or serve to flavor, sweeten, and preserve the drug. Such inert ingredients may be harmless in adults but may, when administered frequently to neonates, result in toxicity (Robertson, 2003b; Committee on Drugs, 1997).

Intravenous Administration

The most effective means of rapid drug delivery in a critically ill neonate is IV administration. As with oral medications, small doses and delivery volumes complicate the delivery of IV medications. Furthermore, IV medication delivery is often delayed, prolonged, or incomplete in the neonatal patient. A slow flow rate, distal drug delivery site, and slow infusion rates delay intravenous drug delivery. A major impact of delayed drug delivery is the potential for subtherapeutic plasma concentrations or even clinical failure with some medications. This is particularly important for medications that may require TDM (El-Chaar, 2003).

Several techniques are currently used to administer IV medications in the neonatal population and include IV push, IV buretrol, IV retrograde, and IV syringe pump. The infusion device, IV tubing, container holding the medication (i.e., syringe, IV bag), dead space at injection ports, and IV in-line filters will affect drug delivery. Patient-specific factors such as body position and vascular occlusion may also affect IV drug delivery (Chen & Martinez, 1998; Jew et al, 1997, Jew, 2002).

Administration of medications using the IV push method allows rapid drug delivery but is not appropriate for many medications. The IV buretrol method is simple and allows easy dilution of a drug in the primary IV fluids. Potential disadvantages of the IV buretrol method include the fact that medications may not reach the patient for a prolonged period of time, particularly if the primary IV flow rate is not high. In addition, part of the dose may be inadvertently discarded with IV tubing changes, and the drug must be compatible with the primary IV fluid to which it is added.

Another technique—one that was started in the early 1970s—is the IV retrograde system, which consists of extension tubing with two 3-way stopcocks (Figure 16-4). When a drug is introduced into the system, the stopcock closest to the patient is turned off to the patient end of the system. The medication is given through the stopcock and forced to move in the direction opposite the usual direction of flow (i.e., retrograde). Simultaneously, the distal stopcock is turned off to the pump end of the system, and a syringe is attached to accept the displaced maintenance fluid, which is discarded. After the drug is in the tubing, the stopcocks are positioned to allow normal flow of maintenance fluid, and the medication is infused at the rate set for the maintenance fluid. This method can yield inconsistent delivery but allows delivery of medications with minimal extra volume.

Drug delivery with a syringe pump and microbore tubing is the preferred method of IV drug administration in the neonatal population. A syringe pump allows absolute control over the rate of drug delivery with minimal IV fluid volume, at a rate that is independent of the primary IV rate (Figure 16-5). The use of microbore tubing allows the use of minimal volumes of flush solution. In addition to intermittent medications, continuous infusion medications such as pressors and inotropes may be administered via a syringe pump. Recently, "smart pump" technology has become available. Smart pumps incorporate computer technology allowing the use of drug libraries, standard drug concentrations, and sophisticated checks for dosing errors. A potential disadvantage of syringe pumps, in particular the smart pumps, is the capital expense required to purchase the pump (Gura, 1999; Jew et al, 1997; Larsen et al, 2005).

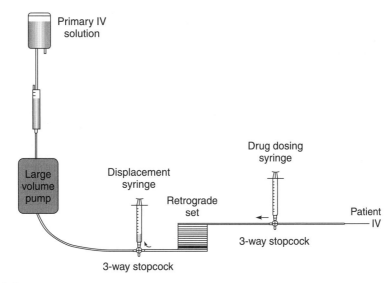

FIGURE **16-4**

Set for retrograde administration of medication. From Jew R et al. Clinical applications of IV drug administration in infants and children. *Critical care nurse* 17(4):69.

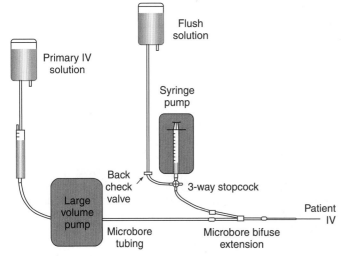

FIGURE **16-5**

Syringe pump delivery of medication for patients with medication volumes, <60 ml. From Jew R et al. Clinical applications of IV drug administration in infants and children. *Critical care nurse* 17(4):69.

Many of the problems that plague commercially available oral medications can also be found in commercial IV medications. IV medications may be available in concentrations that prohibit accurate measurement and administration of small neonatal doses. In selection of parenteral medications, not only drug concentration but also preservatives and other ingredients in the parenteral preparation are factors. Benzyl alcohol is a common preservative added to parenteral drug products. Severe toxicity has been reported in neonates after the use of flush solutions that contain benzyl alcohol. Whenever possible; preservative-free parenteral products should be used in the neonatal population for the first 2 months of life.

The osmolality of a drug solution is an important delivery factor. Tissue irritation or pain at the injection site can occur when a drug solution with an osmolality significantly different from that of the serum (275 to 295 mOsm/kg) is administered intravenously. Infiltration of a hypotonic or hypertonic solution can cause trauma and necrosis of the injection site (Jew et al, 1997; Ramasethu, 2004).

Premature infants typically have fluid restrictions as well as limited intravenous access, and the question of IV drug compatibilities often comes into play. Drug compatibility involves the question of both physical (visual) and chemical (nonvisual) compatibilities. IV drug compatibility is not clearcut. This is true because of the influence of alterations in drug concentration, order of drug infusion, pH, and temperature. For these reasons, reference books and articles may provide conflicting information with regard to drug compatibilities. Two drugs are physically incompatible when turbidity, cloudiness, or a precipitate is formed when two or more drugs are mixed together. An example of a physical incompatibility results when calcium gluconate and sodium bicarbonate–containing or phosphorus-containing solutions are mixed in the same IV solution or IV tubing. Chemical incompatibility implies a loss of potency or formation of a toxic byproduct when two or more substances are mixed. Epinephrine and sodium bicarbonate are chemically incompatible when co-infused (Trissel, 2001; Taketomo et al, 2004; Young & Mangum, 2004).

Extravasation and infiltration are used interchangeably in the literature; both terms reflect a leakage of IV fluid or medication out of a vein and into surrounding tissues (Ramasethu, 2004). Extravasation in neonates with circulatory compromise can lead to significant morbidity, functional impairment, or cosmetic defects. Many medications (i.e., potassium, calcium, parenteral nutrition, and dopamine) that are incorporated into the drug regimens of patients in the neonatal intensive care unit are capable of causing tissue damage if extravasation occurs. The use of small or superficial venous access sites should be avoided for administration of these agents unless absolutely necessary. The degree of cellular injury is often directly related to the physiochemical characteristics of the infusant—including osmolarity, pH, and molecular weight.

TABLE 16-6	Extravasation Treatment
Extravasated Drug/Fluid	**Treatment**
Parenteral nutrition	Topical nitroglycerin, hyaluronidase
Calcium	Topical nitroglycerin, hyaluronidase
Dopamine	Phentolamine, topical nitroglycerin
Dobutamine	Phentolamine
Epinephrine	Phentolamine

Adapted from Ramasethu J (2004). Pharmacology review: prevention and management of extravasation injuries in neonates. Neoreviews 5:491-497.

The treatment of extravasation injuries that result from infiltration of medications and IV solutions involves the use of specific antidotes. Three possible antidotes—hyaluronidase, phentolamine, and topical nitroglycerin—have been studied most extensively in the neonatal population. The mechanism by which IV fluids and medications cause tissue necrosis varies, and optimal treatment choices vary with each extravasated agent (Ramasethu, 2004; Taketomo et al, 2004) (Table 16-6).

Aerosol Administration

The use of aerosolized medications in the neonatal setting has increased with the resurgence of chronic lung disease, and the increased prevalence of pulmonary hypertension. The rationale for aerosol medication delivery includes direct delivery to the target organ (lungs) with decreased systemic adverse drug effects. The therapeutic efficacy of aerosolized medications is dependent on the delivery of an adequate dose of medication to the target sites within the lung. The primary factors that influence lung deposition include particle size, mode of assisted ventilation required, inhaler device, and age of the infant. The available methods to aerosolize medications in the neonate include nebulization either intermittently or continuously or a metered-dose inhaler (MDI) with a spacing device. In addition, the recent advent of Vapotherm further complicates delivery of aerosolized medications, as no stability data exist when nebulizing medications with Vapotherm (Juretschke & Spoula, 2004). Studies have revealed conflicting results with regard to the optimal method and efficacy of aerosol drug delivery in the neonate (Cole, 2000; Hintz, 2003).

Medication Administration in Extracorporeal Membrane Oxygenation

Extracorporeal membrane oxygenation (ECMO) is a highly technical and invasive technique used to treat respiratory failure when conventional means and technologies fail. ECMO is used for a variety of indications in the neonatal population, including those with persistent pulmonary hypertension, meconium aspiration, sepsis, respiratory distress syndrome, pneumonia, or congenital diaphragmatic hernia, and in postoperative congenital heart disease patients. Patients who undergo ECMO receive numerous medications including antibiotics, sedatives, analgesics, inotropes, diuretics, antiepileptics, and medications that are used to maintain the ECMO circuit. Little is known regarding the disposition of drugs in this patient population.

Medications may be administered to ECMO patients either into the ECMO circuit before or after the filter or directly into the patient. Varying pharmacokinetics may be observed, depending on the actual site of injection. Distribution and delivery of medication are more consistent when drugs are injected after the filter. Administration into this site places the patient at risk for development of air emboli, and administration of medications should be done with great caution. Medications injected directly into the reservoir or before the filter usually result in a prolonged time of actual drug delivery to the patient and incomplete drug administration. A large part of the ECMO circuit consists of disposable polyvinyl chloride tubing. The amounts of tubing and other components of the circuit contribute to a large surface area with the potential for drug binding. Therefore increased doses may be required initially when these medications are used or when the circuit is changed during ECMO therapy (Elliott & Buck, 1999).

Interpretation of pharmacokinetic parameters in this type of patient is often difficult because of the influences of the site of injection, flow rate of the ECMO circuit, and clinical status and organ function of the patient. Gentamicin and vancomycin are two antibiotics that are commonly administered to infants on ECMO. Pharmacokinetics for these agents vary, not only with the ECMO circuit but also with the clinical status of the infant—including altered renal function in a sick infant. In addition, pharmacokinetics was found to vary with the infant's gestational age, postnatal age, and weight. Peak effect for these patients is often delayed, thus resulting in false interpretation of serum peak levels for aminoglycoside antibiotics (Buck, 2003).

SUMMARY

The individualization of drug therapy is critical in the neonatal population. The neonatal population presents a unique challenge with regard to both medication dosing and administration. Drug dosing on a mg/kg basis is the most common method because of the ease of calculation. A lack of large, well-controlled trials in this unique patient population results in drug dosing based on extrapolation from the adult literature or anecdotal experience. Furthermore, developmental pharmacokinetics—or the change in absorption, distribution, metabolism, and elimination of drugs—creates a population whose drug dosing is constantly changing. Once an appropriate dosing regimen is determined, the optimal drug administration technique is equally important.

REFERENCES

American Academy of Pediatrics Committee on Drugs (2001). The transfer of drugs and other chemicals into human milk. *Pediatrics* 108(3):776-789.

American Academy of Pediatrics Committee on Drugs and Committee on Hospital Care (2003). Prevention of medication errors in the pediatric inpatient setting. *Pediatrics* 112(2):431-436.

Brent RL (2001). Addressing environmentally caused human birth defects. *Pediatrics in review* 22(5):153-165.

Brummel GL (2001). The FDA drug approval process: focus on pediatric labeling. *Neonatal network* 20(3):49-51.

Buck M (2003). Pharmacokinetic changes during extracorporeal membrane oxygenation. *Clinical pharmacokinetics* 42(5):403-417.

Center for Drug Evaluation and Research (2005). Best Pharmaceuticals Act for Children: Pediatric Exclusivity Provision 2001. Available at: http://www.fda.gov.cder.pediatric. Accessed September 13, 2005.

Chen JL, Martinez CM (1998). Filtration recommendations for IV medications. *American journal of health system pharmacists* 55:1313-1314.

Cole CH (2000). Special problems in aerosol delivery: neonatal and pediatric considerations. *Respiratory care* 45(6):646-651.

Committee on Drugs (1997). "Inactive" ingredients in pharmaceutical products: update (subject review). *Pediatrics* 99(1):268-278.

Committee on Drugs (2002). Uses of drugs not described in the package insert (off-label use). *Pediatrics* 110(1):181-183.

Committee on Fetus and Newborn, American Academy of Pediatrics (AAP) (2002). Postnatal corticosteroids to treat or prevent chronic lung disease in preterm infants. *Pediatrics* 109:330-338.

Committee on Fetus and Newborn, American Academy of Pediatrics (AAP) (2004). Age terminology during the perinatal period. *Pediatrics* 114(5):1326-1364.

El-Chaar G (2003). Pharmaceutical care in premature infants. *US pharmacist*, HS13-HS31.

Elliott ES, Buck ML (1999). Phenobarbital dosing and pharmacokinetics in a neonate receiving extracorporeal membrane oxygenation. *Annals of pharmacotherapy* 33:419-422.

Gura KM (1999). Intravenous drug administration guidelines for pediatric patients 1999. *Journal of pediatric pharmacy practice* 4(2):80-106.

Hale R (2005).Breastfeeding and medication forum. Dr Hale's pharmacology website, http://ibreastfeeding.com. Accessed September 13, 2005.

Hintz SR (2003). Bronchodilator aerosol therapy in the preterm infant. *Neoreviews* 4(9):245-249.

Holdsworth MT (2003). Incidence and impact of adverse drug events in pediatric inpatients. *Archives of pediatric and adolescent medicine* 157:60-65.

Howard CR, Lawrence RA (2001). Xenobiotics and breastfeeding. *Pediatric clinics of North America* 48(2):485-505.

Jew RK et al (1997). Clinical implications of IV drug administration in infants and children. *Critical care nurse* 17(4):62-70.

Jew R et al (2002). Therapeutic drug monitoring in neonates. *Philadelphia College of Pharmacy reports on neonatal pharmacotherapy* 2(2):1-25.

Juretschke R, Spoula R (2004). High flow nasal cannula in the neonatal population. *Neonatal intensive care* 17(6):20-21.

Kaushal R et al (2001). Medication errors and adverse drug events in pediatric inpatients. *Journal of the American Medical Association* 285(16):2114-2120.

Kearns GL et al (2003). Developmental pharmacology—drug disposition, action, and therapy in infants and children. *New England journal of medicine* 349(12):1157-1167.

Larsen GY et al (2005). Standard drug concentrations and smart pump technology reduce continuous-medication-infusion errors in pediatric patients. *Pediatrics* 116(1):21-25.

Levine SA et al (2001). Guidelines for preventing medication errors in pediatrics. *Journal of pediatric pharmacy practice* 6:426-442.

Mestan KK et al (2005). Neurodevelopmental outcomes of premature infants treated with inhaled nitric oxide. *New England journal of medicine* 353(1):23-32.

Raj TN (2005). Research in neonatology for the 21st century: executive summary of the national institute of child health and human development—American Academy of Pediatrics Workshop. Part I: academic issues. *Pediatrics* 115(2):465-474.

Ramasethu J (2004). Pharmacology review: prevention and management of extravasation injuries in neonates. *Neoreviews* 5:491-497.

Robertson AF (2003a). Reflections on errors in neonatology II. The heroic years, 1950 to 1970. *Journal of perinatology* 23(2):54-161.

Robertson AF (2003b). Reflections on errors in neonatology III. The experienced years, 1970 to 2000. *Journal of perinatology* 23(3):240-249.

Shirkey H (1968). Therapeutic orphans. *Journal of pediatrics* 72:119.

Soldin OP et al (2002). Review: therapeutic drug monitoring in pediatrics. *Therapeutic drug monitoring* 24(1):1-8.

Spielberg SP (2001). Pediatric therapy for the new millennium. *Journal of pediatric pharmacology and therapeutics* 6:6-9.

St Onge M et al (2004). Risks associated with medication use in pregnancy. *Drug topics* 84-91.

Taketomo CK et al (2004). *Pediatric dosage handbook*, ed 11. Hudson, OH: Lexi-Comp.

Trissel LA (2001). Drug stability and compatibility issues in drug delivery. In Trissel LA, editor. *Handbook of injectable drugs*, ed 11 (pp 17-22). Bethesda, MD: American Society of Health-System Pharmacists.

Van Meurs KP et al, Preemie Inhaled Nitric Oxide Study (2005). Inhaled nitric oxide for premature infants with severe respiratory failure. *New England journal of medicine* 353(1):13-22.

Woo TM (2004). Pediatric pharmacology update: essential concepts for prescribing. *Advance nursing practice* 12(6):22-27.

Woods TE (2005). Adverse events and preventable adverse events in children. *Pediatrics* 115(1):155-160.

Yaffe S (2003). Pediatric pharmacology: its time has come. *Journal of pediatric pharmacology and therapeutics* 8(1):10-12.

Young TE, Mangum B (2004). *Neofax*, ed 17. Raleigh, NC: Acorn.

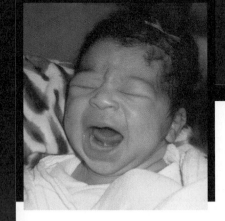

Chapter 17

Pain in the Newborn and Infant

Marlene Walden

Despite advances in neonatal pain assessment and management, nonpharmacologic and pharmacologic analgesic therapies continue to be underutilized to manage both acute and procedural pain (Johnston et al, 1997; Simons et al, 2003a). Untreated acute, recurrent, or chronic pain related to disease or medical care may have significant and lifelong physiologic and psychologic consequences. As with all other medical conditions, the first step in the treatment process is the accurate diagnosis of the problem. Thus pain assessment provides the foundation for all pain treatment. This chapter reviews the developmental neurophysiology of pain, discusses methods to assess pain in infants, highlights factors that influence the pain experience, and discusses evidence-based strategies for managing infant pain.

DEFINING PAIN AND DISTRESS IN INFANTS AND CHILDREN

Pain is defined by the International Association for the Study of Pain (IASP) as "an unpleasant sensory and emotional experience associated with actual or potential tissue damage or described in terms of such damage" (Merskey, 1979). The IASP definition also states that pain is always subjective and is learned through experiences related to injury in early life. This definition is problematic when considering infants who are incapable of self-report and who may not have had previous experience with injury. Anand and Craig (1996) propose that pain perception is an inherent quality of life that appears early in development to serve as a signaling system for tissue damage. This signaling includes behavioral and physiologic responses, which are valid indicators of pain that can be inferred by others. Broadening the definition of pain to include behavioral and physiologic indicators in addition to self-report can benefit preverbal, nonverbal, or cognitively impaired individuals who are experiencing pain by providing objective pain assessment.

DEVELOPMENTAL NEUROPHYSIOLOGY OF PAIN

The basic mechanisms of pain perception in infants and children are similar to those of adults and include (1) transduction and transmission; and (2) perception and modulation. However, because of neurophysiologic and cognitive immaturity, some differences exist. A brief review is presented here and emphasizes the developmental and maturational changes that occur during infancy and childhood (Fitzgerald & Anand, 1993).

Peripheral Transduction and Transmission

Noxious mechanical, thermal, or chemical stimuli excite primary afferent fibers that transmit information about the potentially injurious stimuli from the periphery to the dorsal horn of the spinal cord. A-delta (large, myelinated, and fast-conducting) and C (small, unmyelinated, and slow-conducting) fibers are primarily responsible for pain impulse transmission (nociception). However, these signals can be amplified or attenuated by activation of surrounding neurons in the periphery and spinal cord. For example, tissue injury causes the release of inflammatory mediators (e.g., potassium, bradykinin, prostaglandins, cytokines, nerve growth factors, catecholamines, and substance P) that sensitize A-delta and C fibers and recruit other neurons (silent nociceptors) and result in hyperalgesia. Stimulation of A-beta fibers that signal nonpainful touch and pressure can compete with the transmission of nociception in the dorsal horn of the spinal cord, thus reducing the intensity of the perceived pain.

Central Mechanisms and Modulation

Neurotransmitters in the spinal cord either amplify (e.g., substance P, calcitonin gene-related peptide, neurokinin A) or attenuate (e.g., endogenous opioids, norepinephrine, serotonin, GABA, glycine) pain information from the periphery. Central sensitization occurs when excitatory amino acids act on NMDA receptors to induce prolonged depolarization and windup.

Nociceptive sensory input reaches the thalamus through second-order neurons in the spinothalamic, spinoreticular, and spinomeosencephalic tracts and is then widely distributed throughout the brain. The perception, emotional interpretation, and cognitive meaning of nociceptive stimuli occur within a distributive neuromatrix; no one "pain center" exists. The sensory-discriminative, affective-motivational, and evaluative dimensions of pain perception are mediated by past experience and the context of the painful event. For example, nociceptive stimuli activate areas of the limbic system thought to control emotion, particularly anxiety. Thus differences in physiologic, biochemical, and psychologic factors influence the perception of pain, making it an individual phenomenon.

Descending modulation occurs when efferent projections from supraspinal areas such as the periaqueductal grey, raphe nucleus, and locus coeruleus release inhibitory neurotransmitters. The major neurotransmitters that mediate descending inhibition are norepinephrine, serotonin, endogenous opioids, GABA, and acetylcholine.

Neurodevelopment of Pain Perception

Infants, even prematurely born infants, have the neurologic capacity to perceive pain at birth (Fitzgerald & Anand, 1993). The peripheral and central structures necessary for nociception are present and functional early in gestation (between the first and second trimesters). Functional maturation of the fetal cerebral cortex has been demonstrated by: (1) electroencephalogram (EEG) patterns and cortical evoked potentials; (2) measurement of cerebral glucose use that shows maximal metabolic rates in sensory areas of the brain; and (3) well-defined periods of sleep and wakefulness that are regulated by cortical functioning from 28 weeks of gestation. The newborn infant possesses a well-developed hypothalamic-pituitary-adrenal axis and can mount a fight-or-flight response with the release of catecholamines and cortisol.

Research suggests that some differences in nociceptive processes between infants and adults exist. For example, pain impulse transmission in neonates occurs primarily along nonmyelinated C fibers rather than myelinated A-delta fibers. Less precision also occurs in pain signal transmission in the spinal cord, and descending inhibitory neurotransmitters are lacking (Fitzgerald & Anand, 1993). Thus young infants may perceive pain more intensely than older children or adults because their descending control mechanisms are immature and thus limit their ability to modulate the experience.

Pathophysiology of Acute Pain

Although pain can serve as a warning of injury, the effects of pain are generally deleterious. Pain evokes negative physiologic, metabolic, and behavioral responses in infants (Anand, 1998). These responses include increased heart rate, respiratory rate, and blood pressure and increased secretion of catecholamines, glucagon, and corticosteroids. The catabolic state induced by acute pain may be more damaging to infants, who have higher metabolic rates and fewer nutritional reserves than adults. Pain leads to anorexia and causes poor nutritional intake, delayed wound healing, impaired mobility, sleep disturbances, withdrawal, irritability, and developmental regression. Premature infants who underwent cardiac surgery and who received less anesthesia had more postoperative complications (Anand & Hickey, 1992), and prolonged pain may increase neonatal morbidity and mortality (Anand, 1998; Anand et al, 1999).

Learning about pain occurs with the first pain experience and has profound effects on subsequent pain perception and responses. Memory of pain in infants is evident from differences in responses to painful vaccination in infants who had undergone unanesthetized circumcision in comparison to infants who were uncircumcised or who received analgesia during circumcision (Gunnar et al, 1995; Taddio et al, 1995a; Taddio & Ohlsson, 1997). Findings from two studies suggest that the pain experience in the neonatal intensive care unit (NICU) may alter the normal course of development of pain expression in toddlers and preschoolers (Grunau et al, 1994a, 1994b). A recent study also suggests that prematurely born children and adolescents had more tender points and lower tenderness thresholds than children born at full term (Buskila et al, 2003). Animal research suggests that pain and stress in the neonatal period result in altered pain sensitivity, decreased weight gain, decreased ability to learn, and increased preference for alcohol (Anand & Plotsky, 1995). Humans and animals do not become tolerant to pain and are likely sensitized to the effects of pain over time. Thus recognition and treatment of pain is important for the immediate well-being of infants and for their optimal long-term development.

CLINICAL ASSESSMENT OF PAIN

Presently, no easily administered, widely accepted, uniform technique exists for assessing pain in infants. A multidimensional pain assessment tool that includes measurements for both physiologic and behavioral indicators of pain is preferable given the multifaceted nature of pain (Walden, 2001). A recent systematic integrative review found 17 multidimensional neonatal pain assessment tools, but only 11 have been published (Duhn & Medves, 2004). Since this systematic review was published, at least one more multidimensional pain assessment tool has been published (Cignacco et al, 2004). Selection of an appropriate clinical pain assessment method should be based first on the developmental age of the infant, and second on the type of pain experienced (e.g., for procedural pain or postoperative pain). Validity, reliability, clinical utility, and feasibility are important aspects to consider when choosing a pain assessment tool.

Multidimensional Pain Tools

The most commonly used published multidimensional infant-specific pain assessment tools with psychometric data are listed in Table 17-1. The CRIES (Krechel & Bildner, 1995) and the Pain Assessment Tool (PAT; Hodgkinson et al, 1994) were developed for postoperative pain and the Neonatal Infant Pain Scale (NIPS; Lawrence et al, 1993) and the Scale for Use in Newborns (SUN; Blauer & Gerstmann, 1998) were developed for procedural pain. The Bernese Pain Scale for Neonates (BPSN; Cignacco et al, 2004) was specifically developed to assess the responses of preterm neonates or those who require mechanical ventilation to procedural pain.

The infant pain assessment tool that has been most widely validated in premature and full-term infants during procedural pain is the Premature Infant Pain Profile (PIPP; Stevens et al, 1996). The PIPP is a seven-indicator measure that includes behavioral, physiologic, and contextual indicators. Gestational age and behavioral state of the infant are taken into consideration in the scoring. This measure had initial validity and reliability determined by four retrospective data sets. Clinical validation that included the establishment of interrater and intrarater reliability was determined prospectively (Ballantyne et al, 1999). Clinical utility has been established by comparing the PIPP and the CRIES. The PIPP primarily has been used to evaluate procedural pain in preterm neonates greater than 28 weeks' gestational age, but has also been validated for evaluating postoperative pain in neonates and for determining the efficacy of pain-relieving interventions in premature infants (Eriksson et al, 1999; Stevens et al, 1999).

Factors That Influence Pain

Pain is unique among neurologic functions because of the degree of plasticity in pain neurophysiology. Although structural and functional maturity is reached at an early age, anatomic and functional changes occur throughout life and are related to the effects of each pain experience. This plasticity means that the perception and meaning of pain are unique to each individual and are not determined by maturation alone but are influenced by many individual and contextual factors. Currently available methods to assess pain in infants do not adequately or quantitatively incorporate all aspects of the context of pain that influence the pain experience. Thus the clinician must remain cognizant of the ways in which perception of pain may be positively or negatively influenced

TABLE **17-1**	Multidimensional Pain Assessment Tools in Infants		
Measure	**Age Level**	**Indicators**	**Pain Stimulus**
CRIES	Preterm and full-term infants up to 60 weeks' gestational age	Crying, requires oxygen for saturation >95%, increased vital signs (heart rate and blood pressure), expression, sleepless	Postoperative pain
Bernese Pain Scale for Neonates (BPSN)	Preterm and full-term neonates	Alertness, crying, time to calm, skin color, eyebrow bulge with eye squeeze, posture, breathing pattern, heart rate, oxygen saturation	Procedural pain in neonates with or without ventilation
Neonatal Infant Pain Scale (NIPS)	Preterm and full-term neonates	Facial expression, cry, breathing patterns, arms, legs, state of arousal	Procedural pain
Pain Assessment Tool (PAT)	Full-term neonates	Posture, tone, sleep pattern, expression, color, cry, respirations, heart rate, oxygen saturation, blood pressure, nurses' perception of infant pain	Postoperative pain
Premature Infant Pain Profile (PIPP)	Preterm and full-term neonates	Gestational age, behavioral state, heart rate, oxygen saturation, brow bulge, eye squeeze, nasolabial furrow	Procedural and postoperative pain
Scale for Use in Newborns (SUN)	Preterm and full-term infants	Central nervous system state, breathing, movement, tone, face, heart rate, and blood pressure,	Procedural pain

Adapted from Franck LS et al (2000). Pain assessment in infants and children. Pediatric clinics of North America *47(3):487-512.*

by these factors and subjectively incorporate them into the assessment of pain. These factors do not influence pain in isolation but are listed separately for clarity.

Biologic Factors

Genetic variation leads to differences in the amount and type of neurotransmitters and receptors that are available to mediate pain. Recent advancements in molecular biology have allowed for investigation of the genes responsible for pain perception and modulation. Limited data suggest that gender may also influence pain behaviors, with females expressing increased behavioral responses to acute pain compared to male newborns. It is unknown whether these gender differences are related to pain processing or pain expression (Fuller, 2002; Guinsburg et al, 2000).

Previous pain experience leads to alterations in pain signal processing that may be reversible or permanent. Studies of premature infants (Johnston & Stevens, 1996; Stevens et al, 1999) suggest that previous pain experience is the most important factor accounting for differences in response to the acute pain of heelstick. Infants who were subjected to more frequent painful procedures in the NICU had decreased behavioral and increased cardiovascular responses compared to infants who experienced less pain, even after controlling for gestational age–related differences in pain expression.

Behavioral State

The behavioral state of the infant, ranging from deep sleep to awake and crying, acts as a moderator of behavioral pain responses. The behavioral state of the infant immediately before the painful stimulus affects the robustness of the response. Infants in awake states demonstrate more robust reactions to pain than infants in sleep states. Infants in a deep sleep state will show less vigorous facial expression in response to heelstick than infants who are alert or aroused before the heelstick (Grunau & Craig, 1987; Stevens et al, 1994). Term and healthy preterm newborns who were handled or

immobilized before heelstick exhibited greater physiologic and behavioral reactivity, thus indicating that previous stress may result in greater instability in response to pain (Porter et al, 1998).

Gestational Age

Gestational age affects infant pain responses, with younger infants displaying fewer and less vigorous behavioral responses to pain (Gibbins & Stevens, 2003; Stevens et al, 1994, 1996, 1999). In addition, preterm neonates may demonstrate unique behaviors in response to noxious stimuli. Holsti and colleagues (2004) used the Newborn Individualized Developmental Care and Assessment Program (NIDCAP, Children's Hospital, Boston, MA) to examine responses of preterm neonates to a heelstick procedure and found that preterm neonates may uniquely respond to acute pain by increased flexion and extension of arms and legs, finger splay, fisting, frowning, and hand on face behaviors.

Pain Characteristics

Pain characteristics such as the source or cause of the pain (acute injury, disease), location, and timing of pain influence the perception and response to pain. Most research has focused on the responses to acute pain caused by single noxious stimuli. However, pain commonly occurs over a prolonged period or is recurrent in nature. Because of the tremendous plasticity within pain processing systems, these factors will significantly affect the infant's experience of pain.

Parents

Nurses who care for the infant in pain must care for the infant's family as well. Parents have many concerns and fears about their infants' pain and about the drugs used in the treatment of pain (Gale et al, 2004; Franck et al, 2005). Parents may fear the effects of pain on their children's development. They may also fear that their infant may become "addicted" to the analgesics (Franck et al, 2000). Nurses must be prepared to respond to questions from parents and encourage parent participation in providing nonpharmacologic comfort measures to their infants. Parents must be reassured that they are expected to ask questions about their infants' pain management.

Practitioner Factors

The knowledge, attitudes, and beliefs of health care professionals have played a major factor in the undertreatment of pain in both adults and children, despite emerging scientific evidence. Fear of addiction and disproportionate concern for side effects has resulted in severe underuse of opioid analgesics for acute postoperative pain for infants and children (Sredl, 2003).

Lack of education about pain in nursing and medical education is a major cause of myths and biases that impede appropriate assessment and management of pain in infants. Research has shown that infant pain management is strongly influenced by a nurse's biases, personal experiences with pain, and area of specialization. Nurses must examine closely their own beliefs and attitudes about pain, explore the impact that their attitudes might have on their patient care, and challenge their beliefs to determine whether they are science-based or tradition-based. Hester (1998) describes an "illusion of certainty" in which providers assume they know the level of a patient's pain without having to measure it based on the illness or procedure, without regard to the individual patient's experience. Use of validated pain assessment tools results in greater consistency in provider ratings of pain and may more accurately reflect pain experienced by preverbal infants.

MANAGEMENT OF NEONATAL PAIN

The goals of pain management in infants are (1) to minimize intensity, duration, and physiologic cost of the pain experience; and (2) to maximize the infant's ability to cope with and recover from the painful experience. Depending on duration and severity, pain may be successfully managed with nonpharmacologic and/or pharmacologic therapies.

Nonpharmacologic Management

Painful procedures in the NICU are unavoidable; therefore it is vital that caregivers assist infants to cope with and recover from necessary but painful clinical procedures. Nonpharmacologic strategies can reduce neonatal pain indirectly by reducing the total number of noxious stimuli to which infants are exposed. Strategies to prevent pain should be employed whenever possible, including grouping blood draws to minimize the number of venipunctures per day, establishing central vessel access to minimize vein and artery punctures, and limiting adhesive tape and gentle removal of tape to minimize epidermal stripping.

Nonpharmacologic strategies are hypothesized to directly reduce pain by (1) blocking nociceptive transduction or transmission; (2) activating descending inhibitory pathways; or, (3) activating attention or arousal systems that modulate pain. Nonpharmacologic strategies such as hand or blanket swaddling, nonnutritive sucking, and oral sucrose may help minimize neonatal pain and stress while maximizing the infant's own regulatory and coping abilities.

Swaddling

Several positioning and containment strategies have been investigated as nonpharmacologic strategies to minimize pain in the neonatal population. Although prone positioning of neonates has been demonstrated to promote sleep and improve respiratory function, it has not been found to be helpful in minimizing minor procedural pain in preterm neonates (Grunau et al, 2004; Stevens et al, 1999). Containment strategies to limit excessive, immature motor responses have, however, been demonstrated to be effective in minimizing pain responses in preterm neonates.

Swaddling is thought to reduce pain by providing gentle stimulation across the proprioceptive, thermal, and tactile sensory systems. Several studies have been conducted in the preterm population using different methods of swaddling. A hand swaddling technique known as "facilitated tucking" (holding the infant's extremities flexed and contained close to the trunk), has been shown to reduce pain responses in preterm neonates. In a study by Corff et al (1995), preterm infants undergoing a heelstick procedure demonstrated significantly reduced heart rates and crying, and more stability in sleep-wake cycles, in the hand-swaddled position. Hand-swaddling was also demonstrated to be effective in reducing procedural pain of endotracheal suctioning (Ward-Larson et al, 2004).

A similar containment study conducted by Fearon et al (1997) used blanket swaddling for nesting. The researchers examined the effectiveness of blanket swaddling after a heel lance in younger (<31 weeks' postmenstrual age) and older (at or older than 31 weeks' postmenstrual age) preterm infants. Trends showed that blanket swaddling was effective for reducing heart rate and negative facial displays in the post-heelstick phase for the older infants and increased oxygen saturation levels in younger infants.

Nonnutritive Sucking (NNS)

NNS is the provision of a pacifier into the mouth to promote sucking without the provision of breast milk or formula for nutrition. Franck (1987) found that pacifiers were ranked by NICU as the first choice of pain intervention. NNS is thought to produce analgesia through stimulation of orotactile and mechanoreceptors when a pacifier is introduced into the infant's mouth. NNS is hypothesized to modulate transmission or processing of nociception through mediation by the endogenous nonopioid system (Blass et al, 1987; Gunnar et al, 1988).

NNS has been shown to reduce behavioral pain responses in term infants during immunizations (Blass, 1997) and heel lances in term and preterm infants (Blass & Shide, 1994; Field & Goldson, 1984; Miller & Anderson, 1993). One study found that NNS reduced composite pain responses in preterm infants during heel lances (Stevens et al, 1999). However, pain relief was greater in infants who received both NNS and sucrose. Compared to blanket swaddling (Campos, 1989) or rocking (Campos, 1994) during painful procedures, NNS reduced duration of cry and soothed infants more rapidly. Unlike with blanket swaddling, however, a rebound in distress occurred when the NNS pacifier was removed from the infants' mouths. Therefore the efficacy of NNS is immediate but appears to terminate almost immediately on cessation of sucking.

Sucrose

Sucrose with and without NNS has been the most widely studied nonpharmacologic intervention for infant pain management. Sucrose is a disaccharide that comprises fructose and glucose. A systematic review of 21 randomized control trials of full-term and preterm infants (N = 1616) on the efficacy of sucrose for relieving pain found that sucrose decreased crying time, heart rate, facial action, and composite pain scores during heel lance and venipuncture (Stevens et al, 2004). A pain reduction response is noted with dose volumes ranging from 0.05 ml to 2 ml of a 24% solution administered approximately 2 minutes before the painful stimulus (Stevens et al, 1997). This 2-minute time interval appears to coincide with endogenous opioid release triggered by the sweet taste of sucrose (Stevens et al, 1999). The use of sucrose in combination with other behavioral interventions such as pacifiers, rocking, holding, and skin-to-skin holding may enhance the analgesic effect of sucrose (Stevens et al, 2004).

Two randomized controlled trials evaluated sucrose for immunizations. Two milliliters of 50% to 75% sucrose was effective for immunization pain in infants from 2 to 6 months of age (Lewindon et al, 1998; Ramenghi et al, 2002).

Although relatively few contraindications to the provision of swaddling and nonnutritive sucking for management of pain in neonates exist, the absolute safety of sucrose has not been determined. Rare instances of choking and decreased oxygen saturation, all resolving spontaneously, have been reported (Gibbins & Stevens, 2003; Stevens et al, 2004). Sucrose should be used with caution in extremely preterm neonates, critically ill newborns, neonates with unstable blood glucose levels, and infants at risk for necrotizing enterocolitis. Furthermore, sufficient evidence of the safety of repeated doses of sucrose in neonates to recommend its widespread use for repeated painful procedures is lacking (Stevens et al, 2004; Walden, 2001).

In general, nurses should begin with nonpharmacologic interventions before progressing to pharmacologic agents. However, nonpharmacologic interventions may not be appropriate for situations involving severe or prolonged pain.

Pharmacologic Management

Pharmacologic agents are often required to alleviate moderate to severe procedural, postoperative, or disease-related pain in neonates. Systemic analgesia, epidural anesthesia and analgesia, topical anesthetics, nonopioid analgesia, and adjunctive medications are reviewed.

Opioids

Opioid analgesics are considered the gold standard for pain relief. The most commonly used drugs for analgesia and sedation in neonates are listed in Table 17-2.

Opioids are often the preferred choice to manage moderate to severe pain in neonates. Advantages of opioid therapy include (1) prolonged clinical experience with their use in preterm and full-term neonates; (2) analgesic potency without a ceiling effect; (3) ability to produce sedation in ventilated patients; (4) few hemodynamic side effects; and (5) availability of antagonist drugs such as naloxone to reverse adverse side effects (Anand et al, 2000).

Morphine. Morphine is the most widely studied opioid analgesic in critically ill and postoperative neonates. Mean elimination half-life following single-dose administration of morphine ranges between 2.6 and 14 hours (Bhat et al, 1990, 1994). Differences exist in the pharmacokinetics of morphine administered to premature neonates in the first week of life (Bhat et al, 1990). After bolus administration, neonates of less than 40 weeks' gestation have longer elimination half-lives and delayed clearance of morphine than older neonates. In addition, plasma proteins in premature neonates unbind approximately 80% of morphine. This unbound morphine may account for its increased central nervous system concentrations. When morphine was administered as a continuous infusion, plasma concentrations were three

TABLE 17-2	Commonly Used Drugs for Analgesia and Sedation in Neonates	
Drug	**Intermittent Doses**	**Infusion Dose**
Opioid Analgesics		
Morphine	0.05 to 0.1 mg/kg/dose IV repeated every 4 hours as needed	Loading Dose: 0.1 mg/kg/dose IV infused over $1^1/_2$ hours Maintenance Dose: 0.015 to 0.020 mg/kg/hr IV
Fentanyl	1 to 4 mcg/kg/dose IV repeated every 2 to 4 hours as needed	Loading Dose: 1 mcg/kg IV Maintenance Dose: 0.5 mcg/kg/hr up to 4 mcg/kg/hr IV
Methadone	0.05 to 0.2 mg/kg/dose IV repeated every 6 to 12 hours as needed	
Nonsteroidal Anti-inflammatory Drugs		
Acetaminophen	10 to 15 mg/kg/dose PO repeated every 6 to 8 hours as needed 20 to 25 mg/kg/dose PR repeated every 6 to 8 hours as needed	
Benzodiazepines		
Midazolam	0.05 to 0.1 mg/kg/dose IV every 2 to 4 hours prn	Loading Dose: 0.05 to 0.2 mg/kg IV Maintenance Dose: 0.2 mcg/kg/min up to 0.6 mcg/kg/min
Miscellaneous Agents		
Chloral Hydrate	Intermittent Dose: 20 to 40 mg/kg/dose every 4 to 6 hours as needed PO/PR Single Dose: 30 to 75 mg/kg/dose PO/PR	

Adapted from Zenk KE et al (2003). Neonatal medications & nutrition: a comprehensive guide, ed 3. Santa Rosa, CA: NICU Ink.

times greater, and the elimination half-life was seven times longer, in neonates than in older infants and children.

Effective concentrations of morphine for analgesia and sedation are inconclusive and dependent on the age of the patient, hepatic function, renal function, and clinical condition (Dagan et al, 1993; Faura et al, 1998; Scott et al, 1999). A study by Bouwmeester et al (2003) found that postoperative neonates have a narrower therapeutic window for morphine analgesia than older infants and toddlers.

The effectiveness of morphine for acute pain caused by invasive procedures remains unclear. Although earlier studies supported the effectiveness of morphine analgesia for acute pain (Anand et al, 1999; McCulloch et al, 1995; Scott et al, 1999), more recent studies refute its effectiveness (Anand et al, 2005). No analgesic efficacy of intravenously administered morphine was noted on postoperative pain, endotracheal tube suctioning, or heel lances (Carbajal et al, 2005; Franck et al, 2000; Simons et al, 2003b).

Morphine has few effects on the neonatal cardiovascular system in the well hydrated neonate. Hypotension, bradycardia, and flushing are part of the histamine response to morphine and can be decreased by slow intravenous bolus administration (over 10 to 20 minutes) and optimizing intravascular fluid volume (Anand et al, 2000; Stoelting, 1995). As morphine predisposes patients to hypotension, a recent study by Hall et al (2005) recommends that morphine administration in preterm neonates between 23 and 26 weeks with preexisting hypotension be used with caution, as morphine has been found to be associated with adverse neurologic outcomes including severe intraventricular hemorrhage (IVH) and death. Although relatively uncommon, the effects of histamine release may also cause bronchospasm in infants with chronic lung disease (Anand et al, 2000). Enterohepatic recirculation of morphine may contribute to rebound increases in plasma levels and late respiratory depression (Bhat et al, 1990, 1992). Decreased intestinal motility and abdominal distention may also occur causing a delay in the establishment of enteral feeding in preterm neonates (Saarenmaa et al, 1999). The effect of morphine on gastrointestinal motility is hypothesized to be dose-dependent, and tolerance of enteral feeds may be improved by priming the gut with small volumes of milk and lower doses of morphine (Anand et al, 2000).

Despite relatively few side effects, full-term and especially preterm neonates remain susceptible to morphine toxicity that results from gradually increasing plasma concentrations. Close monitoring and individual titration of the amount and frequency of doses for all neonates receiving morphine therapy is therefore important (Anand et al, 2000).

Fentanyl. Randomized clinical trials in neonates have found that fentanyl is approximately 13 to 20 times more potent than morphine (Saarenmaa et al, 1999). Fentanyl is probably the most widely used analgesic in neonates and offers two distinct advantages over morphine (Anand et al, 2000). First, fentanyl causes less histamine release than morphine and may be more appropriate for infants with hypovolemia or hemodynamic instability, congenital heart disease, or expreterm infants with chronic lung disease (Anand et al, 2000). Second, fentanyl blunts increases in pulmonary vascular resistance. This finding makes it potentially useful in managing pain in neonates with persistent pulmonary hypertension, in neonates during extracorporeal membrane oxygenation, and in neonates after cardiac surgery (Anand et al, 2000).

Fentanyl has a more rapid onset and shorter duration of action compared with morphine and must be administered as a continuous infusion or as an intravenous bolus every 1 to 2 hours. Fentanyl is a highly lipophilic compound that crosses the blood-brain barrier more rapidly and has a longer elimination half-life than morphine (6 to 32 hours after a single-dose administration of fentanyl) (Anand et al, 2000). Accumulation of fentanyl in fatty tissues with extended use may prolong its sedative and respiratory depressant effects and may be responsible for the rebound increase in plasma levels observed following discontinuation of therapy in neonates (Anand et al, 2000). The liver metabolizes more than 90% of fentanyl.

Rarely, fentanyl can significantly reduce chest wall compliance (stiff chest syndrome). This naloxone-reversible side effect can be prevented by slow infusion (as opposed to rapid bolus administration), administration of doses less than 3 mcg/kg, or concomitant use of muscle relaxants.

The administration of fentanyl is associated with a modest increase in intracranial pressure (Anand et al, 2000). Caution is therefore recommended for administration of fentanyl to patients with intracranial pathology.

Increased intra-abdominal pressure can triple the elimination half-life of fentanyl, probably because of reduced hepatic artery blood flow. Although it has only been demonstrated for fentanyl, increased intra-abdominal pressure probably occurs with other opioids that are metabolized by the liver. Because many neonates experience increased intra-abdominal pressure, elimination is an important consideration in administering opioids to neonates.

Prevention of Opioid Withdrawal Symptoms. Neonates who require opioid therapy for an extended period of time may develop physical dependence and withdrawal. Rapid weaning of opioids may lead to withdrawal symptoms such as irritability, crying, increased respiratory rate, jitteriness, hypertonicity, vomiting, diarrhea, sweating, skin abrasions, seizures, yawning, stuffy nose, sneezing, and hiccups. The prevalence of opioid withdrawal is greater in infants after continuous infusions of fentanyl than continuous infusions of morphine (Franck et al, 1998). Dominguez et al (2003) reported a 53% incidence in opioid withdrawal in neonates who received a minimum of 24 hours of fentanyl by continuous infusion. In this study, the most significant risk factors for opioid withdrawal were higher total dose and longer infusion duration. In all neonates with withdrawal, onset of withdrawal symptoms occurred within 24 hours of discontinuation of the fentanyl infusion. Data are insufficient to determine the optimal weaning rate of opioids to prevent withdrawal symptoms in neonates on opioid therapy. Ducharme et al (2005) reported that adverse withdrawal symptoms in children who received continuous infusions of opioids and/or benzodiazepines could be prevented when the daily rate of weaning did not exceed 20% for children who received opioids/benzodiazepines for 1 to 3 days; 13% to 20% for 4 to 7 days; 8% to 13% for 8 to 14 days; 8% for 15 to 21 days; and 2% to 4% for more than 21 days, respectively. Abstinence scoring methods commonly used in the care of the infant with prenatal drug exposure must be used in assessing the infant during opioid weaning (Franck & Vilardi, 1995).

Methadone. Methadone is a synthetic opioid that produces prolonged analgesia and has good oral bioavailability, thus making it an attractive option to treat postoperative pain in neonates (Berde et al, 1991) and prevent neonatal abstinence syndrome (Maas et al, 1990). When an infant is being weaned from opioid therapy to a longer-acting oral medication such as methadone, the starting dose of methadone should be calculated to provide a dose equivalent to the dose of opioid the neonate is receiving (American Academy of Pediatrics et al, 2000). Further weaning should then be accomplished based on frequent reassessment to ensure that the patient is free of pain and withdrawal symptoms. Studies are needed to further establish the pharmacokinetics and dosing requirements of methadone in neonates.

Epidural Anesthesia and Analgesia

Epidural anesthesia and analgesia is a relatively new option available to manage surgical and postoperative pain in many NICUs. Morphine or fentanyl administered alone or in combination with local anesthetics into the epidural space can provide good intraoperative anesthesia and postoperative analgesia after abdominal or lower extremity surgery (Ochsenreither, 1997). Epidural analgesia should not be used in patients with sepsis or local infection at the insertion site, thrombocytopenia or other known coagulopathy, increased intracranial pressure, suspected neurologic disease, or malformations of the vertebral column. It also should not be used in infants who cannot tolerate a decrease in systemic vascular resistance such as those with tetralogy of Fallot (Ochsenreither, 1997).

Use of epidural analgesia may potentially expedite extubation (Murrell et al, 1993; Sethna & Koh, 2000; Valley & Bailey, 1991). Because opioids added to local anesthetic infusions act directly on the neurons in the spinal cord, lower doses of local anesthetic are required for epidural administration, and fewer opioid-related side effects are generally seen. Opioid-related side effects can still occur and require careful monitoring of the patient for side effects such as respiratory depression or urinary retention. Catheter-related side effects include catheter migration, infection, occlusion, neural injury/paresthesia, catheter breakage on removal, or hematoma formation at the site of insertion (Ochsenreither, 1997). Anesthetic-related side effects include injection into the cerebrospinal fluid that results in a high block with muscle paralysis or injection into a blood vessel resulting in seizures, hypotension, dysrhythmia, or cardiac arrest (Ochsenreither, 1997).

Epidural anesthesia and analgesia requires specially trained health care personnel and involves appropriate and close observation (American Academy of Pediatrics et al, 2000). In addition to monitoring for opioid-related, catheter-related, and anesthetic-related side effects, nursing care of neonates who are receiving epidural analgesia includes regular inspection of the catheter site for leakage, drainage, hematoma, and erythema. The infusate, dose, and rate of the infusion should be carefully checked, and the area should be kept clean and dry (Ochsenreither, 1997).

Topical Application of Local Anesthetics

EMLA Cream. EMLA cream (eutectic mixture of local anesthetics, lidocaine, and prilocaine; Astra Pharmaceuticals, London) is approved for use in infants at birth with a gestational age of 37 weeks or greater for a variety of clinical procedures. EMLA produces topical anesthesia when applied as a cream to the surface of intact skin and then covered with an occlusive dressing (Stoelting, 1995). The primary concern

with the use of EMLA is methemoglobinemia caused by prilocaine toxicity (Sethna & Koh, 2000). Neonates, particularly preterm neonates, are at increased risk because of a thinner stratum corneum and less active NADH-dependent methemoglobin reductase enzymes that result in higher plasma levels (Sethna & Koh, 2000). Neonates with anemia, sepsis, hypoxemia, or metabolic acidosis and who are receiving other methemoglobin-inducing drugs such as acetaminophen, phenytoin, phenobarbital, or nitroprusside may also be at increased risk for development of systemic toxicity (Sethna & Koh, 2000). Although it is not routinely recommended for use in preterm neonates, one study found that a single dose of 0.5 g EMLA cream applied for 60 minutes to the intact skin of preterm infants older than 30 weeks' gestation did not result in significant increases in blood methemoglobin concentrations (Taddio et al, 1995b). In addition to the risk of methemoglobinemia, local skin reactions have been noted with EMLA cream and have included blanching, redness, and transient purpuric lesions (Sethna & Koh, 2000). Policies and procedures regarding application of EMLA cream should be established to maximize pain relief while minimizing the potential side effects.

Three primary factors determine the effectiveness of EMLA cream: dose, size of application area, and duration of exposure (Sethna & Koh, 2000). The recommended dose in neonates is 0.5 to 2 g applied to the procedure site 1 hour before the procedure and covered with an occlusive dressing (Anand & International Evidence-Based Group for Neonatal Pain, 2001). Multiple studies document the efficacy of EMLA in reducing pain associated with venipunctures and circumcisions (Anand et al, 2005). EMLA has also been documented to be effective in managing pain associated with lumbar puncture (Kaur et al, 2003). EMLA has not been shown, however, to be effective in managing pain associated with the heelstick procedure (Anand et al, 2005).

Tetracaine 4% Gel. Tetracaine 4% gel (Ametop; Smith & Nephew, London) has also been investigated in neonates for management of procedural pain. Tetracaine gel has been found to be effective in managing pain associated with venipunctures and intravenous cannulation (Jain & Rutter, 2000; Moore, 2001), but ineffective for heel sticks and percutaneous inserted central catheter (PICC) insertions (Jain et al, 2001; Ballantyne et al, 2003).

LMX 4%. Another topical local anesthetic currently used in pediatrics for management of procedural pain is liposomal lidocaine cream (LMX 4%; Ferndale Laboratories, Michigan). Several studies have evaluated the efficacy of LMX and EMLA and found a 30-minute application of LMX to be as effective as a 60-minute application of EMLA for producing topical anesthesia for peripheral intravenous access in older children (Eichenfield et al, 2005; Kleiber et al, 2002; Koh et al, 2004). Similar results were found in a recent study in neonates that found LMX to be equally effective as EMLA in reducing the pain of circumcision in term newborns (Lehr et al, 2005). LMX may offer an improved risk-benefit profile compared to EMLA considering the faster onset of action and no risk of methemoglobinemia. Further studies in neonates are needed to establish the safety and efficacy of LMX for management of procedural pain in neonates.

Nonopioid Analgesics

Acetaminophen. Acetaminophen is a nonopioid analgesic for short-term management of mild to moderate pain in neonates. Acetaminophen has been commonly administered in neonates as an oral or rectal preparation. When acetaminophen is administered concurrently with opioid analgesia, the effect is additive and allows a reduction in dosages of both drugs, resulting in fewer adverse side effects (Menon et al, 1998).

Little information is available on the pharmacokinetics of acetaminophen administration in neonates, especially administration by the rectal route. However, studies in adults have demonstrated greater than 80% bioavailability for orally administered acetaminophen (Depre et al, 1992). In children, peak concentrations of analgesic effect are reached in 30 to 60 minutes. The elimination half-life in newborns is estimated to be less than or equal to 4.9 hours. Acetaminophen is metabolized almost entirely by hepatic conjugation that is then renally eliminated.

Although acetaminophen has been demonstrated to significantly reduce pain responses during skin excision and comfort scores at 6 hours following the circumcision procedure (Howard et al, 1994), other studies have failed to demonstrate efficacy resulting from acute tissue injury of heelstick and postoperative pain relief after cardiac surgery (Shah et al, 1998; Van Lingen et al, 1999). The results from these studies suggest that acetaminophen may be more appropriate for mild to moderate dull, continuous pain resulting from inflammatory conditions than for acute, tissue-damaging, or severe noxious stimuli (Anand et al, 2000).

At therapeutic doses, acetaminophen is well tolerated and has a low toxicity (Olkkola & Hamunen, 2000). Because acetaminophen does not inhibit prostaglandin synthesis in tissues other than the brain, common side effects of nonsteroidal anti-inflammatory drugs—such as inhibition of platelet function, renal insufficiency, and gastrointestinal irritation—do not occur (Anand et al, 2000). The primary concern of acetaminophen is liver damage, but this should not be a concern in neonates if standard doses are used (Berde et al, 1991).

Use of Adjunctive Drugs

In the NICU, the use of sedatives, alone or in combination with analgesics, is controversial. Although sedatives suppress the behavioral expression of pain, they have no analgesic effects and can even increase pain. Sedatives should only be used when pain has been ruled out. When administered with opioids, sedatives may allow more optimal weaning of opioids in critically ill, ventilator-dependent neonates who have developed tolerance from prolonged opioid therapy. No research has been done to determine the safety or efficacy of combining sedatives and analgesics for the treatment of pain in infants.

The most commonly administered sedatives in the NICU are benzodiazepines and chloral hydrate.

Benzodiazepines

Midazolam. Midazolam is a short-acting benzodiazepine that has increasingly been used in the NICU to provide sedation for mechanically ventilated neonates. Midazolam is preferred over other benzodiazepines because of its water solubility, rapid clearance, and shorter elimination half-life (6.5 hours) (Jacqz-Aigrain et al, 1992). Recent concern about the safety of midazolam in neonates has been reported because of the large number of adverse neurologic effects associated with midazolam in term and preterm neonates (Adams et al,

1997; Magny et al, 1994; Ng et al, 2000). Transient neurologic effects after boluses and/or infusions of midazolam include impaired level of consciousness, lack of visual following, hypertonia, hypotonia, choreic movements, dyskinetic movements, myoclonus, epileptiform activity, abnormalities in electroencephalograms, and cerebral hypoperfusion (Ng et al, 2000). A study by Anand et al (1999) also found a higher incidence of poor neurologic outcome as defined by death, severe intraventricular hemorrhage, and periventricular leukomalacia in ventilated preterm neonates treated with midazolam.

Diazepam. Diazepam is not recommended for administration in neonates because of its very prolonged half-life (20 to 50 hours), its long-acting metabolites, and concern about the benzyl alcohol content. The dose of benzyl alcohol preservative in diazepam is, however, below the dose known to cause fatal toxicity in premature neonates (100 to 400 mg/kg/day). Diazepam displaces bilirubin from albumin-binding sites, thereby increasing the neonate's risk of kernicterus (Anand et al, 2000).

Chloral Hydrate.
Chloral hydrate has been used in single doses to sedate neonates during pulmonary function, radiographic, and other diagnostic testing for which the patient must lie still. The onset of action is approximately 30 minutes and the lasts about 2 to 4 hours, depending on the dose (Anand et al, 2000). Although clinically effective, concern has been raised about the potential carcinogenic and genotoxic effects of chloral hydrate administered to animals. Chloral hydrate has also been used in repeated doses to sedate neonates on mechanical ventilation. Alternative sedatives (i.e., benzodiazepines) should be used when possible because chloral hydrate has other gastrointestinal side effects and may be associated with direct hyperbilirubinemia. The extremely long half-life (greater than 72 hours) of chloral hydrate increases the risk of toxicity with repeated administration, which may be manifest as increased agitation.

Management of Specific Pain Types

Pain management techniques may vary based on pain type and clinical situation. This section will review special issues related to procedural pain, postoperative pain, preemptive analgesia for mechanical ventilation, and pain management at end of life.

Procedural Pain.
It has been estimated that newborn infants, particularly those born preterm, are routinely subjected to an average of 61 invasive procedures performed from admission to discharge, with some of the youngest or sickest infants experiencing more than 450 painful procedures during their hospital stays (Barker & Rutter, 1995). Many of the procedures commonly performed in the neonate cause moderate to severe pain, with average pain scores of 5 on a 10-point scale (Simons et al, 2003a). Substantial numbers of failed attempts at procedures dramatically increase the number of painful procedures that neonates are subjected to. Simons et al (2003a) found that the percentages of failed procedures for insertion of central venous catheters, insertion of peripheral arterial catheters, and intravenous cannula insertion were 45.6%, 37.5%, and 30.9%, respectively. These frequent, invasive, and noxious procedures occur randomly in the NICU and many times are not routinely managed with either pharmacologic or nonpharmacologic interventions (Simons et al, 2003a). Anand and the International Evidence-Based Group for Neonatal Pain (2001) provide guidelines for

preventing and treating neonatal procedural pain. Strategies for the management of diagnostic, therapeutic, and surgical procedures commonly performed in the NICU are summarized in Table 17-3.

Local anesthesia may not be sufficient for procedures that affect deeper tissue, such as chest tube insertion or surgical cutdown of vessels. Central analgesia is then required to prevent pain. For the nonventilated patient, in whom concern for the respiratory depressant effects of opioids exists, one half the standard dose may be administered. The infant's respiratory status and responsiveness to pain stimuli can then be

assessed before further drug administration. For the infant who is receiving opioid analgesics on a regular basis, a controlled infusion of a bolus dose may be required to provide adequate analgesia during an invasive procedure.

Postoperative Pain. Adequate analgesia is important during the immediate postoperative period for the optimal recovery of the patient. Unrelieved pain can interfere with ventilation and delay weaning. In general, it is thought that the use of low-dose continuous infusions of opioid analgesics provide more constant, effective pain relief with less medication than intermittent scheduled doses of opioids (Truog &

TABLE 17-3	Suggested Management of Painful Procedures Commonly Performed in the NICU					
Procedures	**Pacifier with Sucrose**	**Swaddling, Containment, or Facilitated Tucking**	**EMLA Cream**	**Subcutaneous Infiltration of Lidocaine**	**Opioids**	**Other**
Diagnostic Procedures						
Arterial puncture	√	√	√	√		
Heel lancing	√	√				Consider venipuncture; skin-to-skin contact with mother; mechanical spring-loaded lance
Lumbar puncture	√		√	√		Use careful physical handling
Venipuncture	√	√	√			
Eye examination	√	√				Consider topical anesthetic
Therapeutic Procedures						
Central venous line placement	√	√	√	√	√	Consider general anesthesia
Chest tube insertion	√			√	√	Anticipate need for intubation and ventilation in neonates spontaneously breathing; consider short-acting anesthetic agents; avoid midazolam
Gavage tube insertion lubrication	√	√				Gentle technique and appropriate lubrication
Intramuscular injection	√	√	√			Give drugs intravenously, whenever it is possible
Peripherally inserted central catheter placement	√	√	√		√	
Endotracheal intubation					√	Various combinations of atropine, ketamine, thiopental sodium, succinylcholine chloride, morphine, fentanyl, nondepolarizing muscle relaxant; consider topical lidocaine
Endotracheal suction	Sucrose optional	√			√	Spray
Surgical Procedures						
Circumcision	√		√			Mogen clamp preferred over Gomco clamp; dorsal penile nerve block, ring block, or caudal block using plain or buffered lidocaine; consider acetaminophen for postoperative pain

Adapted from Anand KJ, the International Evidence-Based Group for Neonatal Pain (2001). Consensus statement for the prevention and management of pain in the newborn. Archives of pediatric adolescent medicine 155:173-180.

Anand, 1989). However, a more recent study by Bouwmeester et al (2003) found no difference in the safety or effectiveness of intermittent doses of morphine compared with continuous infusions of morphine.

Preemptive Analgesia for Mechanical Ventilation.
Opioids are frequently used to sedate, promote respiratory synchrony, produce physiologic stability, and relieve pain or discomfort in ventilated neonates (Anand et al, 1999). A recent Cochrane database systematic review, however, concludes that there is insufficient evidence available to recommend the routine use of opioids in mechanically ventilated neonates (Bellu et al, 2005).

In a multicenter trial of 898 ventilated preterm infants between 23 and 32 weeks' gestation, Anand et al (2004) found that preemptive analgesia using morphine decreased clinical signs of pain but did not reduce the frequency of severe IVH, periventricular leukomalacia, or death in ventilated neonates. This study did, however, demonstrate that additional intermittent boluses of morphine were associated with increased rate of adverse neurologic outcomes.

Several secondary analyses of this data have been published examining hypotension and short-term pulmonary outcomes. Hall et al (2005) found that pre-emptive morphine infusions, additional bolus morphine doses, and lower gestational age were associated with hypotension among preterm neonates. The researchers report that this pre-existing hypotension was associated with the findings of severe IVH and death, but morphine therapy did not contribute to these outcomes. Bhandari et al (2005) demonstrated that infants in the morphine group required significantly longer ventilatory therapy compared to the placebo group and that additional doses of morphine were associated with increased air leaks and longer durations of high-frequency ventilation, nasal continuous airway pressure, and oxygen therapy.

Pain Management at End-of-Life (EOL).
Pain management at end-of-life (EOL) primarily centers on the provision of opioids to minimize pain and nonpharmacologic therapies to enhance the infant's comfort level (Walden et al, 2001). Pain assessment is extremely difficult in neonates at end of life. Therefore caregivers must often consider risk factors for pain and rely on physiologic measures such as increases in heart rate and decreases in oxygen saturation to make pain management decisions.

Continuous infusions of opioid therapy such as morphine and fentanyl are often required to manage pain at EOL and should be titrated to desired clinical response (analgesia) (Anand et al, 2000). Opioid doses well beyond those described for standard analgesia are often required for infants who are in severe pain or who have developed tolerance (decreasing pain relief with the same dosage over time) after the prolonged use of opioids (Partridge & Wall, 1997).

Physiologic comfort measures may palliate pain and distressing symptoms in infants at EOL and include reduction of noxious stimuli, organization of caregiving, and positioning and containment strategies (Walden et al, 2001).

NEONATAL NURSE'S ROLE AND RESPONSIBILITIES

Provision of comfort and relief of pain are two primary goals of nursing care. To accomplish these goals, neonatal nurses must (1) prevent pain when possible; (2) assess pain in their neonatal patients who cannot verbalize their subjective experience of pain; (3) provide relief or reduction of pain through implementation of nonpharmacologic and/or pharmacologic measures; and (4) assist the infant in coping when pain cannot be prevented.

The effective management of infant pain requires nurses to collaborate with each other, with physicians, and with the infant's parents. Nurses must effectively communicate assessments and recommendations in an objective, concise manner and advocate for pain relief strategies with responsible health care team members.

Neonatal nurses must remain informed about professional standards and clinical guidelines related to pain assessment and management in neonates. The nurse should also participate in ongoing pain education and review of new research and scientific developments.

SUMMARY

Pain in neonates is often assessed and managed inadequately in a large proportion of neonates in the NICU. It is clear, however, that caring for infants in pain requires attention not only to the immediate effects but also to the long-term developmental consequences of pain and pain treatment. Through ongoing research, objective assessment, effective collaboration, and systematic application of treatment plans, nurses will achieve greater comfort for individual patients and add to the body of knowledge in this rapidly evolving field.

REFERENCES

Adams MM et al (1997). A series of neonatal patients with paradoxical seizure-like reactions to bolus intravenous injections of midazolam. *Pediatric research* 41:134A.

American Academy of Pediatrics et al (2000). Prevention and management of pain and stress in the neonate. *Pediatrics* 105(2):454-461.

Anand KJ (1998). Neonatal analgesia and anesthesia: introduction. *Seminars in perinatology* 22(5):347-349.

Anand KJ, Craig KD (1996). New perspectives on the definition of pain. *Pain* 67(1):3-6; discussion 209-211.

Anand KJ, Hickey PR (1992). Halothane-morphine compared with high dose sufentanil for anesthesia and post-operative analgesia in neonatal cardiac surgery. *New England journal of medicine* 326(1):1-9.

Anand KJ, the International Evidence-Based Group for Neonatal Pain (2001). Consensus statement for the prevention and management of pain in the newborn. *Archives of pediatric adolescent medicine* 155:173-180.

Anand KJS, Plotsky PM (1995). Repetitive neonatal pain alters weight gain and pain threshold during development in infant rats. *Critical care medicine* 23(Suppl):A22.

Anand KJ et al (1999). Analgesia and sedation in preterm neonates who require ventilatory support: results from the NOPAIN trial: Neonatal Outcome and Prolonged Analgesia in Neonates. *Archives of pediatric adolescent medicine* 153(4):331-338.

Anand KJS et al (2000). Systemic analgesic therapy. In Anand K et al, editors. *Pain in neonates*, ed 2. Amsterdam: Elsevier Science.

Anand KJ et al (2004). Effects of morphine analgesia in ventilated preterm neonates: primary outcomes from the NEOPAIN randomised trial. *Lancet* 363(9422):1673-1683.

Anand KJS et al (2005). Analgesia and local anesthesia during invasive procedures in the neonate. *Clinical therapeutics* 27(6):844-876.

Ballantyne M et al (1999). Validation of the Premature Infant Pain Profile in the clinical setting. *Clinical journal of pain* 15(4):297-303.

Ballantyne M et al (2003). A randomized controlled trial evaluating the efficacy of tetracaine gel for pain relief from peripherally inserted central catheters in infants. *Advances in neonatal care* 3(6):297-307.

Barker DP, Rutter N (1995). Exposure to invasive procedures in neonatal intensive care unit admissions. *Archives of disease in childhood* 72(1):F47-F48.

Bellu R et al (2005). Opioids for neonates receiving mechanical ventilation. *Neonatal modules of the Cochrane database of systematic reviews* [Electronic database].

Berde CB et al (1991). Comparison of methadone and morphine for prevention of postoperative pain in 3-7 year old children. *Journal of pediatrics* 119(1, Part 1):136-141.

Bhandari V et al (2005). Morphine administration and short-term pulmonary outcomes among ventilated preterm infants. *Pediatrics* 116(2):352-359.

Bhat R et al (1990). Pharmacokinetics of a single dose of morphine in preterm infants during the first week of life. *Journal of pediatrics* 117(3):477-481.

Bhat R et al (1992). Morphine metabolism in acutely ill preterm newborn infants. *Journal of pediatrics* 120:795-799.

Bhat R et al (1994). Postconceptual age influences pharmacokinetics and metabolism of morphine in sick neonates. *Pediatric research* 35(4, Part 2):81A.

Blass E (1997). Milk-induced hypoalgesia in human newborns. *Pediatrics* 99:825-829.

Blass E, Shide D (1994). Some comparisons among the calming and pain relieving effects of sucrose, glucose, fructose and lactose in infant rats. *Chemical senses* 19:239-249.

Blass E et al (1987). Interactions between sucrose, pain and isolation distress. *Pharmacology, biochemistry & behavior* 26(3):483-489.

Blauer T, Gerstmann D (1998). A simultaneous comparison of three neonatal pain scales during common NICU procedures. *Clinical journal of pain* 14(1):39-47.

Bouwmeester NJ et al (2003). Age- and therapy-related effects on morphine requirements and plasma concentrations of morphine and its metabolites in postoperative infants. *British journal of anesthesia* 90(5):642-652.

Buskila D et al (2003). Pain sensitivity in prematurely born adolescents. *Archives of pediatric adolescent medicine* 157(11):1079-1082.

Campos RG (1989). Soothing pain-elicited distress in infants with swaddling and pacifiers. *Child development* 60(4):781-792.

Campos RG (1994). Rocking and pacifiers: two comforting interventions for heelstick pain. *Research in nursing & health* 17:321-331.

Carbajal R et al (2005). Morphine does not provide adequate analgesia for acute procedural pain among preterm neonates. *Pediatrics* 115(6):1494-1500.

Cignacco E et al (2004). Pain assessment in the neonate using the Bernese pain scale for neonates. *Early human development* 78(2):125-131.

Corff K et al (1995). Facilitated tucking: a nonpharmacologic comfort measure for pain in preterm neonates. *Journal of obstetric, gynecologic, and neonatal nursing* 24:143-147.

Dagan O et al (1993). Morphine pharmacokinetics in children following cardiac surgery: effects of disease and inotropic support. *Journal of cardiothoracic and vascular anesthesia* 7(4):396-398.

Depre M et al (1992). Tolerance and pharmacokinetics of propacetamol, a paracetamol formulation for intravenous use. *Fundamentals in clinical pharmacology* 6:259-262.

Dominguez KD et al (2003). Opioid withdrawal in critically ill neonates. *Annals of pharmacotherapy* 37(4):473-477.

Ducharme C et al (2005). A prospective study of adverse reactions to the weaning of opioids and benzodiazepines among critically ill children. *Intensive and critical care nursing* 21(3):179-186.

Duhn L, Medves J (2004). A systematic integrative review of infant pain assessment tools. *Advances in neonatal care* 4(3):126-140.

Eichenfield LF et al (2005). A clinical study to evaluate the efficacy of Ela-Max as compared with eutectic mixture of local anesthetics cream for pain reduction of venipuncture in children. *Pediatrics* 109(6):1092-1099.

Eriksson M et al (1999). Oral glucose and venipuncture reduce blood sampling pain in newborns. *Early human development* 55(3):211-218.

Faura CC et al (1998). Systematic review of factors affecting the ratios of morphine and its major metabolites. *Pain* 74(1):43-53.

Fearon I et al (1997). Swaddling after heel lance: age-specific effects on behavioral recovery in preterm infants. *Journal of developmental and behavioral pediatrics* 18:222-232.

Field T, Goldson E (1984). Pacifying effects of nonnutritive sucking on term and preterm neonates during heelstick procedures. *Pediatrics* 74(6):1012-1015.

Fitzgerald M, Anand KJS (1993). Developmental neuroanatomy and neurophysiology of pain. In Schechter NL et al, editors. *Pain in infants, children, and adolescents*, Baltimore: Williams & Wilkins.

Franck LS (1987). A national survey of the assessment of pain and agitation in the national intensive care unit. *Journal of obstetric, gynecologic, and neonatal nursing* 16(6):387-393.

Franck L, Vilardi J (1995). Assessment and management of opioid withdrawal in ill neonates. *Neonatal network* 14(2):39-48.

Franck LS et al (1998). Opioid withdrawal in neonates after continuous infusions of morphine or fentanyl during extracorporeal membrane oxygenation. *American journal of critical care* 7(5):364-369.

Franck LS et al (2000). Plasma norepinephrine levels, vagal tone index, and flexor reflex threshold in premature neonates receiving intravenous morphine during the postoperative period: a pilot study. *Clinical journal of pain* 16(2):95-104.

Franck LS et al (2005). Parent's views about infant pain in neonatal intensive care. *Clinical journal of pain* 21(2):133-139.

Fuller BF (2002). Infant gender differences regarding acute established pain. *Clinical nursing research* 11(2):190-203.

Gale G et al (2004). Parents' perceptions of their infant's pain experience in the NICU. *International journal of nursing studies* 41(1):51-58.

Gibbins S, Stevens B (2003). The influence of gestational age on the efficacy of short-term safety of sucrose for procedural pain relief. *Advances in neonatal care* 3(5):241-249.

Grunau RV, Craig KD (1987). Pain expression in neonates: facial action and cry. *Pain* 28(3):395-410.

Grunau RV et al (1994a). Pain sensitivity and temperament in extremely low-birth-weight premature toddlers and preterm and full term controls. *Pain* 58(3):341-346.

Grunau RVE et al (1994b). Early pain experience, child and family factors, as precursors of somatization: a prospective study of extremely premature and fullterm children. *Pain* 56(3):353-359.

Grunau RE et al (2004). Does prone or supine position influence pain responses in preterm infants at 32 weeks gestational age? *Clinical journal of pain* 20(2):76-82.

Guinsburg R et al (2000). Differences in pain expression between male and female newborn infants. *Pain* 85(1-2):127-133.

Gunnar MR et al (1988). Adrenocortical activity and behavioral distress in human newborns. *Developmental psychobiology* 21(4):297-310.

Gunnar MR et al (1995). Neonatal stress reactivity: predictions to later emotional temperament. *Child development* 66(1):1-13.

Hall RW et al (2005). Morphine, hypotension, and adverse outcomes among preterm neonates: who's to blame? Secondary results from the NEOPAIN trial. *Pediatrics* 115(5):1351-1359.

Hester NO (1998). Assessment: the cornerstone for successful management of intractable pain. *Colorado nurse* 98(1):11.

Hodgkinson K et al (1994). Measuring pain in neonates: evaluating an instrument and developing a common language. *Australian journal of advance nursing* 12(1):17-22.

Holsti L et al (2004). Specific Newborn Individualized Developmental Care and Assessment Program movements are associated with acute pain in preterm infants in the neonatal intensive care unit. *Pediatrics* 114(1):65-72.

Howard CR et al (1994). Acetaminophen analgesia in neonatal circumcision: the effect on pain. *Pediatrics* 93:641-646.

Jacqz-Aigrain E et al (1992). Pharmacokinetics of midazolam during continuous infusion in critically ill neonates. *European journal of clinical pharmacology* 42:329-332.

Jain A, Rutter N (2000). Does topical amethocaine gel reduce the pain of venipuncture in newborn infants? A randomised double blind controlled trial. *Archives of disease in childhood, fetal, neonatal edition* 83(3):F207-F210.

Jain A et al (2001). Topical amethocaine gel for pain relief of heel prick blood sampling: a randomised double blind controlled trial. *Archives of disease in childhood, fetal, neonatal edition* 84(1):F56-F59.

Johnston CC, Stevens BJ (1996). Experience in a neonatal intensive care unit affects pain response. *Pediatrics* 98(2):925-930.

Johnston CC et al (1997). A cross-sectional survey of pain and pharmacologic analgesia in Canadian neonatal intensive care units. *Clinical journal of pain* 13:308-312.

Kaur G et al (2003). A randomized trial of eutectic mixture of local anesthetics during lumbar puncture in newborns. *Archives of pediatric adolescent medicine* 157(11):1065-1070.

Kleiber C et al (2002). Topical anesthetics for intravenous insertion in children: a randomized equivalency study. *Pediatrics* 110(4):758-761.

Koh et al (2004). A randomized, double-blind comparison study of EMLA and ELA-Max for topical anesthesia in children undergoing intravenous insertion. *Pediatric Anesthesia* 14(12):977-982.

Krechel SW, Bildner J (1995). CRIES: a new neonatal postoperative pain measurement score. Initial testing of validity and reliability. *Pediatric anaesthesia* 5:53-61.

Lawrence J et al (1993). The development of a tool to assess neonatal pain. *Neonatal network* 12(6):59-66.

Lehr VT et al (2005). Lidocaine 4% cream compared with lidocaine 2.5% and prilocaine 2.5% or dorsal penile block for circumcision. *American journal of perinatology* 22(5):231-237.

Lewindon PJ et al.,(1998). Randomised controlled trial of sucrose by mouth for relief of infant crying after immunization. *Archives of disease in children* 78(5):453-456.

Maas U et al (1990). Infrequent neonatal opiate withdrawal following maternal detoxification during pregnancy. *Journal of pediatric medicine* 18(2):111-118.

Magny JF et al (1994). Midazolam and myoclonus in neonate. *European journal of pediatrics* 153:389-392.

McCulloch KM et al (1995). Skin blood flow changes during routine nursery procedures. *Early human development* 41(2):147-156.

Menon G et al (1998). Practical approach to analgesia and sedation in the neonatal intensive care unit. *Seminars in perinatology* 22:417-424.

Merskey H (1979). Pain terms: a list with definitions and notes on usage recommended by the IASP Subcommittee on Taxonomy. *Pain* 6(3):249-252.

Miller H, Anderson G (1993). Nonnutritive sucking: effects on crying and heart rate in intubated infants requiring assisted mechanical ventilation. *Nursing research* 42:305-307.

Moore J (2001). No more tears: a randomized controlled double-blind trial of amethocaine gel vs. placebo in the management of procedural pain in neonates. *Journal of advanced nursing* 34(4):475-482.

Murrell D et al (1993). Continuous epidural analgesia in newborn infants undergoing major surgery. *Journal of pediatric surgery* 28(4):548-553.

Ng E et al (2000). Intravenous midazolam infusion for sedation of infants in the neonatal intensive care unit. *Neonatal modules of the Cochrane database of systematic reviews* [Electronic database].

Ochsenreither J (1997). Epidural analgesia in infants. *Neonatal network* 16:79-84.

Olkkola K, Hamunen K (2000). Pharmacokinetics and pharmacodynamics of analgesic drugs. In Anand K et al, editors. *Pain in neonates, ed 2.* Amsterdam: Elsevier Science.

Partridge JC, Wall SN (1997). Analgesia for dying infants whose life support is withdrawn or withheld. *Pediatrics* 99(1):76-79.

Porter FL et al (1998). The effect of handling and immobilization on the response to acute pain in newborn infants. *Pediatrics* 102(6):1383-1389.

Ramenghi LA et al (2002). Intra-oral administration of sweet-tasting substances and infants' crying response to immunization: a randomized, placebo-controlled trial. *Biology of the neonate* 81(3):163-169.

Saarenmaa E et al (1999). Advantages of fentanyl over morphine in analgesia for ventilated newborn infants after birth: a randomized trial. *Journal of pediatrics* 134:144-150.

Scott CS et al (1999). Morphine pharmacokinetics and pain assessment in premature newborns. *Journal of pediatrics* 135(4):423-429.

Sethna N, Koh J (2000). Regional anesthesia and analgesia. In Anand K et al, editors. *Pain in neonates, ed 2.* Amsterdam: Elsevier Science.

Shah V et al (1998). Randomized controlled trial of paracetamol for heel prick pain in neonates. *Archives of disease in childhood, fetal, neonatal edition* 79:F209-211.

Simons SH et al (2003a). Do we still hurt newborn babies? A prospective study of procedural pain and analgesia in neonates. *Archives of pediatric adolescent medicine* 157:1058-1064.

Simons SH et al (2003b). Routine morphine infusion in preterm newborns who received ventilatory support: a randomized controlled trial. *Journal of the American Medical Association* 290(18):2419-2427.

Sredl D (2003). Myths and facts about pain in neonates. *Neonatal network* 22(6):69-71.

Stevens BJ et al (1994). Factors that influence the behavioral pain responses of premature infants. *Pain* 59(1):101-109.

Stevens B et al (1996). Premature Infant Pain Profile: development and initial validation. *Clinical journal of pain* 12:13-22.

Stevens B et al (1997). The efficacy of sucrose for relieving procedural pain in neonates: a systematic review and meta-analysis. *Acta paediatrica* 86:837-842.

Stevens B et al (1999). The efficacy of developmentally sensitive interventions and sucrose for relieving procedural pain in very low birth weight neonates. *Nursing research* 48:35-43.

Stevens B et al (2004). Sucrose for analgesia in newborn infants undergoing painful procedures. *Neonatal modules of the Cochrane database of systematic reviews* [Electronic database].

Stoelting R (1995). *Handbook of pharmacology & physiology in anesthetic practice.* Philadelphia: Lippincott Williams & Wilkins.

Taddio A, Ohlsson A (1997). Lidocaine-prilocaine cream (EMLA) to reduce pain in male neonates undergoing circumcision: *Neonatal modules of the Cochrane database of systematic reviews* [Electronic database].

Taddio A et al (1995a). Effect of circumcision on pain responses during vaccination in male infants. *Lancet* 345:291-292.

Taddio A et al (1995b). Safety of lidocaine-prilocaine cream in the treatment of preterm neonates. *Journal of pediatrics* 127:1002-1005.

Truog R, Anand KJS (1989). Management of pain in the postoperative neonate [review]. *Clinics in perinatology* 16(1):61-78.

Valley RD, Bailey AG (1991). Caudal morphine for postoperative analgesia in infants and children: a report of 138 cases. *Anesthesia and analgesia* 72(1):120-124.

Van Lingen RA et al (1999). Pharmacokinetics and metabolism of rectally administered paracetamol in preterm neonates. *Archives of diseases in childhood, fetal neonatal edition* 80:F59-63.

Walden M (2001). *Pain assessment and management: guideline for practice.* Glenview, IL: National Association of Neonatal Nurses.

Walden M et al (2001). Comfort care for infants in the neonatal intensive care unit at end of life. *Newborn and infant nursing reviews* 1:97-105.

Ward-Larson C et al (2004). The efficacy of facilitated tucking for relieving procedural pain of endotracheal suctioning in very low birthweight infants. *MCN, the American journal of maternal child nursing* 29(3):151-156.

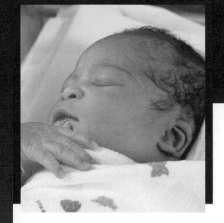

Chapter 18

Fetal Therapy

Jody A. Farrell • Kathy Bergman • Carole Kenner

Throughout recorded history, the fetus has maintained an enigmatic presence, with its development viewed as a mysterious process. To a large extent, ultrasonography and innovations and improvements in diagnostic imaging have unveiled the secrets of the womb, altering our attitudes about the developing fetus and providing a medium to document fetal growth and development. Most important, recent advances and sophistication in fetal imaging and diagnostic equipment and techniques have dramatically improved our ability to identify and manage many prenatally diagnosed malformations. The number of fetal disorders and structural defects that can be identified at a stage early enough to allow thoughtful, timely treatment options, including prenatal intervention, is growing. With improvements in prenatal diagnosis, increasing numbers of patients may choose the option to treat fetuses with major problems either pre- or postnatally (Evans et al, 2002). For many fetal defects, strict selection criteria for in utero intervention have been defined, the anesthetic and tocolytic protocols worked out, and the surgical techniques for hysterotomy and fetal surgery developed. Indeed, the fetus has become a bona fide patient in our lifetime (Harrison, 1996, 2003).

For nurses, fetal therapy presents complex challenges. Nurses offer counseling, educational, organizational, and technical expertise, and skills to the treatment team, patients and families. They also provide significant insight on the ethical considerations that arise in this evolving field. The aims of this chapter are manifold: (1) to provide a historical perspective of fetal treatment, including fetal surgery, and describe some key events of this multifaceted, complex area; (2) to describe in detail the components and dynamics of a collaborative team management of fetal therapy patients; and (3) to outline emerging, future trends in this rapidly evolving field.

HISTORICAL OVERVIEW

Designing a strategy for treating erythroblastosis fetalis, a life-threatening fetal and neonatal complication, prompted the first attempt at amelioration of a fetal condition. In 1963, New Zealand clinician-scientist A. W. Liley performed an in utero, fluoroscopy-guided exchange transfusion of red blood cells into the abdomen of a 32-week fetus (Liley, 1963). This procedure was heralded as paving a new direction and thus initiating a new era in obstetric and pediatric care. Liley's work effectively marked the birth of fetal treatment, the in utero medical intervention or correction of a fetal condition.

Advances in imaging technology have been hallmarks of this evolving field. In the 1950s and 1960s, the use of ultra-sonography as a diagnostic and imaging tool gave rise to farther-reaching implications in health care. Ultrasonography is now reliably and routinely used to determine gestational age, fetal growth patterns, fetal well-being, amniotic fluid levels, and the position of the placenta. It also can detect certain congenital anomalies—a capability that particularly and inextricably links ultrasonography to fetal diagnosis and treatment.

Ultrasonography has also proved to be an adjunct to other diagnostic procedures, such as amniocentesis, chorionic villus sampling, and percutaneous umbilical blood sampling (PUBS) (Laifer & Kuller, 1996). These techniques, with ultra-sonography, laid the groundwork for the new frontier of fetal treatment. Once abnormal fetal conditions could be detected early, many became amenable to prenatal treatment. No longer were management options limited to termination of the pregnancy or postnatal treatment. Table 18-1 summarizes the fetal conditions that often prove amenable to treatment in utero.

In 1981, Michael Harrison and a multidisciplinary team at the University of California, San Francisco, became the first group to clinically attempt in utero correction of urinary tract obstruction. Harrison and his co-investigators hypothesized that if the outlet obstruction could be corrected before birth, then the devastating sequela of fatal pulmonary hypoplasia or renal failure could be averted. The hypothesis was extensively and successfully tested in the fetal sheep model, and the surgical and anesthesia techniques were worked out. This experimental work paved the way for the first attempt at a closed surgical procedure in a human fetus with urinary tract obstruction.

Specifically, in the 1981 case, a catheter needle was passed through the maternal abdominal wall into the fetal bladder. An indwelling bladder catheter then was secured to drain fluid from the bladder into the amniotic sac, and would remain in place until birth. The procedure proved successful. Although the cause of the obstruction was not corrected until the neonatal period, the deleterious effects of the obstruction were prevented while the fetus continued to grow and develop. The promising results of the intervention expanded the possibilities of fetal and neonatal medicine. Other physicians began to consider using this type of surgery for other anomalies.

At about the same time, an international group of physicians, surgeons, and scientists met for an informal exchange of experiences and discussion which resulted in the formation of what is now called the International Fetal Medicine and Surgery Society (Manning, 1986). One of the organization's first tasks was to create an international registry to track the number, type, and outcome of fetal surgical attempts.

TABLE **18-1**	Fetal Conditions Amenable to In Utero Treatment
Condition	**Intervention**
FETAL THERAPY: MEDICAL TREATMENT	
Rh sensitization	Red cell transfusion (into umbilical vessel or intraperitoneal)
Pulmonary immaturity	Betamethasone (transplacental)
Vitamin B_{12} deficiency	Vitamin B_{12} (transplacental)
Carboxylase deficiency	Biotin (transplacental)
Supraventricular tachycardia (SVT)	Digoxin, flecainide, or similar drug (transplacental)
Heart block	Betamimetics (transplacental)
Hypothyroidism	Thyroxine (transplacental)
Adrenal hyperplasia	Steroids
Intrauterine growth restriction (IUGR)	Protein calories (transamniotic)
Severe combined immunodeficiency syndrome (SCID)	Stem cell transplantation into umbilical vessel
FETAL THERAPY: SURGICAL TREATMENT	
Urinary tract obstructions	Closed procedure (i.e., percutaneous catheter placement) or fetal bladder cystoscopy to relieve obstruction
Hydronephrosis	
Lung hypoplasia	
Renal and respiratory failure	
Diaphragmatic hernia	Closed procedure (i.e., temporary tracheal occlusion with a balloon)
Lung hypoplasia	
Respiratory failure	
Cystic adenomatoid malformation of the lung (CCAM)	Closed procedure (i.e., placement of catheter for decompression) or open procedure (i.e., resection of the mass)
Lung hypoplasia	
Respiratory failure	
Sacrococcygeal teratoma	Closed procedure (i.e., interruption of blood flow to the tumor by ablating blood vessels) or open procedure (i.e., resection of tumor)
Heart failure	
Twin-to-twin transfusion syndrome	
Growth restriction of donor	Closed procedure (i.e., laser ablation of intertwin vascular connections)
Heart failure of recipient	

FETUS AS PATIENT: MATERNAL-FETAL RISKS AND BENEFITS

Although prenatal treatment of the fetus presents a formidable yet exciting challenge, fetal surgery is predicated on a profound responsibility to the mother to ensure her safety, because she, along with her unborn child, is a patient. The risk-benefit ratio of antenatal intervention favors the fetus with a lethal malformation, because without intervention, the mortality rate is almost uniformly 100%; with intervention, survival is possible. Justifying risk(s) is more difficult for the mother, whose physical health usually is not jeopardized by her unborn baby's condition. Before clinical application of fetal surgery could be considered, it had to be proved that any intervention through the mother would not imperil her safety or affect her future reproductive potential (Farrell et al, 1999; Wilson et al, 2004). As a result, the safety of fetal surgical procedures was tested first in the most rigorous animal model, the nonhuman primate (monkey), because its anatomy and physiology most closely resembles that of the human pregnancy.

In consideration of preserving the mother's reproductive capability, the ability to deliver subsequent pregnancies was evaluated by a recent, retrospective study (Wilson et al, 2004). Complications were reported in 35% of pregnancies of women who had undergone maternal-fetal surgery. The anticipated risk of certain adverse outcomes has led to several recommen-

dations, including longer interpregnancy intervals and cesarean section. Moreover, it is important to advise the maternal/fetal surgery candidate of the risks both in the present pregnancy and future ones (Wilson et al, 2004). However, maternal results have not been sufficiently measured to permit a full analysis of the efficacy and safety of maternal fetal surgery for patients; thus, both maternal and fetal well-being needs to be measured (Lyerly et al, 2001).

Ethical Considerations

Fetal therapy presents new, often complex ethical dilemmas, rife with challenging questions and controversy, as the very nature of this therapy involves operating on one patient, the fetus, located within another patient, the mother (Caniano, 2004). Balancing is required. The outcomes of fetal surgery have improved over the past decade, yet the neonatal management of anomalies has also advanced (Evans et al, 2002). Thus, the decision-making risk-reward assessment process cannot be taken lightly.

Ethical issues must be addressed carefully in the informed consent process. It is essential that the decision to go ahead with the maternal-fetal surgery be based on informed, autonomous, and voluntary consent (Lyerly et al, 2001). The informed consent process itself can be broken into three discrete elements: (1) disclosure from the physician to the patient of adequate information concerning the patient's condition and its management; (2) the patient's understanding of that information; and (3) a voluntary patient decision to authorize or refuse proposed procedures (Chervenak et al, 2003).

FETAL SURGICAL TECHNIQUES

Open Fetal Surgery

The timing of open fetal surgery depends on the malformation and its pathophysiologic course. Difficulty determining an accurate diagnosis and the fragility of fetal tissue are limiting factors for performing procedures at less than 18 weeks' gestation (Kiatano, 1999). Similarly, after 30 weeks' gestation, manipulation of the uterus is associated with a high risk of premature rupture of the membranes (PROM) and preterm labor. If these events occur, delivery of the fetus and treatment of the malformation with standard postnatal care becomes a more reasonable approach (Kiatano, 1999).

In open fetal surgery, after a general anesthetic is administered to the mother (and transferred to the fetus through the placenta), a low abdominal transverse (Pfannenstiel) incision is made to open the maternal abdomen and visualize the uterus. Intraoperative ultrasound is then used to identify the position of the fetus and the location of the placenta. Depending on the placenta's location, an anterior or posterior hysterotomy is performed with a specially developed, absorbable uterine stapling device that provides hemostasis and seals the membranes to the myometrium. The fetus is given a narcotic and paralytic agent intramuscularly, and the appropriate fetal part(s) is exposed.

Throughout the procedure, warm lactated Ringer's solution is infused around the fetus and open uterus to maintain fetal body temperature. Continuous fetal monitoring during the surgery is done with a sterile pulse oximeter that records the fetal electrocardiogram. After the defect has been repaired, the fetus is returned to the womb and warm saline containing an antibiotic, such as nafcillin, restores amniotic fluid volume. The uterine incision is closed with two layers of absorbable suture, and fibrin glue is used to help seal the incision and prevent leakage of amniotic fluid.

Minimally Invasive Fetal Surgery

Although fetoscopic techniques for direct visualization of the fetus are not new, recent modifications of postnatal endoscopic techniques and the development of new fetoscopic instruments have resulted in minimal access fetal surgery (FETENDO). The FETENDO technique has proved successful at preserving fetal homeostasis by protecting the intrauterine physiologic milieu, while avoiding the maternal morbidity associated with uterine incision (e.g., preterm labor, postoperative bleeding) (Albanese & Harrison, 1998).

For a FETENDO procedure, the mother is placed in a modified lithotomy position; anesthetic techniques, tocolytic therapy, and maternal monitoring are the same as for open fetal surgery. Preoperative and intraoperative sonographies map the position of the placenta and the fetus and guide placement of the trocar. An anterior placenta can require a low transverse abdominal incision to expose the uterus, after which the trocars are placed superiorly and posteriorly. Crucial to optimizing visibility, continuous irrigation is achieved using a pump irrigation system via the sheath of the hysteroscope. This system is superior in that it (1) maintains a constant intrauterine fluid volume; (2) avoids the risk of air embolus

with gas distention of the uterus; (3) ensures a continuously washed operative field; (4) improves visibility by exchanging cloudy amniotic fluid with lactated Ringer's solution; and (5) keeps the fetus warm.

One of the challenges of the FETENDO technique is manipulating the fetus into the correct position that can be maintained for the duration of the procedure. Addressing this frequently frustrating problem is best illustrated by the development of FETENDO tracheal occlusion to treat congenital diaphragmatic hernia. In this procedure, a chin stitch is employed to keep the fetal neck exposed by extending the head (Albanese et al, 1998a; Harrison et al, 1998) until the end of the operation, when the trocars are withdrawn and the puncture sites are closed with absorbable suture and fibrin glue (see Figure 18-1).

Anesthesia

Regardless of the fetal intervention approach (i.e., percutaneous or open surgical procedure), anesthesia is necessary. The anesthesiologist is faced with a complex situation in that two patients are being anesthetized simultaneously. Because the particular hazards of anesthesia during pregnancy are related to physiologic changes in the mother and possible adverse effects on the fetus, anesthetizing a pregnant woman during major surgery requires specially trained anesthesiologists who can provide low-level anesthesia and pain management for the maternal-fetal unit while ensuring the mother's safety and minimal side effects for both patients.

In developing anesthetic techniques for fetal surgery, researchers had to consider the physiologic differences between healthy pregnant women and healthy nonpregnant women. Specifically, pregnancy causes the following:

- Decreased peripheral vascular resistance (cardiac output increases with no increase in blood pressure, resulting in decreased peripheral vascular resistance);
- Decreased functional residual capacity and increased alveolar ventilation (which speeds up induction with inhalation anesthetics);
- Increased oxygen consumption (decreased functional residual capacity combined with increased oxygen consumption predisposes pregnant women to hypoxia); and
- Hypotension as a result of aortocaval compression (lying supine, a pregnant woman in the second and third trimesters experiences reduced blood flow back to the heart because of aortocaval compression by the gravid uterus).

Direct compression of the great vessels by the gravid uterus reduces uterine blood flow. Therefore, the operating table is tilted laterally for all procedures to prevent uterine hypoperfusion. Finally, throughout the procedure, the anesthesiologist and the surgeons must maintain a continuous exchange of information about the status of mother and fetus to ensure both patients' well-being.

As the pregnant uterus grows, the stomach is displaced cephalad and horizontally, changing the angle of the gastroesophageal junction and predisposing the mother to passive regurgitation. This, along with an increase in gastric acid production, makes her more susceptible to regurgitation and aspiration when anesthetized. To reduce the acidity of the gastric juice, oral antacids are administered before general anesthesia is induced.

Pregnant women are also more sensitive to inhalation anesthetics because the endorphin level is elevated; therefore, they are more susceptible to overdosing. Regional anesthetics also require special attention. The increase in femoral venous and intra-abdominal pressure enlarges the epidural veins, which, in turn, decreases the epidural space; thus, less anesthetic is needed.

Fetal oxygenation depends on maternal arterial oxygen content. That is, if the mother's partial pressure of arterial oxygen, partial pressure of arterial carbon dioxide, and uterine blood flow are maintained within normal limits, fetal asphyxia does not occur. Although elevated maternal oxygen tension (a common occurrence during anesthesia) is safe for the fetus, maternal hyperventilation can also cause fetal hypoxia and acidosis. Other causes of fetal asphyxia are maternal hypotension, which causes a decrease in uterine blood flow, as well as uterine vasoconstriction caused by anxiety, insufficient anesthesia, or vasoactive drugs.

When the mother is anesthetized for fetal surgery, the fetus also receives the anesthetic by means of placental transfer. Operating on an unanesthetized fetus results in stimulation of the autonomic nervous system and increases in hormonal and motor activity. For these reasons, general anesthesia is used for all open procedures to provide both maternal and fetal anesthesia.

Anesthesia of the mother and her baby is established with halogenated agents that also provide profound uterine relaxation. Insertion of an epidural catheter enhances postoperative pain control. In the operating room, the mother is placed in the left lateral decubitus position to prevent compression of the inferior vena cava by the gravid uterus. Maternal monitoring is accomplished with standard techniques, including pulse oximetry, a blood pressure cuff, large-bore intravenous catheters, measurement of urine output, and an electrocardiogram.

FETAL MALFORMATIONS AMENABLE TO SURGICAL CORRECTION

Prenatal diagnosis has exposed a "hidden" mortality rate for some lesions (e.g., congenital diaphragmatic hernia, bilateral hydronephrosis, sacrococcygeal teratoma, and congenital cystic adenomatoid malformation of the lung). That is, these lesions, when first evaluated and treated postnatally, demonstrated a favorable selection bias. As a result, mortality rates were skewed, inaccurate, and seemingly lower because the most severely affected fetuses often died in utero or immediately after birth. These deaths, often unaccounted for, represent the hidden, often increased mortality for some anomalies. Although most prenatally diagnosed malformations are best managed by appropriate medical and surgical therapy after maternal transport and planned delivery at a tertiary care center, an expanding number of simple anatomic abnormalities with predictable, lethal consequences have been corrected before birth. Certainly, the development of minimal access fetal surgery techniques, along with improvements in the treatment and prevention of preterm labor, may support a transition from treating life-threatening defects exclusively to including treatment of those non-life-threatening but substantially morbid conditions, such as myelomeningocele and cleft lip or palate.

Obstructive Uropathy

Obstructive uropathy occurs in 1 in 1000 live births. Unilateral urinary obstruction (e.g., ureteropelvic junction obstruction) has a good prognosis and usually does not require fetal intervention. However, fetuses with bilateral obstruction, largely male fetuses with posterior urethral valves, are potential candidates for prenatal intervention based on the degree and duration of the obstruction. Whereas newborns with partial bilateral obstruction may have only mild and reversible hydronephrosis, term infants with a high-grade obstruction may already have advanced hydronephrosis and renal dysplasia, both of which affect survival.

The outcome for patients with urinary tract obstruction depends primarily on whether oligohydramnios develops. Oligohydramnios, a condition characterized by too little amniotic fluid, is the result of decreased fetal urine production and can lead to fatal pulmonary hypoplasia (Potter sequence). Prenatal ultrasound examination reliably detects fetal hydronephrosis and determines the level of the urinary obstruction. When sonography demonstrates bilateral hydronephrosis, initial assessment of fetal renal function consists of quantifying amniotic fluid volume, because most of the amniotic fluid during mid- and late pregnancy is the product of fetal urination. Normal amniotic fluid volume implies production and excretion of urine by at least one functioning kidney. Presence of bilateral hydronephrosis along with diminished amniotic fluid volume demonstrated on serial ultrasound examinations usually indicates deteriorating renal function.

Renal function then can be assessed in two ways: appearance of the renal tissue on ultrasound examination and laboratory analysis of urine obtained by bladder aspiration. The presence of cortical cysts or increased echogenicity is highly predictive of renal dysplasia; however, the absence of these findings does not preclude it. Direct sampling of the fetal urine provides critical information about fetal renal function. Normal fetal urinary chemistry levels are: sodium <100 mEq/dl, chloride <90 mEq/dl, osmolarity <200 mOsm/L, and β_2-microglobulin <4 mg/dl. Higher levels of these components indicate the inability of the fetal kidney to reabsorb these molecules and predict poor postnatal renal function. Three bladder aspirations must be performed, with at least a 24-hour interval separating each succeeding procedure. The first aspiration empties stagnant bladder urine, the second empties stagnant urine in the collecting system, and the third specimen is most reflective of current kidney function.

The crucial question in the treatment of fetal hydronephrosis is how to select those fetuses with dilated urinary tracts and a problem so severe that renal and pulmonary function may be compromised at birth, yet still have sufficient renal function to benefit from prenatal intervention. Candidates for prenatal intervention must (1) have or develop oligohydramnios; (2) have normal renal function (as demonstrated by urine electrolyte and protein values); (3) be less than 30 weeks' gestation; and (4) have no associated anomalies.

The strategy of prenatal intervention for hydronephrosis is to bypass or directly treat the obstruction. If the urinary tract is adequately drained, restoration of amniotic fluid enhances fetal lung growth and prevents further deterioration of renal function. Methods of urinary tract decompression include percutaneous placement of a vesicoamniotic shunt, fetoscopic vesicostomy, open vesicostomy, and fetoscopic fulguration of posterior urethral valves.

Currently the most widely used method of treating bladder outlet obstruction is percutaneous insertion of a double-J vesicoamniotic shunt. The actual surgical procedure itself varies, depending on the specific fetal renal disorder or the surgical team's preference. Posterior urethral valve obstruction may be treated by percutaneous placement of a shunt (catheter) from the fetal bladder to the amniotic sac (closed procedure). In particular, the Harrison French double-reversed pigtail catheter has a stent shaped like a pigtail and has openings at either end. The diameters of the two ends are dissimilar in size, a safety feature in case the catheter becomes dislodged: the larger end is placed in the amniotic cavity, so that the catheter would be more likely to move back into this cavity rather than into the fetal bladder.

A polyethylene catheter is sometimes used because its greater rigidity makes it less likely to bend or kink. The catheter is introduced through the maternal abdomen and uterus into the fetal abdomen and bladder by means of a needle and trocar guidance system, similar to angiocatheters used for intravenous therapy. When the catheter is in place, one end is in the renal pelvis and the other end is in the amniotic sac, providing a means to increase the amount of amniotic fluid in the latter. Once the guidance system is withdrawn, the tubing is left in place. More than one insertion attempt may be necessary for successful placement, as there is a 45% incidence rate of shunt complications, which include catheter migration or malfunction, and abdominal wall disruption (Johnson, 2001). Also during the neonatal period, the fetus must undergo corrective surgery to repair the bladder and abdominal wall and relieve the urethral obstruction.

Advances in the development of smaller instrumentation, fetoscopes, allow relief of the obstruction rather than mere diversion of urine pass the blockage. Fetoscopy with direct fetal cystoscopy may be useful in obstructive uropathy, both diagnostically and therapeutically. It has been used to assess lower urinary tract obstruction etiology, to successfully ablate posterior urethral valves, and to place a transurethral stent. These procedures are technically difficult and the experience is limited; however, this technique avoids the complications of open surgery and may have improved outcomes over vesicoamniotic shunts (Holmes et al, 2001). It should be emphasized that fetal intervention for obstructive uropathy should only be performed in patients who still have residual renal function with severe oligohydramnios, as stated in the criteria previously cited in this section.

To prevent long-term renal and pulmonary problems, treatment must be undertaken early. Fetal surgery for posterior urethral valve obstruction has been performed as early as 18 weeks' gestation and as late as 26 weeks', but the ultimate goal remains the same—to prevent irreversible renal damage and pulmonary hypoplasia.

Congenital Diaphragmatic Hernia

Congenital diaphragmatic hernia (CDH) is a simple anatomic defect in which abdominal viscera herniate into the hemithorax, most often through a posterolateral defect in the diaphragm. Despite advances in prenatal care, maternal transport, neonatal resuscitation, and the availability of extracorporeal membrane oxygenation (ECMO), the devastating physiologic consequences of pulmonary hypoplasia and hypertension are associated with a high neonatal mortality rate and long-term morbidity (Harrison et al, 2001). In the fetal sheep experimental model of CDH, compression of the lungs during the last trimester, either with an intrathoracic balloon or by creation of a diaphragmatic hernia, resulted in fatal pulmonary hypoplasia. Removal of the compression allowed pulmonary growth and development to progress and increased the chances of survival.

Prenatal diagnosis of CDH is established when herniation of abdominal contents (e.g., loops of bowel, the stomach, or the left lobe of the liver) into the fetal thorax is seen on ultrasound examination. The function of certain fetal organs, such as the heart and kidneys, can be assessed in utero, but because the fetal lungs do not exchange gas, function cannot be assessed directly. Several sonographically detectable predictors of the severity of CDH are used routinely. The two most important parameters are the lung to head ratio (LHR) (Lipshutz et al, 1997) and the position of the left lobe of the liver (Albanese et al, 1998b). LHR is the calculated volume of the contralateral lung (the ipsilateral lung cannot be identified with CDH) indexed to head circumference to adjust for gestational age. Fetuses with an LHR of more than 1.4 have a favorable prognosis with tertiary postnatal care and therefore are not candidates for fetal intervention. In addition, fetuses with the liver in the normal abdominal position also tend to do well, and the rate of survival is over 90%. However, on the other end of the spectrum of severity, fetuses with significant herniation of the left lobe of the liver into the hemithorax have an expected survival rate of approximately 50% (Albanese et al, 1998b). Determination of liver position is technically challenging and requires color Doppler ultrasonography to visualize the position of the branches of the left portal vein. Together, these prognostic indicators allow careful selection of severely affected fetuses that may benefit from fetal intervention.

Prenatal treatment of CDH has continued to evolve since the first attempted open CDH repair in 1986 at the University of California at San Francisco. Open fetal surgery, in which a hysterotomy was performed and the diaphragm was repaired directly, presented many technical problems. Specifically, reduction of a herniated lobe of the liver during repair resulted in kinking of the intra-abdominal umbilical vein. As a result, blood flow was cut off from the placenta and led to fetal demise. Data from a 1994 National Institutes of Health (NIH)-sponsored single-center clinical trial at the University of California at San Francisco showed that repair of the diaphragm for fetuses without liver herniation was successful, but that the survival rate did not improve over that for standard postnatal care (Harrison et al, 1997). For the more severe form of CDH (i.e., liver herniation), a redirection in thinking about how to treat was necessary as complete repair was not technically feasible. Serendipity of nature provided a new paradigm for treating these severely affected fetuses. It had long been noted that fetuses with congenital high airway obstruction syndrome (CHAOS) caused by laryngeal or tracheal atresia have large, hyperplastic lungs as a result of overdistention from lung fluid (Fetal Care Center of Cincinnati, 2005). Laboratory studies not only confirmed that a model of CHAOS was reproducible, but also demonstrated that lungs physically larger were also functionally better. Using fetoscopic techniques, this strategy of temporarily occluding the fetal trachea with a balloon to accelerate fetal lung growth was tested (Harrison et al, 1996, 1998) (Figure 18-1). The preliminary data showed this technique to have great promise and, in 1999, formed the basis for a second NIH-sponsored clinical trial of innovative fetal CDH treatment. In this

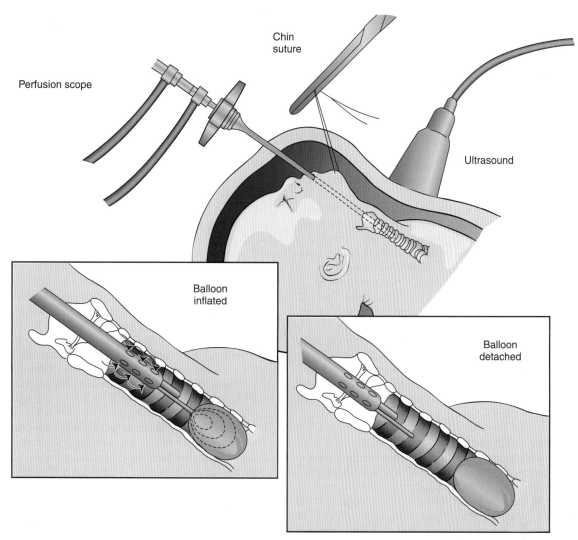

FIGURE **18-1**
Fetal tracheal occlusion with balloon. Courtesy Fetal Treatment Center, University of California, San Francisco.

randomized controlled trial the fetal tracheal occlusion at 26 weeks' gestation was compared with standard postnatal care for fetuses with an LHR less than 1.4 and liver herniation. The primary outcome variable was survival at 90 days. As with the previous trial, there was no demonstrable difference in early mortality between the fetal surgery and standard university postnatal care groups. What was surprising was an unexpectedly high survival rate shown in the standard care group (77%) that resulted in closing enrollment early (Harrison et al, 2003). In addition, the European (EuroFetus Group) experiences with reversible balloon tracheal occlusion shows promise (Deprest et al, 2005). Thus, as tocolytic and surgical methods improve and develop, and the incidence and associated morbidity of prematurity declines, tracheal occlusion may still have a role for managing the most severe cases of CDH, given its documented benefit of inducing pulmonary growth. Investigations are currently underway to examine balloon tracheal occlusion in the most severe cases with a LHR less than 1.

The technique for removing the tracheal balloon is called the "ex utero intrapartum treatment (EXIT)" procedure

(Mychaliska et al, 1997). After hysterotomy is performed, the fetal head and shoulders are delivered, but the cord is not clamped and the fetus remains on placental support. During this period, the pediatric surgeon inserts a bronchoscope, pops the balloon, and removes it with suction. The neonate is intubated; surfactant is administered, and mechanical ventilation (by hand) is begun. Once the oxygen saturation increases, the cord is cut and the infant is delivered.

Congenital Cystic Adenomatoid Malformation

Congenital cystic adenomatoid malformation (CCAM) of the lung is the most common type of fetal thoracic mass that can be detected by prenatal ultrasound examination as early as 16 weeks' gestation. Most cases are diagnosed before 22 weeks' gestation. CCAM is a hamartoma of the lung that usually is unilateral and lobar. The differential diagnoses include pulmonary sequestration, CDH, other congenital cystic malformations (e.g., bronchogenic, enteric, or neurogenic cysts), and CHAOS. CCAMs have a broad spectrum of clinical severity and usually follow one of three courses: they may enlarge significantly, leading to fetal hydrops; they may remain unchanged; or they may shrink and disappear prenatally. These malformations lead to fetal demise in 100% of pregnancies when sufficient cardiac and great vessel compression lead to hydrops. However, the size and degree of mediastinal shift alone is not predictive of hydrops, which occurs in only the minority of prenatally diagnosed CCAMs.

Experimentally, the pathophysiologic consequences and the rationale for in utero treatment of CCAM have been clarified. The only indication for fetal intervention is the presence of hydrops, manifested by fetal ascites, pericardial or pleural effusions, and scalp and integumentary edema. If this condition occurs before 32 weeks' gestation, the fetus may be a candidate for intervention.

Macrocystic lesions can be treated using minimally invasive introduction of a percutaneous thoracoamniotic catheter, which drains and decompresses the mass to allow fetal lung growth. Microcystic lesions have been removed by the open (hysterotomy) technique, with subsequent resolution of hydrops. Solid masses require surgical resection between 21 and 27 weeks' gestation, when lung growth continues and can resume a normal growth pattern for optimal lung development. At this gestational age, as well, type II cells are producing surfactant; therefore the fetus may tolerate the surgical procedure better than at an earlier stage. This fetus-neonate should be delivered at a tertiary care center where ECMO is available, because the possibility of pulmonary hypoplasia still exists. Postnatal radiographic studies are needed to detect any residual or return of the CCAM.

Sacrococcygeal Teratoma

Sacrococcygeal teratoma (SCT) is the most common tumor in newborns, occurring in 1 in 35,000 to 40,000 live births. SCT, a neural tube defect that can be detected by ultrasonography, is the growth of a tumor in the sacral and coccygeal areas of the spinal cord or at the base of the tailbone (coccyx). The natural history of prenatally diagnosed SCT is very different from that of neonatal SCT, and the well-established prognostic indicators for the latter do not apply for fetal SCT. Malignancy is the primary cause of death in neonatal SCT but is rare in these tumors in utero (Graf et al, 1998). The life-threatening consequences of fetal SCT are associated with the development of high output cardiac failure, which results from a "vascular steal" phenomenon through the solid, highly vascular tumors.

Only 10% of fetal SCTs cause hydrops, which left untreated, has an associated mortality rate of 100%. SCT also may lead to a potentially devastating maternal complication called "maternal mirror" (Ballantine's) syndrome, in which the mother experiences progressive symptoms suggestive of preeclampsia, including hypertension, peripheral edema, proteinuria, and pulmonary edema, because of the release of endothelial cell toxins from the edematous placenta. This syndrome is reversed not by removing the SCT prenatally, but only by delivering the fetus and the placenta.

Prenatal sonographic diagnosis of SCT is based on detection of a characteristic sacral and/or intra-abdominal mass, which can be seen as early as 14 weeks' gestation. With widespread use of sophisticated obstetric sonography during midgestation, most SCTs can be diagnosed in utero. Fetal SCTs can be cystic, solid, or mixed in appearance (Westerburg et al, 2000); differential diagnoses include myelomeningocele and obstructive uropathy. Color flow Doppler ultrasonographic examination of large vascular tumors may show markedly increased distal aortic blood flow and shunting of blood away from the placenta to the tumor, a condition that almost uniformly leads to hydrops and makes the fetus a possible candidate for surgical intervention. Of the reported cases undergoing open fetal surgical resection of an SCT, there are few long-term survivors to date (Adzick et al, 1997; Graf et al, 2000).

Fetal surgery for SCT involves tumor resection. Briefly, a maternal hysterotomy is performed, and the fetal buttocks and lower spinal cord are exposed. If the lesion is small, a stapling device is used to apply pressure to the highly vascular tissue, gradually cutting off the blood supply to the tumor; this technique minimizes fetal blood loss. If the tumor is too large to be safely handled by stapling, umbilical tape can be pulled tightly over the tumor mass, binding it and cutting off the blood supply. The surgeon then can remove or resect the tumor with little risk of bleeding. Because these tumors sometimes recur or are not removed completely, further surgery may be required during the neonatal period.

Currently, research efforts are directed toward developing a minimally invasive approach to treatment; rather than debulking the mass, the tumor's blood supply would be interrupted by coagulating the major feeding blood vessels (Westerburg et al, 1998). This approach can be accomplished percutaneously using a radio-frequency ablation device. The UCSF fetal treatment team has used an ultrasonographically guided, percutaneous, minimally invasive technique to coagulate the blood vessels in five fetuses. Two of five fetuses survived in the radio-frequency ablation group, with associated morbidity attributed to burns in adjacent soft tissue (Lam et al, 2002; Paek et al, 2001). Refinement in minimally invasive techniques may allow for future applications that carry less morbidity.

Twin-to-Twin Transfusion Syndrome

Twin-to-twin transfusion syndrome (TTTS) is the most common complication in monochorionic-diamniotic twin pregnancies, occurring in 5% to 35% of these pregnancies. Although associated anomalies are rare, TTTS does carry a high risk of miscarriage, brain damage, perinatal death, and significant morbidity in survivors.

In TTTS, unequal sharing of the monochorionic placenta usually can be visualized sonographically: insertion of the smaller (or donor) twin's placental cord often is marginal or velamentous, whereas the larger (or recipient) twin's cord inserts into the placenta centrally. Vascular connections on the placental surface exist between the twins, and if these are unbalanced, a net shunting of blood occurs as a result of arteriovenous anastomoses, which sometimes can be detected by Doppler ultrasonography.

Ultrasonography commonly demonstrates severe oligohydramnios or anhydramnios in the sac of the donor twin (also known as the "stuck" twin). The differential diagnoses for a "stuck twin" include uteroplacental dysfunction, discordant aneuploidy, structural urinary tract malformations, or congenital infection. The recipient twin, or "pump" twin, on the other hand, develops polyhydramnios, pulmonary hypertension, and cardiomyopathy caused by chronic blood volume overload. The vessels in question are unpaired vessels with flow from the donor fetus to the recipient fetus. Doppler studies demonstrate the characteristic pulsatile arterial blood flow on the donor's side, whereas the vessel shows a continuous venous flow on the recipient's side.

Standard therapy for TTTS varies. Commonly, large-volume amnioreduction of the recipient polyhydramniotic sac is utilized effectively, with survival rates near 60%, but there is significant neurologic and cardiac morbidity (Fisk, 2001). These mechanisms are tailored to minimize perinatal complications secondary to prematurity by reducing polyhydramnios and the likelihood of preterm delivery. Intertwin membrane septostomy has also been performed to restore amniotic fluid dynamics. However, there is risk of fetal demise by cord entanglement or amniotic bands.

More recent, fetoscopic techniques target ablation of intertwin vascular connections using an yttrium aluminum garnet (YAG) laser. The surgical procedure varies—some surgeons coagulate all vessels seen crossing the intertwin septum on the placental surface (Hecher et al, 1999), whereas others coagulate only the unpaired intertwin communicating vessels (Feldstein et al, 2000). Several multicenter, prospective randomized trials are currently in progress to compare the efficacy of laser coagulation vs large-volume amnioreduction for TTTS.

Neural Tube Defects

Myelomeningocele (MMC), or spina bifida, is a midline defect that results in exposure of the contents of the spinal column. The defect usually is located in the lumbosacral portion of the vertebrae. In the United States alone, 1500 to 2000 babies are born with MMC every year. Routine maternal serum alpha-fetoprotein (MSAFP) screening identifies more than 80% of children with MMC. When MSAFP values are outside the normal range, direct sonographic visualization of the fetal spine can be performed by 16 weeks' gestation to confirm the presence of an MMC and other possible associated findings, including frontal bone scalloping (lemon sign), abnormality of the cerebellum (banana sign), Chiari II malformation (hindbrain herniation), hydrocephaly, microcephaly, and encephalocele.

The clinical observation that, in fetuses with MMC, lower extremity function present early in the pregnancy was progressively lost in later gestation provided the rationale for considering prenatal intervention. Creation and repair of the defect in animals showed that intrauterine repair of myelomeningocele may preserve peripheral neurologic function (Meuli et al, 1995a, 1995b; Hutchins et al, 1996). Experimental studies also indicated that the Chiari II malformation, which is nearly always associated with MMC, may be prevented by prenatal repair (Paek et al, 2000).

Recent clinical experience has shown that open fetal surgery may improve neurologic function and more dramatically resolve the hindbrain herniation associated with myelomeningocele (Adzick et al, 1998; Tulipan et al, 1998; Bruner et al, 1999a, 1999b; Sutton et al, 1999). Although this early experience appears promising, the variable natural history of myelomeningocele, the lack of accurate prenatal indicators of neurologic function, and the absence of matched controls and long-term follow-up data hamper assessment of the benefits of prenatal intervention. Given the unclear cost: benefit ratio of fetal vs standard postnatal treatment, there is currently a prospective, multi-institutional, randomized trial ongoing to determine the role of open fetal repair for myelomeningocele. The outcome of this trial will not only define the role for fetal intervention but establish an indication in treating nonlethal defects. How to qualify and quantify fetal benefit to justify the maternal and fetal risk involved remains to be determined.

Congenital High Airway Obstructive Syndrome

Congenital high airway obstruction syndrome usually is caused by laryngeal or tracheal atresia and in rare cases by isolated tracheal stenosis, mucosal web, or extrinsic compression by a large cervical mass (e.g., teratoma or lymphangioma). Regardless of the etiology, fetal upper airway obstruction prevents egress of the fluid produced in the lungs, which normally travels from the airways into the amniotic space. This fluid usually is produced under a pressure that favors movement out through the fetal mouth, partly aided by fetal breathing movements. Sonographic findings of CHAOS include a bilaterally flattened or everted diaphragm; large, overdistended (i.e., fluid filled), echogenic lungs that compress the mediastinum; dilated large airways distal to the obstruction; and fetal ascites or hydrops (or both) resulting from compression of the heart and great vessel or vessels (Hedrick et al, 1994). If hydrops does not develop in utero, a fetus with CHAOS may be treated with the EXIT procedure, which maintains the baby on placental support until an airway is established via orotracheal intubation or tracheostomy (Mychaliska et al, 1997). However, if fetal hydrops develops, early delivery or prenatal tracheostomy is an option for treatment, depending on the gestational age. Three known survivors of prenatally diagnosed CHAOS have been reported in the literature (DeCou et al, 1998; Crombleholme et al, 2000; Paek et al, 2002).

Amniotic Band Syndrome

The incidence of amniotic band syndrome is 1 in 1200 to 15,000 live births. Early rupture of the amnion results in mesodermic bands that emanate from the chorionic side of the amnion and insert onto the fetal body. These bands may lead to amputations, constrictions, and postural deformities that occur secondary to immobilization. Crombleholme and colleagues produced amniotic band syndrome in fetal sheep so as to study the effects of fetoscopic release on morphometric outcome (Crombleholme et al, 1995).

It has been shown that the earlier the band occurs, the more severe is the resulting lesion (Strauss et al, 2000). For example, amniotic rupture in the first weeks of pregnancy may result in craniofacial and visceral defects; with rupture during the second trimester, fetal morbidity ranges from formation of syndactyly to limb amputation. Umbilical cord constriction at any time in gestation may result in fetal death. Given the risks for fetal and maternal morbidity, fetoscopic intervention for mild forms of amniotic band syndrome is not warranted at this time. However, for more severe forms, fetoscopic lysis of the bands may be useful.

INTRAPROFESSIONAL COLLABORATIVE APPROACH TO FETAL THERAPY

The fetus with an anomaly requires the attention of team specialists working together with the mother and fetus. Members of the team include a perinatologist, neonatologist, pediatric surgeon, sonologist, anesthesiologist, operating room and perinatal nurse specialists, physiologist, technicians, a social worker, and a nurse coordinator who can serve as a liaison with the family.

In many instances, time is of the essence with fetal surgery cases; the legal window on the option of pregnancy termination may be closing, and delays can lead to substantial fetal morbidity and even mortality. For maximum possible benefit, fetal surgery candidates should be identified and

BOX 18-1

Sample Care Plan for Women Undergoing Fetal Surgery (Clinical Pathway)

The following care plan is used at the Fetal Treatment Center at the University of California, San Francisco.

1. *Informed consent and counseling:* All members of the team are included (perinatologist, fetal treatment center nurse coordinator, pediatric surgeon, operating room nurse specialist, sonographer, obstetric anesthesiologist, perinatal nurse specialist, perinatal social worker).
2. *Admission:* Evening before procedure.
3. *Preoperative assessment:* Assessment includes baseline cervical examination (digital and by sonogram), baseline maternal vitals and oxygen saturation levels, electronic fetal heart rate, and maternal uterine activity strip.
4. *Tocolysis:* All patients receive tocolysis as follows:
   - Indomethacin: 50 mg by rectum (PR) given at 10 PM before surgery and on call to operating room, then every 4 to 6 hours for at least 24 to 48 hours after procedure.
   - Magnesium sulfate: 2 g/hour given intravenously, initiated intraoperatively and continued until uterine activity has been controlled for 24 to 48 hours.
   - Terbutaline: If the subcutaneous pump is used, it is initiated before the magnesium sulfate is stopped and is continued until delivery.
   - Nifedipine (oral): If used, it is begun when the magnesium sulfate is discontinued and given every 4 to 6 hours until delivery.
5. *Coping and supportive care:* The nurse specialists and the perinatal social worker provide continuity for issues of coping.
6. *Pain management:* All patients undergo general anesthesia for the procedure and have an epidural catheter placed postoperatively for pain management via epidurally administered narcotics and -*caine* anesthetics.
7. *Medications:* Postoperatively patients receive intravenous antibiotics until they are afebrile for 48 hours.
8. *Monitoring:* Patients receive one-to-one care for 24 hours; electronic uterine-fetal monitoring is continuous.
9. *Fluid management:* Strict measurement of intake and output (I&O) measurement and total fluid restriction to 2400 ml in 24 hours are necessary to prevent or limit pulmonary edema. Weighing the patient daily and continuous pulse oximetry help detect pulmonary edema early. Adventitious lung sounds are a late sign.
10. *Oxygen therapy:* Oxygen is provided via nonrebreather mask for the first 2 hours after surgery and then by nasopharyngeal prongs to keep the arterial oxygen saturation above 95%. Incentive spirometer is performed every 3 to 4 hours while awake. Lungs are assessed every 6 hours.
11. *Activity:* Complete bed rest is required until uterine activity is controlled. Thigh-high TEDs and Venodyne boots with a sequential compression device are used while the patient is on complete bed rest to reduce the risk of emboli.
12. *Follow-up:* The patient should return weekly for sonographic evaluation and examination by a perinatologist. Biweekly nonstress test and amniotic fluid index (NST/AFI) should begin a 26 weeks.

The STOP-ROP Multicenter Study Group (2000). Supplemental therapeutic oxygen for prethreshold retinopathy of prematurity (STOP-ROP), a randomized, controlled trial. I: primary outcomes. *Pediatrics* 105:295-310.

referred before 23 weeks' gestation. Early referral allows the fetal surgery team adequate time to consider the clinical situation carefully and to perform appropriately timed interventions. Box 18-1 outlines the multidisciplinary approach to specific interventions developed by the fetal surgery team at the University of California at San Francisco.

Considerations for Collaborative Care Planning

When fetal surgery is chosen, the clinical case may be broken down into six phases: diagnosis, information and decision making, perioperative and postoperative care, home care and follow-up, delivery, and neonatal period.

Diagnosis

The diagnostic phase generally covers the period from referral to the fetal treatment center through the evaluation process. For the families, this typically is a waiting period, first for an appointment and then for the results. For many families this is the most difficult time, and the nurse should provide appropriate information about the process and suggest resources (e.g., social services, support groups, counseling) to help cushion the family against the fears inherent in this situation. The nurse must recognize that the family is enduring the loss of a normal pregnancy and experiencing the anxiety of

an uncertain future. Also, in this phase the family's concerns often center on the diagnosis and cause of the fetal problem and their possible role in the cause. Families need explicit reassurance.

Information and Decision Making

Once the differential diagnoses are established, the family is presented with treatment options. These may include termination of the pregnancy (if still early enough in gestation), surgical intervention, or waiting to term for standard postnatal care. Whether invasive therapy should be offered and recommended or offered but not recommended is posed at this point. Such therapy should be offered and recommended only if two criteria are met: (1) the therapy is judged to have a high likelihood of being life-saving or of preventing serious, irreversible disease, injury, or disability for the fetus and the child to come; and (2) the therapy has a low risk of mortality and a low or manageable risk of disease, injury, or disability to the fetus. Although risk to the mother is expected to be low or manageable, any surgical procedure carries some risk of morbidity and mortality, and this should be stated explicitly in the counseling and informed consent processes.

The decision-making phase often is when the family's worst fears are confirmed. As the grief reaction begins, the family's emotions and feelings may become more intense. They also must face the religious, moral, and ethical implications, as well as financial and practical considerations. The informed consent procedure must seek to minimize family and societal pressures. The individual obtaining the consent should make sure that the woman is alone and that some of the outside pressure is removed (Lyerly et al, 2001).

Before deciding what is best, the family meets with all members of the team. Team members provide detailed information about preoperative, intraoperative, and perioperative care, answer questions, and address concerns. The family also meets privately with the perinatal social worker, who makes a psychosocial assessment and evaluates the family's ability to cope. This evaluation includes assessment of the marital relationship, available support systems, coping strategies used in previous crises, previous experience of loss, current stress factors, unemployment or financial constraints, and other health problems. Collectively, this information assists in the team's assessment of how well the family will cope and what resources may be helpful.

Perioperative and Postoperative Care

If fetal intervention is chosen, nurses help prepare the family for the procedure and provide extensive preoperative teaching. It may also be an appropriate time to suggest and discuss coping strategies, in case fetal loss occurs at any time during the perioperative period.

Postoperative Management. In lieu of direct physical examination in the postoperative stage, daily fetal sonography and echocardiography provide insight and information about fetal status. During this 3- to 7-day period, too, continuous epidural analgesics are given to the mother to ease maternal stress and aid tocolysis. Nurses provide support, encouragement, and education at this critical time, when the mother and family face uncertainty about the survival of their fetus and the possibility of uncontrollable preterm labor. Additional attention to the mother is important, because she must endure the effects of medications that may disrupt her mental status, comfort, and ability to sleep. She also may feel intimidated by the equipment used in postoperative care. The nurse should help promote flexible visiting hours, personalization of the room or bedside, and physical contact with significant others (Howell & Dunphy, 1999).

Preterm Labor. Preterm labor is the Achilles heel of fetal intervention and the primary cause of maternal morbidity and fetal death. Its pathophysiology after hysterotomy is not yet clearly understood, and effective postoperative tocolysis (with minimum side effects) remains a frustrating clinical problem (Albanese & Harrison, 1998). Currently the tocolytic regimen begins with administration of indomethacin to the mother before surgery and over the next several days. Of the available tocolytics, indomethacin was chosen because of its ability to inhibit the synthesis of prostaglandins released during uterine manipulation. In contrast to their value in spontaneous labor, terbutaline, magnesium sulfate, and nifedipine have been relatively ineffective and offer little advantage in the treatment of preterm labor induced by hysterotomy. Outpatient tocolysis consists of oral or subcutaneous terbutaline (administered via a pump) or oral nifedipine. If membranes rupture or labor cannot be controlled, cesarean delivery is performed, usually before 36 weeks' gestation (Harrison et al, 2001).

The mother may be concerned that something she does or fails to do will lead to preterm labor, premature rupture of membranes, or other harm to the fetus. If possible, home care nursing is provided once a week to ensure continuing instruction in self-care, management, and support, if these are not accomplished through outpatient visits.

Home Care and Follow-Up

The discharge to home can be a particularly anxious time. The mother often is restricted to complete bed rest and tocolytic therapy and she may fear that something she does or fails to do will harm the fetus. For this reason, the patient and a family member or friend are encouraged and sometimes required to stay near the medical center so that they can return once or twice a week for fetal evaluation (i.e., nonstress test [NST] and amniotic fluid index [AFI]) and sonographic evaluation and assessment for signs of preterm labor. In some instances plans may be made for patients to stay at a nearby facility, such as a Ronald McDonald House (Harrison et al, 2001). If membranes rupture or shred (i.e., chorioamniotic separation) or if preterm labor cannot be controlled, the mother can be rehospitalized, kept on bed rest, and continuously monitored.

Extended separation from family and friends during this follow-up phase may be a significant emotional strain on the patient, and time away from work may be a financial hardship. The nurse coordinator should remain in daily contact with the family to maintain a sense of their emotional well-being and should suggest or provide whatever resources are appropriate to help ease the burden.

Delivery

Delivery of the infant may take place any time after fetal surgery but most often occurs 4 to 12 weeks after the procedure, depending on a number of factors. The lesion for which the surgery was performed also determines the conditions that must be satisfied in anticipation of delivery.

During this phase, the parents' major concerns focus on the infant's chances of survival, and interestingly, but not surprisingly, on the infant's physical appearance at birth as a result of having undergone a surgical procedure. The parents should have the opportunity to see and touch the infant as soon as possible after birth, regardless of the outcome. If the infant does not survive, one of the nurse specialists should encourage the parents to hold, look at, and take pictures with their infant, because these actions help them accept the outcome and experience closure. If the infant survives, it is equally important for parents to see and touch the baby as soon as possible, to provide reassurance. If the physical conditions of both mother and infant make this contact difficult or impossible, a member of the treatment team should take pictures that can be given to the family immediately.

Neonatal Period

The final phase, the neonatal period, requires the team to work closely with the family's long-term health care providers to ensure appropriate management once the family leaves the fetal treatment center. Even if the infant does not survive, the nurse coordinator should maintain contact so that autopsy results and genetic counseling can be provided. One of the nurse specialists may want to initiate discussion of the various stages of the grief process with the parents. This is also an appropriate time to discuss the reactions of friends and family.

For the family whose infant has survived, the realization that the baby may require further surgery surfaces during this period, or the family may learn that the infant may not live long despite the fetal surgery. Even when the infant is doing well and has minimal risk of further illness, the family may not readily accept the information given. The family may require significant psychosocial support after the discharge to ensure a successful transition to home. This support can be provided through telephone contact, home visits, and clinic visits soon after discharge to assess the family's adjustment. Referrals to support groups, psychologists, or professionals of other disciplines should be made immediately if the family appears to have trouble coping.

As can clearly be seen, the fetus with an anomaly requires the attention of a team of specialists (Harrison et al, 2001). Not only are there ethical issues that require the balancing of risks and benefits, but there are two patients, the mother and the fetus (Spitzer, 2005). Fetal surgery requires a collective approach to caregiving. The multidisciplinary team at a fetal treatment center requires meaningful collaboration involving the pediatric surgeon, perinatal obstetrician, sonographer, anesthesiologist, operating room and obstetrical nurses, geneticist, social worker, ethicist, and nurse coordinator (Taeusch & Ballard, 1998). Various defects require more subspecialties. Despite the multiple talents in the group, the role of the nurse in the team must not be discounted. Nursing represents a source of continuity in maternal-child care sessions; nurses provide care through all stages of fetal surgery and can be critical advocates for maternal and fetal surgery patients.

FETAL THERAPY: NEW HORIZONS

As mentioned previously, treatments for genetic problems in particular are being attempted through fetal therapy. For example, to treat errors of metabolism, the mother receives medication, vitamins, or the substance the infant lacks, to be passed through the placenta to the fetus. Other therapeutic strategies have been aimed at correcting blood incompatibility problems.

One new fetal therapy with exciting potential is the treatment for severe combined immunodeficiency or SCID, a disorder that impels infants and children with essentially nonfunctional immune systems to live in protective bubbles to shield them from exposure to infectious agents. SCID is also associated with a high mortality rate. Fetal stem cell transplantation has been successful in treating this condition in utero, although its application in medicine is in jeopardy as controversy surrounding stem cell research in general mounts. However, perhaps opposition to the use of fetal cells and tissue can be averted and this treatment approach explored, as stem cells can also be harvested from a parent and transfused through the umbilical cord of the fetus. These transplanted cells migrate from the umbilical cord to the fetal bone marrow, where abundant space exists, as the liver is the primary hematopoietic organ during gestational development. Stem cell transplantation takes advantage of the fetus's preimmune state. These transplanted cells (which do not trigger rejection in the fetus because it is in a preimmune state at this stage in gestation) proliferate, replace the fetal stem cells, and become differentiated into the various cell types of the immune system (Wiley, 1996).

In the neonatal period, tests can be performed to identify, in particular, T lymphocytes, which in turn can be tested to determine cell origin. In a successful treatment case at Wayne State Medical Center in Detroit, the cells were paternal in origin and were sufficient in number to suggest a cure for SCID (Flake, 1995). If this therapy continues to be successful, the treatment method may be attempted for all forms of hemoglobinopathies, particularly sickle cell anemia and thalassemia. Already a national network of cord blood banks gives families the opportunity to save cord blood for use later in life in the event that an immune problem arises. The movement to embrace this new therapy brings with it ethical considerations of which the nurse must remain aware (McMillan, 1996).

Future of Fetal Surgery

Increasingly sophisticated techniques for prenatal diagnosis and increasingly innovative, sometimes controversial treatment strategies have revolutionized the field of fetal medicine. The fetus has come a long way from its enigmatic yet impersonal identity as the biblical "seed," the mystical "homunculus," to a unique individual with medical and surgical problems that can be diagnosed and treated. The relatively young but eventful history of fetal surgical intervention offers new hope for the fetus with an isolated congenital malformation. The great promise of fetal therapy is that, for some diseases, the earliest possible intervention (i.e., before birth) produces the best possible outcome (i.e., the best quality of life for the resources expended). However, the potential for cost-effective, preventive fetal therapy can be subverted by misguided clinical applications, such as performing a complex in utero procedure that "half saves" an otherwise doomed fetus for a life of intensive (and financially and emotionally expensive) care. Enthusiasm for fetal intervention must be tempered by reverence for the interests of the mother and her family, by careful study of the disease in experimental fetal animals and untreated human fetuses, and by a willingness to abandon therapy that does not prove both efficacious and cost-effective in properly controlled trials.

Some hospitals, such as Children's Hospital of Philadelphia and the University of California San Francisco Medical Center, have hired nurses with expertise in fetal surgery to work with neonatal intensive care unit (NICU) staff to provide care once the baby is born. Other centers such as Fetal Care Center of Cincinnati chose to locate within a children's hospital to provide continuity of care as well as close proximity of neonatologists, neonatal nurse practitioners, and nursing staff. Short- and long-term clinical follow-up for this population is circumscribed and individualized according to the type of fetal surgery or therapy. While follow-up for the families focuses on general care needs, it must also acknowledge and address the trauma and life-altering effects the fetal treatment itself has had on the family after birth and in the discharge period. This type of specialized care currently is delivered in only a few experienced NICUs, but it is likely to become more widespread as technology and knowledge of genetics expand. Nursing will have a significant role in providing expert input and shaping the future care of these patients.

SUMMARY

The primary goal of this chapter has been to describe fetal treatment and, in particular, fetal surgery. As this field rapidly evolves, expands, and broadens the options for treatment, more neonatal health care professionals will be approached by both colleagues and patients with questions on fetal intervention, including surgery. In this redefined clinical milieu, neonatal nurses must have a basic understanding of this burgeoning area of medicine, including its associated technology and perhaps even the new ethical considerations it poses. This chapter recognizes the critical, complex, and often difficult role nurse specialists fulfill in fetal treatment, acting as both patient advocate and fetal treatment team representative. The responsibilities are complex, and the nurse specialist who fulfills them must be able to weigh, balance, interpret, and act on a variety of issues from a multifaceted, informed perspective. This chapter, then, is an acknowledgment of the talent, intellect, skill, and compassion that nursing professionals bring to the field of fetal treatment.

REFERENCES

Adzick NS et al (1997). A rapidly growing fetal teratoma. *Lancet* 349(9051):538.

Adzick NS et al (1998). Successful fetal surgery for spina bifida. *Lancet* 352(9051):1675-1676.

Albanese CT, Harrison MR (1998). Surgical treatment for fetal disease: the state of the art. *Annals of the New York Academy of Science* 847:74-85.

Albanese CT et al (1998a). Endoscopic fetal tracheal occlusion procedure: evolution of techniques. *Pediatric endosurgery and innovative techniques* 2:47-53.

Albanese CT et al (1998b). Fetal liver position and perinatal outcome for congenital diaphragmatic hernia. *Prenatal diagnosis* 18:1138-1142.

Bruner JP et al (1999a). Endoscopic coverage of fetal myelomeningocele in utero. *American journal of obstetrics and gynecology* 180:153-158.

Bruner JP et al (1999b). Fetal surgery for myelomeningocele and the incidence of shunt-dependent hydrocephalus. *Journal of the American medical association* 282:1819-1825.

Caniano DA (2004). Ethical issues in the management of neonatal surgical anomalies. *Seminars in perinatology* 28:240-245.

Chervenak FA et al (2003). Ethical issues in the management of pregnancies complicated by fetal anomalies. *Obstetrical and gynecological survey* 58:473-483.

Crombleholme TM et al (1995). Amniotic band syndrome in fetal lambs. I. Fetoscopic release and morphometric outcome. *Journal of pediatric surgery* 30:974-978.

Crombleholme TM et al (2000). Salvage of a fetus with congenital high airway obstruction syndrome by ex utero intrapartum treatment (EXIT) procedure. *Fetal diagnosis and therapy* 15:280-282.

DeCou JM et al (1998). Successful ex utero intrapartum treatment (EXIT) procedure for congenital high airway obstruction syndrome (CHAOS) owing to laryngeal atresia. *Journal of pediatric surgery* 33:1563-1565.

Deprest J, FETO Task Group et al (2005). Fetal intervention for congenital diaphragmatic hernia: the European experience. *Seminars in perinatology* 29(2):94-103.

Evans MI et al (2002). Fetal therapy. *Best practice and research clinical obstetrics and gynaecology* 16:671-683.

Farrell JA et al (1999). Maternal fertility is not affected by fetal surgery. *Fetal diagnosis and therapy* 14:190-192.

Feldstein VA et al (2000). Twin-twin transfusion syndrome: the "SELECT" procedure. *Fetal diagnosis and therapy* 15(5):257-261.

Fetal Care Center of Cincinnati (2005). Congenital High Airway Obstruction Syndrome/CHAOS. Available at: http://www.fetalcarecenter.org/medicine/therapies/chaos. Retrieved October 2, 2005.

Fisk NM (2001). The fetus with twin-twin transfusion syndrome. In Harrison MR et al, editors. *The unborn patient: the art and science of fetal therapy* (pp 341-356). Philadelphia: Saunders.

Flake A (1995). Fetal surgery. Presented at the National Association of Neonatal Nurses Regional Conference: From Conception to Kindergarten, October 1995, Chicago.

Graf JL et al (1998). A surprising histological evolution of preterm sacrococcygeal teratoma. *Journal of pediatric surgery* 33:177-179.

Graf JL et al (2000). Successful fetal sacrococcygeal teratoma resection in a hydropic fetus. *Journal of pediatric surgery* 35:1489-1491.

Harrison MR (1996). Fetal surgery. *American journal of obstetrics and gynecology* 174:1255-1264.

Harrison MR (2003). Fetal surgery: trials, tribulations, and turf. *Journal of pediatric surgery* 38:275-282.

Harrison MR et al (1996). Correction of congenital diaphragmatic hernia in utero. VIII. Response of the hyperplastic lung to tracheal occlusion. *Journal of pediatric surgery* 31:1339-1348.

Harrison MR et al (1997). Correction of congenital diaphragmatic hernia in utero. VII. A prospective trial. *Journal of pediatric surgery* 32:1637-1642.

Harrison MR et al (1998). Correction of congenital diaphragmatic hernia in utero. IX. Fetuses with poor prognosis (liver herniation and low lung to head ratio) can be saved by fetoscopic temporary tracheal occlusion. *Journal of pediatric surgery* 33:1017-1022.

Harrison MR et al, editors (2001). *The unborn patient: the art and science of fetal therapy*, ed 3. Philadelphia: Saunders.

Harrison MR et al (2003). A randomized trial of fetal endoscopic tracheal occlusion for severe fetal congenital diaphragmatic hernia. *New England journal of medicine* 349:1916-1924.

Hecher K et al (1999). Endoscopic laser surgery versus serial amniocentesis in the treatment of severe twin-twin transfusion syndrome. *American journal of obstetrics and gynecology* 180:717-724.

Hedrick MH et al (1994). Congenital high airway obstruction syndrome (CHAOS): A potential for perinatal intervention. *Journal of pediatric surgery* 29:271.

Holmes N et al (2001). Fetal surgery for posterior urethral valves: long-term postnatal outcomes. *Pediatrics* 108:1-7.

Howell LJ, Dunphy PM (1999). Fetal surgery: exploring the challenges in nursing care. *Journal of obstetric, gynecologic, and neonatal nursing* 28:427-432.

Hutchins GM et al (1996). Acquired spinal cord injury in human fetuses with myelomeningocele. *Pediatric pathology and laboratory medicine* 16:701-712.

Johnson MP (2001). Fetal obstructive uropathy. In Harrison MR et al, editors. *The unborn patient: the art and science of fetal therapy*, ed 3 (pp 259-285). Philadelphia: Saunders.

Kiatano Y (1999). Open fetal surgery for life-threatening fetal malformations. *Seminars in perinatology* 23:448-461.

Laifer SA, Kuller JA (1996). Percutaneous umbilical blood sampling. In Kuller JA et al, editors. *Prenatal diagnosis and reproductive genetics*. St Louis: Mosby.

Lam YH et al (2002). Thermocoagulation of fetal sacrococcygeal teratoma. *Prenatal diagnosis and therapy* 22:99-101.

Liley AW (1963). Intrauterine transfusion of fetus in haemolytic disease. *British medical journal* 5365:1107-1109.

Lipshutz GS et al (1997). Prospective analysis of lung to head ratio predicts survival for patients with prenatally diagnosed congenital diaphragmatic hernia. *Journal of pediatric surgery* 32:1634-1636.

Lyerly AD et al (2001). Toward the ethical evaluation and use of maternal-fetal surgery. *American college of obstetricians and gynecologists* 98:689-697.

Manning FA (1986). International Fetal Surgery Registry: 1985 update. *Clinical obstetrics and gynecology* 29:551-557.

McMillan MP (1996). Banking on cord blood. *Journal of obstetric, gynecologic, and neonatal nursing* 25:115.

Meuli M et al (1995a). In utero surgery rescues neurologic function at birth in sheep with spina bifida. *Journal of pediatric surgery* 30:342-347.

Meuli M et al (1995b). Creation of myelomeningocele in utero: a model of functional damage from spinal cord exposure in fetal sheep. *Journal of pediatric surgery* 30:1028-1032.

Mychaliska GB et al (1997). Operating on placental support: the ex utero intrapartum treatment (EXIT) procedure. *Journal of pediatric surgery* 32:227-231.

Paek BW et al (2000). Hindbrain herniation develops in surgically created myelomeningocele but is absent after repair in fetal lambs. *American journal of obstetrics and gynecology* 183:1119-1123.

Paek B et al (2001). Radiofrequency ablation of human fetal sacrococcygeal teratoma. *American journal of obstetrics and gynecology* 184(3):305-307.

Paek B et al (2002). Successful fetal intervention for complete high airway. *Fetal diagnosis and therapy* 17(5):272-276.

Spitzer AR (2005). *Intensive care of the fetus and neonate*, ed 2. Philadelphia: Hanley & Belfus.

Strauss A et al (2000). Intrauterine fetal demise caused by amniotic band syndrome after standard amniocentesis. *Fetal diagnosis and therapy* 15:4-7.

Sutton LN et al (1999). Improvement in hindbrain herniation demonstrated by serial fetal magnetic resonance imaging following fetal surgery for myelomeningocele. *Journal of the American Medical Association* 282:1826-1831.

Taeusch HW, Ballard RA, editors (1998). *Avery's diseases of the newborn*, ed 7. Philadelphia: Saunders.

Tulipan N et al (1998). Reduced hindbrain herniation after intrauterine myelomeningocele repair: a report of four cases. *Pediatric neurosurgery* 29:274-278.

Westerburg BW et al (1998). Radiofrequency ablation of the liver in the fetal sheep: a model for treatment of sacrococcygeal teratoma in the fetus. *Surgical forum* 49:461-463.

Westerburg B et al (2000). Sonographic prognostic factors in fetuses with sacrococcygeal teratoma. *Journal of pediatric surgery* 35:322-326.

Wiley JM (1996). Stem cell transplantation for the treatment of genetic disease. In Kuller JA et al, editors. *Prenatal diagnosis and reproductive genetics*. St Louis: Mosby.

Wilson RD et al (2004). Reproductive outcomes after pregnancy complicated by maternal-fetal surgery. *American journal of obstetrics and gynecology* 191:1430-1436.

Chapter 19

Surgical Considerations in the Newborn and Infant

Kaye Spence

Caring for an infant with a surgical condition is an exciting challenge that requires knowledge of pathophysiology and current neonatal care practices, training to recognize and respond to complications, and ability to extend supportive care to the family. Optimum outcome is achieved through the skills of a multidisciplinary team that includes neonatal nurses, neonatologists, pediatric surgeons, radiologists, anesthesiologists, respiratory therapists, and parents. The members of this team must work together, guided by the knowledge that all of principles of neonatal care, as well as additional considerations related to surgical care, apply in each case.

ANTENATAL CONSIDERATIONS

There have been many changes over the past decades in the care and management of newborn infants requiring surgery. Important areas of advancement have been in newborn intensive care and postoperative care. Another area of advancement has been in antenatal diagnosis and the early referral to neonatal intensive care units (NICUs) for information and education regarding the expected course of the treatment and the outcomes of surgical care for newborn infants.

Many congenital surgical defects are diagnosed in utero through routine prenatal screening, providing time for education and emotional support for the family. If possible, a tour of the NICU should be arranged before delivery. Also, the parents should meet with members of the surgical and neonatal teams to discuss the findings and probable prognosis for their infant. Information given to the family should include the natural history of the abnormality, timing of surgery, anticipated surgical outcomes, possible long-term sequelae, and any other possible problems that may be involved with the neonate's course.

TRANSPORTATION OF INFANTS FOR SURGERY

Babies requiring surgery should be born in an appropriate tertiary perinatal center, adjacent to pediatric surgical facilities, in accordance with best practice. For some specific conditions, such as congenital heart disease, transferring the mother for delivery at a high-risk center is preferred (Hellstrom-Westas et al, 2001). Advantages of antenatal referral of babies with congenital anomalies requiring surgery include:
1. Improved neonatal outcomes
2. The opportunity for parents to discuss the following issues with experienced staff:
   - Options for birth
   - Anticipated care of the baby
   - Likely neonatal outcomes
3. The reassurance of access to the best available obstetric and neonatal care
4. Women may also experience a reduction in stress and anxiety as an emergency transfer of the baby resulting in separation of mother and baby is avoided.

Eighty percent of neonates with an antenatal diagnosis of a congenital anomaly require admission to a neonatal intensive care and major surgery (NSW Department of Health, 2005). Emergency Transport Services retrieve neonates to tertiary referral centers for intensive care, diagnostic workup, or surgery. If birth occurs at an appropriate tertiary perinatal center, the potential for an emergency neonatal retrieval to a pediatric facility is avoided.

It is desirable for each maternity unit to have a policy on antenatal referral of mothers with babies known to have a congenital abnormality likely to require surgery. The policy should emphasize antenatal consultation with the appropriate fetal, surgical, and other consultants (e.g., genetics, cardiac) in the preferred facility. It should note that the decision to make an antenatal maternal referral should take into account patient and clinician preferences. The policy should include options and processes for antenatal referral for more detailed fetal assessment and a plan for the optimal place of delivery. This referral will usually occur midpregnancy. If surgery or other critical therapy is likely to be required soon after birth, this plan should include delivery at a perinatal center with direct access to appropriate pediatric surgical services.

SURGICAL NEONATAL INTENSIVE CARE UNITS (SNICUs)

Criteria for neonatal surgical units have been established in several countries to ensure that acceptable standards are met for infants who require surgery during the neonatal period. There are many identified requirements for surgical services that provide operations and general anesthesia for newborn infants. These requirements relate to adequate training for the consultant surgeon and anesthetist with sufficient case loads to maintain skills (Royal College of Surgeons, 2000). In addition, adequately trained and experienced staff to care for the infant postoperatively need to be available in dedicated newborn surgical units.

There are arguments for and against large regional specialist pediatric centers being established for neonatal surgery. Benefits of regionalization include pooling of expertise, appropriate consultants, support services, and staff training. Disadvantages include children and their families having to travel long distances for care, and the loss of expertise at a local level. However, the availability of a neonatal emergency transport service can weigh the benefits against the adverse effects of having to take sick newborn infants to a regional neonatal surgical intensive care center (Arul & Spicer, 1998).

There are trends in some countries to ensure that SNICUs are located in children's hospitals with a colocated perinatal center (NSW Department of Health, 2005). This practice enables the women to deliver with a high-risk obstetric team as well as having a specialist pediatric/neonatal surgical team present to attend to the infant's well-being.

Staffing

The majority of the nursing staff in SNICUs require skills and competence in neonatal intensive care as well the specific management of neonatal surgical patients. Recommendations for staffing ratios vary; however, most infants will require dedicated nursing staff in the immediate postoperative period. During this period many infants will be unstable, and vigilant observation and assessment are required to avert postoperative complications. In addition, the families require additional support and explanation of many of the unique procedures seen in infants who have undergone surgery. A dedicated in-service program that includes a multidimensional approach to various conditions, altered pathophysiology, care paths, techniques, and procedures as well as counseling skills is recommended.

A wide range of subspecialists, including cardiologists, gastroenterologists, endocrinologists, geneticists, infectious disease specialists, respiratory specialists, and anesthetists, are involved in the SNICU; this requires a coordinated effort of team meetings and communication. Nurses are in key positions to coordinate the information and develop care plans to ensure continuity when multiple specialist teams are involved.

The combined skills of the pediatric surgeon, pediatric anesthetist, neonatologist, and neonatal nurse together with the resources available in a regional pediatric center will continue to contribute to the improvements in survival and quality of life of infants requiring neonatal surgery. However, there does need to be continuing debate on the surgical advances for infants with congenital malformations. Issues such as long-term outcomes and future quality of life need to be considered by the team together with the families. Other issues such as resources and cost effectiveness of the treatments need to be part of the community debate for future health care programs (Poley et al, 2001).

Family

Decisions on the management and treatment of the infant require a team approach that includes parents, nurses, obstetricians, pediatric surgeons, neonatologists, nurse practitioners, and radiologists. Supportive services should be provided to the family as indicated to reduce some of the stressors of having their newborn infant undergo surgery.

Parents want comprehensive information, especially during the waiting periods. Parental coping may be greatly enhanced by timely updates from the operating room while the parents are waiting for their infant in surgery. It is also important for the surgeon to speak with the parents immediately after surgery to discuss findings and the infant's condition.

Once the infant is back from the operating room, the parents should be encouraged to visit in a timely manner to reduce anticipatory stress. The nurse should discuss the infant's current condition, the equipment used, and anticipatory care in the short term.

In the postoperative period, parents need to be able to negotiate their parental role with the staff members caring for their infant and should be supported in their attempts to advocate for their infant. Parents should also be encouraged to participate in their child's care to the extent that is comfortable for them. This participation means that parents must be provided with adequate information, guidance regarding their role, coping instructions, and support (Jack, 2004).

CLASSIFICATION OF NEONATAL SURGERY

Neonatal surgery is defined as surgery performed on infants who:
- are less than 28 days old
- weigh less than 2500 g regardless of age
- require care in a neonatal intensive care unit (NICU) regardless of age or weight

Approximately 0.6% of newborn infants undergo surgery in the first 4 weeks of life (Badawi et al, 2003). Some of the most common types of surgical procedures performed are gastrointestinal, cardiovascular, hernia, genitourinary, and neurosurgical.

Neonatal surgery can be classified into three groups for ease of management. Group 1 includes those infants with a life-threatening condition for whom a surgical operation is necessary within the first day of life, such as congenital diaphragmatic hernia, gastroschisis, or esophageal atresia with fistula. In group 2 are those infants with an obvious abnormality but for whom a surgical operation may be deferred for days or months, such as exomphalos minor or cleft lip. Group 3 includes infants who have an obvious abnormality whose management may consist of interventions after due consideration, such as myelomeningocele.

PREPARATION FOR SURGERY

From the time of delivery, the goal is to reduce the likelihood of morbidity and mortality by continually assessing the infant and the responses to treatments instituted. Preparation for surgery starts with discussions with the family and gaining informed consent. The consent process is the responsibility of the surgical team; however, it is good practice for the nurse to be present when these discussions take place. If the parents are from a non–English speaking background, then an interpreter should be present. Often nurses are asked to clarify issues that were discussed, and nurses are in a unique position to communicate misunderstandings back to the surgical team.

Many of the neonatal surgical procedures are performed on emergency operative lists; therefore the preparation needs to be coordinated and the many teams involved aware of the infant's condition prior to surgery. The anesthetist holds a key role in this coordination with multiple subspecialists, and the nurse is pivotal in ensuring the documentation is complete and the family informed and available. Each institution needs to have a clear and comprehensive system of evaluating infants during the preoperative period (Ferrari, 2004) to ensure effective use of operating time and to avoid undue delays and stress on the infant and family.

An understanding of neonatal physiology is necessary to enable the team to provide appropriate care in three areas of homeostasis—temperature regulation, fluid and electrolyte balance, and acid-base balance. In addition, specific practices for preparation for transfer to the operating room are described in this chapter. Each area is discussed in relation to the preparation of the infant for surgery.

Temperature Control

Heat loss can occur during transfer, in the imaging department and in the operating room due to the infant's high ratio of surface area to body weight. It remains important to maintain the core body temperature close to 37° C to minimize oxygen consumption. In the operating room, a low ambient temperature increases heat loss by both convection and radiation. It is ideal that the operating room be warmed to 28° to 30° C for neonatal patients. The infant may be transferred on an open-care bed with a radiant warmer; some surgeons will operate on these beds to minimize the stress of heat loss. The infant undergoing surgical procedures where the organs are exposed is at particular risk of heat loss.

Prevention of hypothermia in the surgical neonate is imperative in the preoperative period. Maintaining a neutral thermal environment is a constant challenge. In a neutral thermal environment, metabolic activity is minimal because body temperature is kept stable. Oxygen consumption is reduced, and acidosis is prevented. Any prolonged deviations from the neutral thermal environment further stress the infant's already limited thermoregulatory abilities. Strategies such as wrapping the infant's head and limbs in cotton webbing can be useful in reducing some of the inevitable heat loss.

Heat loss occurs through evaporation, conduction, convection, and radiation. Evaporative heat loss occurs with exposure of the intestinal contents of a ruptured omphalocele or gastroschisis. In the case of an encephalocele or a myelomeningocele, the unprotected spinal cord may allow heat loss. The exposed bladder mucosa in exstrophy of the bladder also contributes to heat loss. This type of heat loss can be prevented by applying warm dressings to the defects and then covering these areas with plastic wrap.

Conductive heat loss occurs with direct skin contact with a cold surface, such as cold or wet linens, an operating table, radiographic plates, or an unwarmed bed. To prevent this type of heat loss, linens should be prewarmed as the bed or incubator is warmed. Operating or radiography tables can be warmed with heat lamps before and during procedures. Linens that become wet should be replaced with dry, warmed linens; radiographic plates and scales should be covered with warmed linens before the infant is placed on them.

Heat loss by convection occurs when air blows over the infant. Use of warmed oxygen in head hoods and ventilators can reduce this type of heat loss. Also, it is essential that the incubator door not be open for prolonged periods. Insertion of nasogastric tubes, placement of intravenous lines, radiographic studies, physical examinations, and phlebotomy procedures should be performed through the incubator portholes to reduce heat loss. An additional heat source may be placed over the incubator when the door must be open.

Heat loss by radiation is the most difficult to control. This type of heat loss occurs during transportation of the neonate in cold hallways, or in the cold operating room. To prevent this cold stress, the infant should be covered with warmed linens or wrapped during transport. Operating rooms should be prewarmed to well above the "comfortable" temperature.

Nursing care that focuses on the thermoregulatory process of the neonate is vital to the prevention of complications related to poor temperature control. It is also beneficial to use warmed solutions for suctioning and dressing changes. Frequent monitoring of the infant's temperature is extremely important. Consistency in the method of measuring temperature and appropriate documentation are also essential.

Fluid and Electrolyte Balance

Adequate fluid volume is required to ensure adequate perfusion of all organ systems. An inadequate vascular volume interferes with the oxygen supply to peripheral tissues, resulting in cellular damage and acidosis. Precision in fluid management is essential; there is little margin for error. Particular care needs to be taken to ensure excessive volumes are not delivered with additional drugs used during the anesthesia.

All fluid losses must be measured accurately to ensure adequate replacement. Estimation of insensible fluid losses is essential, including those caused by humidification through ventilation and radiant heating. Unexpected fluid losses and inadequate fluid replacement delay preoperative stabilization of the neonate's condition.

Infants with an esophageal atresia may have continuous losses of saliva suctioned from the esophageal pouch which must be measured and replaced. The large exposed intestinal area seen with a ruptured omphalocele or gastroschisis results in large volumes of fluid losses. Replacement of these losses may involve up to twice the normal maintenance fluids of a neonate. If a membranous sac protects an omphalocele, the fluid requirement is less.

Gastrointestinal obstructions cause fluid losses from vomiting and from the suctioning required for gastric decompression. Peritonitis, such as occurs with perforations in necrotizing enterocolitis, midgut volvulus, or ruptured meconium ileus, causes third-spacing of fluid (capillary leak syndrome) or fluid shifts into the bowel, necessitating increased fluid replacement. Infants with open neural tube defects also have increased fluid losses. A leaking myelomeningocele requires increased fluid administration to keep up with the loss of cerebrospinal fluid.

Third-spacing of fluids, or capillary leak syndrome, is the result of trauma to the gastrointestinal system. The capillary membrane's permeability is changed. This phenomenon may be due to natural fibronectin, a glycoprotein secreted by epithelial cells in the pulmonary and gastrointestinal trees. It is secreted in response to stimulation of the immune system to heal a wound. Fibronectin alters capillary permeability, shifting fluid and resulting in a "leaky capillary" and the third-spacing of fluid. The body's compensatory response to any gastrointestinal trauma, then, can result in a movement of fluid across this "leaky" membrane. Fluid moves out of the vascular compartment and into the tissues, and the infant develops generalized edema. Abdominal swelling exerts pressure on the thoracic cavity, increasing the work of breathing. Gas exchange and ventilation are compromised as a result of (1) the pressure; (2) the decreased circulation; (3) the increased workload of the heart, which delivers oxygen to the tissues; and (4) the increasing loss of the buffer system through the mechanisms of diminished kidney perfusion and gastric losses.

The immediate reaction of inexperienced health professionals may be to restrict fluids in this edematous infant, even though the vascular compartment is severely depleted of fluids. The infant is hypotensive, which increases cardiopulmonary compromise. Liberalization of fluids, therefore, is necessary to avoid total vascular collapse.

Diagnostic enemas with hyperosmolar solutions can have catastrophic results in a neonate who is not properly hydrated. Adequate intravenous access and good hydration are essential. Vascular collapse and even shock can occur rapidly if the fluid is shifted from the vascular bed to the bowel and is extracted with the enema and not appropriately replaced.

The numerous conditions that affect the surgical neonate may result in imbalances of serum electrolytes, especially sodium and potassium. Fluid losses and inadequate intake result in hypokalemia and hyponatremia.

Hyperkalemia occurs with acidosis, excessive potassium intake, and renal failure. Renal failure may result from genitourinary obstructions or from sepsis and poor perfusion, as is seen with necrotizing enterocolitis with perforation or peritonitis.

The causes of hypernatremia generally are iatrogenic. An excessive intake of sodium occurs with administration of hypertonic solutions, intravenous flushes with normal saline or heparinized normal saline, or sodium bicarbonate for treatment of acidosis. Therapy with antibiotics such as ampicillin enhances the risk of hypernatremia. Return to a fluid and electrolyte balance is needed to improve the neonate's ability to tolerate any necessary operative procedure and to reduce the likelihood of complications.

Maintenance of Glucose Levels

Fluctuation in the glucose level is a major indication of stress and infection. Preoperative hyperglycemia can result from sepsis or excessive intravenous administration of glucose. Hypoglycemia may result from a multitude of problems. For example, reduced glycogen stores are seen in premature infants and in infants with intrauterine growth restriction. Excessive insulin production occurs in the infant of a diabetic mother and with sudden or prolonged cessation of glucose infusions, as may occur with difficult or delayed insertion of intravenous lines. Abnormalities in glucose metabolism are evident with sepsis, shock, and asphyxia, as well as with various central nervous system (CNS) abnormalities. Glucose infusions must be carefully titrated to provide adequate hydration while the serum glucose is slowly restored to an acceptable concentration, avoiding extremes in the serum glucose level.

Acid-Base Balance

A variety of factors can alter the acid-base balance in the surgical neonate. Major conditions that can result in acidosis include inadequate respiratory support and fluid or electrolyte imbalances. The effects of sepsis and tissue necrosis are also significant causes of acidosis. Acidosis in the surgical neonate can be the respiratory, metabolic, or mixed type.

Respiratory acidosis could occur with decreased ventilation, resulting in an increased partial pressure of carbon dioxide (PCO_2) and a decreased pH. An overproduction of acids may occur with any condition that causes a decrease in oxygenation or perfusion. Impaired kidney function, such as that which occurs in acute renal failure or renal tubular necrosis, reduces elimination of hydrogen ions, contributing to the development of metabolic acidosis. Bicarbonate losses are increased with severe diarrhea, intestinal fistulas, vomiting, and gastric drainage, resulting in metabolic acidosis.

The neonate with a diaphragmatic hernia is at great risk for the development of respiratory acidosis or metabolic acidosis, or both. Such an infant requires aggressive ventilation and administration of a buffering agent (e.g., sodium bicarbonate, tromethamine [Tham, Abbott Labs, Abbot Park, IL]) to prevent acidosis, which could contribute to the development of persistent pulmonary hypertension.

Poor tissue perfusion causes acidosis, as is seen with multiple gastrointestinal anomalies that are accompanied by large fluid losses. These anomalies include tracheoesophageal fistula with esophageal atresia, ruptured omphalocele and gastroschisis, bowel obstruction, and necrotizing enterocolitis. Adequately replenishing fluid or blood volume usually corrects this metabolic acidosis. When necrosis or perforation occurs, however, the acidosis may not be correctable until the necrotic bowel has been removed and any resulting sepsis treated.

Drugs

The role of prophylactic antibiotics remains controversial. However, with suspected gastrointestinal obstruction, antibiotics may be needed to treat peritonitis or enterocolitis. The progression of necrotizing enterocolitis may be slowed with vigorous antibiotic therapy. Treatment of omphalocele and gastroschisis may include antibiotics to protect the exposed gastrointestinal contents and to help prevent ischemic injury to the abdominal contents. If pneumonia accompanies an esophageal atresia with tracheoesophageal fistula, aggressive antibiotic therapy should be instituted to clear the pneumonia and promote optimum surgical repair of the defect. The infant with a myelomeningocele requires antibiotic treatment to prevent meningitis.

Inotropic agents may be necessary to improve cardiac function and thus improve organ perfusion impaired by sepsis and stress. The most frequently used agents are dobutamine and dopamine. Dobutamine hydrochloride achieves organ perfusion by increasing cardiac output. Dopamine hydrochloride, used in low to moderate doses, causes vasodilation with resultant improvement in cardiac, renal, gastrointestinal, and cerebral blood flow. Use of dopamine hydrochloride at high doses, however, causes vasoconstriction of renal and gastrointestinal vessels. This vasoconstriction could worsen the condition of a renal system affected by obstruction or poor flow status, as well as the gastrointestinal system already compromised by necrotizing enterocolitis, omphalocele, gastroschisis, or obstruction. Doses of dobutamine hydrochloride and dopamine hydrochloride, therefore, must be carefully calculated and continually titrated to achieve the desired effect. Furthermore, these medications are incompatible with many other drugs. For example, alkaline solutions (e.g., sodium bicarbonate, ampicillin, gentamicin, and furosemide) can inactivate dobutamine and dopamine. These inotropic agents are also irritating to vessels, and close monitoring of intravenous sites for infiltration is essential.

A buffering agent may be required to treat the acidosis that may accompany a diaphragmatic hernia, necrotizing enterocolitis, omphalocele, gastroschisis, or obstruction with resulting ischemic injury. Adequate ventilation and tissue perfusion must be established and maintained before medication is used to treat acidotic conditions.

Monitoring

Infants will require preoperative monitoring that continues during the operation into the postoperative period. At a minimum, cardiorespiratory monitoring is essential. The electrodes and leads should be placed with consideration of the operative area; this will enable the monitoring leads to be used during the surgery without the necessity of tissue damage from removal and re-siting. A pulse oximeter on an upper limb will enable the oxygen saturation levels to be monitored. The nurse needs to be mindful that some monitoring, such as transcutaneous oxygen, may be ineffective because of changes in skin perfusion during the procedure. The placement of a temperature probe can assist the anesthetist in monitoring the temperature during surgery.

Intravascular Lines

Ideally a central venous catheter (CVC) will be required postoperatively if multiple drug infusions or parental nutrition will be required. It may be opportune for the CVC to be inserted during the operative procedure; this may be negotiated with the surgeon and anesthetist.

In addition, a peripheral arterial line will be required for the continuing measurement of the acid-base balance during the operation and in the postoperative period. It is best if this is inserted before the infant is transferred to the operating room. Precautions should be taken to ensure that all connections are Luer-lok to avoid accidental disconnection when covered with surgical drapes.

Nurse's Role

Adequate and thorough preparation of the infant can minimize stress during the process and help reduce the preparation and time of the surgery. Being prepared and anticipating the time and call for surgery can ensure that the infant is adequately prepared for transfer and surgery. If the nurse accompanies the infant to the operating room, continuing monitoring and a smooth handover can occur. In some institutions the neonatal nurse can remain in the operating room assisting the infant and helping with the monitoring of the oxygenation and temperature. This is, however, a contentious issue for some institutions and operating room staff.

Preoperative Assessment

A checklist maybe helpful in ensuring that all the relevant information is available.
- Record infant's weight and gestational age
- Determine that preoperative condition is stable and optimal
- Identify associated conditions such as heart or lung disease, renal abnormalities
- Review preoperative investigations
- Ensure that venous access has been established
- Ensure that consent has been obtained
- Reassure the parents

DURING SURGERY

Anesthesia

The intraoperative period places the infant at risk of fluctuations in vital signs as well as stress and complications. Many neonates will arrive at the operating room already intubated and ventilated. The endotracheal tube needs to be secure to ensure that accidental extubation does not occur.

This is the responsibility of the anesthetist, who may elect to re-intubate prior to the surgery.

The choice of anesthetic agent will depend on the type of operation, the defect, and the infant's status. Muscle relaxants are commonly used together with controlled ventilation and humidified gases for neonates. Inhalation anesthetic agents are commonly administered in 100% oxygen during the anesthesia, and the use of opioid can limit episodes of hypoxic pulmonary vasoconstriction (Golianu & Hammer, 2005). How infants are positioned during surgery can predispose them to hypoxia. For example, when positioned in the lateral decubitus position for thoracic surgery, infants are at significant risk of hypoxia due to their increased consumption of oxygen (Golianu & Hammer, 2005). This type of information is useful when nurses are challenged to care for recovering infants in the postoperative period.

Anesthetic agents can cause respiratory depression, as can narcotic and sedative medications. The neonate has a limited capacity to tolerate prolonged anesthesia. Residual effects of anesthesia can delay recovery from the surgical procedure, as seen by the infant's diminished respiratory effort and apnea. For these reasons it remains unwise to extubate the infant in the immediate postoperative period. At least 24 hours of postoperative ventilation enables more control of the infant's condition and stability as well as enabling adequate postoperative pain management.

Thermoregulation

Concerns regarding temperature regulation continue during the intraoperative period. Although achieving a normal core temperature in the infant before surgery is always helpful, it is not always possible. Body temperature should be monitored throughout the procedure using either a skin or a rectal probe. A radiant warmer should be used during line placement, preparation, draping, and induction of anesthesia. A warming blanket under the infant can also be used to achieve constant temperature control. In addition, the room temperature should be increased to help compensate for the neonate's inability to stabilize temperature. Another mechanism for improving temperature control is humidification and warming of anesthetic gases. Slightly warming blood products, irrigation fluids, and intravenous fluids also assists in temperature maintenance. Surgical drapes should be replaced, if possible, when they become wet.

Another challenge in temperature maintenance is encountered during transport of the neonate to and from the operating room. To ensure temperature stability, the infant should be covered with warmed linen during transport. During the operative procedure, the transfer bed should be warmed to allow for some warmth during transport postoperatively.

Fluid and Electrolyte Balance

The goal of intraoperative fluid management is to replace the fasting fluid deficit, maintenance and third-space fluid losses, and blood loss to maintain homeostasis. Constant monitoring of fluid balance should continue throughout the surgical procedure. During the operative procedure, the fluid choice reflects the most dominant fluid loss. Early treatment of hypovolemia is essential. Intravenous fluid administration rates must be monitored to prevent fluid boluses, which could compromise fluid and electrolyte balance. Fluid loss from the surgical defect and blood loss during the operative procedure must be monitored and replaced. The metabolic response to surgery may also alter the infant's fluid and electrolyte balance. Hyperglycemia is a common response to surgical stress. Cold stress adds to this metabolic response and consequent fluid needs.

Monitoring

The trends of the infant's vital signs of heart rate, oxygenation, and gases are useful indicators for the anesthetist. Continuous monitoring during the operative phase can be useful in reviewing the infant's course during the surgery.

POSTOPERATIVE CARE

Oxygenation and Ventilation

Respiratory care in the postoperative period can present a great challenge to the caregiver. Intubation, anesthetic gases, and the stress of the procedure can traumatize the infant's respiratory tract. Depression of respiratory drive may be seen as a residual effect of anesthesia, and airway clearance may be difficult to maintain. These alterations in respiratory mechanics may lead to respiratory insufficiency and the need for prolonged mechanical support. Although specific respiratory needs may vary depending on the surgical procedure, a conservative approach to respiratory care is essential to maintain optimum oxygenation. An aggressive plan of weaning may cause recurring acidosis, hypoxia, or damage to the surgical repair.

Postoperative care of the neonate with necrotizing enterocolitis includes aggressive ventilation. Many of these infants are small, premature, or of low birth weight and have lung function that is already compromised. The stress of severe infection and the surgical procedure itself, as well as the prematurity of the lungs, may necessitate prolonged ventilation with a slow weaning process.

Pain Management

The assessment of the infant for postoperative pain is an important component of nursing care. Nurses need to have a good knowledge base for the physiologic responses, pharmacokinetics, and behavioral responses of the infant in pain. The use of a validated pain assessment tool and the reliability of the use of the tool between clinicians are important if postoperative pain is to be adequately managed (Spence et al, 2005). Most infants will have a narcotic infusion in the immediate postoperative period. The use of narcotics is encouraged; however, the assessment of their effect is important. There remains a lack of information on the effectiveness of pain management strategies and outcomes of infants managed for pain with narcotics.

Fluid and Electrolyte Balance

The goal of postoperative care is to provide fluid and electrolyte balance without overhydration. Hypovolemia is a major cause of hypotension and must be resolved quickly to ensure adequate perfusion to all organ systems and to combat acidosis. However, extreme care must be taken in administering fluids because premature infants are susceptible to third-spacing and edema. Neonates are also very easily overloaded with excessive fluids.

Vital signs should be monitored frequently, as changes in heart rate or blood pressure could indicate shock or undetected fluid loss for which the body is trying to compensate. Assess-

ment of temperature continues to be an important factor and must be considered when evaluating fluid needs. The serum electrolyte and glucose levels should be evaluated immediately postoperatively and then intermittently until the infant's condition is stable. The frequency of laboratory evaluation should be individualized to the neonate's condition. Sodium losses may continue through wound drainage as well as through gastric decompression. Thus re-evaluation of intravenous fluids, both maintenance and replacement, is required to achieve and maintain electrolyte balance. Glucose metabolism may be altered as a response to surgery. Serum glucose levels should be monitored every 1 to 2 hours after surgery.

Replacement fluid therapy is designed to make up for abnormal fluid and electrolyte losses during therapy to reduce vomiting and for losses incurred through diarrhea, nasogastric tube drainage, stoma output, wound drainage, pleural fluid, and fistula losses. Because the constituents of these losses frequently are quite different from the composition of maintenance fluids, it may be hazardous to simply increase the volume of maintenance fluids in an attempt to compensate for these losses. In some cases, it is preferable to actually measure and analyze the electrolyte content of these losses and replace them milliequivalent for milliequivalent and milliliter for milliliter. Samples may be sent to the laboratory as needed for exact determination of the electrolyte content of these various body fluids.

The rate at which abnormal losses are replaced depends on the rate at which the fluid is lost and the patient's size. In small infants, even modest abnormal losses should be replaced every 2 to 4 hours.

Overzealous attempts to correct glucose or electrolyte problems can produce a rebound effect. The neonate may change from being hyperglycemic to being hypoglycemic without intervention over a period of minutes or hours. The neonate moves from a catabolic to an anabolic state fairly rapidly compared with an older child or adult. These phases may occur over a few days or weeks in the infant instead of over months as in the adult. Therefore it is best to obtain baseline serum electrolyte and glucose levels. These values should be obtained every 1 to 4 hours, depending on how extreme the levels are. When intervention is needed, the sodium, potassium, or other electrolyte should be increased or decreased slowly and in small increments. These incremental changes should be followed by repeated measurement of serum levels, which must be closely monitored.

Third-spacing of fluids (capillary leak syndrome) that causes edema in the first few postoperative days is an additional consideration. The infant's weight, renal function, and nutritional needs must continue to be evaluated, and nursing care must include measures to maintain skin integrity during this period of edema and fluid mobilization.

Nutrition

Feeding is usually commenced as soon as possible after surgery. This is largely controlled by the type of surgery performed and the responsiveness of the individual infant. Infants who have undergone surgery on the gastrointestinal tract may take several days or indeed weeks before full enteral feeds are tolerated.

For some surgical neonates there may be concern during the convalescent period that goes beyond fluid and electrolyte balance. The nutritional needs of infants with altered function of the gastrointestinal tract present unique problems. A small stomach size with altered emptying ability, as is sometimes seen with a diaphragmatic hernia, gastroschisis, omphalocele, and bowel resection, may present paramount problems in providing proper nutrition when feedings are started. Use of continuous feedings may help with these problems.

Gastroesophageal reflux (GER) may present challenges in feeding. Assessments of vomiting and large gastric aspirates must be made. Treatment of reflux may include positioning the infant prone or in an upright position after feedings and thickening the feeding. Pharmacologic treatment may be initiated in the immediate postoperative period in anticipation of GER, or it may be started once symptoms appear.

The neonate who has had a bowel resection after perforation (as in necrotizing enterocolitis) can present a significant challenge. Concerns should center on vomiting, diarrhea, distention, or the presence of glucose or blood in the stool. The infant may not tolerate standard formulas, and an alternative formula, such as an elemental formula, may be required.

Wound Care

Surgical neonates are vulnerable to infection throughout their hospital course. To prevent infection, the nurse must provide careful wound care. Wound infections can occur during or after the surgical procedure. They are related to the duration of the procedure and factors at operation and can be a complicating factor (Allpress et al, 2004; Duque-Estrada et al, 2003). Infection occurs more often after "contaminated" surgeries, such as an intestinal perforation, compared with "clean" surgeries, such as ductal ligation. These wound infections often require treatment with antibiotics.

Nursing assessment of the site must be continual, because these observations may provide the first indication of poor healing or wound infection. The neonatal or surgical team (or both) should be made aware of any changes. If any suspicion of infection exists, blood cultures should be taken before treatment is started with broad-spectrum antibiotics that target anaerobes, aerobes, and gram-positive and gram-negative organisms. Consideration should be given to pain relief during potentially painful removal of surgical and wound dressings. The use of oral sucrose for pain relief is recommended if given 2 minutes prior to the procedure. The small volume given is not contraindicated when the infant is ordered nothing by gastrointestinal tract.

Outcomes

Long-term consequences of neonatal surgery have been identified in several studies. Peters et al (2005) concluded that prior tissue damage can contribute to long-term neurobiologic differences. Sternberg et al (2005) reported that early exposure to noxious or stressful stimuli such as surgery may induce long-lasting pain behavior changes into adulthood. However, Peters and colleagues (2003) found that major surgery in combi-

nation with preemptive analgesia within the first months of life does not alter response to subsequent pain exposure in childhood. They found that greater exposure to early hospitalization influences the pain responses after prolonged time (Peters et al, 2003).

Neurodevelopmental outcomes in school-age children were found to be reduced in children who underwent an arterial-switch operation; however, there was no cognitive dysfunction (Hovels-Gurich et al, 2002). The deleterious effects of severe preoperative acidosis and hypoxia, and postoperative hemodynamic instability contribute to the risk of developmental impairment (Hovels-Gurich et al, 2002).

These outcomes need to be considered when following infants who have undergone neonatal surgery. It appears that the experience of surgery, neonatal intensive care, and hospitalization can be deleterious for sick infants and their families. Care needs to be taken to ensure that the stressors encountered are kept to a minimum, and nurses are in key positions to provide a quality focus to the care of these infants and families.

REFERENCES

Allpress AL et al (2004). Risk factors for surgical site infections after pediatric cardiovascular surgery. *Pediatric infectious disease journal* 23(3):231-234.

Arul GS, Spicer RD (1998). Where should paediatric surgery be performed? *Archives of diseases in childhood* 79:65-72.

Badawi N et al (2003). Neonatal surgery in New South Wales, what is performed where? *Journal of pediatric surgery* 38(7):1025-1031.

Duque-Estrada EO et al (2003). Wound infections in pediatric surgery: a study of 575 patients in a university hospital. *Pediatric surgery international* 19(6):436-438.

Ferrari L (2004). Preoperative evaluation of pediatric surgical patients with multisystem considerations. *Anesthesia analog* 99:1058-1069.

Golianu B, Hammer GB (2005). Pediatric thoracic anesthesia. *Current opinion in anaesthesiology* 18:5-11.

Hellstrom-Westas L et al (2001). Long-distance transports of newborn infants with congenital heart disease. *Pediatric cardiology* 22:380-384.

Hovels-Gurich HH et al (2002). Long-term neurodevelopmental outcomes in school-aged children after neonatal arterial switch operation. *Journal of thoracic cardiovascular surgery* 124:448-458.

Jack P (2004). Children born with cyanotic congenital heart disease: effects on the family. *Journal of neonatal nursing* 10(6):191-195.

NSW Department of Health (2005). Selected speciality and statewide service plans: Neonatal Intensive Care Plan to 2006. Available at: http://www.health.gov.au.

Peters JWB et al (2003). Major surgery within the first 3 months of life and subsequent biobehavioral pain responses to immunization at later age: a case comparison study. *Pediatrics* 111(1):129-135.

Peters JW et al (2005). Does neonatal surgery lead to increased pain sensitivity in later childhood? *Pain* 114(3):444-454.

Poley MJ et al (2001). The cost-effectiveness of neonatal surgery and subsequent treatment for congenital anorectal malformations. *Journal of pediatric surgery* 36(10):1471-1478.

Royal College of Surgeons of England (2000). *Children's surgery: a first class service: report of the Paediatric Forum of the Royal College of Surgeons for England.* London: Author.

Spence K et al (2005). A clinically reliable pain assessment tool for use in neonates. *Journal of obstetric, gynecologic, and neonatal nursing* 34(1):80-86.

Sternberg WF et al (2005). Long-term effects of neonatal surgery on adulthood pain behaviour. *Pain* 113(3):347-353.

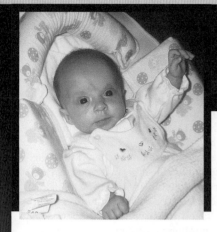

Chapter **20**

Newborn or Infant Transplant Patient

Linda MacKenna Ikuta

Transplantation is not a common procedure in the neonatal period. The ability to perform various transplants has risen as technology has improved and knowledge of the physical processes has increased. Solid organ transplants such as liver, kidney, and heart are the most usual procedures. The use of stem cells is an exciting prospect for treating many limiting and sometimes fatal congenital diseases, but this therapy is surrounded by controversy regarding the ethics of its use. The ethics of transplantation in general is muddled when a child's life is at stake. However, it is not always in the infant's best interest to do these procedures. In this chapter, common types of transplants are discussed. Procurement of organs and cells is addressed. The procedure descriptions are meant to provide an overview.

LIVER TRANSPLANTATION IN INFANTS AND CHILDREN

Liver transplantation in recent years has become a viable solution to many destructive liver diseases. In infants and small children, especially those weighing less than 15 pounds, a liver from a larger donor is "trimmed" to fit the small recipient. This has reduced the wait for an ideal matching donor. The technique is applied in living-related liver transplants when a segment of liver from a relative is removed and transplanted into the recipient. By using reduced size and related donors, mortality has been reduced to as little as 4% in some transplant centers. Increase in survival has been coupled by reduced stay and a greater number of transplants being done for infants and children.

Etiology

In neonates acute liver failure (ALF) is a rare but often a fatal event. Infants and younger children do not display the main symptom of ALF, hepatic encephalopathy, as do adults and older children. It is hard to diagnose and prove. Causes of ALF include congenital malformations, metabolic liver disease, hepatotoxins, idiopathic liver failure, malignant and benign neoplasms of the liver, infections, ischemic injury, congenital vascular or heart anomalies, and drugs.

Recognition of liver disease in a newborn is difficult because biochemical findings, such as hyperbilirubinemia and coagulopathy, may be due to various physiologic and pathophysiologic processes:

1. Hepatic encephalopathy is difficult to identify in any infant and almost impossible to distinguish from other metabolic encephalopathies in an ill neonate, especially if the infant requires ventilation support.
2. Because infants are so young, all neonatal liver failure tends to be labeled as "acute," which is consistent with the adult definition of a duration of less than 8 weeks. However, some infants clearly have liver failure from end-stage liver disease with cirrhosis due to liver damage that occurred during gestation (Jackson & Roberts, 2001).

Biliary Atresia

A progressive inflammatory process beginning shortly after birth is the hallmark of biliary atresia. Extrahepatic biliary atresia is the most common form. Biliary atresia occurs in one in 15,000 live births. The cause of the disease is unknown, but about 10% of the cases have other associated congenital defects of heart, blood vessels, intestine, and/or spleen involvement.

The Kasai procedure or Roux-en-Y hepatoportojejunostomy is the treatment for biliary atresia. Of newborns under 3 months of age undergoing this procedure, 80% will have re-establishment of their bile flow. The 20% remaining infants will not be helped by the procedure. A liver transplant is their only other treatment option.

Errors of Metabolism

Inherited errors of metabolism contribute greatly to liver failure and must be diagnosed promptly in the neonatal period. Galactosemia, hereditary fructose intolerance, and tyrosinemia are the most common metabolic diseases. Newborn screening by tandem mass spectrometry in many states tests for many metabolic diseases. These infants are being identified at a much earlier age than in previous years and treated when possible. An associated metabolic disease with acute liver disease is neonatal hemochromatosis (NH). It is the most common cause of liver failure in infancy, linked with massive intra- and extrahepatic iron disposition sparing the reticuloendothelial system (Dhawan & Mieli-Vergani, 2005). Despite chelation therapy, many severely affected infants will require transplantation.

CONTRAINDICATIONS FOR LIVER TRANSPLANTATION

There are many contraindications or reasons why transplantation should not be performed: (1) positive test for acquired immunodeficiency syndrome (AIDS) or human immunodeficiency virus (HIV); (2) cancer outside the liver; (3) infection outside the liver; (4) technical infeasibility; and (5) other medical problems such as heart disease, lung failure, or epilepsy that would interfere with the success of the transplant (Esquivel, 2005).

TRANSPLANT SELECTION

The advent of partial liver transplant and the use of living liver donors has eased transplant selection. Not all patients can receive a transplant. A liver function test based on the hepatic conversion of lidocaine to monoethylglycinexylidide (MEGX) can give prognostic information. This test has been used because of its rapid turnaround for real-time assessment of hepatic function in transplantation. The MEGX test is a useful tool that can improve the decision-making process with respect to the selection of transplant candidates. Patients with a MEGX 15- or 30-minute test value less than 10 mcg/L have a particularly poor 1-year survival rate. Serial monitoring of liver graft recipients early after transplantation with the MEGX test may initially alert the clinician to a major change in liver function; if used with other tests, such as serum hyaluronic acid concentrations, it may become more discriminatory. In critically ill patients, several studies have shown that an initially rapid decrease in MEGX test values is associated with an enhanced risk for the development of multiple organ dysfunction syndromes and a poor outcome. Further, this decrease appears to be associated with an enhanced systemic inflammatory response (Oellerich & Armstrong, 2001).

ESTIMATION SCALES OF LIVER ALLOCATION

The Model for End-Stage Liver Disease (MELD) and Pediatric End-Stage Liver Disease (PELD) are numerical scales that are currently used for liver allocation. The MELD and PELD scores are based on a patient's risk of dying while waiting for a liver transplant and are based on objective and verifiable medical data. UNOS (2005) uses the PELD for patients who are under 12 years old. The PELD score is calculated using:

    Albumin (g/dl)
    Bilirubin (mg/dl)
    International Normalized Ratio (INR)
    Growth failure (based on gender, height and weight ratio)
    Age at listing

Nutritional Support

Nutrition is best achieved enterally. Effective enteral administration is not always possible with patients with liver failure because of impaired absorption. Total parenteral nutrition (TPN) may be needed to support hepatocellular function and improve altered metabolism and absorption. A thorough assessment of nutritional status can be difficult because of metabolic disturbances. The balanced dietary approach moderated to replenishment of substrates and calories as needed helps prevent complications. Protein is needed to maintain lean body mass and preserve organ function (Pomposelli et al, 2002).

PRETRANSPLANT MANAGEMENT

Management of infants and children before the transport is paramount for success. So-called spiffing up to improve the clinical status of the patient before surgery could include normalizing electrolyte imbalances, nutrition, decreasing ascites and edema, improving diuresis, and giving blood transfusions if indicated.

TYPES OF LIVER TRANSPLANTS

The orthotopic approach requires replacing the recipient liver with the donor liver. After the donor liver is removed, preserved, and packed for transport, it must be transplanted into the recipient within 12 to 18 hours. The surgery begins by removing the diseased liver from the four main blood vessels and other structures that hold it in place in the abdomen. After the recipient's liver is removed, the new healthy donor liver is then connected and blood flow is restored. The final connection is made to the bile duct, a small tube that carries bile made in the liver to the intestines.

HETEROTOPIC LIVER TRANSPLANTATION

In heterotopic liver transplantation, the recipient's liver is left in place and a donor liver is sewn into an ectopic site (UNOS, 2005). The advantage to this transplant is that the patient retains the original liver with the donor liver helping. It is not as common as other types of liver transplantation in recent years.

REDUCED-SIZE LIVER TRANSPLANTATION

In reduced-sized liver transplantation, allografts of donor liver are divided into eight pieces, each supplied by a different set of blood vessels. Two of these pieces have been enough to save a patient in liver failure, especially if the patient is a child. It is therefore possible to transplant one liver into at least two patients. Liver tissue grows to accommodate its job so long as there is initially enough of the organ to use. Patients have survived with only 15% to 20% of their original liver, provided that the 15% to 20% was healthy (Carter et al, 2006).

LIVING DONOR TRANSPLANTATION

Living donor liver transplantation (LDLT) is a procedure in which a healthy, living person donates a portion of his or her liver to another person. The feasibility of LDLT was first demonstrated in the United States in 1989. The recipient was a child, who received a segment of his mother's liver. In the pediatric experience, survival of the recipient child and function of the transplanted liver (graft) at 1 year is about 90%. The transplanted liver grows to almost full size within 6 to 8 weeks and begins to function fully.

AUXILIARY LIVER TRANSPLANTATION

There are three levels of cells in the hepatic lineage that respond to injury: the mature hepatocyte, the ductular "bipolar" progenitor cell, and a putative periductular stem cell. Hepatocytes are numerous and respond rapidly to liver cell loss by one or two cell cycles. The ductular progenitor cells are less numerous, may proliferate for more cycles than hepatocytes, and are generally considered "bipolar," that is, they can give rise to biliary cells or hepatocytes. Periductular stem cells, although rare in the liver, can proliferate for a long time. Extrahepatic (bone marrow) origin of the periductular stem cells is supported by recent data showing that hepatocytes may express genetic markers of donor hematopoietic cells after bone marrow transplantation.

These different regenerative cells with variations in potential for proliferation and differentiation may provide different sources of cells for liver transplantation: hepatocytes for treatment of acute liver damage, liver progenitor cell lines for liver-directed gene therapy, and bone marrow-derived cells for chronic long-term liver replacement. A limiting factor in the success of liver cell transplantation is the condition of the hepatic microenvironment in which the cells must proliferate and set up housekeeping (Sell, 2001).

Few liver stem-cell transplantations have taken place. Cases of mold and other infections have been associated with liver stem-cell transplantations. Further evaluation is warranted before such transplantation is accepted as a therapy in end-stage liver disease.

PORTAL HYPERTENSION

Portal hypertension is abnormally high blood pressure in the portal vein, the primary vein that brings blood from the intestine to the liver. When this vein clots or when the liver develops scar tissue from disease and compresses the vein, the blood pressure in the vein goes up and portal hypertension develops. In most patients portal hypertension develops regardless of primary disease process with progressive cirrhosis.

The liver normally filters blood from the abdominal organs. Portal hypertension can prohibit the liver from doing its job by causing the growth of collaterals that connect blood flow from the intestine to the general circulation, bypassing the liver. When this occurs, substances that are normally removed by the liver pass into general circulation. If not treated, portal hypertension can be progressive and cause serious complications. Pharmacologic management with medications such as vasopressin and octreotide has been used for acute portal hypertension. Complications of portal hypertension can include esophageal varices complicated by hemorrhage and hypersplenism. Treatment with endoscopic sclerotherapy has emerged as an effective treatment for bleeding esophageal varices. Sclerotherapy is the ideal, safe, and effective treatment for bleeding esophageal varices; it prevented bleeding in 88.1% of patients after variceal eradication (Zargar et al, 2004). Though rarely used; the Sengstaken-Blakemore tube can achieve direct balloon tamponade of bleeding varices or transthoracic ligation of the bleeding.

Splenectomy is used for older children when hypersplenism and splenic sequestration of blood components is noted (leukopenia, thrombocytopenia, or anemia). In neonates and small children splenectomy is rarely done, as fatal sepsis is a major complication; functional disorders, such as ascites and thrombocytopenia, should be treated with a more conservative approach.

INFECTION

Infants and children are compromised, as their immune system is still developing. End-stage liver disease decreases further their ability to fight off any infections. They are especially vulnerable to infections normally seen during childhood such as colds, flu, and other childhood diseases (e.g., meningitis, otitis media, and pneumonia). Nosocomial exposure in the hospital from invasive procedures (liver biopsy, intravenous lines) and handling by the health care team further jeopardize the patient for infections. Standard precautions must be followed. According to the indications from the Centers for Disease Control and Prevention (CDC), infection can be decreased by as much as half with attention to handwashing, draping for procedures, rubbing IV hubs with alcohol before using them by at least 30 seconds, use of disinfectant before invasive events, and discontinuance of lines on a timely basis. Antibiotics are used when indicated by culture and sensitivity.

Vaccinations should be given to infants and children on a routine, scheduled basis when possible. Other immunizations advised before transplantation include hepatitis B, hepatitis A, and influenza for older children. Respiratory syncytial virus (RSV) is the most common cause of bronchiolitis and pneumonia among infants and children under one year of age. RSV is highly infectious and almost all babies get it before the age of two. Palivizumab (Synagis; MedImmune, Gaithersburg, MD) is given for neonates at risk for RSV before transplant on a monthly basis.

POSTTRANSPLANT MANAGEMENT

Posttransplant management would include care given to any postoperative patient. Blood gases, laboratory reports, fluid balance, urinary output (1 to 2 ml/kg), and intravenous access are as usual watched closely. Drainage from the liver transplant is closely observed. Dark, black, bloody discharge can mean that the circulation to the transplant is not working, and the liver may be dead.

Prophylactic antibiotics are given before, during, and after surgery. Antifungal and anti–herpes virus prophylaxis is also given.

Immunosuppressive Management

Immunosuppressive management usually starts with prednisone in infants and children. The calcineurin inhibitors cyclosporine and tacrolimus are also used; they have distinct advantages and drawbacks. It is important to tailor their use to the patient's tolerance. In some patients, the need to ameliorate the adverse effects of tacrolimus may necessitate a switch to cyclosporine-based therapy and vice versa. Some centers use azathioprine as part of an initial cyclosporine immunotherapy program. It is usually discontinued early in the posttransplant period.

Rejection is treated with steroid pulses, steroid recycling, or the monoclonal anti-T-cell antibody muromonab-CD3 (Orthoclone OKT3). Daily monitoring of immunosuppressive medications is necessary for proper dose adjustment in infants and children. Rescue therapy with a cyclosporine microemulsion (Neoral, Novartis Pharmaceuticals Corporation, East Hanover, NJ)–based regimen for transplant patients intolerant of tacrolimus has been evaluated to assess the best method of switching and determine the initial and maintenance doses in children. Transplant centers are evaluating this therapy at present.

Drugs used for immunosuppression have been implicated in causing numerous long-term side effects including nephrotoxicity, glucose intolerance, and hyperlipidemia. Calcineurin inhibitors are known to cause nephrotoxicity, which is of concern in pediatric liver transplant recipients. Almost all patients will require antihypertensive therapy. Posttransplant malignancies are among the most important complications in organ transplantation.

POSTOPERATIVE COMPLICATIONS

Most complications after liver transplantation are heralded by an increase in hepatocellular enzymes, often associated with malaise, fever, leukocytosis, and jaundice. The clinical picture defines hepatic allograft dysfunction, but it does not separate allograft rejection from other allograft complications such as primary nonfunction, bile duct abnormalities, hepatic artery thrombosis, or allograft infection. The use of real-time and Doppler ultrasonography to assess hepatic vasculature and the use of computed tomography (CT) and magnetic resonance imaging (MRI) are often necessary. Allograft biopsy is definite when the cause of the graft abnormality is rejection; it can strongly support the diagnosis of viral infection or cholangitis when the characteristic histologic markers and microscopic appearance are seen. Definitive diagnosis of the cause of the allograft dysfunction should precede immunologic manipulation.

HEART TRANSPLANT

With advents in surgical techniques younger and smaller patients are having heart transplants. The availability of organs is limited for small children. Many centers try to wait till the child is larger to accommodate a larger heart. Developmental studies have shown that young infants and children are at risk for growth failure, developmental delays, and serious neurologic sequelae.

Bridge to Transplant

Heart failure due to congenital defects and organ deterioration affects the entire body. Many patients in waiting for a heart transplant are so debilitated that they may not be able to receive it. To assist the body and improve the patients' physical status several modalities are used to help the patient gain strength while awaiting transplant hence a "bridge-to-transplant." Devices commonly used for bridge-to-transplant are the left ventricular assist device (LVAD), extracorporeal membrane oxygenation (ECMO), and on a limited basis the Berlin Heart.

Left Ventricular Assist Device (LVAD)

The LVAD is an implantable mechanical device to pump blood through the body. It takes over the work of the failing heart. Bridge-to-transplant facilities that have an aggressive approach to implantable LVAD placement may substantially improve the survival rate of patients with postcardiotomy heart failure.

Extracorporeal Membrane Oxygenation (ECMO)

ECMO currently comes in two varieties: venoarterial (VA), and venovenous (VV). VA ECMO takes deoxygenated blood from a central vein or the right atrium, pumps it past the oxygenator, and then returns the oxygenated blood, under pressure, to the arterial side of the circulation (typically to the aorta). This form of ECMO partially supports the cardiac output as the flow through the ECMO circuit is in addition to the normal cardiac output. VV ECMO takes blood from a large vein and returns oxygenated blood back to a large vein. VV ECMO does not support the circulation. VA ECMO helps support the cardiac output and delivers higher levels of oxygenation support than does VV ECMO. VA ECMO carries a higher risk of systemic emboli than does VV.

The normalization of left heart filling pressures allowed the resolution of pulmonary edema and improves the child's physical status.

Berlin Heart

The Berlin Heart (Berlin Company, Berlin, Germany) has been used for infants and small children who can utilize neither LVAD nor ECMO. Named after the company in Berlin, Germany, that manufactures it, the Berlin Heart is a ventricular assist device. The device works by helping the right ventricle of the heart pump blood to the lungs and the left ventricle to pump blood to the rest of the body. The bulk of the Berlin Heart is located on the outside of the body, with only the pumps connected to the heart emerging from the body. The device is run by a laptop computer. The Berlin Heart comes in various sizes for a range of patients and is the only mechanical heart small enough to be used in very young children. It currently is not approved for use by the United States Food and Drug Administration (FDA). In each case where it has been used, the FDA has been petitioned.

PHYSIOLOGY OF THE TRANSPLANTED HEART

The physiology of the transplanted heart is distinctive. Both the recipient and donor atria are present but function separately. This results in decreased atrial input that does not contract together but independently. The transplanted heart does not experience angina because of denervation. Low cardiac output can result.

Postoperative Management

Care of the heart transplant patient is similar to any other cardiac surgery. Perfusion with adequate gas exchange and hemodynamic stability are goals after transplantation. Normal perfusion is evidenced by normalized blood gases, urinary output, and adequate blood pressure.

A major complication from surgery is hemorrhage. This can be due to anticoagulation therapy secondary to end-stage heart disease, reoperation (prior cardiac surgery), cardiopulmonary bypass during surgery, and clotting related to hepatic congestion secondary to severe right heart failure. The donor heart is smaller than the diseased heart it replaced. This results in the pericardial space acting as a reservoir for blood, resulting in cardiac tamponade. Frequent milking of the chest tubes is warranted to decrease the blood volume in the pericardial space and clotting off the chest tubes.

RENAL TRANSPLANTATION IN INFANTS AND CHILDREN

Renal transplantation in infants and children has been the most successful modality of all transplants. Recent advances in the techniques of dialysis and the management of end-stage renal disease (ESRD) in neonates have allowed many patients with complex urologic or hereditary abnormalities to reach the age and size at which transplantation is possible. These advances have allowed the implementation of renal transplantation, along with dialysis, as a complementary treatment in the care of infants with irreversible renal dysfunction.

Etiology

Acute renal failure in infants is most often the consequence of hemodynamic instability, hypoxia, or malperfusion, resulting in acute tubular necrosis. Most of these infants either recover sufficient function for normal long-term survival or die of multisystem failure. Chronic renal failure is uncommon in infants. Congenital nephrosis, dysplasia-hypoplasia, and other anatomic abnormalities associated with complex urogenital malformations are the common causes of ESRD in infants. In children younger than 5 years of age who have glomerulonephritis, 46% have a congenital cause for ESRD. Lupus nephritis and recurrent pyelonephritis, which are more common in older patients, are uncommon causes of ESRD in the infant. Hereditary causes of renal failure are important to identify in planning the appropriate overall treatment strategy; evaluation of other family members and provision of genetic counseling, when needed, must also be considered. Appropriate identification of the cause of the ESRD also allows assessment of the potential for recurrence within a transplant allograft and consideration of living related-donor transplantation.

Pretransplant Management

Pretransplant tests are done to evaluate the patient's physical status and also identify potential problems. The tests help determine whether transplantation is truly the best option and increase the likelihood of success. Transplant feasibility consists of histocompatibility laboratory tests of tissue typing, panel reactive antibody (PRA), cross-match testing, and blood typing.

Dialysis

Dialysis is indicated in infants as in older children, if complications of medical management of ESRD occur, namely hyperkalemia, volume overload, acidosis, intractable hypertension, and uremic symptoms, such as vomiting. Dialysis can be accomplished by hemodialysis or peritoneal dialysis. Dialysis centers can take older children until a transplant is available. In neonates and small children, peritoneal dialysis is frequently utilized because (1) it avoids the multiple transfusions associated with hemodialysis; (2) it allows smoother gradual correction of electrolyte abnormalities, preventing cerebral disequilibrium syndrome in small infants; and (3) it is easier to perform.

For long-term peritoneal dialysis, parents are taught how to care for the infant. This allows the parent to take the child home and be a family. The infant is given time to grow and normalize as much as possible. Glucose and electrolytes can be enhanced via peritoneal dialysis to give extra nutrients.

Nutritional Support

Nutritional support is a primary concern for the renal patient. Growth retardation is a major problem. The cause of this growth disturbance is multifactorial and includes both protein and calorie insufficiency, renal osteodystrophy, aluminum toxicity, acidosis, impaired somatomedin activity, and insulin resistance. A registered dietitian will need to constantly monitor nutritional needs of the infant and child. The most intense period of growth occurs during the first 2 years of life. Head circumference is the key to monitoring growth.

INTESTINAL TRANSPLANT

Since 1985, data compiled by the international Intestinal Transplant Registry show that 55 intestinal transplant programs have performed 601 transplants, of which 402 were in children. Although not many infants and children have had intestinal transplants, the numbers are growing.

Intestinal Transplant Considerations

Patients with poor intestinal function who cannot be maintained on TPN via intravenous routes are potential candidates for transplantation. In some patients most of the bowel has been surgically removed to treat the disease, or it became diseased. This produces the short-gut syndrome, which is the most common cause of intestinal failure. For some infants and children, the entire intestine is present, but it is unable to absorb enough fluids and nutrients. Transplantation is a potentially life-saving option for patients with intestinal failure who cannot tolerate TPN. Because patients' survival rates are better after isolated bowel transplants, this is the preferred type of transplant. Combined intestinal-liver transplants or cluster transplants are options for patients who have developed liver failure on TPN or for patients who have large, local tumors that can only be removed by removing several organs.

Diseases leading to intestinal transplantation include:
- Short-gut syndrome caused by volvulus, gastroschisis, trauma, necrotizing enterocolitis (NEC), ischemia, Crohn's disease
- Poor absorption caused by microvillus inclusion, secretory diarrhea, autoimmune enteritis
- Poor motility caused by pseudo-obstruction, aganglionosis (Hirschprung's disease), visceral neuropathy
- Tumor or cancer such as desmoid tumor, familial polyposis (Gardner's disease)
- Congenital intestinal atresia
- Poor intestinal absorption
- Autoimmune disorders
- Brush-border element assembly problems
- Microvillus inclusion disease
- Severe disorders of motility resulting from intestinal pseudo-obstruction (congenital or acquired)
- Tumors
- Gardner's disease (intestinal polyposis)
- Desmoid tumors
- Serious complications of TPN therapy
- Thrombosis (blockage due to a blood clot) of two or more major central veins (subclavian, jugular, femoral)
- Repeated episodes of line sepsis or line infections
- The decision to proceed with intestinal transplantation is made only after careful evaluation determines that the surgery is the child's most promising treatment option.

Donor Options

Most intestinal grafts come from cadaver donors—people who have been declared dead in a hospital while attached to a ventilator (artificial breathing machine). Consent is given by the next of kin for organ removal and transplant. Occasionally, a portion of the bowel is taken from a living donor—a relative such as a parent or sibling.

Intestinal Transplant Evaluation

Small-intestine transplant evaluation is similar to liver transplant evaluation. It is important that the child have a good history of central line placement, IV access, upper gastrointestinal studies, number of gastrointestinal resections, and length of bowel to ensure that transplantation is the best medical option.

Studies done for evaluation include:
- Blood tests
- Chemistry panel

- Liver panel
- Hematology group
- Coagulation studies
- Blood typing and antibody screen
- Infectious diseases: hepatitis B, hepatitis C, HIV, cytomegalovirus, Epstein-Barr virus
- Imaging studies and other tests
- Ultrasound of the liver in combined intestinal-liver transplants
- CT scan
- MRI to map abdominal vasculature
- Endoscopy (EGD)
- Mobility studies
- Colonoscopy
- Liver biopsy for combined liver-intestinal patients to determine whether TPN damage is reversible
- Psychosocial and developmental evaluations
- Social worker
- Child development expert

If the child is a candidate for intestinal transplantation, his or her name is added to the transplant waiting list for an isolated intestinal transplant or for a combined liver and intestinal transplant, based on the severity of organ damage and dysfunction. Transplant waiting lists are maintained by the United Network of Organ Sharing (UNOS).

Postoperative Management

After the procedure, patients are placed on immunosuppressive drugs to prevent rejection of the transplanted organ. The doctors perform biopsies (take tissue samples of the intestine) at various intervals to check for signs of rejection. Rejection may be managed by adding immunosuppressive drugs or increasing dosages. Patients who have received intestinal transplants remain on immunosuppressive drugs indefinitely.

Since patients on immunosuppressive drugs are vulnerable to infections by bacteria and viruses, they are monitored for signs and symptoms of infection. Particular attention is paid to wound care issues and fluid management. The multidisciplinary team performs a nutritional assessment to determine the child's caloric needs.

Intestinal Transplantation Survival

Improved antirejection drugs, refined surgical procedures, and a greater understanding of immunology have contributed to successful intestinal transplants. Short-term survival is now comparable to lung transplantation results. Most of the patients in the international Intestinal Transplant Registry have been followed for a brief time; it will take several years to obtain reliable data on long-term results.

Until a few years ago, cyclosporine was used most often to prevent organ rejection. Tacrolimus (Prograf, Astellas Pharma US, Deerfield, IL) has been given to most intestinal transplant patients over the past 4 years. As of June 1995, 49% of all intestinal patients had died, usually from sepsis (42%) or multiple organ system failure (30%). Four patients (5%) died of rejection. Of the surviving patients, 78% had stopped total parenteral nutrition (TPN) and had resumed a normal, oral diet.

To become the standard treatment for intestinal failure, transplantation must offer better survival, better quality of life, and lower costs than TPN. Considerable progress has been made toward these goals, but further refinements are needed before bowel transplantation becomes a routine surgical procedure.

Despite improved immunosuppression, the intestine offers more rejection than other organs. Rejection of the intestine is also difficult to diagnose since there are no biochemical (blood) tests to indicate rejection. To prevent intestinal rejection, patients require higher doses of immunosuppression than with other types of transplantation. Now, because of new, more specific antirejection medications, the success of intestinal transplant has improved dramatically (Intestinal Transplant Registry, 2005).

ORGAN PROCUREMENT

Organ procurement is facilitated by the United Network for Organ Sharing, a nonprofit, scientific and educational organization that administers the nation's only Organ Procurement and Transplantation Network (OPTN) and was established by the U.S. Congress in 1984. Functions of OPTN include the following:

- Collects and manages data about every transplant event occurring in the United States
- Facilitates organ matching and placement process using UNOS-developed data technology and the UNOS Organ Center
- Brings together medical professionals, transplant recipients, and donor families to develop organ transplantation policy

UNOS was awarded the initial OPTN contract on September 30, 1986. UNOS is the only organization to ever manage the OPTN and has continued to administer the contract for more than 16 years and four successive contract renewals.

PEDIATRIC CRITICAL PATHWAY

After brain death has been declared, and consent granted for organ donation, pediatric specialists and organ procurement professionals should work together to care for the organ donor and family members. The United Network for Organ Sharing (UNOS) (2005) (Figure 20-1), describes optimal care for the pediatric organ donor and maps the process to improve the outcome for successful organ transplantation.

STEM CELL TRANSPLANTATION

Human umbilical cord blood in recent years has become a source of hematopoietic progenitor cells. These so-called stem cells are used to treat a variety of diseases such as malignancies, hemoglobinopathies, immunodeficiencies, and inborn errors of metabolism.

Umbilical cord blood (CB) was used until recently to assess infants' health status. Otherwise, cord blood was discarded with all the other biologic tissues of birth: placenta, amniotic fluid, birth sac, and umbilical cord. These biologic tissues have been shown to be useful medically for other purposes. For example, it was found that a specific lung lipid isolated from amniotic fluid could ascertain the lung maturity of the fetus in the last trimester of pregnancy: the lecithin/sphingomyelin ratio.

Physiology

Umbilical cord blood is extremely rich in stem cells. Stem cells differ from other kinds of cells in the body. Regardless of their source, they have three general properties:

Critical Pathway for Donation After Cardiac Death

AOPO — Association of Organ Procurement Organizations   AST — AMERICAN SOCIETY OF TRANSPLANTATION   ASTS — American Society of Transplant Surgeons   NATCO   UNOS — UNITED NETWORK FOR ORGAN SHARING — DONATE LIFE

Collaborative Practice	Phase I Identification and Referral	Phase II Preliminary Evaluation	Phase III Family Discussion and Consent	Phase IV Comprehensive Evaluation and Donor Management	Phase V Withdrawal of Support/Pronouncement of Death/Organ Recovery
The following health care professionals may be involved in the Donation After Cardiac Death (DCD) donation process: Check all that apply: ○ Physician (MD) ○ Critical Care RN ○ Nurse Supervisor ○ Medical Examiner/ Coroner ○ Respiratory Therapy (RT) ○ Laboratory ○ Pharmacy ○ Radiology ○ Anesthesiology ○ OR/Surgery Staff ○ Clergy ○ Social Worker ○ Organ Procurement Coordinator (OPC) ○ Organ Procurement Organization (OPO)	Prior to withdrawing life support, contact local OPO for any patient who fulfills the following criteria: ○ Devastating neurologic injury and/or other organ failure requiring mechanical ventilatory or circulatory support ○ Family and/or care giving team initiate conversation about withdrawal of support Following referral, additional evaluation is done collaboratively to determine if death is likely to occur within 1 hour (or within a specified timeframe as determined by care giving team and OPO) following withdrawal of support Patient conditions might include the following: ○ **Ventilator dependent for respiratory insufficiency:** apneic or severe hypopneic; tachypnea ≥ 30 breaths/ min after DC ventilator ○ **Dependent on**	Physician ○ Supportive of withdrawal of care and has communicated grave prognosis to family ○ Review DCD procedure with OPC ○ Will be involved in withdrawal/ pronouncement ○ Will designate a person to be involved with withdrawal and/or pronouncement Family ○ Has received grave prognosis ○ Understands prognosis ○ In conjunction with care giving team, decide to withdraw support Patient ○ Age ___ ○ Weight ___ ○ Height ___ ○ ABO ___ ○ Medical Hx ___ ○ Surgical Hx ___ ○ Social Hx ___ ○ Death likely < 1 hour following withdrawal (determined collaboratively by	○ Support services offered to family ○ OPC/hospital staff approach family about donation options ○ Legal next-of-kin (NOK) fully informed of donation options and recovery procedures ○ Legal NOK grants consent for DCD following withdrawal of support ○ Family offered opportunity to be present during withdrawal of support ○ OPC obtains ___ Witnessed consent from legal NOK for DCD ___ Signed consent Time ___ Date ___ Detailed med/soc history ___ Notification of donation ○ Hospital supervisor ○ ME/coroner notified ___ ME/coroner releases for donation ___ ME/coroner has restrictions	○ MD, in collaboration with OPO, implements management guidelines ○ Establish location and time of withdrawal of support ○ Review plan for withdrawal to include: – Pronouncing MD (should be in attendance for duration of withdrawal of support, determination of death, and may not be a member of the transplant team) – Comfort care – Extubation and discontinuation of ventilator support – Establish plan for continued supportive care if pt survives > 1 hour or predetermined time interval after withdrawal of support ○ Notify OR/Anesthesia ___ Review patient's clinical course, withdrawal plan, and potential organ recovery	○ Withdrawal occurs in ___ OR ___ ICU ___ Other ___ ○ Family present for withdrawal of support ___ Yes ___ No ○ OR/room prepared and equipment set up ○ Transplant team in the OR (not in attendance during withdrawal) ○ Care giving team present ○ Administration of preapproved medication (e.g., heparin/Regitine) ○ **Withdrawal of support according to hospital/MD practice guidelines** Time ___ Date ___ ○ **Vital signs are monitored and recorded every minute (see attached sheet)** ○ **Pt pronounced dead and appropriate documentation completed**

			Time _____ Date _____ MD _____
mechanical circulatory support: LVAD; RVAD; V-A ECMO; pacemaker with unassisted rhythm < 30 beats/min ○ **Severe disruption in oxygenation:** PEEP ≥ 10 and SaO$_2$ ≤ 92%; FiO$_2$ ≥0.50 and SaO$_2$ ≤ 92%; V-V ECMO requirement ○ **Dependent upon pharmacologic circulatory assist:** norephinephrine, epinephrine, or phenylephrine ≥ 0.2 mcg/kg/min; dopamine ≥ 15 mcg/kg/min ○ **IABP and inotropic support:** IABP 1:1 and dobutamine or dopamine ≥ 10 mcg/kg/min and CI ≤ 2.2 L/min/M², IABP 1:1 and CI ≤ 1.5 L/min/M²	evaluating injury, level of support, respiratory drive assessment) Stop pathway if — ○ Family, ME/coroner denies consent ○ Patient determined to be unsuitable candidate for DCD ○ Patient progresses to brain death during evaluation — refer to brain dead pathway	procedures _____ Schedule OR time _____ ○ Notify recovery teams ○ Prepare patient for transport to prearranged area for withdrawal of support ○ Patient transported to prearranged area ○ Note: Should the clinical situation require premortum femoral cannulation, the following should be reviewed: – Family consent or understanding – MD inserting cannula – Time and location of cannula insertion – If death does not occur, determine if cannula should be removed	○ **Transplant team initiates surgical recovery** at prescribed time following pronouncement of death ○ Allocation of organs per OPTN/UNOS policy ○ *If cardiac death not established within 1 hour or predetermined time interval after withdrawal of support – Stop pathway Patient moved to predetermined area for continuation of supportive care* ○ *Postmortem care administered*
Labs/Diagnostics	○ ABO ○ Electrolytes ○ LFTs ○ PT/PTT ○ CBC with Diff ○ Beta HCG (female pts) ○ ABG	Repeat full panel of labs additionally: ○ Serology testing ○ Infectious disease profile ○ Blood cultures X2 ○ UA and urine culture ○ Sputum culture ○ Tissue typing	
Respiratory	○ Maintain ventilator support ○ Pulmonary toilet PRN	○ Respiratory drive assessment RR _____ VT _____ VE _____ NIF _____	○ ABGs as requested ○ Notify RT of location and time of withdrawal of support	○ Transport with mechanical ventilation using lowest FiO$_2$ possible while maintaining the SaO$_2$ >90%

Continued

FIGURE **20-1**
Critical pathway for donation after cardiac death. Reprinted with permission of United Network for Organ Sharing (UNOS), Richmond, VA.

		Minutes off ventilator _____ ○ Hemodynamics while off ventilator _____ HR _____ BP _____ SaO$_2$ _____		○ Postmortem care at conclusion of case
Treatments/Ongoing Care	Maintain standard nursing care to include: ○ Vital signs q 1 hour ○ I and O q 1 hour			
Medications			○ Provide medications as directed by MD in consult OPC	○ Heparin and other medications prior to withdrawal of support
Optimal Outcomes	The potential DCD donor is identified, and a referral is made to the OPO	The donor is evaluated and found to be a suitable candidate for donation	The family is offered the option of donation, and their decision is supported	Optimal organ function is maintained, withdrawal of support plan is established, and personnel are prepared for potential organ recovery	Death occurs within 1 hour of withdrawal of support and all suitable organs and tissues are recovered for transplant

FIGURE **20-1, cont'd**
Critical pathway for donation after cardiac death. Reprinted with permission of United Network for Organ Sharing (UNOS), Richmond, VA.

1. They are capable of dividing and renewing themselves for long periods
2. The cells are unspecialized
3. They give rise to specialized cells

There is controversy regarding where stem cells and progenitor cells originate in the yolk sac or aorta-gonad-mesonephros region/intraembryonic splanchnopleura region. Cells move through the fetal liver and then the fetal circulation, where the numbers are high at birth.

In October 1988 the first cord blood transfusion was performed for a patient with Fanconi anemia: a sibling donor contributed the HLA-matched cells. Since this time several diseases have been treated with stem cells. In a number of genetic, hematologic, and oncologic disorders, infusion of cord blood can be a potentially lifesaving procedure. Allogenic (related or unrelated) or autologous (self) bone marrow is the usual source of hematopoietic progenitor cells. One child in 2700 might eventually benefit from an autologous stem cell transplant. Bone marrow is not always readily available. Umbilical cord blood can be a viable alternative for certain conditions (Table 20-1).

Collection of Cord Blood

Cord blood can be collected from the placenta in situ during the third stage of labor or immediately after delivery of the placenta. About 50% to 70% of donated units are ineligible for storage, mainly because of low volume. Each unit should contain more than 40 ml of cord blood for a child weighing up to 30 kg. Maximal storage time is unknown, but under stable conditions the cells are likely to remain viable for decades.

Cord blood is collected according to directions for the particular bank. In general the samples are obtained from normal full-term deliveries under orders from the health care provider (physician, midwife, or nurse practitioner). Once labor has been established, the nurse will label the tubes, place them in a plastic zip-closure bag, and return them to the kit's Styrofoam box per instructions. The Styrofoam box will then be labeled with time, date, name, and initials of collector. The tops of the heparin vials are cleansed with alcohol and 5 ml is drawn. The heparin is injected into 60-ml syringes. Each syringe is labeled.

After the infants' birth, cord blood is collected within 10 minutes. Cord blood is drawn from the umbilical vein with as much blood as possible. The syringes are inverted back and forth for 1 to 2 minutes to mix the blood and heparin well. The syringes are capped and put into the provided plastic bag. Then they are packaged into the Styrofoam box with provided absorbent pad. Blood should remain at room temperature to ensure viability of stem cells. Cord blood is not refrigerated. It is usually the families' responsibility to ship the blood in a timely manner to the cord blood bank.

Cord Blood Banks

Private banks such as the Cord Blood Registry in San Bruno, California, offer collection kits to families. Private banks are companies that are accredited by the American Association of Blood Banks (AABB). Typical fees range from $1000 to $1500 for registration and collection. Storage is charged $100 a year, but there are no additional fees for retrieving the cells for use. The costs are born by the families.

Public cord banks accept collections only from affiliated hospitals. Units stored in them are available for any patient in need who is medically eligible for transplantation therapy. In the unlikely event that the donor or a member of his family develops an indication for a stem cell transplant, the stored cells could be traced and used. Public blood cord banks charge no fees for donation, but may charge $15,000 or more if the blood is actually used. The number of public banks is limited.

The American Academy of Pediatrics (AAP) recommends that institutions or organizations (private or public) involved in cord blood banking should consider the following recommendations:

- Recruitment practices should be developed with an awareness of the possible emotional vulnerability of pregnant women and their families and friends. Efforts should be made to minimize the effect of this vulnerability on recruitment decisions.
- Accurate information about the potential benefits and limitations of allogenic and autologous cord blood banking and transplantation should be provided.

TABLE 20-1	**Conditions for Which Umbilical Cord Blood Can Be a Viable Alternative**	
Disease	**Indication**	**Blood Cell Transplantation**
Leukemia, lymphomas	Engraftment of healthy cells	Effective
Bone and soft tissue sarcomas, Wilms' tumor, brain tumors	Very rarely indicated	Effectiveness unproven
Hematologic diseases	The new donor cells will produce normal white cells, red cells, and platelets	Effective
Immunodeficiency diseases	Engraftment of healthy allogenic cells	Effective
Hemoglobinopathies	The new donor cells will produce normal white cells, red cells, and platelets	Effective
Metabolic storage disorders	Donor cell will eventually produce the deficient enzyme	Controversial; may be effective in select patients
Genetic conditions	Cells from umbilical cord blood can be isolated, transduced, and engrafted to produce mature hematopoietic and lymphoid cells for at least several years	Effective in select diseases

From Baggott C, Fochtman D (2002). Nursing care of children and adolescents with cancer. Philadelphia: Saunders; Hockenberry-Eaton MJ, editor (1998). Essentials of pediatric oncology nursing: a core curriculum. Glenview, Ill: Association of Pediatric Oncology Nurses.

- A policy should be developed regarding disclosing to the parents any abnormal findings in the harvested blood.
- Specific permission for maintaining demographic medical information should be obtained, and the potential risks of breaches of confidentiality disclosed.
- Written permission should be obtained during prenatal care, and before the onset of labor. The practice of collecting blood first and obtaining permission afterward is considered unethical and should be discouraged.
- Consultation with the institutional review board or hospital ethics committee about recruitment strategies and the wording of consent forms is recommended.
- Cord blood collection should not be done in complicated deliveries, and the cord blood stem collection program should not alter routine practice for the timing of umbilical cord clamping.
- Because of the investigational status of cord blood banking and the high risk for its potential abuse, the regulatory agencies (e.g., U.S. Food and Drug Administration, Federal Trade Commission, state equivalent of these federal agencies) are encouraged to have an active role in providing oversight for the safety and welfare of the population.

Cord Blood Transfusion in Neonate

There are two types of cord stem cell transfusions: frozen and fresh. Each type of transfusion is discussed in regard to considerations, side effects, and nursing care needed for the neonate.

Frozen stem cells are used in autologous (collected from the patient) cord blood transplants. A preservative, dimethyl sulfoxide (DMSO) is added to the cells just prior to cryopreservation. It acts to coat the cells and prevent their lysis during the process of freezing and thawing. DMSO is infused to the patient with the transfusion of the cells. The garlic-like odor of DMSO is very distinctive and unpleasant. DMSO is excreted primarily through the respiratory system. DMSO is smelled and tasted as soon as it is infused, which can result in the baby having nausea and vomiting. Other side effects commonly seen are bradycardia and shortness of breath. Volume overload can occur as each bag of cells contains 50 to 100 ml. Hypertension may require medication with antihypertensives and diuretics. Giving the transfusion over a 2- to 4-hour time period and in two different sessions may help lessen side effects. A significant reaction to DSMO may occur even without volume overload. The transfusion is thawed to break the ice crystals, so it is advised to keep the infant's environment as thermally neutral as possible with the use of a radiant warmer, isolette, or warm blankets. Monitor the temperature frequently. Stem cells should not be warmed as they may be damaged. After the transfusion, red urine may be seen as some of the cells will be excreted in the urine. Red urine will diminish over time. Hydration should be provided following infusion.

Fresh stem cells are given for allogenic transplants (related or unrelated) transplants within 48 hours of collection. Side effects may include hemolytic transfusion reactions, volume overload, pulmonary microemboli, and infection (as the transfusion is neither irradiated nor filtered).

Assess the family's understanding of cord blood transfusion prior to the procedure and provide information and or education. For either transfusion type, careful monitoring of intake and output, oxygenation saturation, heart and respiratory rates, and blood pressures is warranted. Vital signs are taken before, during, and after the infusion. Interventions are based on the type of transfusion used (Table 20-2).

Umbilical cord blood transfusions offer hope to families of infants with various diseases requiring hematopoietic progenitor cells. It is not a common procedure as yet. In neonatal units affiliated with cord blood banks, study of benefits vs. ineffectiveness is occurring. It is still an uncommon procedure that can have far-reaching consequences. Thorough education of the family is required to deal with potential complications associated with stem cell infusion. Neonatal nurses need to be aware of the immediate, delayed, and late effects to give prompt intervention and treatment as needed.

SUMMARY

In the past decade, transplantation has become more common but is more the exception than the rule. Transplants with solid organs were the mainstay but stem cell transplants are beginning to be explored. Transplants are a tertiary treatment that is not irreversible. It is the last, best option for many patients. The next few years will change indications for transplant, with earlier treatments and procedures.

TABLE 20-2	Possible Complication Sequence for Cord Blood Transfusion	
Immediate	**Delayed (First Month)**	**Late Effects (After First Month)**
Nausea/vomiting	Bone marrow suppression	Immunosuppression
Diarrhea	Mucositis	Chronic graft-vs-host disease
Red urine	Hemorrhagic cystitis	Cataracts
Parotitis	Anorexia	Endocrine dysfunction
Hypertension	Capillary leak syndrome	Pulmonary restrictive disease
Volume overload	Veno-occlusive disease	Genetic disease recurrence
Apnea/bradycardia	Graft failure	Secondary malignancies
Tachypnea	Graft-vs-host disease	Bacterial infections
Respiratory distress	Acute renal failure	Cytomegalovirus infection
	Bacterial infection	*Varicella zoster* infection
	Viral infections (herpes simplex, cytomegalovirus)	Latent virus infections
	Fungal infection	*Pneumocystis carinii* pneumonia

From Baggott C, Fochtman D (2002). Nursing care of children and adolescents with cancer. *Philadelphia: Saunders; Hockenberry-Eaton MJ, editor (1998). Essentials of pediatric oncology nursing: a core curriculum. Glenview, Ill: Association of Pediatric Oncology Nurses.*

REFERENCES AND SUGGESTED READINGS

Abramowicz M (2001). Cord blood banks. *Medical letter* 43:1114.

Alonso EM (2004). Long-term renal function in pediatric liver and heart recipients. *Pediatric transplantation* 8(4):381-385.

American Academy of Pediatrics (1999). Cord blood banking for potential future transplantation (RE9860). *Pediatrics* 104:116-118.

Amir G et al (2005). Neonatal brain protection and deep hypothermic circulatory arrest: pathophysiology of ischemic neuronal injury and protective strategies. *Annals of thoracic surgery* 80(5):1955-1964.

Baggott C, Fochtman D (2002). *Nursing care of children and adolescents with cancer.* Philadelphia: Saunders.

Ballen K (2005). New trends in umbilical cord blood transplantation. *Blood* 105(10):3786-3792.

Broxmeyer HE (1998). *Cellular characteristics of cord blood and cord blood transplantation.* Bethesda, MD: AABB Press.

Carter BA et al (2006). History of pediatric liver transplantation. Available at: http://www.emedicine.com/ped/topic2840.htm. Retrieved August 17, 2006.

Chin C et al, editors (2005). Induction therapy for pediatric and adult heart transplantation: comparison between OKT3 and daclizumab. *Transplantation* 80(4):477-481.

Chrisant MRK et al (2005). Fate of infants with hypoplastic left heart syndrome listed for cardiac transplantation: a multicenter study. *Journal of heart and lung transplantation* 24(5):576-582.

Coulthard M, Crosier JJ (2002). Outcome of reaching end-stage renal failure in children under 2 years of age. *Archives of disease in childhood fetal and neonatal edition* 87(6):511-517.

Dhawan A, Mieli-Vergani G (2005). Acute liver failure in neonates. *Early human development* 81(12):1005-1010.

Domínguez-Bendala J et al (2002). Stem cells and their clinical application. *Transplantation proceedings* 34(5):1372-1375.

Eisen H, Ross H (2004). Optimizing the immunosuppressive regimen in heart transplantation. *Journal of heart and lung transplantation* 23(5, Suppl 1):S207-S213.

Esquivel C (2005). *Liver transplantation in children.* Stanford University Medical School. Available at: http://med.stanford.edu/shs/txp/livertxp/HTML/selection.pediatric.html. Retrieved November 23, 2005.

García Meseguer C et al (2002). Renal transplantation in children under 2 years. *Transplantation proceedings* 34(1):350-351.

Hockenberry-Eaton MJ, editor (1998). *Essentials of pediatric oncology nursing: a core curriculum.* Glenview, Ill: Association of Pediatric Oncology Nurses.

Humar A et al (2001). Kidney transplantation in young children: should there be a minimum age? *Pediatric nephrology* 16(12):941-945.

Intestinal Transplant Registry (2005). The Intestinal Transplant Registry. Available at: http://www.intestinaltransplant.org. Retrieved August 4, 2006.

Jackson R, Roberts E (2001). Identification of neonatal liver failure and perinatal hemochromatosis in Canada. *Paediatrics & child health* 6(5):229-231.

Kadner A et al (2000). Heterotopic heart transplantation: experimental development and clinical experience. *European journal of cardio-thoracic surgery* 17(4):474-481.

Kanter KR et al (2004). Cardiac retransplantation in children. *Annals of thoracic surgery* 78(2):644-649.

Kirby G (2004). Nutritional problems in liver transplantation. *Hospital medicine* 65(12):710-711.

Lawlor GF et al (2002). Enriched levels of erythropoietin in human umbilical cord blood stimulate hematopoietic progenitor cells. *Journal of biochemistry, molecular biology, and biophysics* 6(1):65-70.

Loebe M et al (2000). Extracorporeal support: the Berlin Heart. In Goldstein et al, editors. *Cardiac assist devices.* Armonk, NY: Futura Publishing

Luikart H (2001). Pediatric cardiac transplantation: management issues. *Journal of pediatric nursing* 16(5):320-331.

Mahle WT et al (2005). Cardiac retransplantation in childhood: analysis of data from the United Network for Organ Sharing. *Journal of thoracic and cardiovascular surgery* 130(2):542-546.

Mandalam RK, Smith AK (2002). Ex vivo expansion of bone marrow and cord blood cells to produce stem and progenitor cells for hematopoietic reconstitution. *Military medicine* 167(2 suppl):78-81.

Mitka M (2005). Cord blood stem cell network proposed. *Journal of the American Medical Association* 293(19):2332.

National Institutes of Health (2004). *Stem cell information.* Available at: http://stemcells.nih.gov. Retrieved August 17, 2006.

Oellerich M, Armstrong VW (2001). The MEGX Test: a tool for the real-time assessment of hepatic function. *Therapeutic drug monitoring* 23(2):81-92.

Pomposelli J et al (2002). Nutrition support in the liver transplant patient. *Nutrition in clinical practice* 17(6):341-349.

Potapov EV et al (2005). Bridging to transplantability with a ventricular assist device. *Journal of thoracic and cardiovascular surgery* 130(3):930.

Sell S (2001). The role of progenitor cells in repair of liver injury and liver transplantation. *Wound repair and regeneration* 9(6):467-482.

Shapiro C (2005). Organ transplantation in infants and children—necessity or choice: the case of K'aila Paulette. *Pediatric nurse* 31(2):121-122.

Taegtmeyer AB et al (2004). Reduced incidence of hypertension after heterotopic cardiac transplantation compared with orthotopic cardiac transplantation: evidence that excision of the native heart contributes to post-transplant hypertension. *Journal of the American College of Cardiology* 44(6):1254-1260.

United Network for Organ Sharing (UNOS) (2005). Critical pathway for pediatric organ donation. Available at: http://www.unos.org/resources/donorManagement.asp?index=2. Retrieved August 17, 2006.

Utterson ES et al, Split Research Group (2005). Biliary atresia: clinical profiles, risk factors, and outcomes of 755 patients listed for liver transplantation. *Journal of pediatrics* 8(147):180-185.

Warady B, Bradley A (2002). Neurodevelopment of infants with end-stage renal disease: is it improving? *Pediatric transplantation* 6(1):5-7.

Watt SM, Contreras AM (2005). Stem cell medicine: umbilical cord blood and its stem cell potential. *Seminars in fetal and neonatal medicine* 10(3):209-220.

Zargar SA et al (2004). Fifteen-year follow-up of endoscopic injection sclerotherapy in children with extrahepatic portal venous obstruction. *Journal of gastroenterology and hepatology* 19(2):139-145.

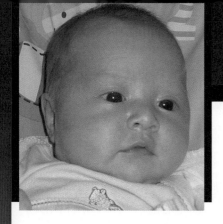

Chapter 21

Substance-Exposed Newborn

Deborah L. Fike

Substance abuse during pregnancy has become a major health problem over the past two decades, reaching epidemic proportions in North America. In 2003, 4.3% of pregnant women aged 15 to 44 used illicit drugs, 4.1% reported binge alcohol use, and 18% reported smoking cigarettes (United States DHHS, 2005a). These numbers are most likely underestimated because they were based on maternal report. Maternal reporting of drug use has been shown to be far from accurate. Many users will tend to deny or underreport drug use because they fear legal consequences or are embarrassed to admit to substance use (Bar-Oz et al, 2003).

There is a documented association between perinatal substance abuse and a significant increased incidence of perinatal morbidity and mortality. Generally, the consequences of fetal exposure include poor intrauterine growth, prematurity, fetal distress, spontaneous abortion, stillbirth, cerebral infarctions and other vascular accidents, malformations, and neurobehavioral dysfunction (El-Mohandes et al, 2003; Martinez et al, 2005; Rao & Desai, 2002). In addition to the effects of drug exposure, these infants also have multiple risk factors for compromised intellectual, social, and behavioral development due to a poor postnatal environment. Disorganized households that may include parental criminal involvement, drug dealing, passive exposure to drugs, and parents who are ill, absent, depressed, or stressed are common (Butz et al, 2001; Martinez et al, 2005). This chapter outlines the most common substances used during pregnancy and their effects on the fetus and newborn.

OVERVIEW

Pregnant women who are substance users often show a general inattention to their health and to that of their fetus. They often have inadequate nutrition and adverse environmental conditions leading to poor general prepregnancy health. Many have erratic, late, or no prenatal care, and interventions may not occur until late in the pregnancy or at the time of delivery. These women are more likely to have low income and limited education, and they are more likely to receive welfare support. They are less likely to be married, and many live in the inner cities. Domestic violence is also a significant factor. Furthermore, there is an increased incidence of sexually transmitted infections, hepatitis, and human immunodeficiency virus (HIV) (Askin & Diehl-Jones, 2001; Bauer et al, 2002; Campbell, 2003; D'Apolito & Hepworth, 2001; Hurt, 2005; Martinez et al, 2005).

Polydrug use (concurrent use of three or more drugs) is common among pregnant women, with a documented link between illicit drug use, alcohol, and cigarettes. This polydrug use makes it difficult to assess the effects of isolated drugs. There have been a limited number of studies that address the effects of polydrug exposure. Early studies suggested that tremors and startles, increased muscle tone, greater irritability, difficulty being consoled, and decreased interactive behavior were among the most frequent symptoms of polydrug exposure (Bauer et al, 2002; D'Apolito & Hepworth, 2001; Lewis & Weiss, 2003; Greene & Goodman, 2003; Lester et al, 2001). A study by D'Apolito and Hepworth (2001) provided data about the most prominent symptoms of withdrawal found in a group of infants exposed to a variety of both legal and illegal drugs during pregnancy. Results indicate that infants exposed to combinations of opiates, depressants, sedatives, and stimulants prenatally may experience more prominent symptoms of increased tone, increased respiratory rates, disturbed sleep, fever, excessive sucking, and watery or loose stools during withdrawal.

Additional studies suggest that prenatal drug exposure may result in abnormal structural organization and vascular injury of the fetal brain. The drugs appear to change the activity of neurons by altering the brain's neurochemistry. As the mechanisms underlying drug effects are beginning to be understood, their impact on drug-exposed infants is becoming more apparent, including a variety of neurobehaviors not typically seen. One of the problems in understanding how initial neurobehavioral risks may influence infant outcomes has been the lack of adequate assessments that are tailored to the characteristics of these infants (Lewis & Weiss, 2003).

An organized infant is capable of regulating physiologic and behavioral systems in order to achieve smooth, purposeful movements and steady autonomic states during interactions with the environment. In contrast, infants who are drug-exposed are frequently disorganized and show diminished interactive behaviors, poor state organization, atypical sensory responses and motor behaviors, impaired attention and orientation, and abnormal reflexes. If this disorganized behavior is not resolved, the infant's systems for modulating stimulation become further compromised, contributing to later cognitive and socioemotional problems. Thus, it is necessary to identify these infants and begin appropriate interventions as quickly as possible (Lewis & Weiss, 2003).

A study by Lewis and Weiss (2003) refined and tested the validity and reliability of a risk assessment developed specifically for evaluation of the neurobehavioral status of drug-exposed infants. This assessment, the Lewis Neurobehavioral Assessment Scale (LNAS) was first developed as a clinical tool to identify and describe the neurobehaviors of infants with prenatal drug exposure in an early intervention program.

Results of this study suggest that the LNAS has the potential to play an important role in identifying initial neurobehavioral risk of infants exposed to drugs prenatally. Such an assessment can be a valuable resource to health care workers both in the identification of drug-exposed infants and in planning appropriate early interventions. However, further studies with larger samples need to occur to determine its long-term predictive validity for developmental outcomes.

A review of the literature often reveals contradictory results when addressing studies of substance-exposed infants. There are four important issues that must be considered when interpreting these studies. First, there is great variation in amount of exposure between children. Many studies categorize infants as exposed vs nonexposed and have not attempted to quantify exposure to illicit drugs. If exact amounts cannot be obtained, even broad categories of usage would be more informative than simply labeling an infant as exposed or not. Second, there is variation across trimesters for the same child. Drug use is not necessarily consistent throughout each trimester of the pregnancy. If researchers use data from only one trimester, there will be substantial error in measurements. Exposure should be assessed separately for each trimester. Third, many infants are exposed to multiple drugs. If a study focuses only on one drug, then outcomes may be attributed to that drug when actually, they may be a result of a different drug or a combination of drugs. For example, early research on cocaine exposure may have mistakenly attributed the effects of alcohol to cocaine because of inadequate documentation of heavy alcohol use. Fourth, there is an issue with consistency across multiple sources of exposure data. Studies that do not use multiple sources of drug exposure data can have contaminated comparison groups. For example, when children of known drug exposure are compared with children who are thought to be drug free, they may in fact be undetected drug-exposed children. Thus, research must include multiple forms of data (Bergin et al, 2001).

Substance use by pregnant women remains one of the most frequently missed diagnoses in perinatal medicine. Legal, social, attitudinal, operational, and logistical barriers often inhibit open communication between the patient and physician. These barriers often result in a low rate of prenatal screening or intervention for substance use. In spite of evidence that screening improves identification of substance abusing patients, there is a lack of screening in primary care settings (Chasnoff et al, 2001, 2005; Ebrahim & Gfroerer, 2003). Reluctance to screen pregnant women for substance use stems from several factors. These include concerns and misconceptions about the liability and risks associated with treating substance users, a lack of knowledge about addiction and referral options, and a lack of confidence in treatment programs (Chasnoff et al, 2001; Kopcha, 2005). However, to reduce the risk for the pregnancy and the infant, it is essential that women be identified early in pregnancy and that treatment, intervention, and prevention services be made available (Chasnoff et al, 2001, 2005; Hurt, 2005; Martinez et al, 2005).

It is important that public education campaigns focus on pre- as well as postconceptional health. Several studies have demonstrated that many of the complications associated with the prenatal use of alcohol or illicit drugs are preventable with early identification and referral to treatment. Infants whose alcoholic mothers are alcohol free by the third trimester have been shown to have substantially improved outcome at birth.

Cessation of cocaine by the third trimester significantly reduces the rate of prematurity and low birth weight. It has also been documented that educational input provided by the prenatal care provider significantly increases the woman's likelihood to make healthy decisions during pregnancy as well as those in subsequent pregnancies (Chasnoff et al, 2005; El-Mohandes et al, 2003; Holl & Lussky, 2003).

SCREENING FOR MATERNAL SUBSTANCE USE

Over the past few years, there has been an emerging emphasis for the health care provider to identify the pregnant substance user and to refer these women for further assessment and treatment. Therefore, there needs to be a screening instrument that can easily be used in the clinical setting. Ideally, this instrument would be brief, easily administered and scored, sensitive, and inexpensive to administer. It should also build on the principle that one begins with questions respondents are unlikely to find threatening and then moves on to those that may be more threatening (Chang, 2001; Chasnoff et al, 2001).

Historically, substance use and abuse have been viewed as problems specific to men. As a result, screening, intervention, and treatment protocols have been developed with language and approaches that are not necessarily appropriate for addressing these problems in women, especially those who are pregnant. A study by Chasnoff and associates looked at the 4P's Plus (NTI Publishing, Chicago, IL) screen to determine the prevalence of substance use among pregnant women in five diverse communities. The 4P's Plus consists of five questions specifically designed to quickly identify obstetric patients in need of in-depth assessment or follow-up monitoring for risk of alcohol, tobacco, or illicit drug use. It takes less than 1 minute, is easily integrated into the initial prenatal visit, and can be used for follow-up screening throughout the pregnancy. In the evaluation of clinical experience with the 4P's Plus, identification of women at risk for substance use can be accomplished within the context of routine prenatal care. Using this screen, they were able to effectively identify pregnant women at the highest risk for substance use in pregnancy.

When discussing alcohol consumption during pregnancy, there are two separate patients, the mother and the fetus, who may suffer from two separate disorders. Thus, screening is needed for two problems, maternal alcohol dependence and fetal alcohol exposure (Savage et al, 2003). Numerous self-report, alcohol dependence screening tools are in use, but not all meet the needs of the pregnant woman and their fetus. The Cut-Down, Annoyance, Guilt, Eye-Opener (CAGE) and Michigan Alcohol Screening Test (MAST) are alcohol-screening questionnaires but are less effective in identifying drinking problems among women than among men (Chang, 2001). The Tolerance, Annoyance, Cut-Down, and Eye-Opener (T-ACE) and Tolerance, Worried, Eye-Openers, Amnesia, Cut-Down (TWEAK) are screening tools that are superior to the CAGE and MAST in identifying pregnancy risk drinking. However, these focus only on alcohol dependence (Chang, 2001; Savage et al, 2003). Savage and associates have proposed a two-step process, the Time Line Followback (TLFB) (Figure 21-1). The first step is to screen for fetal exposure to alcohol, and the second step is to screen mothers who report alcohol use for alcohol dependence. This process allows both the fetus and the mother to be addressed so that appropriate interventions can be initiated for both.

Administration of the TLFB takes about 10 minutes during the first prenatal visit. Subsequent screenings take only 3 to 5 minutes and should be completed at each prenatal visit. At the end of the prenatal period, there will be a record of the total amount of alcohol to which the fetus has been exposed, when the exposure occurred, and at what points during fetal growth and development the fetus was exposed to higher doses of alcohol (Savage et al, 2003).

The two most common methods of determining drug exposure are maternal self-report and urine toxicology screens. The advantage of self-report is that mothers can provide information about quantity and frequency of drug use throughout the pregnancy. However, it has been shown that self-report is far from accurate. Self-protection from fear of legal consequences or embarrassment from admission of illicit substance use leads many to underreport or deny substance use. Currently, there are 25 states that have laws permitting the commitment of pregnant women who abuse illicit drugs during pregnancy (Bar-Oz, 2003; Bergin et al, 2001; Hulsey, 2005; Lester et al, 2001; Ostrea, 2001). Appropriate interviewing techniques are critical in obtaining a comprehensive substance abuse history. Confidentiality is essential, and the most useful information will be obtained in an atmosphere of mutual trust and comfort. The interview must be done in a respectful, nonjudgmental, and nonpunitive manner. Interviews should be conducted in a private office and should start with generic questions regarding factual information (e.g., name, address), progressing to the most sensitive information at the end of the interview (e.g., substance use). Questions should be open-ended and phrased in a manner to permit discussion. In return, the interviewer should expect the woman to be open and honest. This attitude is subtly conveyed to the woman and becomes a self-fulfilling prophecy (Box 21-1). The tobacco, alcohol, and drug use patterns of a woman resemble those of her partner, and past use parallels current practices. The interview should begin by saying that the following questions are asked of everyone. Additionally, the ordering of questions is important and should begin with questions regarding the partner's use, the woman's past use, and last, the woman's current use (Box 21-2) (Bergin et al, 2001; Hurt, 2005; Kulig et al, 2005).

BOX 21-1

Effective Interview Techniques

- Create a comfortable atmosphere
- Conduct interview in a private office/area
- Use open-ended questions
- Phrase questions in a manner to permit discussion
- Begin with generic questions regarding factual information (e.g., name, address)
- Progress to most sensitive questions at end of interview (e.g., substance use)
- Use nonjudgmental questions
- When discussing substance use, begin with questions regarding partner's use, followed by woman's past use, ending with woman's current use
- Interviewer should expect the woman to be open and honest; the attitude of the interviewer is subtly conveyed to the woman and becomes a self-fulfilling prophecy

---

BOX 21-2

Effective Interview Questions for the Substance-Using Mother

"I would like to begin by asking a few questions about your partner's habits."
- "How many packs/day of cigarettes does your partner smoke?"
- "How often does your partner drink beer, wine coolers, malt liquor, or hard liquor?" (NOTE: Several alcoholic beverages are itemized, as many individuals do not realize that wine coolers and beer contain enough alcohol to harm the fetus.)
- "How many drinks does your partner have at one time?"
- "Does he party?"

If yes, ask
- "Does he ever do pot, crack/cocaine or other drugs when he's out with his friends?"

If yes, ask
- "What do you do when he is partying?"

If no to the party question, ask
- "When was the last time he used pot, crack/cocaine, or other drugs?" (NOTE: Women whose partners use are more likely to use themselves. Questions about partner's behaviors should be explored to identify women at risk for substance use.)
- "Considering the last six months before you knew you were pregnant could you answer the following questions?" (NOTE: If women admit to use prior to pregnancy, then they may have continued use before they realized they were pregnant or may still be using but not disclosing.)
- "How many packs of cigarettes/day do you smoke?"
- "How often do you drink beer, wine cooler, whiskey, or other drinks containing alcohol?"
- "Do you have 3 or 4 drinks at a time?" (NOTE: By asking about large amounts of drinking, the woman may feel comfortable disclosing that she has one or two drinks per night.)
- "When was the last time you used pot, crack/cocaine, or other drugs?"

These questions are more likely to elicit accurate information than the question "Do you drink?" or "You don't drink, do you?"

The recommended questions are nonjudgmental and give the woman permission to report drinking and the use of drugs. If the woman is drinking two drinks per day and she is asked if she drinks three or four, then she will feel more comfortable self-reporting drinking. It is also phrased so that the answer will be more than yes or no, and prompt some discussion. If the woman responds to any of the questions with ambiguous answers such as "I'm a social drinker" or "I use crack for recreation," the responses need to be clarified with respect to amount and frequency of use.

If a woman becomes angry about the questions or refuses to answer, it may be because the questions have become uncomfortably close to her personal use and she is not willing to discuss this. She may also react out of shock at being questioned. Her response should be noted and evaluated. If the interviewer feels that the mother is perhaps using substances and not disclosing it, the subject can be brought up again later in the course of her care.

The American Academy of Pediatrics (AAP) recommends that a comprehensive medical and psychosocial history that includes specific information concerning maternal drug use should be included in every newborn evaluation. Although maternal self-reporting frequently underestimates exposure, and maternal urine screening during pregnancy fails to identify many cases of drug use, laboratory screening should be seen as only a potential adjunct to a thorough history. However, the AAP also suggests that screening is needed when there are certain maternal characteristics present. These include limited or no prenatal care, previous unexplained fetal demise, precipitous labor, abruptio placentae, hypertensive episodes, severe mood swings, cerebrovascular accidents, myocardial infarction, and repeated spontaneous abortions. Infant characteristics that may suggest maternal drug use include prematurity, unexplained intrauterine growth restriction (IUGR), neurobehavioral abnormalities, urogenital anomalies, and atypical vascular incidents, such as cerebrovascular accidents, myocardial infarction, and necrotizing enterocolitis in otherwise healthy full-term infants (AAP Policy Statement, 1998).

LABORATORY TESTS
Blood Analysis

Blood, serum, or plasma can be analyzed for drugs, although it is rarely used for illicit drug testing. There are several disadvantages to blood analysis. Blood collection is invasive and requires trained personnel. The amount of drug in blood is affected by the metabolism or distribution of the drug in the body; thus the drug concentration may be too low to be detected by ordinary screening methods. Also, the serum drug level is dependent on the interval between the last drug intake by the mother and testing in the infant. The time difference can be substantial (Ostrea, 2001).

Urine Analysis

Urine has been the most commonly used specimen for neonatal drug testing because the collection is easy and is noninvasive. Additionally, drug concentration is higher in the urine than in serum because of the concentrating ability of the kidneys. Urine is easier to process than blood because it is devoid of protein and cellular constituents, and urine can be tested by most drug testing methods. However, there are several limitations to this method. Drugs in the infant's urine represent recent drug use by the mother; thus the specimen must be collected from the infant as close to birth as possible. There is a high incidence of false negative tests in urine testing, as high as 63%. The urine may test negative if the mother is an infrequent or inconsistent user of drugs, or if she abstained from use within a week of delivery. Premature infants may test positive for a longer period of time because of the possibility of lower plasma and liver cholinesterase activity and reduced renal function. If a positive result is obtained, it is important to do confirmatory testing because there are other substances such as over-the-counter medications and herbal preparations that can lead to positive results (Askin & Diehl-Jones, 2001; Hurt, 2005; Johnson et al, 2003a; Lester et al, 2001; Ostrea, 2001; Rosen & Bateman, 2002).

Urine testing for cotinine, a metabolite of nicotine, has been suggested as a way to quantify maternal tobacco use. A study by England and colleagues (2001) examined the relationship between self-reported number of cigarettes smoked and urine cotinine concentration during pregnancy. The researchers were unable to demonstrate a close correlation between self-report and urine cotinine levels. Possible explanations include inaccurate maternal reporting and individual differences in inhalation, absorption, and metabolism. Additionally, previous studies have suggested differences in cotinine concentration among different ethnic groups. Although this study also found higher levels in African-American women, the difference was not significant after adjustment for potential confounders. Thus, the additional expense and inconvenience of collecting urine and measuring cotinine as a measure of tobacco use may not be warranted.

Meconium Analysis

The presence of drugs or drug metabolites in meconium can provide a long-term, semiquantitative measure of fetal exposure. In the fetus, drugs are metabolized into water-soluble products in the liver and are then excreted in the urine or bile. These metabolites accumulate in the meconium either by direct deposition from bile or by ingestion of metabolites present in amniotic fluid. Meconium is not normally excreted in utero, allowing for concentration of the metabolite in the sample (Ostrea, 2001; Rosen & Bateman, 2002).

There are several advantages in using meconium for drug testing. There is a high sensitivity and specificity, and the collection of meconium is noninvasive and poses no risk to the infant. Also, metabolites in meconium reflect maternal drug intake during the second and third trimesters of pregnancy, giving a wide window of time for detecting intrauterine exposure. On the other hand, meconium is only available for the first few days of life, leaving a smaller time frame for collection. Meconium analysis can be performed by most hospital laboratories, and the overall cost is comparable to that of urine analysis. Because of the high sensitivity and the ease of collection, meconium analysis is the best test for perinatal drug screening (Askin & Diehl-Jones, 2001; Bar-Oz et al, 2003; Koren et al, 2003; Lester et al, 2001; Ostrea, 2001; Ostrea et al, 2001; Rosen & Bateman, 2002).

In the past, the determination of fetal alcohol exposure has largely depended on maternal interview, but laboratory testing is becoming more widely used. Fatty acid ethyl esters (FAEEs) are metabolic products that result from the interaction between fatty acids and alcohol. FAEEs accumulate in adipose tissue after ethanol has been eliminated from the body and can be found in blood, hair, placenta, cord blood, and meconium. As a result, it has been suggested that FAEE detection in meconium may be a potential biomarker of fetal exposure to alcohol, and their detection may serve as a diagnostic tool to assess the extent of fetal exposure. Further study is needed to determine if this will be a reliable, cost-effective method of screening for alcohol exposure (Bearer, 2001; Moore et al, 2003; Ostrea, 2001).

Hair Analysis

Hair analysis is a sensitive method for detection of prenatal drug use. Drugs and their metabolites accumulate in hair in proportion to their concentration in the blood nourishing the hair root. Once the drug is deposited in the hair shaft, it remains for an indefinite period of time. As the hair grows, the deposited drugs follow the growth of the hair shaft, with the hair closest to the scalp being the most recently exposed.

Therefore, sectional analysis can provide information on the duration and time of drug use. Another advantage of using hair analysis is that it may be available for up to 3 months, whereas meconium is only available for the first few days. However, there are several drawbacks that limit its usefulness. First, hair levels of drugs are affected by the amount of melanin in the shaft. Coarse black hair incorporates more of the drug than brown or blond hair, necessitating the need for differential scaling by hair color. Second, in an infant, the growth of hair occurs only during the latter part of pregnancy, so drug use in early pregnancy is not detected. Additionally, hair sampling is invasive, and even if the infant has enough hair to collect an adequate sample, the mother may be reluctant to allow the infant's hair to be cut (Askin & Diehl-Jones, 2001; Bar-Oz et al, 2003; Ebrahim & Gfroerer, 2003; Koren et al, 2003; Ostrea, 2001; Ostrea et al, 2001; Rosen & Bateman, 2002).

Ostrea and associates (2001) compared the sensitivity and specificity of maternal interview, meconium analysis, and maternal hair analysis in detecting perinatal exposure to cocaine, opiates, and cannabinoid. The maternal interview showed the lowest sensitivity in detecting cocaine and opiate exposure but the highest in detecting cannabinoid exposure. Maternal hair analysis had the highest sensitivity to detection of cocaine (100%) and opiates (80%). The sensitivity of meconium analysis was 87% for cocaine and 77% for opiates. However, hair analysis had a high false positive rate for cocaine and opiates when compared to meconium, most likely due to passive exposure to drugs. Also noted were increased false positive rates for meconium to opiates. This is most likely a result of cross-reactivity to various opiates, perhaps those used during labor and delivery. The incidence of false positive rates with any type of analysis clearly reinforces the need for confirmation by a second test (Lester et al, 2001; Ostrea, 2001; Ostrea et al, 2001). Currently, there is an ongoing legal battle related to hair analysis. For more information, see the Evolve website. **evolve**

Other Methods of Analysis

Other specimens that have been used for drug testing include saliva, perspiration, and nail clippings. In the newborn, tests of amniotic fluid and gastric aspirates have been reported. However, the antenatal collection of amniotic fluid is extremely invasive. Gastric aspirates have reportedly been tested for cocaine and its metabolites, although results are uncertain. It is thought that collection and analysis shortly after birth allows earlier diagnosis of drug exposure, especially in premature infants whose passage of urine or meconium may be delayed. However, further testing and refinement are needed in order to improve reliability (Ostrea, 2001).

ETHICAL CONSIDERATIONS

Screening of pregnant women or their offspring for substance poses several ethical dilemmas for health care personnel. Studies have shown that many drug-using mothers are unable to properly care for their infants, or that their environments are unsafe for them. As a result, many institutions have taken measures to identify these infants, and child protective agencies have acted to separate them from the mothers. The American Academy of Pediatrics (AAP) considers the practice of performing drug screening for the primary purpose of detecting illegal use as unethical. They suggest that criminal prosecution and incarceration are unjustified and that it is more important to have effective drug treatment programs available. Their recommendation is that drug screening should be done only as part of a medical evaluation in order to assist in diagnosis of drug exposure, thus ensuring prompt and proper treatment (AAP Policy Statement, 1998; Askin & Diehl-Jones, 2001).

DRUGS AND THE INTERNET

The explosive growth of the Internet in recent years has provided a wealth of information on recreational drugs. Internet access greatly facilitates the free and easy exchange of ideas, opinions, and unedited and unsupervised information. Many of the websites present mixed messages. Although the risks and problems of the recreational drugs are discussed, they are downplayed. Accessible information includes items such as effects of different doses (including the pleasurable effects) and the price one should expect to pay. Recommendations for use for the drugs can also be found, including advice to start at lower doses when first using a particular drug (Wax, 2002). Please refer to the Evolve website for additional information. **evolve**

TOBACCO
History

Cigarette smoking remains the leading preventable cause of death in the United States. In 2003, approximately 21.6% of adults in the United States were current smokers. Although this prevalence is lower than the previous 2 years, the rate of decline is not sufficient to meet the national health objective target of 12% by 2010 (CDC, 2005a; United States DHHS, 2005b). The prevalence of smoking is higher among women with a General Educational Development (GED) diploma than among women with 16 or more years of education, and is most frequent among those living below the poverty level. Smoking prevalence is highest among American Indians/ Alaska Natives, followed by whites, then African Americans (CDC, 2004a, 2004c).

For the first time since 1991, the overall prevalence of cigarette smoking among women declined below 20%, to 19.2% (CDC, 2005b). However, the rate of smoking among women peaked between 25 and 44 years of age, a period of childbearing age. Despite increased knowledge about the dangers of smoking, many women who smoke have difficulty abstaining from tobacco use during pregnancy. An estimated 18% of pregnant women aged 15 to 44 years smoke cigarettes, with the highest rate of use in the younger women. Of the pregnant women who smoke, 38% report being heavy smokers (more than one pack per day) (Albrecht, 2004; U.S. Department of Health and Human Services [USDHHS], 2005a, 2005b).

A common consequence of tobacco use is addiction to nicotine. One puff on a cigarette results in peak nicotine levels in the brain within 10 seconds, activating the circuitry of the brain that regulates pleasure. The acute effects of nicotine dissipate in a few minutes, causing the smoker to continue dosing throughout the day to maintain the pleasurable effects and prevent withdrawal. Most smokers report a true enjoyment, associated with a sense of relaxation during stress, especially with the first cigarette of the day (AAP Policy Statement, 2001d; NIDA, 2001). Nicotine dependence is a primary, chronic disease with psychosocial, environmental, and genetic factors influencing its development and manifestations, and is common after smoking as few as 100 cigarettes (AAP Policy Statement, 2001d).

Mechanism of Action

Tobacco in cigarettes primarily consists of leaves from the plant *Nicotiana tabacum* L. The smoke from tobacco contains more than 4000 compounds, many of which are pharmacologically active, mutagenic, and carcinogenic. Tobacco smoke acts in two ways: centrally and peripherally. Central action occurs when the smoker inhales on a cigarette. This smoke is produced at high temperatures and only pollutes the environment after having been inhaled through the cigarette, filtered through the lungs of the smoker, and, finally, exhaled. It is the primary source of exposure among active smokers. Peripheral smoke is produced at lower temperatures during the slow spontaneous combustion at the end of the cigarette, between puffs. This is what is inhaled by passive smokers and is responsible for 85% of cigarette smoke released directly to the environment. Peripheral smoke differs from central smoke in that it is not filtered and the nicotine is in a gaseous state (Nakamura et al, 2004).

There are multiple compounds found in cigarette smoke that have been associated with adverse health effects. Among these compounds are nicotine and carbon monoxide.

Nicotine is a pale yellow alkaloid that is both water- and lipid-soluble. It has a low boiling point; therefore it is vaporized as tobacco is smoked. Because of its short half-life of 2 hours, measures of nicotine in the serum or saliva reflect exposures only from the past day.

The liver metabolizes nicotine to cotinine within hours. Cotinine can be found in a number of body fluids, including urine, blood, and saliva, and has been found to accumulate in the fetal compartment as early as 7 weeks' gestation. Levels of cotinine are indicative of exposure during the preceding few days because of a longer half-life of 15 to 30 hours (DiFranza et al, 2004).

Nicotine acts on the cardiovascular system, causing the release of catecholamines into the mother's circulation, resulting in tachycardia, peripheral vasoconstriction and reduction of placental blood flow. This leads to poor nutritional and oxygenation rates for the fetus. Cotinine enhances the vasoconstrictive action of prostaglandin E2. The accumulation of cotinine in the fetal bloodstream may contribute to the onset of premature labor and spontaneous abortions among pregnant smokers (Nakamura et al, 2004).

Carbon monoxide, a colorless and odorless gas, is produced when cigarettes are incompletely burned. Compared to oxygen, it has a 200-fold affinity for hemoglobin. Carbon monoxide binds hemoglobin to form carboxyhemoglobin, which then reduces the oxygen carrying capacity of blood. Also, it increases the binding of hemoglobin to oxygen, impairing its ability to release oxygen into the tissues. It has been reported that a carboxyhemoglobin concentration of 10% observed in heavy smokers (40 cigarettes per day) resulted in a 60% reduction in fetal blood flow, thereby affecting the transportation of oxygen, leading to chronic hypoxia. Therefore, carbon monoxid interferes in tissue oxygenation in two ways. It reduces the blood oxygen transportation capacity and alters the oxyhemoglobin saturation curve to the left, thus favoring hypoxemia and resulting in growth restriction (Horne et al, 2002; Nakamura et al, 2004; NIDA, 2001; Wisborg et al, 2001).

Risk Factors

Cigarette smoking has been associated with a variety of perinatal complications, including spontaneous abortions, prematurity, stillbirth, and fetal growth restriction. It represents the most influential and most common factor adversely affecting perinatal outcomes (Hofhuis et al, 2003; Law et al, 2003; Martinez et al, 2005; Nakamura et al, 2004).

The nicotine in cigarette smoke acts as a neuroteratogen that interferes with fetal development, specifically the developing nervous system. Nicotine targets nicotinic acetylcholine receptors in the fetal brain to change the pattern of cell proliferation and differentiation. The nicotinic cholinergic receptor binding sites are upregulated by nicotine exposure. This causes abnormalities in the development of synaptic activity. This leads to cell loss and ultimately, neuronal damage. Additionally, because nicotine concentrations on the fetal side of the placenta generally reach levels 15% higher than maternal levels, even a small amount of cigarette smoking may expose the fetus to harmful amounts of nicotine. Preclinical studies have shown that doses of nicotine that do not cause low birth weight may still produce deficits in fetal brain development (Buka et al, 2003; DiFranza et al, 2004; Horne et al, 2002; Law et al, 2003).

The presence of tobacco-specific metabolites in fetal blood and amniotic fluid, as well as in newborns of women who smoke, suggests a possible genotoxic effect of smoking during pregnancy. Although there are several cytogenetic studies that have demonstrated the existence of an increased incidence of chromosomal aberrations in adult smokers, no data regarding a possible genotoxic effect on the fetus are available. A study by Ana de la Chica and associates (2005) examined amniocytes which were obtained by amniocentesis, looking for genotoxic effects expressed as an increased chromosomal instability. In addition, they analyzed whether any chromosomal regions were especially affected by tobacco exposure. Results showed an association between maternal smoking during pregnancy and an increased chromosomal instability in amniocytes. Band 11q23, known to be involved in leukemogenesis, appeared to be particularly sensitive to the genotoxic compounds in tobacco, suggesting a possible increased risk of pediatric hematopoietic malignancies. At this time, these findings should be viewed as highly preliminary. However, if the results of this study can be substantiated with further research, there would be important implications for the immediate and long-term health effects of children born to mothers who smoke (DeMarini & Preston, 2005).

Smoking during pregnancy increases the risk factor for maternal colonization of group B streptococcus. The colonization rate for smokers is 33% vs 16% for nonsmokers. Although there is no proven association between smoking during pregnancy and an increased risk of chorioamnionitis, group B streptococcus is a key pathogen. Because chorioamnionitis is responsible for a significant number of placental abruptions, spontaneous abortions, preterm deliveries, and neonatal infection, a relationship between smoking and perinatal complications as a direct result of chorioamnionitis must be considered (Hofhuis et al, 2003). Please refer to the Evolve website for additional information. **evolve**

Fetal Effects
Low Birth Weight (LBW)
Maternal smoking has been documented as responsible for reduced birth weight and fetal growth restriction. Mothers who smoke are almost twice as likely to have a LBW infant, and smoking during pregnancy is responsible for 20% to 30%

of all LBW infants. These infants weigh an average of 150 to 250 g less than infants born to nonsmoking mothers. The effect on fetal growth is significant, affecting growth in a dose-dependent manner. Lower birth weights have been associated with exposure as measured by cotinine levels as well as by the number of cigarettes smoked. The mechanism for growth restriction is uncertain, but may include direct effects of nicotine on placental vasoconstriction and decreased uterine blood flow. As the metabolites of cigarette smoke pass through the placenta to the fetus, they act as vasoconstrictors, reducing uterine blood flow by up to 38%. Thus the fetus is deprived of nutrients and oxygen, resulting in fetal hypoxia-ischemia and malnutrition. Also implicated are increased levels of carboxyhemoglobin, adverse maternal nutrition, and altered maternal and placental metabolism (DiFranza et al, 2004; Goel et al, 2004; Hurt, 2005; Jauniaux et al, 2001; Kalinka et al, 2005; Law et al, 2003; Martinez et al, 2005; Ventura et al, 2003; Wang et al, 2002).

The developing fetus is dependent on the supply of amino acids from the maternal blood for protein synthesis. Higher amino acid concentrations in the umbilical vein compared with maternal venous blood is thought to indicate active transport systems within the placenta. A study by Jauniaux and associates (2001) assessed the influence of chronic active maternal smoking on cord blood amino acid and enzyme levels at term. Levels of several amino acids were decreased, confirming that tobacco exposure has a marked effect on fetoplacental metabolism. These findings suggest that the metabolism of some amino acids is altered by tobacco and that this will be associated with a chronic amino acid deficit for protein synthesis by the fetus, which may contribute to fetal growth restriction in mothers who smoke.

A study by England and colleagues (2001) examined the relation between self-reported number of cigarettes smoked and urine cotinine concentration during pregnancy and the relation between these two measures of exposure and birth weight. The comparison between number of cigarettes smoked and cotinine levels is discussed earlier in this chapter. Additional results demonstrated a decrease in birth weight as tobacco exposure increased. However, this relationship was not linear. Instead, the sharpest declines in birth weight were found at low levels of exposure. Thus, there appears to be no "safe" level of prenatal smoking.

In a review of birth certificate data by Ventura and associates (2003), it was found that even among those infants delivered to the lightest smokers (i.e., 1 to 5 cigarettes per day), the percentage of LBW infants was substantially higher than for nonsmokers. However, women who quit smoking before or during pregnancy reduced the risk for adverse pregnancy outcomes, including premature rupture of membranes, preterm delivery, and low birth weight (DiFranza et al, 2004).

Neurobehavioral Effects

Although the effects of maternal smoking during pregnancy are well known, little is known about how such effects affect newborn neurobehavior. Multiple studies have reported increases in hypertonicity, tremors, and startles among infants prenatally exposed to tobacco. In older children, there appeared to be an association with negativity and externalizing behavior problems (DiFranza et al, 2004).

A study by Law and associates (2003) found tobacco-exposed infants to be highly aroused and reactive as indicated by higher excitability and handling scores on the NICU

Network Neurobehavioral Scale (NNNS). On exam, they were also found to be more hypertonic. Furthermore, there was a dose-response relationship demonstrated between smoking and neurobehavior as increasingly negative neurobehavioral effects were related to more tobacco exposure.

Studies of children prenatally exposed to tobacco have consistently demonstrated higher rates of behavior problems when compared to those whose mothers did not smoke. Increased rates of child behavior problems and attention-deficit/hyperactivity disorder–like behaviors have been documented, even after controlling for potential confounders (DiFranza et al, 2004; Hofhuis et al, 2003; Law et al, 2003).

Infants exposed to tobacco prenatally have decreased rates of auditory habituation and increased sound thresholds. By ages 3 and 4 years, language development has been found to be adversely affected by tobacco exposure. These findings are dose related and have persisted through 12 years of age (DiFranza, 2004). Additional information can be found on the Evolve website. **evolve**

Cardiovascular System

Prenatal exposure to cigarette smoke inhibits cardiac DNA synthesis and impairs vascular smooth muscle function. In infants, cardiac cell damage is a consequence of concurrent, repeated exposures to nicotine and hypoxia; nicotine and cotinine appear to play a major role in the failure of vascular reconstruction. Additional deleterious effects on the heart including reduced platelet activation, increased resting sympathetic nerve activity, and hypertension. Severe wall damage of umbilical vessels has also been associated with maternal tobacco use during pregnancy. Evidence suggests that these effects are attributable to numerous smoke constituents, rather than a single component (Mone et al, 2004).

Both prenatal and neonatal exposure to second-hand smoke have been found to have a harmful effect on vascular smooth muscle function in infant rats as evidenced by abnormal vasoconstrictor and vasodilator responses. Endothelial cell function abnormalities were found in adult rabbits that were exposed to second-hand smoke as was left ventricular hypertrophy. However, thus far, these findings have not been replicated in humans (Mone et al, 2004).

Intrauterine Lung Growth

Animal studies have demonstrated that exposure to cigarette smoke during pregnancy leads to a reduction in fetal breathing movements. Prolonged impairment or absence of fetal breathing movements is likely to result in hypoplasia of the lungs with fewer saccules, resulting in a reduced surface potentially available for gas exchange. Additionally, in utero cigarette smoke exposure decreased alveolar attachment points to the airways and caused changes in airway dimensions. These observations may be applicable to humans since nicotine has been found to cause a reduction in the incidence of fetal breathing movements in normal and abnormal human pregnancies. As a result, the reduced lung growth found in children of mothers who smoke may begin antenatally. How long this impaired lung function that results from in utero exposure continues to be significant is still not known (Elliot et al, 2003; Hofhuis et al, 2003).

Nicotine Withdrawal

Maternal drug use during pregnancy is associated with fetal addiction and neonatal withdrawal. Because cigarette smoking is associated with addiction and withdrawal in adults, it has been suggested that exposure to heavy maternal smoking during pregnancy may cause withdrawal in these newborns. A study by Law and associates (2003) examining the effects of prenatal tobacco exposure on newborn neurobehavior found that these infants showed stress and abstinence signs consistent with what has been reported in other drug-exposed infants. Although they could not conclude these symptoms indicated neonatal withdrawal from nicotine, it opened the door for further research.

A study by Godding and colleagues (2004) found significantly lower neurologic scores in infants born to heavy smokers when compared to infants of nonsmokers. Additionally, the Finnegan withdrawal score was significantly higher in newborns of heavy smokers. Fetal exposure was confirmed by the presence of cotinine in the cord blood and the infants' urine. There was significant improvement in the neurologic score of the nicotine-exposed infants between days 1 and 5, which was felt to be due to the short half-life of nicotine. Normalization of withdrawal scores were not seen by day 5. However, the infants were discharged on the fifth day of life and no follow-up evaluations were completed. Although results of this study strongly suggest that nicotine withdrawal symptoms, even discrete, are present in infants born to heavy smokers, there is no information about the length of time symptoms persist.

Although some researchers are confident that nicotine withdrawal has been demonstrated, in reality it is difficult to determine whether symptoms are indeed withdrawal or due to acute toxicity or more permanent central nervous system (CNS) damage. Withdrawal requires the study of patterns, not single scores, and most studies to date have not studied the infants for prolonged periods of time. Thus, nicotine withdrawal is an area in which further research is needed (García-Algar et al, 2004; Lester et al, 2004).

Fetal Death and Neonatal Mortality

A study by Wisborg and associates (2001) looked at the association between prenatal exposure to tobacco smoke and the risk of stillbirth and infant death. Compared with nonsmokers, women who smoked had about twice the risk of stillbirth and of infant death. However, when women stopped smoking before 16 weeks' gestation, the risk of stillbirth and infant death was comparable to that in infants born to women who had not smoked during the pregnancy.

Risk Factors in Infancy and Childhood
Gastrointestinal Dysregulation

Throughout the first 6 months of life, infants typically double their birth weights. During this time of intense growth, the gastrointestinal (GI) tract needs to be able to function optimally. It is important to identify modifiable precursors of GI tract dysfunction in order to identify effective interventions, and, most importantly, for developing early prevention and health promotion strategies. One such precursor appears to be maternal smoking, both during and after pregnancy.

Recent evidence suggests that exposure to cigarette and its metabolites may be linked to infantile colic. Additionally, studies of the GI system provide corroborating evidence suggesting that smoking is linked to increased plasma and intestinal motilin levels. Higher-than-average intestinal motilin levels have been associated with elevated risks of infantile colic. Colic potentially has long-lasting effects on

both the mother-infant dyad and the entire family. Infants with colic may have more sleep difficulties as well as more feeding difficulties. If, as suspected, exposure to cigarette smoke increases the incidence of colic, then there is additional incentive for infants to be protected from cigarette smoke, both during pregnancy and from environmental exposure after birth. However, these findings are preliminary and further studies are needed to prove such a relationship (Shenassa & Brown, 2004).

Risk of Obesity

Several studies have reported an association between maternal smoking during pregnancy and offspring obesity (Toschke et al, 2003). It was hypothesized that smoking during the first trimester could mimic fetal malnutrition because of reduced food intake by the mother or reduced blood supply because of vasoconstrictive effects on maternal and uteroplacental vasculature. Nutritional deprivation might affect differentiation of hypothalamic centers regulating food intake, growth, and number of filled adipocytes. Additionally, inhaled tobacco may have a potentiating effect on hypothalamic structures, resulting in impaired insulin signaling and metabolism. Refer to the Evolve website for additional information. **evolve**

Sudden Infant Death Syndrome

Sudden infant death syndrome (SIDS) is the primary cause of death during the first year of life. The incidence of SIDS has declined dramatically after public health campaigns advising parents to place sleeping infants on their backs. As a result, maternal smoking is the major suspected risk factor for SIDS. Numerous studies have identified maternal smoking during pregnancy as a risk factor. The consistency of the findings and the strength of the statistical association suggest a causal relationship. Maternal smoking appears to double the risk of SIDS and a significant dose-response relationship has been suggested. However, the exact mechanism by which smoking affects the incidence of SIDS has not yet been determined (DiFranza, 2004; Hofhuis, 2003; Horne et al, 2002; Sawnani et al, 2004; Tong et al, 2005).

A key feature of the apnea theory of SIDS is that the arousal mechanism of smoke exposed infants has been altered. The arousal response is a protective mechanism by which infants increase activity to prevent life-threatening asphyxia. Early studies reported that infants born to smoking mothers have a higher arousal threshold to auditory stimuli during REM sleep. Subsequent studies have substantiated this finding and have showed that maternal smoking leads to impairment of both stimulus-induced arousal and spontaneous arousal. Additionally, an increase in the frequency and duration of obstructive apnea in infants born to mothers who smoked has also been documented (Chang et al, 2003; Sawnani et al, 2004).

Respiratory Effects

Maternal cigarette smoking during pregnancy is known to cause altered lung function in the women's infants. Although it has been suggested that altered lung and airway development in utero may result in altered lung function, the exact mechanism is unknown. Elliot and associates (2003) examined the lung structure of infants who died from SIDS, looking at airway dimensions, alveolar attachment points, and parenchymal elastin content. They found a significantly greater difference between alveolar attachments in intraparenchymal airways in infants exposed to cigarette smoke in utero, but did not find these changes in infants exposed only postnatally. Possible causes for the decreased number of attachment points include destruction of existing alveoli or abnormal growth of alveoli. An increased thickness of the inner airway wall was found in those infants exposed postnatally to cigarette smoke. These outcomes suggest that changes in airway thickness may be associated with postnatal smoke exposure while the increase in attachment point distances may be related to in utero or both in utero and postnatal exposure. There were no differences in the elastin content among the study groups.

Environmental tobacco smoke (ETS) exposure among children can begin before birth, continue throughout childhood, and is a preventable cause of morbidity. Mannino and associates (2001) examined the effects of prenatal and postnatal smoke exposure on the respiratory health of children in the United States. They found that children of all ages exposed to ETS had health effects potentially related to this exposure, and that recent exposure was important no matter whether there was prenatal exposure or not. Generally, observed effects were stronger in younger children. The younger children were felt to have greater exposure because they are inherently more home-bound than older children, "trapped" within the smoking environment (Rieves, 2002).

It has been suggested that suboptimal development of the respiratory system during fetal life or early childhood may adversely influence airway function throughout life. Diminished respiratory function in the first few months of life appears to precede and be predictive of wheezing in early childhood. Dezateux and associates (2001) examined the association of diminished premorbid airway function, wheezing, and maternal smoking with airway function at 1 year of age. They found that maternal smoking and diminished airway function measured early in life are independently associated with lower levels of airway function at the end of the first year, suggesting that this association may reflect impaired growth and development during fetal and early life. These findings add to the growing body of evidence supporting the association between maternal smoking and impaired respiratory function.

Although evidence has been conflicting, there is a "fetal origins hypothesis" of association between birth weight and adult lung function. It has been proposed that an adverse environment in utero can decrease weight gain of the fetus which, in turn, can restrict the growth of the airways with effects that persist into late adulthood. A study by Edwards and colleagues (2003) found that LBW predicts lower lung function at mean age 47 years after controlling for potential confounders, thus supporting the fetal origins hypothesis. Refer to the Evolve website for more information about the effects of tobacco exposure on older children. **evolve**

Tobacco Dependence

Earlier studies have reported high rates of smoking among the offspring of women who smoke during pregnancy. A physiologic link between maternal smoking and smoking among offspring is plausible because nicotine and other substances in cigarette smoke cross the placental barrier, causing direct and long-term effects. Nicotine passes from mother to fetus and stimulates nicotinic receptors that are present from the early stages of fetal development, possibly causing permanent abnormalities in the brain's dopaminergic regulation. These effects may result in a greater liability to nicotine

dependence than in those who were not exposed to tobacco smoke in utero. The researchers also found no correlation between smoking during pregnancy and marijuana use in offspring (Buka, 2003). Refer to the Evolve website for more information. **evolve**

Second-Hand Smoke

Environmental tobacco smoke (ETS) has been described as passive smoking, involuntary smoking, or second-hand smoke, and is recognized as a major health hazard. ETS is a combination of side-stream smoke that is emitted from the burning end of a cigarette and the mainstream smoke that is exhaled by the smoker. More than 4000 chemical compounds are generated during the burning of tobacco products. Side-stream smoke constitutes about 85% of the smoke present in a room and contains several potentially toxic gases in higher concentrations than mainstream smoke. The smoke produced from a single cigarette in a large room causes the air to fail the national minimum standard set by the Clean Air Act of 1994.

Multiple studies have shown that infants and children exposed to ETS are adversely affected, especially their respiratory health. It has been estimated that passive smoke exposure among children results in direct medical expenditures of $4.6 billion annually in the United States. However, because women who smoke during pregnancy are likely to continue smoking after delivery, it is difficult to study the independent effects of in utero exposure to maternal smoking and postnatal ETS exposure (Emmons, 2001; Gilliland et al, 2001; Matt et al, 2004; McMillen et al, 2003; Goel et al, 2004).

Vapor-phase components of ETS deposit and are absorbed onto walls, furniture, clothes, toys, and other objects within 10 minutes to hours after tobacco smoke has been emitted. From there, they are re-emitted into the air over time, from hours to months. ETS particulate matter can deposit on surfaces within hours after the cigarette was smoked, from where it may be resuspended or react with vapor-phase compounds. Thus, ETS can contaminate house dust, carpets, walls, furniture, and other household objects for weeks and months after ETS was initially emitted. Infants of smoking parents are at a particular risk of second-hand smoke exposure through these contaminated surfaces. During the first year of life, infants spend much time indoors, are in close proximity to contaminated dusts and objects, and are in close physical contact with their smoking parents. Their dust ingestion rate is estimated to be more than twice that of adults, and because of their developmental stage, infants exhibit a higher frequency of hand-to-mouth contacts and ingestion of nonfood items. Additionally, considering that an infant has a higher respiratory rate and a lower body weight than an adult, this relatively low dose of ETS exposure may accumulate over the course of weeks to levels equivalent to several hours of active adult smoking. Can parents protect their infants from second-hand smoke by smoking outside and away from the child? Studies by Matt and associates (2004) and Leung and associates (2004) demonstrated that smoking outside the home and away from the infant is of some help, but does not completely protect a smoker's home from ETS contamination and a smoker's infant from ETS exposure. In addition to exposure to contaminated surfaces, including a smoker's finger, ETS may find its way into the home through windows and doors if cigarettes are smoked outside, and through contaminated clothes, skin, and dust carried into the home if cigarettes were smoked elsewhere (Blackburn et al, 2003).

It is well known that maternal smoking during pregnancy is a major cause of LBW, altered lung function, and most likely, SIDS. Goel and colleagues (2004) examined the effects of passive smoking on pregnancy outcomes. They found exposure to ETS during pregnancy to be associated with more than twofold higher risk of small-for-gestational-age (SGA) infants, even after adjusting for all possible confounders. There also appeared to be a dose-response relationship with a higher risk of premature birth and SGA infants with increasing cumulative exposure. These results were confirmation of an earlier study by Jaakkola and associates (2001), which also demonstrated a higher incidence of low-birth-weight infants and premature delivery (Perera et al, 2004).

A causal relationship has been found between parental smoking and an increased risk of acute lower respiratory illness in infancy. Most likely this is due to both prenatal and postnatal passive smoking, but it is difficult to distinguish the independent contributions. There appears to be a positive dose-response relationship, which is stronger with maternal smoking. There is a higher degree of postnatal exposure from the mother as the principal caregiver. In addition, intrauterine lung growth might already have been affected as a result of in utero exposure. In the first 2 years of life, passive smoking is associated with a higher incidence of respiratory infections, including respiratory syncytial virus bronchiolitis. Passive smoking is also a risk factor for developing tuberculosis immediately following an infection and is a risk factor in meningococcal disease. This could possibly be the result of a direct effect of cigarette smoke on host defenses, given that smoking is negatively associated with cell mediated and humoral immunity, and smoking increases bacterial adherence and the risk of inflammation and other infections (Hofhuis et al, 2003; Schuster et al, 2002).

There is most likely a causal relationship between parental smoking and both acute and chronic middle ear disease in children. Chronic middle ear disease is 20% to 50% more frequent in children exposed to ETS. There are also reports that children of smokers are more likely to have a tonsillectomy/adenoidectomy although these findings have not been substantiated (Emmons et al, 2001; Hofhuis et al, 2003; Schuster et al, 2002).

Breastfeeding

Nicotine is present in breast milk in concentrations between 1.5 and 3.0 times the simultaneous maternal plasma concentration, and elimination half-life is similar, 60 to 90 minutes. At this time, there is no concrete evidence to document whether the amount of nicotine in breast milk presents a health risk to the nursing infant. Although pregnancy and lactation are ideal occasions for physicians to urge cessation, it is recognized that there are mothers who are unable to stop smoking. An earlier study reported that among women who continued to smoke during breastfeeding, the incidence of respiratory illness was decreased among their infants, compared with infants of smoking mothers who were bottle feeding. The conjecture is that breastfeeding and smoking may be less detrimental to the infant. The AAP has placed emphasis on increasing breastfeeding in the United States. Because of this recommendation as well as the lack of evidence of harmful effects of nicotine and breastfeeding, the Committee on Drugs has not placed nicotine (and thus smoking) on the list of contradicted drugs during breastfeeding (AAP Policy Statement, 2001c; Buka et al, 2003).

Smokeless Tobacco

The use of smokeless tobacco has become more popular and widespread, especially among young adults. Tobacco in smokeless form contains several carcinogenic and toxic substances that have been shown to cross the placental barrier. Although there are assumptions that using smokeless tobacco may be as detrimental to fetal health as cigarette smoking, there has been little research data to substantiate these opinions. One study in India examined the use of smokeless tobacco during pregnancy and the effects on birth weight and gestational age at birth. The researchers found that maternal use of smokeless tobacco decreased both weight and gestational age after adjusting for the confounders of low socioeconomic and educational status, maternal weight, and less than optimal antenatal care (Gupta & Sreevidya, 2004).

Recommendations

The AAP calls on all health care professionals to routinely inquire about household smoking history, advise as to the adverse effects of ETS on child health, and offer smoking cessation services to parents who smoke (AAP Policy Statement, 2001b, 2001d; Leung, 2004; Schuster et al, 2002; Tong et al, 2005; Winickoff et al, 2003a, 2003b). Hospitalization has been found to be significantly higher among infants exposed to ETS if it was accompanied by poor smoking hygiene, such as smoking in the immediate vicinity of the infant (Leung, 2004). Although recommendations are for complete cessation, proper smoking hygiene practices for those unable to quit smoking will help somewhat reduce exposure.

Many parental smokers often see their child's health care provider much more frequently than their own. Therefore, pediatricians are in a key position to influence parental smoking behavior. Reviews of physician-patient counseling have found that one-time interventions are marginally efficacious at best, but that repeated minimal interventions by physicians and nurses can lead to higher rates of smoking cessation. There also appeared to be more success when the issue was addressed at their child's clinic visit (AAP Policy Statement, 2001d; Emmons et al, 2001; Schuster et al, 2002; Winickoff et al, 2003b, 2003c). More information can be found on the Evolve website. *evolve*

A five-step intervention program, referred to as the "5 A's" model, has been successfully used for smoking cessation. The five steps are: (1) ask—about tobacco use; (2) advise—to quit; (3) assess—willingness to make a quit attempt; (4) assist—in quit attempt; and (5) arrange—follow-up. Success in quitting is facilitated by a patient, persevering, nonjudgmental, empathic approach on the part of the health care professional (Albrecht et al, 2004; AAP Policy Statement, 2001d; Winickoff et al, 2003c).

ALCOHOL

History

Since the beginning of recorded history, people have consumed alcohol beverages for the purposes of religious ceremony, celebration, medicinal therapy, recreation, and pleasure. Although the consumption of alcohol can be traced to Biblical times, it was not until more than 200 years ago that adverse effects in offspring from excessive alcohol consumption during pregnancy were suspected. In the early 1970s, the features and problems of fetal alcohol syndrome (FAS) were first described by Jones and colleagues (AAP Policy Statement, 2001a; Eustace et al, 2003; Jones & Bass, 2003).

Although the overall rate of alcohol use among pregnant women has declined since 1995, frequent and binge drinking continues to occur. In order to determine alcohol consumption patterns among all women of childbearing age, the Centers for Disease Control and Prevention (CDC) monitors the prevalence of alcohol use through the Behavioral Risk Factor Surveillance System survey. From data analysis of women 18 to 44 years, CDC found that approximately 10% of pregnant women used alcohol, and approximately 2% engaged in binge drinking or frequent use of alcohol. Results further indicated that more than half of women who did not use birth control and therefore might become pregnant reported alcohol use, and 12.4% reported binge drinking. Frequent drinking is considered seven or more drinks per week and binge drinking is five or more drinks on any one occasion (CDC, 2004b, 2005c; United States DHHS, 2005a).

Women who abuse alcohol usually have friends or family members who are problem drinkers and often live with men who are heavy drinkers. These women frequently have late prenatal care or a complete lack of care. They are often malnourished with poor weight gain and may have a severe, unexplained anemia during pregnancy. Addicted women tend to engage in risky behaviors such as sex with multiple partners or unprotected sex. Polydrug use is common. There is often a history of abuse in the family, and Child Protective Services may be involved with other children (CDC, 2004b; Jones & Bass, 2003; May & Gossage, 2001).

Mechanism of Action

Ethyl alcohol (ethanol) is an analgesic with a depressant effect on the CNS. Because of its small molecular size and fat solubility, alcohol readily crosses the placenta and the fetal blood-brain barrier, leading to nearly equal fetal and maternal alcohol levels. Fetal elimination is dependent on the maternal liver to metabolize alcohol and is therefore, regulated primarily by maternal elimination. After birth, alcohol levels are higher in the infant than in the mother, and alcohol is eliminated more slowly because the infant has an immature liver with a limited ability to metabolize alcohol. Thus these infants with high ethanol levels may appear intoxicated until the liver can complete metabolism (Hurt, 2005; Jones & Bass, 2003; Rosen & Bateman, 2002; Welch-Carre, 2005).

Fetal Effects

Prenatal alcohol exposure is the leading preventable cause of birth defects, mental retardation, and neurodevelopmental disorders. Alcohol is a potent teratogen, capable of causing severe damage to the fetus. Alcohol is also classified as a neurobehavioral teratogen because of its harmful effects on the CNS. The effects of prenatal alcohol exposure on a fetus can vary from subtle to profound, with FAS and perinatal death constituting the most severe outcomes (Hankin, 2002; Jones & Bass, 2003; Maier & West, 2001; Rosen & Bateman, 2002; Welch-Carre, 2005).

Studies have shown that the impact of alcohol on the fetus varies throughout pregnancy and may depend on the drinking pattern of the mother. Binge drinking appears to have a greater effect on the fetus compared with regular drinking in small amounts. Because the mother is ingesting several alcoholic drinks on one occasion, binge drinking exposes herself and her fetus to considerably higher blood alcohol levels, thereby increasing the risk of alcohol-related damage to the fetus. The fetus is especially vulnerable to alcohol-induced brain injury during specific stages of brain development, many of which occur early in pregnancy, often before a pregnancy is known. More recent studies have suggested that the impact of alcohol on the developing brain may be most pronounced during the last trimester of pregnancy, the period coincident with brain growth spurt. However, autopsies performed on infants with FAS have shown a wide array of brain abnormalities involving almost every stage of brain development (Beblo et al, 2005; Holl & Lussky, 2003; Jones & Bass, 2003; Maier & West, 2001; Sokol et al, 2003).

Alcohol can lead to cell death by both necrosis and apoptosis, or programmed cell death, in the developing embryo and fetus. Cells in the CNS have a lower threshold for alcohol. As a result, these cells experience more rapid cell death than any other cells in the developing embryo. Once a particular cell line has been damaged, the production, migration, and differentiation of future cell lines are affected (Jones & Bass, 2003; Welch-Carre, 2005).

Oxidative stress is also thought to play a role in fetal alcohol syndrome. Oxidative stress occurs when the free-radical production exceeds the ability of the cells to eliminate them. There are two means by which this may occur. First, a byproduct of alcohol is free radicals, particularly oxygen-containing free radicals. Second, alcohol consumption suppresses antioxidants that are necessary for free-radical elimination. The combination of increased production and decreased elimination can cause toxic levels of free-radical exposure, causing mitochondrial dysfunction, cell damage, and death (Welch-Carre, 2005).

Imaging studies have found the overall size of the brain to be decreased in children with FAS. Specific regions affected by alcohol are the basal ganglia, corpus callosum, cerebellum, and hippocampus. These areas affect motor and cognitive skills, learning, memory, and executive function. Additionally, electroencephalographic (EEG) findings suggest there may be deficits in information processing (Hurt, 2005; Jones & Bass, 2003; Martinez et al, 2005; Mattson et al, 2001; Rosen & Bateman, 2002; Welch-Carre, 2005).

A study by De Los Angeles Avaria and associates (2004) examined nerve conduction velocity to determine the effect of prenatal alcohol exposure on the peripheral nervous system. Prenatal alcohol exposure is known to affect the sensory nervous system as demonstrated by abnormal visual and auditory evoked potentials. Thus, they hypothesized that there were most likely changes in the developing peripheral nervous system. Children prenatally exposed to alcohol showed a significant reduction in both nerve-conduction velocity and amplitude in the newborn period that persisted at 1 year of age. Because the differences remained at 1 year of age, it was suggested that alcohol can cause permanent, or at least persistent, damage to developing nerves, unlike temporary damage that is seen in nerves already developed. Although further research is needed with larger sample sizes, health care personnel should be aware of possible nerve conduction abnormalities resulting from prenatal alcohol exposure.

Fetal Alcohol Syndrome

Fetal alcohol syndrome (FAS) refers to a group of physical, behavioral, and cognitive abnormalities that result from consumption of alcohol during pregnancy. It is the leading known cause of mental retardation and is 100% preventable (Eustace et al, 2003). CDC estimates that among the approximately 4 million infants born each year, an estimated 1000 to 6000 will be born with FAS. However, the actual prevalence of FAS is unknown as health care providers have not consistently recognized the effects of prenatal alcohol exposure on infants and children. In fact, up to 89% of cases are not diagnosed until a child is 6 years old. Disadvantaged groups, Native Americans, and other minorities have rates as high as 3 to 5 children with FAS per 1000 children. Mothers of children with FAS have a greater risk of having more children with FAS. If mothers continue to drink with successive pregnancies, children born later frequently have more profound effects of FAS (CDC, 2004d; Kvigne et al, 2003; Martinez et al, 2005; Stokowski, 2004).

The National Center on Birth Defects and Developmental Disabilities at the CDC, in collaboration with the National Task Force on Fetal Alcohol Syndrome (FAS) and Fetal Alcohol Effects (FAE) has developed a new set of guidelines for diagnosis and referral of infants and children with FAS. The primary goal of these guidelines was to provide standard diagnostic criteria so that consistency in the diagnosis can be established for clinicians, scientists, and service providers. The guidelines are based on scientific research, clinical expertise, and family input regarding the physical and neuropsychologic features of FAS (CDC, 2004d; Stokowski, 2004).

The guidelines state that a diagnosis of FAS requires the presence of three criteria: (1) documentation of all three facial abnormalities (smooth philtrum, thin vermillion border, and small palpebral fissures); (2) documentation of growth deficits (height, weight, or both at or below the 10th percentile); and (3) documentation of CNS abnormalities (structural, neurologic, or functional, or combination thereof) (Box 21-3) (CDC, 2004d; Stokowski, 2004).

FAS is diagnosed from maternal history and physical findings of the infant or child. No laboratory tests are available for clinical use to quantify the extent of prenatal alcohol exposure. Additionally, there are no clinical methods for validating maternal self-reporting of alcohol use, quantifying the level of fetal exposure, or predicting future disability after fetal exposure. The CDC recommends that developmental screening be implemented to improve children's health and help them reach their full potential. A framework was developed to provide an overview of the entire process, including the identification, referral, diagnosis, and treatment process (Figures 21-1 and 21-2) (CDC, 2004d; Martinez et al, 2005).

Fetal Alcohol Spectrum Disorders

The term *fetal alcohol effects* was originally used to describe children who had some, but not all, of the characteristics of FAS. This description was problematic because it could not be proved or disproved in any given case. Additionally, it was vague, allowing for broad interpretation by clinicians, making it clinically useless. More recently, the term *fetal alcohol spectrum disorder* (FASD) has been used to include all categories of prenatal alcohol exposure, including FAS. However, FASD is an umbrella term describing the range of effects that can occur in an individual exposed prenatally to alcohol and is not

---

BOX 21-3

Brief Outline of Diagnostic Criteria for Fetal Alcohol Syndrome

Facial Dysmorphia
Based on racial norms, individual exhibits all three characteristic facial features:
- Smooth philtrum (University of Washington Lip-Philtrum Guide rank 4 or 5)
- Thin vermillion border (University of Washington Lip-Philtrum Guide rank 4 or 5)
- Small palpebral fissures (at or below 10th percentile)

Growth Problems
Confirmed prenatal or postnatal height or weight, or both, at or below the 10th percentile, documented at any one point in time (adjusted for age, sex, gestational age, and race or ethnicity).

Central Nervous System Abnormalities
I. Structural
1. Head circumference (OFC) at or below the 10th percentile adjusted for age and sex.
2. Clinically significant brain abnormalities observable through imaging.

II. Neurological
Neurological problems not due to a postnatal insult or fever, or other soft neurological signs outside normal limits.

III. Functional
Performance substantially below that expected for an individual's age, schooling, or circumstances, as evidenced by:
1. *Global cognitive or intellectual deficits representing multiple domains of deficit (or significant developmental delay in younger children) with performance below the 3rd percentile (2 standard deviations below the mean for standardized testing)*
   or
2. *Functional deficits below the 16th percentile (1 standard deviation below the mean for standardized testing) in at least three of the following domains:*
   a. cognitive or developmental deficits or discrepancies
   b. executive functioning deficits
   c. motor functioning delays
   d. problems with attention or hyperactivity
   e. social skills
   f. mother, such as sensory problems, pragmatic language problems, memory deficits, etc.

Maternal Alcohol Exposure
I. Confirmed prenatal alcohol exposure
II. Unknown prenatal alcohol exposure

Criteria for FAS Diagnosis
Requires all three of the following findings:
1. Documentation of all three facial abnormalities (smooth philtrum, thin vermillion border, and small palpebral fissures)
2. Documentation of growth deficits
3. Documentatation of CNS abnormality

From National Center on Birth Defects and Developmental Disabilities (July 2004). *Fetal alcohol syndrome: guidelines for referral and diagnosis* (p 20). Atlanta: Centers for Disease Control and Prevention, Department of Health and Human Services.

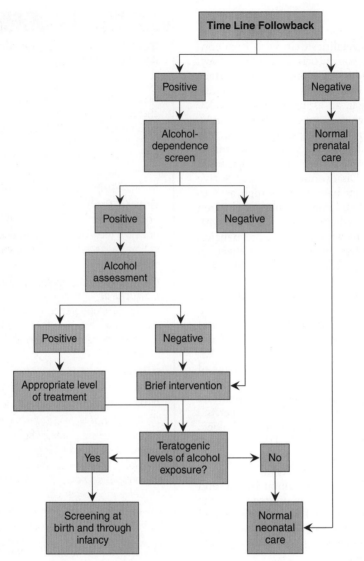

FIGURE **21-1**
Screening for alcohol consumption during pregnancy and the time line followback calendar (TLFC). From Savage C et al (2003). Current screening instruments related to alcohol consumption in pregnancy and a proposed alternative method. *Journal of obstetric, gynecologic, and neonatal nursing* 32(4):437-446.

meant to be used as a clinical diagnosis. Research is ongoing in an attempt to further refine the FAS criteria and potentially delineate additional diagnostic categories and criteria for alcohol-related conditions (CDC, 2004d; Hoyme et al, 2005; Warren & Foudin, 2001; Welch-Carre, 2005). Refer to the Evolve website for additional information. **evolve**

Neurobehavioral Effects

Adverse behavioral effects in children exposed prenatally to alcohol have been well documented. A study by Sood and associates (2001) evaluated the dose-response effect of prenatal alcohol exposure for adverse behavior outcomes at 6 to 7 years of age. Using the Achenbach Child Behavior Checklist, they found that externalizing (aggression and delinquent) behaviors were most significantly affected. Effects were observed at levels of exposure as low as one drink per week. Effects on the Delinquent behavior and Total Problem scores were not observed until there was moderate/heavy levels of exposure.

Children with any prenatal alcohol exposure were 3.2 times as likely to have increased Delinquent behavior scores. The adverse behaviors persisted after controlling for any potential confounders. These results suggest that adverse effects of prenatal alcohol exposure are evident at much lower levels than previously reported.

Infants exposed prenatally to alcohol also demonstrate areas of delay in various areas of development, including language and fine and gross motor development. Head banging and body rocking are often seen. They do not do well with changes and transitions. Also seen is habituation, the lessening of response to repetitive stimuli (Jones & Bass, 2003; Sokol, 2003).

Effects on Children and Adults

Effects of prenatal alcohol exposure present in various forms as these children grow. The effects on older children and adults are discussed in greater detail on the Evolve website. **evolve**

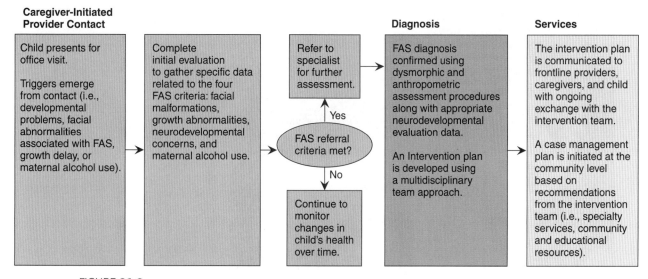

Caregiver-Initiated Provider Contact

Child presents for office visit.

Triggers emerge from contact (i.e., developmental problems, facial abnormalities associated with FAS, growth delay, or maternal alcohol use).

Complete initial evaluation to gather specific data related to the four FAS criteria: facial malformations, growth abnormalities, neurodevelopmental concerns, and maternal alcohol use.

Refer to specialist for further assessment.

FAS referral criteria met?

Yes

No

Continue to monitor changes in child's health over time.

Diagnosis

FAS diagnosis confirmed using dysmorphic and anthropometric assessment procedures along with appropriate neurodevelopmental evaluation data.

An Intervention plan is developed using a multidisciplinary team approach.

Services

The intervention plan is communicated to frontline providers, caregivers, and child with ongoing exchange with the intervention team.

A case management plan is initiated at the community level based on recommendations from the intervention team (i.e., specialty services, community and educational resources).

FIGURE **21-2**
Framework for FAS diagnosis and services. From National Center on Birth Defects and Developmental Disabilities (July 2004). *Fetal alcohol syndrome: guidelines for referral and diagnosis*, Atlanta: Centers for Disease Control and Prevention, Department of Health and Human Services.

Physical characteristics associated with fetal alcohol syndrome and alcohol exposure include microcephaly and prenatal and postnatal growth deficiency. Craniofacial abnormalities include the following: short palpebral fissures, maxillary hypoplasia with relative prognathism, and epicanthal folds (Figures 21-3, 21-4, and 21-5). As a child reaches puberty, these physical characteristics become less noticeable. However, behavioral, emotional, and social problems become more obvious. The foremost deficits are memory impairment and problems with judgment and abstract reasoning (Eustace et al, 2003; Jones & Bass, 2003; Sokol, 2003).

Studies have shown that removing children with FAS from homes with alcoholic parents and placing them into foster or

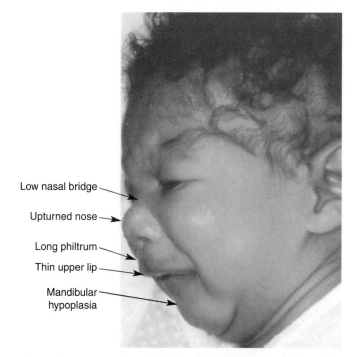

Low nasal bridge

Upturned nose

Long philtrum

Thin upper lip

Mandibular hypoplasia

FIGURE **21-3**
Facial features of a 1-month-old infant (side view). Note low nasal bridge, upturned nose, long philtrum, thin upper lip, and mandibular hypoplasia. From Jones MW, Bass WT (2003). Fetal alcohol syndrome. *Neonatal network* 22(3):64.

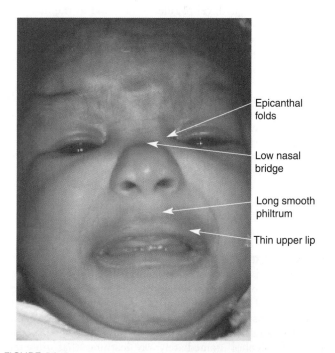

Epicanthal folds

Low nasal bridge

Long smooth philtrum

Thin upper lip

FIGURE **21-4**
Facial features of a 1-month-old infant (front view). Note epicanthal folds, low nasal bridge, long smooth philtrum, and thin upper lip. From Jones MW, Bass WT (2003). Fetal alcohol syndrome. *Neonatal network* 22(3):64.

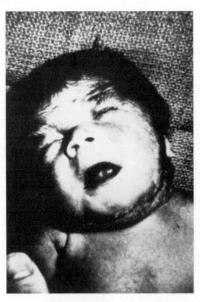
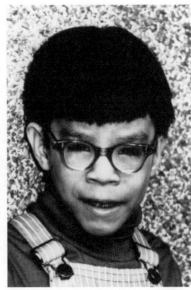
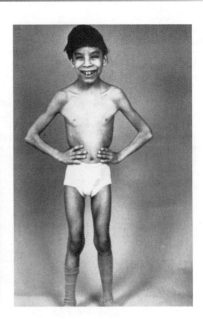

FIGURE **21-5**
Fetal alcohol syndrome (FAS). From Streissguth AP et al (1985). Natural history of the fetal alcohol syndrome: a 10-year follow-up of eleven patients. *Lancet* 2(8445):85-91.

adoptive homes did not improve their intellectual or cognitive outcomes. However, there appeared to be an improvement in their social and emotional development when their home environments became more stable (Eustace et al, 2003; Jones & Bass, 2003).

Breastfeeding
When a lactating woman consumes alcohol, less than 2% of the alcohol dose reaches her milk. Alcohol is not stored in breast milk, but its level parallels that found in the maternal blood. Thus, as long as the mother has substantial blood alcohol levels, the breast milk will also contain alcohol. Pumping the breasts and discarding the milk immediately after drinking alcohol does not speed up the disappearance of alcohol. The newly produced breast milk will still contain alcohol as long as the mother has measurable blood levels. Peak alcohol levels occur approximately one-half hour to an hour after drinking and decrease thereafter. Therefore, mothers should not attempt to nurse for several hours after drinking. Instead, they should wait until their blood alcohol levels have declined. Currently, the American Academy of Pediatrics considers maternal alcohol use to be compatible with breastfeeding, although it recognizes that adverse effects can occur (American Academy of Pediatrics Policy Statement, 2001c; Mennella, 2001).

Recommendations
No threshold for alcohol's detrimental effects on the developing fetal brain has been established. Therefore, the American Academy of Pediatrics and the American College of Obstetricians and Gynecologists (ACOG) recommend complete abstinence during pregnancy. Women should cease to drink alcohol immediately on learning that they are pregnant. Ideally, women who are contemplating pregnancy should consider changing their drinking habits even before conception. Accordingly, educational efforts should be directed particularly toward young women who may engage in

binge-drinking patterns that might lead to unplanned pregnancies (Chang et al, 2005; Maier & West, 2001).

A study by Chang and colleagues (2005) tested the effectiveness of a brief intervention in the reduction of prenatal alcohol consumption by women when their partners were included. They found that brief interventions most significantly reduced alcohol consumption for those women with the highest consumption initially. Furthermore, the effects were significantly enhanced with the participation of the woman's partner.

FAS can be devastating to society both financially and emotionally, yet it is 100% preventable. It is imperative that physicians receive comprehensive education in this field, not only to help prevent FAS, but also in early detection, which can lead to interventions that can improve the quality of life of these affected children. Refer to the Evolve website for additional recommendations. **evolve**

COCAINE
History
Cocaine, the primary alkaloid extract from the leaves of the *Erythroxylon coca* plant, is a highly psychoactive stimulant with a long history of abuse. The leaves of the coca plant, indigenous to the mountains of Central and South America, has been chewed or made into a stimulant tea for centuries by the natives of these areas to decrease fatigue and hunger. The euphoria-producing effect of cocaine was exploited extensively in the United States in the late 19th and early 20th centuries when it was an active ingredient in numerous over-the-counter elixirs and tonics used to treat a wide variety of illnesses. Before the adverse effects were recognized, it was a major ingredient in the original Coca-Cola (The Coca-Cola Company, Atlanta, GA) (Askin & Diehl-Jones, 2001; Hurt, 2005; Martinez et al, 2005; NIDA, 2005b).

Until the mid-1980s, cocaine was considered an expensive and exotic drug used primarily by the affluent as well as a performance enhancer by those in the sports and entertainment fields. Its reputation as a glamour drug, the widely held misconception that cocaine is nonaddicting, and the development and marketing of crack; a cheap version of cocaine, were key factors in the resurgence of drug use.

In 2002, the National Survey on Drug Use and Health (USDHHS, 2005a) estimated 1.5 million Americans could be classified as dependent on or abusing cocaine in the past 12 months. The same survey estimated there were 2 million current (past-month) users. Adults 18 to 25 years old had the highest rate of current cocaine use, with an estimated 13% of women using cocaine regularly (NIDA, 2004; Hurt, 2005; Martinez et al, 2005). Additional history can be found on the Evolve website. **_evolve_**

Mechanism of Action

Cocaine is a central nervous system stimulant that inhibits postsynaptic reuptake of norepinephrine, dopamine, and serotonin neurotransmitters by sympathetic nerve terminals, allowing higher concentrations of neurotransmitters to interact with receptors. Higher levels of norepinephrine lead to vasoconstriction, tachycardia, and hypertension while increased levels of dopamine produce euphoria or enhanced feeling of well-being, hyperactivity, decreased appetite, and sexual excitement. However, the prolonged use of cocaine leads to dopamine depletion, dysphoria, depression, and drug craving (Martinez et al, 2005; Hurt, 2005; Rosen & Bateman, 2002). Tryptophan uptake is similarly inhibited, altering serotonin pathways. This affects the sleep-wake cycle, leading to a diminished need for sleep (Askin & Diehl-Jones, 2001; Martinez et al, 2005; Rosen & Bateman, 2002).

Cocaine is metabolized by enzymes in the liver and plasma, called cholinesterases. These enzymes transform cocaine into two main derivatives: benzoylecgonine and ethyl methylecgonine. Both are water-soluble and are excreted in urine and sweat. Crack cocaine is metabolized into anhydroecgonine methyl ester and is also detectable in urine (Askin & Diehl-Jones, 2001; Rosen & Bateman, 2002).

Norcocaine, another metabolite of cocaine, is produced in the liver by the cytochrome P450 system. Although norcocaine is produced in minor quantities, it has significant toxic effects and has been implicated in neurologic damage and macrophage dysfunction. Additionally, norcocaine causes hepatic damage, thus compromising the further metabolism of cocaine by liver enzymes (Askin & Diehl-Jones, 2001; Rosen & Bateman, 2002).

It has been estimated that as many as 90% of cocaine users concomitantly consume alcohol. The human liver combines cocaine and alcohol, producing a third substance, cocaethylene. Cocaethylene is pharmacologically similar to cocaine but is reported to be 10 times more potent than cocaine alone, which suggests that it is more toxic in its effects on the growing fetus. Cocaethylene has a much longer duration of action and even greater physiologic effects, particularly on heart rate and blood pressure. As a result, the euphoric effects of cocaine are intensified but the risk of sudden death is potentially increased (Askin & Diehl-Jones, 2001; NIDA, 2005b; Rosen & Bateman, 2002; Weiner & Finnegan, 2002).

Routes of Administration

Basically, there are two chemical forms of cocaine: the hydrochloride salt and the "freebase." Cocaine hydrochloride is a water-soluble white powder that can be used orally, intranasally, or intravenously. Freebase refers to the compound that has not been neutralized by an acid to make the hydrochloride salt. Crack cocaine, the most widely available form of freebase, is processed with ammonia or baking soda and heated to remove the hydrochloride, resulting in a paste that, once dried, forms a hard, rocklike substance that can be smoked. The term "crack" is derived from the crackling sound that is generated when it is prepared or smoked (Askin & Diehl-Jones, 2001; Martinez et al, 2005; NIDA, 2005b).

The euphoric effects of cocaine include hyperstimulation, reduced fatigue, and mental clarity. The duration of these effects depends on the route of administration; the faster the absorption, the more intense the high. On the other hand, the faster the absorption, the shorter the duration of effects (NIDA, 2005b).

Snorting is the process of inhaling cocaine powder through the nostrils, where it is absorbed into the bloodstream through the nasal tissues. The high achieved from snorting cocaine may last 15 to 30 minutes. Intravenous, also called _mainlining_ or _injecting_, releases the drug directly into the bloodstream and heightens the intensity of its effects. Smoking involves the inhalation of cocaine vapor or smoke into the lungs. Crack is almost pure cocaine. When it is smoked, it quickly enters the bloodstream, producing levels similar to those achieved by intravenous use. The user experiences a high in less than 10 seconds while the high may last 5 to 10 minutes. This almost immediate and euphoric effect is one of the reasons crack has become so popular. However, because the high is so short-lived, crack use becomes more frequent and quickly leads to addiction. Furthermore, a tolerance to the "high" may develop. Many addicts report that they fail to achieve the same degree of pleasure as they did with their first exposure. Thus, some users will increase their doses or add additional drugs to intensify and prolong the euphoric effects and alleviate the unpleasant down periods as the drug effects wear off (Askin & Diehl-Jones, 2001; Martinez et al, 2005; NIDA, 2005b; Rosen & Bateman, 2002).

Adverse Effects of Cocaine

Use of cocaine in a binge, during which the drug is taken repetitively and at increasingly high doses, can lead to a state of increasing irritability, restlessness, and paranoia. This can lead to full-blown paranoid psychosis, where the user loses touch with reality and experiences auditory hallucinations (Martinez et al, 2005; NIDA, 2005b).

Cocaine has also been associated with cardiac arrhythmias, cardiac arrest, myocardial infarction, cerebral hemorrhage, seizures, headaches, and intestinal ischemia. Chronic cocaine use is associated with anorexia and poor nutrition (Martinez et al, 2005; NIDA, 2005b).

Different means of cocaine administration can produce different adverse effects. Regularly snorting cocaine can cause a loss of sense of smell, nosebleeds, difficulty swallowing, hoarseness, and a chronically runny nose. Ingestion of cocaine can cause intestinal gangrene due to decreased blood flow. People who inject cocaine can have allergic reactions and are at increased risk for contracting HIV and other blood borne diseases (NIDA, 2005b).

Effects on Pregnancy

Cocaine easily and rapidly crosses the placenta by simple diffusion because it is of low molecular weight and lipophilic.

However, it is not significantly metabolized during maternal-fetal transfer. As a result, once it is in the fetal circulation, cocaine and its metabolites are widely distributed and are detectable in a variety of human fetal tissues. Although studies indicate that fetal brain and plasma levels of cocaine are approximately one-third those of the mother, it is clear that the fetus is at considerable risk of exposure through maternal consumption (Askin & Diehl-Jones, 2001; Hurt, 2005; Martinez et al, 2005; Rosen & Bateman, 2002).

Maternal cardiovascular adaptation to pregnancy appears to influence the physiologic responses to cocaine, and pregnancy appears to increase the toxicity of cocaine. Animal studies demonstrated changes in maternal and fetal blood pressure, uterine blood flow, and uterine vascular resistance after cocaine was administered to a pregnant ewe. There was a dose-dependent decrease in uterine blood flow and an increase in uterine vascular resistance shortly after the ewe was injected with cocaine. The maternal systolic blood pressure increased within 1 minute and returned to baseline in about 10 minutes. Fetal blood pressure also increased, lagging behind the maternal changes by several minutes. Of greater concern, significant fetal hypoxemia was associated with these changes (Askin & Diehl-Jones, 2001; Hurt, 2005; Martinez et al, 2005; Rosen & Bateman, 2002).

After maternal ingestion, the fetus showed hypoxemia, tachycardia, and hypertension. On the other hand, direct administration of cocaine to the fetus caused an increase in heart rate and blood pressure, but no changes in fetal oxygenation. Thus, it appears that the hypoxemic effects related to uterine artery vasoconstriction may make maternal ingestion more detrimental to fetal health than if the drug were given directly to the fetus (Askin & Diehl-Jones, 2001; Rosen & Bateman, 2002).

Animal studies have also shown decreased cholinesterase levels during pregnancy in both mother and fetus, resulting in a slower rate of metabolism of cocaine. Additionally, the N-demethylation pathway is more active during pregnancy, leading to a higher concentration of norcocaine in the urine. It is also thought that amniotic fluid may serve as a reservoir for cocaine and its metabolites, thus prolonging exposure to vasoactive compounds (Martinez et al, 2005; Rosen & Bateman, 2002).

Maternal use of cocaine has been associated with several complications, including a higher risk for stillbirths, spontaneous abortions, abruptio placentae, IUGR, anemia, and malnutrition. There is also an increased risk of maternal death from intracerebral hemorrhage, most likely due to acute hypertensive events. Cocaine directly stimulates uterine contractions because of its alpha-adrenergic, prostaglandin, or dopaminergic effects, resulting in greater risks for fetal distress and premature births. Abruptio placentae appears to be related to cocaine only when the drug is used shortly before delivery (Bauer et al, 2002; Campbell, 2003; Martinez et al, 2005; Rosen & Bateman, 2002).

Effects on the Fetus and Newborn

Although numerous clinical studies have linked prenatal cocaine use with a variety of adverse fetal effects, methodologic limitations have made it difficult to establish a causal relationship between these effects and maternal cocaine use. Not only are the timing, frequency, and dose of cocaine difficult to determine, but also, harmful effects related to low socioeconomic status, poor nutrition, polydrug use, infections, and a lack of prenatal care are difficult to dissociate from effects of cocaine use alone.

Consequently, the issue of how much risk to the fetus is associated with cocaine use during pregnancy is unresolved. Over the years, the results of clinical studies have produced somewhat conflicting outcomes. It is well documented that initial predictions of catastrophic effects of prenatal cocaine exposure were exaggerated. Current research suggests that the effects of cocaine on development are inconsistent and subtle and need to be understood in the context of polydrug use and the caregiving environment. However, the media has portrayed the so-called "crack kids" as inevitably and permanently damaged cognitively, as well as morally and emotionally troubled. Despite recent studies that have failed to show catastrophic effects of prenatal cocaine exposure, attitudes and public policies still reflect the belief that cocaine is a uniquely dangerous teratogen. This has led to some children being unfairly stigmatized by the public, including educators and health care professionals (Bandstra et al, 2001; Bauer et al, 2002; Behnke et al, 2001; Frank et al, 2001; Lester et al, 2002; Zuckerman et al, 2002).

Cocaine-exposed infants are about twice as likely to require admission to the NICU. These infants have a higher incidence of low birth weight, smaller head circumference, and prematurity with associated complications. The adverse effects of cocaine are thought to result primarily from vascular disruptive events due to the vasoconstrictive effects of cocaine on both the maternal and fetal vasculature, with the most consistently found fetal effect being growth retardation. Additionally, poor maternal nutritional status and decreased nutritional intake, decreased placental nutrient transfer associated with diminished uterine artery perfusion, interference with placental amino acid transport, and direct inhibition of cell differentiation and proliferation, particularly in the central nervous system, most likely act in conjunction with the vasoconstriction to cause these effects (Askin & Diehl-Jones, 2001; Hurt, 2005; Martinez et al, 2005; Rosen & Bateman, 2002; Ward et al, 2002).

Premature Birth

Generally, cocaine-exposed infants are born 1 to 2 weeks earlier than unexposed infants. The earlier delivery may be related to the direct alpha-adrenergic effect of cocaine causing uterine contractions, to placental abruption, or to increased rates of maternal infection (Rosen & Bateman, 2002). However, not all studies have been able to demonstrate a clear-cut link between cocaine use and premature delivery, instead suggesting that a more precise explanation would be a combination of polydrug use and environmental factors. In populations studied where the mother received good prenatal care in association with drug treatment, the incidence of prematurity was low. In the presence of poor prenatal care and no drug treatment, the frequency of prematurity was high (Askin & Diehl-Jones, 2001; Martinez et al, 2005).

Cerebral Effects

There have been conflicting reports regarding the effects of prenatal cocaine exposure on the developing brain. Studies using cranial ultrasonography and computed tomography scans have demonstrated a greater incidence of hemorrhagic infarcts, cystic lesions, intraventricular hemorrhages, and echodensities, especially in infants whose mothers were heavy users of cocaine. These defects are possibly related to the vascular disruptive effects of cocaine. Increased cerebral arterial blood flow has been described during the first few days of life that has been thought to place the infant at greater risk. However, other studies have failed to prove an association between cocaine exposure and these abnormalities. Given that the results have been inconsistent, further research is needed (Hurt, 2005; Rosen & Bateman, 2002).

Smith and colleagues (2001) used proton magnetic resonance spectroscopy in an attempt to identify possible neurotoxic effects of prenatal cocaine on the developing brain. They found increased creatine levels in the frontal white matter with normal N-acetyl-containing compounds in the absence of structural changes or atrophy. These findings suggest biochemical alterations at the cellular level in response to cocaine exposure, although their implications for long-term outcomes are unclear. Additional studies are needed to explore the significance of these abnormalities in energy metabolism in the brain.

Abnormal electroencephalograms (EEGs) and visual evoked potentials have been documented in cocaine-exposed infants, although follow-up EEGs were within normal limits after 2 to 12 months. Clinical seizures have also been reported, possibly due to toxicity from cocaine metabolites. Subsequent studies, however, were unable to confirm a relationship. In the clinical setting, neonatal seizures stemming directly from maternal use of cocaine are rare, and if they occur, are most likely due to complications associated with maternal abuse (Hurt, 2005; Martinez et al, 2005; Rosen & Bateman, 2002).

A study by Lester and associates (2003) examined the auditory brainstem response (ABR) of cocaine-exposed infants at 1 month of age. The ABR provides an index of brainstem transmission time and reflects the functional integrity of the central nervous system (CNS). After adjusting for covariates of alcohol, marijuana, tobacco, gestational age at birth, and social class, the results demonstrated changes in interpeak latencies, indicating prolongation in neural transmission and delayed brainstem maturation with heavy cocaine exposure. Although it is not clear if these effects are transient, even transient trauma to the functional integrity of the CNS could have long-term consequences by disrupting emerging behavioral processes.

Tan-Laxa and colleagues (2004) also demonstrated prolonged peak latencies in the ABRs of infants exposed prenatally to cocaine, reflecting an abnormality in the peripheral auditory system. These results reflect delayed or desynchronized transmission of auditory information along the brainstem auditory pathway. It is possible that cocaine may have a direct and indirect effect on the auditory system resulting in the abnormal ABR. Animal studies have demonstrated a direct toxic effect on the organ of Corti, causing damage during critical periods of development, resulting in the prolonged latencies. Human studies have shown that cocaine induced a toxic effect on the brainstem auditory neurons, causing impairment in synaptic efficiency and prolongation of interpeak latencies. Conversely, other studies have reported no apparent effects of cocaine on the auditory system in otherwise healthy, term infants.

It has also been hypothesized that the abnormalities in the fetal auditory system may be secondary to the vasoconstrictive effects of cocaine, leading to placental insufficiency and ischemic injury to the developing brain and the auditory system, which is especially sensitive to oxygen deprivation. Currently, it is not known whether these abnormalities are transient or permanent. Nonetheless, cocaine-exposed infants should be considered high-risk for auditory system dysfunction (Tan-Laxa et al, 2004)

Intrauterine Growth Restriction (IUGR)/ Low Birth Weight (LBW)

In utero exposure to cocaine is reported to be associated with increased incidence of LBW. A decrease in uterine blood flow together with fetal hypoxemia is regarded as the cause of IUGR in cocaine-exposed infants. However, some investigators suggest that the growth restriction is more likely multifactorial. As discussed earlier, other sources most likely include poor maternal nutritional status, decreased placental nutrients, interference with placental amino acid transport, and direct inhibition of cell differentiation and proliferation (Askin & Diehl-Jones, 2001; Bada et al, 2002b; Hurt, 2005; Martinez et al, 2005; Rosen & Bateman, 2002; Ward et al, 2002).

Frank and associates (2001) reviewed outcomes in early childhood after prenatal cocaine exposure. After controlling for confounders, there was no consistent negative association between cocaine and physical growth. Most of their findings could be explained in part by other factors, including multi-drug exposure and environmental quality.

In opposition, results of a study by Bandstra and associates (2001) reported cocaine-associated growth deficits in full-term infants. These deficits were not seen in the drug-free neonates or those exposed prenatally only to tobacco, alcohol, or marijuana. Evidence showed that some of the cocaine effects on fetal growth were direct while some were indirect via the influence of cocaine on gestational age.

Behnke and colleagues (2001) examined the association between prenatal cocaine exposure and identifiable abnormalities. Although they were unable to identify a pattern of malformations, they did find that the cocaine-exposed infants were significantly smaller in birth weight, length, and head circumference. They did not differ on remaining anthropometric measurements.

As part of the Maternal Lifestyle Study, Bada and colleagues (2002b) looked at the effects of cocaine exposure on intrauterine growth. They concluded that in utero cocaine exposure is associated with fetal growth restriction involving all birth measurements, becoming more pronounced with advancing gestation. Bada's study found that growth measurements were significantly decreased in those mothers with poor socioeconomic status. Higher growth measurements were noted in infants born after 32 weeks' gestation whose mothers had adequate prenatal care, although an inverse relationship was found between prenatal care and growth during gestations of less than 32 weeks. Maternal weight gain during pregnancy was not significantly related to growth measurements.

Shankaran and associates (2004) studied the effects of maternal substance use on growth parameters at birth. They found that infant birth weight, length, and head circumference were lower in the presence of multidrug use, with tobacco having the greatest effect on all three parameters. Cocaine appeared to affect only birth weight and head circumference. Low cocaine use throughout pregnancy was associated with a negative effect on birth weight that was similar to that of high tobacco use.

Although results are conflicting, growth restriction due to prenatal cocaine exposure continues to be an accepted consequence. It is felt that this growth restriction occurs later in gestation and may be reversible with catch-up growth occurring by 12 to 18 months (Askin & Diehl-Jones, 2001; Rosen & Bateman, 2002).

Cardiac Effects

Arrhythmias are frequently seen with cocaine exposure. Ventricular tachycardia and conduction disturbances are the most common and are often markedly resistant to conventional therapy (Behnke et al, 2001; Hurt, 2005; Martinez et al, 2005; Mone et al, 2004; Rosen & Bateman, 2002). Refer to the Evolve website for additional information. **evolve**

Gastrointestinal Effects

Prenatal cocaine exposure has been associated with several gastrointestinal problems, including necrotizing enterocolitis and intestinal perforation. Because of the vasoconstrictive effects of cocaine, there is an alteration of fetal intestinal blood flow resulting in ischemic/hypoxic events. Alpha-2 adrenergic receptors are thought to play a role in the autoregulatory mechanism in the newborn intestine that responds to hypoxia and ischemia (Hurt, 2005; Martinez et al, 2005). Ward and associates (2002) examined the expression of this receptor in embryonic rats exposed to high and low dose cocaine in utero. They found a significant decrease in the α-2 receptor expression in the intestine of both the low-dose and high-dose rats. These changes may limit the normal adaptation to vasoconstriction, thus exacerbating the already insufficient compensatory mechanisms for responding to ischemic injury, and may predispose the cocaine-exposed infant to necrotizing enterocolitis (Askin & Diehl-Jones, 2001).

Ophthalmic Effects

Alterations in the visual system have been observed after prenatal exposure to cocaine. Ocular abnormalities include retinopathy, persistent hyperplastic vitreous, dilated and tortuous iris blood vessels, delayed visual maturation, and palpebral edema as well as structural abnormalities. All defects are thought to be a consequence of the hypertensive, vasoconstrictive, ischemic, hemorrhagic effects of cocaine (Martinez et al, 2005).

Cocaine as a Teratogen

Cocaine has been implicated as a potential teratogen when ingested during pregnancy. Although it is difficult to document this definitively because of confounding variables such as polydrug use, correlations between the use of cocaine and congenital anomalies must be considered. Animal studies have described fetal vascular disruption, believed to be secondary to an interruption of blood flow. If the blood supply is compromised by vasoconstriction during a critical period of organogenesis, impaired oxygenation and nutrition of fetal tissue may result. This impairment during a critical time in organ formation may restrict the growth and development of developing cells, with resultant disruption or absence of growth (Askin & Diehl-Jones, 2001; Behnke et al, 2001; Hurt, 2005; Martinez et al, 2005).

Cardiovascular abnormalities have been associated with prenatal cocaine exposure. These abnormalities, which include congenital cardiovascular malformations, abnormalities of ventricular structure and function, arrhythmias, and intracardiac conduction abnormalities, persist beyond the period of cocaine exposure. They may be associated with congestive heart failure, cardiorespiratory arrest, and death in some children (Behnke et al, 2001; Hurt, 2005; Martinez et al, 2005; Mone et al, 2004; Rosen & Bateman, 2002).

Cardiomyocytes are highly differentiated cells that rarely replicate after birth. Therefore, any agent that harms these cells during the fetal period can cause lasting damage. Loss of cardiomyocytes before birth may permanently decrease the number of functioning units in the heart, predisposing the myocardium to alterations that can lead to heart failure (Mone et al, 2004).

Cocaine has a direct cytotoxic effect in the fetal rat heart, inducing apoptosis ("cell suicide") in myocardial cells in a time- and dose-dependent manner. Although no similar data have been reported for humans, these findings in rats suggest that maternal cocaine use may permanently impair heart function even in children who do not develop frank anomalies (Mone et al, 2004).

Other anomalies include structural malformations of the eye, genitourinary malformations, limb reduction, and abdominal wall defects. However, at this time, no well-defined cocaine-associated syndrome has been identified and the teratogenic potential of cocaine remains controversial. The association between congenital malformations and fetal exposure may be confounded by polydrug use, including alcohol, tobacco, and marijuana. Overall, multiple studies have failed to demonstrate higher rates of anomalies associated with cocaine only (Behnke et al, 2001; Hurt, 2005; Martinez et al, 2005; Mone et al, 2004; Rosen & Bateman, 2002).

Long-Term Outcomes

As discussed earlier in this chapter, methodologic limitations have made it difficult to establish a causal relationship between adverse fetal effects and maternal cocaine use. Researchers continue to study children who were exposed prenatally to cocaine, looking for neurobehavioral and developmental changes.

Several studies performed over the past several years have been a part of the Maternal Lifestyle Study. The Maternal Lifestyle Study (MLS) is a multisite study by the National Institute of Child Health and Human Development (NICHD) Neonatal Intensive Care Unit Research Network. The purpose of the study is to examine the effects of prenatal drug exposure on child outcome. Thus far, the MLS is the largest clinical, prospective, longitudinal study of acute neonatal events and long-term health and developmental outcomes associated with cocaine use during pregnancy.

The Neonatal Intensive Care Unit Network Neurobehavioral Scale (NNNS) was developed for the NICHD as a part of the study because of concerns that existing instruments were not sensitive to the neurobehavioral effects of prenatal drug exposure and infants at risk. The NNNS will be discussed in greater detail later in this chapter.

Singer and associates (2001) studied children at 1 year of age who were exposed to cocaine prenatally, looking for an association of level of fetal cocaine exposure to developmental precursors of speech-language skills. Their results documented significant behavioral teratogenic effects on attentional abilities underlying auditory comprehension skills considered to be precursors of receptive language. Children who were more heavily exposed were more likely to be classified as mildly delayed in language skills. Most often delayed were localizing to sounds, visually following an object, attending to toys or books, and playing social games, all of which can easily be evaluated by parents or health care workers.

Another study by Singer and colleagues (2002) examined cocaine-exposed infants up to 24 months' corrected age in an attempt to assess the effects of cocaine on child developmental outcomes. The study found significant cognitive deficits, with cocaine-exposed children twice as likely to have significant delays throughout the first 2 years of life. The percentage of children with mild or greater delays requiring intervention was almost double the rate of the high-risk non-cocaine but polydrug-exposed comparison group. Cognitive delays could not be attributed to polydrug exposure or to other potentially confounding variables. Furthermore, poorer cognitive outcomes were related to higher amounts of cocaine metabolites in meconium as well as to maternal self-report of cocaine use. Because 2-year Mental Development Index scores are predictive of later cognitive outcomes, it is likely that these children will continue to have learning difficulties at school age.

A follow-up study by Singer and colleagues (2004) assessed the effects of prenatal cocaine exposure as well as the quality of the caregiving environment on 4-year cognitive outcomes. After controlling for confounding variables, prenatal cocaine exposure was not associated with lower full-scale, verbal, or performance IQ scores, but was associated with an increased risk of specific cognitive impairments and lower likelihood of IQ above the normative mean at 4 years. However, higher concentrations of cocaine metabolites in infant meconium were significantly related to lower verbal IQ and arithmetic scores. These results are consistent with other studies of preschool cocaine-exposed children in which specific, but not global, IQ deficits were found. Also negatively affected was the acquisition of general knowledge. It is hypothesized that cocaine may affect later learning by negatively regulating neuronal path finding and ultimately, synaptic activity through the disruption of dopaminergic and noradrenergic systems prenatally.

Of significant interest is the influence of the caregiving environment on the performance of cocaine-exposed children. When covariates were examined, the quality of the environment was the strongest independent predictor of outcomes. The children in foster or adoptive care had higher scores than those in biologic maternal or relative care. Results showed that the children in foster or adoptive care lived in more stimulating home environments and their caregivers had better vocabulary scores when compared with children living with their families. The children in foster or adoptive care also demonstrated verbal, performance, and full-scale IQs equivalent to those of nonexposed children, whereas those in biologic maternal or relative care had lower full-scale and performance IQ scores than nonexposed children, in spite of the fact that children in foster or adoptive care had twice the severity of cocaine exposure. Additionally, children in foster or adoptive care had the lowest occurrence of IQ scores in the range of mental retardation and were similar to nonexposed children. These findings underscore the beneficial effects of environmental intervention in the prevention of mental retardation for cocaine-exposed children. Drug treatment and education for pregnant, drug-abusing women along with intensive intervention for their infants are essential to help maximize the future well-being of these families (Singer et al, 2004).

As part of the MLS, Lester and associates (2002) studied the effects of prenatal cocaine exposure on neurobehavioral outcomes in term and preterm infants at 1 month of age. They found that cocaine exposure was related to lower arousal and higher excitability, resulting in poor self-regulation. Poor regulation and higher excitability appeared to be attributable to heavy cocaine exposure, and the lowest arousal scores were in the some-cocaine-exposure but not in the heavy-exposure group, suggesting that specific neurobehavioral syndromes may be related to level of exposure. Higher doses of cocaine may produce excitable infants, whereas, lower doses may lead to lethargic infants. Also found were infants with poorer quality of movement, more hypertonia, and more nonoptimal reflexes with most effects maintained after adjustment for covariates. No effects of stress or abstinence were found to be attributable to cocaine exposure.

In earlier studies, acoustical analysis of cry has been related to prenatal polydrug use, including cocaine. Measures of cry acoustics reflect mechanisms that mediate cry production, including central nervous system reactivity, respiratory control, and sound characteristics related to neural control of the vocal tract (Lester et al, 2004). A study by Lester and associates (2002) found a louder, higher pitched cry with less resonance in the upper vocal tract in cocaine-exposed infants and more turbulence in the cry signal with heavy exposure. However, after adjusting for covariates, these effects were not observed, suggesting they are not attributable to cocaine only, but are a product of polydrug exposure.

Subtle effects of prenatal cocaine exposure were also demonstrated in this study. Although small reliable differences were attributable to drug exposure, they are not necessarily deficits. Although these findings do not provide evidence of a clinically significant disorder, they do have short-term and long-term implications. The short-term importance of these findings is that they reflect neurobehavioral vulnerability that may be exacerbated by the caregiving environment. Because many drug-exposed infants grow up in nonoptimal environments, small differences can become exaggerated and develop into significant deficits. If these infants are considered "at risk," interventions can be initiated that may help prevent more serious deficits later in life. The long-term implications are that cocaine may affect areas of the brain that are not evident until these children reach school age. Therefore, it is imperative that children exposed prenatally to drugs continue to be followed, and that health care professionals remain open to the possibility that even subtle findings in infancy may be a indication of more serious long-term deficits (Lester et al, 2002).

Bada and associates (2002a) studied infants exposed to cocaine and opiates to determine the risk for central nervous system/autonomic nervous system (CNS/ANS) changes. Although there was a lower prevalence of CNS/ANS signs than in other reports, they did find that cocaine exposure was associated with increased likelihood of manifesting a constellation of CNS/ANS signs, an effect independent of opiate exposure. The infants with confirmed cocaine exposure were more likely to have jitteriness, tremors, irritability, hypertonia, and high-pitched cry and were difficult to console, findings that are consistent with other studies.

A study by White-Traut and associates (2002) compared responses of nonexposed and drug-exposed newborns to auditory, tactile, visual, and vestibular (ATVV) intervention. They hypothesized that this multisensory stimulation would improve behavioral state organization and autonomic function in infants exposed prenatally to illicit drugs, including cocaine. Results suggest that autonomic and behavioral function is disrupted in cocaine-exposed infants. However, the ATVV intervention appeared to modify the behavioral responses of the drug-exposed infants to be similar to those seen in non-exposed infants, both during and for 31 minutes after the intervention was applied, suggesting that even a short-term delivery of the ATVV intervention modified the behavior. Although results from this study are encouraging, only a small sample of infants was used and the intervention occurred during early postnatal life when many physiologic and behavioral adjustments are normally occurring. However, it provides a basis for further research to determine whether the ATVV intervention throughout the early neonatal period could improve neurobehavioral function and have a positive impact on physiologic and behavioral function on a long-term basis.

Frank and colleagues (2001) reviewed multiple studies of cocaine-exposed infants, studying outcomes in early childhood in five domains, including physical growth, cognition, language skills, motor skills, and behavior, attention, affect, and neurophysiology. Their conclusions were that after controlling for confounders, there is no convincing evidence that prenatal cocaine exposure is associated with developmental toxicity different in severity, scope, or kind from the sequelae of many other risk factors among children aged 6 years or younger. Many findings once thought to be specific effects of cocaine can be explained in whole or in part by other factors such as polydrug use or quality of the environment.

Neurobehavioral

A variety of neurobehavioral changes have been reported in cocaine-exposed infants. Using the Brazelton Neonatal Behavioral Assessment Scale (NBAS), these infants were found to have decreased state organization, abnormal reflexes, and decreased habituation and are less able to orient to their environment. These infants are also described as being hypertonic, irritable, and tremulous, and they may have abnormal crying, sleep, and feeding patterns (Askin & Diehl-Jones, 2001; Campbell, 2003; Hurt, 2005; Martinez et al, 2005; Rosen & Bateman, 2002).

A study by Frank and associates (2002) looked at whether there is an independent association between the level of prenatal cocaine exposure and infants' developmental test scores after controlling for confounding variables and, if an association exists, what social and biologic variables may modify it. They found that heavier prenatal exposure is not an independent risk factor for depressed scores of the Bayley Scales of Infant Development (BSID) up to 24 months of age when compared to term infants with lighter or no exposure. However, they did find that cocaine-exposed infants with birth weight below the 10th percentile for gestational age and gender, as well as those placed with kinship caregivers, are at risk for less optimal developmental outcomes. Several possible factors may influence these findings. Clinical experience suggests that children in kinship care receive intervention only after more severe impairments have manifested themselves. Kinship caregivers usually receive less financial support and less monitoring from social service agencies than unrelated foster families, which is a potential factor in later intervention. Also, infants with heavier cocaine exposure experienced the greatest number of changes in caregivers and were most likely to be removed from the biologic mother's custody and placed with unrelated foster parents. These babies were most likely to have earlier developmental intervention, perhaps due to closer supervision and evaluation, leading to improved developmental outcomes. The findings of this study were consistent with those of previous studies that showed a beneficial impact of such interventions on cocaine-exposed infants.

Lester and associates (2004) presented the most recent descriptive statistics from the Maternal Lifestyle Study based on data from 1388 1-month-old infants. Results showed that prenatal cocaine exposure was related to lower arousal, poorer quality of movement and regulation, higher excitability, more hypertonia, and more nonoptimal reflexes, with most effects remaining after adjustment for covariates. Although this study has the advantage of a large sample size, there are limitations. The data are limited to the population studied and may not represent all drug-exposed infants. Also, there is no true unexposed group as a comparison group. This study is best thought of as a sample of infants at varying degrees of biologic or social risk. The results provide a reference on the neurobehavioral organization of drug-exposed infants and may be useful for researchers and clinicians as they further study this population and develop appropriate treatment programs.

LaGasse and associates (2003) evaluated feeding difficulties and maternal behavior of 1-month-old infants exposed prenatally to cocaine and/or opiates. Their goal was to test the hypothesis that these infants have abnormal sucking patterns and increased feeding problems, and that their mothers are less responsive. Previous research has described poor and disorganized feeding in infants exposed prenatally to cocaine. However, these results were not replicated in a second study with a larger sample. In this study, cocaine exposure was not associated with poor sucking or feeding, and exposed infants did not show disorganized, nonoptimal sucking rhythms or increased feeding problems. However, mothers of cocaine-exposed infants were less warm or engaged with their infants, showed less flexibility in response to their infants' cues, and had a shorter feeding session, suggesting less sensitivity and involvement with the infant during the feeding session. Feeding problems with cocaine-exposed infants appear to be related to the feeding interaction between mother and infant rather than to actual feeding problems in the infant. It is important for health care personnel to observe early feeding interactions in order to identify problems in the mother-infant relationship that could have long-term implications for poor weight gain and subsequent relationship difficulties.

Motor Development

The effects of prenatal cocaine exposure on motor function are controversial and varied. However, recent studies have suggested motor problems across the first 2 years of life in infants with in utero cocaine exposure. During the newborn period, problems such as coordination and hypertonicity were seen. Later in the first 2 years, significantly poorer gross and fine motor skills were found. A study by Miller-Loncar and associates (2005) examined the pattern of motor development across the first 18 months of life to determine how prenatal cocaine exposure related to motor development. They found that infants showed low motor skills at their initial assessment at 1 month of age but displayed significant increases over time with recovery to normal functioning by 18 months of age. This pattern suggests an early neurotoxic effect that recovers.

Although the most recent studies have failed to demonstrate the predictions of catastrophic effects of prenatal cocaine exposure, results suggest there are long-term neurobehavioral changes, although there is not a definitive consensus as to what the exact problems entail. Several things are becoming clear. Most of the abnormalities found in cocaine-exposed infants cannot be isolated to cocaine, but appear to be related more to polydrug use. Also, the influence of the environment is significant as evidenced by improved scores from children living with nonbiologic caregivers and from those receiving more stimulation and intervention. Continued efforts are needed to provide services, not only to the children, but also to their parents, in order to improve the child's nurturing environment and decrease the rates of parenting failure.

The results of multiple studies looking at cocaine-exposed infants have been contradictory and inconclusive. Although the ominous forecast from early studies has not come about, much is still not known about the long-term results of prenatal cocaine exposure. A "cocaine baby syndrome," which includes abnormal arousal and attentional processing, has been suggested and is currently an active area of investigation by many researchers.

Recommendations

The AAP recommends that pediatricians provide developmental monitoring through the process of surveillance in which performing skilled, longitudinal observations is emphasized. Because even the relatively small effects on attention and auditory comprehension documented in this study can have large population effects on the numbers of children needing long-term intervention services, increased developmental surveillance of cocaine-exposed infants by pediatricians is needed (Singer et al, 2001).

Current studies emphasize how important it is for practitioners, as well as researchers, to consider postnatal factors, particularly the adequacy of the home environment, in their evaluation and treatment of children with a history of prenatal drug exposure. Also, it is essential that as a risk factor for atypical motor development, prenatal drug exposure be considered as a marker for other potential problems that can have a negative impact on a child's development. Therefore, it is vital for practitioners, caregivers, educators, and researchers to monitor the progress of these children, examining all areas of risk, so that appropriate interventions can be put into place that will enhance optimal performance.

Breastfeeding

Cocaine readily enters breast milk because of its low molecular weight and high fat solubility, and has been detected up to 36 hours after its use. Cocaine intoxication has been reported in infants consuming milk containing cocaine. These infants demonstrated tremors, irritability, seizures, and diarrhea lasting up to 48 hours. Both breast milk and the infants' urine tested positive for cocaine and its metabolites. Also, seizures, tremors, and ataxia have been reported in infants and toddlers seemingly intoxicated by passive inhalation of crack smoke in poorly ventilated "crack dens" (Rosen & Bateman, 2002).

Sudden Infant Death Syndrome (SIDS)

The incidence of SIDS in infants exposed prenatally to cocaine is three to seven times higher than normal, although, after controlling for other risk factors for SIDS, cocaine was not found to be an independent risk factor. Abnormalities of respiratory pattern and abnormal hypoxic arousal responses have been described in studies of cocaine-exposed infants as well as animal studies. However, many of these infants are also exposed to multiple drugs, including opiates and nicotine. Thus, it is difficult to attribute these respiratory changes solely to cocaine. Although assumptions have been made that an increased risk of SIDS must be considered, a causal relationship has not been supported (Frank et al, 2001; Rosen & Bateman, 2002).

Clinical Management

In contrast to infants exposed to opioids in utero, an abstinence syndrome for infants exposed prenatally to cocaine has not been identified. Instead, it is believed that the manifestations seen at birth reflect ongoing toxic effects of the drug itself. Pharmacologic therapy is recommended for narcotic withdrawal, but infants exposed solely to cocaine do not usually require such treatment. Decreasing environmental stimulation and using techniques such as swaddling and flexed positioning are effective strategies to manage signs of CNS irritation (Askin & Diehl-Jones, 2001).

HEROIN

History

Derivatives of opium have been used as analgesics for centuries, most likely dating back about 6000 years. Opium is derived from the seed of the unripe poppy plant, *Papaver somniferum*. Its derivatives include meperidine, heroin, methadone, morphine, and codeine (Hurt, 2005; Martinez et al, 2005).

Hippocrates, who mentioned "uterine suffocation" as possibly secondary to opium use, made one of the earliest references to complications of opium in the perinatal period. By the late 1800s, perinatal problems associated with opium were being reported while morphine's potential for abuse and addiction was first documented in the mid-1800s. Even so, opium derivatives remain the most effective analgesics available (Hurt, 2005; Martinez et al, 2005).

Heroin (diacetylmorphine), an illegal, highly addictive drug, is both the most abused and most rapidly acting of the opiates. Heroin is processed from morphine, one of the naturally occurring substances extracted from the poppy seed. Although the abuse of heroin has trended downward during the past several years, its prevalence is still higher than in the early 1990s (NIDA, 2005d).

The 2003 National Survey on Drug Use and Health (USDHHS, 2005a) reported that an estimated 3.7 million people had used heroin at some time in their lives, and more than 119,000 has used heroin within the month preceding the survey. An estimated 314,000 Americans had used heroin in the past year, and the group with the highest number of users included those 26 years of age or older. In 2003, 57.4 % of past-year users were classified with dependence or abuse of heroin, with an estimated 281,000 receiving treatment. In recent years, the availability of higher purity heroin and decreases in prices have increased the appeal of heroin for new users. Additionally, it has been appearing in more affluent communities (NIDA, 2005d; Rosen & Bateman, 2002).

Mechanism of Action

Heating morphine with acetyl anhydride produces heroin. The result is an off-white or pale brown powder that can be sniffed, smoked, or injected parenterally. Heroin is more potent than morphine and has a faster action. It is lipophilic and of low molecular weight, allowing the drug to cross the placenta easily. It is present in fetal tissue within 1 hour of administration. Once in the fetus, heroin is distributed widely throughout the fetal tissues and body compartments (Hurt, 2005; NIDA, 2005d; Rosen & Bateman, 2002).

The most common route for heroin use is by intravenous injection, known as "mainlining." This route provides the greatest intensity and the most rapid onset of euphoria, within 7 to 8 seconds. This brief but intense high is followed by a drowsy, detached, peaceful period of several hours that is followed by an intense craving for more of the drug. Typically, a heroin abuser may inject up to four times a day to satisfy this craving. Intramuscular injection produces a slower onset of euphoria, 5 to 8 minutes. Sniffing or smoking heroin does not produce a "rush" as quickly or as intensely as intravenous injection, with peak effects felt within 10 to 15 minutes. Nonetheless, NIDA researchers have confirmed that all three forms of administration are addictive (NIDA, 2005d).

Heroin injection is reportedly on the rise while inhalation is declining. However, certain groups such as Caucasian suburbanites report smoking or inhaling heroin because they believe that these routes of administration are less likely to lead to addiction (NIDA, 2005d).

Risk Factors

Many heroin-addicted women have poor general health with multiple medical problems associated with the drug abuse lifestyle. They are at high risk for human immunodeficiency virus (HIV) and viral hepatitis as the result of both needle sharing and unsafe sexual practices. Infections account for a high percentage of complications. Those most frequently seen are types A, B, and C hepatitis, tuberculosis, bacterial endocarditis, septicemia, cellulitis, and sexually transmitted infections (Hurt, 2005; Martinez et al, 2005; NIDA, 2005d; Wilbourne et al, 2001).

Although purer heroin is becoming more common, most "street" heroin is mixed with other drugs such as amphetamines or lidocaine, or with substances such as sugar, starch, powdered milk, or quinine. Heroin may also be cut with strychnine or other poisons. These substances, in and of themselves, can have deleterious effects on the fetus (NIDA, 2005d).

Because heroin abusers do not know the actual strength of the drug or its true contents, they are at risk of overdose or death. Also, the sterility of heroin is unclear and the drug may be tainted with bacteria, fungi, or virus. A separate risk factor that can jeopardize the health of the fetus is whether the mother has contacted HIV or viral hepatitis resulting in an increased risk of transmission to the fetus and neonate (Martinez et al, 2005; NIDA, 2005d).

Narcotic Antagonists

Narcotic antagonists such as naloxone should not be administered to a newborn of a narcotic-addicted mother as it may cause abrupt drug withdrawal. A case of apparent naloxone-induced seizures was reported in an infant whose mother had taken methadone 8 hours prior to delivery. The infant, apneic and intubated, was given intramuscular naloxone. Within 2 minutes seizures developed that did not respond to administration of diazepam, paraldehyde, or phenobarbital, but finally terminated with a bolus of morphine. For that reason,

health care personnel need to be aware of any history of opiate use during pregnancy. However, the history is not always immediately available, so, if using naloxone, personnel must be aware of the potential risk of rapid withdrawal and be prepared to treat withdrawal in the delivery room (AAP Policy Statement, 1998; Beauman, 2005).

Effects on the Fetus and Newborn

Infants born to heroin-addicted women have a higher incidence of being born prematurely, having LBWs, and being small for gestational age (SGA). Postmortem studies of placentas of heroin-addicted mothers demonstrated a high rate of chorioamnionitis and other maternal infections, which may be a causal factor in the increased incidence of prematurity. The mechanism by which heroin inhibits growth is not known. However, autopsies of infants who were SGA and born to narcotic-addicted mothers revealed that their organs were small and consisted of decreased numbers of normal-sized cells. These results differ from those obtained from malnourished infants born to nonaddicted mothers, whose organs demonstrated a decrease in both the number and the size of their cells. Thus, it has been suggested that maternal undernutrition is not the only factor responsible for the growth retardation seen in infants born to narcotic addicts. In reality, heroin may have a direct growth-inhibiting effect on the fetus. However, heroin does not appear to be associated with congenital malformations or a specific dysmorphic syndrome (NIDA, 2005d; Rosen & Bateman, 2002; Weiner & Finnegan, 2002).

Prenatal heroin exposure has been reported to accelerate fetal lung maturity. The incidence of respiratory distress syndrome is lower in these exposed infants. However, it is not known whether this occurs as a direct effect of heroin exposure or from the growth restriction and chronic stress (Martinez et al, 2005; Weiner & Finnegan, 2002).

Withdrawal of opiates in pregnant women can be associated with significant fetal distress and even fetal death. Fetal withdrawal usually coincides with the mother's withdrawal. Fetal withdrawal results in an increased risk of intrauterine seizures, hyperactivity, and an increase in catecholamines. This, in turn, increases oxygen consumption of the fetus that can lead to asphyxia. Because of the risks associated with fetal withdrawal, detoxification of women during pregnancy is rarely attempted. Instead, the mother can be placed on methadone maintenance and given prenatal care, nutritional assistance, and counseling (Ballard, 2002; Dashe et al, 2002; Hurt, 2005; Wilbourne et al, 2001).

Methadone

Methadone maintenance has been found to be the most effective treatment for opioid dependence. Studies have shown that methadone maintenance decreases illicit opioid use, criminal activity, and mortality rates in heroin-addicted adults. Methadone use during pregnancy was also reported to improve perinatal outcomes (Berghella et al, 2003; Dashe et al, 2002; Hurt, 2005).

Methadone readily crosses the placenta and is much longer lasting than heroin, with effects that can last up to 24 hours. The half-life of methadone is relatively long, 24 to 36 hours. Methadone is stored in body fat, and withdrawal is more severe and prolonged in the term newborn when compared to the premature infant. This is most likely due to the amount of total body fat in term infants that is available to store the drug, allowing it to be released slowly over time. Typically, it takes 10 to 14 days to withdraw from methadone, compared to 3 to 5 days to withdraw from heroin (Beauman, 2005; Dashe et al, 2002; Wilbourne et al, 2001).

The goal of methadone treatment is to prevent withdrawal, reduce or eliminate drug craving, and block the euphoric effect of narcotics. As pregnancy progresses, there is an accelerated clearance of methadone from the maternal circulation due to a larger maternal blood volume, increased metabolism related to increasing progestins, and higher fetal tissue concentrations. Therefore, in order to prevent symptoms of withdrawal in the mother, increased doses are usually required as gestation nears term (Ballard, 2002; Berghella et al, 2003).

There has been much controversy as to the effects of maternal methadone doses on neonatal abstinence, resulting in two different recommendations for treatment. One viewpoint is that treatment of heroin addicts should aim to detoxify and lower doses during pregnancy because there is a relationship between the severity of withdrawal and maternal methadone dose. Studies have reported that higher doses lead to longer neonatal hospitalization, higher abstinence scores, and increased need for treatment. This group recommends that the maternal methadone dose be kept at less than 20 mg per dose in an attempt to prevent neonatal abstinence. Other studies have challenged these results, finding no relationship between neonatal withdrawal incidence and severity and methadone dosage, even in pregnancies in which doses of greater than 80 mg per dose are used. An effective dose for methadone maintenance in nonpregnant adults is in the range of 50 mg to 120 mg. It has been hypothesized that nontherapeutic maternal dosage may promote illicit drug use and increase the risk to both mother and fetus. Thus, methadone should be given to pregnant addicts at the "most effective dose," which must be "individually determined" and "adequate to prevent maternal withdrawal symptoms." Effective methadone maintenance within a comprehensive program that includes prenatal care will result in a lower incidence of neonatal morbidity and mortality (Berghella et al, 2003; Dashe et al, 2002; Johnson et al, 2003b; Martinez et al, 2005; Sharpe & Kuschel, 2004; Wilbourne et al, 2001).

Breastfeeding

The AAP has approved breastfeeding for women taking methadone. Although there is transfer of methadone into breast milk, the amount is thought to be minimal. Studies have estimated that the dose of methadone the infant receives is approximately 2.8% of the maternal dose (Philipp et al, 2003).

Ongoing research is examining the possibility that breast milk from methadone-treated mothers may help alleviate symptoms of neonatal abstinence in their infants. Some studies have suggested that breastfeeding may be beneficial. However, additional studies have been unable to substantiate these findings. The excretion of methadone in human milk is variable but is not thought to be significant enough to prevent abstinence. Also, most infants who needed treatment were started on it within 48 hours, when milk production was still being established; again making it unlikely the infant would receive enough methadone to prevent symptoms. Continued research is needed to clarify the role of breastfeeding in the treatment of neonatal abstinence (Ballard, 2001; Kuschel, 2004; Philipp et al, 2003).

OxyContin

OxyContin, a controlled-release oxycodone hydrochloride, is a long-acting synthetic narcotic indicated for pain control in postoperative patients, cancer patients, and those with painful conditions such as osteoarthritis. The primary therapeutic effect is analgesia, although euphoria and feelings of relaxation have also been reported. Effects of OxyContin may be mediated through the opioid receptors in the CNS and spinal cord.

In the past few years, OxyContin has become a popular substitute for street drugs such as heroin. It is available as an oral preparation, but the tablet can be crushed to be illicitly used for inhalation or dissolved in solution for intravenous injection. At this time there are few data on the effects of OxyContin on a pregnant woman and her fetus. However, there have been numerous case reports of neonatal withdrawal symptoms following maternal OxyContin use. Symptoms reportedly improved when the infants were treated for neonatal abstinence syndrome. Clinical management of infants exposed to OxyContin is of particular concern because OxyContin and its metabolites are unlikely to be detected by methods used for urine and meconium opiate screens. The effect of prenatal exposure to OxyContin on newborns is an emerging problem that requires further study to determine the best treatment plans for these infants (Rao & Desai, 2002).

NEONATAL ABSTINENCE SYNDROME (NAS)

NAS can occur in two ways: (1) by the passive exposure to opioids in utero as a consequence of maternal addiction to heroin, methadone, and other narcotic analgesics; and (2) iatrogenically, by the administration of opiates such as fentanyl and morphine to the infant for the purpose of analgesia and sedation (Weiner & Finnegan, 2002). For the remainder of this chapter, the focus is on NAS due to passive exposure.

Neonatal abstinence is described as a generalized disorder characterized by CNS hyperirritability, gastrointestinal dysfunction, respiratory distress, and autonomic dysfunction manifested by vague symptoms such as yawning, hiccups, sneezing, mottled color, and fever (Martinez et al, 2005; Weiner & Finnegan, 2002). The origin of neonatal abstinence syndrome is the abnormal uterine environment. The continuing or episodic transfer of addictive substances from the maternal to fetal circulation, during which time the fetus goes through a biochemical adaptation to the drugs, threatens the growth and survival of the fetus. At delivery, the abrupt removal of the drug precipitates the onset of symptoms. The infant continues to metabolize and excrete the drug so that withdrawal signs occur when critically low tissue levels have been reached (Weiner & Finnegan, 2002).

The onset of withdrawal symptoms usually occurs within the first 72 hours after birth, often within the first 24 to 48 hours. However, there is a variance dependent on several factors such as the type of substance and amount used by the mother, the time and duration of drug exposure, the drug elimination half-life, and the routes of drug metabolism and excretion in both the mother and fetus (Table 21-1). Other factors that may also affect the rate and extent of drug transfer to the fetus include lipid solubility, molecular mass, protein binding, and placental blood flow and permeability (D'Apolito & Hepworth, 2001; Greene & Goodman, 2003; Hurt, 2005; Rosen & Bateman, 2002; Weiner & Finnegan, 2002).

Signs of neonatal abstinence occur in 50% to 85% of infants born to narcotic-addicted mothers. Heroin is not stored in

TABLE 21-1	Neonatal Neurobehavioral Symptoms After Fetal Drug Exposure			
Drug	**Onset (days)**	**Peak (days)**	**Duration**	**Relative Severity**
Alcohol	0-1	1-2	1-2 days	Mild
Cocaine	0-3	1-4	? months	Mild-moderate
Amphetamine	0-3		2-8 weeks	Mild-moderate
Heroin	0-3	3-7	2-4 weeks	Mild-moderate
Phencyclidine	0-2	5-7	2-6 months	Moderate-severe
Methadone	3-7	10-21	2-6 weeks	Mild-severe

From Taeusch HW (2005). Avery's diseases of the newborn, ed 8, St Louis: Saunders.

appreciable amounts by the fetus, so signs of heroin withdrawal appear quickly, usually within 24 to 48 hours after birth. However, methadone is stored in the fetal lung, liver, spleen, and body fat, facilitating the slower decline of methadone levels, resulting in a later onset of symptoms, possibly as late as 4 weeks (AAP Policy Statement, 1998; Beauman, 2005; Weiner & Finnegan, 2002).

Withdrawal may be mild, transient, and delayed in onset. Symptoms may be intermittent or follow a biphasic course characterized by acute NAS symptoms, improvement, and then the onset of a subacute withdrawal. Withdrawal appears to be more severe in infants exposed to large amounts of drugs for an extended period. Generally, the closer to delivery a mother takes a drug, the more severe the symptoms and the longer the delay in onset. Symptoms may last up to 4 to 6 months. The prolonged symptoms are usually milder than the initial ones and consist of irritability, tremors, hypertonicity, sneezing, hiccups, and regurgitation. This persistence is related directly to the initial severity and is more prolonged in infants with severe withdrawal (Hurt, 2005; Rosen & Bateman, 2002; Weiner & Finnegan, 2002).

Neurologic Signs of NAS

Neurologic signs are the most common symptoms of NAS and appear early. These include those of CNS excitability, such as hyperactivity, irritability, tremors, and hypertonicity (D'Apolito & Hepworth, 2001; Weiner & Finnegan, 2002). Initially, the infant may appear only to be restless. Tremors develop, which are mild and only occur with the infant is disturbed, but progress to the point where they occur spontaneously without any external stimulation. High-pitched cry, increased muscle tone, and further irritability progress to the point of inconsolability. When the infant is examined, there is a tendency to have increased deep tendon reflexes and an exaggerated Moro reflex (Greene & Goodman, 2003; Hurt, 2005; Rosen & Bateman, 2002; Weiner & Finnegan, 2002).

Abstinence-associated seizures have been reported to occur in about 1% to 2% of heroin-exposed infants and about 7% of methadone-exposed infants. Onset occurs most often around 10 days of age. These seizures are most likely to be generalized motor seizures or myoclonic jerks and may occur even during NAS treatment. Abnormal EEGs tend to occur only during the active seizure, and prognosis is favorable (Hurt, 2005; Martinez et al, 2005; Rosen & Bateman, 2002; Weiner & Finnegan, 2002).

These infants have seriously disturbed sleep patterns. Studies have shown that narcotics obliterate REM sleep in infants and withdrawal prevents normal adequate periods of deep sleep.

However, appropriate therapy will allow the return of REM and sleep cycles (Hurt, 2005; Martinez et al, 2005; Rosen & Bateman, 2002; Weiner & Finnegan, 2002).

Gastrointestinal Signs of NAS

Infants with NAS have an abnormal feeding pattern. Previous research has reported less sucking with reduced sucking pressure resulting in lower nutrient consumption. However, LaGasse and associates (2003) found that these infants did not suck less during the feeding session. Instead, they showed prolonged sucking with fewer pauses, which is consistent with greater energy intake. They also documented more feeding problems such as spitting up and refusal, as well as increased arousal, all of which are consistent with opiate withdrawal.

These infants appear incessantly hungry and suck frantically on their fists or fingers. However, they often have difficulty feeding because of uncoordinated and ineffectual suck and swallow reflexes, resulting in poor nutrient intake, excessive weight loss, and suboptimal weight gain. Also common are vomiting and diarrhea that can be severe enough to cause not only profound weight loss, but alterations in electrolytes and pH, as well as dehydration (Greene & Goodman, 2003; Hurt, 2005; LaGasse et al, 2003; Martinez et al, 2005; Rosen & Bateman, 2002; Weiner & Finnegan, 2002).

Respiratory Signs of NAS

Respiratory signs most common in NAS include tachypnea, irregular respirations, rhinorrhea, a stuffy nose, nasal flaring, chest retractions, intermittent cyanosis, and apnea. Increased severity of these symptoms may develop if the infant regurgitates, aspirates, or develops aspiration pneumonia. There has been some evidence of transient abnormalities of lung compliance and tidal volume in opiate-exposed infants, suggesting that opioids may alter the fetal development of the respiratory system. Alkalosis may be seen that is due to hyperventilation and may cause decreased levels of ionized calcium, which could lead to tetany (Hurt, 2005; Martinez et al, 2005; Rosen & Bateman, 2002; Weiner & Finnegan, 2002).

Signs of Autonomic Dysfunction in NAS

Infants undergoing withdrawal exhibit signs such as frequent sneezing, yawning, mottling of skin, tearing, and excessive generalized sweating. Sweating may be caused by the predominantly central-neurogenic stimulation of sweat glands induced by heroin withdrawal. Occasionally, fever may be seen with the increased neuromuscular activities of tremors (Hurt, 2005; Martinez, 2005; Rosen & Bateman, 2002; Weiner & Finnegan, 2002).

Diagnosis of Neonatal Abstinence

The diagnosis of NAS is dependent on a thorough maternal history, including medication/drug use and social habits, maternal and infant toxicology screens, and clinical presentation of the infant. However, differentiating signs of drug withdrawal from infections or metabolic disorders may be difficult. No clinical signs should be attributed only to withdrawal without appropriate assessment and diagnostic tests to rule out other causes such as hypoglycemia, hypocalcemia, hypomagnesemia, and hypothermia (AAP Policy Statement, 1998; Hurt, 2005; Rosen & Bateman, 2002; Weiner & Finnegan, 2002).

There are several scoring tools available to assist the caregiver in evaluation and treatment of neonatal abstinence. The Neonatal Intensive Care Unit Network Neurobehavioral Scale (NNNS) was developed for the National Institute of Child Health and Human Development (NICHD) Neonatal Intensive Care Unit Research Network as a part of the Maternal Lifestyle Study. The NNNS, an "offspring" of the Neonatal Behavioral Assessment Scale (NBAS), was developed because of concerns that existing instruments were not sensitive to the neurobehavioral effects of prenatal drug exposure and infants at risk. It was designed to provide a comprehensive assessment of both neurologic integrity and behavioral function, including withdrawal and general signs of stress. It is applicable to term, normal healthy infants, premature infants, and infants at risk because of factors such as prenatal substance abuse. The NNNS includes three parts: (1) the more classic neurologic items that assess active and passive tone and primitive reflexes as well as items that reflect CNS integrity; (2) behavioral items including state and sensory and interactive responses; and (3) stress/abstinence items especially appropriate for high-risk infants. The stress/abstinence portion of the examination is a checklist that includes traditional items that reflect neonatal abstinence described by Loretta Finnegan. Additional signs of stress that have been described in cocaine-exposed infants as well as signs of stress typical of other high-risk infants have also been added.

The NNNS should be performed on infants who are medically stable, preferably in an open crib or incubator. The complete examination is probably not appropriate for infants less than 30 weeks' gestation, although a precise lower gestational age cannot be set. The upper age limit may vary depending on the developmental maturation of the infant, although a reasonable upper limit is 46 to 48 weeks (corrected or conceptional age) (Boukydis et al, 2004; Lester et al, 2004; Lester & Tronick, 2004).

Although this tool provides a comprehensive evaluation of drug-exposed infants, its use requires certification of the examiner. It is extremely useful as a basis for consultation between clinician and parent, enabling them to mutually evaluate the infant and arrive at an appropriate plan of care, including parental needs and anticipatory guidance, but may be too time consuming to be used as a bedside tool (Boukydis et al, 2004; Lester, 2004; Lester & Tronick, 2004).

The Neonatal Drug Withdrawal Scoring System, also known as the Lipsitz tool, consists of assigning scores to 11 categories. Scores of 0, 1, 2, or 3 are assigned for each of the following: tremors, irritability, reflexes, stools, muscle tone, skin abrasions, and tachypnea. Additionally, the following are assigned a yes (1) or no (0) score: repetitive sneezing, repetitive yawning, and vomiting or fever. The highest possible score of 20 reflects severe withdrawal. The goal is to maintain a score no greater than 4 (AAP Policy Statement, 1998; Beauman, 2005; Jackson et al, 2004).

Loretta Finnegan's system, The Neonatal Abstinence Scoring System, monitors the infant in a comprehensive and objective way. It can be used to assess the onset, progression, and resolution of symptoms, and can also be used to monitor the infant's response to pharmacotherapy used to control the symptoms of NAS. This system uses 31 items most commonly observed in withdrawal, rated on a 1 to 5 point scale based on their clinical significance. Infants are initially assessed 2 hours after birth and every 4 hours afterwards. If scores increase to 8 or higher, every-2-hour scoring is instituted. The need for medication is indicated when the total score is 8 or higher for three consecutive scorings, or when the average of any three consecutive scores is 8 or higher. Medication is not needed if consecutive scores or the average of any three consecutive scores continues to be 7 or less during the first 4 days of life. Finnegan's system continues to be one of the most comprehensive and widely used tools (Beauman, 2005; Weiner & Finnegan, 2002). Refer to the Evolve website for additional NAS assessment methods. **evolve**

Treatment of Neonatal Abstinence

Infants with confirmed drug exposure who do not have signs of withdrawal do not require pharmacologic treatment. Furthermore, not all infants with NAS will require pharmacologic treatment. All infants with withdrawal symptoms should receive supportive care. This includes swaddling, providing sucking opportunities with a pacifier, decreasing external stimulation such as light and noise, and maintaining a calm, quiet environment. If these infants begin to show worsening symptoms of withdrawal, then medication must be considered (AAP Policy Statement, 1998; D'Apolito & Hepworth, 2001; Martinez et al, 2005; Weiner & Finnegan, 2002).

Pharmacologic Therapy

The goal of treatment of NAS is to minimize physiologic effects of central and autonomic system dysfunction. The decision to begin drug therapy must be individualized, based on the severity of withdrawal symptoms and an assessment of the risks versus benefits. Although drug therapy is known to decrease symptoms of withdrawal, the effects on long-term morbidity are unknown (AAP Policy Statement, 1998; Greene & Goodman, 2003; Weiner & Finnegan, 2002).

Approximately 50% to 60% of opiate-exposed infants will present with symptoms significant enough to require pharmacologic agents. Indications for the initiation of drug therapy include the presence of seizure activity, poor feeding, severe diarrhea and vomiting that results in excessive weight loss and dehydration, inability to sleep, and fever unrelated to infection, as well as elevated scores on Finnegan's scoring system (AAP Policy Statement, 1998; Rosen & Bateman, 2002; Weiner & Finnegan, 2002).

If pharmacologic management is needed, selection of a drug from the same class as the drug causing the withdrawal symptoms is recommended as it is more physiologic. A study by Jackson and associates (2004) demonstrated that for opiate withdrawal, opiate replacement therapy was superior for management of symptomatic NAS. They found a more rapid resolution of symptoms resulting in a shorter treatment, and a significantly reduced requirement for higher intensity nursing care (AAP Policy Statement, 1998; Beauman, 2005; Coyle et al, 2002; Greene & Goodman, 2003; Lifshitz, 2001).

Guides to adequate therapy include a normal temperature curve, the ability of the infant to sleep between feedings and medications, a decrease in activity and crying, a decrease in motor instability, and weight gain. Several pharmacologic agents have been used for therapy (Table 21-2) (AAP Policy Statement, 1998; Beauman, 2005; Coyle et al, 2002; Greene & Goodman, 2003; Jackson et al, 2004; Lifshitz, 2001).

Paregoric

Paregoric, a product that contains anhydrous morphine (0.4 mg/ml), was one of the first drugs used to treat NAS. Infants treated with paregoric had improved sucking patterns resulting in increased nutrient consumption and better weight gain, as well as better seizure control than phenobarbital or diazepam. Despite the beneficial effects, the use of paregoric has declined during recent years because of the known and potential toxic effects of its ingredients. Paregoric contains

TABLE 21-2	Pharmacologic Management of Neonatal Abstinence Syndrome	
Drug	**Advantages**	**Disadvantages**
Paregoric (0.4 mg/ml anhydrous morphine)	Improved sucking patterns, better seizure control, diminished bowel motility and loose stools	Large doses and long duration of therapy are required to control symptoms. Drug contains toxic ingredients that can cause serious side effects in the neonate.
Tincture of opium (10 mg/ml)	Limited toxic effects; when used as a 25-fold dilution with water, contains the same concentration of morphine equivalent as paregoric and is stable for 2 weeks	Drug does not control loose stools.
Morphine sulfate	Lower alcohol content and fewer additives than paregoric	Drug contains additives that have been associated with adverse effects in infants, although the amounts may not be large enough to cause significant side effects. No reported studies are available about use for neonatal abstinence syndrome (NAS). No current comparison studies with paregoric are available.
Methadone	Has been used effectively to treat NAS	Infants are not discharged from the hospital while undergoing methadone therapy because of the potential for maternal abuse; therapy must be tapered and discontinued before discharge. Long half-life makes dose titration difficult. Use of drug results in prolonged hospitalization.
Phenobarbital	Has been used extensively for treatment of opiate or barbiturate withdrawal; effective in controlling irritability and insomnia; serum levels easily obtained	At high doses drug impairs sucking reflex. Tolerance to sedation develops. Induction of enhanced drug metabolism occurs. Drug is effective only for control of CNS symptoms. No effect is seen on gastrointestinal symptoms.
Chlorpromazine	Effective in controlling gastrointestinal and CNS symptoms	Adverse effects can include cerebellar dysfunction, lower seizure threshold, and hematologic abnormalities. Elimination is slow; half-life is 3 days. Titration is difficult.
Clonidine	Used effectively in treatment of withdrawal symptoms in opiate-addicted adults; small trials show effective reduction in most symptoms, except poor sleep, with no adverse effects; duration of treatment is significantly shorter	Drug has limited use in neonates; additional studies are needed in infants before routine use can be recommended.
Diazepam	Effective when used in conjunction with paregoric or phenobarbital; helps control symptoms of tremulousness, abnormal sucking, and irritability	Drug is not effective as a single agent. Elimination of drug and metabolites is lengthy (takes >1 month). Late-onset seizures are common. Drug contains additives that may result in cerebral and hepatic dysfunction and hyperosmolarity.

the isoquinoline derivatives noscapine and papaverine, which are antispasmodics. It also contains other potentially toxic compounds that include camphor, a CNS stimulant that is eliminated from the body slowly. There is a high concentration of ethanol, 44% to 46%, a CNS depressant, and anise oil, which may cause habituation. Benzoic acid, an oxidative product of benzyl alcohol, is present and may compete for bilirubin binding sites or cause "gasping baby syndrome," characterized by severe acidosis, CNS depression, respiratory distress, hypotension, kidney failure, and death in small premature infants. Glycerin is also present and may cause severe diarrhea. In addition, large doses of paregoric and a long duration of use may be needed to control symptoms (AAP Policy Statement, 1998; Beauman, 2005; Johnson et al, 2003b; Langenfeld et al, 2005; Lifshitz et al, 2001; Martinez et al, 2005; Weiner & Finnegan, 2002).

Tincture of Opium

Tincture of opium (10 mg/ml) has been preferred to paregoric for treatment of opiate withdrawal. It is effective for controlling withdrawal symptoms but is very concentrated. Therefore, a small error in dosing can lead to a significant overdose to the infant. A 25-fold dilution of tincture of opium contains the same concentration of morphine equivalent as paregoric and, once it is diluted, is stable for 2 weeks. Tincture of opium does not control diarrhea as well as paregoric does (AAP Policy Statement, 1998; Beauman, 2005; Greene & Goodman, 2003; Langenfeld et al, 2005).

Phenobarbital

Although phenobarbital has been used for acute opiate withdrawal, it does not reduce significant physiologic signs of withdrawal such as diarrhea and seizures. Large doses of phenobarbital may significantly depress the CNS of the infant, impairing the suck reflex and causing excessive sedation, as well as delaying bonding between mother and infant. On the other hand, it is especially effective in controlling irritability and insomnia. If phenobarbital is used, measuring plasma concentrations 24 to 48 hours later is important with the goal of 20 to 30 mg/L (AAP Policy Statement, 1998; Beauman, 2005; Coyle et al, 2002, 2005; Martinez et al, 2005).

Current recommendations are that opiate withdrawal be treated with an opiate. Many clinicians are giving phenobarbital in combination with tincture of opium or morphine in an attempt to decrease the severity of symptoms of withdrawal. A study by Coyle and associates (2002) demonstrated that a combination of tincture of opium and phenobarbital resulted in a shorter duration of hospitalization, less severe withdrawal, and reduced hospital cost when compared to treatment with tincture of opium alone. Another study by Coyle and colleagues (2005) examined neurobehavioral scores of infants treated with the combination compared with those treated with tincture of opium alone. Results showed that infants treated with the combination of tincture of opium and phenobarbital were more interactive, had smoother movements, were easier to handle, and were less stressed. This improved neurobehavioral organization during the first 3 weeks of life was felt to indicate a more rapid recovery from opiate withdrawal.

Morphine

An oral preparation of morphine is available in concentrations of 2 mg/ml and 4 mg/ml. It has several advantages compared with paregoric in that it contains less alcohol and fewer additives. The parenteral form of morphine contains bisulfite and phenol, both of which have been associated with adverse effects in infants. However, the amount of additives in standard doses of morphine are most likely not large enough to affect the newborn significantly (AAP Policy Statement, 1998; Beauman, 2005).

Although some clinicians are using morphine to treat NAS, thus far, there have been few studies about its effectiveness in relieving symptoms of withdrawal. Using a randomized double-blind controlled trial, Langenfeld and associates (2005) compared tincture of opium with morphine drops in the treatment of NAS. Results showed no significant differences in the duration of therapy or the abstinence scores, although weight gain was better in the morphine group. Thus, their conclusion was that morphine was as suitable as tincture of opium for treatment of NAS, but avoided the potential effects of the alcoholic extracts and various alkaloids found in tincture of opium.

Methadone

Methadone has been used extensively to reduce withdrawal symptoms in adults and to help them abstain from heroin use. It has also been used effectively in the treatment of NAS, although its use may be limited because of several factors. Methadone has a long half-life, making dose titration difficult. Infants are not usually discharged from the hospital while taking methadone because of the potential for maternal abuse; therefore therapy is generally tapered and discontinued before the addicted infant is discharged. This results in prolonged hospitalization for the infant. Although there are methadone treatment centers where adults can receive treatment, there are few that will treat infants after discharge (AAP Policy Statement, 1998; Beauman, 2005; Martinez et al, 2005).

Chlorpromazine

Chlorpromazine has been shown to be effective in controlling gastrointestinal and CNS symptoms of NAS. However, its use has been limited because of adverse effects such as cerebellar dysfunction, decreased seizure threshold, and hematologic abnormalities. Also, the drug is eliminated very slowly in the neonate, with a reported half-life of 3 days, making dose titration very difficult (AAP Policy Statement, 1998; Beauman, 2005; Johnson et al, 2003b).

Clonidine

Clonidine, a nonnarcotic medication, has been used effectively in the adult population for treatment of withdrawal from substances of abuse. Treatment duration is significantly shorter with clonidine than with other medications. It is frequently used in the treatment of hypertension and attention deficit hyperactivity disorder, working by modulating the release of norepinephrine and dopamine. With its use, there are risks of oversedation and cardiovascular effects. However, the use of clonidine in neonates is limited. There have been limited studies evaluating treatment value and safety in infants. Also, the drug is available in tablet and transdermal patch forms, which may lead to difficulty with neonatal dosing. Because supportive evidence in the neonate is lacking, current recommendations are that clonidine should be used only for randomized clinical trials in the neonatal population (AAP Policy Statement, 1998; Beauman, 2005).

Diazepam

Diazepam has been effective for the treatment of NAS in opiate-exposed infants when used in conjunction with a second medication, usually an opiate. However, it has never been successful as a single agent. It is rarely used to treat NAS for several reasons. First, since newborns have a limited capacity to metabolize and excrete diazepam, the elimination of the drug and its metabolites are prolonged, as long as 1 month. Second, adverse effects such as respiratory depression, an impaired metabolic response to cold stress, and late-onset seizures have been documented. Finally, the parenteral formulation contains benzyl alcohol, sodium benzoate, ethyl alcohol, and propylene glycol, which may result in cerebral and hepatic dysfunction and hyperosmolarity in infants (AAP Policy Statement, 1998; Beauman, 2005; Johnson et al, 2003a).

METHAMPHETAMINE

In recent years, methamphetamine, also known as "ice," "crank," "crystal," or "speed," has become a highly prevalent drug of abuse. In 2003, the National Survey on Drug Use and Health (USDHHS, 2005a) reported that 12.3 million Americans age 12 and older had tried methamphetamine at least once in their lifetimes, 5.2% of the population, with the majority of past-year users between 18 and 34 years old. The drug is a derivative of amphetamine and is easily made in clandestine laboratories through the reduction of ephedrine or pseudoephedrine. The ease of its synthesis, its availability, and its affordability, as well as a prolonged high, have made it an increasingly popular drug of choice (NIDA, 2002, 2005a).

Methamphetamine is a powerfully addictive stimulant that causes a massive release of dopamine in the brain. It dramatically affects the CNS, producing increased alertness, sleeplessness, euphoria, and exhilaration. It can be smoked or used intravenously, intranasally, or orally. Immediately after smoking or intravenous injection, the user experiences an intense sensation, a "rush," which lasts only a few minutes and is described as extremely pleasurable. Oral or intranasal use produces euphoria and a high but not a rush. Intranasal use produces effects within 3 to 5 minutes, whereas oral ingestion produces effects within 15 to 20 minutes. Tolerance develops quickly, requiring higher and more frequent doses. Methamphetamine metabolizes slowly, the "high" lasting 10 to 24 hours. The "high" is followed by a "crash" that may last 4 to 5 days (NIDA, 2005a; Rosen & Bateman, 2002; Smith et al, 2003).

Central nervous system effects of methamphetamine include increased wakefulness, increased physical activity, increased respiration, hyperthermia, and euphoria. Additional effects include irritability, confusion, tremors, seizures, paranoia, aggressiveness, and extreme anorexia. Methamphetamine causes tachycardia and increased blood pressure and can cause irreversible damage to blood vessels in the brain, producing strokes (NIDA, 2005a; Rosen & Bateman, 2002).

Currently, little is known about the effects and mechanism of action on the fetus and neonate. Much of what is known is a result of animal studies. Studies with methamphetamine in the pregnant ewe have demonstrated rapid transfer and distribution in the fetus. Peak concentration was higher in the mother, but elimination from the fetus was slower. The highest concentration of methamphetamine was found in the fetal lung. The brain and heart had the lowest concentration, but the concentration was still three to four times that of the plasma. Amniotic fluid appears to act as a reservoir for the drug. After IV administration of methamphetamine, the fetal ewe demonstrated a 20% to 37% increase in blood pressure, an increase in heart rate, and a decrease in pH, oxygen partial pressure, and oxygen saturation (Rosen & Bateman, 2002; Wouldes et al, 2004).

Infants prenatally exposed to methamphetamine have been found to be premature and small for gestational age and to exhibit hypersensitivity to sound, abnormal sleeping patterns, and increased tone. Cranial ultrasound scans have demonstrated cystic and echodense areas and hemorrhages, most likely related to the vasoconstrictive properties. Animal studies have also found a variety of effects including increased maternal and offspring mortality, retinal defects, cleft palate, rib malformations, decreased rate of physical growth, and delayed motor development. Neurotoxic effects of prenatal exposure on serotoninergic neurons produce neurochemical alterations in the CNS thought to be associated with learning impairment, behavioral deficits, increased motor activity, and enhanced conditioned avoidance responses (Rosen & Bateman, 2002; Wouldes et al, 2004).

Smith and associates (2003) retrospectively studied infants exposed prenatally to methamphetamine. Their preliminary findings suggest methamphetamine use is associated with growth restriction in infants born at term with restriction seen during all three trimesters.

ECSTASY/MDMA

The drug 3,4-methylenedioxymethamphetamine (MDMA), also known as "ecstasy," is a "designer" drug that has become increasingly popular over the past two decades. It was first used in the late 1970s as an adjunct to psychotherapy and gained popularity among adolescents and young adults in the nightclub scene. It is a synthetic, psychoactive drug with both stimulant and hallucinogenic properties. Street names for MDMA include "XTC," "hug," "beans," "Adam," and "love drug." In 2003, an estimated 470,000 people in the United States age 12 or older had used MDMA in the past 30 days, a substantial decrease from 2002 (NIDA, 2005c).

MDMA can affect the brain by altering the activity of neurotransmitters, which enable nerve cells in the brain to communicate with one another. Animal research has shown that MDMA can be toxic to nerve cells that contain serotonin, causing long-lasting damage. MDMA can also interfere with the body's ability to control its temperature, which has led to severe medical consequences, including death. It also causes the release of norepinephrine, which is likely what causes the increase in heart rate and blood pressure often seen with MDMA use (NIDA, 2005c).

There have been few studies on the effects of MDMA on the fetus and neonate. However, early studies have suggested a significantly increased risk of congenital defects, with a predominance of cardiovascular and musculoskeletal anomalies (Hurt, 2005).

A study by Broening and associates (2001) using neonatal rats suggests that MDMA may pose a risk to the developing brain by inducing long-term deleterious effects on learning and memory.

Meyer and associates (2004) studied newborn rat pups after repeated treatment with MDMA. Findings indicated that MDMA stimulated apoptotic cell death in the brain, produced deficits in serotoninergic markers, and subsequently led to a reorganization of the forebrain serotoninergic innervation. Considering that the neonatal period in rats is thought to model the third trimester of fetal brain development in humans, these results suggest that infants whose mothers take MDMA during late pregnancy are at risk for multiple neuro-developmental abnormalities.

Kelly and colleagues (2002) used neonatal rats to demonstrate relatively widespread changes in cerebral function related to prenatal MDMA exposure, which persist into adult life. The underlying mechanism was not determined, but the results further highlight the potentially harmful effects of MDMA.

SUMMARY

Even if the teratogenicity of a specific substance has not been well established, a number of maternal-fetal health problems as well as psychosocial risks accompany addictions to drugs. Clinical monitoring of infants, social services for families to ensure a safe home environment, and addiction services for the mother are appropriate standards of care. However, there is an attitude that women who use illegal substances are morally unfit and intentionally abusive, which may alter how care is provided. There is a need to identify and reduce exposures to all harmful agents during pregnancy, whether legal or not. Also needed are intervention services to all children with develop-mental risks, whether due to prenatal exposure of harmful substances or social/environmental causes. Health care professionals must be aware of any attitudinal biases that may affect clinical treatment (Zuckerman et al, 2002).

Studies have shown that effective follow-up interventions result in improved outcomes for drug-exposed infants. A study by Butz and colleagues (2001) examined child behavioral problems and parenting stress in drug-exposed children after receiving in-home intervention. The home-based intervention focused on parenting education and skills as well as caregiver emotional support. Results showed that with the home-based intervention, these infants had significantly fewer perceived behavioral problems compared with infants receiving no home intervention. There was also a trend toward lower parenting stress. A more aggressive home-based intervention may have a greater impact on drug-using mothers and their children and should be considered as a treatment option with these families.

Schuler and associates (2003) evaluated the effects of a home intervention on the developmental outcome of drug-exposed infants. Findings demonstrated improved scores on the Bayley Scales of Infant Development when a home intervention was in place. Scores were higher in infants whose mothers reported no ongoing drug use, but were lower in the presence of continued drug use. However, scores decreased by 18 months of age, leading the researchers to conclude that environmental factors of inner-city homes and low socio-economic status had a significant impact on developmental outcomes.

For the neonatal nurse, infants who have been exposed to substances in utero present a challenge. They require accurate assessments to anticipate and plan for potential problems. Although research is ongoing, much is still not known about the long-term risks. The complexity of care of substance-expose infants is increased because of the pattern of maternal polydrug use; thus, each neonate may present with different clinical manifestations. The information in this chapter will assist health care personnel in providing better care for these infants and their families.

REFERENCES

Albrecht SA et al (2004). Smoking cessation counseling for pregnant women who smoke: scientific basis for practice for AWHONN's success project. *Journal of obstetric, gynecologic, and neonatal nursing* 33(3):298-305.

American Academy of Pediatrics Policy Statement (1998). Neonatal drug withdrawal. *Pediatrics* 101(6):1079-1088.

American Academy of Pediatrics Policy Statement (2001a). Alcohol use and abuse: a pediatric concern. *Pediatrics* 108(1):185-189.

American Academy of Pediatrics Policy Statement (2001b). Improving substance abuse prevention, assessment, and treatment financing for children and adolescents. *Pediatrics* 108(4):1025-1029.

American Academy of Pediatrics Policy Statement (2001c). The transfer of drugs and other chemicals into human milk. *Pediatrics* 108(3):776-789.

American Academy of Pediatrics Policy Statement (2001d). Tobacco's toll: implications for the pediatrician. *Pediatrics* 107(4):794-798.

Ana de la Chica R et al (2005). Chromosomal instability in amniocytes from fetuses of mothers who smoke. *Journal of the American Medical Association* 293(10):1212-1222.

Askin DF, Diehl-Jones B (2001). Cocaine: effects of in utero exposure on the fetus and neonate. *Journal of perinatal and neonatal nursing* 14(4):83-102.

Bada HS et al (2002a). Central and autonomic system signs with in utero drug exposure. *Archives of disease in childhood, fetal and neonatal edition* 87:F106-F112.

Bada HS et al (2002b). Gestational cocaine exposure and intrauterine growth: Maternal Lifestyle Study. *Obstetrics and gynecology* 100(5):916-924.

Ballard JL (2002). Treatment of neonatal abstinence syndrome with breast milk containing methadone. *Journal of perinatal and neonatal nursing* 15(4):76-85.

Bandstra ES et al (2001). Intrauterine growth of full-term infants: impact of prenatal cocaine exposure. *Pediatrics* 108(6):1309-1319.

Bar-Oz B et al (2003). Comparison of meconium and neonatal hair analysis for detection of gestational exposure to drugs of abuse. *Archives of disease in childhood, fetal and neonatal edition* 88:F98-F100.

Bauer CR (2002). The maternal lifestyle study: drug exposure during pregnancy and short-term maternal outcomes. *American journal of obstetrics and gynecology* 186(3):487-495.

Bearer CF (2001). Markers to detect drinking during pregnancy. *Alcohol research and health* 25(3):210-218.

Beauman SS (2005). Identification and management of neonatal abstinence syndrome. *Journal of infusion nursing* 28(3):159-167.

Beblo S et al (2005). Effects of alcohol intake during pregnancy on docosahexaenoic acid and arachidonic acid in umbilical cord vessels of black women. *Pediatrics* 115(2):194-203.

Behnke M et al (2001). The search for congenital malformations in newborns with fetal cocaine exposure. *Pediatrics* 107(5):e74. Available at: http://www.pediatrics.org/cgi/content/full/107/5/e74. Retrieved May 22, 2005.

Berghella V et al (2003). Maternal methadone dose and neonatal withdrawal. *American journal of obstetrics and gynecology* 189(2):312-317.

Bergin C (2001). Measuring prenatal drug exposure. *Journal of pediatric nursing* 16(4):245-255.

Blackburn C et al (2003). Effects of strategies to reduce exposure of infants to environmental tobacco smoke in the home: cross sectional survey. *British medical journal*, 327. Available at: http://bmj.com/cgi/content/full/327/7409/257. Retrieved June 26, 2005.

Boukydis CFZ et al (2004). Clinical use of the neonatal intensive care unit network neurobehavioral scale. *Pediatrics* 111(3):679-689.

Broening HW et al (2001). 3,4-Methylenedioxymethamphetamine (Ecstasy)-induced learning and memory impairments depend on the age of exposure during early development. *Journal of neuroscience* 21(9):3228-3235.

Buka SL et al (2003). Elevated risk of tobacco dependence among offspring of mothers who smoked during pregnancy: a 30-year prospective study. *American journal of psychiatry* 160(11):1978-1984.

Butz AM (2001). Effectiveness of a home intervention for perceived child behavioral problems and parenting stress in children with in utero drug exposure. *Archives of pediatrics and adolescent medicine* 155:1029-1037.

Campbell S (2003). Prenatal cocaine exposure and neonatal/infant outcomes. *Neonatal network* 22(1):19-21.

Centers for Disease Control and Prevention (2002). National task force on fetal alcohol syndrome and fetal alcohol effect. *MMWR Morbidity and mortality weekly report*, 51(RR14), 9-12. Retrieved July 9, 2005 from http://www.cdc.gov/mmwr/preview/mmwrhtml/rr5114a2.htm.

Centers for Disease Control and Prevention (2004a). *Adult cigarette smoking in the United States: Current estimates—fact sheet.* Available at: http://www.cdc.gov/tobacco/factsheets/AdultCigaretteSmoking_Factsheet. htm. Retrieved July 10, 2005.

Centers for Disease Control and Prevention (2004b). Alcohol consumption among women who are pregnant or who might become pregnant—United States, 2002. *MMWR Morbidity and mortality weekly report* 53(50):1178-1181. Available at: http://www.cdc.gov/mmwr/preview/mmwrhtml/mm5350a4.htm. Retrieved July 9, 2005.

Centers for Disease Control and Prevention (2004c). *Women and tobacco—fact sheet.* Available at: http://www.cdc.gov/tobacco/factsheets/WomenTobacco_Factsheet.htm. Retrieved July 10, 2005.

Centers for Disease Control and Prevention, National Center on Birth Defects and Developmental Disabilities (2004d). *Fetal alcohol syndrome: guidelines for referral and diagnosis.* Available at: http://www.cdc.gov/ncbddd/fas/documents/FAS_guidelines_accessible.pdf. Retrieved July 10, 2005.

Centers for Disease Control and Prevention (2005a). Cigarette smoking among adults—United States, 2003. *MMWR Morbidity and mortality weekly report* 54(20):1-6. Available at: http://www.ncadi.samhsa.gov/govpubs/mmwr/vol54/mm5420a3.aspx. Retrieved July 11, 2005.

Centers for Disease Control and Prevention (2005b). *Pattern of tobacco use among women and girls—fact sheet.* Available at: http://www.cdc.gov/tobacco/sgr/sgr_forwomen/factshet_tobaccouse.htm. Retrieved July 10, 2005.

Centers for Disease Control and Prevention, National Center on Birth Defects and Developmental Disabilities (2005c). *Preventing alcohol-exposed pregnancies.* Available at: www.cdc.gov/ncbddd/fas/fasprev.htm. Retrieved July 10, 2005.

Chang AB et al (2003). Altered arousal response in infants exposed to cigarette smoke. *Archives of disease in childhood* 88:30-33.

Chang G (2001). Alcohol-screening instruments for pregnant women. *Alcohol research and health* 25(3):204-209.

Chang G et al (2005). Brief intervention for prenatal alcohol use: a randomized trial. *Obstetrics and gynecology* 105(5):991-998.

Chasnoff IJ et al (2001). Screening for substance use in pregnancy: a practical approach for the primary care physician. *American journal of obstetrics and gynecology* 184(4):752-758.

Chasnoff IJ et al (2005). The 4P's Plus screen for substance use in pregnancy: clinical application and outcomes. *Journal of perinatology* 25:368-374.

Coyle MG et al (2002). Diluted tincture of opium (DTO) and phenobarbital versus DTO alone for neonatal opiate withdrawal in term infants. *Journal of pediatrics* 140(5):561-564.

Coyle MG et al (2005). Neurobehavioral effects of treatment for opiate withdrawal. *Archives of disease in childhood, fetal and neonatal edition* 90:F73-F74.

D'Apolito K, Hepworth JT (2001). Prominence of withdrawal symptoms in polydrug-exposed infants. *Journal of perinatal and neonatal nursing* 14(4):46-60.

Dashe JS et al (2002). Relationship between maternal methadone dosage and neonatal withdrawal. *Obstetrics and gynecology* 100(6):1244-1249.

De Los Angeles Avaria M et al (2004). Peripheral nerve conduction abnormalities in children exposed to alcohol in utero. *Journal of pediatrics* 144:338-343.

DeMarini DM, Preston RJ (2005). Transplacental mutagenesis of the fetus by tobacco smoke [Editorial]. *Journal of the American Medical Association* 293(10):1264-1265.

Dezateux C et al (2001). Airway function at one year: association with premorbid airway function, wheezing, and maternal smoking. *Thorax* 56:680-686.

DiFranza JR et al (2004). Prenatal and postnatal environmental tobacco smoke exposure and children's health. *Pediatrics* 113(4):1007-1015.

Ebrahim SH, Gfroerer J (2003). Pregnancy-related substance use in the United States during 1996-1998. *Obstetrics and gynecology* 101(2):374-379.

Edwards CA et al (2003). Relationship between birth weight and adult lung function: controlling for maternal factors. *Thorax* 58:1061-1065.

Elliot JG et al (2003). Airway alveolar attachment points and exposure to cigarette smoke in utero. *American journal of respiratory and critical care medicine* 167:45-49.

El-Mohandes A et al (2003). Prenatal care reduces the impact of illicit drug use on perinatal outcomes. *Journal of perinatology* 23:354-360.

Emmons KM et al (2001). A randomized trial to reduce passive smoke exposure in low-income households with young children. *Pediatrics* 108(1):18-24.

England LJ et al (2001). Measures of maternal tobacco exposure and infant birth weight at term. *American journal of epidemiology* 153(10):954-960.

Eustace LW et al (2003). Fetal alcohol syndrome: a growing concern for health care professionals. *Journal of obstetric, gynecologic, and neonatal nursing* 32(2):215-221.

Frank DA et al (2001). Growth, development, and behavior in early childhood following prenatal cocaine exposure. *Journal of the American Medical Association* 285(12):1613-1626.

Frank DA et al (2002). Level of prenatal cocaine exposure and scores on the Bayley scales of infant development: modifying effects of caregiver, early intervention, and birth weight. *Pediatrics* 110(6):1143-1152.

García-Algar Ó et al (2004). Effects of maternal smoking during pregnancy on newborn neurobehavior: neonatal nicotine withdrawal syndrome [Letter to the Editor]. *Pediatrics* 113(3):623-624.

Gilliland FD et al (2001). Effects of maternal smoking during pregnancy and environmental tobacco smoke on asthma and wheezing in children. *American journal of respiratory and critical care medicine* 163:429-436.

Godding V et al (2004). Does in utero exposure to heavy maternal smoking induce nicotine withdrawal symptoms in neonates? *Pediatric research* 55(4):645-651.

Goel P et al (2004). Effects of passive smoking on outcome in pregnancy. *Journal of postgraduate medicine* 50(1):12-16.

Greene CM, Goodman MH (2003). Neonatal abstinence syndrome: strategies for care of the drug-exposed infant. *Neonatal network* 22(4):15-25.

Gupta PC, Sreevidya S (2004). Smokeless tobacco use, birth weight, and gestational age: population based, prospective cohort study of 1217 women in Mumbai, India. *BMJ*, dol:10.1136/bmj.38113.687882.EB. Available at: www.bmj.com/cgi/content/full/328/7455/1538. Retrieved May 29, 2005.

Hankin JR (2002). Fetal alcohol syndrome prevention research. *Alcohol research and health* 26(1):58-65.

Hofhuis W et al (2003). Adverse health effects of prenatal and postnatal tobacco smoke exposure on children. *Archives of disease in childhood* 88:1086-1090.

Holl JA, Lussky RC (2003). Assessing the educational and resource informational needs of health care providers in the area of prenatal alcohol exposure: the first step in the development of a comprehensive fetal alcohol syndrome curriculum. *Neonatal intensive care* 16(2):10-16.

Horne RSC et al (2002). Effects of maternal tobacco smoking, sleeping position, and sleep state on arousal in healthy term infants. *Archives of disease in childhood, fetal and neonatal edition* 87:F100-F105.

Hoyme HE et al (2005). A practical clinical approach to diagnosis of fetal alcohol spectrum disorders: clarification of the 1996 institute of medicine criteria. *Pediatrics* 115(1):39-47.

Hulsey T (2005). Prenatal drug use: the ethics of testing and incarcerating pregnant women. *Newborn and infant nursing reviews* 5(2):93-96.

Hurt H (2005). Substance use during pregnancy. In Spitzer AR, editor. *Intensive care of the fetus and neonate*, ed 2 (pp 317-326). Philadelphia: Elsevier Mosby.

Jaakkola JJK et al (2001). Fetal growth and length of gestation in relation to prenatal exposure to environmental tobacco smoke assessed by hair nicotine concentration. *Environmental health perspectives* 109(6):557-561.

Jackson L et al (2004). A randomized controlled trial of morphine versus phenobarbitone for neonatal abstinence syndrome. *Archives of disease in childhood, fetal and neonatal edition* 89:F300-F304.

Jauniaux E et al (2001). Chronic maternal smoking and cord blood amino acid and enzyme levels at term. *Obstetrics and gynecology* 97(1):57-61.

Johnson K et al (2003a). Substance misuse during pregnancy [Editorial]. *British journal of psychiatry* 183:187-189.

Johnson K et al (2003b). Treatment of neonatal abstinence syndrome. *Archives of disease in childhood, fetal and neonatal edition* 88:F2-F5.

Jones MW, Bass WT (2003). Fetal alcohol syndrome. *Neonatal network* 22(3):63-70.

Kalinka J et al (2005). Impact of prenatal tobacco smoke exposure as measured by midgestation serum cotinine levels, on fetal biometry and umbilical flow velocity waveforms. *American journal of perinatology* 22(1):41-47.

Kelly PAT et al (2002). Functional consequences of perinatal exposure to 3,4-methylenedioxymethamphetamine in rat brain. *British journal of pharmacology* 137(7):963-970.

Kopcha J (2005). Would you recognize a problem drinker? *The clinical advisor* June:49-51.

Koren G et al (2003). Fetal alcohol spectrum disorder. *Canadian medical association journal* 169(11):1181-1185.

Kulig JW et al (2005). Tobacco, alcohol, and other drugs: the role of the pediatrician in prevention, identification, and management of substance abuse. *Pediatrics* 115(3):816-821.

Kuschel CA et al (2004). Can methadone concentrations predict the severity of withdrawal in infants at risk of neonatal abstinence syndrome? *Archives of disease in childhood, fetal and neonatal edition* 89:F390-F393.

Kvigne VL et al (2003). Characteristics of mothers who have children with fetal alcohol syndrome or some characteristics of fetal alcohol syndrome. *Journal of the American board of family practice* 16(4):296-303.

LaGasse LL et al (2003). Prenatal drug exposure and maternal and infant feeding behavior. *Archives of disease in childhood, fetal and neonatal edition* 88:F391-F399.

Langenfeld S et al (2005). Therapy of the neonatal abstinence syndrome with tincture of opium or morphine drops. *Drug and alcohol dependence* 77:31-36.

Lavoie, D. (2005). Suit kindles debate on testing hair for drugs. *Dayton daily news*, August 25.

Law KL et al (2003). Smoking during pregnancy and newborn neurobehavior. *Pediatrics* 111(6):1318-1323.

Lester BM et al (2001). The maternal lifestyle study: drug use by meconium toxicology and maternal self-report. *Pediatrics* 107(2):309-317.

Lester BM, Tronick EZ (2004). History and description of the neonatal intensive care unit network neurobehavioral scale. *Pediatrics* 113(3):634-640.

Lester BM et al (2002). The Maternal Lifestyle Study: effects of substance exposure during pregnancy on neurodevelopmental outcomes in 1-month-old infants. *Pediatrics* 110(6):1182-1192.

Lester BM et al (2003). The Maternal Lifestyle Study (MLS): effects of prenatal cocaine and/or opiate exposure on auditory brain response at one month. *Journal of pediatrics* 142:279-285.

Lester BM et al (2004). Summary statistics of neonatal intensive care unit network neurobehavioral scale scores from the Maternal Lifestyle Study: a quasinormative sample. *Pediatrics* 113(3):668-675.

Leung GM (2004). Secondhand smoke exposure, smoking hygiene, and hospitalization in the first 18 months of life. *Archives of pediatrics and adolescent medicine* 158:687-693.

Lewis KD, Weiss SJ (2003). Psychometric testing of an infant risk assessment for prenatal drug exposure. *Journal of pediatric nursing* 18(6):371-378.

Lifshitz M et al (2001). A four year survey of neonatal narcotic withdrawal: evaluation and treatment. *Israel Medical Association journal* 3(1):17-20.

Maier SE, West JR (2001). Drinking patterns and alcohol-related birth defects. *Alcohol research and health* 25(3):168-174.

Mannino DM et al (2001). Health effects related to environmental tobacco smoke exposure in children in the United States: data from the third national health and nutrition examination survey. *Archives of pediatrics and adolescent medicine* 155:36-41.

Martinez A et al (2005). Perinatal substance abuse. In Taeusch HW et al, editors. *Avery's diseases of the newborn*, ed 8 (pp 106-126). Philadelphia: Elsevier Saunders.

Matt GE et al (2004). Households contaminated by environmental tobacco smoke: sources of infant exposures. *Tobacco control* 13:29-37.

Mattson SN et al (2001). Teratogenic effects of alcohol on brain and behavior. *Alcohol research and health* 25(3):185-191.

May RA, Gossage JP (2001). Estimating the prevalence of fetal alcohol syndrome. *Alcohol research and health* 25(3):159-167.

McMillen RC et al (2003). U.S. adult attitudes and practices regarding smoking restrictions and child exposure to environmental tobacco smoke: changes in the social climate from 2000–2001. *Pediatrics* 112(1):e55-60. Available at: http://www.pediatrics.org/cgi/content/full/112/1/e55. Retrieved June 25, 2005.

Mennella J (2001). Alcohol's effect on lactation. *Alcohol research and health* 25(3):230-234.

Meyer JS et al (2004). Neurotoxic effects of MDMA ("ecstasy") administration to neonatal rats. *International journal of developmental neuroscience* 22:261-271.

Miller-Loncar C (2005). Predictors of motor development in children prenatally exposed to cocaine. *Neurotoxicology and teratology* 27:213-220.

Mone SM et al (2004). Effects of environmental exposures on the cardiovascular system: prenatal period through adolescence. *Pediatrics* 113(4):1058-1069.

Moore C et al (2003). Prevalence of fatty acid ethyl esters in meconium specimens. *Clinical chemistry* 49(1):133-136.

Nakamura MU et al (2004). Obstetric and perinatal effects of active and/or passive smoking during pregnancy. *São Paulo medical journal* 122(3):94-98.

National Institute on Drug Abuse, National Institutes of Health (2001). *Research report series—nicotine addiction*. Available at: http://www.drugabuse.gov/researchreports/nicotine/nicotine.html. Retrieved July 31, 2005.

National Institute on Drug Abuse, National Institutes of Health. (2002). Prenatal exposure to ecstasy may impair memory and cognition. *NIDA*

Notes 17(3). Available at: http://www.drugabuse.gov/NIDA_Notes/NNVol17N3/Prenatal.html. Retrieved July 10, 2005.

National Institute on Drug Abuse, National Institutes of Health. (2004). *NIDA InfoFacts: Methamphetamine*. Available at: http://www.drugabuse.gov/infofacts/methamphetamine.html. Retrieved July 10, 2005.

National Institute on Drug Abuse, National Institutes of Health (2005a). *Message from the Director on methamphetamine abuse*. Available at: http://www.drugabuse.gov/about/welcome/messagemeth405.html. Retrieved July 10, 2005.

National Institute on Drug Abuse, National Institutes of Health (2005b). *NIDA InfoFacts: Crack and cocaine*. Available at: http://www.nida.nih.gov/Infofacts/cocaine.html. Retrieved August 9, 2005.

National Institute on Drug Abuse, National Institutes of Health (2005c). *NIDA InfoFacts: MDMA (Ecstasy)*. Available at: http://www.drugabuse.gov/infofacts/ecstasy.html. Retrieved July 10, 2005.

National Institute on Drug Abuse, National Institutes of Health (2005d). *Research report series—heroin abuse and addiction*. Available at http://www.drugabuse.gov/PDF/RRHeroin.pdf. Retrieved November 9, 2006.

Ostrea EM (2001). Understanding drug testing in the neonate and the role of meconium analysis. *Journal of perinatal and neonatal nursing* 14(4):61-82.

Ostrea EM et al (2001). Estimates of illicit drug use during pregnancy by maternal interview, hair analysis, and meconium analysis. *Journal of pediatrics* 138(3):344-348.

Perera FP et al (2004). Molecular evidence of an interaction between prenatal environmental exposures and birth outcomes in a multiethnic population. *Environmental health perspectives* 112(5):626-630.

Philipp BL et al (2003). Methadone and breastfeeding: new horizons [Commentary]. *Pediatrics* 111(6):1429-1430.

Rao R, Desai NS (2002). OxyContin and neonatal abstinence syndrome. *Journal of perinatology* 22:324-325.

Rieves D (2002). Suffer the children [Editorial]. *Chest* 122(2):394-396.

Rizzi M et al (2004). Environmental tobacco smoke may induce early lung damage in healthy male adolescents. *Chest* 125(4):1387-1393.

Rosen TS, Bateman DA (2002). Infants of addicted mothers. In Fanaroff AA, Martin RE, editors. *Neonatal-perinatal medicine: diseases of the fetus and infant*, ed 7 (pp 661-673). St Louis: Mosby.

Savage C et al (2003). Current screening instruments related to alcohol consumption in pregnancy and a proposed alternative method. *Journal of obstetric, gynecologic, and neonatal nursing* 32(4):437-446.

Sawnani H et al (2004). The effects of maternal smoking on respiratory and arousal patterns in preterm infants during sleep. *American journal of respiratory and critical care medicine* 169:733-738.

Schuler ME et al (2003). Drug-exposed infants and developmental outcome: effects of a home intervention and ongoing maternal drug use. *Archives of pediatrics and adolescent medicine* 157:133-138.

Schuster MA et al (2002). Smoking patterns of household members and visitors in homes with children in the United States. *Archives of pediatrics and adolescent medicine* 156:1094-1100.

Shankaran S et al (2004). Association between patterns of maternal substance use and infant birth weight, length, and head circumference. *Pediatrics* 114(2):e226-e234. Available at: http://www.pediatrics.org/cgi/content/full/114/2/e226. Retrieved June 25, 2005.

Sharpe C, Kuschel C (2004). Outcomes of infants born to mothers receiving methadone for pain management in pregnancy. *Archives of disease in childhood, fetal and neonatal edition* 89:F33-F36.

Shenassa ED, Brown M-J (2004). Maternal smoking and infantile gastrointestinal dysregulation: the case of colic. *Pediatrics* 114(4):e497-e505. Available at: http://www.pediatrics.org/cgi/content/full/114/4/e497. Retrieved June 25, 2005.

Singer LT et al (2001). Developing language skills of cocaine-exposed infants. *Pediatrics* 107(5):1057-1064.

Singer LT et al (2002). Cognitive and motor outcomes of cocaine-exposed infants. *Journal of the American Medical Association* 287(15):1952-1960.

Singer LT et al (2004). Cognitive outcomes of preschool children with prenatal cocaine exposure. *Journal of the American Medical Association* 291(20):2448-2456.

Smith LM et al (2001). Brain proton magnetic resonance spectroscopy and imaging in children exposed to cocaine in utero. *Pediatrics* 107(2):227-231.

Smith L et al (2003). Effects of prenatal methamphetamine exposure on fetal growth and drug withdrawal symptoms in infants born at term. *Developmental and behavioral pediatrics* 24(1):17-23.

Sokol RJ et al (2003). Fetal alcohol spectrum disorder. *Journal of the American Medical Association* 290(22):2996-2999.

Sood B et al (2001). Prenatal alcohol exposure and childhood behavior at age 6 to 7 years: I. dose-response effect. *Pediatrics* 108(2):34. Available at: http://www.pediatrics.org/cgi/content/full/108/2/e34. Retrieved June 25, 2005.

Stokowski LA (2004). Fetal alcohol syndrome: new guidelines for referral and diagnosis. *Advances in neonatal care* 4(6):324.

Svanes C et al (2004). Parental smoking in childhood and adult obstructive lung disease: results from the European community respiratory health survey. *Thorax* 59:295-302.

Tan-Laxa MA et al (2004). Abnormal auditory brainstem response among infants with prenatal cocaine exposure. *Pediatrics* 113(2):357-360.

Tong EK et al (2005). Changing conclusions on secondhand smoke in a sudden infant death syndrome review funded by the tobacco industry. *Pediatrics* 115(3):e356-e366. Available at: http://www.pediatrics.org/cgi/content/full/115/3/e356. Retrieved June 25, 2005.

Toschke AM et al (2003). Early intrauterine exposure to tobacco-inhaled products and obesity. *American journal of epidemiology* 158(11):1068-1074.

U.S. Department of Health and Human Services Substance Abuse and Mental Health Services. (2005a). The national survey on drug use and health report. *Substance use during pregnancy: 2002 and 2003 update*. Available at: www.oas.samhsa.gov/2k5/pregnancy/pregnancy.pdf.

U.S. Department of Health and Human Services and SAMHSA's National Clearinghouse for Alcohol & Drug Information (2005b). Cigarette smoking among adults—United States 2003. *MMWR Morbidity and mortality weekly report* 54(20):509-513. Available at: http://ncadi.samhsa.gov/govpubs/mmwr/vol54/5420a3.aspx. Retrieved July 10, 2005.

Ventura SJ et al (2003). Trends and variations in smoking during pregnancy and low birth weight: evidence from the birth certificate, 1990–2000. *Pediatrics* 111(5):1176-1180.

Wang X et al (2002). Maternal cigarette smoking, metabolic gene polymorphism, and infant birth weight. *Journal of the American Medical Association* 287(2):195-202.

Ward LP et al (2002). Alpha-2A adrenergic receptor subtype gene expression in the intestines of cocaine-exposed rat embryos. *Pediatric research* 52(4):504-508.

Warren KR, Foudin LL (2001). Alcohol-related birth defects—the past, present, and future. *Alcohol research and health* 25(3):153-158.

Wax PM (2002). Just a click away: recreational drug web sites on the Internet. *Pediatrics* 109(6):96. Available at: http://www.pediatrics.org/cgi/content/full/109/6/e96. Retrieved June 25, 2005.

Weiner SM, Finnegan LP (2002). Drug withdrawal in the neonate. In Merenstein GB, Gardner SL, editors. *Handbook of neonatal intensive care*, ed 5 (pp 163-178). St Louis: Mosby.

Welch-Carre E (2005). The neurodevelopmental consequences of prenatal alcohol exposure. *Advances in neonatal care* 5(4):217-229.

White-Traut R et al (2002). Pulse rate and behavioral state correlates after auditory, tactile, visual, and vestibular intervention in drug-exposed neonates. *Journal of perinatology* 22:291-299.

Wilbourne P et al (2001). Clinical management of methadone dependence during pregnancy. *Journal of perinatal and neonatal nursing* 14(4):26-45.

Winickoff JP et al (2003a). A smoking cessation intervention for parents of children who are hospitalized for respiratory illness: the stop tobacco outreach program. *Pediatrics* 111(1):140-145.

Winickoff JP et al (2003b). Intervention with parental smokers in an outpatient pediatric clinic using counseling and nicotine replacement. *Pediatrics* 112(5):1127-1133.

Winickoff JP et al (2003c). Addressing parental smoking in pediatrics and family practice: a national survey of parents. *Pediatrics* 112(5):1146-1151.

Wisborg K et al (2001). Exposure to tobacco smoke in utero and the risk of stillbirth and death in the first year of life. *American journal of epidemiology* 154(4):322-327.

Wouldes R et al (2004). Maternal methamphetamine use during pregnancy and child outcome: what do we know? *New Zealand medical journal* 117(1206):1-10. Available at: http://www.nzma.org.nz/journal/117-1206/1108/. Retrieved July 31, 2005.

Zuckerman B et al (2002). Cocaine-exposed infants and developmental outcomes: "Crack kids" revisited [Editorial]. *Journal of the American Medical Association* 287(15):1990-1991.

Chapter 22

Extremely Low Birth (ELBW) Weight Infant

Shahirose Premji

The extremely low birth weight (ELBW) infant, one who is born weighing less than 1000 g, is a frequent resident of most neonatal intensive care units (NICUs) these days. The survival rate for ELBW infants has improved as a result of advances in technology and organization of perinatal care (Roze & Breart, 2004). Greater survival, however, has not always been associated with increased quality-adjusted survival (Kilbride, 2004). We must look to the future in anticipation, not of change in the limit of viability, but rather of evidence-based strategies to improve the quality of perinatal, neonatal, and postdischarge care with the goal to improve the long-term outcome of ELBW (Roze & Breart, 2004).

EVIDENCE-BASED NEONATAL NURSING CARE

Many years ago, all preterm infants were viewed as "low birth weight or small infants," and their care usually reflected a variation on general pediatric care. Over the past 45 years, it has become clear that preterm infants are a heterogeneous population who require very specialized treatment depending on their birth weight. The definition of low birth weight now includes very low birth weight (VLBW), as an infant who is born weighing less than 1500 g, and ELBW. Whatever the reasons for the ELBW status, these neonates require highly specialized care if they are to survive and thrive. In the 1950s and 1960s health care professionals realized that neonates, especially those who were sick and premature, required care based on an understanding of the disorders and disease and identification of rigorously evaluated treatment (Silverman, 1992). Examples such as retrolental fibroplasias (ROP) secondary to the introduction of unrestricted oxygen therapy and kernicterus resulting from the use of sulfisoxazole underscore the importance of evidence-based practice.

IMPACT OF BIRTH OF EXTREMELY LOW BIRTH WEIGHT INFANTS

Decision Making in the Delivery Room

At ELBW, particularly between 400 and 600 g defined as the zone of "uncertain viability," issues related to moral status (Smith, 2005), survival, and quality of life achieved by these immature infants poses a dilemma for health care professionals, parents, and society (Kraybill, 1998). An ELBW infant gains status as a patient and in a social sense as a member of a family once the infant is born. Health care professionals owe the ELBW infant a duty of ethical treatment and care because of this status (Smith, 2005). Whether to resuscitate and to initiate and continue intensive care raises questions related to the primacy of the newborn's best interest, respect for persons and legal rights, and the health care providers' consideration of ethical principles of beneficence, nonmaleficence, autonomy, justice, and futility. Ethical principles are difficult to implement in practice (Kraybill, 1998; Lorenz, 2003; Wilder, 2000). Ideally a resuscitation plan should be in place prior to delivery. An individualized approach is recommended in management decisions regarding the aggressive resuscitation of ELBW infants. Ethical decisions regarding the extent of resuscitation efforts should be based on multiple factors including gestational age, birth weight, sex of the fetus, the infant's condition at birth, survival and morbidity data, and the parents' wishes. Information should be provided in a consistent manner, and a multidisciplinary approach will ensure that a range of concerns and areas of clinical care are addressed (American College of Obstetricians and Gynecologists, 2002). The plan should be based on consensus decision making by parents and all health care professionals involved in the provision of care to the mother and ELBW infant (Kraybill, 1998; Wilder, 2000).

In many instances though, there is often little time to make informed decisions about the reasonableness of resuscitation and initiation of intensive care. Three systematic approaches have been identified reflecting varying opinions to the proper approach to resuscitation and initiation of intensive care in ELBW infants: provisional intensive care for all, limited care based on probability of survival, and continued intensive care for all (Kraybill, 1998). In the provisional intensive care for all approach, all necessary life support is initiated at least temporarily, to permit assessment of the harm-to-benefit ratio based on projected suffering and burden as determined by current data or "best guess" (Kraybill, 1998; Smith, 2005). Advantages of this approach include an opportunity for survival while minimizing risk of long-term disability if the child is incorrectly judged to be nonviable and survives (Kraybill, 1998; Wilder, 2000); provision of time to more accurately assess the viability of the infant; ability to opt for withdrawal to avoid futile prolongation of life of an infant considered nonviable or one who is considered viable but has suffered a catastrophic complication; and opportunity for parents to discuss the option to reject intensive care in favor of basic care (warmth, supplemental oxygen, and appropriate hydration) (Kraybill, 1998).

In the second approach, statistical prognostic strategy, limited care is provided based on probability of survival (Kraybill, 1998; Lorenz, 2003). Criteria such as gestational age, birth weight, Apgar scores, and possibly others are applied to subjectively identify the upper limit of survival probability. Basic supportive care is provided for those infants whose survival probability is determined to be below that limit in order to avoid prolonged, costly interventions. In the last approach, continued intensive care is provided for all infants from birth until the infant dies. Although this wait-until-certain strategy (Lorenz, 2003) offers the greatest opportunity for survival, the unrestricted use of technology has the potential for causing harm to the infant, parents, and health care professionals responsible for providing care to the infant (Kraybill, 1998).

A single approach or philosophy to care that is appropriate for all countries, cultures, or communities is an unreasonable expectation. Individual and societal values, long-term outcomes and associated physical, psychologic, emotional and financial costs, and finite resources will play a significant role in decision making regarding whether or not to resuscitate and continue care in ELBW infants. The marked variation in the frequency with which aggressive resuscitation is initiated in the zone of uncertainty is not surprising given the various ways in which competing values may be balanced by different individuals, cultures, and societies (Lorenz, 2003).

Survival of Extremely Low Birth Weight Infants

Data based on gestational age are more appropriate than those based on birth weight for projecting survival and future disability in infants. However, unreliable gestational age estimates, and earlier reporting practices of rounding off gestational age to the nearest week of gestation, can have a significant impact on survival statistics (Ho & Saigal, 2005). Population-based studies examining survival by gestational age report marked variation in survival rates among different geographic areas. Differences in survival rates reported in the literature are likely a reflection of approach to resuscitation and initiation of intensive care in ELBW infants, and duration of survival considered in the study (Hack & Fanaroff, 1999; Ho & Saigal, 2005; Lorenz, 2004). Hack & Fanaroff (1999), based on a review of the world literature and personal experience, report survival ranges from 2% to 35% at 23 weeks' gestational age, from 17% to 58% at 24 weeks' gestational age, and from 35% to 85% at 25 weeks' gestational age. At lower ranges of gestational age, with each additional week of gestational age, a large improvement in survival rate is evident (American College of Obstetricians and Gynecologists, 2002; Ho & Saigal, 2005). At comparable gestational age and birth weight, mortality rates are higher for males compared to females (American College of Obstetricians and Gynecologists, 2002).

Morbidity in Extremely Low Birth Weight Infants

Chronic lung disease, necrotizing enterocolitis, retinopathy of prematurity, and disabilities in mental and psychomotor development, neuromotor function, or sensory and communication function are major neonatal morbidities associated with ELBW (American College of Obstetricians and Gynecologists, 2002; Hakansson et al, 2004; Ho & Saigal, 2005). The proportion of ELBW survivors with adverse outcomes has increased (Tyson & Saigal, 2005) and morbidity has increased with decreasing gestational age and birth weight (Hack & Fanaroff, 1999). Variability in morbidity reported in the literature is striking (Lorenz, 2003) and may be due to differences in center demographics, antenatal interventions, and neonatal clinical practice or interventions (Vohr et al, 2004). At comparable gestational age and birth weight, disability rates (e.g., cerebral palsy) are higher for males than for females (American College of Obstetricians and Gynecologists, 2002).

Chronic Lung Disease

Chronic lung disease, the most prevalent morbidity in ELBW infants, occurs in 57% to 70% of infants at 23 weeks' gestational age. At 24 weeks' gestational age rates of chronic lung disease range from 33% to 89%, and at 25 weeks' gestational age ranges from 16% to 71%. Chronic lung disease is a major morbidity influencing later development, given its association with poor nutrition and growth, poor feeding skills, prolonged hospitalization, and episodes of nosocomial infection. The "new BPD" (chronic lung disease) that occurs primarily in ELBW infants is thought to have a qualitatively different pathogenesis marked by immaturity and alveolar hypoplasia rather than the hyperoxic barotrauma or volutrauma typically seen in surfactant deficient lungs (Narendran et al, 2003).

Early delivery room or prophylactic stabilization with continuous positive airway pressure regardless of respiratory status has been proposed as a strategy to improve respiratory outcomes such as development of chronic lung disease in ELBW infants. The effectiveness of this strategy, particularly with respect to neurodevelopmental outcomes, remains to be determined (Lindner et al, 1999; Subramaniam et al, 2005). Dexamethasone treatment has been found to have no effect on chronic lung disease and is associated with gastrointestinal perforation and decreased growth in ELBW infants (Stark et al, 2001). More importantly, a systematic review reported dramatic increase in neurodevelopmental impairment in preterm infants treated with glucocorticoids in the postnatal period (Barrington, 2001).

Necrotizing Enterocolitis

Necrotizing enterocolitis, an acquired gastrointestinal disease that complicates the neonatal course of survivors, affects 1 to 3 infants per 1000 live births (Guthrie et al, 2003; Lee & Polin, 2003). ELBW infants are particularly susceptible and have a higher incidence of NEC; however, the clinical presentation is relatively similar to that for other affected neonates. The cause of necrotizing enterocolitis remains unclear but most likely represents a complex interaction of factors with a final common pathway of intestinal ischemia. In epidemiologic studies prematurity is consistently identified as an independent determinant of necrotizing enterocolitis (Lee & Polin, 2003). Other factors include feeding practices, intestinal ischemia, and bacterial colonization (Kliegman, 1990). Hallmarks of necrotizing enterocolitis include pneumatosis intestinalis, hepatic portal venous gas, perforation and pneumoperitoneum; these are evident on abdominal x-ray (Meerstadt & Gyll, 1994; Snapp, 1994). Manifestations of necrotizing enterocolitis include abdominal distention, residuals, vomiting, bloody stools, metabolic acidosis, cellular destruction, and gut necrosis. Treatment focuses on medical stabilization, and interventions include bowel rest, gastric decompression, broad-spectrum systemic antibiotics, and parenteral nutrition. Infants with perforation either are operated on or have a peritoneal drainage (Lee & Polin, 2003). The catastrophic nature of necrotizing enterocolitis and the fragility of ELBW infants are evident in the overall mortality of the disease, which is approximately 50% (Blakely et al, 2005). Once necrotizing enterocolitis develops, the long-term consequences may include growth delay and severe neurodevelopmental delay (Salhab et al, 2004).

Foster and Cole (2004) conducted a systematic review of studies in which oral immunoglobulin was used in an attempt to prevent necrotizing enterocolitis in premature infants. They found no significant difference in the incidence of necrotizing enterocolitis between infants who received oral immunoglobulin and those who did not. Standardized feeding regimens have been introduced in an attempt to reduce incidence of necrotizing enterocolitis by minimizing variations in enteral feeding practices. A systematic review and meta-analysis of observational studies ("before" and "after") reported a reduced incidence of necrotizing enterocolitis after the introduction of a standardized feeding regimen (Patole & de Klerk, 2005).

Retinopathy of Prematurity

Retinopathy of prematurity (ROP), a vascular proliferative disorder of the immature retina (i.e., abnormal growth of retinal capillaries during vascularization), causes acuity defects, refractive errors (particularly myopia), gaze abnormalities, and blindness (Andersen & Phelps, 2005). Retinopathy of prematurity varies in rate from 33% to 50% at 23 weeks' gestational age. At 24 weeks' gestational age the rate of severe ROP ranges from 13% to 23%, and at 25 weeks' gestational age, from 9% to 17% (Hack & Fanaroff, 1999). The incidence and severity of retinopathy of prematurity is inversely related to gestational age (Palmer et al, 2005; Subhani et al, 2001). Cryotherapy and laser therapy are standard care for threshold ROP (Cryotherapy for Retinopathy of Prematurity Cooperative Group, 2005).

Given the substantial proportion of eyes treated with cryotherapy that developed retinal detachment and unfavorable distance visual acuity, current research is focusing on early treatment for ROP (Early Treatment for Retinopathy of Prematurity Cooperative Group, 2004; Subhani et al, 2001). A systematic review by Andersen and Phelps (2005) has reported early treatment with peripheral retinal ablation to be effective for treating eyes determined to be at high risk for a poor outcome or prethreshold ROP. Treatment resulted in reduced risk of adverse structural outcome at 12 months and $5\frac{1}{2}$ years with corresponding reduction in adverse acuity. Further research is required to assess whether the benefits of treatment will persist into adult life.

To facilitate earlier identification and timely intervention for prethreshold retinopathy of prematurity, it is recommended that in ELBW infants the guidelines of chronologic age of 4 to 6 weeks rather than 31 to 33 week postconceptional age be used (Subhani et al, 2001). Subsequent eye examinations, depending on the results, occur at least every 2 weeks until the retina is fully vascularized. Continued ophthalmologic follow-up of ELBW infants with severe ROP is essential: ROP may represent a lifelong disease, as evidenced by the number of eyes, both cryotherapy-treated and non-cryotherapy-treated, that developed retinal detachment,

blindness, and other related complications between ages 10 and 15 years (Cryotherapy for Retinopathy of Prematurity Cooperative Group, 2005; Palmer et al, 2005).

Vascularization of the retina is complete by 40 weeks' gestational age. In premature infants factors such as change in oxygen exposure have been proposed to cause distribution in this vascularization. In a systematic review, supplementation with vitamin E, an antioxidant agent, was not supported given that there was an increased risk of sepsis and reduced risk of severe retinopathy and blindness among VLBW infants who were given vitamin E supplements (Brion et al, 2005). Supplementation with vitamin A, the precursors of which have antioxidant properties, has been shown in a systematic review to be a potential protective therapy for ROP in VLBW infants (Darlow & Graham, 2005). Darlow and Graham (2005) found a reduction in oxygen requirement at 1 month of age and in ELBW infants and a reduction in oxygen requirement among survivors at 36 weeks' postmenstrual age in infants who received such supplementation. Askie and Henderson-Smart (2001) performed a systematic review of studies of unrestricted oxygen use and outcomes in premature infants. They found that if oxygen levels were not monitored closely, morbidity in this population rose. Oxygen levels, therefore, must be watched and controlled carefully.

Neurodevelopment

Much is still unknown about the long-term neurodevelopmental outcomes of ELBW infants (Ho & Saigal, 2005). Major neurologic impairments include cerebral palsy, motor impairment, visual and hearing impairments, and cognitive deficits. (Ho & Saigal, 2005; Hack & Fanaroff, 1999; Wood et al, 2000). Because of varying criteria for defining and reporting neurologic impairments, as well as differences in age of assessment, it has been challenging to compile disability rates in ELBW infants (Ho & Saigal, 2005). Infants have been reported to have developmental lags without defined impairment (Ho & Saigal, 2005).

A study of 219 ELBW survivors admitted between 1992 and 1995 to Rainbow Babies and Children's Hospital in Cleveland, Ohio and assessed at 8 years of age reported the following outcomes: (1) major neurosensory impairment including cerebral palsy, deafness, and blindness (16%); (2) asthma requiring therapy (21%); (3) functional limitations including delay in growth or development, mental or emotional delay, need to reduce or inability to participate in physical activities, difficulty seeing, hearing, speaking, or communicating, and inability to play or socialize with others (64%); (4) one or more compensatory dependence needs including prescribed medication, life-threatening allergic reactions, prescribed special diet, special equipment to see, hear, or communicate, and need for help or special equipment for walking, feeding, dressing, washing, and toileting (48%); and (5) services needed above routine, including visiting a physician regularly for a chronic condition, nursing care or medical procedures, occupational or physical therapy, special school arrangements, or an individualized education program (65%). The findings of this study may not be representative of all ELBW survivors as this was not a population-based study. Severe disability, measured at a median age of 30 months corrected for gestational age, was reported to be common among ELBW in a population-based study (Wood et al, 2000).

Severe brain injury as evidenced by abnormal cerebral ultrasound findings is another major morbidity that affects long-term outcomes, and rates vary from 10% to 83%, 17% to 64%, and 10% to 22% at 23, 24, and 25 weeks' gestational age, respectively. Interventions such as prophylactic indomethacin therapy have been used in clinical practice to reduce the occurrence of severe interventricular hemorrhage or periventricular leukomalacia, which are significant short-term predictors of neurodevelopmental morbidity in ELBW infants. Although prophylactic administration of indomethacin reduces the incidence of severe intraventricular hemorrhage, it does not improve neurodevelopmental outcomes (Fowlie & Davis 2005; Schmidt et al, 2001). Among other contributing factors, the neurodevelopmental morbidity has been partially attributed to the stressful nature of the intensive care unit (Gorski, 1991). Neurodevelopment can be promoted if the potential impact of the environment is recognized and interventions including one or more elements such as control of external stimuli (e.g., light, noise, minimal stimulation), clustering of care activities, and positioning or swaddling are implemented. There is evidence that this broad category of interventions, referred to as developmental care, offers the following benefits to preterm infants: improved short-term growth and feeding outcomes, decreased respiratory support, decreased length and cost of hospital stay, and improved neurodevelopmental outcomes to 24 months corrected age (Symington & Pinelli, 2005).

COMPLICATIONS OF BEING BORN AT EXTREMELY LOW BIRTH WEIGHT

In the immediate neonatal period ELBW infants are more susceptible to all the possible complications of premature birth because of their very vulnerable state of development. The balance of this chapter is an overview, a quick reference for typical problems experienced by ELBW infants and some of the outcomes for these infants. The chapter also addresses the key areas for care where nurses need to contribute to the scientific basis for practice.

Thermoregulation

Cold stress is associated with increased mortality and morbidity (e.g., hypoglycemia, respiratory distress, and metabolic acidosis) in premature infants. Provision of warmth is the first step in the resuscitation of the newborn because the risk of cold stress is greatest at birth (Knobel et al, 2005). The impaired ability of premature infants to prevent heat loss because of a high body surface area-to-body weight ratio (Lyon et al, 1997), and their decreased ability to produce heat because of decreased brown fat stores and decreased glycogen supply, makes them particularly vulnerable to hypothermia (defined as <36.5° C) (Knobel et al, 2005; McCall et al, 2005; Sauer et al, 1984). A systematic review (McCall et al, 2005) found that early intervention in the delivery room, particularly the application of plastic wraps (for infants <28 weeks' gestational age), skin-to-skin contact (for infants 1200 to 2199 g birth weight), or transwarmer mattresses (infants <1500 g) within 10 minutes after birth, prevents hypothermia, keeping infants warmer on admission to the NICU. These early interventions are in addition to "routine" care implemented immediately after birth such as drying the infant thoroughly, especially the head, removing any wet blankets, wrapping infant in a prewarmed blanket, and prewarming any contact surfaces. Further

research is required to facilitate firm recommendations of these early interventions in clinical practice.

The "gold standard" for nursing preterm infants in incubators or under radiant warmers is to maintain the body temperature at which the metabolic rate reaches the minimum or thermoneutral temperature (Rieger-Fackeldey et al, 2003). In the first week of life this thermoneutral temperature is dependent on gestational age and postnatal age, after which time it depends on body weight and postnatal age (Sauer et al, 1984). However, for ELBW infants, this optimal body temperature is not known (Rieger-Fackeldey et al, 2003). A study of ventilator-dependent ELBW infants in the early postnatal age (day 2 to 14) reported pronounced and consistent changes in spontaneous breathing secondary to minor changes in core body temperature within a range commonly accepted in routine clinical care in the NICU. The observed changes to body temperature are of uncertain clinical significance (Rieger-Fackeldey et al, 2003).

Respiratory Distress Syndrome

Respiratory distress syndrome (RDS), a common problem among ELBW infants, has a pathogenesis dominated by surfactant deficiency. Surfactant deficiency leads to decreased lung compliance, reduced alveolar ventilation, atelectasis, and alveolar hypoperfusion, which clinically manifests as grunting respirations, retractions, nasal flaring, cyanosis, and increased oxygen requirement shortly after birth. Clinical management includes supplemental oxygen and ventilatory support, and the clinical course may be complicated by air leaks, significant shunting through the patent ductus arteriosus, or bronchopulmonary dysplasia (Rodriguez et al, 2002). Prophylactic (delivery room) and rescue (after established RDS) administration of surfactant reduces mortality associated with RDS in preterm infants (Soll & Morley, 2005). Prophylactic administration of surfactant has been reported to decrease the incidence of pneumothorax, the risk of pulmonary interstitial emphysema, and the risk of bronchopulmonary dysplasia (Soll & Morley, 2005). Prophylactic administration of synthetic surfactant, however, has been noted to show a more variable response with no significant difference in risk of bronchopulmonary dysplasia and increased risk of developing patent ductus arteriosus and pulmonary hemorrhage (Soll, 2005).

Endotracheal suctioning for mechanically ventilated patients in the NICU is customary nursing practice aimed at reducing buildup of secretions and tube obstruction, which can cause discomfort, hypoxemia, hypercapnia, and lobar collapse. There is currently a paucity of research with respect to procedures such as preoxygenation, endotracheal suctioning without disconnection from the ventilator, increased mechanical ventilation, manual ventilation, and use of normal saline instillation for suctioning, which are part of the protocols for endotracheal suctioning. The potential serious side effects associated with these procedures warrant development of evidence-based protocols for endotracheal suctioning (Pritchard et al, 2001; Woodgate & Flenady, 2005).

Hyperbilirubinemia

High levels of bilirubin are associated with kernicterus, a form of brain damage with sequelae such as deafness, mental retardation, and cerebral palsy. Given that studies have indicated that kernicterus can occur in ELBW infants at low levels of serum bilirubin, many clinicians have been inclined to initiate phototherapy at low serum bilirubin levels (less than 7 to 10 mg/dl). These studies, however, may be biased toward overestimating bilirubin toxicity because most problems that cause developmental delay are also associated with hyperbilirubinemia (Ambalavanan & Whyte, 2003). In VLBW infants, phototherapy may increase insensible water loss (Bell et al, 1979) secondary to heat generated by the phototherapy equipment (Kjartansson et al, 1992), thereby complicating fluid management. Other known harmful effects of phototherapy include an increase in the incidence of patent ductus arteriosus (Rosenfeld et al, 1986), as well as a potential increase in the incidence of retinopathy of prematurity (Yeo et al, 1998). The benefits and known and unknown adverse effects of phototherapy need to be weighed in decision making regarding initiation of phototherapy at low serum bilirubin levels (Ambalavanan & Whyte, 2003).

Apnea of Prematurity

There is uncertainty about the long-term consequence of apnea (Martin et al, 2004; Stokowski, 2005). Apnea, generally defined as periodic pauses in respirations lasting greater than 15 seconds duration, are considered clinically significant if associated with cyanosis, pallor, hypotonia, or bradycardia. There are multiple etiologic factors such as intracranial hemorrhage, infection, gastroesophageal reflux, anemia or hypoxemia, metabolic disorder, drug therapy, and temperature instability that may contribute to apnea. Apnea of prematurity (AOP) is a diagnosis of exclusion (Martin et al, 2004; Stokowski, 2005). A proposed pathophysiologic mechanism thought to contribute to apnea of prematurity involves immaturity of reflex pathways initiated by hypercapnia, hypoxia, and upper airway afferents (Martin et al, 2004). Clinical interventions for apnea include tactile stimulation, provision of thermoneutral environment, methylxanthine therapy, continuous positive airway pressure or ventilatory support (Martin et al, 2004; Stokowski, 2005), and, more recently, olfactory stimulation (Marlier et al, 2005). Although the use of methylxanthines and nasal intermittent positive pressure ventilation have been shown in a systematic review to be effective in reducing the number of apneic and bradycardic episodes, more research is required before these interventions can be recommended as standard therapy (Henderson-Smart & Steer, 2005; Lemyre et al, 2005).

Nurses spend a significant amount of time monitoring, assessing, and managing apneic and bradycardic episodes, given that nearly all ELBW infants experience AOP. The incidence of apnea of prematurity increases as gestational age decreases. In ELBW infants, apneic and bradycardic episodes persist beyond term gestation, most likely secondary to the higher incidence of chronic lung disease. These persistent apneic and bradycardic episodes complicate and contribute to variability in management decisions related to discharge planning and may prolong hospital stay (Eichenwald et al, 1997). There is a need to develop evidence-based criteria for minimal safe observation period between the time of last apneic episode and hospital discharge (Eichenwald et al, 1997). Furthermore, a clear understanding of the impact of use of technology (e.g., home monitoring) on hospital discharge, subsequent rehospitalization, postdischarge morbidities (Eichenwald et al, 1997), and family functioning and coping is required.

Patent Ductus Arteriosus

Premature infants, particularly ELBW infants, have a significant incidence of persistent patent ductus arteriosus (PDA), a vascular connection between the aorta and pulmonary artery. As a result, these infants experience increases in mortality and morbidities such as more prolonged and severe respiratory distress syndrome, chronic lung disease, and necrotizing enterocolitis (Dollberg et al, 2005). Reliable diagnosis of patent ductus arteriosus in the first 4 days of life depends on echocardiography because of poor specificity of clinical signs (e.g., murmur, wide pulse pressure, bounding pulses, and increased precordial activity) (Skelton et al, 1994). A cardiac murmur is more reliable after this time (Skelton et al, 1994). Treatment decisions for a diagnosed patent ductus arteriosus are based on the clinical significance or clinical effect, the criteria for which vary among neonatologists (Wyllie, 2003).

Prophylactic treatment circumvents the challenges of deciding whether a patent ductus arteriosus is significant or not (Wyllie, 2003). Prophylactic administration of indomethacin reduces the incidence of symptomatic patent ductus arteriosus, and the need for surgical duct ligation.

Adverse effects of indomethacin including necrotizing enterocolitis, excessive bleeding, or sepsis were no different between preterm infants receiving prophylactic indomethacin and controls. The incidence of oliguria was increased; however, this was not associated with major renal impairment. Although prophylactic administration of indomethacin reduces the incidence of severe intraventricular hemorrhage, it does not improve neurodevelopmental outcomes (Fowlie & Davis, 2005; Schmidt et al, 2001). Furthermore, approximately 64% of preterm infants will be medicated unnecessarily (Wyllie, 2003). Values attached by health care providers and parents to the benefits and risks of prophylactic treatment with indomethacin will guide the implementation of this intervention (Fowlie & Davis, 2005).

Ibuprofen has been reported to have similar efficacy to indomethacin (Shah & Ohlsson, 2005), with potentially fewer adverse effects, as it does not reduce blood flow velocity to the brain, gastrointestinal system, or kidneys (Wyllie, 2003). Further evidence of short-term side effects (e.g., pulmonary hypertension) and long-term neurodevelopmental outcomes is required before its use can be recommended. Other interventions include fluid restriction and use of diuretics; however, there is little evidence to support their routine use in clinical practice (Wyllie, 2003). Surgical closure is undertaken when medical intervention fails or is contraindicated (Malviya et al, 2005; Wyllie, 2003). At present there is a paucity of research to determine with certainty whether surgical closure is preferable to medical treatment with cyclooxygenase inhibitors for symptomatic patent ductus arteriosus in preterm infants (Malviya et al, 2005).

Hypotension

Hypotension affects one-third of VLBW infants (Subhedar et al, 2005) and may reduce perfusion of organs such as the brain, heart, kidneys, and gastrointestinal system. It is unclear what drop in blood pressure constitutes hypotension in ELBW infants (Ambalavanan & Whyte, 2003). Hypotension clinically manifests as low blood pressure, reduced cutaneous perfusion, and metabolic acidosis (Osborn & Evans, 2005a, 2005b). Hypotension predisposes premature infants to intraventricular hemorrhage (Watkins et al, 1989) and is associated with increased risk for cerebral palsy (Murphy et al, 1997). Strategies for management of hypotension include inotropes, volume expansion, or corticosteroids (Osborn & Evans, 2005a, 2005b). In preterm infants without cardiovascular compromise, evidence does not support the routine use of early volume expansion (Osborn & Evans, 2005a). Dopamine has been shown to be more effective than albumin (Osborn & Evans, 2005b) and dobutamine (Subhedar et al, 2005), but no firm recommendations can be made as there is a paucity of evidence regarding the long-term benefit of dopamine (Osborn & Evans, 2005b; Subhedar et al, 2005). Generally, corticosteroids are used as a last-chance therapy in managing hypotension. Use of corticosteroids is supported based on our current understanding of pathophysiology (e.g., adrenocortical insufficiency, lower levels of cortisol concentration) (Sasidharan, 1998; Subhedar et al, 2005).

Fluid and Electrolytes

In ELBW the first days after delivery are characterized by fluid shifts resulting from both physiologic changes and pathophysiologic events. "Physiologic weight reduction," the contraction of the extracellular compartment of body water, can be exacerbated as a result of insensible water loss (water lost from skin surface and the respiratory tract) and sensible water loss (water lost through the urine and stool). Insensible water losses are extremely high and variable, making it challenging to predict total fluid intake. Given that the ELBW infant's kidneys have limited ability to compensate for varying water and solute intake (i.e., to adjust the concentration of urine), dehydration, fluid overload, and electrolyte imbalance are common events during the immediate postnatal period (Bell & Acarregui, 2005; Gaylord et al, 2001; Lorenz et al, 1995). Fluid requirements must be monitored closely, as fluid disturbances can affect overall risk of death (Bell & Acarregui, 2005) and exacerbate morbidities such as patent ductus arteriosus, congestive heart failure (Bell et al, 1980), necrotizing enterocolitis, and bronchopulmonary dysplasia (Bell & Acarregui, 2005). Daily weights, regular monitoring of electrolytes, strict documentation of fluid intake and output, cumulative fluid balance recordings, and graphic trends of growth facilitate decisions related to fluid management in ELBW infants. A retrospective study revealed that using humidified incubators in ELBW infants led to improved fluid management (Gaylord et al, 2001). Some NICUs use swamping (piping highly humidified air into the isolette) when the infant is under a radiant warmer in an effort to reduce insensible water losses and promote thermoregulation. Innovative strategies that facilitate fluid management warrant further research.

Metabolic Considerations

In ELBW infants, maintaining normoglycemia is difficult because of insufficient glycogen stores, stress, high metabolic rates, and variability in fluid requirements. Additionally, what constitutes normoglycemia in ELBW infants is controversial as low blood glucose concentrations may reflect the normal process of metabolic adaptation to extrauterine life, the infant may be asymptomatic, symptoms (e.g., lethargy, apnea, tachypnea, seizures) if present are nonspecific, and long-term sequelae of asymptomatic hypoglycemia have not been shown (Cornblath et al, 2000; Kalhan & Parimi, 2001). At present there is no consensus regarding cutoff values for hypoglycemia. A blood glucose concentration persistently less than 36 mg/dl (2.0 mmol/L) or, in a symptomatic infant, a blood glucose concentration less than 45 mg/dl (2.5 mmol/L) is considered an indication for clinical intervention (Cornblath et al, 2000; Kalhan & Parimi, 2001). Rapid or high-concentration boluses are not advisable, because rebound hypoglycemia can occur. Clinical management of hypoglycemia and hyperglycemia with devices such as the continuous glucose monitoring sensor may prove beneficial in ELBW infants (Beardsall et al, 2005).

Nutrition

In ELBW infants endogenous nutritional stores are limited as their bodies are primarily water. These endogenous nutritional stores are quickly depleted under conditions of starvation as metabolic needs are high. Early nutrition is imperative to ensure the infants' continued survival. Nourishing ELBW infants is an important clinical concern as nutritional management, particularly in the first weeks of life, has an impact on growth, neurologic development, and health indices (Lucas, 1990; Morley & Lucas, 2000). ELBW infants are at an increased risk of poor somatic growth, with the poorest growth being seen in those infants who have comorbidities (e.g., feeding problems, respiratory illness, neurologic and developmental difficulties) (Wood et al, 2003).

Given that ELBW infants may be slow to tolerate introduction of enteral feeds because of delayed gastric emptying and immaturity of intestinal motor activity, parenteral nutrition should be established soon after birth. Generally, infants are gradually started on parenteral nutrition with amino acids and intralipid being increased over a period of several days to a maximum of 3.5 g/kg per day and 3 g/kg per day, respectively. Aggressive intake of amino acids and intralipid, administration of 3.5 g/kg per day of amino acids and 3 g/kg per day of intralipid, is being advocated immediately after birth (within 1 hour) in VLBW infants (Ibrahim et al, 2004). Numerous detrimental effects of total parenteral nutrition are cited in the literature, including necrotizing enterocolitis, infection, and changes in the structural integrity and function of the gastrointestinal system. Refinement of feeding strategies that facilitate quick transition from parenteral to enteral nutrition and that meet the specific needs of ELBW infants should be the focus of future research.

Use of minimal enteral nutrition (MEN) (small-volume feeding of <24 ml/kg per day) shortly after birth to achieve a biologic effect on the gastrointestinal system is well supported based on evidence from a systematic review (Tyson & Kennedy, 2005) and our understanding of the anatomic and physiologic disadvantages of delaying feeding (Premji et al, 2002). The optimum timing of minimal enteral nutrition is unclear, as initiation ranged from day 1 to day 8 in studies included in the systematic review. Initiating MEN within 48 hours of birth permits assessment of physiologic stability in ELBW infants (Premji et al, 2002). For ELBW infants, the continuous tube feeding method may be more energy efficient, as a subgroup analysis of infants included in a systematic review suggested that infants weighing less than 1000 g gained weight significantly faster when fed by this method (Premji & Chessell, 2005). Further research is required to discern the benefits and risk of continuous tube feeding methods in ELBW infants.

Human milk is considered the best feeding substrate for premature infants as it confers biologic (e.g., easier to digest and absorb), immunologic (e.g., lower rate of infection and incidence of NEC), and developmental (e.g., improved intelligence quotient) advantages (Schanler, 1995; Lucas & Cole, 1990; Lucas et al, 1992). However, preterm human milk does not have sufficient quantities of protein, sodium, phosphate, and calcium to meet estimated needs for growth. Fortification of human milk is therefore essential to maintain adequate growth, nutrient retention, and biochemical homeostasis (Atkinson, 2000; Schanler, 1995). Commercially available fortifiers come in liquid or powder form. Potential complications of fortification include distended abdomen, increased osmolarity, and bacterial contamination. In a systematic review, protein supplementation of human milk in relatively healthy preterm infants resulted in short-term growth; however, the adverse effects of protein supplementation could not be discerned (Kuschel & Harding, 2005).

Currently there is controversy with respect to concurrent feeding and indomethacin therapy. The reduced mesenteric diastolic blood flow associated with indomethacin therapy may be counteracted by minimal enteral nutrition, thereby exerting a protective influence on the gastrointestinal system. However, clinical practice varies between units, with some following the conventional wisdom of withholding enteral feeding during indomethacin therapy in order to prevent necrotizing enterocolitis (Premji et al, 2002).

Rapid advancement in feedings (40 to 60 ml/kg per day) has been implicated as one factor that puts stressed premature infants at greater risk for developing necrotizing enterocolitis. Rapid advancement in feeding offers the advantage of overall reduction in days to full enteral feedings and days to regain birth weight (Kennedy & Tyson, 2005). Given that information regarding safety is unclear, a feeding advancement of not more than 30 ml/kg per day has been advocated (Premji et al, 2002).

Patole and de Klerk (2005) propose that clinical variation in practice determines risk of necrotizing enterocolitis. Nursing management of tube feeding is inconsistent, and variability in the practice of withdrawing feeding and management of feeding residuals has been shown (Hodges & Vincent, 1993). A better understanding is required of nursing practice related to tube feeding in order to facilitate a standardized systematic evidence-based approach founded on the current state of scientific knowledge (Premji, 2005).

Physiologic, behavioral, and neurologic immaturity contribute to feeding problems experienced by ELBW infants. A prerequisite to safe and successful oral feeding is effective sucking behaviors and intact gag and cough reflexes (Shaker, 1990; Medoff-Cooper & Ray, 1995). Transitioning ELBW infants from tube feeding to oral feeding is a major challenge for nurses, as no criteria exist to guide practice (Hawdon et al, 2000; Pickler & Reyna, 2003), and hence the practice is variable and based on custom (McCain et al, 2001). An evidence-based neonatal oral feeding protocol has been developed to create positive feeding experiences while assisting high-risk infants to achieve full oral feedings (Premji et al, 2004). Infant characteristics (not postconceptional age) are the primary determinants used to plan physiologically appropriate feeding experiences for each stage—preoral stimulation, nonnutritive sucking, and nutritive sucking—of progression to oral feeding. The mainstay of this protocol is

a professional resocialization in the way nurses view and engage in feeding interactions, with emphasis on the quality of the feeding interaction rather than the quantity of milk consumed by the infant. The extent to which this protocol is adopted in practice will determine its efficacy and safety. A study is currently in progress to determine this. For continued improvement in nutritional management of ELBW infants, it is imperative that nurses engage in protocol appraisal and self-appraisal of practice, and that they review new evidence.

Gastroesophageal Reflux

Another complication related to digestion is gastroesophageal reflux (GER), a maturational phenomenon caused by transient lower esophageal sphincter relaxation (Ambalavanan & Whyte, 2003; Omari et al, 2004). Placement of a feeding tube across the gastroesophageal junction has been shown to increase the incidence of GER (Peter et al, 2002b). Although GER is regarded as a risk factor for apnea, no temporal relationship has been demonstrated between apnea and GER in preterm infants (Peter et al, 2002a). GER is also considered a risk factor for aspiration and subsequent pneumonia (Ambalavanan & Whyte, 2003). The association between chronic lung disease and GER is thought to be due to greater diagnostic suspicion in infants with chronic lung disease (Fuloria et al, 2000). GER does not appear to increase the risk of delayed growth (<10th percentile) or development (Bayley Mental Developmental and Psychomotor Developmental Indices of <70) in VLBW infants (Fuloria et al, 2000).

At present, there is lack of consensus with regard to optimal management of GER in ELBW infants, as there are few randomized controlled trials to guide practice. Therapies used in clinical practice include nonpharmacologic measures (e.g., positioning and thickening of feedings), and pharmacologic measures (e.g., metoclopramide, domperidone) (Ambalavanan & Whyte, 2003). A study by Ewer, James, and Tobin (1999) reported that prone and left lateral positioning reduced the number and duration of reflux episodes. GER is difficult to diagnose, as current techniques of esophageal pH monitoring cannot reliably detect GER in preterm infants. This is because frequent feeding causes esophageal acidification to pH less than 4 (Grant & Cochran, 2001; Omari et al, 2004). Consequently, the contribution of GER to neonatal morbidity and the efficacy of therapies for gastroesophageal reflux are difficult to evaluate.

Anemia

The primary cause of anemia, particularly in the first 2 weeks of life, is phlebotomy losses resulting from intensive laboratory testing. Other causes include inability to increase erythropoietin concentration and erythropoiesis, and severely limited blood volume based on body weight (Ohls, 2002). In the preterm infant typically there is a physiologic fall in hemoglobin and hematocrit levels by approximately 6 weeks of age. The decline in hematocrit in ELBW infants is associated with clinical findings necessitating packed red blood cell transfusion, and hence is not considered "physiologic" (Aher & Ohlsson, 2005). It is uncertain what hematocrit levels precipitate clinical signs of anemia of prematurity and what is the minimal acceptable level for infants requiring ventilatory support (Ohls, 2002). Low hemoglobin and hematocrit levels often guide decisions regarding blood transfusion (Aher & Ohlsson,

2005). As a result of more stringent transfusion guidelines, the numbers of blood transfusions have decreased over the past decade (Maier et al, 2000); however, ELBW infants continue to receive numerous transfusions (Aher & Ohlsson, 2005). Plasma erythropoietin with iron supplementation (to reduce the risk of the development of iron deficiency) has also been used in the prevention and treatment of anemia of prematurity (Aher & Ohlsson, 2005; Kotto-Kome et al, 2004). A retrospective study of ELBW infants revealed that the number of blood transfusions was significantly associated with severity of retinopathy of prematurity (Englert et al, 2001). Other benefits of reducing the number of packed red blood cell transfusions include reduced risk of transmission of viral infections, reduced risk of incompatibility, and reduced cost (Aher & Ohlsson, 2005). Consequently, strategies or interventions that reduce phlebotomy losses and blood transfusions throughout the infant's hospital stay warrant further investigation.

Point-of-care devices, that is, laboratory blood testing using bedside devices may potentially contribute towards reducing phlebotomy losses and blood transfusions (Madan et al, 2005; Moya et al, 2001) and warrant further investigation. Additionally, the nurse must act as an advocate to eliminate unnecessary laboratory monitoring. A meta-analysis reported that administration of recombinant erythropoietin in the first week of life resulted in moderate reduction in the proportion of VLBW infants requiring blood transfusion. Subgroup analysis revealed that ELBW infants were less likely to avoid transfusion if treated with recombinant erythropoietin (Kotto-Kome et al, 2004).

Infection

Infections are frequent complications of ELBW with approximately 65% of infants having at least one infection during hospitalization. Infection rates increase with decreasing birth weight and gestational age and are associated with increased mortality and poor neurodevelopmental and growth outcomes in childhood (Stoll et al, 2004). Early-onset infection (before 72 hours) is due to maternal factors (congenital) and is uncommon, but can be life-threatening (Ambalavanan & Whyte, 2003). Risk of early onset sepsis (e.g., group B streptococcal) may be decreased with intra-partum antibiotic prophylaxis, but there is concern that it may mask infection, with onset of signs of sepsis taking longer. In almost all ELBW infants, antibiotics (ampicillin or penicillin and aminoglycoside) for suspected sepsis are initiated after birth, and if the infant is asymptomatic and culture is negative, antibiotic therapy is discontinued after 48 to 72 hours. It is unclear what impact the frequent and empiric use of antibiotics has on incidence and resistance pattern of late-onset bacterial infection (Ambalavanan & Whyte, 2003).

Late-onset sepsis (after 72 hours), referred to as nosocomial infection, is an acquired infection with coagulase-negative staphylococci being the most common cause of bacteremia. It is treated with vancomycin (Craft et al, 2005). The risk of acquired infection is high, because ELBW infants have an immature immune system; they often lack the protection of passive immunity, they have poor epidermal and gastrointestinal barrier function, and they may have central arterial or venous catheters (e.g., umbilical lines and percutaneous central venous catheters). There are multitudes of nonspecific signs and symptoms of sepsis, namely, temperature instability, apnea and bradycardia, feeding intolerance, abdominal distension, lethargy, septic shock, and increased need for oxygen or ventilatory support (Craft et al, 2005).

Skin breakdown, another pathway for infection, occurs more frequently in ELBW infants, and it is proposed that topical ointment therapy may serve as a protective barrier leading to improved skin integrity and decrease risk of nosocomial infection (Conner et al, 2005). Application of preservative-free emollient ointment improves skin condition and reduces transepidermal water loss, but is associated with adverse outcomes. The risk of coagulase-negative staphylococcal infection and any nosocomial infection (e.g., bacterial and fungal organism) was increased with application of ointment (Conner et al, 2005). Other potential strategies to minimize skin breakdown, thereby reducing risk of infection, include use of as little tape as possible, and changing the infant's position frequently to prevent abrasions and pressure areas. It is important to remember that other treatments, procedures, and conditions may aggravate the problem (e.g., steroid therapy; use of blood products, leading to thrombocytopenia or lymphocytopenia; invasive procedures; changes in the pH of the skin as a result of bathing practices). Renal function is compromised in ELBW infants. It is imperative that nurses give medications (particularly drugs that are nephrotoxic such as gentamicin) with careful consideration of renal function. If renal function is compromised, a toxic level of this drug can be reached quite quickly, leading to permanent renal and auditory damage. The nurse should consider where the drug is metabolized and cleared through the body. If the site is the renal system and if output is severely diminished, use of the medication may need to be suspended temporarily.

Given the spectrum of issues that may be encountered by an ELBW infant, an individualized approach to care is crucial. Consistent and sound clinical reasoning based on history and physical examination, comprehensive data (e.g., essential laboratory findings), and knowledge (e.g., research evidence) should guide nursing practice decisions. Moreover, parents' wishes should be considered in making judgments about best practices, as they hold the ultimate moral and legal authority to make decisions about the infant's treatment. The ethical imperative is shared decision making (Penticuff & Arheart, 2005).

FAMILIES OF EXTREMELY LOW BIRTH WEIGHT INFANTS

The birth of an ELBW infant generates a cascade of parental emotions and fears beginning with decisions related to resuscitation, to uncertainty regarding survival of the infant, the numerous complications and variability in treatment decisions, the technology in the NICU, appearance of the child, and unfamiliar people (Sydnor-Greenberg & Dokken, 2000). Parental grief over the death of an ELBW infant, loss of a desired child, loss of pregnancy, or past losses may be adversely influenced by nursing behaviors (Golish & Powell, 2003; Sydnor-Greenberg & Dokken, 2000). Effective communication that incorporates support (physical or social) and teaching will assist parents to find their own unique paths to meaningful involvement (Sydnor-Greenberg & Dokken, 2000). It is important that nurses realize that there will be individual differences depending on the race, religion, nationality, and cultural background of the families. Although it may seem daunting at times, nurses should attempt to accurately interpret and respond to various behaviors by parents to facilitate meaningful involvement in caring for their infant (Sydnor-Greenberg & Dokken, 2000). Principles of family-centered care provide an excellent framework to encourage families to participate as fully as possible in caring for and making decisions about their infant, and to form mutually beneficial and supportive partnerships in the NICU (Harrison, 1993).

A crucial element in caring for ELBW infants is to engage families to participate collaboratively in deciding appropriate care. The ability of the families to understand accurately their infant's medical condition, prognosis, and treatment options is dependent on the health care professional's ability to take a participatory approach to care (Penticuff & Arheart, 2005). Interventions that facilitate effective communication, collaborative care, and shared decision making warrant closer scrutiny by evaluating their efficacy.

SUMMARY

This chapter presented a brief overview of the mortality and morbidities associated with being born ELBW, care required for the problems encountered by ELBW infants, and potential areas for future research. There are many unknowns; however, there is hope . . . a trust in the future of life. Nurses, physicians, other health care providers, and parents can make a difference if they are aware of the potential problems and know how to detect or recognize them early.

REFERENCES

Aher S, Ohlsson A (2005). Late administration of erythropoietin for preventing red blood cell transfusion in preterm and/or low birth weight infants (Protocol). In *The Cochrane library*, vol 3. Oxford: Update Software.

Ambalavanan N, Whyte RK (2003). The mismatch between evidence and practice. Common therapies in search of evidence. *Clinics in perinatology* 30:305-331.

American College of Obstetricians and Gynecologists (ACOG) (2002). Perinatal care at the threshold of viability. ACOG Practice Bulletin No 38. *International journal of gynecology and obstetrics* 79:181-188.

Andersen CC, Phelps DL (2005). Peripheral retinal ablation for threshold retinopathy of prematurity in preterm infants (Cochrane Review). In *The Cochrane Library*, vol 3. Oxford: Update Software.

Askie LM, Henderson-Smart DJ (2001). Restricted versus liberal oxygen exposure for preventing morbidity and mortality in preterm or low birth weight infants (Cochrane Review). In *The Cochrane Library*, vol 3. Oxford: Update Software.

Atkinson SA (2000). Human milk feeding of the micropremie. *Clinics in perinatology* 27:235-247.

Barrington KJ (2001). The adverse neuro-developmental effects of postnatal steroids in the preterm infant: a systematic review of RCTs. *BMC pediatrics* 1(1):e1.

Beardsall K et al (2005). The continuous glucose monitoring sensor in neonatal intensive care. *Archives of disease in childhood: fetal and neonatal edition* 90:F307-F310.

Bell EF, Acarregui MJ (2005). Restricted versus liberal water intake for preventing morbidity and mortality in preterm infants (Cochrane Review). In *The Cochrane library*, vol 3. Oxford: Update Software.

Bell EF et al (1980). Effect of fluid administration on the development of symptomatic patent ductus arteriosus and congestive heart failure in premature infants. *New England journal of medicine* 302:598-604.

Bell FB et al (1979). Combined effect of radiant warmer and phototherapy on insensible water loss in low-birth-weight infants. *Journal of pediatrics* 94:810-813.

Blakely ML et al, NEC Subcommittee of the NICHD Neonatal Research Network (2005). Postoperative outcomes of extremely low birth-weight infants with necrotizing enterocolitis or isolated intestinal perforation: a prospective cohort study by the NICHD Neonatal Research Network. *Annals of surgery* 241:984-999.

Brion LP et al (2005). Vitamin E supplementation for prevention of morbidity and mortality in preterm infants (Cochrane Review). In *The Cochrane Library*, vol 3. Oxford: Update Software.

Conner JM et al (2005). Topical ointment for preventing infection in preterm infants (Cochrane Review). In *The Cochrane library*, vol 3. Oxford: Update Software.

Cornblath M et al (2000). Controversies regarding definition of neonatal hypoglycemia: suggested operational thresholds. *Pediatrics* 105:1141-1145.

Craft AP et al (2005). Vancomycin for prophylaxis against sepsis in preterm neonates (Cochrane Review). In *The Cochrane library*, vol 3. Oxford: Update Software.

Cryotherapy for Retinopathy of Prematurity Cooperative Group (2005). 15-year outcomes following threshold retinopathy of prematurity: final results from the multicenter trial of cryotherapy for retinopathy of prematurity. *Archives of ophthalmology* 123:311-318.

Darlow BA, Graham PJ (2005). Vitamin A supplementation for preventing morbidity and mortality in very low birth weight infants (Cochrane Review). In *The Cochrane library*, vol 3. Oxford: Update Software.

Dollberg S et al (2005). Patent ductus arteriosus, indomethacin and necrotizing enterocolitis in very low birth weight infants: a population-based study. *Journal of pediatric gastroenterology and nutrition* 40:184-189.

Early Treatment for Retinopathy of Prematurity Cooperative Group (2004). Multicenter trial of early treatment for retinopathy of prematurity: study design. *Controlled clinical trials* 25:311-325.

Eichenwald EC et al (1997). Apnea frequently persists beyond term gestation in infants delivered at 24 to 28 weeks. *Pediatrics* 100:354-359.

Englert JA et al (2001). The effect of anemia on retinopathy of prematurity in extremely low birth weight infants. *Journal of perinatology* 21:21-26.

Ewer AK et al (1999). Prone and left lateral positioning reduce gastro-oesophageal reflux in preterm infants. *Archives of disease in childhood, fetal and neonatal edition* 81:F201-F205.

Foster J, Cole M (2004). Oral immunoglobulin for preventing necrotizing enterocolitis in preterm and low birth weight neonates (Cochrane Review). In *The Cochrane Library*, vol 3. Oxford: Update Software.

Fowlie PW, Davis PG (2005). Prophylactic intravenous indomethacin for preventing mortality and morbidity in preterm infants (Cochrane Review). In *The Cochrane library*, vol 3. Oxford: Update Software.

Fuloria M et al (2000). Gastroesophageal reflux in very low birth weight infants: association with chronic lung disease and outcomes through 1 year of age. *Journal of perinatology* 4:235-239.

Gaylord MS et al (2001). Improved fluid management utilizing humidified incubators in extremely low birth weight infants. *Journal of perinatology* 21:438-443.

Golish TD, Powell KA (2003). 'Ambiguous loss': managing the dialectics of grief associated with premature birth. *Journal of social and personal relationships* 20:309-334.

Gorski PA (1991). Promoting infant development during neonatal hospitalization: critiquing the state of the science. *Children's health care* 20:250-257.

Grant L, Cochran D (2001). Can pH monitoring reliably detect gastro-esophageal reflux in preterm infants? *Archives of disease in childhood, neonatal and fetal edition* 85:F155-F157.

Guthrie SO et al (2003). Necrotizing enterocolitis among neonates in the United States. *Journal of perinatology* 23:278-285.

Hack M, Fanaroff AA (1999). Outcomes of children of extremely low birthweight and gestational age in the 1990's. *Early human development* 53:193-218.

Hakansson S et al (2004). Proactive management promotes outcomes in extremely preterm infants: a population-based comparison of two perinatal management strategies. *Pediatrics* 114(1):58-64.

Harrison H (1993). The principles of family-centered neonatal care. *Pediatrics* 92(5):643-650.

Hawdon J et al (2000). Identification of neonates at risk of developing feeding problems in infancy. *Developmental medicine and child neurology* 42:235-239.

Henderson-Smart DJ, Steer P (2005). Methylxanthine treatment for apnea in preterm infants (Cochrane Review). In *The Cochrane library*, vol 3. Oxford: Update Software.

Ho S, Saigal S (2005). Current survival and early outcomes of infants of borderline viability. *NeoReviews* 6(3):e123-e132.

Hodges C, Vincent P (1993). Why do NICU nurses not refeed gastric residuals prior to feeding by gavage? *Neonatal network* 12:37-40.

Ibrahim HM et al (2004). Aggressive early total parental nutrition in low-birth-weight infants. *Journal of perinatology* 24:482-486.

Kalhan SC, Parimi PS (2001). Disorders of carbohydrate metabolism. In Fanaroff AA, Martin RJ, editors. *Neonatal-perinatal medicine: diseases of the fetus and infant*, ed 7 (pp 3-12). St Louis: Mosby.

Kennedy KA, Tyson JE (2005). Rapid versus slow rate of advancement of feedings for promoting growth and preventing necrotizing enterocolitis in parenterally fed low-birth-weight infants (Cochrane Review). In *The Cochrane library*, vol 3. Oxford: Update Software.

Kilbride HW (2004). Effectiveness of neonatal intensive care for extremely low birth weight infants. *Pediatrics* 114:1374.

Kjartansson S et al (1992). Insensible water loss from the skin during phototherapy in term and preterm infants. *Acta paediatrica* 81:764-768.

Kliegman RM (1990). Models of the pathogenesis of necrotizing enterocolitis. *Journal of pediatrics* 117:S2-S5.

Knobel RB et al (2005). Heat loss prevention for preterm infants in the delivery room. *Journal of perinatology* 25:304-308.

Kotto-Kome AC et al (2004). Effect of beginning recombinant erythropoietin treatment within the first week of life, among very-low-birth-weight neonates, on "early" and "late" erythrocyte transfusions: a meta-analysis. *Journal of perinatology* 24:24-29.

Kraybill EN (1998). Ethical issues in the care of extremely low birth weight infants. *Seminars in perinatology* 22:207-215.

Kuschel CA, Harding JE (2005). Protein supplementation of human milk for promoting growth in preterm infants (Cochrane Review). In *The Cochrane library*, vol 3. Oxford: Update Software.

Lee JS, Polin RA (2003). Treatment and prevention of necrotizing enterocolitis. *Seminars in neonatology* 8:449-459.

Lemyre B et al (2005). Nasal intermittent positive pressure ventilation (NIPPV) versus nasal continuous positive airway pressure (NCPAP) for apnea of prematurity (Cochrane Review). In *The Cochrane library*, vol 3. Oxford: Update Software.

Lindner W et al (1999). Delivery room management of extremely low birth weight infants: spontaneous breathing or intubation? *Pediatrics* 103:961-967.

Lorenz JM (2003). Management decisions in extremely premature infants. *Seminars in neonatology* 8:475-482.

Lorenz JM (2004). Proactive management of extremely premature infants. *Pediatrics* 114:264.

Lorenz JM et al (1995). Phases of fluid and electrolyte homeostasis in the extremely low birth weight infant. *Pediatrics* 96:484-489.

Lucas A (1990). Does early diet program future outcome? *Acta paediatrica Scandinavica* 365:58-67.

Lucas A, Cole TJ (1990). Breast milk and neonatal necrotizing enterocolitis. *Lancet* 336:1519-1523.

Lucas A et al (1992). Breast milk and subsequent intelligence quotient in children born preterm. *Lancet* 339:261-264.

Lyon AJ et al (1997). Temperature control in very low birthweight infants during first five days of life. *Archives of disease in childhood* 76:F47-F50.

Madan A et al (2005). Reduction in red blood cell transfusions using a bedside analyzer in extremely low birth weight infants. *Journal of perinatology* 25:21-25.

Maier RF et al (2000). Changing practices of red blood cell transfusions in infants with birth weights less than 1000 g. *Journal of pediatrics* 136(2):220-224.

Malviya M et al (2005). Surgical versus medical treatment with cyclooxygenase inhibitors for symptomatic patent ductus arteriosus in preterm infants (Cochrane Review). In *The Cochrane library*, vol 3. Oxford: Update Software.

Marlier L et al (2005). Olfactory stimulation prevents apnea in premature newborns. *Pediatrics* 115:83-88.

Martin RJ et al (2004). Apnoea of prematurity. *Pediatric respiratory reviews* 5:S377-S382.

McCain GC et al (2001). A feeding protocol for healthy preterm infants that shortens time to oral feeding. *Journal of pediatrics* 139:374-379.

McCall EM et al (2005). Interventions to prevent hypothermia at birth in preterm and/or low birthweight babies (Cochrane Review). In *The Cochrane library*, vol 3. Oxford: Update Software.

Medoff-Cooper R, Ray W (1995). Neonatal sucking behaviors. *Image—journal of nursing scholarship* 27:195-200.

Meerstadt PWD, Gyll C (1994). *Manual of neonatal emergency x-ray interpretation*. London: Saunders.

Morley R, Lucas A (2000). Randomized diet in the neonatal period and growth performance until 7.5-8 y of age in preterm children. *American journal of clinical nutrition* 71:822-828.

Moya MP et al (2001). The effect of bedside blood gas monitoring on blood loss and ventilator management. *Biology of the neonate* 80:257-261.

Murphy DJ et al (1997). Neonatal risk factors for cerebral palsy in very preterm babies: case-control study. *BMJ* 314:404-408.

Narendran V et al (2003). Early bubble CPAP and outcomes in ELBW preterm infants. *Journal of perinatology* 23:195-199.

Ohls RK (2002). Erythropoietin treatment in extremely low birth weight infants: blood in versus blood out. *Journal of pediatrics* 141:3-6.

Omari TI et al (2004). Paradoxical impact of body positioning on gastroesophageal reflux and gastric emptying in the premature neonate. *Journal of pediatrics* 145:194-200.

Osborn DA, Evans N (2005a). Early volume expansion for prevention of morbidity and mortality in very preterm infants (Cochrane Review). In *The Cochrane library*, vol 3. Oxford: Update Software.

Osborn DA, Evans N (2005b). Early volume expansion versus inotrope for prevention of morbidity and mortality in very preterm infants (Cochrane Review). In *The Cochrane library*, vol 3. Oxford: Update Software.

Palmer EA et al (2005). Cryotherapy for Retinopathy of Prematurity Cooperative Group. 15-year outcomes following threshold retinopathy of prematurity: final results from the multicenter trial of cryotherapy for retinopathy of prematurity. *Archives of ophthalmology* 123:311-318.

Patole S, de Klerk N (2005). Impact of standardised feeding regimens on incidence of neonatal necrotising enterocolitis: a systematic review and meta analysis of observational studies. *Archives of disease in childhood, neonatal and fetal edition* 90:F147-F151.

Penticuff JH, Arheart KL (2005). Effectiveness of an intervention to improve parent-professional collaboration in neonatal intensive care. *Journal of perinatal and neonatal nursing* 19:187-202.

Peter CS et al (2002a). Gastroesophageal reflux and apnea of prematurity: no temporal relationship. *Pediatrics* 109:8-11.

Peter CS et al (2002b). Influence of nasogastric tubes on gastroesophageal reflux in preterm infants: a multiple intraluminal impedance study. *Journal of pediatrics* 141:277-279.

Pickler RH, Reyna BA (2003). A descriptive study of bottle-feeding opportunities in preterm infants. *Advances in neonatal care* 3:139-146.

Premji SS (2005). Standardised feeding regimens: hope for reducing the risk of necrotizing enterocolitis. *Archives of disease in childhood* 90:192-193.

Premji S, Chessell L (2005). Continuous nasogastric milk feeding versus intermittent bolus milk feeding for premature infants less than 1,500 grams (Cochrane Review). In *The Cochrane library*, vol 3. Oxford: Update Software.

Premji SS et al (2002). Evidence-based feeding guidelines for very-low-birth-weight infants. *Advances in neonatal care* 2(1):5-18.

Premji SS et al (2004). Regional neonatal oral feeding protocol: changing the ethos of feeding preterm infants. *Journal of perinatal and neonatal nursing* 18(4):371-384.

Pritchard M et al (2001). Preoxygenation for tracheal suctioning in intubated, ventilated newborn infants (Cochrane Review). In *The Cochrane library*, vol 3. Oxford: Update Software.

Rieger-Fackeldey E et al (2003). Effect of body temperature on the pattern of spontaneous breathing in extremely low birth weight infants supported by proportional assist ventilation. *Pediatric research* 54:332-336.

Rodriguez RJ et al (2002). Part 3: Respiratory distress syndrome and its management. In Fanaroff AA, Martin RJ, editors. *Neonatal-perinatal medicine* (pp 1001-1011). St Louis: Mosby.

Rosenfeld W et al (1986). Phototherapy effect on the incidence of patent ductus arteriosus in premature infants: prevention with chest shielding. *Pediatrics* 78:10-14.

Roze JC, Breart G (2004). Care of very premature infants: looking to the future. *European journal of obstetrics, gynecology, and reproductive biology* 117:S29-S32.

Salhab WA et al (2004). Necrotizing enterocolitis and neurodevelopmental outcome in extremely low birth weight infants < 1000 g. *Journal of perinatology* 24:534-540.

Sasidharan P (1998). Role of corticosteroids in neonatal blood pressure homeostasis. *Clinics in perinatology* 25:723-740.

Sauer PJ et al (1984). New standards for neutral thermal environment of healthy very low birthweight infants in week one of life. *Archives of disease in childhood* 59:18-22.

Schanler RJ (1995). Suitability of human milk for the low-birth weight infant. *Clinics in perinatology* 22:207-222.

Schmidt B et al, and the TIPP investigators (2001). Long-term effects of indomethacin prophylaxis in extremely-low-birth-weight infants. *New England journal of medicine* 344:1966-1972.

Shah SS, Ohlsson A (2005). Ibuprofen for the prevention of patent ductus arteriosus in preterm and/or low birthweight infants (Cochrane Review). In *The Cochrane library*, vol 3. Oxford: Update Software.

Shaker CS (1990). Nipple feeding preterm infants: a different perspective. *Neonatal network* 8:9-17.

Silverman W (1992). Foreword. In Sinclair JC, Bracken MB, editors. *Effective care of the newborn.* New York: Oxford University Press.

Skelton R et al (1994). A blinded comparison of clinical and echocardiographic evaluation of the preterm infant for patent ductus arteriosus. *Journal of paediatrics & child health* 30:406-411.

Smith L (2005). The ethics of neonatal care for the extremely preterm infant. *Journal of neonatal nursing* 11:40-58.

Snapp B (1994). NEC and NIBD similar but distinct. *NANN central lines* 10:1, 13.

Soll RF (2005). Prophylactic synthetic surfactant for preventing morbidity and mortality in preterm infants (Cochrane Review). In *The Cochrane library* vol 3. Oxford: Update Software.

Soll RF, Morley CJ (2005). Prophylactic versus selective use of surfactant in preventing morbidity and mortality in preterm infants (Cochrane Review). In *The Cochrane library* vol 3. Oxford: Update Software.

Stark AR et al (2001). Adverse effects of early dexamethasone in extremely-low-birth-weight infants. National Institute of Child Health and Human Development Neonatal Research Network. *New England journal of medicine* 344:95-101.

Stokowski LA (2005). A primer on apnea of prematurity. *Advances in neonatal care* 5:155-170.

Stoll BJ et al (2004). National Institute of Child Health and Human Development Neonatal Research Network. Neurodevelopmental and growth impairment among extremely-low-birth-weight infants with neonatal infection. *Journal of the American Medical Association* 292(19):2357-2365.

Subhani M et al (2001). Screening guidelines for retinopathy of prematurity: the need for revision in extremely low birth weight infants. *Pediatrics* 107:656-659.

Subhedar NV et al (2005). Corticosteroids for hypotension in preterm infants (Protocol). In *The Cochrane library*, vol 3. Oxford: Update Software.

Subramaniam P et al (2005). Prophylactic nasal continuous positive airway pressure for preventing morbidity and mortality in very preterm infants (Cochrane Review). In *The Cochrane library*, vol 3. Oxford: Update Software.

Sydnor-Greenberg N, Dokken D (2000). Coping and caring in different ways: understanding and meaningful involvement. *Pediatric nursing* 26:185-190.

Symington A, Pinelli J (2005). Developmental care for promoting development and preventing morbidity in preterm infants (Cochrane Review). In *The Cochrane library* vol 3. Oxford: Update Software.

Tyson JE, Kennedy KA (2005). Minimal enteral nutrition in parenterally fed neonates (Cochrane Review). In *The Cochrane library*, vol 3. Oxford: Update Software.

Tyson JE, Saigal S (2005). Outcomes for extremely low-birth-weight infants. *Journal of the American Medical Association* 294:371-373.

Vohr BR et al, and the Neonatal Research Network (2004). Center differences and outcomes of extremely low birth weight infants. *Pediatrics* 113:781-789.

Watkins AMC et al (1989). Blood pressure and cerebral haemorrhage and ischaemia in very low birthweight infants. *Early human development* 19:103-110.

Wilder MA (2000). Ethical issues in the delivery room: resuscitation of extremely low birth weight infants. *Journal of perinatal and neonatal nursing* 14:44-57.

Wood NS et al (2000). Neurologic and developmental disability after extremely preterm birth. *New England journal of medicine* 343:378-384.

Wood NS et al, for the EPICure Study Group (2003). The EPICure study: growth and associated problems in children born at 25 weeks of gestational age or less. *Archives of disease in childhood neonatal and fetal edition* 88:492-500.

Woodgate PG, Flenady V (2005). Tracheal suctioning without disconnection in intubated ventilated neonates (Cochrane Review). In *The Cochrane library*, vol 3. Oxford: Update Software.

Wyllie J (2003). Treatment of patent ductus arteriosus. *Seminars in neonatology* 8:425-432.

Yeo KL et al (1998). Outcomes of extremely premature infants related to their peak serum bilirubin concentrations and exposure to phototherapy. *Pediatrics* 102:426-431.

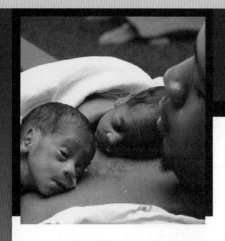

Chapter **23**

Neurobehavioral Development

Diane Holditch-Davis • Susan Tucker Blackburn

The care of high-risk infants, both those born prematurely and those with medical, surgical, or developmental problems, has long been a major focus of nursing. Efforts to increase the understanding of the pathophysiologic problems encountered by these infants, along with new management strategies and technologies, have markedly improved the outcome of these infants. Much of the focus of the neonatal intensive care unit (NICU) has been on meeting the physiologic needs of these infants, with less attention, until recently, on the social interactive consequences of the NICU environment. Thus the advances in neonatal care have been accompanied by increasing concerns about the impact of the NICU environment on the infant's physiologic and neurobehavioral functioning, the lack of sensory input geared to meet the individual infant's needs and current level of developmental function, and the effects of stress and overstimulation.

Although tremendous progress has been made in reducing mortality and morbidity in high-risk infants, these infants, especially those born prematurely, are still vulnerable to a wide variety of neurodevelopmental problems. These problems have been referred to as the "new morbidities of low birth weight infants" and include behavioral disorganization, attention deficit disorders, hyperexcitability, language problems, sensory/perceptual and higher-order cognitive problems, regulatory disorders, and school dysfunction (Bennett, 2005; Bhutta et al, 2002; Marlow et al, 2005; McGrath et al, 2005). Adverse outcomes of high-risk infants may be related to a variety of factors, including immaturity, perinatal trauma, the early NICU environment, the home environment in which the child is raised, and parent-child interactions. The development of many of these infants is characterized by an unevenness that can lead to later difficulties. This unevenness may be as much the result of the impact of the early NICU environment as the effects of perinatal stress.

Immature infants differ in two important ways from healthy full-term infants. First, these infants are born early and therefore must adapt to the extrauterine environment with bodily systems, including a central nervous system (CNS), that are not yet mature. Second, this interruption of intrauterine life significantly modifies the environment of the infant

(Blackburn, 1998). Thus the preterm infant spends the last weeks or months of gestation in an environment—the NICU—that is very different from that of the uterus or the home of a healthy full-term infant. The NICU environment has similar implications for the more mature, although still vulnerable, ill full-term infant. For these infants, this environment is also abnormal and quite different from that experienced by healthy infants who go home with their parents soon after birth.

Neonatal nurses are very familiar with interpreting the physiologic status of infants and basing their interventions on physiologic changes. Nurses have placed increased emphasis on the importance of understanding the behaviors of infants under their care because behavior is the only way infants can communicate their needs and their responses to nursing interventions (Als, 1986; Catlett & Holditch-Davis, 1990). However, two factors make this understanding difficult. First, newborn infants have very limited behavioral repertoires. The same behavior may have different meanings in different situations, but busy neonatal nurses may not have the time necessary to correctly interpret infants' behaviors by comprehensively assessing both the infants' actions and the environmental stimulation. Second, the behaviors of critically ill infants are even more difficult to interpret because they lack the energy to display characteristic behavioral responses. Thus neonatal nurses can never rely totally on infants' behaviors to determine infants' needs, but in combination with physiologic parameters, understanding infant behavior enriches both nursing assessment and the evaluation of nursing interventions.

In considering the vulnerabilities of ill and immature infants, it is useful to examine the implications of the state of central nervous system and sensory system development, neonatal neurobehavioral development, and to examine sleeping and waking states—and their relevance for neonatal nursing.

FETAL AND NEONATAL CENTRAL NERVOUS SYSTEM DEVELOPMENT

As noted in Chapter 12, the development of the CNS can be divided into six overlapping stages (Table 12-1). These stages are important to consider in examining the effects of the NICU environment because the stage of development influences the effect of any insult. In addition, several areas of the CNS continue to undergo significant changes during the period when preterm infants are in the NICU, increasing their vulnerability to insult. The stage of development is also reflected by the behaviors characteristic of immature infants (Box 23-1). The first three stages of CNS development (dorsal induction, ventral induction, and neurogenesis) are completed before the fourth month of gestation. The last three stages (neuron migration, organization, including synaptogenesis and arborization, and myelinization) continue during the time many infants are in the NICU (Volpe, 2001) and have implications for the effects of the NICU environment and care.

Areas of development during the last part of gestation that are particularly critical in considering neurobehavioral vulnerabilities of ill or immature infants include (1) autonomic homeostatic control; (2) alterations in the germinal matrix and migration of neurons and glial cells; (3) CNS organizational processes; and (4) growth of the cortex and cerebellum. From about 28 to 32 weeks' gestational age, preterm infants begin to achieve some degree of physiologic homeostasis, with increasing control of the sympathetic system over their autonomic functioning. With increasing autonomic control, the infant develops greater autonomic stability. This autonomic stability can be seen, for example, in the decreasing incidence of apnea and bradycardia. As these infants move to greater cortical control over the next months, their development is characterized by periods of temporary organization followed by periods of disorganization as new levels of maturation and control are achieved. These periods of disorganization are reflected in the infant's sleep-wake patterns, proportion of transitional or indeterminate sleep, and fragmented behavioral responses and reflexes.

The germinal matrix in the periventricular subependymal area is a site of origin for neuronal and glial cells. Neurons and glial cells migrate from the germinal matrix to their eventual loci within the CNS, where they further differentiate and take on unique and individual functions (Moore & Persaud, 2003). Initially the neurons migrate to areas deep within the cortex; later neurons migrate further toward the surface of the cortex. Thus neurons formed early come to lie in deeper layers of cortex and subcortex; those formed later are found in more superficial layers. The cortex generally has a complete component of neurons by 33 weeks' gestation. Until 32 to 34 weeks' gestational age, the fragile, poorly supported blood vessels in this area receive a significant proportion of cerebral blood flow (Volpe, 2001). Insults to this area before this period may lead to germinal matrix and intraventricular hemorrhage (Chapter 12).

Organization, or "the processes by which the nervous system takes on the capacity to operate as an integrated whole" (Blackburn, 2003), begins during the sixth month of gestation and extends many years after birth. Neuron growth and connections lead to development of brain sulci and gyri. A brain growth spurt occurs from 26 to 30 weeks, leading to more complex behaviors (Als, 1999; Volpe, 2001). Organization of the CNS is critical for cortical and cognitive development. These processes may be particularly vulnerable to insults from the effects of the NICU environment (Bhutta & Anand, 2002; Sizun & Westrup, 2004).

Subplate neurons differentiate early and migrate to cortex from the germinal matrix to serve as guides for ascending and descending projections to target neurons. The subplate neurons provide critical connection sites for axons ascending from thalamus and other sites, until the neurons that these axons will eventually connect with have migrated from the germinal matrix. The subplate reaches its peak from 22 to 34 weeks, a time of particularly high vulnerability to perinatal brain injury in preterm infants (McQuillen & Ferriero, 2005; Volpe, 2001). Once cortical neurons have reached their eventual loci, they become arranged in layers and develop dendrites and axons that undergo extensive branching. The pattern of dendritic connections between neurons is a critical growth process that constitutes the "wiring" of the brain (also called arborization). These interconnections are critical for processing of impulses, cell-to-cell communication, and communication throughout the nervous system. Lack of connections can result in hypersensitivity, poorly modulated behaviors, and all-or-nothing responses, which can often be observed in preterm infants in the NICU (see Box 23-1). Similar behavior patterns can also be seen in some children in later infancy and childhood.

Another component of organization is the formation of connections or synapses between neurons and development of intracellular structures and enzymes for neurotransmitter production. Synaptogenesis is critical for integration across all areas of the nervous system. Synapses continue to restructure throughout development, and this process is thought to be the basis for memory and learning. Synaptogenesis is

---

BOX 23-1

Neurodevelopmental Limitations of the Very-Low-Birth-Weight Infant and Related Behavioral Manifestations

Limitations in Neurologic Function
Sparse myelin
Lung refractory period
Weak transmission
Decreased inhibitory potential
Decreased functional validation (ability to utilize various systems)
Slow nerve conduction
Slow synaptic potential
Unable to sustain high firing rates
Incomplete cell differentiation
Decreased synaptogenesis and dendritic arborization

Behaviors of Immature Infants
Irregular state regulation
Increased and decreased tone
Alterations in primitive reflexes
Easily exhausted
Irritable, difficult to soothe
Inability to inhibit
Jerky movements
Low arousal, inability to sustain an alert state
Poor coordination
Altered autonomic regulation
Asymmetrical, uncoordinated posture and movement

mediated by excitatory neurotransmitters such as glutamate. Glutamate acts on N-methyl-D-aspartate (NMDA) receptors to enhance neuronal proliferation, migration, and synaptic plasticity (Ikonomidou et al, 2001; Sanchez & Jensen, 2001). Another component of organization is reduction in the number of neurons and their connections through the death of many neurons and regression of dendrites and synapses. Neuronal death assists in elimination of errors within the nervous system, such as neurons that are improperly located, that fail to achieve adequate connections, or that are underused (Koizumi, 2004). For example neuronal density in the visual cortex decreases from 620,000 neurons/mm^3 at 7 months gestation to 1000,000 at term and 40,000 in the adult (Koizumi, 2004).

Organizational processes and modification of neurons continue into adulthood but are particularly vulnerable during infancy. The ability of a neuron to change structure and function has been called plasticity (Huttenlocher, 2002).

> The more immature the infant at birth the greater the impact of neural plasticity. There is considerable evidence in animal studies that sensory input influences later neuronal structure and function; for instance, an enriched environment during infancy improves developmental outcome by maximizing brain potential. This plasticity is both an advantage and a liability. Although sensory input may increase cellular processes and interconnections, the sensory environment may also produce undesired changes in structure and function (Blackburn, 2003).

Thus the preterm infant in the NICU may be particularly vulnerable to these alterations. Adverse neonatal experiences may alter brain development during this vulnerable time and thus later development (Als et al, 2004; Anand & Scalzo, 2000; Philbin et al, 2000).

Neuronal differentiation and organization are controlled by the interaction of genes with the environment. Each neuron has many synaptic connections that allow the brain to integrate and organize information. There is initially an overproduction of neurons and nerve connections. Many of these neurons and connections are later eliminated. Whether a connection is retained or eliminated is influenced by the infant's early environment and experiences (Black, 1998; DiPietro, 2000). For example, the brain is more likely to strengthen and retain connections that are used repeatedly and to eliminate underused connections. Improper sensory input (too much or too little) or input that is inappropriate in terms of timing may alter brain development (Black, 1998). Thus the environment of the immature infants in the NICU and in the early months following discharge is critical for brain development and later cognitive function (Lickliter, 2000a, 2000b; Sizun & Westrup, 2004). Animal models demonstrate permanent alterations in neuronal networks, wiring, function, and behavior with exposure to early inappropriate sensory input (Graven, 2004; Lickliter, 2000a, 2000b; Sizun & Westrup, 2004). Preterm infants in the NICU are experiencing a very different pattern and type of sensory input than they would encounter in utero, and different from what the brain is expecting at any given gestational age. This creates a mismatch between the sensory environment of the infant and the requirements of the central nervous system for growth and development (Als & Lawhon, 2004). Brain function and structures are reported to be

different, even in healthy preterm infants, compared to term infants of similar post conceptional age (Als et al, 2004).

Greenough and Black have postulated that there are two types of neural plasticity: experience-expectant and experience-dependent (Black, 1998; Greenough et al, 1987). Experience-expectant plasticity is linked to the brain's developmental timetable. Thus specific sensory experiences and input are needed at specific times for neural development and maturation. Altered sequences or types of sensory input can alter or disrupt development. Experience-dependent plasticity involves interaction with the environment to develop specific skills for later use. This form of plasticity involves memory and learning and allows development of flexibility, adaptation, and individual differences in social and intellectual development (Black, 1998; Greenough et al, 1987).

The cerebellum is also vulnerable to insults from the early environment. The cerebellum is primarily concerned with control of muscles and coordination of movements; it undergoes a critical growth spurt at 30 to 32 weeks' gestation. This spurt includes an increase in dendritic arborization, which is complete earlier than many other areas of the brain. Insults may lead to the altered sequences of motor development seen in some preterm infants (Volpe, 2001).

Neonatal Sensory Development

The sensory systems develop in a specific sequence: somatosensory (tactile and proprioceptive), vestibular, chemoreceptive, auditory, and visual. During fetal life there is a lack of competing stimuli during rapid maturation of each system. For example, the infant develops chemoreception before the structures for hearing and vision are in place and after somatosensory and vestibular function has matured. Similarly, the hearing maturation in the fetus is most rapid during a time when vision is still immature and in an environment where vision is not being stimulated by light. Animal studies have demonstrated that out-of-sequence stimulation of one system interferes with development of not only that system but also other systems that are still immature (Graven, 2000; Lickliter, 2000a, 2000b). For example, in animal models inappropriate visual stimulation while hearing and vision are still developing may alter not only vision but also hearing development (Glass, 2005; Graven, 2004; Lickliter, 2000a, 2000b).

Somatosensory and vestibular sensations mature early. The fetus responds to touch around the mouth by 2 months of gestational age; hands become touch sensitive by 10 to 11 weeks. Receptors and an intact cortical pathway are present throughout the fetal body by 20 to 24 weeks (Glass, 2005). Vestibular stimulation is mediated by receptors in the ear that detect changes in directions and rate of head movement and rotation. Vestibular system maturation reaches structural maturation by 14 to 20 weeks' gestation with responses to vestibular stimulation seen as early as 25 weeks' gestation (Glass, 2005). Oral (taste) and nasal (smell) chemoreception develop during the second trimester. The taste buds appear by 8 to 9 weeks and receptors by at least 16 weeks. By term the infant has adult numbers of receptors. Nasal chemoreceptors develop from 7 to 20 weeks' gestation and respond to the fragrant molecules in amniotic fluid. The composition of amniotic fluid varies with maternal diet and bathes both oral and nasal chemoreceptors. Fetal swallowing rates have been reported to change with exposure to different taste in amniotic fluid (Mennella et al, 2001). Preterm infants respond to different tastes and smells by at least 28 weeks' gestation (Bartocci et al, 2001; Bingham et al, 2003; Lecanuet & Schaal, 1996). Nutrient odor may influence non nutritive sucking in preterm infants (Bingham et al, 2003). Term infants are able to detect, localize, and discriminate a variety of distinct odors and tastes. They respond preferentially to breast odors, their mothers' scents, and other odors associated with positive reinforcements (Schaal et al, 2004).

The structures of the auditory system, including the inner ear and cochlea, are mature enough to support hearing by approximately 20 to 25 weeks' gestation. Fetal hearing is thought to begin at 24 to 25 weeks. In preterm infants, auditory evoked potentials can be recorded and responses to sound observed as early as 25 to 26 weeks (Hall, 2000). Auditory cortex development begins by the second trimester but is not mature until later in childhood (Moore, 2002). Between 28 and 34 weeks, the preterm infant develops the ability to begin to orient to sound, turning the head in the direction of an auditory stimulus and showing evidence of arousal and attention (Glass, 2005; Gray & Philbin, 2004). During the third trimester the cochlea continues to mature and develop its ability to hear sounds across frequencies. The hearing threshold decreases with gestational age. Infants have a preference for their own mothers' voices even before birth (Kisilevsky et al, 2003). Anatomic and functional development of hearing in preterm and term infants is summarized in Table 23-1.

The eyes begin to develop early in the embryonic period but continue anatomic and functional maturation into the third trimester and early infants (Graven, 2004). Vision is the least mature sense at birth, and even full-term infants undergo significant continued maturation during infancy. By 22 weeks' gestation, the layers of the retina have formed rod differentiation, and retinal vascularization begins by 25 weeks' gesta-tional age; myelinization of the optic nerve begins at 24 weeks. By 26 weeks, visual cortex neurons are in place with rapid development of visual neuronal connections and processes between 28 and 34 weeks' gestation (Glass, 2005). See Table 23-2.

NEONATAL NEUROBEHAVIORAL DEVELOPMENT

To provide developmentally supportive, family-focused care for high-risk infants in the NICU, the nurse must understand behavioral and developmental issues as they affect the infant and the family. The term *neurobehavioral* "recognized bidirectionality—that biologic and behavioral systems dynamically influence each other and that the quality of behavior and physiologic processes is depending on neural feedback" (Lester & Tronick, 2004). In the past 20 years, our knowledge of early childhood development has been dramatically altered by an avalanche of new research in neurobiologic, behavioral, and social sciences that has led to major advances in understanding the conditions that influence the well-being and early development of infants and young children. A deeper understanding of the importance of early life experience and the highly interactive influences of genetics and the environment on the developing brain has deepened our understanding of the early years. Attention to the powerful influence of the role of early relationships and the capabilities of the development of emotions in young children has finally taken center stage. Add to this the changes in our social structures and changes in our families, culturally and economically—including the shifting of parenting roles, along with changes in the workplace and in child care services for the very youngest, and the continuing high levels of economic hardship in many families—and it becomes clear that a professional review and rethinking of policy and practice required dedicated attention and a thoughtful response (Shonkoff & Phillips, 2000).

TABLE **23-1**	Development of Hearing in Preterm and Term Infants
Age	**Anatomic and Functional Development**
Preterm infants <28 weeks	Fetal hearing begins by 23 to 24 weeks
	Threshold about 65 dB, 500 to 1000 Hz
	Auditory brainstem responses by 26 to 28 weeks
Preterm infants 28 to 30 weeks	Rapid maturation of cochlea and auditory nerve
	Responses rapidly fatigue
	Initial auditory processing by 30 weeks
	Threshold 40 dB with an increased frequency range
Preterm infants 32 to 34 weeks	Outer hair cells mature by 32 weeks
	Rapid maturation of cochlea and auditory nerve
Preterm infants >34 weeks	Increased speed of conduction
	Ossicles and electrophysiology complete by 36 weeks
	Hearing threshold 30 dB, increasing range
	Increasing ability to localize and discriminate
Term infants	Ability to localize and discriminate sounds
	Hearing threshold 25 dB
	Range 500 to 4000 Hz

From Glass P (2005). The vulnerable neonate and the neonatal intensive care environment. In MacDonald MG et al, editors. Avery's neonatology: pathophysiology and management of the newborn, ed 5 (pp 111-128). Philadelphia: Lippincott Williams & Wilkins; Hall JW (2000). Development of the ear and hearing. Journal of perinatology 20:S12; Lecanuet JP, Schaal B (1996). Fetal sensory competencies. European journal of obstetrics and gynecology 68:1; and Philbin MK, Klaas P (2000). Hearing and behavioral responses to sound in full-term newborns. Journal of perinatology 20:S68.

TABLE 23-2	Development of Vision in Preterm and Term Infants
Age	**Anatomic and Functional Development**
Preterm infants 24 to 28 weeks	Eyelids: unfuse at 24 to 26 weeks Lens: cloudy, second of four layers forming Cornea: hazy until 27 weeks Retina: rod differentiation by 25 weeks, vascularization begins Visual cortex: rapid dendritic growth No pupillary response Eyelid tightening to bright light but quickly fatigues VER to bright light but quickly fatigues Very myopic
Preterm infants 30 to 34 weeks	Lens: clearing, second layer complete, third forming Retina: rod complete except for fovea by 32 weeks, cone differentiation begins Visual cortex: rapid dendritic and synapse development VER more complex, latency decreases Bright light causes sustained pupil closure Abrupt reduction may cause eye opening Pupillary response sluggish but more mature Spontaneous eye opening, brief fixation in low light
Preterm infants 34 to 36 weeks	Pupils: complete pupillary reflex by 36 weeks Retina: cone numbers in fovea increase Blood vessels reach nasal retina Visual cortex: morphologically similar to term Increased alertness, less sustained than term VER resembles that of term infant with longer latency Spontaneous orientation toward soft light Beginning to track, show visual preferences Less myopic
Term infants	Still immature with much development from 0 to 6 months Retinal vessels reach periphery of temporal retina Lens transmits more short-wave light than adult Acuity approximately 20/200 to 20/1600 Attend to form, object, face, track horizontally and some vertically See objects to at least 2 feet, attend best at 8 to 12 inches

Compiled from Glass P (2005). The vulnerable neonate and the neonatal intensive care environment. In MacDonald MG et al, editors. Avery's neonatology: pathophysiology and management of the newborn, ed 5 (pp 111-128). Philadelphia: Lippincott Williams & Wilkins.

One of the first requirements of early development is the process of acquiring the capacity to self-regulate. This capacity refers to the mastery of tasks that were in the beginning carried out and accomplished by the mother's body while the infant was in the womb; after birth and the transition out of the womb, the task becomes the infant's job. This transition from external regulation to the ability to accomplish regulation on one's own is a lengthy process in infant development. The tasks involved initially include physiologic regulation such as maintaining normal body temperature, regulating day-night cycles, and learning to calm oneself and relax after basic needs are met. Later, self-regulation means controlling one's own emotions and managing to keep one's attention focused (Shonkoff & Phillips, 2000).

Shonkoff and Phillips (2000) refer to this process as reacting and regulating one's range of developmental function. The process is deeply related to one's relationships with others. Parents become the "co-regulators" or extensions of the infant's internal regulatory systems working to regulate function in the young child just as he or she is working toward the same. This requires of caregivers the ability to read and understand the infant's needs and the sensitivity, knowledge, and energy to respond in helpful, satisfying ways. Parents must establish "regulatory connections" with young children and then shift the independent task of regulation gradually over to them, one domain and one day at a time, being forever watchful that the balance in the child is not seriously disrupted. The ways that infants and young children learn about self-management involves behavioral, emotional, and cognitive self-control, which must evolve for competent functioning.

During early child development (birth to 6 years) children become consistently independent and develop the ability to manage their own behavior. Two concerns related to these developmental processes that have been thoroughly covered in developmental literature are sleep behavior and crying behavior. Infants with serious medical conditions that require intensive care nursery stays, including preterm or medically fragile infants, have more difficult transitions to regulatory competence. Immature sick newborns are much less able to organize and stabilize sleep, waking, and feeding. They tend to be unpredictable, to cry more, and to be fussier. They tend to make less eye contact, smile less, vocalize less, and show less positive affect, and they are generally more difficult and harder for parents to read (Barnard, 1999; Beckwith & Rodning, 1992). During the first 3 months after birth for a full-term newborn, the infant depends on the relationship with the primary caregiver. The infant takes on an extensive undertaking that requires that he or she learn to get to sleep without help, stop crying when consoled, respond to the caregiver, and establish day-night, wake-sleep rhythms. Once the rapid developmental changes of the first 3 months of life after full-term birth accomplish its developmental changes, the infant faces another level of regulation in controlling his or her emotions and behavior. Followed by the regulation of attention and the regulation of mental processes, a process known as executive function emerges and involves the ability to think, retrieve, and remember information, solve problems, and engage in complex activities, which involve oral language, reading and writing, math, and social behavior.

A key concept that is emerging from this synthesis of the most recent research reveals that early experiences clearly affect the development of the brain. Development begins during early fetal life and lays a foundation for all that is to follow. Als and colleagues (Als, 1982, 1986) have developed a model, the synactive theory of development, for understanding the organization of neurobehavioral capabilities in the development of the fetus and newborn infant. This model describes emerging behavioral organizational abilities of the neonate. This model is based on the assumption that infants actively communicate via their behavior, which becomes an important route for understanding thresholds of stress or stability. Behavior of the infant not only is the main route of communication but also provides the basis for the structure of developmental assessment and provision of developmentally appropriate care (Als, 1986).

This synactive theory of development (Als, 1982) provides a model through which one can specify the degree of differentiation of behavior and the ability of infants to organize and control their behavior. The focus is not on assessment of skills but on the unique way each individual infant deals with the world around her or him. The synactive theory of development specifies the range of neonatal behavior as the infant matures as well as the ability of the infant to regulate behavior. This model is based on the assumption that the infant's primary route of communicating both functional stability and the limits for stress is through behavior (Als, 1986). For example, infants who extend their limbs after being turned to supine to have their diaper changed may be communicating that they cannot control their limbs and movement in that position. Containing the limbs of these infants helps them to develop control and reduces stress over the loss of control.

Infants are seen as being in continual interaction with their environment via five subsystems: autonomic/physiologic; motor; state/organizational; attentional/interactive; and self-regulatory. These subsystems mature simultaneously, and within each subsystem a developmental sequence can be observed. Thus at each stage of development, new tasks and organizations are learned against the backdrop of previous development. The subsystems are interdependent and interrelated. For example, physiologic stability provides the foundation for motor and state control; the infant cannot respond socially to caregivers until motor and state control is achieved. The loss of integrity in one subsystem can influence the organization of other subsystems in response to environ-

mental demands. In the preterm, less organized infant, the systems interplay, continuously influencing each other. In the healthy full-term infant, these systems are synchronized and function smoothly. Thus full-term infants can regulate their autonomic, motor, state, and attentional systems with ease and without apparent stress. However, less mature infants tend to be able to tolerate only one or minimal activity at a time and may easily lose control if their individual thresholds are exceeded.

Instability in the autonomic system can be seen in the pattern of respiration (pauses, tachypnea), color changes (red, pale, dusky, mottled), and various visceral signs (regurgitation, twitching, stooling). Organization of the motor system is assessed by observing the infant's tone and posture (flexed, extended, hyperflexed, flaccid); specific movement patterns of the extremities, head, trunk, and face; and level of activity. The development of motor responses is closely linked to state organization (Als, 1986, 1996).

The state system is understood by noting the available range of states of consciousness (sleep to arousal, awake to alert, crying), how well each state is defined (in terms of behavioral and physiologic parameters), transitions between states, and the quality of organization of these states. States may be poorly defined at first, especially in the immature infant. For example, jerky body twitches and fussing may accompany sleep and wake states. In addition, the immature infant may not be able to achieve clearly defined states as seen in the mature infant (Als, 1982).

Initially, preterm infants tend to be unstable and fragile, with sudden changes in their autonomic, motor, and state systems. These infants often have minimal response to handling or other sensory input until a threshold is reached, then quickly develop a cascade of responses, ending in several color changes, flaccidity, bradycardia, and apnea. As the infant matures, the responses are more variable, and the infant is less likely to totally decompensate (Als, 1986, 1999). Changes within the autonomic, motor, and state systems at all stages of development not just are reactions to stress and overstimulation but can signal that the infant's tolerance threshold has been exceeded. By recognizing these signs early, the nurse can intervene to prevent mild to severe decompensation.

The attentional/interactive system involves the infant's ability to orient and focus on sensory stimuli, such as faces, sounds, or objects—that is, the external environment. This system also includes the range of abilities in states of consciousness: how well periods of alertness are defined and how transitions into and out of alertness are handled. At first, this alertness may be very brief, with a dull look or glassy-eyed stare. As this system matures, the infant is able to interact with greater ease and for longer periods. Social responsiveness requires that the infant have enough state control to sustain some awake and alert states (Als, 1982).

The self-regulatory system includes behaviors the infant uses to maintain the integrity and balance of the other subsystems, to integrate the other systems, and to move smoothly between states. For example, some infants can tuck their limbs close to their body in an effort to gain control when stressed, whereas others seem to relax if they can brace a foot against the side of the crib.

In summary, the process of development appears to be that of stabilization and integration of some subsystems, which allows the differentiation and emergence of others that in turn feed back on the integrated system. In this process the whole system is reopened and transformed to a new level of more differentiated integration, from which the next newly emerging subsystem can further differentiate and press to actualization and realization (Als, 1982, 1996). By observing and assessing the newborn infant's responses to the caregiver and other aspects of the environment across these five subsystems of behavioral functioning, one can develop and implement a plan of care to support the infant's emerging neurodevelopmental organization and reduce stress.

The NICU staff—especially nurses—play a significant role in shaping the environment and making caregiving more responsive to infants. This requires as careful observation and documentation of infant behavior as is given to physiologic status and development of an individualized plan of care (Box 23-2). Infant responses to the environment will be influenced by factors such as state; basic needs (e.g., hunger); sensory threshold; parameters of the animate and inanimate environment, including readability, predictability, and responsivity; infant health status; and level of neurobehavioral maturity (Blackburn, 1998). Infant behavioral responses include specific autonomic, motoric, and state cues, which indicate disorganization and stress and the need for immediate

intervention, and stability and self-regulatory cues, which indicate that the infant is coping positively. Tables 23-3 and 23-4 summarize infant stability/self-regulatory and instability/disorganization cues. Examples of selected cues are illustrated in Figures 23-1 and 23-2.

ASSESSMENT OF NEONATAL NEUROBEHAVIORAL DEVELOPMENT

Developmental assessment of newborn functioning emerged with the awareness of the amazing capabilities of neonates. The newborn infant, who for years was thought to be nonreactive and incapable of social participation, is now seen as an active participant in social interaction and capable of self-regulation (Als, 1984, 1996; Brazelton & Nugent, 1995). Even with a greater understanding of newborn capabilities, researchers and clinicians have been unable to accurately predict the future course of an infant's development from early neurologic or behavioral assessments.

Historically, two types of neonatal assessments have evolved—the neurologic examination and the behavioral examination. The neurologic examination assesses the function of the CNS and typically includes assessment of motor tone and reflex behaviors within the context of infant state.

BOX 23-2

Outline of Components for Direct Caregiving (Derived from VandenBerg, 1999)

Preparation for Care

Assess your readiness to begin:
- Are my materials appropriate? (Gather all items needed.)
- Is the room appropriate? (Check light, noise, temperature, and traffic.)
- Am I ready?
- Is the baby in a good state to begin?
- Are self-regulatory supports in place? (Does the baby have something to suck? Something against which to brace its feet? Something to grasp and hold onto? [or whatever else the baby needs])

During Care

As you begin:
- Gently introduce yourself.
- Observe the baby's state as you begin.
- Plan to be vigilant of the baby's reactions—watch for the following:

State changes

RR, HR, O₂, color changes

Changes in position, or remains in flexed position

Baby's use of self-regulatory supports (e.g., sucks pacifier, holds finger, braces feet)
- If these happen as stress reactions, stop, break, and provide support until the baby returns to stable levels.
- If the infant loses control, stop and resupport (if possible).

Important: Note the following:
- How does the baby manifest stress?
- How can you prevent onset of stress reactions?

- What strategies work best?
- How far can you go with care and pace?
- Where does the baby become disorganized? How is this manifested?
- What can be done to help avoid these stress behaviors? To minimize them?
- How much stress is exhibited? What behaviors are seen? What stability is seen?

Recovery

Energy:
- Assess level of fatigue, tolerance, and energy.
- Can I get the baby's energy to return? How?
- Is the baby exhausted or tired? Or fatigued, with some energy left?
- How could we avoid loss of energy or work at a successful level for the baby?

Environment:
- Adjust noise or light to support resting or waking position.
- Reposition and add supports.
- What supports go in place to support transition to sleep or wakefulness?

Transition to stability:

Transitions are events in themselves. Do not underestimate the energy they may take from the baby!
- Make the transition to sleep (reposition first, adjust environment and room).
- Stay with the baby until transition is complete (organized state).

Note: Transitioning to an organized state means to organized calm sleep or an awake state, which is deep sleep or quiet alert.

Developed by Kathleen VandenBerg. From Presentation (1999): Management of difficult behaviors. Developmental interventions in neonatal care conference. Dublin, CA: Contemporary Forums.

TABLE 23-3	Signs of Stability in Intensive Care Nursery Infants			
Autonomic System	**Motor System**	**State System**	**Attentional Interaction System**	**Self-Regulatory System**
Smooth, regular respirations	Smooth, controlled posture	Clear, well-defined sleep states	Responsivity to auditory and visual stimuli bright and of long duration	Infant has sophisticated, well-differentiated repertoire of successful strategies to maintain each system, autonomic, motor, state, and attention, such as:
Pink, stable color	Smooth movements extremities of and head seen in: • hand clasp	Good self-quieting and consolability Robust crying	Actively seeks out auditory and shifts attention smoothly on his or her own from one stimulus to another	• autonomic: sucking, grasping • motor: tucking, foot bracing • state: visual tracking, sucking • attention: hand to mouth, hand holding
Stable viscera with **no** evidence of: • seizures • gagging • emesis • grunting • tremors • startles • twitches • coughing • sneezing • yawning • sighing	• leg/foot brace • foot clasp • finger folding • hand to mouth • grasping • sucking • tucking • hand holding Good, consistent tone throughout body	Focused, clear alertness with animated expressions such as: • frowning • cheek softening • "ooh" face • cooing • smiling	Face demonstrates bright-eyed, purposeful interest varying between arousal and relaxation	
Interventions				
Interventions not necessary to reduce stress, but to enhance and facilitate normal development				

From VandenBerg KA, Franck LS (1990). Behavioral issues for infants with BPD. In Lund C, editor. BPD: strategies for total patient care (p 125). Santa Rosa, CA: Neonatal Network. Reprinted by permission of NICU Ink®, Santa Rosa, CA. Derived from Assessment of Preterm Infant Behavior, Als, 1982.

The behavioral examination complements and elaborates on the neurologic assessment. An assumption underlying the behavioral examination is that the observable behavior of an infant is a reflection of his or her underlying neurologic status. The behavioral examination seeks to describe the quality of behavioral performance. More recently, these two forms of assessment have been combined into the neurodevelopmental or neurobehavioral assessment.

The neurodevelopmental examination is important because it yields a large pool of early observable behavior, including information about the infant's neurologic status and abilities to cope and interact with the environment. In addition, data from this examination can assist the clinician in estimating maturity and in identifying and evaluating problems that could be precursors to later developmental problems. Because the neurodevelopmental examination provides an immediate basis for determining the status of the infant's development, the results can be used for planning intervention strategies as well as for screening for infants in need of further diagnostic assessments.

Who Needs to Be Assessed?

All neonates and their caregivers can benefit from ongoing neurobehavioral assessment. These assessments provide information on the infant's behavioral capabilities, interactive qualities, and adaptations to the extrauterine environment.

This information can be used in planning care, developing individualized intervention strategies, modifying care as the infant matures, and parent teaching and other activities to promote parent-infant interaction. However, for some infants, neurodevelopmental assessment is critical for documentation of neurodevelopmental status, screening, and early case finding.

Certain groups of infants are at increased risk for developmental disabilities and later cognitive impairment (Bennett, 2005). Infants that fall into the highest risk category include very-low-birth-weight (VLBW) infants and those with significant intracranial hemorrhages. Preterm infants with known sensory impairment and chronic illness are also at risk for later cognitive dysfunction. Infants with respiratory distress syndrome (RDS) are at greater risk if they also develop chronic lung disease. Severe bronchopulmonary dysplasia (BPD) is generally associated with a prolonged and complicated hospital course, increasing the risk for later neurodevelopmental problems. Preterm infants as a group are at greater risk than term infant of comparable postconceptional ages (Als et al, 2004; Glass, 2005). Preterm infants often exhibit manifestations of altered brain organization, including disrupted sleep, difficult temperament, both hyperresponsivity and hyporesponsivity to sensory input, prolonged attention to redundant information, inattention to novel stimuli, and poor quality of motor function. These precursors of learning

TABLE 23-4	Signs of Disorganization and Stress in Intensive Care Nursery Infants			
Autonomic System	**Motor System**	**State System**	**Attentional Interaction System**	**Self-Regulatory System**
Respiration: • Pauses • Tachypnea • Gasping Color Changes: • Paling around nostrils • Perioral duskiness • Mottled • Cyanosis • Gray • Flushed • Ruddy Visceral: • Hiccups • Gagging • Grunting • Spitting up • Straining as if actually producing a bowel movement Motor: • Tremors–startles • Twitching • Coughing • Sneezing • Yawning • Sighing	Fluctuating tone: Flaccidity of: • Trunk • Extremities • Face Hypertonicity: • Leg extensions • Salutes • Airplaning • Sitting on air • Arching • Finger splays • Tongue extensions • Fisting Hyperflexions: • Trunk • Extremities • Fetal tuck • Frantic, diffuse activity	Diffuse states: Sleep: • Twitches • Sounds • Jerky moves • Irregular respirations • Whimpers • Grimacing • Fussy in sleep Awake: • Eye floating • Glassy eyed • Strained/fussy • Staring • Gaze aversion • Panicked, worried or dull look • Weak cry • Irritability • Abrupt state changes	May demonstrate stress signals of other systems: • Irregular respirations • Color changes • Visceral responses • Coughing, twitches • Sneezing • Yawning • Sighing • Eye floating • Glassy eyed • Staring • Straining • Gaze aversion • Panicked, worried, or dull look • Weak cry • Irritability • Abrupt state changes • Fluctuating tone • Frantic diffuse activity • Becomes more stressed with more than one mode of stimuli	May use the following to attempt to gain balance: • Lower state • Postural changes • Motoric strategies: leg/foot bracing, hand clasping, foot clasping, finger folding, hand to mouth, sucking, grasping, hand holding, tucking • Good self-quieting and consolability • Rhythmic, robust crying • Clear sleep states • Focused alertness with shiny-eyed and focused expression, frowning, cheek softening, "ooh" face, cooing, smiling
		Intervention Strategies to Reduce Stress		
Modify environment (light, noise, traffic) Positioning Minimal handling Swaddling, covering	Positioning Handling to contain limbs Handling slow/gentle Blanket rolls Containment, nesting	Clustering care Primary nursing to accurately read infant cues Appropriate timing of activities and daily routines Autonomic and motoric subsystems must have reached stability	Modulate interactions to infant's tolerance level Provide supports necessary to bring out best alertness Offer one mode of stimulation at a time Use modulated voice, face, rattle, face and voice together (Baby responds best to animate stimuli)	

Adapted from VandenBerg KA, Franck L (1990). Behavioral issues for infants with BPD. In Lund C, editor. BPD: strategies for total patient care (p 124). Santa Rosa, CA: Neonatal Network, p 124. Reprinted by permission of NICU Ink®, Santa Rosa, CA. Derived from Assessment of Preterm Infant Behavior, Als, 1982.

problems in school are not fully explained by either the severity of illness among preterm infants or by later conditions in the home environments (Glass, 2005).

Neurobehavioral Assessment in the NICU and Early Infancy

Neurobehavioral assessment can be performed at several different levels and is an essential part of comprehensive care of the high-risk infant in the NICU. Individuals such as Brazelton, Als, and their colleagues have sought to assess preterm and full-term newborn behavior and adaptations. Their work is based on an understanding of newborns as competent individuals with emerging developmental processes who are engaged in dynamic interactions and negotiations with their environment. As a result, several tools have been developed to describe and quantify neurobehavioral

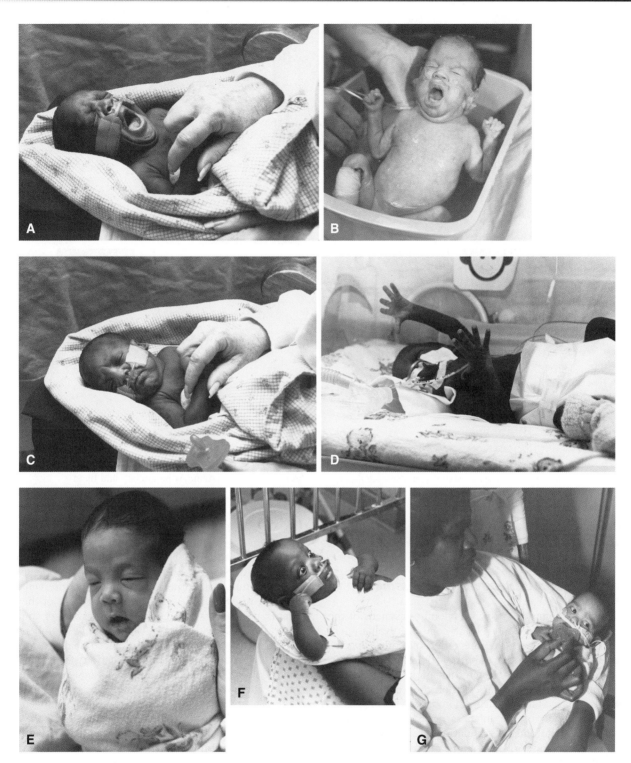

FIGURE **23-1**
Examples of selected disorganization and instability cues. From the autonomic system: **A,** yawning; **B,** mottling. From the motor system: **B,** fussing; **C,** straining; **D,** finger splay; **E,** facial hypotonia. From the state system: **F,** glassy-eyed hyperalertness; **G,** gaze aversion. (Courtesy Children's Hospital, Oakland, CA.)

organization of both preterm and full-term newborns. The tools that are described here are the Brazelton Neonatal Behavioral Assessment Scale (NBAS) (Brazelton & Nugent, 1995); the Assessment of Preterm Infant Behavior (APIB) (Als et al, 1982), which is a component of the neonatal individualized development care and assessment program (NIDCAP Boston: Children's Hospital) (Als, 2002); the NICU Network Neurobehavioral Scale (NNNS) (Lester & Tronick, 2004; Salisbury et al, 2005); Family and Infant Relationship Support Training (FIRST) (Browne, 1996); and

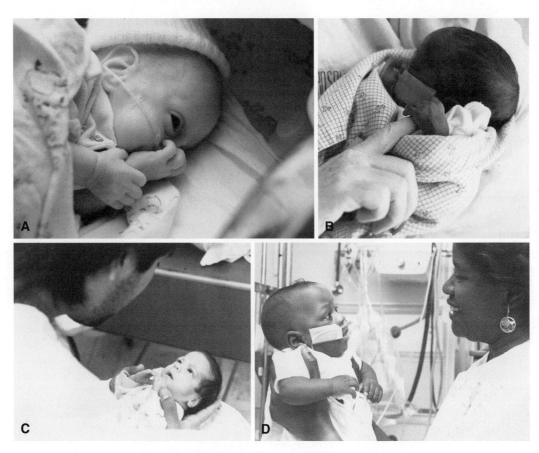

FIGURE **23-2**
Examples of selected stability and self-regulatory cues. From the motor system: **A,** hand clasp and hand-to-mouth activity; **B,** grasping; **C,** hands together at midline. From the state system: **A,** active self-quieting; **C** and **D,** focused, shiny-eyed alertness. (Courtesy Children's Hospital, Oakland, CA.)

the Neurobehavioral Assessment of the Preterm Infant (NAPI) (Korner et al, 2000).

Brazelton Neonatal Behavioral Assessment Scale (NBAS)

The NBAS is a comprehensive behavioral assessment of the healthy full-term neonate. The NBAS combines evaluation of basic reflex responses with the integration of motor capacity, state regulation, and interactive abilities (Brazelton & Nugent, 1995). Infants are followed through the various states of sleep, arousal, and wakefulness and assessed on their ability to self-regulate in the face of increasingly vigorous activity. A primary focus is observation of the infant's individual and unique ability to respond to outside stimulation while regulating responses to and coping with pleasurable or stressful situations. The infant's best performance is scored. The results are an assessment of the infant's ability to (1) organize states; (2) habituate to external stimulation; (3) regulate motoric activity in the face of increasing sensory input; (4) respond to reflex testing; (5) alert and orient to visual and auditory stimuli; (6) interact with a caregiver; and (7) self-console. Individuals planning to use the NBAS for clinical or research purposes must establish reliability with a recognized trainer. Training in the use of the NBAS is provided in various locations (http://www.brazelton-institute.com/intro.html).

The NBAS has been used in numerous studies of neonatal behavior, including investigations of cross-cultural differences,

characteristics of drug-addicted infants, effects of obstetric medication, and aspects of maternal-infant interaction (Brazelton & Nugent, 1995). An especially valuable use of the NBAS for nurses and other clinicians is as an intervention. For example, when an NBAS is performed in front of the infant's parents, the parents become increasingly aware of and amazed at the remarkable abilities of their infant. An understanding of their newborn's capacity to interact visually, turn to their voices, regulate state and motor activity, and self-console expands the parent's perception of the infant as a unique, competent individual and enhances parent-infant interaction (Als, 1999; Blackburn & Kang, 1991; Brazelton & Nugent, 1995; Das Eiden & Reifman, 1996).

In response to a need to identify the preterm infant's neurobehavioral repertoire, the NBAS was expanded and modified for use with low-birth-weight infants. Items were added to the original scale, including difficulty of elicitation of alerting, degree of facilitation necessary to support the infant, control over stimulation, robustness, endurance, degree of exhaustion, quality of alertness, and balance of tone (Brazelton & Nugent, 1995). These subscales are also useful in describing at-risk full-term infants, such as drug-exposed infants.

Assessment of Preterm Infant Behavior (APIB)

The APIB was developed to respond to the need for a more discrete assessment of preterm infant functioning. Als (1984) felt that the additional items on the NBAS encompassed only the range of behavior close to that of the full-term infant and did not provide a comprehensive description of the subtler differences seen in less mature neonates. The APIB is based on the synactive theory of development, which describes the early behavioral organization and development of the neonate. The APIB is particularly useful for the preterm and full-term high-risk infant from birth to 44 weeks' postconceptional age. The purpose of this assessment is to determine organization of the CNS and how infants cope with the intense environment of the NICU. The focus of the APIB is not only assessment of skill performance or specific responses to various stimuli but also the unique way each individual infant deals and interacts with the world around him or her. As described previously, infants are seen as being in continual interaction with their environment and as communicating their responsiveness via five subsystems (autonomic, motor, state, attentional, and self-regulatory) (Als, 1986; Als et al, 2005).

The APIB consists of six packages or sets of maneuvers adapted from the NBAS. The packages are organized to provide increasing input with which the infant must react, starting with stimulation while the infant is asleep to assess habituation. Subsequent packages move through maneuvers ranging from low and medium tactile manipulations to high tactile and vestibular handling. Throughout the assessment, the infant is continually observed for responses related to each of the five subsystems. Thus the infant is observed and scored on each of the five subsystems and for examiner facilitation (ability to use support) before, during, and after administration of the items in each package. These responses are called the system scores and range on a 9-point scale from organized (1) to disorganized (9).

The APIB has been used for research and clinical purposes. As a research tool, it has been used to describe and identify neonatal behavioral organization in preterm and other high-risk infants (Als, 1986; Als et al, 2005). Clinically, psychologists, neonatologists, neurologists, nurses, developmental specialists, and therapists have used the APIB in providing consultation in the NICU regarding developmental interventions for specific infants. The APIB is useful in determining an infant's degree of fragility and ability to tolerate different caregiving parameters. By measuring maturity of the five subsystems, one can determine maturity of each system and tolerance for handling as well as generate developmental care plans specific to each infant at that stage of development. The APIB is also useful in assessing infant readiness for changes in caregiving routines and in the physical and social environment. Assessing the degree of fragility and tolerance for activities can provide an invaluable piece of information about the infant's functional level and assist staff in making decisions about whether to protect the infant or to advance to the next level of care, as is illustrated in the following case.

A 28-week preterm infant had just been extubated and graduated to oxygen by nasal cannula and moved from the open bed to the incubator. An APIB revealed a responsive infant but one who was working extremely hard to regulate his system amid two major changes: extubation and change of physical environment. Although successful regulation was noted, it was also apparent that the infant was at maximal capacity in organizing himself. He showed efforts to tuck and maintain hand to mouth; however, he could not maintain these postures for long without help. It was apparent that the infant's threshold had been reached and that any more change

or stress would have caused a loss of control in his system's integrity. Immediately after the assessment, the neonatologists ordered nipple feedings once a day. With this new demand, the examiner felt that this infant would exceed his threshold and be unable to regulate himself. The developmental specialist recommended waiting 1 week for the infant to stabilize and to integrate his new experiences before taking on any new demands. This recommendation was not followed, and feeding continued. Two days later, the developmental specialist returned and noted that the infant had a trial of nippling. He had desaturated, become bradycardic, required bag-and-mouth ventilation, and was considered to have "flunked" nippling. The order was terminated, with the plan to try again in a week. When feeding was reordered a week later, the infant tolerated it well.

Training in the APIB (http://www.nidcap.com/) is extensive and requires knowledge of the NICU, including care practices and routines, staffing patterns, and typical infant experiences in that setting as well as physiologic limitations and medical problems. Interrater reliability, and concurrent and construct validity have been reported (Als et al, 2005).

Neonatal Individualized Development Care and Assessment Program

The NIDCAP (Boston: Children's Hospital) incorporates several levels of developmental training in assessment techniques and intervention planning for high-risk preterm and full-term infants. Included in this program is an observation tool (level 1 NIDCAP naturalistic behavioral observation), which is extremely useful for the NICU nurse. This assessment involves an observation of the infant before, during, and after a routine caregiving episode. It provides the NICU nurse with information on the infant's individual cues for both stress and stable, organized function. The nurse can then structure the infant's experiences, including caregiving interventions and the physical and social environment, to support the infant at the current level of tolerance. This support includes an awareness of the timing of caregiving events, sequencing events and interventions to prevent or reduce stress as well as to enhance stable behavior. Support for parents in understanding their infant's unique behavior and needs is also provided. Parents have reported more satisfaction with NIDCAP-based care than with traditional care (Wielenga et al, 2006).

NIDCAP training (http://www.nidcap.com/) involves didactic sessions and clinical demonstration of the observational tool, after which the trainee completes a specified number of observations on infants of different gestational age, postbirth age, and health status. This observation period is followed by an assessment of reliability for certification by the trainer. Individualized developmentally supportive care (see Chapter 25) as a total care concept, with care provided by NIDCAP certified or trained staff, has been demonstrated to result in a number of positive outcomes in various studies including fewer medical complications, reduced hospital stay and costs, lower parental stress and improved organization and neurobehavior (Als et al, 1994, 2003; Becker et al, 1991b, 1993; Buehler et al, 1995; Fleisher et al, 1995; Kleberg et al, 2000, 2002; Peters, 2004; Westrup et al, 2000, 2004).

NICU Network Neurobehavioral Scale

The NICU Network Neurobehavioral Scale (NNNS™) (Baltimore, MD: Brooks Publishing) was developed for use with preterm and other at-risk infants such as those with perinatal drug exposure to measure the process of neurobehavioral organization, capturing both the normal range of behaviors and those present in high-risk infants (Salisbury et al, 2005). The NNNSTM builds on several earlier assessments including the Neurological Examination of the Fullterm Newborn Infant (Prechtl & Beintema, 1968), abstinence syndrome scoring, and several of the assessments described in this section (NBAS, APIB, and NAPI) (Lester & Tronick, 2004). The NNNSTM can be used with infants from about 30 weeks' gestation to 46 to 48 weeks postconceptional age and assesses 115 items in three areas that examine both behavioral function and neurological integrity: (1) neurologic status (active and passive muscle tone, primitive reflexes, and central nervous system integrity); (2) behavioral state, sensory, and interactive responses; and (3) stress/abstinence scale. Items are administered only if the infant is in an appropriate state for that item. Administration of the assessment takes about 30 minutes (Lester & Tronick, 2004; Salisbury et al, 2005).

Normative data are available for comparison to other samples, and cross-cultural studies have been done (Lester et al, 2004; Tronick et al, 2004). The scale can be applied for clinical use (Boukydis et al, 2004) as well as research. Training (http://www.infantdevelopment.org/trainingandedu cation.htm) includes didactic content and observation of an examination (both of which can be done via telemedicine and video conferencing for trainees in remote locations), practice and reliability certification by a trainer.

Neurobehavioral Assessment of the Preterm Infant

The Neurobehavioral Assessment of the Preterm Infant (NAPI) is an assessment developed at Stanford University to assess differential maturity of infants between 32 weeks' postconceptional age and term (Korner & Thom, 1990; Korner et al, 2000). Components include assessment of behavioral states, active tone, strength, reflexes, excitation and inhibition proneness, and orientation to visual and auditory stimuli (Korner et al, 2000; Pressler et al, 2004; Senn & Espy, 2003).The NAPI has been used to monitor the developmental progress, to identify persistent lags in development, as an outcome measure in intervention studies and other studies, to describe individual differences in preterm infant development, and to identify infants with neurobehavioral alternations (Korner et al, 2000). The reliability and validity of this test and normative data have been established. Training is available to learn to achieve reliability in administration and scoring of the examination (http://www.med.stanford.edu/school/pediatrics/NAPI).

Family Infant Relationship Support Training (FIRST)

The FIRST, adapted from the NIDCAP (Boston: Children's Hospital), is an observation of the high-risk newborn infant and caregiver behavior in the context of their relationship immediately after discharge from the intensive care nursery (Browne, 1996). The FIRST is used with infants and caregivers in the home and community up to 8 months of age. Once the observation can be completed, provision of appropriate developmentally supportive care is outlined by observing typical routine caregiving events such as diaper changing or feeding. Developmentally supporting the newborn

and caregiver during the transition from hospital to home and through these early crucial stages of recovery from intensive care not only smoothes the transition but also supports the emerging relationship between infants and parents.

Training (http://www.uchsc.edu/cfii/first1.htm) involves a workshop followed by a practicum in which observations are practiced with extensive videotapes and clinical practice utilizing supportive developmental strategies. After practice trainees return for a skills check evaluation to determine independent use of the tool.

Assessment Beyond Neonatal Development

As the infant matures, moves out of the neonatal period, and becomes a "long termer" in the NICU with chronic respiratory or other problems, neurodevelopmental assessments continue to provide important information. For the infant who requires prolonged hospitalization, a developmental assessment at the bedside can provide information on how the infant interacts with objects and people, organizes behavior, and copes with the environment as well as on the infant's neurologic status. No formal developmental assessments have been standardized for these NICU populations. Most developmental psychologists or specialists adapt items from other examinations such as the Bayley Scales of Infant Development II (Bayley, 1993) or the recent Bayley Scales of Infant and Toddler Development (Bayley, 2005).

Because of the nature and severity of their illnesses, these infants may not be able to tolerate a complete examination at one session. To learn about the infant's behavioral capabilities and coping abilities adequately, the examiner must consider events that occurred for several hours before the assessment and be aware of the environment in which the infant normally lives and of his or her usual types of sensory experiences. Important areas of assessment include (1) availability of alerting; (2) ability to use interventions for consoling or developmental activities; (3) self-soothing capacity; (4) motor activities and strengths; (5) tolerance for handling (how long? with whom?); (6) degree of fragility; (7) degree of distractibility; (8) hand use; (9) parts of body available for use; and (10) respiratory capacity and tolerance.

Sleep-Wake States

Another aspect of neurobehavioral development that is considered as part of any developmental program is sleep-wake states and how they affect responses to stimuli. Sleeping and waking states are clusters of behaviors that tend to occur together and represent the level of arousal of the individual, the individual's responsivity to external stimulation, and the underlying activation of the central nervous system. Three states have been identified in adults: wakefulness, non-REM (rapid eye movement) sleep, and REM sleep. In infants, it is also possible to identify states within waking and states that are transitional between waking and sleeping because infants are less able to make rapid changes between states than are adults. Infants also have more difficulty sustaining alertness when awake. Because the electrophysiologic patterns associated with sleeping and waking states in infants are somewhat different from those in adults, the sleep states are usually designated active and quiet sleep, rather than REM and non-REM sleep.

Neonatal nurses need to be aware of the infant's present sleep-wake state and typical sleep-wake patterns when making assessments because infant behavior and physiology are affected by state. The functioning of cardiovascular, respiratory, neurologic, endocrine, and gastrointestinal systems differ in different states. Moreover, sleeping and waking states affect the infant's ability to respond to stimulation. Thus infant responses to nursing interventions and to parental interactions depend to a great deal on the infant's state when the stimulation begins (Johnston et al, 1999b; Oehler et al, 1988). Timing routine interventions to occur when the infant is most responsive is an important aspect of some current systems of individualized nursing care (Als et al, 1986; Becker et al, 1991b). Finally, studies have indicated that sleeping and waking patterns are closely related to neurologic status (Halpern et al, 1995; Thoman, 1982). Thus aberrant sleep-wake patterns could potentially be used to identify infants at risk for neurologic complications or poor developmental outcome.

STATE SCORING SYSTEMS

In adults, sleeping and waking are usually scored by electroencephalography (EEG). However, because of the neurologic immaturity of infants, EEG is less reliable and needs to be combined with observation. When EEG and behavioral scoring of states in preterm infants are compared, there is a high degree of agreement (Sahni et al, 1995). Thus by directly observing infants, whether full-term or preterm, and identifying global categories that are made up of a number of specific behaviors that tend to occur together and reflect a similar level of arousal and responsiveness to the environment, nurses can validly score sleeping and waking states in newborn infants. The behaviors that seem to be most important for scoring are respiration and eye movements (Brandon & Holditch-Davis, 2005).

Nurse researchers currently use four standardized systems for scoring behavioral observations of sleep-wake states. The systems were developed by Brazelton (1984), Thoman (1990), Als et al (1982), and Anderson (1999). These systems define states in very similar ways and are probably equally useful for clinical purposes. Figure 23-3 presents a comparison of the state definitions used in these systems.

Clinicians and researchers differ in the ways they use these scoring systems. Neonatal nurses spend a lot of time observing infants and altering their care in response to infant behavioral changes. Experienced clinicians are undoubtedly already familiar with the characteristics of sleeping and waking states in these infants, even though they may be unable to name specific states. Thus all they need to do to include judgments of sleeping and waking states is to use the state definitions of any standardized scoring system to systematize their clinical impressions.

For research, however, it is essential that the investigator receive training in the use of a particular scale so that it is used reliably. Clinicians reading research need to understand the differences among the scoring systems so that they can better interpret the findings and understand reports using different names for the same sleep-wake state.

Early State Scoring Systems

Sleeping and waking scoring systems for infants originated in the work of neurologists, pediatricians, and behaviorists in the 1960s. The neurologists needed a way to systematize the observations they made along with EEG studies, and

behaviorists and pediatricians were particularly interested in the waking states and the effect of state on responsiveness to stimulation. Wolff (1959, 1966), a pediatrician, conducted extensive observations of newborn infants in the hospital and at home. As the result of his observations, he proposed a seven-state system. Prechtl and Beintema (1968), pediatric neurologists, proposed a simple five-state system that could be used either to score observations made along with EEG or to ensure that motor reflexes were elicited under optimal conditions. Finally, a team of pediatricians and neurologists at the University of California at Los Angeles (UCLA) developed a manual to define the behavioral and EEG criteria for sleeping and waking (Anders et al, 1971). Each of the state scoring systems currently in use is a refinement of these earlier systems.

Brazelton's State Scoring System

T. Berry Brazelton is a pediatrician from Harvard University in Cambridge, Massachusetts. He and his colleagues developed a state scoring system to be used as part of a behavioral evaluation of newborn infants, the Neonatal Behavioral Assessment Scale or NBAS (Brazelton, 1984; Brazelton & Nugent, 1995). The purpose of this tool was to assess the individuality of the infant within the interactional process. This state scale was derived both from Dr. Brazelton's clinical experiences and from the existing state systems of Prechtl and Beintema (1968) and Thoman (1975). Brazelton's state scoring system consists of six states: deep sleep, light sleep, drowsy, alert, considerable motor activity, and crying. During the administration of the NBAS, this scoring system is used to identify predominant states, state transitions, and the quality of the alertness. However, it can also be used for scoring sleep-wake states during other situations. By 1983, more than 100 papers had been published using the NBAS and Brazelton's state scale (Brazelton, 1984), and many more have been published since then.

Brazelton's state scoring system has a number of advantages that make it the scoring system of choice for clinicians and also useful for researchers. This state system is easy to learn because the differences between the states are fairly obvious and there are only six states. Because of the widespread use of Brazelton's state scoring system, individuals experienced with this scale are located in virtually every part of the United States. In addition, there are reliability-training centers located throughout the country for those who want to use the entire NBAS or plan to use the state scoring system in research. Thus obtaining training in this scoring system is relatively easy. Finally, most researchers and experienced clinicians are familiar with the state definitions from this scale so that findings of sleeping and waking observations made with this scoring system are readily understood.

On the other hand, this state scoring system does have some limitations for use in research. First, because of the small number of states, it is not always sensitive enough to identify differences between normal full-term infants and infants with perinatal complications. Moreover, the NBAS state scoring system is appropriate for use only with infants between 36 and 44 weeks' gestational age (GA). The sleeping and waking states of infants born before 36 weeks' gestation and those born after 44 weeks' gestation will not be completely captured with this system. For example, older infants frequently are motorically active and alert during play, but in Brazelton's system, alertness is scored only when the infant is motorically quiet. Young preterm infants are frequently unable to make much sound when crying; thus their cry periods would be scored as considerable motor activity.

Thoman's State Scoring System

Evelyn B. Thoman is a psychobiologist who worked at the University of Connecticut. Although trained as an experimental psychologist to work with animals, she became interested in the interactions between human infants and their mothers when she went to work with Dr. Anneliese Korner at Stanford University in 1969 and has been studying them ever since. She developed her first state scoring system in 1975 (Thoman, 1975) based on the work of Wolff (1966) and Korner (1972). Although some researchers continue to use this system today, it has undergone considerable revision (Thoman, 1990). The Thoman state scoring system consists of 10 sleeping and waking states: alert, nonalert waking activity, fuss, cry, daze, drowse, sleep-wake transition, active sleep, active-quiet transitional sleep, and quiet sleep. Dr. Thoman and others have shown that both acceptable interrater reliability and test-retest reliability can be obtained with her system (Holditch-Davis et al, 2004b; Holditch-Davis and Edwards, 1998a; Holditch-Davis & Thoman, 1987; Thoman et al, 1987). Predictive validity is demonstrated by evidence that early sleeping and waking behaviors scored on Thoman's scale are related to later developmental outcome (Holditch-Davis et al, 2005; Thoman et al, 1981).

Thoman's state scoring system has a number of advantages. The documented reliability and validity of this system is of value to researchers. The sleeping and waking states are differentiated enough that they can be used with infants with perinatal complications (Holditch-Davis et al, 2004b; Holditch-Davis & Thoman, 1987; Thoman et al, 1988). This system has been used with preterm infants (Holditch-Davis et al, 2004b) and with infants older than 1 month after term (Holditch-Davis et al, 2000). The states in this system can also be combined when an investigator does not need such fine discriminations.

This scoring system has two disadvantages. First, a 10-state system is somewhat more difficult to learn than a 6-state system because it requires more subtle discriminations. However, individuals experienced in using a 6-state system, such as Brazelton's, can readily learn this system. Also, because this state scoring system is not as widely used as Brazelton's, it is more difficult to obtain training in its use.

Als' State Scoring System

Heidelise Als is a psychologist working at Harvard Medical School with Dr. Brazelton and his colleagues. For a number of years, she has worked with these colleagues to modify the NBAS (Brazelton, 1984) to make it more appropriate for use with premature infants. The Assessment of Preterm Infants' Behavior (APIB) is administered in much the same way as the NBAS, but the infant's behavior is scored in much greater detail so as to quantify not only the infant's skills but also the infant's reactivity and stress in response to environmental stimulation (Als et al, 1982; Pressler & Hepworth, 2002). Like the NBAS, the APIB is best administered to infants between 36 and 44 weeks' GA, but the observational portion of the tool can be used with younger preterm infants (Als, 1986). The state scale from the NBAS has been expanded into a 13-state system by subdividing each of the 6 states so that the immature

and unclear sleeping and waking states of premature infants can be more adequately described. These 13 states are very still deep sleep, deep sleep, light sleep, "noisy" light sleep, drowsy with more activity, drowsy, awake and quiet, hyper-alert, bright alert, active, considerable activity, crying, and lusty crying. The state subscale of the APIB has been shown to differentiate between premature and full-term infants after term (Als et al, 1988; Mouradian et al, 2000) and to correlate with electrophysiologic measures of brain activity (Duffy et al, 1990). In addition, the APIB and the state subscale are used to provide assessments that are the basis for planning individualized interventions as part of the Neonatal Individualized Developmental Care and Assessment Program (NIDCAP) (Als, 1986; Als et al, 1986; Pressler & Hepworth, 2002).

The Als' state scoring system has a number of advantages and disadvantages for clinicians and researchers. First, a 13-state system is more difficult to learn than a 6-state system such as Brazelton's (Brazelton & Nugent, 1995). However, since the Als system was developed from the Brazelton states, individuals familiar with the Brazelton system should have no difficulty learning it, and when the complexity of the 13 states is not needed they can be collapsed to the 6 states from the NBAS. Second, inasmuch as the APIB, like the NBAS, was never intended for use with infants older than 1 month after term, the state scale may not adequately capture the states of older infants.

Anderson's State Scoring System

Gene Cranston Anderson is a doctorally prepared nurse researcher who worked at Case Western Reserve University in Cleveland, Ohio. She has long been interested in interventions that keep mother and infant together after birth, reduce infant crying, and promote feeding. She developed a 12-state scoring system, the Anderson Behavioral State Scale (ABSS), to be used with preterm infants based on her own observations of these infants (Anderson, 1999) and on the work of Parmelee and Stern (1972). Parmelee was one of the contributors to the UCLA state manual (Anders et al, 1971). The ABSS consists of very quiet sleep, quiet sleep with irregular respirations, restless sleep, very restless sleep, drowsy, quiet awake, alert inactivity, restless awake, very restless awake, fussing, crying, and hard crying. The states are arranged so that there is a linear relationship between the states and heart rate and energy consumption, with the states with the lowest numbers having the lowest mean heart rates. The ABSS has been used to show the effects of prefeeding nonnutritive sucking (Gill et al, 1988) and kangaroo care (Ludington, 1990) on preterm infant state patterns.

As with the other scoring systems, the ABSS has a number of advantages and disadvantages for clinicians and researchers. As the newest state scoring scale, it has had only limited use outside of nursing. Because the ABSS was designed for use with preterm infants, the utility of this scale for full-term infants and older infants is unknown, although its similarity to other state scoring systems suggests that it should be applicable for healthy full-term newborn infants. The ABSS may also be difficult to learn because of the complexity of 12 states. As Figure 23-3 illustrates, the sleep states in this system differ markedly from the sleep states defined in other state scoring systems, so this is not a good scoring system to use if one is primarily interested in studying sleep states and wants to compare findings with other studies. Finally, the linear

Brazelton	Thoman	Als	Anderson
6. Crying	Cry	6B. Lusty crying	12. Hard crying
		6A. Crying	11. Crying
5. Considerable motor activity	Fuss	5B. Considerable activity	10. Fussing
	Nonalert waking activity	5A. Active	9. Very restless awake
			8. Restless awake
4. Alert	Alert	4B. Bright alert	7. Alert inactivity
		4AH. Hyperalert	
		4AL. Awake and quiet	
3. Drowsy	Daze	3B. Drowsy	6. Quiet awake
	Drowse		5. Drowsy
	Sleep-wake transition	3A. Drowsy with more activity	4. Very restless sleep
2. Light sleep	Active sleep	2B. "Noisy" light sleep	3. Restless sleep
	Active-quiet transitional sleep	2A. Light sleep	2. Quiet sleep: irregular respiration
1. Deep sleep	Quiet sleep	1B. Deep sleep	1. Very quiet sleep
		1A. Very still deep sleep	

FIGURE **23-3**

Approximate equivalence of the four major sleep-wake state scoring systems. Note: Because the criteria used by these systems differ and because they are based on different conceptual frameworks, exact equivalence among them is not possible. Isolated instances of infant behavior may be scored quite differently than suggested by this table.

relationship between the states in this system and heart rate may make it the ideal choice for researchers who are primarily interested in studying the energy consumption of infants. However, this feature means the ABSS has a very different theoretical basis than the other state scales. The other state scoring systems differentiate among states based on qualitatively different aspects of the infant's behavior, but the ABSS emphasizes quantitative differences among the states, although more recently Anderson emphasized qualitative differences between states.

Description of Individual States

Because the definitions of sleep-wake states are so similar among these scoring systems (see Figure 23-3), it is possible to describe in general the sleeping and waking states displayed by infants. For clarity's sake, generic state names will be used in all further descriptions. When they are not available, the state names from the Thoman system will be used. Each sleeping and waking state is made up a different constellation of behaviors and serves a different function for the infant. Physiologic functioning is also different in each of these states.

Infants are most responsive to the environment when in the waking states, and, in particular, when alert. When the infant is alert, the eyes are open and scanning. Motor activity is typically low, particularly in full-term newborns, but premature infants and infants older than 1 month after term may be motorically active. Alertness is the state in which the infant exhibits focused attention on sources of stimulation (Brazelton & Nugent, 1995). Thus this is the best state in which to test reflexes (Prechtl & Beintema, 1968). Alertness has been suggested to be the optimal state for feeding (McCain et al, 2001; White-Traut et al, 2005). This state is also the one in which infants are most receptive to interactions with their parents and other adults. Yet alertness rarely occurs in the preterm period (Holditch-Davis, 1990a; Holditch-Davis & Edwards, 1998a) and occurs relatively infrequently during the first month after term, only about 10% to 15% of the total day (Colombo & Horowitz, 1987).

Crying, another waking state, serves a communication function. However, the meaning of cries differs in different situations and may depend on their intensity (Fuller, 1991). Although crying that occurs when the infant is alone may elicit parental attention, crying that occurs during social exchanges may actually disrupt the parent-infant relationship. In full-term infants, crying during social interactions is related to the overall amount of maternal stimulation and to consistency in the patterning of maternal activities over weeks (Acebo & Thoman, 1995; Thoman et al, 1983). Studies have indicated that the intensity of crying is directly related to the heart rate of the infant (Ludington, 1990), and the higher the heart rate the greater the energy consumption of the infant (Woodson et al, 1983). In addition, this state is associated with decreased oxygenation in the bloodstream (Levesque et al, 2000) and brain (Brazy, 1988).

The final waking state, nonalert waking activity, is characterized by periods when the infant is motorically active but not alert or crying. Usually the infant's eyes are open. One study of nonalert activity found that excess amounts of this state in full-term infants are associated with inconsistency in the patterning of states over weeks (Becker & Thoman, 1982), and, in turn, inconsistency in state patterning is related to poor developmental outcome (Thoman

et al, 1981). Premature infants, after term, exhibit elevated levels of this state (Holditch-Davis & Thoman, 1987) and are known to be at increased risk of poor developmental outcome (Bhutta et al, 2002; Marlow et al, 2005; McGrath et al, 2005). However, whether there is a relationship between these findings is unknown.

The states transitional between sleeping and waking have rarely been studied. In fact, the Prechtl scoring system omits them altogether on the grounds that they are not true states but just transitions between states (Prechtl & Beintema, 1968). However, newborn infants, both term and preterm, actually spend significant amounts of time in them, ranging from about 6% of the day at 29 weeks' GA to 14% in the first month after term (Holditch-Davis, 1990a; Holditch-Davis & Thoman, 1987). Thoman (1990) describes three states transitional between waking and sleeping: drowse, when the infant is quiet and appears sleepy with eyes opening and closing slowly; daze, when the infant is quiet with eyes that are open but dazed in appearance; and sleep-wake transition, when the infant exhibits mixed signals of waking and sleeping, is motorically active, and may appear to be waking up. Drowse and daze typically occur in the midst of periods of waking or as the infant is falling asleep. Sleep-wake transition typically occurs at the end of sleeping as the infant is awakening but may also occur in the middle of sleep, particularly in premature infants. Drowse, daze, and sleep-wake transition are often combined in research reports. However, studies have indicated that these states have different patterns of correlations with other states (Thoman et al, 1987). During the first month after term, premature infants have been found to spend significantly more time in sleep-wake transition and less time in drowse or daze than full-term infants (Holditch-Davis & Thoman, 1987). If these three states had been combined, these differences would have been missed. In addition, hospitalized preterm infants spend more time in sleep-wake transition when they are with nurses rather than parents but do not differ in the amount of drowsiness that occurs with these different caregivers (Miller & Holditch-Davis, 1992). They also exhibit more sleep wake-transition and less drowsiness during procedural care than during feeding and changing (Brandon et al, 1999).

There are two major sleep states—active sleep and quiet sleep—although some state systems define a transitional state between them. In active sleep, the infant's respiration is uneven and primarily costal in nature. Sporadic motor movements occur, but muscle tone is low between these movements. Most behaviors, including hiccups, yawns, jitters, negative facial expressions (frowns and grimaces), and large movements, are less frequent in active sleep than waking but more frequent than in quiet sleep, but startles and jerks occur most frequently in active sleep (Holditch-Davis et al, 2003). The most distinct characteristic of this state is rapid eye movements that occur intermittently.

Active sleep is the most common state from birth throughout infancy, but it occurs during only about 20% of sleep in adults. Because of this dramatic developmental decrease and the frequent movements seen in infants during active sleep, many clinicians think of active sleep as a disorganized and primitive state. Surprisingly, this state has relatively recent phylogenetic origins, occurring only in birds and mammals. Thus it has been hypothesized to be necessary for brain development (Roffwarg et al, 1966). This hypothesis has received support in full-term infants (Denenberg & Thoman,

1981). In animal studies, prolonged deprivation of active sleep in infancy permanently altered brain functioning and resulted in hyperactivity, distractibility, and altered sexual performance (Mirmiran, 1986). Inasmuch as respiratory patterns are relatively unstable in active sleep (Holditch-Davis et al, 2004a; Vecchierini et al, 2001) and oxygenation is lower and more variable (Gabriel et al, 1980; Martin et al, 1979), the large amount of active sleep seen in young preterm infants (Holditch-Davis et al, 2004b; Holditch-Davis & Edwards, 1998a) may contribute to their respiratory difficulties.

The other sleep state, quiet sleep, is characterized by a lack of body movements and the presence of regular respiration. A tonic level of motor tone is maintained in this state. Most behaviors, including hiccups, yawns, mouth movements, jitters, negative facial expressions, and large movements, are less frequent in quiet sleep than in waking or active sleep; the exception is sighs, which occur most frequently in quiet sleep (Holditch-Davis et al, 2003). The major purpose of quiet sleep seems to be rest and restoration. This state has been hypothesized to be necessary for healing (Adam & Oswald, 1984). Quiet sleep may also be needed for growth because it is in this state that growth hormone is secreted in adults. However, a study of full-term infants did not find any relationship between growth hormone secretion and quiet sleep (Shaywitz et al, 1971). Oxygenation is higher during this sleep state; thus quiet sleep may be beneficial for infants with respiratory problems (Gabriel et al, 1980; Martin et al, 1979).

The amount of quiet sleep is also very sensitive to the environment. Infant stimulation studies, for example, have found that quiet sleep is the state most likely to be increased by vestibular and kinesthetic interventions (Ingersoll & Thoman, 1994; Johnston et al, 1997). The stimulation provided by routine nursing care, on the other hand, results in significantly less quiet sleep as compared with times when the preterm infant is undisturbed (Brandon et al, 1999; Holditch-Davis, 1990b), and the amount of this state is further reduced when the infant experiences painful or uncomfortable procedures (Holditch-Davis & Calhoun, 1989). Thus this is the state most likely to be affected by the NICU environment.

EFFECT OF PHYSIOLOGIC PARAMETERS ON STATE

Physiologic functioning varies in different states. In turn, abnormalities in physiologic functioning can alter the sleeping and waking states of infants. This discussion focuses on the interrelationship of sleeping and waking and four areas of physiologic functioning of interest to neonatal nurses—perinatal illness, the central nervous system, circulatory system, and respiration.

Perinatal Illness

The state patterns of infants who experienced perinatal complications may differ markedly from the state patterns of healthy full-term infants. Small-for-gestational-age full-term infants, for example, have more disorganized sleep as evidenced by more active sleep without rapid eye movements than healthy full-term infants (Watt & Strongman, 1985). They also exhibited poorer responsiveness during alertness as measured by the NBAS (Lester et al, 1986).

The sleep of premature infants after term is known to differ from that of full-term infants of the same corrected ages, in that there is a decreased total amount of sleep, longer episodes of quiet sleep, more body movements, more frequent REM episodes, and somewhat lower correlation among the various behavioral criteria of the sleep states (Ellingson & Peters, 1980; Holditch-Davis & Thoman, 1987; Watt & Strongman, 1985). Premature infants show day-night differentiation in their sleeping and waking patterns at the same or an earlier postmenstrual age than full-term infants (Shimada et al, 1993; Whitney & Thoman, 1994). In addition, their EEG patterns differ from those of full-term infants. Premature infants display longer bursts during trace alternans, earlier sleep spindle appearance, more immature EEG patterns, and poorer phase stability for EEG frequencies (Ellingson & Peters, 1980; Karch et al, 1982). Premature and full-term infants also differ on architectural, phasic, continuity, spectral, and autonomic measures (Curzi-Dascalova et al, 1988; Scher et al, 1992, 1994b, 1994c).

The ways in which the waking states differ between full-term and premature infants of similar postmenstrual ages are less well established. Over prolonged observation periods, premature infants exhibited more alertness and nonalert waking activity and less drowsiness than full-term infants (Holditch-Davis & Thoman, 1987).

The severity of illness that the infant experiences during the perinatal period has relatively small additional effects on sleeping and waking. In general, critical illness has immediate effects on sleeping and waking patterns, but these effects disappear after the infant recovers as long as there are no neurologic complications and as long as infants are observed at same ages corrected for GA at birth. Karch and colleagues (1982) studied healthy and ill preterm infants at comparable ages and found that ill infants exhibited more quiet sleep, more indeterminate sleep, and less wakefulness. The ill infants in this study were examined while on mechanical ventilation. Thus the state differences reflect the immediate influence of critical illness and mechanical ventilation. Preterm infants ill with respiratory distress syndrome have been found to exhibit delayed state development but show state patterns comparable to those of healthy preterm infants once they recover (Holmes et al, 1979). Doussard-Roosevelt et al (1996) found that preterm infants with more medical complications showed more active sleep during brief sleep observations at 33 to 35 weeks than healthier preterm infants. Curzi-Dascalova et al (1993) found that the longest sleep cycle of mechanically ventilated preterm infants was shorter than that of nonventilated infants. Holditch-Davis and Hudson (1995) used changes in sleep-wake states to identify a wide variety of acute medical complications in preterm infants, including hydrocephalus, sepsis, and cold stress. Infant medical complications also affected the scores of infants on standardized neurobehavioral assessments, but only on items requiring vigorous responses (e.g., vigor of crying, irritability, and motor development) and not on other state items, including alertness and percent sleeping (Korner et al, 1994).

Studies of infants who have recovered from their illnesses have found fewer differences. High and Gorski (1985) did not find any differences in the sleeping and waking patterns of convalescent premature infants differing in the severity of their previous illness. Likewise, Holditch-Davis (1990a) found that the only difference in the development of sleeping and waking states in convalescent preterm infants was that more severely ill infants showed less fussing and somewhat poorer organization of quiet sleep. However, Holditch-Davis et al

(2004b) found that longer mechanical ventilation was associated with more active sleep and less active sleep without REMs and that infants with lower birth weights had more regularity of respiration in quiet sleep. On the other hand, Brandon et al (2005) found that longer mechanical ventilation was associated with less active sleep. Als et al (1988) found no difference in the state organization of premature infants born at less than 33 weeks' GA and premature infants born between 33 and 37 weeks' GA when state organization was measured 2 weeks after term. In addition, scores on the NBAS state scale did not differ significantly between sick and healthy full-term infants at the time of hospital discharge (Holmes et al, 1982).

Infants with chronic lung disease are more likely than other premature infants to have oxygen desaturations when sleeping (Zinman et al, 1992). Yet it is unclear whether this illness has any effect on sleeping and waking patterns. Holditch-Davis and Lee (1993) compared high-risk preterm infants with and without chronic lung disease from 32 to 36 weeks' postmenstrual age on sleep-wake states and sleep organization exhibited over 4-hour observations in the intermediate care unit. The only difference between the infants with and without chronic lung disease was that infants with chronic lung disease had more irregular respiration in quiet sleep. Despite the fact that many clinicians believe that infants with chronic lung disease are more sensitive to stimulation, there were also no differences in sleeping and waking when the infants with and without chronic lung disease were with caregivers (Holditch-Davis, 1995). However, at term age, premature infants with chronic lung disease had less active sleep, more frequent arousals, and more frequent body movements in sleep than premature infants who never experienced any respiratory illnesses and performed more poorly on the interactive and motor clusters of the NBAS (Myers et al, 1992).

Treatments for perinatal illnesses also may affect the sleeping and waking states of preterm infants. In addition, supplemental oxygen was associated with increased quiet sleep and total sleep time (Simakajornboon et al, 2002). Prenatal magnesium sulfate affected the organization of sleep states leading to dysmaturity (a combination of accelerated and delayed state organization), whereas antenatal steroids had no effect (Black et al, 2006). Preterm infants whose mothers received antenatal phenobarbital did not differ in heart rate or sleep-wake states in the first 3 days of life from infants not receiving the medication, suggesting that the antenatal dosage was not sedating (McCain et al, 1999).

Neurologic System

Because sleeping and waking states are assumed to reflect the underlying activation of the central nervous system (CNS), it is not surprising that close relationship exists between sleep-wake states and CNS functioning. Four factors illustrate this interrelationship. First, sleeping and waking exhibit a large amount of development in the first year of life, the time of the most rapid CNS development. Sleeping and waking state affect neurologic responses. Infants with neurologic abnormalities exhibit abnormal sleeping and waking patterns. Finally, sleeping and waking states can be used to predict developmental outcome.

Development of Sleeping and Waking States

Infants exhibit definite developmental changes in their sleeping and waking state patterns throughout the first year

of life. The age at which sleep-wake states first appear is unknown. The earliest study of sleeping and waking in preterm infants younger than 30 weeks' GA found that these infants had only a single active sleep-like state (Dreyfus-Brisac, 1968), but these findings are questionable because all of the infants in this study were dying at the time of the state recordings. More recent studies of preterm infants have found that by 24 weeks' GA, cycling between waking and sleeping can be identified by EEG in some preterm infants (Hellstrom-Westas et al, 1991). By 25 to 27 weeks' GA (the earliest age studied), infants exhibit distinct waking and sleeping states (Curzi-Dascalova et al, 1988, 1993; Holditch-Davis et al, 2004b; Holditch-Davis & Edwards, 1998a; Scher et al, 2005). However, before 30 weeks' GA, the various behaviors associated with sleep and waking—eye movements, body movements, respiration, and muscle tone—are not well coordinated; not until at least 36 weeks' GA do preterm infants exhibit the same degree of correlation between these parameters as do full-term infants (Curzi-Dascalova et al, 1988; Parmelee & Stern, 1972). Studies of sleeping and waking states in fetuses conducted using observations made during ultrasound examinations have had similar findings (DiPietro et al, 1996).

Infants exhibit greater amounts of active sleep and indeterminate states during the preterm period and lower amounts of waking states than after term (High & Gorski, 1985; Holditch-Davis, 1990a; Holditch-Davis et al, 2004b; Holditch-Davis & Edwards, 1998a). Active sleep occupies as much as 60% to 70% of the day for young preterm infants (High & Gorski, 1985; Holditch-Davis et al, 2004b; Holditch-Davis & Edwards, 1998a). The major developmental change during the preterm period is a decrease in the amount of sleep due to a decrease in active sleep (High & Gorski, 1985; Holditch-Davis et al, 2004b; Holditch-Davis & Edwards, 1998a; Ingersoll & Thoman, 1999). In addition, quiet sleep and waking states, especially crying, increase (High & Gorski, 1985; Holditch-Davis et al, 2004b; Holditch-Davis & Edwards, 1998a; Vles et al, 1992). The organization of the sleep states, as measured by the percentages of the state with typical state criteria or by the correlation between criteria, also increases throughout the preterm period (Curzi-Dascalova et al, 1988; Holditch-Davis et al, 2004b; Holditch-Davis & Edwards, 1998a). The mean duration and frequency of episodes of each state also change over the preterm period: quiet waking, active waking, and sleep-wake transition episodes occurred more frequently than active waking and quiet sleep, but length of these periods increased over age (Holditch-Davis & Edwards, 1998b; Ingersoll & Thoman, 1999).

The sleeping and waking states of infants in the first month after term differ dramatically from those of preterm infants. Healthy full-term neonates sleep about $13\frac{1}{2}$ hours a day (Thomas & Foreman, 2005) and spend approximately 40% of the daytime in active sleep and 20% in quiet sleep (Holditch-Davis & Thoman, 1987). Slightly higher amounts of sleep states occur at night (Thoman & Whitney, 1989; Whitney & Thoman, 1994). Waking states make up the rest of the day, with alertness (14%) and drowsiness (13%) being the most common (Holditch-Davis & Thoman, 1987).

The major developmental trends exhibited by full-term infants in the first month are a decrease in active sleep and an increase in the amount of alertness (Denenberg & Thoman, 1981; Kohyama & Iwakawa, 1990). Moreover, the mean lengths of episodes of the sleep states change, with active sleep decreasing and quiet sleep increasing (Thoman & Whitney, 1989). Similar trends occur for premature infants during this period (Ariagno et al, 1997; Mirmaran et al, 2003; Whitney & Thoman, 1994). In addition, both full-term and premature infants begin to show entrainment to a day-night schedule of sleeping and waking by about a month after term (Ariagno et al, 1997; Shimada et al, 1999).

Sleeping and waking states continue to develop throughout the first year. Waking periods become longer and more consolidated (Holditch-Davis et al, 1999; Louis et al, 1997). The infant spends an increasing proportion of wakefulness in the alert state. The amount of time spent crying decreases (Michelsson et al, 1990; St. James-Roberts & Plewis, 1996). In addition, total sleep time decreases, with almost all of this decrease due to a decrease in active sleep time (Holditch-Davis et al, 1999; Kohyama & Iwakawa, 1990; Louis et al, 1997; St. James-Roberts & Plewis, 1996). The amount of quiet sleep remains the same or increases from term age on; thus by about 6 months of age, the amount of quiet sleep exceeds the amount of active sleep (Louis et al, 1997). The nature of these changes depends somewhat on feeding type, as breastfed infants exhibit less total sleep, longer sleep latency, more non-REM sleep, and shorter duration of REM sleep than formula-fed infants do (Butte et al, 1992; Quillin & Glenn, 2004). In addition, the number of sleep episodes decreases and becomes consolidated primarily into nighttime, although most infants continue to exhibit some amount of night waking (Ottaviano et al, 1996; Scher, 1991). By 1 year, the infant is taking about two daytime naps (Weissbluth, 1995) and sleeping about 10 to 12 hours through the night. Prematurely born infants may display shorter night sleep and more night awakenings than full-term infants (Ju et al, 1991).

Other developmental changes during the first year affect the organization of sleep. The cycling between active and quiet becomes more consistent over the first few months, and by 4 months of age, the complete sleep cycle first exhibits a standard length of about 1 hour (Harper et al, 1981). Many preterm infants display hour-long sleep cycles by 36-week postmenstrual age (Borghese et al, 1995). The sleep states also develop the EEG patterns typical of adults. By 3 months of age, the EEG stages within quiet sleep can be identified, and this sleep state can now be called non-REM sleep (Ellingson & Peters, 1980).

Neurologic Responses

Infants exhibit different neurologic responses in different sleeping and waking states. The magnitude of neurologic reflexes is known to differ greatly in different states (Prechtl & Beintema, 1968). Therefore standardized infant assessments and neurologic examinations specify which states are optimal for testing each reflex (Brazelton & Nugent, 1995; Prechtl & Beintema, 1968). The amplitude, wave form, and latency of visual evoked potentials are different in different sleeping and waking states, with the greatest differences being between sleep and waking (Apkarian et al, 1991).

Neurologic Problems

The state patterns of infants with neurologic insults differ markedly from those of healthy infants. Infants with Down syndrome have been found to spend more time awake and to have abnormally long periods of quiet sleep (Prechtl et al, 1973). At term, using the NBAS, premature infants with intraventricular hemorrhage have been found to have lower

arousal than healthy full-term infants (Anderson et al, 1989). Full-term infants with hyperbilirubinemia show decreased amounts of wakefulness (Prechtl et al, 1973). As compared to full-term infants with only mild bilirubin elevations, infants with moderately elevated bilirubin values exhibit significantly lower scores in state regulation and range on the NBAS and exhibit minor neurologic abnormalities as shown by increased latency of brain-stem auditory evoked potentials (Vohr et al, 1990). Abnormal cry patterns have been found in infants who have neurologic injuries or hyperbilirubinemia or are at risk for sudden infant death syndrome (SIDS)(Corwin et al, 1995).

In addition, infants exposed prenatally to drugs or alcohol exhibit abnormalities in their state patterns, possibly as the result of neurologic insults caused by the drugs. For example, alcohol-exposed infants exhibit sleep disruptions and abnormal cries (Nugent et al, 1996; Scher et al, 1988). Newborn infants of mothers who smoked during pregnancy had higher cries than did infants whose mothers did not smoke (Nugent et al, 1996). Infants exposed to marijuana have shorter, higher cries with more variation in frequency (Lester & Dreher, 1989) and exhibit a decrease in quiet sleep time (Scher et al, 1988). Methadone-exposed infants exhibit abnormal cries with short first expirations and are more irritable and less able to sustain a high-quality alert state (Huntington et al, 1990; Jeremy & Hans, 1985). Infants experiencing opiate withdrawal exhibit more waking, more sleep fragmentation, and less quiet sleep (O'Brien & Jeffery, 2002). Infants who were exposed to cocaine or opiates during pregnancy showed more alertness and less quiet sleep than nonexposed infants (White-Traut et al, 2002). Infants who were prenatally exposed to cocaine showed less active sleep and more indeterminate sleep; they also showed less orientation and poorer state regulation, including more jitters, high-pitched cries, and hyperalertness, than drug-free infants (Bauer et al, 2005; Black et al, 1993; Regalado et al, 1995). On the other hand, Woods and colleagues (1993) did not find any differences on the NBAS between cocaine-exposed and drug-free infants (Chapter 21).

Prediction of Developmental Outcome

Finally, the organization of sleeping and waking, as indicated by individual state criteria or the overall patterning of states, can be used to predict the developmental outcome of infants. Greater amounts of quiet sleep in the preterm period relate to better alertness and orientation, less irritability, and better orientation to inanimate visual and auditory stimulation on the Neurobehavioral Assessment of the Preterm Infant (Korner et al, 1991), an assessment similar to the APIB, at 32 and 36 weeks' postmenstrual age (Brandon et al, 2005). In healthy preterm infants, lower spectral EEG energies predicted lower neurodevelopmental performance at 12 and 24 months (Scher et al, 1994a). Low levels of trace alternans, an EEG pattern seen during quiet sleep in neonates, is predictive of lower intelligence quotients (IQs) in premature infants (Beckwith & Parmelee, 1986), and delayed maturity of EEG patterns of preterm infants was found to be associated with poor neurologic outcome (Ferrari et al, 1992; Hahn & Tharp, 1990). More sleep-wake transition, shorter sleep periods, and fewer arousals from quiet sleep during the first day of life in full-term infants are associated with lower developmental scores at 6 months (Freudigman & Thoman, 1993). Elevated amounts of intense bursts of rapid eye movements and long sleep-cycle lengths at 6 months are associated with developmental problems in full-term infants (Becker & Thoman, 1982; Borghese et al, 1995). Acoustic characteristics of infant cries have been used to predict developmental outcome in preterm infants and infants who were prenatally exposed to drugs (Huntington et al, 1990). Measures of sleep-wake states during the preterm period—including the total amount of sleep, the overall quality of state organization as compared with other infants, and sleep cycle length—have been found to predict Bayley scores at 6 months to 3 years corrected age (Borghese et al, 1995; DiPietro & Porges, 1991; Fajardo et al, 1992; Gertner et al, 2002; Holditch-Davis et al, 2005; Whitney & Thoman, 1993). However, the amount of indeterminate sleep—any period not meeting the criteria for one of the five states defined by Prechtl and Beintema (1968)—in premature infants at term was not related to developmental status at 2 years (Maas et al, 2000). In apparently normal full-term infants, the stability of state patterns in the first month has been found to predict developmental outcome (Thoman et al, 1981). This finding has been replicated in premature infants after term (Whitney & Thoman, 1993) and in siblings of infants who died from SIDS (Thoman et al, 1988).

Circulatory System

Sleeping and waking states affect the infant's circulatory system. Overall, heart rate is higher in waking than sleeping states, and particularly during crying (Ludington, 1990; van Ravenswaaij-Arts et al, 1989). Mean heart rates in the two sleep states are very similar, but heart rate is more variable in active sleep (Galland et al, 2000). This difference in variability is large enough that it is possible to differentiate between the two sleep states on the basis of heart rate variability (DeHaan et al, 1977). Thus neonatal nurses need to be aware of the infant's state when determining heart rate, and routine vital signs probably should not be obtained while the infant is crying.

Sleeping and waking states also affect the infant's circulation. Cerebral blood flow is highest in waking (Greisen et al, 1985). It is significantly higher in active sleep than in quiet sleep in full-term infants (Milligan, 1979), but not in infants less than term age (Greisen et al, 1985). Variability in cerebral blood flow velocity is lowest in quiet sleep, whereas marked fluctuations occur in active waking (fussing and nonalert waking activity; Ramaekers et al, 1989). Blood pressure is slightly higher when the infant is awake than when asleep (van Ravenswaaij-Arts et al, 1989).

Respiration

The effect of sleeping and waking states on the respiratory system is even greater than on the circulatory system. The nervous system controls of breathing differ in different states (Phillipson, 1978). During wakefulness, breathing is regulated by metabolic controls, general stimulation from the reticular activating system, and voluntary activities. In quiet sleep, metabolic controls predominate, and maintaining acid-base and oxygen homeostasis is the primary stimulus for breathing. Medullary respiratory center activity varies during active asleep depending on whether the infant is experiencing rapid eye movements and motor activity (phasic active sleep) or not (tonic active sleep), indicating that these two types of active sleep include different controls on breathing. During phasic active sleep, behavioral controls, similar to the vol-

untary controls in waking, predominate. In tonic active sleep, the major respiratory control results from direct stimulation of the state in a manner similar to the reticular stimulation of respiration during wakefulness. As a result of these different controls, infants exhibit higher respiratory rates and lower tidal volumes in phasic active sleep than in tonic active sleep (Haddad et al, 1982). In addition, the Hering-Breuer reflex is strong in active sleep in preterm infants (Hand et al, 2004).

Respiratory activity responds differently to chemical stimulation in different states. Baseline arterial oxygen and carbon dioxide levels are lower in active sleep than in either waking or quiet sleep (Gabriel et al, 1980; Martin et al, 1979; Mok et al, 1988), possibly because of hypoventilation or ventilation-perfusion inequalities in this state. Arousal in response to hypoxia differs in quiet sleep and active sleep, with some studies finding that it is slower in quiet sleep (Parslow et al, 2004) and others finding it slower in active sleep (Fewell & Baker, 1987). Response to hypercapnia is also different in different states. There is a shift to the right in the carbon dioxide response curve in quiet sleep as compared to waking (Cohen et al, 1991; Phillipson, 1978). This response is further reduced in tonic active sleep and is absent in phasic active sleep (Sullivan, 1980).

As a result of these differing neurologic controls on breathing, a number of respiratory variables in both full-term and preterm infants are influenced by sleep and waking states. Respiration rates are higher and more variable in active sleep (Holditch-Davis et al, 2004a; Patzak et al, 1999). Active sleep has also been shown to result in hypoventilation in preterm infants because of central inhibition of spinal motoneurons (Schulte et al, 1977) and poor coordination between chest and abdominal muscles (Gaultier, 1990). Thus paradoxical movements of the chest wall and abdominal muscles during breathing are common during active sleep in preterm infants. However, it is not clear whether lung volume is decreased in active sleep in full-term infants. Expiratory volumes and flow rates are larger in waking than in sleeping infants (Lodrup et al, 1992).

The frequency of central apnea also differs between the two sleep states. Central apnea rarely occurs during waking. Most studies indicate that brief apneic pauses of less than 20 seconds in length occur more frequently in active sleep than quiet sleep in both full-term and preterm infants (Curzi-Dascalova et al, 2000; Holditch-Davis et al, 1994, 2004a; Vecchierini et al, 2001). However, the frequency of periodic respiration (cyclic breathing alternating with brief apneic pauses) does not appear to differ between the sleep states (Holditch-Davis et al, 1994, 2004a). The mean length of apneic pauses is longer in quiet sleep (Holditch-Davis et al, 1994, 2004a). In addition, a variety of stresses, including an increase in body temperature and sleep deprivation, have been shown to increase apnea frequency, primarily in active sleep (Gaultier, 1994).

However, it cannot be concluded from these studies that pathologic apneas (apneic episodes longer than 20 seconds and usually associated with bradycardia and hypoxemia) are more common in active sleep because these studies rarely included episodes of pathologic apnea. Pathologic apnea is often too rare to permit statistical analyses comparing states (Holditch-Davis et al, 1994, 2004a). Yet some association may exist between active sleep and pathologic apnea inasmuch as the methylxanthines, caffeine and theophylline, used to treat this condition are generally found to increase the amount of wakefulness and decrease the amount of sleep in addition to their direct effects on respiration (Brandon et al, 2005; Thoman et al, 1985). Infants have also been found to have greater respiration regularity in active sleep occurred during treatment with theophylline and caffeine (Holditch-Davis et al, 2004a). On the other hand, other studies have found that theophylline and caffeine had minimal effects on sleep-wake development (Curzi-Dascalova et al, 2002; Holditch-Davis & Edwards, 1998a).

EFFECT OF HEALTH CARE INTERVENTIONS ON STATE

Sleeping and waking states are also affected by the types and timing of stimulation that the infant receives from the environment. Thus health care interventions have the potential either to promote state organization or to disrupt it. The effects of four common nursing interventions—routine NICU care, painful procedures, social interaction, and infant stimulation—on infant sleeping and waking are examined in this section.

Effect of Environmental Stimulation

The hospital provides stimulation that may be inappropriate for the development of premature infants and is likely to result in disorganized sleeping and waking patterns. The NICU provides infants with an extremely bright and noisy environment with little diurnal variation and frequent interventions for technical procedures, but little positive handling (Duxbury et al, 1984; Gottfried & Gaiter, 1985; Zahr & Balian, 1995). The sickest infants actually receive the most handling (High & Gorski, 1985; Zahr & Balian, 1995), even though they lack the physiologic reserves to cope with it. Premature infants may become hypoxic in response to virtually any form of stimulation. The severity of the negative physiologic responses to one procedure, endotracheal suctioning, has been related to the infant's state during the procedure (Bernert et al, 1997). Preterm infants who cried during suctioning had greater changes in oxygenation and heart rate than infants who slept through suctioning. Convalescent infants are handled less than ill infants but do experience social interactions as a greater percent of their care (High & Gorski, 1985).

Several of the aspects of routine NICU care are known to contribute to disruption of infant sleeping and waking patterns. Nursing and medical interventions frequently result in state changes. The frequency of these interventions in the NICU has been found to be as high as five times per hour (Duxbury et al, 1984). Preterm infants change their sleep-wake states about six times per hour, and 78% of these changes are associated with either nursing interventions or NICU noise (Zahr & Balian, 1995). Preterm infants are rarely able to sustain quiet sleep during nursing interventions (Brandon et al, 1999; Holditch-Davis, 1990b) and usually awaken with each intervention. Inasmuch as infants fall asleep in active sleep, frequent nursing interventions are particularly likely to reduce the amount of quiet sleep that the infant experiences. Preterm infants normally spend only a small percentage of their time in waking states (High & Gorski, 1985; Holditch-Davis, 1990a), but this percentage increases significantly when they are with nurses (Brandon et al, 1999; Holditch-Davis, 1990b). Also, developmental changes in the amount of waking occur only over the time infants are with

nurses, and the distribution of states differs depending on the nursing activity, with active waking more common and drowsiness less common during more intrusive care (Brandon et al, 1999). On the other hand, preterm infants showed more quiet sleep after nursing interventions than before them (Symanski et al, 2002), and bathing did not affect sleep-wake patterns (Lee, 2002).

Moreover, neonatal nurses and physicians often do not consider infant sleep-wake states and other infant cues when choosing the time for routine interventions. Although two studies found relationships between nursing care and sleeping and waking for groups of preterm infants (Barnard & Blackburn, 1985; Lawson et al, 1985), these results probably represent infant reactions to nursing care or infants conditioned to anticipate regular nursing procedures rather than nurses responding to infant states. Infant activity has been found to decrease after nursing interventions (Blackburn & Barnard, 1985). Gottfried (1985) found that nurses responded to fewer than half the cries of convalescent premature infants. Yet a lack of responsiveness to infant cues may serve to slow the development of stable diurnal patterns of sleeping and waking that several investigators have suggested is the first task of infancy (Barnard & Blackburn, 1985). Full-term infants receiving responsive care develop day-night differentiation in their sleeping and waking in 5 to 7 days, whereas this differentiation is delayed when the care is not responsive (Sander et al, 1979).

In light of the recommendation by the American Academy of Pediatrics (AAP) (1992) that infants be placed on their backs to sleep, the effects of positioning on infant sleep-wake states also need to be considered. Full-term infants in the supine position show greater wakefulness, less quiet sleep, lower heart rates, higher rates of brief respiratory pauses, and better airway protection during sleep than when prone (Jeffery et al, 1999; Skadberg & Markestad, 1997). Similar effects on sleeping and waking, heart rate, and oxygenation have been found in growing preterm infants and in preterm infants with chronic lung disease (Ariagno et al, 2003; Chang et al, 2002; Goto et al, 1999; Horne et al, 2002; McEvoy et al, 1997; Myers et al, 1998). Thus supine positioning may not be appropriate for preterm infants with respiratory compromise. Moreover, in preterm infants who are no longer acutely ill, positioning decisions will require balancing infant needs for rest and oxygenation with the need to provide an example for parents. Although prone sleeping has decreased after discharge for preterm infants, mothers of very low birth weight infants still tend to place their infants on their sides, rather than supine (Vernacchio et al, 2003).

Finally, the lighting of the NICU, as discussed earlier in this chapter, contributes to sleeping and waking problems in infants. Lighting in most NICUs is continuous, high-level, and fluorescent. The frequency of eye opening and waking states is related to the level of illumination in the NICU; less eye opening occurs when the lights are brightest (Moseley et al, 1988; Robinson et al, 1989). Sudden decreases in lighting result in increased eye opening (Moseley et al, 1988). This finding supports the common nursing and parental intervention of shading infant eyes with one's hand to elicit alertness. In addition, infants exposed to NICUs that vary the intensity of lighting on a diurnal pattern open their eyes significantly more than those exposed to continuous illumination (Robinson et al, 1989).

In view of the problems with routine NICU care, several researchers have attempted to alter this environment to promote better sleeping and waking patterns in infants. When Gabriel and associates (1981) consolidated nursing care so that convalescent premature infants were disturbed less often, the infants were awake less often and had longer sleep episodes. Fajardo et al (1990) cared for premature infants in a quiet, private room with a day-night cycle, demand feedings, and social interactions by the nurses. These babies showed an increase in the mean length of active sleep and an increase in the organization of sleep states as evidenced by a decreased number of state changes and increased number of enduring state episodes.

Als and colleagues (1986) developed a system of individualized interventions for preterm infants that included sensitivity to infant cues and careful avoidance of sleep disruptions. Their experimental infants did not exhibit different state patterns compared to the control infants, but the experimental infants did have fewer medical complications and improved performance on the APIB. A replication found improved state regulation and state stability as measured on the APIB (Buehler et al, 1995). Using a modification of Als' intervention system, Becker and associates (1991a) also found improvements in infant morbidity but did not find differences in state behaviors on the NBAS at the time of hospital discharge; however, the experimental infants showed higher oxygen saturations, fewer disorganized movements, and more alertness during nursing care than did controls (Becker et al, 1993). Later studies found that infants receiving the intervention slept more than infants receiving traditional handling (Becker et al, 1997; Bertelle et al, 2005). However, other studies using Als' intervention system did not find that it had any effect on sleep-wake states, either in the preterm period or after discharge (Ariagno et al, 1997; Westrup et al, 2002).

A number of researchers altered NICU lighting patterns. Mann et al (1986) cared for preterm infants in a nursery in which light and noise intensities were reduced between 7:00 AM and 7:00 PM. As compared with infants from a control nursery, the experimental infants were found to sleep more, but not until after hospital discharge. Blackburn and Patteson (1991) compared preterm infants in a nursery with continuous lighting with infants in a nursery with lighting that was dimmed at night. Infants in cycled light exhibited less motor activity during the night and lower heart rates over the entire day than the control infants. When preterm infants in the intermediate care unit were given four half-hour nap periods a day during which their incubators were covered and they received no nursing or medical procedures, they exhibited less quiet waking and longer uninterrupted sleep bouts than preterm infants without naps (Holditch-Davis et al, 1995), and they experienced a more rapid decline in apnea and more rapid weight gain (Torres et al, 1997). Brandon and colleagues (2002) compared preterm infants who received care in near darkness with infants who received cycled light. Although there were no differences in state patterns (Brandon et al, 2005), the infants receiving cycled light showed more rapid weight gain (Brandon et al, 2002). In another study, preterm infants receiving cycled light showed earlier day-night patterning of activity than infant cared for in dim light (Rivkees et al, 2004). However, a third study found no differences in sleep or circadian patterns after discharge in infants exposed to dim lighting or cycled lighting (Mirmaran et al, 2003). All together, these findings suggest that neonatal nurses need to examine their routine practices to see if changes could be made to better promote stable sleeping and waking patterns in infants.

Painful Procedures

Infants in intensive care inevitably experience painful procedures. Neonatal nurses need to be alert to the effects of these procedures on infant sleeping and waking states. During painful procedures, infants are more likely to be awake and less likely to be in quiet sleep than during routine nursing care (Fearon et al, 1997; Van Cleve et al, 1995). All but the youngest and sickest preterm infants are likely to cry (Johnston et al, 1999b; Van Cleve et al, 1995), although the length of time until the cry begins depends on the infant's sleeping and waking state at the beginning of the procedure (Grunau & Craig, 1987). Healthy full-term infants have the longest latency to cry when in quiet sleep, and young, preterm infants who are asleep at the beginning of the procedure and have recently undergone another painful procedure are the most likely to show only a minimal behavioral response to a painful procedure (Johnston et al, 1999a; Stevens et al, 1994). Immediately after the painful procedure, full-term infants are likely to remain awake (Anders & Chalemian, 1974). However, in preterm infants, this tendency is not any greater than the tendency to stay awake after routine handling (Holditch-Davis & Calhoun, 1989).

Nursing comfort measures have the potential to minimize some of these state effects. Yet how frequently practicing nurses actually use them is unclear. In one study, nurses were not found to use positive touches or talking any more frequently during painful procedures than during routine care (Holditch-Davis & Calhoun, 1989). Franck (1987) identified nine different comfort measures that nurses reported using to soothe infants who were receiving painful procedures (Chapter 17). To date, only a few of them have been studied. Tactile stimulation, music, and intrauterine sounds were found ineffective for both preterm and full-term infants when given during painful procedures (Beaver, 1987; Marchette et al, 1989). However, pacifiers were found to reduce crying and arousal in full-term and preterm infants when given during and after the procedure (Fearon et al, 1997). A sucrose-flavored pacifier was found to be even more effective than a plain pacifier in reducing the amount of crying by full-term and preterm infants during blood drawing and circumcision (Abad et al, 1996; Johnston et al, 1997, 1999b). Swaddling has been shown to reduce arousals in sleep and increase REM sleep in full-term infants (Gerard et al, 2002). Facilitated tucking—a modified form of swaddling in which the infant's arms and legs are contained in a flexed position next to the trunk—was effective in reducing responses to heelsticks (Corff et al, 1995). Preterm infants who received facilitated tucking during and after heelsticks exhibited less crying, less sleep disruption, and fewer state changes after the heelstick than without tucking. Rocking was not effective in reducing cry facial expressions in preterm infants in response to a heelstick, although the infants were in quiet sleep more (Johnston et al, 1997). Thus there is evidence that use of swaddling and pacifiers with sucrose can help reduce the sleeping and waking changes caused by painful procedures. However, additional research is needed to determine the effects of other comfort measures and how comfort measures affect more severe pain, such as post-operative pain.

Social Interaction

Sleeping and waking states are known to influence the interactions between full-term and premature infants and their mothers after term age, and in turn maternal interactions alter infant sleep-wake patterns. For example, infant crying may lead the mother to pick up the infant. At another time, a mother may awaken a sleeping infant for a feeding, thereby altering the infant's sleeping and waking patterns. Mothers have been found to exhibit different patterns of interactions when infants are in different states (Rosenthal, 1983). Aspects of the infant's state organization, including the degree to which he or she shows different patterns of crying and alertness in different situations, are related to the overall quality of the mother-infant interaction (Acebo & Thoman, 1995). A responsive style of mothering results in infants developing day-night differentiation in their sleeping and waking patterns sooner (Sander et al, 1979). In addition, maternal emotional stress has been found to relate to the amount of night sleeping that full-term infants exhibit at 4 and 12 months (Becker et al, 1991a).

Social interaction is known to affect sleep-wake patterns of premature infants after hospital discharge. At 4 to 6 weeks corrected age, breastfed premature infants exhibited more crying, especially during daytime, than formula-fed infants did (Thomas, 2000). At 6 months corrected age, premature infants were more likely to be drowsy or asleep during feeding and alert during nonfeeding periods, and the behaviors of mothers differed during feeding and nonfeeding (Holditch-Davis et al, 2000). Mothers were more likely to engage in behaviors that involved close contact during feeding, such as holding, having body contact, and rocking their infants, whereas during non-feeding periods, they were more likely to engage in more distal behaviors, such as gesturing and playing with the infant.

Less is known about the effect of social interaction in the hospital on infant sleeping and waking states. Minde et al (1983) found that ill preterm infants exhibited less eye opening—and thus probably less waking—when they were interacting with their mothers than did healthier preterm infants. Mothers report being aware of the sleeping and waking behaviors of their preterm infants—especially eye movements, orientation, and body movements—when they attempt to interact; they also report having used specific infant responses as guides to increase or decrease their interactive activity (Oehler et al, 1993). Waking, eye opening, increased body movements, positive facial expressions, and calming encouraged increased interaction; body movements, negative facial expressions, and withdrawing discouraged maternal interaction. However, preterm infants exhibited the positive interactive behaviors rather small portions of the time with their mothers (Oehler, 1995).

Moreover, social stimulation affects the physiologic status of preterm infants. The variation in infant oxygen saturation during parent touching was related to behavioral state and gestational age, such that infants who were more aroused and awake at the beginning of touch and had younger gestational ages at birth showed greater variation in their oxygen saturations (Harrison et al, 1991). Using a standardized protocol of social stimulation, Eckerman and colleagues (1994) found that preterm infants of at least 33 weeks' post-conceptional age responded to talking by eye opening and arousal, but when touching was added to the talking, the infants showed increased periods of closed eyes and negative facial expressions. Infants with more neurologic insults showed even greater negative responses to touching. This finding suggests that preterm infants are responsive to social stimulation of low intensity but that if the intensity of social stimulation is increased, they are no longer able to cope with it. Furthermore, medical complications further decrease infants' ability to cope with moderate-intensity social stimulation.

Preterm infants have also been found to respond differently to nurses and parents. In one study, preterm infants opened their eyes more when interacting with parents than when interacting with nurses (Minde et al, 1975). In another study with sicker infants, preterm infants spent more time in active sleep and less time in sleep-wake transition when with their parents than when with nurses (Miller & Holditch-Davis, 1992). In both of these studies, parents and nurses behaved differently toward infants, with nurses more likely to engage in routine nursing and medical procedures and parents more likely to hold infants and provide positive social stimulation. These findings suggest that preterm infants respond to the less active, more social stimulation provided by parents at first by sleeping and then, as they mature, by awakening to engage in interaction. The early sleeping may serve to conserve energy consumption and promote growth.

Kangaroo care, a recent nursing intervention to promote mothers' holding their preterm infants in skin-to-skin contact, has been found, in many studies, to increase amount of sleeping—and especially quiet sleep—and decrease crying as compared with periods when the infant is alone in the incubator (Chwo et al, 2002; Ludington, 1990; Ludington et al, 1992; Ludington-Hoe et al, 1994, 1999; Messmer et al, 1997). A few researchers, however, have not found any changes in state patterns during kangaroo care (de Leeuw et al, 1991) or have found a decrease in active sleep and an increase in transitional sleep, but no change in quiet sleep (Bosque et al, 1995). Studies using historical controls or allowing mothers to choose whether they wanted to provide kangaroo care found that infants receiving kangaroo care had more rapid maturation of sleep-wake states (longer bouts of quiet sleep and alertness and shorter bouts of active sleep) and higher orientation and state scores on the NBAS (Feldman & Eidelman, 2003; Ohgi et al, 2002).

Infant Stimulation

A number of the stimulation interventions used with infants are known to affect sleeping and waking states. In some cases, the goal of the intervention is to alter sleeping and waking states either to lower the infant's arousal so as to provide more energy for growth or to promote more mature state patterns. In other cases, the state effects are side effects of interventions that were designed to alter other aspects of the infant's functioning. This section examines the effects of several different types of infant stimulation interventions currently in use in NICUs.

Nonnutritive sucking is an intervention that has been variously used to soothe irritable infants and to promote feedings and growth. It is known to decrease restlessness and increase sleep time in full-term and preterm infants (Schwartz et al, 1987; Woodson et al, 1985). The NBAS state scores were not altered in preterm infants offered regular nonnutritive sucking during tube feedings as compared to control infants (Field et al, 1982). Nonnutritive sucking is effective in reducing crying after painful procedures and promoting either alertness or sleeping (Fearon et al, 1997). When given to preterm infants just before feedings, nonnutritive sucking helps them to arouse into a quiet, waking state and then maintain this state, in which they are most likely to feed effectively (Gill et al, 1988; McCain, 1992, 1995; Pickler et al, 1996). Nonnutritive sucking is more effective in this arousal than stroking (McCain, 1992). When nonnutritive sucking was used as an intervention to bring preterms to a waking state before feeding, infants receiving the intervention took 5 fewer days to achieve full oral feedings than control infants (McCain et al, 2001). Other researchers did not find a change of state with nonnutritive sucking but did find that preterm infants who received nonnutritive sucking before feedings had higher feeding performance scores and more sleep after feedings (Pickler et al, 1993).

Waterbeds are another common infant stimulation intervention known to affect the sleeping and waking states of preterm infants. The purpose of this intervention is to provide compensatory vestibular-proprioceptive stimulation for preterm infants who are largely deprived of this form of stimulation in the NICU. Infants on waterbeds exhibit increased amounts of active and quiet sleep, less irritability, fewer state changes, and decreased crying (Deiriggi, 1990; Korner et al, 1990). These effects are enhanced if the waterbed oscillates (Korner et al, 1990), but even infants on plain waterbeds exhibit more sleep than they do on regular incubator mattresses (Deiriggi, 1990). When infants have been on waterbeds for prolonged periods of time, state effects continue even during periods when the infant is off the waterbed, as evidenced by decreased irritability and increased alertness during a standardized assessment of preterm infant behavior (Korner et al, 1983). It has also been suggested that waterbeds reduce apnea (Korner et al, 1978). However, it is unlikely that this effect has clinical significance. When infants treated with theophylline for apnea of prematurity were placed on waterbeds, they showed the same state effects as found in infants without this complication, but they did not exhibit decreased apnea (Korner et al, 1982).

Gentle touching is another form of infant stimulation. Harrison et al (1996) provided 15 minutes of daily gentle human touch to preterm infants in the first 2 weeks of life. Infants had significantly less active sleep and motor activity during the periods of gentle touching. When the frequency of this intervention was increased to three times a day, preterm infants exhibited less active sleep, motor activity, and distress during gentle touching periods but did not differ from control infants on any outcome variable (Harrison et al, 2000).

Infant massage is another common infant stimulation technique. It provides both tactile and kinesthetic stimulation because it is necessary to move the infant to provide tactile stimulation to different parts of the body. The purpose of this type of stimulation is primarily to promote growth and augment development, but it also affects infant sleeping and waking states. White-Traut and Pate (1987) used the Rice Infant Sensomotor Stimulation, a 10-minute structured massage of the infant's entire body from head to toe, to provide extra stimulation for growing preterm infants. They found that during massage infants were more alert. In this study, however, infants were taken out of the incubator for the massage, so

the state changes might have been the result of changes in the thermal environment. In another study, the intervention protocol was altered to be more contingent to infant cues (White-Traut et al, 1993). Again, the experimental infants showed increased alertness during the intervention and continued to be alert for 30 minutes afterward. In another study, the massage intervention was compared with auditory stimulation alone; auditory stimulation along with massage; and auditory, massage, and rocking combined (White-Traut et al, 1997). Infants showed increasing alertness during the intervention in the massage and massage plus auditory groups, whereas the auditory group showed more quiet sleep. The massage, auditory, and rocking group showed minimal changes during the intervention but sustained alertness for 30 minutes afterward. The combined auditory, massage, and rocking intervention was then tested on preterm infants with periventricular leukomalacia (White-Traut et al, 1999). Infants who received this combined intervention showed an increase in alertness over the intervention period and were hospitalized for 9 fewer days. Increased alertness also resulted from this intervention when it was used with infants with prenatal substance exposure (White-Traut et al, 2002).

In other studies, stroking of the infant's body followed by passive flexion and extension of the extremities for 15 minutes 3 times a day for 5 to 10 days was shown to result in increased weight gain in preterm infants (Dieter et al, 2003; Scafidi et al, 1990, 1986). During massage treatments, infants exhibited more active sleep (Scafidi et al, 1990), but whether these state effects persisted after the treatment period is less clear. In two studies, massage-treated infants exhibited better scores on the NBAS and spent less time asleep (Dieter et al, 2003; Scafidi et al, 1986), whereas in another, no differences in the state organization of treated and control infants were found (Scafidi et al, 1990). Infants receiving moderate pressure massage from their mothers showed a greater decrease in active sleep, less agitated behavior, and less crying than infants receiving a light pressure massage (Field et al, 2004).

Rocking is a form of infant stimulation usually performed in order to soothe the infant. It has been administered either directly while holding the infant or by placing the infant in special cribs or incubators modified to rock at specific speeds. The immediate effects of rocking are reduced crying (Byrne & Horowitz, 1981). However, the rhythm and direction of rocking are important in determining which of the other states the infant was most likely to exhibit (Byrne & Horowitz, 1981). Exposing preterm infants to rocking over a 2-week period had longer-lasting results (Cordero et al, 1986). They exhibited increased quiet sleep and decreased active sleep.

In yet another study, preterm infants were placed in a nonrigid reclining chair twice a day for 3 hours from about 30 weeks' postmenstrual age until hospital discharge (Provasi & Lequien, 1993). Sleeping and waking states were observed for a 2-hour period for control infants and two 2-hour periods for the experimental infants (once in their beds and once in the infant seat) shortly before discharge. Experimental infants spent more time in quiet sleep and active sleep and less time in quiet and agitated waking than the control infants, but no differences were found in the state patterns of the experimental infants when in their beds and in the infant seat.

In a final type of infant stimulation, Thoman and Graham (1986) placed a "breathing" stuffed bear in the incubator with a preterm infant. The goal of this intervention was to provide a form of rhythmic stimulation that would help the infant organize his or her sleeping and waking patterns. In addition, this form of stimulation was voluntary. Because the bear took up only a small part of the incubator and babies were usually put to sleep in positions in which they were not in physical contact with the bear, infants could choose whether or not to remain in contact with the bear whenever their random movements brought them into contact with it. As compared with controls, experimental infants spent a much greater percentage of time in contact with the area of the incubator with the bear. By the end of the intervention period, experimental infants exhibited significantly increased quiet sleep time. This study has been replicated with two additional samples, and both have shown increased contact with the breathing bear as well as more quiet sleep and less active sleep than infants given a nonbreathing bear (Ingersoll & Thoman, 1994; Thoman et al, 1991).

USEFULNESS OF NEONATAL SLEEP-WAKE STATES FOR ASSESSMENT

Sleeping and waking states are ubiquitous characteristics of neonates. The infant's behavioral and physiologic responses are filtered through neural controls mediated by the sleeping and waking states. Although it is certainly possible to give competent nursing care to high-risk infants without considering their sleep-wake states, recognizing specific states will enable the nurse to better interpret both physiologic and behavioral changes. By observing sleeping and waking, the nurse will be able to determine whether physiologic parameters are consistent with those expected in a particular state. Changes in sleeping and waking patterns can be used to help the nurse identify the need for interventions and to aid the evaluation of these interventions. Most importantly, by observing sleeping and waking behaviors, the nurse will come to know each infant better and thus be better able to provide individualized care. This knowledge of individual infants can then be shared with parents to help them develop positive interactions with their children.

SUMMARY

High-risk infants are both dependent on and vulnerable to their early environment—the NICU and intermediate nursery—to maintain their physiologic function, to promote growth and development, and to provide opportunities for the organization of state, behavioral, and social responsiveness. The immaturity and physiologic and neurobehavioral instability of these infants make them particularly vulnerable to environments that do not support their emerging organization and patterns or that do not attend to their cues and respond appropriately. Nurses can and do play a big role in controlling sleep in the NICU environment. It is important that parents be included in these efforts to promote positive sleep-wake patterns in the NICU and once the infant is home.

In summary, the goals in addressing the neurobehavioral needs of high-risk infants are the following:

1. Provide an environment that enhances and supports the infant's developing capabilities.
2. Protect the infant from sensory overload and minimize stressors.
3. Assist parents in understanding their infant's unique abilities.
4. Help parents interact with their infant in ways appropriate to the infant's health status, sleep-wake state, and level of maturity.

REFERENCES

Abad F et al (1996). Oral sweet solution reduces pain-related behaviour in preterm infants. *Acta paediatrica* 85:854-858.

Acebo C, Thoman EB (1995). Role of infant crying in the early mother-infant dialogue. *Physiology and behavior* 57(3):541-547.

Adam K, Oswald I (1984). Sleep helps healing [Editorial]. *British medical journal (clinical research edition)* 289(6456):1400-1401.

Als H (1982). Toward a synactive theory of development: promise for the assessment and support of infant individuality. *Infant mental health journal* 3:229-243.

Als H (1984). Newborn behavioral assessment. In Burns WJ, Lavigne JV, editors. *Progress in pediatric psychology*. New York: Grune & Stratton.

Als H (1986). A synactive model of neonatal behavioral organization: framework for assessment of neurobehavioral development in the premature infant and for support of infants and parents in the neonatal intensive care environment. part 1: theoretical framework. *Physical and occupational therapy in pediatrics* 6(3-4):3-53.

Als H (1996). *The very immature infant—environmental and care issues*. Paper presented at The Physical and Developmental Environment of the High Risk Neonate. Clearwater Beach, FL: University of South Florida College of Medicine.

Als H (1999). Reading the premature infant. In Goldson E, editor. *Nurturing the premature infant: developmental interventions in the neonatal intensive care nursery* (pp. 18-85). New York: Oxford University Press.

Als H (2002). *Program guide: Newborn Individualized Developmental Care and Assessment Program (NIDCAP®): an education and training program for health care professionals*, rev 11. Boston: NIDCAP Federation International.

Als H, Lawhon G (2004). Theoretical perspective for developmentally supportive care. In Kenner C, McGrath JM, editors. *Developmental care of newborns and infants. A guide for health professionals* (pp 47-63). St Louis: Mosby.

Als H et al (1982). Manual for the assessment of preterm infants' behavior (APIB). In Fitzgerald HE et al, editors. *Theory and research in behavioral pediatrics*, vol. 1 (pp 65-132). New York: Plenum.

Als H et al (1986). Individualized behavioral and environmental care for the very-low-birth-weight preterm infant at high risk for bronchopulmonary dysplasia: neonatal intensive care unit and developmental outcome. *Pediatrics* 78(6):1123-1132.

Als H et al (1988). Behavioral differences between preterm and full term newborns as measured on the APIB System scores. *Infant behavior and development* 11(3):305-318.

Als H et al (1994). Individualized developmental care for the very-low-birth-weight preterm infants: medical and neurofunctional effects. *Journal of the American Medical Association* 272(11):853-858.

Als H et al (2003). A three-center, randomized, controlled trial of individualized developmental care for very low birth weight preterm infants: medical, neurodevelopmental, parenting, and caregiving effects. *Journal of developmental and behavioral pediatrics* 24:399-408.

Als H et al (2004). Early experience alters brain function and structure. *Pediatrics* 113:846-857.

Als H et al (2005). The Assessment of Preterm Infants' Behavior (APIB): furthering the understanding and measurement of neurodevelopmental competence in preterm and full-term infants. *Mental retardation and developmental disabilities research review* 11:94-102.

American Academy of Pediatrics. Task Force on Infant Positioning and SIDS (1992). Positioning and SIDS. *Pediatrics* 89:1120-1126.

Anand KJS, Scalzo FM (2000). Can adverse neonatal experiences alter brain development and subsequent behavior? *Biology of the neonate* 77:69-82.

Anders T et al (editors) (1971). *A manual of standardized terminology, techniques and criteria for scoring of states of sleep and wakefulness in newborn infants*. Los Angeles: UCLA Brain Information Service/BRI Publications Office.

Anders TF, Chalemian RJ (1974). The effects of circumcision on sleep-wake states in human neonates. *Psychosomatic medicine* 36(2):174-179.

Anderson GC (1999). Kangaroo care of the premature infant. In Goldson E, editor. *Nurturing the premature infant: developmental interventions in the neonatal intensive care nursery* (pp 131-160). New York: Oxford University Press.

Anderson LT et al (1989). Behavioral characteristics and early temperament of premature infants with intracranial hemorrhage. *Early human development* 18(4):273-283.

Apkarian P et al (1991). Effects of behavioural state on visual processing in neonates. *Neuropediatrics* 22(2):85-91.

Ariagno RL et al (1997). Developmental care does not alter sleep and development of premature infants. *Pediatrics* 100(6): e9. Available at: http://www.pediatrics.org/cgi/content/full/100/6/e9. Retrieved January 15, 2003.

Ariagno RL et al (2003). Effect of position on sleep, heart rate variability, and QT interval in preterm infants at 1 and 3 months' corrected age. *Pediatrics* 111(3):622-625.

Barnard KE (1999). *Beginning rhythms: the emerging process of sleep-wake behaviors and self-regulation.* Seattle, WA: AVENUW.

Barnard KE, Blackburn S (1985). Making a case for studying the ecological niche of the newborn. In Raff BS, Paul NW, editors. *NAACOG Invitational Research Conference. Birth defects: original article series,* 21(3):71-88.

Bartocci M et al (2001). Cerebral hemodynamic response to unpleasant odors in the preterm newborn measured by near-infrared spectroscopy. *Pediatric research* 50:324-330.

Bauer CR et al (2005). Acute neonatal effects of cocaine exposure during pregnancy. *Archives of pediatric and adolescent medicine* 159(9):824-834.

Bayley N (1993). *Bayley Scales of Infant Development,* ed 2. San Antonio, TX: The Psychological Corporation.

Bayley N (2005). *Bayley Scales of Infant and Toddler Development,* ed 3. San Antonio, TX: Harcourt Assessment.

Beaver PK (1987). Premature infants' response to touch and pain: can nurses make a difference? *Neonatal network* 6(3):13-17.

Becker PT, Thoman EB (1982). Waking activity: the neglected state of infancy. *Brain research* 256(4):395-400.

Becker PT et al (1991a). Correlates of diurnal sleep patterns in infants of adolescent and adult single mothers. *Research in nursing and health* 14(2):97-108.

Becker PT et al (1991b). Outcomes of developmentally supportive nursing care for very low birth weight infants. *Nursing research* 40(3):150–155.

Becker PT et al (1993). Effects of developmental care on behavioral organization in very-low-birth-weight infants. *Nursing research* 42(4):214-220.

Becker PT et al (1997). Behavioral state organization of very low birth weight infants: effects of developmental handling during caregiving. *Infant behavior and development* 20:503-514.

Beckwith L, Parmelee AH, Jr. (1986). EEG patterns of preterm infants, home environment, and later IQ. *Child development* 57(3):777-789.

Beckwith L, Rodning C (1992). Evaluating effects of intervention with parents of preterm infants. In Friedman SI, Sigman MD, editors. *The psychological development of low-birth-weight children.* Norwood, NJ: Ablex.

Bennett FC (2005). Developmental outcomes. In MacDonald MG et al, editors. *Avery's neonatology: pathophysiology and management of the newborn,* ed 5 (pp 1632-1651). Philadelphia: Lippincott Williams & Wilkins.

Bernert G et al (1997). The effect of behavioural states on cerebral oxygenation during endotracheal suctioning of preterm babies. *Neuropediatrics* 28:111-115.

Bertelle V et al (2005). Sleep of preterm neonates under developmental care or regular environmental conditions. *Early human development* 81(7):595-600.

Bhutta AT, Anand KJ (2002). Vulnerability of the developing brain. Neuronal mechanisms. *Clinics in perinatology* 29:357-372.

Bhutta AT et al (2002). Cognitive and behavioral outcomes of school-aged children who were born preterm: a meta-analysis. *Journal of the American Medical Association* 288:728-737.

Bingham PM et al (2003). A pilot study of milk odor effect on nonnutritive sucking by premature newborns. *Archives of pediatric and adolescent medicine* 157:72-75.

Black JE (1998). How a child builds its brain: some lessons from animal studies of neural plasticity. *Preventative medicine* 27:168-171.

Black B et al (2006). Effects of antenatal magnesium sulfate and corticosteroid therapy on sleep states of preterm infants. *Research in nursing and health* 29(4):269-280.

Black M et al (1993). Prenatal drug exposure: neurodevelopmental outcome and parenting environment. *Journal of pediatric psychology* 18(5):605-620.

Blackburn ST (1998). Environmental impact of the NICU on developmental outcomes. *Journal of pediatric nursing* 13:279-289.

Blackburn ST (2003). *Maternal, fetal and neonatal physiology: a clinical perspective,* ed 2. Philadelphia: Saunders.

Blackburn S, Barnard KE (1985). Analysis of caregiving events in preterm infants in the special care unit. In Gottfried A, Gaiter J, editors. *Infants under stress: environmental neonatology* (pp 113-129). Baltimore: University Park.

Blackburn S, Kang RE (1991). *Early parent-infant relationships* (ed 2), White Plains, NY: March of Dimes.

Blackburn S, Patteson D (1991). Effects of cycled lighting on activity state and cardiorespiratory function in preterm infants. *Journal of perinatal and neonatal nursing* 4(4):47-54.

Borghese IF et al (1995). Sleep rhythmicity in premature infants: implications for developmental status. *Sleep* 18:523-530.

Bosque EM et al (1995). Physiologic measures of kangaroo versus incubator care in a tertiary-level nursery. *Journal of obstetric, gynecologic, and neonatal nursing* 24(3):219-226.

Boukydis CF et al (2004). Clinical use of the Neonatal Intensive Care Unit Network Neurobehavioral Scale. *Pediatrics* 113:679-689.

Brandon DH, Holditch-Davis D (2005). Validation of an instrumented sleep-wake state assessment against biobehavioral assessment. *Newborn and infant nursing reviews* 5(3):109-115.

Brandon DH et al (1999). Nursing care and the development of sleeping and waking behaviors in preterm infants. *Research in nursing and health* 22:217-229.

Brandon DH et al (2002). Preterm infants born at less than 31 weeks' gestation have improved growth in cycled light compared with continuous near darkness. *Journal of pediatrics* 140(2):192-199.

Brandon DH et al (2005). Factors affecting early neurobehavioral and sleep outcomes in preterm infants. *Infant behavior and development* 28(2):206-219.

Brazelton TB (1984). *Neonatal behavioral assessment scale,* ed 2. Philadelphia: Spastics International Medical Publications, in association with William Heinemann Medical Books and Lippincott.

Brazelton TB, Nugent JK (1995). *Neonatal behavioral assessment scale,* ed 3. London: MacKeith.

Brazy JE (1988). Effect of crying on cerebral volume and cytochrome aa_3. *Journal of pediatrics* 112(3):457–461.

Browne JV (1996). *Family Infant Relationship Support Training.* Denver: The Center for Family and Infant Interaction.

Buehler DM et al (1995). Effectiveness of individualized developmental care for low-risk preterm infants: behavioral and electrophysiological evidence. *Pediatrics* 96:923-932.

Butte NF et al (1992). Sleep organization and energy expenditure of breast-fed and formula-fed infants. *Pediatric research* 32(5):514-519.

Byrne JM, Horowitz FD (1981). Rocking as a soothing intervention: the influence of direction and type of movement. *Infant behavior and development* 4(2):207-218.

Catlett AT, Holditch-Davis D (1990). Environmental stimulation of the acutely ill preterm infant: physiological effects and nursing implications. *Neonatal network* 8(6):19-26.

Chang YJ et al (2002). Effects of prone and supine positions on sleep state and stress responses in mechanically ventilated preterm infants during the first postnatal week. *Journal of advanced nursing* 40(2):161-169.

Chwo MJ et al (2002). A randomized controlled trial of early kangaroo care for preterm infants: effects on temperature, weight, behavior, and acuity. *Journal of nursing research* 10(2):129-142.

Cohen G et al (1991). Ventilatory response of sleeping newborn to CO_2 during normoxic rebreathing. *Journal of applied physiology* 71(1):168-174.

Colombo J, Horowitz FD (1987). Behavioral state as a lead variable in neonatal research. *Merrill-Palmer quarterly* 33(4):423–437.

Cordero L et al (1986). Effects of vestibular stimulation on sleep states in premature infants. *American journal of perinatology* 3(4):319-324.

Corff KE et al (1995). Facilitated tucking: a non-pharmacologic comfort measure for pain in preterm neonates. *Journal of obstetric, gynecologic and neonatal nursing* 24:143-147.

Corwin MJ et al (1995). Newborn acoustic cry characteristics of infants subsequently dying of sudden infant death syndrome. *Pediatrics* 96:73-77.

Curzi-Dascalova L et al (1988). Development of sleep states in normal premature and fullterm newborns. *Developmental psychobiology* 21(5):431-444.

Curzi-Dascalova L et al (1993). Sleep state organization in premature infants of less than 35 weeks' gestational age. *Pediatric research* 34:624-628.

Curzi-Dascalova L et al (2000). Physiological parameters evaluation following apnea in healthy premature infants. *Biology of the neonate* 77:203-211.

Curzi-Dascalova L et al (2002). Sleep organization is unaffected by caffeine in premature infants. *Journal of pediatrics* 140:766-771.

Das Eiden R, Reifman A (1996). Effects of Brazelton demonstrations on later parenting: a meta-analysis. *Journal of pediatric psychology* 21:857-868.

DeHaan R et al (1977). Definition of sleep state in the newborn infant by heart rate analysis. *American journal of obstetrics and gynecology* 127(7):753-758.

Deiriggi PM (1990). Effects of waterbed flotation on indicators of energy expenditure in preterm infants. *Nursing research* 39(3):140-146.

de Leeuw R et al (1991). Physiological effects of kangaroo care in very small preterm infants. *Biology of the neonate* 59(3):149-155.

Denenberg VH, Thoman EB (1981). Evidence for a functional role for active (REM) sleep in infancy. *Sleep* 4(2):185-191.

Dieter JN et al (2003). Stable preterm infants gain more weight and sleep less after five days of massage therapy. *Journal of pediatric psychology* 28(6):403-411.

DiPietro JA (2000). Baby and the brain: advances in child development. *Annual review of public health* 21:455-471.

DiPietro JA, Porges SW (1991). Relations between neonatal states and 8-month developmental outcome in preterm infants. *Infant behavior and development* 14(4):441-450.

DiPietro JA et al (1996). Fetal neurobehavioral development. *Child development* 67:2553-2567.

Doussard-Roosevelt J et al (1996). Behavioral sleep states in very low birth-weight preterm neonates: relation to neonatal health and vagal maturation. *Journal of pediatric psychology* 21:785-802.

Dreyfus-Brisac C (1968). Sleep ontogenesis in early human prematurity from 24 to 27 weeks of conceptional age. *Developmental psychobiology* 1:162-169.

Duffy FH et al (1990). Behavioral and electrophysiological evidence for gestational age effects in healthy preterm and fullterm infants studied two weeks after expected due date. *Child development* 61(4):271-286.

Duxbury ML et al (1984). Caregiver disruptions and sleep of high-risk infants. *Heart and lung* 13(2):141-147.

Eckerman CO et al (1994). Premature newborns as social partners before term age. *Infant behavior and development* 17(1):55-70.

Ellingson RJ, Peters JF (1980). Development of EEG and daytime sleep patterns in low risk premature infants during the first year of life: longitudinal observations. *Electroencephalography and clinical neurophysiology* 50(1-2):165-171.

Fajardo B et al (1990). Effect of nursery environment on state regulation in very-low-birth-weight premature infants. *Infant behavior and development* 13(3):287-303.

Fajardo B et al (1992). Early state organization and follow-up over one year. *Journal of developmental and behavioral pediatrics* 13(2):83-88.

Fearon I et al (1997). Swaddling after heel lance, age-specific effects on behavioral recovery in preterm infants. *Journal of developmental and behavioral pediatrics* 18:222-232.

Feldman R, Eidelman AI (2003). Skin-to-skin contact (Kangaroo Care) accelerates autonomic and neurobehavioural maturation in preterm infants. *Developmental medicine and child neurology* 45(4):274-281.

Ferrari F et al (1992). Bioelectric maturation in fullterm infants and in healthy and pathological preterm infants at term post-menstrual age. *Early human development* 28(1):37-63.

Fewell JE, Baker SB (1987). Arousal from sleep during rapidly developing hypoxemia in lambs. *Pediatric research* 22(4):471-477.

Field T et al (1982). Nonnutritive sucking during tube feedings: effects on preterm neonates in an intensive care unit. *Pediatrics* 70(3):381-384.

Field T et al (2004). Massage therapy by parents improves early growth and development. *Infant behavior and development* 27:435-442.

Fleisher BE et al (1995). Individualized developmental care for very-low-birth-weight premature infants. *Clinical pediatrics* 34:523-529.

Franck LS (1987). A national survey of the assessment and treatment of pain and agitation in the neonatal intensive care unit. *Journal of obstetric, gynecologic, and neonatal nursing* 16(6):387-393.

Freudigman KA, Thoman EB (1993). Infant sleep during the first postnatal day: an opportunity for assessment of vulnerability. *Pediatrics* 92:373-379.

Fuller BF (1991). Acoustic discrimination of three types of infant cries. *Nursing research* 40:156-160.

Gabriel M et al (1980). Sleep induced pO_2 changes in preterm infants. *European journal of pediatrics* 134(2):153-154.

Gabriel M et al (1981). Sleep-wake pattern in preterm infants under two different care schedules during four-day polygraphic recording. *Neuropediatrics* 12(4):366-373.

Galland BC et al (2000). Factors affecting heart rate variability and heart rate responses to tilting in infants aged 1 and 3 months. *Pediatric research* 48:360-368.

Gaultier C (1990). Respiratory adaptation during sleep in infants [Review]. *Lung* 168(Suppl):905-911.

Gaultier CL (1994). Apnea and sleep state in newborns and infants [Review]. *Biology of the neonate* 65(3-4):231-234.

Gerard CM et al (2002). Spontaneous arousals in supine infants while swaddled and unswaddled during rapid eye movement and quiet sleep. *Pediatrics* 110(6):e70. Available at: http://www.pediatrics.org/cgi/content/full/110/6/e70. Retrieved January 15, 2003.

Gertner S et al (2002). Sleep-wake patterns in preterm infants and 6 month's home environment: Implications for early cognitive development. *Early human development* 68:93-102.

Gill NE et al (1988). Effect of nonnutritive sucking on behavioral state in preterm infants before feeding. *Nursing research* 37(6):347-350.

Glass P (2005). The vulnerable neonate and the neonatal intensive care environment. In MacDonald MG et al, editors. *Avery's neonatology: pathophysiology and management of the newborn*, ed 5 (pp 111-128). Philadelphia: Lippincott Williams & Wilkins.

Goto K et al (1999). More awakenings and heart rate variability during supine sleep in preterm infants. *Pediatrics* 103:603-609.

Gottfried AW (1985). Environment of newborn infants in special care units. In Gottfried AW, Gaiter JL, editors. *Infant stress under intensive care: environmental neonatology* (pp 23–54). Baltimore: University Park.

Gottfried AW, Gaiter JL (editors) (1985). *Infant stress under intensive care: environmental neonatology*. Baltimore: University Park.

Graven SN (2000). Sound and the developing infant in the NICU: conclusions and recommendations for care. *Journal of perinatology* 20:S88-S93.

Graven SN (2004). Early sensory visual development of the fetus and newborn. *Clinics in perinatology* 31:199-216.

Gray L, Philbin MK (2004). Effects of the neonatal intensive care unit on auditory attention and distraction. *Clinics in perinatology* 31:243-260.

Greisen G et al (1985). Sleep-waking shifts and cerebral blood flow in stable preterm infants. *Pediatric research* 19(11):1156-1159.

Greenough WT et al (1987). Experience and brain development. *Child development* 58:539-559.

Grunau RV, Craig KD (1987). Pain expression in neonates: facial action and cry. *Pain* 28(3):395-410.

Haddad GG et al (1982). Determination of ventilatory pattern in REM sleep in normal infants. *Journal of applied physiology: respiratory, environmental and exercise physiology* 53(1):52-56.

Hahn JS, Tharp BR (1990). The dysmature EEG pattern in infants with bronchopulmonary dysplasia and its prognostic implications. *Electroencephalography and clinical neurophysiology* 76(2):106-113.

Hall JW (2000). Development of the ear and hearing. *Journal of perinatology* 20:S12-S20.

Halpern LF et al (1995). Infant sleep-wake characteristics: relation to neurological status and the prediction of developmental outcome. *Developmental review* 15:255-291.

Hand IL et al (2004). Hering-Breuer reflex and sleep state in the preterm infant. *Pediatric pulmonology* 37(1):61-64.

Harper RM et al (1981). Temporal sequencing in sleep and waking states during the first 6 months of life. *Experimental neurology* 72(2):294-307.

Harrison LL et al (1991). Preterm infants' physiologic responses to early parent touch. *Western journal of nursing research* 13(6):698-713.

Harrison L et al (1996). Effects of gentle human touch on preterm infants: pilot study results. *Neonatal network* 15(2):35-42.

Harrison LL et al (2000). Physiologic and behavioral effects of gentle human touch on preterm infants. *Research in nursing and health* 23:435-446.

Hellstrom-Westas L et al (1991). Cerebral function monitoring during the first week of life in extremely small low birthweight (ESLBW) infants. *Neuropediatrics* 22(1):27-32.

High PC, Gorski PA (1985). Recording environmental influences on infant development in the intensive care nursery: womb for improvement. In Gottfried AW, Gaiter JL, editors. *Infant stress under intensive care: environmental neonatology* (pp 131-155). Baltimore: University Park.

Holditch-Davis D (1990a). The development of sleeping and waking states in high-risk preterm infants. *Infant behavior and development* 13(4):513-531.

Holditch-Davis D (1990b). The effect of hospital caregiving on preterm infants' sleeping and waking states. In Funk SG et al, editors. *Key aspects of recovery: improving nutrition, rest, and mobility* (pp 110-122). New York: Springer.

Holditch-Davis D (1995). Behaviors of preterm infants with and without chronic lung disease when alone and when with nurses. *Neonatal network* 14(7):51-57.

Holditch-Davis D, Calhoun M (1989). Do preterm infants show behavioral responses to painful procedures? In Funk SG et al, editors. *Key aspects of comfort: management of pain, fatigue, and nausea* (pp 35-43). New York: Springer.

Holditch-Davis D, Edwards L (1998a). Modeling development of sleep-wake behaviors: II. results of 2 cohorts of preterms. *Physiology and behavior* 63(3):319-328.

Holditch-Davis D, Edwards L (1998b). Temporal organization of sleep-wake states in preterm infants. *Developmental psychobiology* 33:257-269.

Holditch-Davis D, Hudson DC (1995). Using preterm infant behaviors to identify acute medical complications. In Funk SG et al, editors. *Key aspects of caring for the acutely ill: technological aspects, patient education, and quality of life* (pp 95-120). New York: Springer.

Holditch-Davis D, Lee DA (1993). The behaviors and nursing care of preterm infants with chronic lung disease. In Funk SG et al, editors. *Key aspects of caring for the chronically ill: hospital and home* (pp 250-270). New York: Springer.

Holditch-Davis D, Thoman EB (1987). Behavioral states of premature infants: implications for neural and behavioral development. *Developmental psychobiology* 20(1):25-38.

Holditch-Davis D et al (1994). Pathologic apnea and brief respiratory pauses in preterm infants: relation to sleep state. *Nursing research* 43(5):293-300.

Holditch-Davis D et al (1995). The effect of standardized rest periods on convalescent preterm infants. *Journal of obstetric, gynecologic and neonatal nursing* 24(5):424-432.

Holditch-Davis D et al (1999). Early interactions between mothers and their medically fragile infants. *Applied developmental science* 3:155-167.

Holditch-Davis D et al (2000). Feeding and non-feeding interactions of mothers and prematures. *Western journal of nursing research* 22(3):320-334.

Holditch-Davis D et al (2003). Development of behaviors in preterm infants: relation to sleeping and waking. *Nursing research* 52(5):307-317.

Holditch-Davis D et al (2004a). Respiratory development in preterm infants. *Journal of perinatology* 24(10):631-639.

Holditch-Davis D et al (2004b). Sleeping and waking state development in preterm infants. *Early human development* 80(1):43-64.

Holditch-Davis D et al (2005). Prediction of 3-year developmental outcomes from sleep development over the preterm period. *Infant behavior and development* 28(2):118-131.

Holmes DL et al (1982). Early influences of prematurity, illness, and prolonged hospitalization on infant behavior. *Developmental psychology* 18(5):744-750.

Holmes GL et al (1979). Central nervous system maturation in the stressed premature. *Annals of neurology* 6(6):518-522.

Horne RS et al (2002). Effects of age and sleeping position on arousal from sleep in preterm infants. *Sleep* 25(7):746-750.

Huntington L et al (1990). The relations among cry characteristics, demographic variables, and developmental test scores in infants prenatally exposed to methadone. *Infant behavior and development* 13:533-538.

Huttenlocher PR (2002). *Neural plasticity. The effects of environment on the development of the cerebral cortex.* Cambridge, MA: Harvard University Press.

Ikonomidou C et al (2001). Neurotransmitters and apoptosis in the developing brain. *Biochemical pharmacology* 62:401-405.

Ingersoll EW, Thoman EB (1994). The breathing bear: effects on respiration in premature infants. *Physiology and behavior* 56(5):855-859.

Ingersoll EW, Thoman EB (1999). Sleep/wake states of preterm infants: stability, developmental change, diurnal variation, and relation with caregiving activity. *Child development* 70:1-10.

Jeffery HE et al (1999). Why the prone position is a risk factor of sudden infant death syndrome. *Pediatrics* 104:263-269.

Jeremy RJ, Hans SL (1985). Behavior of neonates exposed in utero to methadone as assessed on the Brazelton Scale. *Infant behavior and development* 8(3):323-336.

Johnston CC et al (1997). Effectiveness of oral sucrose and simulated rocking on pain response in preterm neonates. *Pain* 72:193-199.

Johnston CC et al (1999a). Do cry features reflect pain intensity in preterm neonates? *Biology of the neonate* 76:120-124.

Johnston CC et al (1999b). Factors explaining lack of response to heelstick in preterm newborns. *Journal of obstetric, gynecologic and neonatal nursing* 28:587-594.

Ju SH et al (1991). Maternal perceptions of the sleep patterns of premature infants at seven months corrected age compared to full-term infants. *Infant mental health journal* 12(4):338-346.

Karch D et al (1982). Behavioural changes and bioelectric brain maturation of preterm and fullterm newborn infants: a polygraphic study. *Developmental medicine and child neurology* 24(1):30-47.

Kisilevsky BS et al (2003). Effects of experience on fetal voice recognition. *Psychological science* 14:220-224.

Kleberg A et al (2000). Developmental outcome, child behavior and mother-child interaction at 3 years of age following Newborn Individualized Developmental Care and Intervention Program (NIDCAP) intervention. *Early human development* 60:123-135.

Kleberg A et al (2002). Indications of improved cognitive development at one year of age among infants born very prematurely who received care based on the Newborn Individualized Developmental Care and Assessment Program (NIDCAP). *Early human development* 68:83-91.

Kohyama J, Iwakawa Y (1990). Developmental changes in phasic sleep parameters as reflections of the brain-stem maturation: polysomnographical examinations of infants, including premature neonates. *Electroencephalography and clinical neurophysiology* 76(4):325-330.

Koizumi H (2004). The concept of "developing the brain": a new natural science for learning and education. *Brain development* 26:434-441.

Korner AF (1972). State as variable, obstacle, and as mediator of stimulation in infant research. *Merrill-Palmer quarterly* 18(2):77-94.

Korner AF, Thom VA (1990). *Neurobehavioral assessment of the preterm infant* Orlando, FL: The Psychological Corporation, Harcourt, Brace & Jovanovich.

Korner AF et al (1978). Reduction of sleep apnea and bradycardia in preterm infants on oscillating water beds: a controlled polygraphic study. *Pediatrics* 61(4):528-533.

Korner AF et al (1982). Effects of water beds on the sleep and motility of theophylline-treated preterm infants. *Pediatrics* 70(6):864-869.

Korner AF et al (1983). Effects of vestibular-proprioceptive stimulation on the neurobehavioral development of preterm infants: a pilot study. *Neuropediatrics* 14(3):170-175.

Korner AF et al (1990). Sleep enhanced and irritability reduced in preterm infants: differential efficacy of three types of waterbeds. *Journal of behavioral and developmental pediatrics* 11(5):240-246.

Korner AF et al (1991). Establishing the reliability and developmental validity of a neurobehavioral assessment for preterm infants: a methodological process. *Child development* 62(5):1200-1208.

Korner AF et al (1994). Preterm medical complications differentially affect neurobehavioral functions: results from a new neonatal medical index. *Infant behavior and development* 17(1):37-43.

Korner AF et al (2000). *Neurobehavioral Assessment of the Preterm Infant revised*, ed 2. Van Nuys, CA: Child Development Media.

Lawson KR et al (1985). Infant state in relation to its environmental context. *Infant behavior and development* 8(3):269-281.

Lecanuet JP, Schaal B (1996). Fetal sensory competencies. *European journal of obstetrics, gynecology and reproductive biology* 68:1-23.

Lee HK (2002). Effects of sponge bathing on vagal tone and behavioural responses in premature infants. *Journal of clinical nursing* 11:510-519.

Lester BM, Dreher M (1989). Effects of marijuana use during pregnancy on newborn cry. *Child development* 60(4):765-771.

Lester BM, Tronick EZ (2004). History and description of the Neonatal Intensive Care Unit Network Neurobehavioral Scale. *Pediatrics* 113:634-640.

Lester BM et al (1986). Effects of atypical patterns of fetal growth on newborn (NBAS) behavior. *Child development* 57(1):11-19.

Lester BM et al (2004). Normative neurobehavioral performance of healthy infants on the Neonatal Intensive Care Unit Network Neurobehavioral Scale. *Pediatrics* 113:676-678.

Levesque BM et al (2000). Pulse oximetry: what's normal in the newborn nursery? *Pediatric pulmonology* 30:406-412.

Lickliter R (2000a). The role of sensory stimulation in perinatal development: insights from comparative research for care of the high-risk infant. *Journal of behavioral and developmental pediatrics* 21:437-447.

Lickliter R (2000b). Atypical perinatal sensory stimulation and early perceptual development: insights from developmental psychobiology. *Journal of perinatology* 20:S45-S54.

Lodrup KC et al (1992). Lung function measurements in awake compared to sleeping newborn infants. *Pediatric pulmonology* 12(2):99-104.

Louis J et al (1997). Sleep ontogenesis revisited: a longitudinal 24-hour home polygraphic study on 15 normal infants during the first two years of life. *Sleep* 20(5):323-333.

Ludington SM (1990). Energy conservation during skin-to-skin contact between premature infants and their mothers. *Heart and lung* 19(5, Part 1):445-451.

Ludington SM et al (1992). Efficacy of kangaroo care with preterm infants in open-air cribs. *Neonatal network* 11(6):101.

Ludington-Hoe SM et al (1994). Kangaroo care: research results, and practice implications and guidelines; findings of two research projects. *Neonatal network* 13(1):19-27, 29-34.

Ludington-Hoe SM et al (1999). Birth-related fatigue in 34-36-week preterm neonates: rapid recovery with very early kangaroo (skin-to-skin) care. *Journal of obstetric, gynecologic and neonatal nursing* 28:94-103.

Maas YGH et al (2000). Predictive value of neonatal neurological tests for developmental outcome of preterm infants. *Journal of pediatrics* 137:100-106.

Mann NP et al (1986). Effect of night and day on preterm infants in a newborn nursery: randomised trial. *BMJ (clinical research edition)* 293(6557):1265-1267.

Marchette L et al (1989). Pain reduction during neonatal circumcision. *Pediatric nursing* 15(2):207–210.

Marlow N et al, the EPICure Study Group (2005). Neurologic and developmental disability at six years of age after extremely preterm birth. *New England journal of medicine* 352(1):9-19.

Martin R et al (1979). Changes in arterial oxygen tension during quiet and active sleep in the neonate. *Birth defects: original article series* 15(4):493-494.

McCain GC (1992). Facilitating inactive awake states in preterm infants: a study of three interventions. *Nursing research* 41(3):157-160.

McCain GC (1995). Promotion of preterm infant nipple feeding with nonnutritive sucking. *Journal of pediatric nursing* 10:3-8.

McCain GC et al (1999). Preterm infant behavioral and heart rate responses to antenatal phenobarbital. *Research in nursing and health* 22:461-470.

McCain GC et al (2001). A feeding protocol for healthy preterm infants that shortens time to oral feeding. *Journal of pediatrics* 139:374-379.

McEvoy C et al (1997). Prone positioning decreases episodes of hypoxemia in extremely low birth weight infants (1000 grams or less) with chronic lung disease. *Journal of pediatrics* 130:305-309.

McGrath MM et al (2005). Early precursors of low attention and hyperactivity in a preterm sample at age four. *Issues in comprehensive pediatric nursing* 28(1):1-15.

McQuillen PS, Ferriero DM (2005). Perinatal subplate neuron injury: implications for cortical development and plasticity. *Brain pathology* 15:250-260.

Mennella JA et al (2001). Prenatal and postnatal flavor learning by human infants. *Pediatrics* 107:E88.

Messmer PR et al (1997). Effect of kangaroo care on sleep time for neonates. *Pediatric nursing* 23:408-414.

Michelsson K et al (1990). Crying, feeding and sleeping patterns in 1- to 12-month-old infants. *Child: care, health and development* 16(2):99-111.

Miller DB, Holditch-Davis D (1992). Interactions of parents and nurses with high-risk preterm infants. *Research in nursing and health* 15(3):187-197.

Milligan DWA (1979). Cerebral blood flow and sleep state in the normal newborn infant. *Early human development* 3(4):321-328.

Minde K et al (1975). Interactions of mothers and nurses with premature infants. *Canadian Medical Association journal* 113(8):741-745.

Minde K et al (1983). Effect of neonatal complications in premature infants on early parent-infant interactions. *Developmental medicine and child neurology* 25(6):763-777.

Mirmiran M (1986). The importance of fetal/neonatal REM sleep. *European journal of obstetrics, gynecology, and reproductive biology* 21(5-6):283-291.

Mirmiran M et al (2003). Circadian and sleep development in preterm infants occurs independently from the influences of environmental lighting. *Pediatric research* 53(6):933-938.

Mok JY et al (1988). Effect of age and state of wakefulness on transcutaneous oxygen values in preterm infants: a longitudinal study. *Journal of pediatrics* 113(4):706-709.

Moore JK (2002). Maturation of human auditory cortex: implications for speech perception. *Annals of otolaryngology, rhinology and laryngology* 189:7-10.

Moore KL, Persaud TVN (2003). *The developing human: clinically oriented embryology,* ed 7. Philadelphia: Saunders.

Moseley MJ et al (1988). Effects of nursery illumination on frequency of eyelid opening and state in preterm infants. *Early human development* 18(1):13-26.

Mouradian LE et al (2000). Neurobehavioral functioning of healthy preterm infants of varying gestational ages. *Journal of developmental and behavioral pediatrics* 21:408-416.

Myers BJ et al (1992). Prematurity and respiratory illness: Brazelton Scale (NBAS) performance of preterm infants with bronchopulmonary dysplasia (BPD), respiratory distress syndrome (RDS), or no respiratory illness. *Infant behavior and development* 15(1):27-42.

Myers MM et al (1998). Effects of sleeping position and time after feeding on the organization of sleep/wake states in prematurely born infants. *Sleep* 21:343-349.

Nugent JK et al (1996). The effects of maternal alcohol consumption and cigarette smoking during pregnancy on acoustic cry analysis. *Child development* 67:1806-1815.

O'Brien CM, Jeffery HE (2002). Sleep deprivation, disorganization and fragmentation during opiate withdrawal in newborns. *Journal of paediatrics and child health* 38(1):66-71.

Oehler JM (1995). Development of mother-child interaction in very low birth weight infants. In Funk SG et al, editors. *Key aspects of caring for the acutely ill: technological aspects, patient education, and quality of life* (pp 120-133). New York: Springer.

Oehler JM et al (1988). Social stimulation and the regulation of premature infants' state prior to term age. *Infant behavior and development* 11(3):333-351.

Oehler JM et al (1993). Maternal views of preterm infants' responsiveness to social interaction. *Neonatal network* 12(6):67-74.

Ohgi S et al (2002). Comparison of kangaroo care and standard care: behavioral organization, development, and temperament in healthy, low-birth-weight infants through 1 year. *Journal of perinatology* 22(5):374-379.

Ottaviano S et al (1996). Sleep characteristics in healthy children from birth to 6 years of age in the urban area of Rome. *Sleep* 19:1-3.

Parmelee AH Jr, Stern E (1972). Development of states in infants. In Clemente CD et al, editors. *Sleep and the maturing nervous system* (pp 200-215). New York: Academic Press.

Parslow PM et al (2004). Effects of sleep state and postnatal age on arousal responses induced by mild hypoxia in infants. *Sleep* 27(1):105-109.

Patzak A et al (1999). Rhythms and complexity of respiration during sleep in pre-term infants. *Clinical physiology* 19:458-466.

Peters KL (2004). *A research project—NIDCAP—The Edmonton, Alberta experience.* Paper presented at Developmental Interventions in Neonatal Care. Seattle, Washington.

Philbin MK et al (2000). Sensory experience and the developing organism: a history of ideas and view to the future. *Journal of perinatology* 20:S2-S5.

Phillipson EA (1978). Control of breathing during sleep. *American review of respiratory disease* 118(5):909-939.

Pickler RH et al (1993). The effect of nonnutritive sucking on bottle-feeding stress in preterm infants. *Journal of obstetric, gynecologic and neonatal nursing* 22(3):230-234.

Pickler RH et al (1996). Effects of nonnutritive sucking on behavioral organization and feeding performance in preterm infants. *Nursing research* 45:132-138.

Prechtl HF et al (1973). Behavioural state cycles in abnormal infants. *Developmental medicine and child neurology* 15(5):606-615.

Prechtl HFR, Beintema J (1968). *The neurological examination of the full-term newborn infant.* Philadelphia: Spastics International Medical Publications, in association with William Heinemann Medical Books and Lippincott.

Pressler JP, Hepworth JT (2002). A quantitative use of the NIDCAP tool. *Clinical nursing research* 11(1):89-102.

Pressler JL et al (2004). Developmental care: an overview. In Kenner C, McGrath JM, editors. *Developmental care of newborns and infants. A guide for health professionals* (pp 1-34). St Louis: Mosby.

Provasi J, Lequien P (1993). Effects of nonrigid reclining infant seat on preterm behavioral states and motor activity. *Early human development* 35(2):129-140.

Quillin SIM, Glenn LL (2004). Interaction between feeding method and co-sleeping on maternal-newborn sleep. *Journal of obstetric, gynecologic and neonatal nursing* 33(5):580-588.

Ramaekers VT et al (1989). The influence of behavioural states on cerebral blood flow velocity patterns in stable preterm infants. *Early human development* 20(3-4):229-246.

Regalado MG et al (1995). Sleep disorganization in cocaine-exposed neonates. *Infant behavior and development* 18:319-327.

Rivkees SA et al (2004). Rest-activity patterns of premature infants are regulated by cycled lighting. *Pediatrics* 113(4):833-839.

Robinson J et al (1989). Eyelid opening in preterm neonates. *Archives of disease in childhood* 64(7, Spec. No.):943–948.

Roffwarg HP et al (1966). Ontogenetic development of the human sleep-dream cycle. *Science* 152:604–619.

Rosenthal MK (1983). State variations in the newborn and mother-infant interaction during breast feeding: some sex differences. *Developmental psychology* 19(5):740-745.

Sahni R et al (1995). Methodological issues in coding sleep states in immature infants. *Developmental psychobiology* 28(2):85-101.

Salisbury AL et al (2005). Neurobehavioral assessment from fetus to infant: the NICU Network Neurobehavioral Scale and the Fetal Neurobehavior Coding Scale. *Mental retardation and developmental disabilities research review* 11:14-20.

St. James-Roberts I, Plewis I (1996). Individual differences, daily fluctuations, and developmental changes in amounts of infant waking, fussing, crying, and sleeping. *Child development* 67:2527-2540.

Sanchez RM, Jensen FE (2001). Maturational aspects of epilepsy mechanisms and consequences for the immature brain. *Epilepsia* 42:577-585.

Sander LW et al (1979). Changes in infant and caregiver variables over the first two months of life: regulation and adaptation in the organization of the infant-caregiver system. In Thoman EB, editor. *Origins of the infant's social responsiveness* (pp 349-407). Hillsdale, NJ: Lawrence Erlbaum Associates.

Scafidi FA et al (1986). Effects of tactile/kinesthetic stimulation on the clinical course and sleep/wake behavior of preterm neonates. *Infant behavior and development* 9(1):91-105.

Scafidi FA et al (1990). Massage stimulates growth in preterm infants: a replication. *Infant behavior and development* 13:167-168.

Schaal B et al (2004). Olfaction in the fetal and premature infants: functional status and clinical implications. *Clinics in perinatology* 31:261-286.

Scher A (1991). A longitudinal study of night waking in the first year. *Child: care, health and development* 17(5):295-302.

Scher MS et al (1988). The effects of prenatal alcohol and marijuana exposure: disturbances in neonatal sleep cycling and arousal. *Pediatric research* 24(1):101-105.

Scher MS et al (1992). Comparisons of EEG sleep measures in healthy full-term and preterm infants of matched conceptional ages. *Sleep* 15(5):442-448.

Scher MS et al (1994a). Lower neurodevelopmental performance at 2 years in healthy preterm neonates. *Pediatric neurology* 11:121.

Scher MS et al (1994b). Comparison of EEG sleep state specific spectral values between healthy full-term and preterm infants at comparable postconceptional ages. *Sleep* 17(1):47-51.

Scher MS et al (1994c). Comparisons of EEG spectral and correlation measures between healthy term and preterm infants. *Pediatric neurology* 10(2):104-108.

Scher MS et al (2005). Cyclicity of neonatal sleep behaviors at 25 to 30 weeks' postconceptional age. *Pediatric research* 57(6):879-882.

Schulte FJ et al (1977). Rapid eye movement sleep, motoneurone inhibition, and apneic spells in preterm infants. *Pediatric research* 11(6):709-713.

Schwartz R et al (1987). A meta-analysis of critical outcome variables in nonnutritive sucking in preterm infants. *Nursing research* 36(5):292-295.

Senn TE, Espy KA (2003). Effects of neurobehavioral assessment on feeding and weight gain in preterm neonates. *Journal of developmental and behavioral pediatrics* 24:85-88.

Shaywitz BA et al (1971). Growth hormone in newborn infants during sleep–wake periods. *Pediatrics* 48(1):103–109.

Shimada M et al (1993). Development of the sleep and wakefulness rhythm in preterm infants discharged from a neonatal intensive care unit. *Pediatric research* 33(2):159-163.

Shimada M et al (1999). Emerging and entraining patterns of sleep-wake rhythm in preterm and term infants. *Brain and development* 21:468-473.

Shonkoff JP, Phillips DA (2000). *From neurons to neighborhoods: the science of early childhood development*. Washington, DC: National Academy Press.

Simakajornboon N et al (2002). Effect of supplemental oxygen on sleep architecture and cardiorespiratory events in preterm infants. *Pediatrics* 110:884-888.

Sizun J, Westrup B (2004). Early developmental care for preterm neonates: a call for more research. *Archives of diseases in children, fetal and neonatal edition* 89:F384-F388.

Skadberg BT, Markestad T (1997). Behavior and physiological responses during prone and supine sleep in early infancy. *Archives of disease in childhood* 76:320-324.

Stevens BJ et al (1994). Factors that influence the behavioral pain responses of premature infants. *Pain* 59:101-109.

Sullivan CE (1980). Breathing in sleep. In Orem J, Barnes CD, editors. *Physiology in sleep* (pp 213-272). New York: Academic Press.

Symanski ME et al (2002). Patterns of premature newborns' sleep-wake states before and after nursing interventions on the night shift. *Journal of obstetric, gynecologic and neonatal nursing* 31(3):305-313.

Thoman EB (1975). Early development of sleeping behaviors in infants. In Ellis NR, editor. *Aberrant development in infancy: human and animal studies* (pp 122-138). New York: Wiley.

Thoman EB (1982). A biological perspective and a behavioral model for assessment of premature infants. In Bond LA, Joffee JM, editors. *Primary prevention of psychopathology: facilitating infant and early childhood development*, vol 6 (pp 159-179). Hanover, NH: University Press of New England.

Thoman EB (1990). Sleeping and waking states in infancy: a functional perspective. *Neuroscience and biobehavioral reviews* 14(1):93-107.

Thoman EB, Graham SE (1986). Self-regulation of stimulation by premature infants. *Pediatrics* 78(5):855-860.

Thoman EB, Whitney MP (1989). Sleep states of infants monitored in the home: individual differences, developmental trends, and origins of diurnal cyclicity. *Infant behavior and development* 12(1):59-75.

Thoman EB et al (1981). State organization in neonates: Developmental inconsistency indicates risk for developmental dysfunction. *Neuropediatrics* 12(1):45-54.

Thoman EB et al (1983). Infant crying and stability in the mother-infant relationship: a systems analysis. *Child development* 54(3):653–659.

Thoman EB et al (1985). Theophylline affects sleep-wake state development in premature infants. *Neuropediatrics* 16(1):13-18.

Thoman EB et al (1987). The sleeping and waking states of infants: correlations across time and person. *Physiology and behavior* 41(6):531-537.

Thoman EB et al (1988). Infants at risk for sudden infant death syndrome (SIDS): differential prediction for three siblings of SIDS infants. *Journal of behavioral medicine* 11(6):565-583.

Thoman EB et al (1991). Premature infants seek rhythmic stimulation, and the experience facilitates neurobehavioral development. *Journal of behavioral and developmental pediatrics* 12(1):11-18.

Thomas KA (2000). Differential effects of breast- and formula-feeding on preterms' sleep-wake patterns. *Journal of obstetric, gynecologic and neonatal nursing* 29:145-152.

Thomas KA, Foreman SW (2005). Infant sleep and feeding pattern: effects on maternal sleep. *Journal of midwifery and women's health* 50(5):399-404.

Torres C et al (1997). Effect of standardized rest periods on apnea and weight gain of convalescent preterm infants. *Neonatal network* 16(8):35-43.

Tronick EZ et al (2004). Normative neurobehavioral performance of healthy infants on the Neonatal Intensive Care Unit Network Neurobehavioral Scale. *Pediatrics* 113:676-678.

Van Cleve L et al (1995). Pain responses of hospitalized neonates to venipuncture. *Neonatal network* 14(6):31-36.

van Ravenswaaij-Arts CM et al (1989). Influence of behavioural state on blood pressure in preterm infants during the first 5 days of life. *Acta paediatrica Scandinavica* 78(3):358-363.

Vecchierini M-F et al (2001). Patterns of EEG frequency, movement, heart rate, and oxygenation after isolated short apneas in infants. *Pediatric research* 49:220-226.

Vernacchio L et al (2003). Sleep position of low birth weight infants. *Pediatrics* 111(3):633-640.

Vles JS et al (1992). State profile in low-risk pre-term infants: a longitudinal study of 7 infants from 32-36 weeks of postmenstrual age. *Brain and development* 14(1):12-17.

Vohr BR et al (1990). Behavioral changes correlated with brain-stem auditory evoked responses in term infants with moderate hyperbilirubinemia. *Journal of pediatrics* 117(2, Part 1):288-291.

Volpe JJ (2001). *Neurology of the newborn*, ed 4. Philadelphia: Saunders.

Watt JE, Strongman KT (1985). The organization and stability of sleep states in fullterm, preterm, and small-for-gestational-age infants: a comparative study. *Developmental psychobiology* 18(2):151-162.

Weissbluth M (1995). Naps in children: 6 months–7 years. *Sleep* 18(2):82-87.

Westrup B et al (2000). A randomized, controlled trial to evaluate the effects of the Newborn Individualized Developmental Care and Assessment Program in a Swedish setting. *Pediatrics* 105:66-72.

Westrup B et al (2002). No indication of increased quiet sleep in infants receiving care based on the Newborn Individualized Developmental Care and Assessment Program (NIDCAP). *Acta paediatrica* 91:318-322.

Westrup B et al (2004). Preschool outcome in children born very prematurely and cared for according to the Newborn Individualized Developmental Care and Assessment Program (NIDCAP). *Acta paediatrica* 93:498-507.

White-Traut RC, Pate CM (1987). Modulating infant state in premature infants. *Journal of pediatric nursing* 2(2):96-101.

White-Traut RC et al (1993). Patterns of physiologic and behavioral response of intermediate care preterm infants to intervention. *Pediatric nursing* 1(6):625-629.

White-Traut RC et al (1997). Response of preterm infants to unimodal and multimodal sensory intervention. *Pediatric nursing* 23:169-175, 193.

White-Traut RC et al (1999). Developmental intervention for preterm infants diagnosed with periventricular leukomalacia. *Research in nursing and health* 22:131-143.

White-Traut R et al (2002). Pulse rate and behavioral state correlates after auditory, tactile, visual, and vestibular intervention in drug-exposed neonates. *Journal of perinatology* 22:291-299.

White-Traut RC et al (2005). Feeding readiness in preterm infants: the relationship between preterm behavioral state and feeding readiness behaviors and efficiency during transition from gavage to oral feeding. MCN, *American journal of maternal child nursing* 30(1):52-59.

Whitney MP, Thoman EB (1993). Early sleep patterns of premature infants are differentially related to later developmental disabilities. *Journal of developmental and behavioral pediatrics* 14(2):71-80.

Whitney MP, Thoman EB (1994). Sleep in premature and full term infants from 24-hour home recordings. *Infant behavior and development* 17:223-234.

Wielenga JM et al (2006). How satisfied are parents supported by nurses with the NIDCAP(R) model of care for their preterm infant? *Journal of nursing care quality* 21:41-48.

Wolff PH (1959). Observations on newborn infants. *Psychosomatic medicine* 21:110-118.

Wolff PH (1966). The causes, controls, and organization of behavior in the neonate. *Psychological issues* 5(1):1-105.

Woods NS et al (1993). Cocaine use during pregnancy: maternal depressive symptoms and infant neurobehavior over the first month. *Infant behavior and development* 16(1):83-98.

Woodson R et al (1983). Estimating neonatal oxygen consumption from heart rate. *Psychophysiology* 20(5):558–561.

Woodson R et al (1985). Effects of nonnutritive sucking on state and activity: term-preterm comparisons. *Infant behavior and development* 8(4):435-441.

Zahr LK, Balian S (1995). Responses of premature infants to routine nursing interventions and noise in the NICU. *Nursing research* 44(3):179-185.

Zinman R et al (1992). Oxygen saturation during sleep in patients with bronchopulmonary dysplasia. *Biology of the neonate* 61(2):69-75.

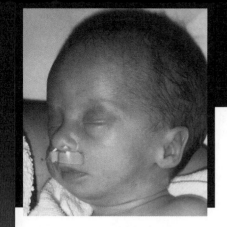

Chapter 24

The Neonatal Intensive Care Unit (NICU) Environment

Leslie Altimier

The management of premature infants has advanced over the past three decades to the point that infants born as early as 23 weeks' gestation now have a chance of survival in part due to technologic advances. With this technology growth the neonatal intensive care unit (NICU) environment has become increasingly stressful. From the first moments of life the premature infant is subjected to excessive noise, constant bright lights, and a multitude of painful procedures along with excessive handling. As we strive to continue to improve our morbidity and mortality rates, we are challenged to enhance the developmental potential of these infants, thus demonstrating the need for an appropriately and developmentally supportive environment in which to care for the fragile preterm infant. Infants have demonstrated markedly improved outcomes when the stress of environmental overstimulation is reduced. This is accomplished through a reduction of noxious stimuli (light, sound, activity) and the promotion of proper positioning and handling (Blackburn, 1998).

The high-risk infant in the NICU lives in a markedly different environment from the home environment of the healthy full-term neonate. Neurologic development begins in the third week of gestation with the formation of the neural plate, neural folds, and neural tube during dorsal introduction. Once the tube is formed and becomes a closed system, different regions of the brain begin to develop (McGrath, 2000). As these different regions of the brain begin to form, the development of the central nervous system (CNS) is characterized by the following distinct overlapping processes: neuronal proliferation, migration, organization, and myelination (Blackburn, 2002). The forebrain, thalamus, hypothalamus, cerebral hemispheres, and basal ganglia are the first areas to develop in the fetal brain (Moore & Persaud, 2003; Volpe, 2001). Although this development begins before birth, it does not fully mature until adulthood. (For more detailed information on neurobehavioral development and the neurologic system, see Chapters 12 and 23.)

The neonate's neurologic system needs to perform at birth. Understanding how we can better support the infant's fragile neurologic system can be the beginning of helping the infant to manage within the extrauterine environment. A part of this support is the adoption of the conceptual framework and philosophy of developmental care. The pioneering work by researchers Sameroff, Brazelton, and Als found that assessing the individual infant's ability to cope with excessive stimulation provides the caregiver with information to modify each infant's environment and treatment strategies. When preterm infants were assessed and provided with developmentally supportive individualized care, Als (1986) saw significant outcome improvements, as shown by the following factors:

- Fewer days on the ventilator
- Earlier feeding success
- Shorter hospital stay
- A marked reduction in the number of complications
- Improved neurodevelopmental outcomes during the first 18 months of life

Improvements in medical outcomes as well as hospital costs were demonstrated by Altimier et al (2005) and Hendricks-Munoz et al (2002) in two separate studies when developmental education and subsequent change of care practices were implemented. Altimier et al's (2005) results showed that a change in the physical NICU environment, as well as a comprehensive developmental care training program can be effective in improving the NICU environment, improving medical outcomes, decreasing length of stay (LOS), and decreasing hospital costs. The results by Hendricks-Munoz et al (2002) showed that an alternative model of developmental care training can be effective in initiating immediate change in a NICU.

Improved short-term medical outcomes, decreased length of hospitalization, and decreased hospital costs were all associated with developmental education and an improved NICU environment. A recent study by Louw and Maree (2005) demonstrated statistically significant improvement in the neonatal nurses' handling and positioning of preterm infants after formal exposure to developmental care principles and hands-on experience in the format of a workshop. Reports of young adult outcomes of very low birth weight (<1.5 kg) children who survived the initial years of neonatal intensive care reveal that the neurodevelopmental sequelae and poor educational achievement evident during childhood persist into adulthood (Hack et al, 2002). The increase in psychopathology among very low birth weight survivors as young adults indicates a need for anticipatory guidance as well as early intervention that might help to prevent potential psychopathology (Hack et al, 2004).

The full-term healthy infant has a consistent nurturing caregiver as well as an appropriate variety of stimulation. The full-term infant with 40 weeks of intrauterine development is ready for a variety of sensory experiences, including visual, tactile, auditory, olfactory, and gustatory. Appropriate patterns of adaptation, cognitive learning, and motor control are formed when sensory information interacts with experience. On the other hand, a premature infant typically has numerous caregivers and is exposed to high levels of inappropriate sensory input that can alter adaptation patterns (Holditch-Davis et al, 2003).

The NICU is often a stressful environment for infants, parents, and staff. Sources of stress for infants in NICU include the physical environment, caregiver interventions, medical and surgical procedures, pain, distress, pathologic processes, temperature changes, handling, and multiple modes of stimulation (Blackburn, 1998). Consequences of neonatal stress include energy expenditure, altered healing and recovery, altered growth, and altered organization. Stress can also affect interactions and parenting. In the NICU the infant may experience significant stress during a period of critical development. An infant's stress tolerance may be reached or exceeded repeatedly, contributing to short- and long-term morbidity (Anand & Scalzo, 2000; DiMaggio & Gibbons, 2005).

To better understand the correlation of early environmental factors to the developmental problems associated with prematurity and other high-risk events, it is essential to examine the environment in which these infants spend the critical period of their development. The neurologic and sensory systems do not exist as separate entities, but are interdependent and comprise the neurobehavioral and neurosensory development of the infant. Every sensory experience is recorded in the brain, leading to a behavioral response, thereby leading to yet another sensory experience. This cyclic interdependent action and reaction is the basis for neurobehavioral and neurosensory development. This chapter briefly reviews the neurologic development of the infant. It highlights aspects of developmental care and the impact of the extrauterine (NICU) environment on neurologic development.

INTRAUTERINE VS EXTRAUTERINE ENVIRONMENT

The intrauterine environment is recognized as optimal to foster fetal growth and development. The environment provides a variety of stimuli to the fetus while modifying the intensity and nature of the sensory input. Types of auditory input include maternal bowel sounds, blood flow through the umbilical cord, and muffled sounds from the extrauterine environment. Vestibular and tactile stimuli come from maternal and fetal movements and from contact with warm amniotic fluid as well as from contact with body parts or the wall of the uterus. Maternal movement and buoyant amniotic fluid provide vestibular stimulation, and noise in utero is conducted through fluid rather than air, which attenuates the sound and modulates its intensity (Holditch-Davis et al, 2003). Intrauterine sounds also tend to be low frequency and low intensity compared to extrauterine sounds. Less than 2% of external light is transmitted into the uterus (Glass, 1999).

When an infant is born premature, the still-developing brain and sensory systems are affected by the continuous interplay of interactions in the NICU. A principle of sensory interference may occur when immature sensory systems are stimulated out of turn or with inappropriate stimuli.

DIMENSIONS OF NEUROBEHAVIORAL ORGANIZATION

Ideally, the early environment of preterm infants should create a situation in which infant maturation can take place with minimal interference. The ideal NICU environment will support and promote the premature infant's adaptability to extrauterine life, known as neurobehavioral organization. The five dimensions of neurobehavioral organization are autonomic, motor, state, attention/interaction, and self-regulatory (Als, 1986). Infants are in continual interaction with their environment via these five subsystems. The goal for each dimension is an "organized" infant, who responds to environmental demands without disruption in physiologic and behavioral responses.

Autonomic Dimension

The first dimension the infant must tackle is the autonomic dimension. The premature infant's physiologic parameters vacillate greatly. With age, infants gain physiologic stability. An autonomically organized infant maintains autonomic stability despite disturbances from the environment. Instability in the autonomic system can be seen in the pattern of respiration (pauses, tachypnea), color changes (red, pale, dusky, mottled), and various visceral signs (regurgitation, twitching, stooling) (Holditch-Davis et al, 2003).

Motor Dimension

The motor system includes behaviors associated with muscle tone, posture, and generalized body movements (Als, 1986). Random, disorganized body movements are signs of motor disorganization, as are losing tone and becoming limp. Premature infants often lack the motor maturity to respond to environmental stimuli with the smooth, coordinated movements exhibited by the well newborn. A goal of developmental care is to support the infant to alleviate random, disorganized movements in order to conserve energy and promote normal motor development.

State Dimension

The state organization system incorporates the different ranges of sleep-wake states. Neonatal researcher T. Berry Brazelton developed a state scoring system that consists of the following six states:

1. Deep sleep
2. Light sleep
3. Drowsy
4. Alert
5. Considerable motor activity
6. Crying

A state-organized infant can transition between states appropriately and has the physiologic and behavioral conditions to reach or withdraw from any state. Brazelton's state scoring system is advantageous because it is easy to learn and the six states are fairly obvious (Holditch-Davis, 2003). Individualized developmental care based on this Synactive model of development does show benefits. Als et al (1994) reported improved medical status and developmental outcomes, including earlier discharge from the NICU.

For the premature infant who is overstimulated in the NICU environment, 60% to 70% of sleep time is active sleep (Holditch-Davis, 2003). Interventions that increase sleep and maximize quiet sleep are needed to protect the infant from environmental stimulants and foster motor control.

Deep sleep is characterized by regular breathing, no evidence of rapid eye movements, relaxed facial expression, any spontaneous motor activity, and occasional startles. Light sleep, on the other hand, is characterized by rapid eye movements under closed eyelids, periods of irregular and regular breathing, and low-level activity. In addition, occasional startles, whimpers, smiles, mouthing, and sucking behaviors may be observed. If the infant is receiving too much or too little stimulation, he or she may demonstrate behaviors of state disorganization, including fussing, yawning, frowning, and involuntary eye movements. If the infant's behavioral cues are not addressed and stimulation modified, further signs of physiologic and motoric disorganization may result (Als & Duffey, 1996).

Attention/Interaction Dimension

The attention/interaction dimension incorporates attentiveness. This system involves the infant's ability to orient and focus on sensory stimuli such as faces, sounds, or objectives (Holditch-Davis et al, 2003). Nurses need to be knowledgeable about sleep-wake states because infant behavior is affected by state. Timing routine interventions to occur when infants are most responsive is important when planning individualized care. Infant responses to nursing interventions and to parental interactions are affected by the infant's state. Learning takes place in the alert state. Alertness is an exciting milestone. An organized infant has the ability to attain, maintain, and withdraw from attentiveness. Preterm infants have difficulty maintaining their attention and become easily overwhelmed with the environment. These infants may avert their gaze, close their eyes, or become glassy-eyed. These are signs of overstimulation of the attention/interactive dimension.

Self-Regulatory Dimension

The self-regulatory dimension is associated with the infant's ability to achieve and maintain a balance of all neurobehavioral dimensions through use of self-consoling behaviors, such as sucking or hand-to-mouth maneuvers (Als, 1986). Since premature infants are often unable to maintain homeostasis of their autonomic, motoric, and state dimensions, it is very difficult for them to self-regulate and maintain a balance of all the dimensions.

Infants can achieve self-regulation when a developmentally appropriate setting is provided for the infants and families. By assessing the infant's behavioral responses to caregivers and other aspects of the physical environment, one can support the infant's neurodevelopment and can decrease stress. The bedside caregiver must ensure that the infant is comfortable, so as not to cause the infant to burn excess calories in an effort to get comfortable. All medical equipment should be well supported, so as not to place undue stress on the infant's musculoskeletal system.

The birth process brings new experiences to infants. The ability to adapt to the extrauterine environment is poorly developed in the premature infant. The goal of the NICU environment is to support the infant in the new extrauterine life. Advances in the medical management of premature infants have resulted in decreased infant mortality, especially among extremely low birth weight infants. NICUs and special care nurseries (SCNs) are in a unique position to support the infant's continued neurobehavioral development by modifying the high-risk neonatal environment.

ENVIRONMENTAL FACTORS/MACROENVIRONMENT

Light

Exposure of infants in NICUs to high-intensity light is disconcerting. Preterm infants are at risk for structural and growth alterations of the eye (such as retinopathy of prematurity, also known as ROP, amblyopia, myopia, strabismus, and astigmatism), as well as alterations in visual function that may reflect alterations in the visual cortex (Fielder & Moseley, 2000).

Lighting in the NICU needs to be balanced between dimmed ambient lighting, natural lighting, and brighter task lighting. Premature infants are photophobic; however, they will open their eyes with dim lights. Lighting in most NICUs is continuous, high-level, and fluorescent. Continuous bright lights in the NICU can disrupt sleep/wake states. If the light levels never change, infants never experience the diurnal rhythm necessary for development. Studies have demonstrated benefits to NICU infants exposed to diurnal variations in ambient lighting that reduces nighttime levels to as low as 0.5 foot-candles. NICUs should provide ambient lighting at levels recommended by the Illuminating Engineering Society (10 to 20 foot-candles), especially entrainment through cycled lighting during the last 2 weeks before discharge (Illuminating Engineering Society of North America, 1995; Rivkees et al, 2004). Ambient light levels need to be adjustable at each bedside at a level of 1 to 60 foot-candles (Martin, 2003). Reducing light levels may facilitate rest and subsequent energy conservation, and promote organization and growth.

Both natural and electric light sources need to have controls that allow immediate, sufficient darkening of any bed space for transillumination when necessary (Figure 24-1). Use

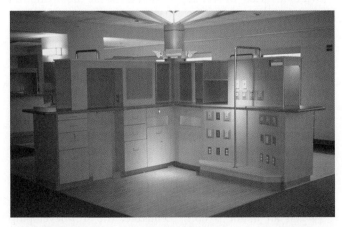

FIGURE **24-1**
Lighting. Courtesy Good Samaritan Hospital, Cincinnati, Ohio.

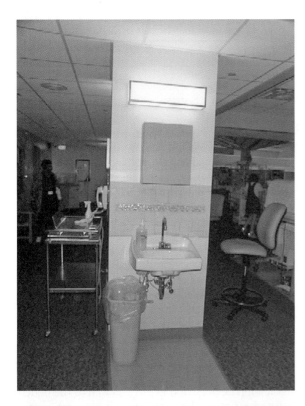

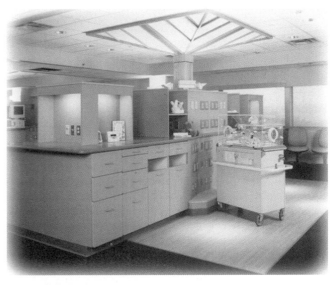

FIGURE **24-3**
Procedural lighting. Courtesy Good Samaritan Hospital, Cincinnati, Ohio.

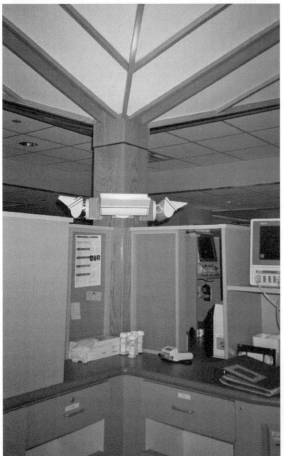

FIGURE **24-4**
Illumination of support area. Courtesy Good Samaritan Hospital, Cincinnati, Ohio.

of multiple switches with individual dimmers to allow different levels of illumination is helpful (Figure 24-2). Procedural lighting should be available at each bedside to allow caregivers to evaluate a baby or to perform a procedure (Figure 24-3). This increased illumination should not increase light levels of adjacent babies. Illumination of support areas such as charting areas, medication preparation areas, and reception areas should be adequate to allow important or critical tasks to be performed (Figure 24-4). This light level should conform to Illuminating Engineering Society specifications (Illuminating Engineering Society of North America, 1995). When possible, independent controls should be used to accommodate sleeping infants and working nurses.

At least one source of daylight should be visible from the patient care area. Windows provide a psychologic benefit to

FIGURE **24-2**
Different levels of illumination on multiple switches. Courtesy Good Samaritan Hospital, Cincinnati, Ohio.

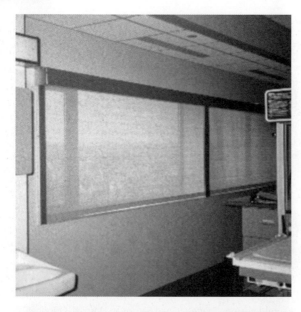

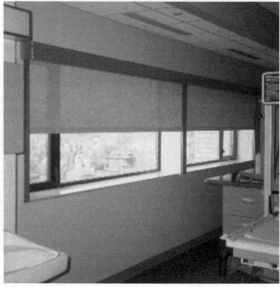

FIGURE **24-5**
Shading devices. Courtesy Good Samaritan Hospital, Cincinnati, Ohio.

TABLE **24-1**	Decibel Levels of NICU Equipment	
Equipment	**dB Level**
IV pump alarm	60-78
Tapping incubator with fingers	70-95
Closing incubator drawer	70-95
Bubbling water in ventilator/hood tubing	62-87
Closing a solid plastic porthole	80-111
Pulse oximeter alarm	86

Sound

Sound and noise levels in the NICU may cause damage to the developing cochlea resulting in hearing loss and arousal. Arousal is important with premature infants who are unable to inhibit responses. High noise levels in NICUs affect infants as well as staff and families. Excessive noise can damage delicate auditory structures and can have adverse physiologic effects such as hypoxia, increased intracranial pressure, increased blood pressure, apnea, bradycardia, and color changes (Bremmer et al, 2003). These high noise levels are often a result of equipment, alarms, ceiling and flooring material, communication devices, and talking, as well as the underlying heating and air conditioning ventilation system. Personnel and equipment also generate transient sounds. NICU sound levels vary based on the hour of day and is often related to activities such as shift change and medical rounds (Krueger et al, 2005).

Sound levels in NICUs have been documented to range from 50 to 90 decibels (dB) with peaks up to 120 dB. The decibel levels of various NICU equipment are shown Table 24-1 (Thomas, 1989). Safety standards for sound exposure in adults have long been established; for the neonate, more evidence is mounting to support standards that go beyond the recommendations from the NICU Design Committee under Dr. Robert White's leadership. The latest recommendations (White, 2006) now used worldwide are available at www.nd.edu/~nicudes. Adult, work-related errors have been noted to be more frequent in the noisy NICU environment (Thomas & Martin, 2000).

Both intensity and duration of sound exposure should be considered when evaluating the noise level in a NICU. Awareness of the impact of increased census and equipment on sound levels can influence health care personnel's ability to provide environmentally appropriate care to premature infants (Byers et al, 2005). Equipment should be selected with a noise criterion rating of less than 40 dB. Infant bed areas should be situated to produce minimal background noise and to contain and absorb as much transient noise as possible. Many sound control features should be considered when designing a NICU. Evidence-based sound-reducing strategies have been shown to decrease decibel levels by 4 to 6 dB when planning environment management as part of a developmental, family-centered NICU (Byers et al, 2006). The current air duct and ventilation system should be evaluated for noise as well as dust. Acoustic ceiling tiles in direct patient care areas with a noise reduction coefficient (NRC) rating of at least 0.90 should be considered (American Society for Testing and Materials, 1992). Raised ceilings can be used to create an open atmosphere. Porcelain

NICU staff as well as families. Daylighting is desirable for charting as well as the evaluation of infant skin tone. Exterior windows provide the recommended natural light and assist with diurnal cycling. However, serious problems with radiant heat loss or gain and glare can occur if infants are placed too close to external windows. External windows should be at least 2 feet away from the infant's bed and may be placed away from direct patient areas—for example, high up on the walls, as skylights, or in other locations that provide indirect light to the patient area. The latter might be a window in a hallway that secondarily allows light to pass into the NICU. All windows, including skylights, should have retractable covers for times when light is not desired. These windows should be insulated and have shading devices (Figure 24-5) in a neutral color to minimize color distortion from transmitted light (Martin, 2003).

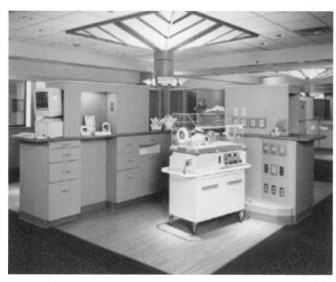

FIGURE **24-6**
Vinyl flooring at the bedside. Courtesy Good Samaritan Hospital, Cincinnati, Ohio.

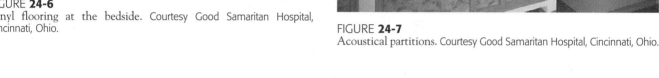

FIGURE **24-7**
Acoustical partitions. Courtesy Good Samaritan Hospital, Cincinnati, Ohio.

sinks rather than stainless steel sinks can also minimize noise. Carpet decreases the noise level and promotes a homelike environment, yet vinyl flooring material directly at the bedside can ease the routine cleaning (Figure 24-6).

Despite concerns over carpet use in NICUs, no documented studies or evidence to support increased infection rates exist. One important issue is the noise created by the equipment used to clean the carpet. When industrial-sized vacuum cleaners are used, the noise level exceeds the recommended sound level in the immediate area of the infants and decreases the dust level. On the other hand, a centralized vacuum system limits noise level and decreases the dust level. Acoustical partitions may be used to additionally minimize noise (Figure 24-7) (Altimier, 2001).

Background sound levels in the NICU may interfere with an infant's ability to discriminate speech of parents and other caregivers. Neonates are also exposed to vibration and noise when transported and when on high-frequency ventilation. Noise and vibration combined may have a synergistic effect. Noise can be limited through use of a wireless phone system that each health care provider carries, rather than using bedside phones. The ringer can be set to vibrate to minimize the noise level (Figure 24-8). Some units are placing microphones (Decibel Systems) in the ceiling above or on walls adjacent to infant care areas to determine the sound levels that are transmitted to the infant. These microphones are wired to an alarm device that feeds a signal to a ceiling light or light panel if the sound level exceeds a predetermined level. This system helps alert staff and parents to sounds that exceed a reasonable level. A decibel-monitoring limit should be set at 65 dB and can then be strategically dialed down as staff changes their behavior (Figure 24-9).

The following acoustical design guidelines should be considered:
- Background noise 50 dB (EPA)
- Transient noise <70 dB (AAP)
- Equipment with NC rating <40 dB

- Incubator motor noise <50 dB (AAP)
- Voice levels 60 to 70 dB
- Noise levels (work-related) 90 dB (OSHA)

Air ventilation systems are a challenge in a unit that attempts to provide private, separate areas that require a full ceiling-to-floor separation. From a budgetary perspective, it may substantially increase the cost of the unit renovation or construction. Those units that have met the fiscal and physical challenges of providing adequate ventilation have done so in an attempt to provide a more homelike atmosphere. Music therapy is used in some units to calm and soothe the environment. This therapy works for infants, families, and staff alike. However, the sound must be monitored for safe and reasonable levels.

Other guidelines include environmental factors that should also be considered throughout renovation:
- Temperature 75° to 79° F (23.8° to 26.1° C)
- Humidity 30% to 60%
- Air exchange six per hour (two with outside air exchange)
- All air filtered at 90% efficiency

Activity

For the premature infant, the nurse in the NICU is usually the primary caregiver. The unborn infant lives in a warm, cushioned, amniotic fluid environment. Once born, the infant is exposed to a multitude of intrusive and stress-producing activities. Infants may exhibit adverse physiologic symptoms to this stimulation, such as tachycardia, bradycardia, color changes, and oxygen desaturations. More profound infant distress signals such as retractions, vomiting, or seizure activity may occur with overstimulation (Graven et al, 1992). A principle termed "activity-dependent development" refers to the influence of usage and repetition in formation of neural connections and pathways in the brain. It is hypothesized that if specific neurons are consistently fired together, they are strengthened and become dominant, causing a hard wiring for

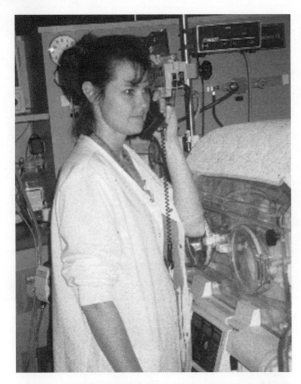

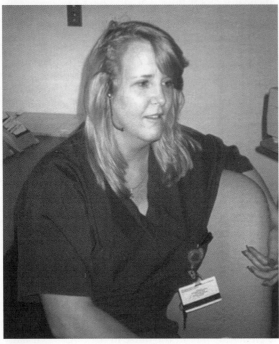

FIGURE **24-8**
Wireless phone system. Courtesy Good Samaritan Hospital, Cincinnati, Ohio.

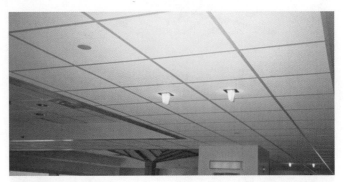

FIGURE **24-9**
Decibel-monitoring system. Courtesy Good Samaritan Hospital, Cincinnati, Ohio.

environment, however, does not lend itself to consistent responses like that of the womb. The principle of activity-dependent development is important to consider with the constant repetitive activities done in the NICU by the bedside caregiver. This principle encourages the bedside caregiver to adapt all caregiving behaviors to alleviate as much aversive or negative sensory input from caregiving activities as possible.

Neonates' sense of smell is stimulated primarily by unpleasant odors. Betadine (Purdue-Frederick, Stamford, CT), skin preps, and alcohol smells are often present in the typical NICU environment. Additionally, the neonate is exposed to fragrances worn by staff members. Infants may respond to olfactory stimuli with altered respirations, increased heart rate, and physical movements to push away from the unpleasant stimulus (Merenstein & Gardner, 1989). Behaviorally, staff should be educated on this topic to prevent olfactory overstimulation.

Developmental care is often associated with clinical bedside caregiving activities such as positioning, handling, cobedding, environmental modifications, and skin-to-skin care (Altimier & Lutes, 2000). Limiting developmental care to these activities alone, however, does not encompass the breadth of developmental care. Developmental care is a frame of reference on which to base all caregiving in the NICU. Developmental care principles include the ability to individualize care based not only on a given diagnosis or gestational age, but also on the individual capabilities and needs of the infant.

CAREGIVING FACTORS/MICROENVIRONMENT

Gestational age, gravity, medical equipment, hard and flat surfaces, medications, and improper positioning are all factors that contribute to the altered development of the NICU infant. However, with appropriate positioning, caregiving, and handling, these factors may be minimized and outcomes enhanced.

The majority of caregiving experienced by infants in NICUs involves medical or other caregiving interventions associated with high levels of sensory input. Infants should be handled gently without sudden changes in movement. Pharmacologic as well as nonpharmacologic comfort measures should be provided with painful procedures. Infants should be placed in a position of comfort with well-defined boundaries to promote flexion. Patterns of caregiving in the NICU can profoundly affect the development of infant state organization and biologic rhythms.

that response. In contrast, neurons that are not used or fired develop a weak neuronal connection, or may even disappear (Penn & Schatz, 1999). Therefore, the consistency of the environment can strengthen or weaken a neuronal response. The womb allows for this consistency as the fetus stretches and moves and is always met with a boundary, giving the resting posture of flexion and midline for the fetus. The NICU

Caregiving based on infant cues is an integral part of providing developmentally appropriate care. These cues provide communication about an infant's needs and status at any given time. Caregiving based on infant cues involves attention to messages from the infant that may indicate timing for interventions or opportunities for sensory input and interaction. These cues also indicate how the infant tolerates stimuli and stimulation.

Positioning

In utero, the infant is confined to an enclosed space with relatively well-defined boundaries. As the infant grows, his or her available space for free movement decreases and his or her body becomes more flexed (physiologic flexion). The developing infant has the opportunity to extend the arms and legs, meet resistance, and pull extremities back into a gentle flexion (Hunter, 2005). Physiologic flexion is believed to be vital for the development of normal body movement and control. Additionally, prone flexion may promote physiologic subsystem stability as evidenced by improved oxygenation and stable heart rate and respirations (Als, 1986).

After delivery, the infant is placed supine on a flat surface with limited physical boundaries to enhance or support flexion. Providing opportunities for both flexion and extension is essential in helping the infant achieve motor stabilization and may decrease the incidence of musculoskeletal abnormalities (Hunter, 2005). The head shape of the very low birth weight premature infant is often referred to medically as dolicocephalic. "Premie head" and "toaster head" are two terms often used casually by NICU caregivers to refer to the typical head shape seen in very premature infants. This flattening of the sides, with an elongated, narrow head shape, occurs as a result of the constant pressure and position of the infant's head as well as the molding that takes place after birth. The infant's head is often turned to one side or the other, regardless of whether the infant is prone, supine, or side lying. Right-sided flattening is often worse than left-sided because infants are more often placed on the right side to assist with gastric emptying. In addition, right-handed caregivers tend to position infants on their right side, allowing for ease with handling and caregiving activities from this direction. Flattening of the sides of the head does not diminish at discharge and can lead to long-term dolicocephaly. This has the potential to affect parent bonding, self-image, and possibly even the shape of the hard palate (Waitzman, 2007).

Hypotonia is normal for extremely preterm infants, and muscle tone in preterm infants gradually increases with age (Hunter, 2005). The premature infant often makes repeated, yet unsuccessful attempts to seek boundaries by extending his or her arms and legs. In addition, he or she may try to return to a tucked and flexed position. These repeated motoric efforts could exhaust the infant, using much of an already limited energy supply.

Developmental support in the form of environmental and caregiving modifications is provided in the NICU because preterm and sick infants lack the maturity, health, or competence necessary to cope easily with life in the NICU (Hunter, 2005). Developmentally supportive caregiving is aimed at minimizing energy expenditure while promoting a balance between flexion and extension for any infant. Proper positioning and handling have been shown to affect many physiologic and neurobehavioral parameters in the preterm infant. Appropriate positioning—such as midline orientation, hand-to-mouth activity, flexion, self-soothing, and self-regulatory abilities—contributes to neurobehavioral development. Occupational therapists working in NICUs frequently make positioning recommendations to optimize self-regulation. Grenier and colleagues (2003) found that infants performed the fewest stress behaviors in prone nested, prone unnested, or side-lying nested positions. Correct body positioning can prevent postural deformities such as hip abduction and external rotation, ankle eversion, retracted and abducted shoulders, increased neck hyperextension and shoulder elevation, and cranial molding. An infant with an extended neck caused by shortening of the trapezius and occipital muscles may have difficulty putting the head in neutral for feeding. Prone positioning increases oxygenation, tidal volume, and the compliance of the lungs.

The short- and long-term effects of improper positioning can be very expensive for parents and the taxpayer. In proper positioning and alignment (regardless of prone, supine, or side-lying position), the knees and nipples should be in the same plane. If the hips are unsupported, gravity will pull the knees apart, and the infant will exhibit "froglike" positioning, which enables the gluteus muscles (muscles in the buttock) and latissimus dorsi (muscles in the lower back) to shorten, thus decreasing the ability of those muscles to elongate in a sitting position. Diapers that do not fit appropriately can also cause this damage. Scapular retraction can occur if the shoulder girdle is not supported in a fixed position. In summary, the healthy term newborn infant is able to maintain physiologic flexion independently while moving against gravity. The premature or sick newborn infant has low muscle tone and is either unable to move against gravity or uses much of his or her energy in doing so.

Containment

Containment refers to the 360 degrees of surface pressure the fetus is provided in utero. Body containment is an important factor because it increases the infant's feelings of security and self-control and decreases stress. Infants who are contained tend to be calmer, require less medication, and gain weight more rapidly. The premature infant at term age differs from a full-term newborn; however, those premature infants that have the benefit of boundaries and containment to maintain postures similar to in utero position develop patterns more similar to those of term infants. Parents should be encouraged to provide gentle touch and containment by cupping the infant's head and buttocks rather than lightly stroking his skin.

Handling

Although positioning is very important in the NICU, the astute bedside caregiver realizes that it is not just static position that affects neurodevelopmental outcomes, but handling of the infant as well. Therefore, developmental care includes not just positioning, but also all handling and caregiving activities. Handling of infants should be done with slow, modulated movements, with the infant's extremities flexed and contained.

Frequent handling and touching disturbs sleep, which leads to decreased weight gain and decreased state regulation. In one study, premature infants were found to be disturbed an average of more than 23 times in 24 hours (Altimier et al, 1999). The premature infant in the NICU achieves an average of 5 to

15 minutes of deep, undisturbed sleep within a 24-hour day (Altimier et al, 1999). Routine procedures often result in significant hypoxia. Most episodes of hypoxemia happen during handling by caregivers. The extent of hypoxemia was greatly reduced when caregiving was modified.

The idea of clustering care came from developmental care literature in an effort to allow infants longer undisturbed sleep. This means limiting the frequency of interruptions of the infant by performing more required caregiving activities at one time. The developmentally supportive caregiver identifies the importance of clustering care as well as providing the appropriate quality and intensity of stimulation during wakefulness.

Kangaroo Care

Kangaroo care is the practice of holding a diaper-clad newborn or preterm infant on a parent's bare chest in an upright prone position. The infant is tucked inside a parent's shirt or gown while maintaining connections to life-sustaining medical equipment (Johnston et al, 2003). The practice first originated in Bogotá, Colombia, and is analogous to marsupials' care of their young, hence the name "kangaroo care" (Chandra & Baumgart, 2005). In Bogotá, multiple infants commonly shared isolettes, which increased infection and contributed to a high mortality rate of up to 70% for premature infants (Eichel, 2001). By comparison, the mortality rate in the United States in 1983 for very low birth weight infants was 39% (Ludington-Hoe & Golant, 1993). Parents were also reluctant to bond to their infant because of the increased mortality, which increased maternal abandonment. Rey and Martinez consequently introduced kangaroo care in an effort to save these premature infants. Infection, mortality, morbidity, and abandonment were all reduced with the new practice (Anderson, 1999). Kangaroo care spread to western European NICUs and the United States by the late 1980s. The practice of kangaroo care has now been established and is increasing dramatically. One important reason for this is the numerous physiologic and emotional benefits noted for both the infant and the parent. Kangaroo care decreases purposeless motor activity thereby conserving energy, diminishes infection and morbidity, improves weight gain, and decreases an infant's length of stay resulting in possible financial gain for the hospital (Kenner & McGrath, 2004; Aucott et al, 2002; McGrath & Brock, 2002).

Parental benefits from kangaroo care have also been studied. Benefits include improved bonding, a greater feeling of control and confidence with infant care, greater self-esteem, and an increased eagerness to take their infant home (Feldman et al, 2002; Gardner & Goldson, 2002). Parents who "kangaroo" their infants visit them more frequently and work through the experience of having a premature birth (Dodd, 2005; Gardner & Goldson, 2002). Offering parents the opportunity to kangaroo their infant may help facilitate the family's psychologic healing, enhance parent-infant bonding, improve lactation, and promote positive growth (Anderson et al, 2003; Beal & Wood, 2005) (Figure 24-10).

As with any nursing practice, benefits and risks must be considered. Thermoregulation is always an issue when discussing NICU nursing. Kangaroo care has the potential risk of hyperthermia or hypothermia. Many studies have found sufficient support for adequate thermoregulation, but each infant-parent team is unique, and monitoring of the infant's

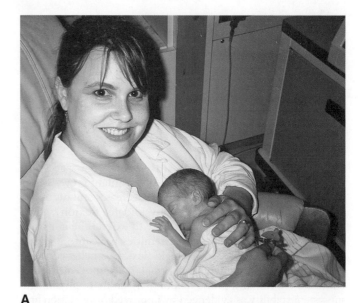

A

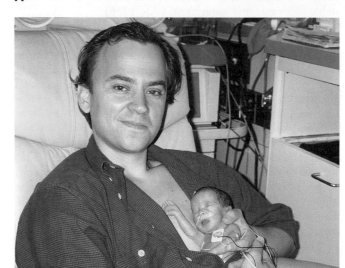

B

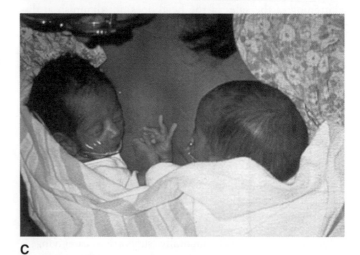

C

FIGURE **24-10**
Kangaroo care with mother (**A**), father (**B**), and mother holding twins (**C**). **A** and **B,** Courtesy Kristin Geen, St Louis, MO. **C,** Courtesy Good Samaritan Hopital, Cincinnati, OH.

temperature during kangaroo care is required according to each unit's policy and procedure. Ludington-Hoe and Golant (1993) have also suggested the possible lack of thermo-regulation among fathers, with resulting hyperthermia of the infant. Mothers, however, seem to synchronize temperatures more effectively and can even regulate different temperatures for each breast as needed as in the case of simultaneous twin kangarooing (Ludington-Hoe et al, 2006).

Browne (2004) and Johnson (2005) suggest implications for the nursing profession that include envisioning the parent's body as an ideal environment for an infant's NICU stay and to help facilitate the use of kangaroo care to strengthen the parent-infant bond and to maximize the long-term benefits.

FAMILY-CENTERED CARE

The admission of an infant to the NICU frequently is a crisis for the family. The delivery is often unexpected and the family unit is now separated (Hunter, 2005). Family-centered care in the NICU offers a philosophy of care that acknowledges that the family has the greatest influence over an infant's health and well-being. All families, even those that are struggling with difficulties, bring important strengths to their infant's experiences in the NICU. Key principles in the practice of family-centered care include respect for the infant and parents, promotion of shared information, and parent planning and participation. True family-centered care creates a collaborative partnership between the health care team and the family. Parenting can have a profound impact on long-term outcomes. Parents are not visitors to the NICU, rather partners (McGrath, 2005). Partnerships should begin as soon as the infant enters the NICU and continue as long as it is in the best interest of the child (Gates et al, 2004). The NICU is a difficult place to establish family-professional partnerships. However, because families are the constant in the infant's environment, assisting families to have a positive outcome from their NICU experience should be a priority when providing care (Gates et al, 2004). Open communication between parents and the NICU team is the foundation for family-centered caregiving decisions.

TOUCH AND MASSAGE IN THE NEONATAL INTENSIVE CARE UNIT

Massage is a hot topic in health care, especially in the NICU. What used to be thought of as purely an alternative therapy has become more accepted by medical professionals in various health care settings. Traditionally, massage has not been part of neonatal care. However, with the advancement of develop-mentally supportive care and family-centered care, massage is being considered more frequently. As massage seems to both decrease stress and provide tactile stimulation, it has been recommended as an intervention to promote growth and development of preterm and low-birth weight infants (Vickers et al, 2006). In fact, the core principles of developmental and family-centered care are easily translated through massage.

Vandenberg (1997) identified four principles of develop-mental care. These principles identified that care should be (1) relationship based, (2) cure based, (3) individualized, and (4) family centered. Infant massage inherently has these four principles. Massage in the NICU can be taught to parents to enhance their relationship with their infant. It is a wonderful activity that can support positive opportunity for interaction and relationship building between parents and their infant.

SUMMARY

As the preterm infant matures and the ill preterm or full-term infant recovers, the provision of sensory input is important for neurologic development. Caregivers must be cautious when providing sensory input and must be sensitive to infant responses and abilities to tolerate stimuli. High-risk infants are both dependent on and vulnerable to their early environment, the NICU, to maintain their physiologic function and to promote growth and development. Developmentally sup-portive care is sometimes perceived as "nice," yet optional. Consistent acceptance, practice, and accountability must be established to provide high-quality care for infants and families. Use of established guidelines, policies, and procedures to guide neonatal practice is critical (Altimier et al, 2006). To provide developmentally supportive care and optimize the experience of neonates in intensive care, an understanding of their behavioral capabilities as well as their surrounding physical environment is essential. Changes in developmental care can often begin with a few caregivers altering the way they care for premature infants. Role modeling, mentoring, and collaboration are all useful in promoting optimal developmental care. High-tech and high-touch care can be provided with low lighting and acoustic levels. The production of an efficient, peaceful, and satisfying environment for both administering and receiving care is an optimal goal for each high-risk infant.

REFERENCES

Als H (1986). A synactive model of neonatal behavioral organization: framework for the assessment of neurobehavioral development in the premature infant and for support of infants and parents in the neonatal intensive care environment. *Physical and occupational therapy in pediatrics* 6(3/4):3-53.

Als H, Duffy F (1996). Effectiveness of individualized neurodevelopmental care in the newborn intensive care unit (NICU). *Acta paediatrica supplemental* 416:21-30.

Als H et al (1994). Individualized developmental care for the very low-birthweight preterm infant. *Journal of the American Medical Association* 272(11):853-858.

Altimier L (2001). High-tech, high-touch care. *Nursing management* 32(7):40-43.

Altimier L, Lutes L (2000). Changing units for changing times: the evolution of a NICU. *Neonatal intensive care* 13(6):23-27.

Altimier L et al (1999). Neonatal thermoregulation: bed surface transfers. *Neonatal network* 18(4):35-37.

Altimier L et al (2005). Developmental care: changing the NICU physically and behaviorally to promote patient outcomes and contain costs. *Neonatal intensive care* 18(4):12-16.

Altimier L et al (2006). NANN guidelines for neonatal nursing policies, procedures, competencies, and clinical pathways. Available at www.NANN.org/publications.

American Society for Testing and Materials (1992). *Standard definitions of terms relating to environmental acoustics*. Publication ASTM C-634. Philadelphia: American Society for Testing and Materials.

Anand KJ, Scalzo FM (2000). Can adverse neonatal experiences alter brain development and subsequent behavior? *Biology of the neonate* 77:60.

Anderson GC (1999). Kangaroo care of the premature infant. In Goldson E, editor, *Nurturing the premature infant: developmental interventions in the neonatal intensive care nursery* (pp 131-160). New York: Oxford University Press.

Anderson GC et al (2003). Mother-newborn contact in a randomized trial of kangaroo (skin-to-skin) care. *Journal of obstetrics, gynecologic, and neonatal nursing* 32(5):604-611.

Aucott S et al (2002). Neurodevelopmental care in the NICU. *MRDD Research Reviews* 8:298-308.

Beal JA, Wood SH (2005). Implications of kangaroo care for growth and development in preterm infants. *American journal of maternal child nursing* 30(5):338.

Blackburn ST (1998). Environmental impact of the NICU on developmental outcomes. *Journal of pediatric nursing* 13:279-289.

Blackburn ST (2002). *Maternal, fetal, and neonatal physiology: a clinical perspective*, ed 2. St Louis: Saunders.

Bremmer P et al (2003). Noise and the premature infant: physiological effects and practice implications. *Journal of obstetric, gynecologic, and neonatal nursing* 32:447-454.

Browne J (2004). Early relationship environments: physiology of skin-to-skin contact for parents and their preterm infants. *Clinical perinatology* 31:287-298.

Byers JF et al (2006). Sound level exposure of high-risk infants in different environmental conditions. *Neonatal network* 25(1):25-32.

Byers JF et al (2005). Neonatal intensive care unit sound levels, environment, and infant responses. *Neonatal intensive care* 18(3):48-53.

Chandra S, Baumgart S (2005). Fetal and neonatal thermoregulation. In Spitzer AR, editor. *Intensive care of the fetus & neonate*, ed 2 (pp 495-513). Philadelphia: Elsevier.

DiMaggio TJ, Gibbons ME (2005). Neonatal pain management in the 21st century. In Taeusch HW et al, editors, *Avery's diseases of the newborn*, ed 8 (pp 438-446). Philadelphia: Elsevier.

Dodd VL (2005). Implications of kangaroo care for growth and development in preterm infants. *Journal of obstetric, gynecologic and neonatal nursing* 34(2):218-232.

Eichel P (2001). Kangaroo care: expanding our practice to critically ill neonates. *Newborn and infant nursing reviews* 1(4):224-228.

Feldman R et al (2002). Comparison of skin-to-skin (kangaroo) and traditional care: parenting outcomes and preterm infant development. *Pediatrics* 110(1):16-26.

Fielder AR, Moseley MJ (2000). Environmental light and the preterm infant. *Seminars in perinatology* 24:291-298.

Gardner SL, Goldson E (2002). The neonate and the environment: impact on development. In Merenstein GB, Gardner SL, editors. *Handbook of neonatal intensive care* (p 240). St Louis: Mosby.

Gates et al (2004). Family issues professional partnerships. In Kenner C, McGrath JM, editors. *Developmental care of newborns and infants: a guide for health professionals*. St Louis: Mosby.

Glass P (1999). The vulnerable neonate and the neonatal intensive care environment. In Avery GB et al, editors. *Neonatology: pathophysiology and management of the newborn*, ed 5. Philadelphia: Lippincott.

Graven S et al (1992). The high-risk infant environment. Part 1. *Journal of perinatology* 12(2):164-172.

Grenier IR et al (2003). Comparison of motor self-regulatory and stress behaviors of preterm infants across body positions. *American journal of occupational therapy* 57(3):289-297.

Hack MB et al (2002). Young adult outcomes of very low birth weight children. *New England journal of medicine* 346:149-157.

Hack MB et al (2004). Behavioral outcomes and evidence of psychopathology among very low birth weight infants at age 20 years. *Pediatrics* 114(4):932-940.

Hendricks-Munoz K et al (2002). Developmental care: the impact of Wee Care developmental care training on short-term infant outcomes and hospital costs. *Newborn and infant nursing reviews* 2(1):39-45.

Holditch-Davis D (2003). The development of sleeping and waking states in high-risk preterm infants. *Infant behavior & development* 13:513-531.

Holditch-Davis D et al (2003). Newborn and infant neurobehavioral development. In Kenner C, Lott J, editors. *Comprehensive neonatal nursing*, ed 3 (pp 236-284). St Louis: Saunders.

Hunter J (2005). Neonatal intensive care unit. In Case-Smith J, editor. *Occupational therapy for children*, ed 5. St Louis: Mosby.

Illuminating Engineering Society of North America (1995). *Lighting for healthcare facilities*. RP29. New York: Illuminating Engineering Society of North America.

Johnson AN (2005). Kangaroo holding beyond the NICU. *Pediatric nursing* 21(1):53-56.

Johnston CC et al (2003). Kangaroo care is effective in diminishing pain response in preterm neonates. *Pediatric adolescent medicine* 157(11):1084-1088.

Kenner C, McGrath JM (2004). *Developmental care of newborns and infants*. St Louis: Mosby.

Krueger C et al (2005). Elevated sound levels within a busy NICU. *Neonatal network* 24(6):33-37.

Louw R, Maree C (2005). The effect of formal exposure to developmental care principles on the implementation of developmental care positioning and handling of preterm infants by neonatal nurses. *S. Africa* 10(2):24-32.

Ludington-Hoe SM, Golant SK (1993). *Kangaroo care: the best you can do to help your preterm infant*. New York: Bantam Books.

Ludington-Hoe SM et al (2006). Breast and infant temperatures with twins during shared kangaroo care. *Journal of obstetric, gynecologic, and neonatal nursing* 35(2):223-231.

Martin G (2003). Recommended standards for newborn ICU design. Report of the Fifth Consensus Conference by the Committee to Establish Recommended Standards for Newborn ICU Design. *Journal of perinatology* 23(1):S3-S24.

McGrath J (2005). Partnerships with families: a foundation to support them in difficult times. *Journal of perinatal and neonatal nursing* 19(2):94-96.

McGrath J (2000). Developmental physiology of the neurological system. *Central lines* 16(4):1-16.

McGrath JM, Brock N (2002). Efficacy and utilization of skin-to-skin care in the NICU. *Newborn and infant nursing reviews* 2(1):17-26.

Merenstein G, Gardner S (1989). *Handbook of neonatal intensive care*, ed 2. St. Louis: Mosby.

Moore K, Persaud TVN (2003). *The developing human*, ed 7. Philadelphia: Saunders.

Penn AA, Schatz CJ (1999). Brain waves and brain wiring: the role of endogenous and sensory-driven neural activity in development. *Pediatric research* 45(4):447-458.

Rivkees SA et al (2004). Rest-activity patterns of premature infants are regulated by cycled lighting. *Pediatrics* 113(4):833-839.

Thomas K (1989). How the NICU environment sounds to a preterm infant. *American journal of maternal child nursing* 14:249-251.

Thomas KA, Martin PA (2000). Differential effects of breast- and formula-feeding on preterms' sleep-wake patterns. *Journal of perinatology* 20:S94-S99.

Vandenberg K (1997). Basic principles of developmental caregiving. *Neonatal network* 6:69-71.

Vickers A et al (2006). Massage for promoting growth and development of preterm and/or low-birth-weight infants. *Cochrane database of systematic reviews* (CD000390).

Volpe JJ (2001). *Neurology of the newborn*, ed 4. St Louis: Saunders.

Waitzman K (2007). Neuromotor development. In Altimier L, editor. *Mosby's neonatal nursing course*. St Louis: Mosby.

White R (2006). *Recommended standards for newborn ICU design*. Available at http://www.nd.edu/~nicudes/. Retrieved July 10, 2006.

Chapter 25

Family: Essential Partner in Care

Jacqueline M. McGrath

Parents and families often enter the bewildering, unfamiliar environment of the neonatal intensive care unit (NICU) for the first time while still exhausted from delivery and emotionally drained by the unexpected birth experience they have just encountered. It is at this moment that a partnership must be formed between the family and professionals caring for their infant and continue as long as it is in the best interest of the child (McGrath, 2005a; Gates et al, 2004). Partnerships exist when there is a relationship between two or more parties that have a shared goal. Effective partnerships between professionals and families are based on mutual respect, valuing of family expertise, fully shared information, and joint decision making (Brazy et al, 2001). If parents were consistently well informed and involved as partners with the NICU team, ethical dilemmas might be lessened and care decisions might be optimized in the best interest of the infant and their family (Bruns & McCollum, 2002). These partnerships are essential and are the crux of the discussion within this chapter.

Change is the most certain event in life. A family experiencing the birth of an infant faces many changes. Some variations in lifestyle occur in the areas of employment, financial security, daily activities, relationships with others, and role. These changes have a major impact on each of the parents and on the family as a whole. When medical needs require admission of the infant to the neonatal intensive care unit (NICU), the changes become even more significant because, for the most part, the needs of this "different" child or "different" birth have not been planned for or expected (Doering et al, 2000). For the family, the changes can be devastating and challenging to manage without integration into the NICU caregiving team. During this difficult time parents need more than support; they need to be a true partner and an integral part of the process of caring for and parenting their child (Holditch-Davis & Miles, 2000).

In the NICU, it is wholly impossible to provide excellent health care to the infant without partnering with the parents or family, or preferably both, in every aspect of the care (Beveridge et al, 2001). Families provide the foundation for health concepts and are the child's portal to the health care system. Family beliefs and individual health values are highly correlated. Families are the constant for the child. The provision of individualized developmentally supportive care, of which family-centered care is a core principle, is pivotal to the long-term medical and developmental outcomes of the child (Aita & Snider, 2003). For these reasons, understanding the many influences of the context of family on each of its members is important for those caring for infants and children (Weiss & Chen, 2002) (Box 25-1). Most professionals who work with children and families believe that a family-centered approach is the best option, because this type of care likely will produce benefits for the child beyond those derived from high-quality professional and technical care (Ahmann et al, 2003).

Clear definitions of family and the philosophy of family-centered care are critical to the foundation of the concepts presented in this chapter. Role theory is used to explain the issues that families face during this challenging time. Factors that influence parenting behaviors include personal experiences, medical and nursing staff expectations, environmental conditions, and peer relationships; these factors can either promote or interfere with the development of an intact family unit. A critically ill newborn complicates the attachment process and the learning of parenting skills, and thus, a framework is provided for understanding what families need in the neonatal setting. The chapter concludes with family-centered care strategies that help the family unit function at its best during the NICU experience and that promote the discharge of intact families after the crisis has resolved. These strategies also cover issues related to sibling adaptation and involvement of extended family members in the care and decision making related to the infant.

FAMILY-CENTERED CARE

Family-centered care (FCC) is a philosophy of care in which the pivotal role of the family in the lives of children is recognized and respected (Johnson, 2003). According to this philosophy, families are supported in their natural caregiving and decision-making roles by building on their unique strengths as persons, and then as a family unit. Family-centered care recognizes and promotes the normal patterns of a family's life at home and in the community. Rather than expecting the family to take on the medical culture of the institution, health care professionals recognize and reinforce the family's culture through a partnership formed in the best interests of the child. Parents and professionals are equals in a partnership committed to the child and to the development of optimum quality in the delivery of all levels of health care (Johnson, 2003, 2004). Family-centered care strengthens the family unit through empowerment and by enabling the family to nurture and support their child's development (Institute for Family-

---

BOX 25-1

Key Elements of Family-Centered Care

The practice of family-centered care involves the following:

1. Recognizing the family as the constant in a child's life, whereas the service systems and those who work in them change.
2. Facilitating family-professional partnership and collaboration at all levels of health care.
3. Providing care for the child and recognizing he is an individual.
4. Parent participation in program development, implementation, and evaluation.
5. Contributing to policy formation that enhances the family.
6. Honoring the racial, ethnic, cultural, religious, and socioeconomic diversity of families.
7. Recognizing family strengths and individuality and respecting different methods of coping.
8. Sharing with families, on a continuing basis and in a supportive manner, complete and unbiased information.
9. Encouraging and facilitating family-to-family support and networking.
10. Understanding and incorporating the developmental needs of infants and their families into health care systems.
11. Implementing comprehensive policies and programs that provide emotional and financial support to meet the needs of families.
12. Designing accessible health care systems that are flexible, culturally competent, and responsive to family-identified needs.

Adapted from Johnson BH (2003). Patient and family-centered care. In *AHA news*. Bethesda, MD: Institute of Family-Centered Care.

BOX 25-2

Two Principles That Form the Foundation of Family-Centered Care

Enabling: Creating opportunities and ways for families to use the abilities and competencies they already have to learn new ones as necessary to meet child and family needs.

Empowering: Acknowledging and respecting the fact that the family has existing strengths and capabilities, and the professional builds on those strengths by supporting the family in meaningful decision making about issues that affect their welfare. Professionals who empower families interact and form partnerships with families in ways such that the family keeps or develops a sense of control over their own lives and attributes positive changes to their own strengths, abilities, and actions.

Adapted from Johnson BH (2003). Patient and family-centered care. In *AHA news*. Bethesda, MD: Institute of Family-Centered Care; Johnson BH (2004). Families are allies for enhancing quality, patient safety. In *AHA news*. Bethesda, MD: Institute of Family-Centered Care.

Centered Care, 2002) (Box 25-2). From the child's perspective, family-centered care is safe and familiar; the infant/child is immediately a member of a family and thus needs their special support. When the framework of family-centered care is the foundation of caregiving, the family is visible, available, and supportive of their infant's needs. The family also is an empowered partner in the caregiving of their child within the health care setting. It is important to remember that families are not replaceable at any level in the overall development of the child. Their impact will always supersede that of the health care system.

DEFINITION OF FAMILY

The concept of who and what comprises a family in North America has changed significantly in recent years. Families expand, contract, and realign at a rapid pace to keep up with the rapidly changing demands of our world. In modern times, dual-career families, permanent single-parent households, unmarried couples, homosexual couples, remarried couples, and sole-parent adoptions have emerged as other models of family, in addition to the family units seen as "traditional" a century ago.

"Family" is a broad term that is best defined by the individual; however, in general, a family is made up of those people, both related and unrelated, who provide support, structure beliefs, and define values. Family has also been defined as a social system composed of two or more people who coexist in the context of some expectations of reciprocal affection, mutual responsibility, and temporal duration (Hanson & Boyd, 2001). Families provide the framework through which individuals enter and interact with society at large. For infants and children, families are the means to resources, education, and society. Again, it is important to remember that families bring their children to the health care system for care, and no matter how an infant comes to us, they come with a family.

A family is defined by its members; "family" is an internal concept of how that particular group defines itself. It may be composed of family or friends; it may not depend on a blood bond but on the emotional tie or closeness felt among its members. It also may be an extended family that includes parents, grandparents, other relatives, and friends. Families nowadays are not necessarily defined as they have been in the past and not according to gender-specific roles. Families also can be defined by considering the degree to which the following five attributes are present (keeping in mind that these attributes also depend on the family's societal and cultural orientation) (Hanson & Boyd, 2001):

1. A family is a social system or unit.
2. Family members may or may not be related by birth, adoption, or marriage.
3. A family may or may not include dependent children.
4. Families involve commitment and attachment.
5. Family members usually have roles and caregiving functions (e.g., protection, nourishment, and socialization).

ROLE THEORY

Role theory, which appeared in the literature in the 1930s, offers a framework for understanding families and identifying the roles that individuals play within the family. As a broad term, role theory represents a collection of concepts, sub-theories, and research that addresses aspects of social behavior relevant to families. Over the years role theory has come to include two major theoretical perspectives: symbolic interaction and social structural role (Hanson & Boyd, 2001). Within both perspectives, role is a basic concept in the attempt to explain social order and interpersonal relationships within family and society.

The symbolic interaction theory relates to individuals who create and construct their personal environment as they interact with, shape, and adapt to their own social environment. These individual behaviors aid in constructing the meaning of roles. In contrast, social structural role theory has a broader base. It focuses on the ways in which society, social structure, and other social systems shape and determine an individual's behavior. Roles are social facts with patterned behaviors that develop over time, and they are predetermined by social forces.

The term *role* has diverse uses. One definition of a role is overt and covert goal-directed patterns of behavior that result from individuals interacting with, shaping, and adapting to their social environment. Roles are dynamic, interactional, and reciprocal relationships among individuals; therefore values, attitudes, and behaviors influence these relationships. Each role has specific behaviors and expectations placed on it by society, and these expectations guide individuals as to when, where, and in what manner they are to perform the role.

Each role also has specific demands. An individual learns these demands by maturing and advancing through the middle to later stages of the life cycle: (1) adolescence, (2) adulthood, (3) marriage and parenthood, and (4) middle and old age. Individuals respond to the demands of a role differently based on their maturity and current stage in the life cycle. For example, a single, adolescent girl would be expected to perform the maternal role differently from a married, adult woman.

Concepts within role theory identify seven areas of distress associated with roles: (1) role ambiguity, (2) role conflict, (3) role incongruity, (4) role overload, (5) role underload, (6) role overqualification, and (7) role underqualification. These terms are defined in Table 25-1. These areas of distress are responsible for producing role stress and strain. Role stress is defined as either internal or external pressure that generates role strain. As a consequence, feelings of frustration, tension, or anxiety are produced in either the individual or the reciprocal partners. More information on this topic can be found on the Evolve website. **evolve**

PARENTAL ROLE

Certain behaviors that are specific to both mother and father define the role of the parent. Several factors influence these behaviors: cultural background, personality, previous parenting and life experiences, degree of attachment to the infant, and expectations parents have of themselves and the infant or child. A child changes everything in the close-knit relationship of the couple. Both must take on a new role; they are not just wife and husband, they are now mother and father as well. Feelings of inadequacy, conflict, and fatigue are often apparent during the transition and may adversely affect both existing relationships and those just developing between the parent and child. Parenting remains the only major role for which there is little preparation in our society; difficulties encountered in the early stages of parenting may adversely affect all relationships but most especially the marital relationship. These difficulties can arise even if the new child is not the first child; each additional member of the family brings unique joys and challenges.

TABLE 25-1	Potential Role Problems
Role	**Potential Problems**
Role ambiguity	Role expectations are vague or lack clarity.
Role conflict	Role expectations are incompatible (conflicts exist between reality and expectations).
Role incongruity	Self-identity and subjective values are grossly incompatible with role expectations.
Role overload	Too much is expected in the time available.
Role underload	Role expectations are minimal and underuse the role occupant's abilities.
Role overqualification	Role occupant's motivation, skills, and knowledge far exceed those required.
Role underqualification	Role incompetence; the role occupant lacks one or more necessary resources (commitment, skill, knowledge).

Data from Hardy M, Conway ME (1988). Role theory: perspectives for health professionals, ed 2. Norwalk, CT: Appleton & Lange.

The situation in which a person must parent also influences behaviors. Parents faced with a crisis state must modify their roles and adapt to the necessary changes. Role and behavior changes can cause considerable stress, especially if these changes occur abruptly. Parents suffering from mental or physical illness or those who are chemically dependent can have limited coping abilities and social supports. Single, adolescent, or first-time parents also are at a disadvantage. They may lack maturity and coping skills because of limited life experiences and unavailable or inappropriate social support systems. These situations may inhibit the development of the parent-infant relationship and thus impair parenting behaviors. In addition, mothers and fathers parent differently and take on the role differently (Hynan, 2005; Sydnor-Greenberg & Dokken, 2000). These differences are not wrong or right; they are just differences that need to be acknowledged and accepted. In the NICU, mothers are often the focus and fathers can be easily overlooked and not well supported (Davis et al, 2003; O'Shea & Timmins, 2002).

Infant-related factors can also interfere with parental attachment and subsequent parenting behaviors. An example is an infant born with a congenital anomaly. Many of these infants may be mentally or physically disabled for a lifetime, which interferes with the parents' expectations of their infant. A visible anomaly is particularly difficult for parents because society places such emphasis on appearance. An infant with an easily correctable anomaly is tentatively unacceptable to society, until the anomaly has been corrected. A visible, noncorrectable anomaly has a greater impact on the parents and other family members. This stigma may include preterm infants who have deficits related to their untimely birth, such as blindness, deafness, or severe respiratory compromise. These parents may suffer from "chronic sorrow," and the child may grow up hindered by "vulnerable child syndrome" (Major,

2003). It may be helpful to connect these families to support groups or other families with children with similar disabilities or diagnoses (Carvajal, 2002).

A life-threatening or terminal illness in a child is another situation that may interfere with parenting attachment and behaviors. Parents may "hold back" their feelings for the child to try to protect themselves from loss and pain if the child dies. This inability to attach to their infant interferes with the parenting experience and may affect the child's development if the child lives past the previously expected life span. More information can be found on the Evolve website. **evolve**

At any birth or interaction between a parent and their child, the nurse must identify adaptive and maladaptive parenting behaviors. Adaptive behaviors indicate that both the infant's and parent's needs are met, and thus the parent-child relationship can be established. Mothers and fathers have different ways of expressing their parental roles based on gender differences alone (Hynan, 2005; Sydnor-Greenberg & Dokken, 2000). Tables 25-2 and 25-3 identify mothering and fathering behaviors the nurse can use in assessing adaptive or maladaptive behavior. It is important to remember that these are guidelines and must be adapted to each parent based on his or her personality and the specific situation.

Parenting During Crisis

Taking on the parenting role is a major life task for a couple. The crisis of having a critically ill newborn in the NICU compounds the stress of that task. Whether the family unit attains growth from a positive resolution of this crisis or splinters because of a maladaptive adjustment largely depends on the partnership formed with caregiving and the quality of support provided (Carter, 2002). The memory of what happens in the first days after a traumatic birth often stays with a family forever; just ask a mother to describe her birth experience, and she will talk for hours, explaining every detail (VandeVusse, 1999). Consequently, the relationships formed and interventions provided during the initial trauma can be critical to the adjustment and continued growth of the family unit.

Parents' Reactions

Crisis can be defined as an upset of a steady state. It is a period of disequilibrium precipitated by an inescapable demand to which the person is temporarily unable to respond adequately. The birth of a critically ill infant represents two types of crises for parents. The birth of any infant is a developmental crisis, a natural transitional phase in the lives of a couple. When the infant is premature or ill, parents also experience an accidental and unexpected crisis. The meaning of the event for the family and the resources available to deal with the event are variables that determine the scope of the crisis (Spear et al, 2002). With the technologic advances that have been made in medicine, some families now are able to better prepare for and make decisions about their child's prognosis and medical needs before birth. For example, many infants with gastroschisis or other anomalies are diagnosed during a prenatal ultrasound examination. In such cases, families have the opportunity to better plan for the birth and to make decisions with the health care team in a more conducive and supportive environment. The ability to anticipate the needs of the child reduces the sense of crisis for these families with the birth of the child.

Families of a premature or sick newborn react in different and individual ways. Some common reactions are anxiety, guilt,

fear, resentment, and anger. During the illness of a newborn, the parents must face many charged issues; two important ones are the loss of the perfect child they have anticipated and a fear that their infant may die (Higgins & Dullow, 2003).

In general, excitement and a flurry of preparation surround the birth of a child. Family celebrations help parents share the anticipation of a new infant with friends and extended family members. Parents spend much time imagining what this child will look like and dreaming about the joys of parenting. The couple experience disappointment when the infant or pregnancy is not as anticipated. They may feel a sense of isolation from other couples who have had a normal pregnancy or infant. They may even have feelings of isolation from each other or from close family members. The inability to produce a healthy infant or to protect the infant from the invasive and painful environment necessary to sustain the child's life may cause feelings of inadequacy. For many parents, the role the couple had thought they would assume seems impossible to attain in the environment of the NICU, where often it seems everyone else is making decisions about the fate of their infant (Higgins & Dullow, 2003). Parents seldom have had experience with the NICU before the intensity of the situation is heightened even more by the fact that they and their infant are center stage.

Parents must reconcile their idealized image of the child with the actual infant. They mourn the loss of the perfect child that was expected and feel anticipatory grief for the infant whose life may now be in jeopardy (Hulac, 2001). (For more information see Chapter 27 and the Evolve website.) The birth of an ill or a premature infant often places parents in a state of disequilibrium; nothing is as it was before. Mothers of premature infants have had the emotional work of pregnancy cut short and thus are often psychologically unprepared for the birth (Higgins & Dullow, 2003; Partridge et al, 2005). If the mother had felt ambivalent about the pregnancy, she may believe that the infant's illness is somehow punishment for those emotions. A mother may also feel guilty that she could not carry the infant to term, even if no reason can be found for the baby's premature birth. **evolve**

Many parents of sick newborns go through identifiable stages of grief and loss with very emotional reactions (Spear et al, 2002). The initial response usually is one of overwhelming shock, characterized by irrational behavior, crying, and feelings of helplessness and despair. Families at this stage have difficulty with organization because their lives have been disrupted by the unexpected birth. They may feel as if everything is in chaos and the situation is out of their control. Substance abuse, teenage pregnancy, clinical depression, and domestic violence can increase the chaos and vulnerability of these families (Loo et al, 2003). Parents also may feel guilt over the premature delivery or the infant's illness. Self-blame often characterizes these feelings ("If only I had stayed home that day I noticed the spotting"). Parents may try to escape the situation by using denial ("Everything will all be fine in just a few days."). At the bedside in these initial days, parents may focus on facts they can understand and avoid issues they do not understand. To health care providers, this may seem as if the parents aren't listening or that they are unwilling to hear the information provided, yet the parents are trying to cope with what to them is an overwhelming situation (Higgins & Dullow, 2003).

Intense feelings of resentment and anger follow denial. Parents may direct these feelings at themselves, the infant,

TABLE 25-2	Guidelines for Assessing Adaptive and Maladaptive Mothering Behaviors
Adaptive Behavior	**Maladaptive Behavior**

DELIVERY

Adaptive Behavior	Maladaptive Behavior
Attempts to position head to see infant as soon as delivered and while infant is on warming table.	Does not position head to see baby.
When shown infant:	When shown infant:
Smiles	Frowns
Keeps eyes on infant, looking at all parts exposed	Stares at ceiling
Attempts en face position	Stares at baby without expression
Uses fingertip touch on face and extremities	Does not assume en face position
Asks to hold baby	Does not touch baby
Partly opens blanket to see more of infant	Does not ask to hold baby
Talks to baby	Declines offer to hold baby
Asks questions about baby	If infant is placed in her arms, lies still and does not touch or stroke baby's face or extremities
	May not look at infant
	Does not talk to baby
	Asks few or no questions
Makes positive statements about baby: "She's so cute!" "He's so soft!"	Makes no comments or makes only negative statements: "She looks awful." "He's ugly."
May cry out of joy or relief that infant is normal or of desired sex.	May cry, appearing unhappy or depressed.
May smile and cry at the same time. (To differentiate from crying out of disappointment, note facial expressions and verbal statements.)	When asked why she is crying, states she is disappointed in baby.
Expresses satisfaction with or acceptance of infant's gender: "We really wanted a girl, but it's more important that he's healthy."	Expresses dissatisfaction with baby's gender: "Not another girl. I should have known better than to try again for a boy." "I don't even want to see him." May use profanity when told gender.
"I can't believe it; a boy, at last!"	
Predominant affect: appears pleased and happy.	Predominant affect: appears sad, angry, or expressionless.
Suddenly decides she wants to breastfeed.	Suddenly decides against breastfeeding.

FIRST WEEK

Adaptive Behavior	Maladaptive Behavior
Initially uses fingertips on head and extremities. Progresses to using fingers and palm on infant's trunk. Eventually draws infant toward her, holding infant against her body.	Uses fingertip touch without progressing to palm on trunk or drawing infant toward her body
Snuggles infant to neck and face.	Does not hold infant to neck or face.
Makes spontaneous movements, kissing, stroking, and rocking.	Makes few or no spontaneous movements with infant.
Attempts to establish eye contact by moving infant, assuming en face position, or shielding infant's eyes from light.	Does not use en face position or attempt to establish eye-to-eye contact.
Handles and holds baby at times other than when giving direct care	Handles baby only as necessary to feed or change diapers.
Talks to infant.	Does not talk to infant.
Smiles at baby frequently; changes affect appropriately, such as when infant cries.	Rarely smiles at baby, or smiles all the time without change in affect.
Makes many specific observations of infant: "Her eyes look like they might turn brown." "One foot turns in just a bit."	Makes no observations.
	Makes few observations that are either general or negative.
Discusses infant's characteristics, attempting to relate them to others in the family: "He has my ears but his daddy's chin." "She really doesn't look like either of us, she just looks like herself."	Does not discuss infant's characteristics in relation to characteristics of family members.
With a positive manner, uses animal characteristics to describe baby: "She's just like a cuddly little kitten." "His hair feels like down."	In a negative or hostile manner, uses animal characteristics to describe baby: "She looks awful, just like a drowned rat." "He looks like an ape to me."
Asks questions about caring for infant after discharge.	Asks no questions about care.

Continued

TABLE 25-2 Guidelines for Assessing Adaptive and Maladaptive Mothering Behaviors—cont'd	
Adaptive Behavior	**Maladaptive Behavior**

FIRST FEW WEEKS (IF INFANT REMAINS HOSPITALIZED AFTER MOTHER HAS BEEN DISCHARGED)

Adaptive Behavior	Maladaptive Behavior
Calls every day or every other day.	Calls less frequently than every other day or not at all.
Visits a minimum of twice a week.	Visits less frequently than twice a week or not at all.
Visits for a minimum of 30 minutes.	Visits for less than 30 minutes.
Asks specific questions about infant's condition.	Asks no specific questions.
Asks appropriate questions frequently.	Asks inappropriate questions.
Spends most of visit looking at and handling infant.	Spends most of visit observing unit activities and other infants (this may be normal behavior for the first one or two visits); has little or no interaction with infant during visits.
Becomes involved with care when encouraged and supported by staff.	When encouraged by staff to participate in care, refuses, terminates visit, or performs only minimal care.
Although visits are frequent and last longer than 30 minutes, says she misses infant at home or that she wishes she could visit more often and stay longer.	Makes no statements about missing infant, or states that she misses infant at home and wishes she could visit more often, but comments are not validated by frequent or lengthy visits.
Expresses reluctance to terminate visit.	Leaves nursery with little hesitation.
Waits until infant is asleep before leaving; touches or talks to baby just before leaving; may stand outside window and look at baby before leaving unit.	Frequently asks nurse to complete feeding or to change and settle infant.

FIRST MONTHS

Adaptive Behavior	Maladaptive Behavior
Holds infant close to her body.	Does not hold infant securely against her body.
Supports infant's trunk and head in position of comfort.	Head and body of infant are not well supported.
Muscles in her arms and hands are relaxed and conform to curvature of infant's body.	Shoulder, arm, and hand muscles appear tense; hands and fingers do not conform to infant's body.
During feedings, holds infant in well-supported position against her body.	Holds infant away from her body during feedings or props infant or bottle.
Positions during feeding so eye-to-eye contact can occur.	Position during feeding prevents eye-to-eye contact.
Minimizes talking to infant while baby is sucking.	Continues talking to infant during feeding even though infant is distracted and stops sucking.
Refers to infant using given or affectionate name.	Refers to infant in impersonal way (e.g., "the baby," "she," or "it").
Plays with infant at times unrelated to direct care.	Handles infant mainly during caretaking activities.
When infant is in infant seat, playpen, or crib, frequently interacts with baby.	Leaves infant for long periods in infant seat, playpen, or crib, interacting only after infant becomes fussy.
Places infant, when awake, in an area where baby can observe and interact with others.	Leaves infant, when awake, alone for long periods in bedroom or isolated area.
Occasionally leaves infant with someone else.	Frequently leaves baby with someone else or refuses to leave baby with someone else.
Uses discretion in selecting baby-sitter and provides instructions on baby's routines, likes, and dislikes.	Does not use good judgment in selecting baby-sitter; provides inadequate or no instructions for care.
Provides infant with routine well-baby care. Carries out medical plan for management of specific problems or conditions (e.g., thrush, anemia, or ear infection).	Fails to provide infant with well-baby care, seeking medical assistance only after problems, or keeps all appointments and makes additional phone calls or additional visits to physician to emergency room for imagined or insignificant problems.
Remains close to infant during physical examinations and attempts to soothe baby if infant becomes distressed.	Remains seated at a distance from the examination table; does not soothe infant during examination; frequently arranges for someone else to take infant for medical appointments.
Makes positive statements about mothering role.	Makes negative statements about mothering role.

From Hall-Johnson S (1986). *Nursing assessment and strategies for the family at risk, ed 2. Philadelphia: JB Lippincott.*

members of the health care team, God, or even each other as parents. They may also experience feelings of ambiguity and may fear the infant's physical and mental outcome. For these reasons, they may avoid emotional involvement with the infant to protect themselves from the pain of possible loss. A lessening of the intense emotional reactions and an increased ability to begin caring for their infant's emotional and physical needs are characteristic of adaptation and of taking on the parenting role. Reorganization is the final stage; at this point,

parents come to terms with their infant's problems. This can take a few days to several months. In some cases, these feelings of loss and grief may never be resolved (Spear et al 2002).

Factors That Affect Parenting Skills

Certain factors affect a couple's ability to acquire parenting skills during the NICU experience (Box 25-3). Parents are unable to attach and detach at the same time; these two tasks are incongruent. Parents need time to detach or grieve for the

TABLE 25-3	Guidelines for Assessing Adaptive and Maladaptive Fathering Behaviors	
Situation	**Adaptive Behavior**	**Maladaptive Behavior**
Touches child	Freely, uses whole hand	Infrequent, uses fingertips, rough
Holds child	Holds child close to his body, relaxed posture	Holds child distant from his body, tense posture
Talks to child	Shows positive manner and tone; uses appropriate language, speech, content	Uses curt, loud, inappropriate language or content
Facial expression	Makes eye contact, expresses spectrum of emotions	Makes limited eye contact, little change in expression
Listens to child	Active listener, gives feedback	Inattentive or ignores child
Demonstrates concern for child's needs	Active, involves others, seeks information	Indifferent, asks few questions
Aware of own needs	Expresses feelings about self in relation to child	Gives no expression about self
Responds to child's cues	Responds promptly to verbal, nonverbal cues	Has limited awareness and response
Relaxed with child	Shows relaxed posture, muscle tone	Shows rigid posture, tension, fidgeting
Disciplines child	Initiates reasonable, appropriate discipline	Does not initiate discipline or uses measures too severe or too lax
Spends time with, visits child	Routinely, uses time so that child is involved	Has no routine, no emphasis on child during time spent
Plays with child	Uses appropriate level of play, active, both enjoy interaction	Uses inappropriate play, no obvious enjoyment
Gratification after interaction with child	Father states he is, appears gratified	Gives no statement or display of gratification
Initiates activity with child	Frequently	Infrequently
Seeks information and ask questions about child	Concerned, asks frequent, appropriate questions	Asks few questions, needs prompting
Responds to teaching	Positive, reinforces instructor, seeks more information	Has little interest
Knowledge of child's habits	Knowledgeable	Has little knowledge
Participates in physical care	Feeds, bathes, dresses child	Allow others to perform tasks
Protects child	Aware of environmental hazards, actively protects	Protective behaviors not exhibited
Reinforces child	Gives verbal-nonverbal responses to child's positive behaviors	Does not notice or acknowledge child's behavior
Teaches child	Initiates teaching	Shows no teaching behavior
Verbally communicates with mother about child	Uses positive, frequent verbal encounters	Gives negative, infrequent communication
Verbally and nonverbally supports mother	Demonstrates support; reassures, touches	Support not obvious
Mother supports father, father responds	Gives positive response	Responds negatively or gives no response
Speaks of other children	Responds when asked, initiates	Shows no interest, no initiation

From Hall-Johnson S (1986). Nursing assessment and strategies for the family at risk, ed 2. Philadelphia: Lippincott.

lost perfect child before they can begin to attach to the ill infant. This adjustment may take days or even weeks, and for some parents attachment may never occur.

Parents in the NICU environment face physical and mechanical as well as psychologic and emotional obstacles during this difficult time. Miles and associates have developed a parental stressor scale for the parent with an infant in the NICU. Its purpose is to measure parental perceptions of stressors inherent to the NICU environment. This tool has found that an infant's appearance and experience of painful procedures, as well as the perceived severity of the child's illness, all contribute to the degree of stress experienced by parents (Miles & Brunssen, 2003; Franck et al, 2005). A nurse who can properly identify the specific stressors with each parent or family has the opportunity to assist them in reducing those stressors and promoting adaptation for the family unit (Callahan & Hynan, 2002).

BOX 25-3

Factors That Influence Family Reactions to a Child's Hospitalization or Illness

- Severity of the illness and the threat to the child
- Previous experience with illness or hospitalization (or both)
- Familiarity with the medical procedures involved in diagnosis and treatment
- Available support systems
- Coping strategies of family members
- Other family stresses
- Cultural or religious beliefs
- Communication patterns of family members

However, the nurse is still potentially the principal barrier to parenting in the NICU, because the nurse can be seen as the gatekeeper of the infant (Hegedus, 1999; Sudia-Robinson & Freeman, 2000). The baby must in every aspect belong to the family and not to the medical team. For parents to attach to their infant, a welcoming, calming environment in which they feel comfortable is essential in the NICU (Box 25-4). This kind of environment encourages parents in their primary caregiver role so they can develop skills to be advocates for their child. This advocacy is essential for the infant's continuing development, especially if the child has special needs (Franck et al 2005).

Mothers and fathers react to stress and grief in different ways (O'Shea & Timmins, 2002; Sydnor-Greenberg & Dokken, 2000). A father may become engrossed in his work and may not share his feelings with the mother. A father often tries to be strong for the mother and may become protective, shielding her from painful information (Hynan, 2005). The mother may view the husband's stoic behavior as cold and unfeeling. Both may have difficulty discussing the child because of guilt feelings. Normal postpartum blues can increase the mother's sensitivity and depression (Callahan & Hynan, 2002). She may cry for no real reason and feel embarrassed about irrational behavior. Existing weaknesses in a relationship may be magnified. Parents are separated at this time, and the fear may arise that their relationship will fall apart. Lack of communication can lead to isolation and feelings of resentment. Each may make assumptions about the other's feelings, resulting in misconceptions; these misconceptions, along with gender differences in coping, may continue for a lifetime if they are not recognized in this neonatal period, especially if the child has special needs or a developmental disability (Amankwaa, 2005; Heaman, 1995).

BOX 25-4

Creating a Welcoming Environment in the Hospital for Families

1. When the opportunity presents before the birth, prepare the family for the infant's admission to the neonatal intensive care unit and hospital course.
2. Give a special orientation for families who have undergone an emergency admission.
3. Provide for the needs of families who travel long distances.
4. Make fathers as welcome as mothers.
5. Meet the needs of siblings and other family members.
6. Enable families to be together as much as possible; have open visiting hours 24 hours a day.
7. Encourage families to bring things from home that make their child feel more at home.
8. Provide privacy for family visiting.
9. Encourage family participation in the child's care.
10. Help the family stay in touch with extended family members and support givers in the community; isolation at the hospital is not helpful for the continued growth of the family.

Adapted from Johnson BH (2003). Patient and family-centered care. In *AHA news*. Bethesda, MD: Institute of Family-Centered Care; Johnson BH (2004). Families are allies for enhancing quality, patient safety. In *AHA news*. Bethesda, MD: Institute of Family-Centered Care.

Other stressors in the family, such as the needs of other children, financial concerns, illness of family members, or marital stress, can complicate the situation (Doucette & Pinelli, 2004). For example, factors that can influence the degree of stress perceived by the family include the availability of appropriate emotional and psychologic support among family members and from friends and the availability and use of community resources (Pinelli, 2000). Maintaining a support system and using community resources and professional assistance are ways of dealing with the crisis. Coping abilities shown during previous crises often can predict how parents will cope with the current crisis. In an acute crisis, the family may be unable to use the resources available adequately because of lowered self-esteem, reduced family cohesiveness, and impaired family communication. Communication patterns could be impaired because of anger or emotion derived from the crisis situation (Sudia-Robinson & Freeman, 2000). Therefore, at times when the family may require outside assistance, they may be unable to use or maintain the community resources required (Patterson, 1995).

A stressful situation has a specific meaning for each family and for each member of the family because of previous experiences and the family's perceptions of their demands and capabilities. Certain personality types thrive on stress and deal effectively with any crisis. Others are unable to deal with even the smallest crisis. For example, if a family acknowledges a stressor as a "challenge" or can bestow meaning on the situation, such as believing that "it is the Lord's will," adaptation will be successful. Maladaptation results if the family interprets the stressor as threatening or undesirable. According to McCubbin and Patterson (1983), a stressful event has three levels of meaning within a family: the meaning of the stressful situation itself, the values inherent in the family identity, and the family's overall worldview (Patterson, 1995). The family's expectations for themselves and this new child affect parenting skills. The couple draws on childhood experience for parenting role models. The meaning the stressor has to the family also depends on the family's identity, cultural beliefs, and worldview. The family's identity comprises the values of the family, which are seen in the routines and rituals that develop in individual families. Stressors may disrupt these routines and rituals, threatening the development, maturation, and stability of the family system (Patterson, 1995). The family's worldview is based on how the family interprets reality, its core belief system (religious and cultural beliefs), and its purpose in life. The way a family handles its problems or deals with change often is based on the family identity and worldview. The family' worldview is the most stable of the three levels of meaning, but even it can be shattered by a severe crisis (Patterson, 1995).

The coping strategies are cognitive and behavioral components of the effort to handle the stressful event: that is, what the family "does" to handle the stress. These strategies can be emotion focused (i.e., strategies for controlling the emotions the crisis has engendered, such as denial or anger) or problem focused (i.e., action-oriented strategies to manage the crisis). Coping behaviors are learned, and families can use any or all of the major coping functions. Emotion-focused strategies are used mostly in the adjustment phase of a crisis, and problem-focused strategies are used more in the adaptation phase (Sudia-Robinson & Freeman, 2000; Doucette & Pinelli, 2004).

CULTURAL PERSPECTIVES

Definitions

Some key definitions are important to an understanding of cultural perspectives.

- Ethnicity: A common ancestry through which individuals have evolved shared values and customs.
- Culture: Socially inherited characteristics, such as rituals; the thoughts, beliefs, behavior patterns, and traits inherent within a certain racial, religious, or social group.
- Acculturation: Changing one's cultural patterns and assimilating behaviors consistent with those of the society in which one lives. This task can be done by learning the language, intermingling socially, or developing friendships, or through marriage or relationships formed in school or work places.
- Religion: A belief in divine powers; a system of beliefs, practices, and rituals.

The family has always been seen as the critical social unit for passing on beliefs and values in our society. Health care professionals must recognize and be sensitive to the influence of culture and ethnicity on a child's development and the family's response to illness or a chronic condition (Lipson et al, 1996). The family's cultural ties provide support and a sense of stability during times of upheaval and stress.

The meaning of family varies with the ethnic or cultural background of the family (Lipson et al, 1996). The concept of immediate family in Anglo-Americans means the nuclear family of mother, father, and children. For African American families, this usually means extended family within the community. For Italians, family means a very strongly knit group of family and friends extending over three or four generations. The Chinese family consists of all their ancestors and all their descendants. Understanding and appreciating the differences in cultures and ethnic groups can assist the health care professional in promoting the family's health and supporting the family in times of illness or debilitating conditions.

Ethnic or cultural groups differ in the meaning of illness and disability and in when they seek health care (Lipson et al, 1996). In general, Italians rely on the family for help when ill and seek medical help only as a last resort. They use words and emotion to convey the meaning of an experience to others. The close-knit family is of vital importance, and the nurse must respect the family as a cohesive unit. African Americans have an underlying distrust of the health care system. To effectively work with African American families, the nurse must help the family or empower the family to solve their own problems. Racism and oppression have left their marks on these families, and health care providers must enable the family to be the advocate for the ill child, to cope constructively with problems, and to deal with an unknown future if disabilities persist.

Some ethnic groups (e.g., Irish, African Americans, and Norwegians) consider illness to be the result of an individual's own sins, actions, or inadequacies. Native American Indians consider illness or disability the result of misconduct, for which the family is being punished (Lipson et al, 1996). The illness is part of the whole person. Native American Hawaiians view illness as an imbalance in the energy or harmony within the family. The illness is part of wellness, and this disharmony is a normal part of life. Anglo-Americans view illness as stemming from a scientific cause that is outside the family. The illness is foreign and intrusive to the individual and the family.

When a child is hospitalized, several important issues must be discussed with the family:

- What support the family wants
- Their preferences regarding language, food, holidays, religion, and kinship
- Their beliefs with regard to health, illness, and technologic advances
- Their health practices (e.g., immunizations, annual physical examinations)
- Their habits, customs, and rituals, which could affect their health

An understanding of family cultural differences can help the nurse provide care, determine the meaning of the illness or disability to the family, and assist the family in interventions appropriate to their culture. This understanding also shapes parent and staff expectations of each other and of the ways in which care is provided.

PARENT AND STAFF EXPECTATIONS

When parents have a sick infant in the NICU, they have expectations. They expect excellent medical and nursing care (Cescutti-Butler & Gavin, 2003). They expect accurate and timely information throughout their child's illness, and they expect to be involved in decision making about the infant's care (Ward, 2001). They expect this relationship that is developing will be a partnership and that the partnership will be honored in every interaction. The medical and nursing staff members, working as a team and supporting each other, have the ability to instill confidence in parents through this partnership. Parents develop advocacy skills through these types of communications with the nursing and medial team (Sudia-Robinson & Freeman, 2000).

Conversely, members of the medical and nursing staffs have expectations of the infants and families within this partnership related to the care of the infant. Expectations for the family may include visiting regularly, respecting the routines of the NICU setting, and sharing information that may be helpful in the care of the infant. Sometimes these expectations are unrealistic. For example, the staff may expect parents to visit more often, even though the parents live far from the hospital, have other children, must return to work, and have other responsibilities that may prevent more frequent visits (Franck & Spencer, 2003). Parents may also feel there is no role for them in the NICU if the partnership has not been established and the environment is not welcoming. Staff expectations for the infant may include wanting them to nipple-feed more often or be weaned from oxygen faster. It can be distressing to parents to think that the medical staff is not pleased with their infant's progress, even though this attitude may not be verbalized. For this reason, incongruities should be avoided both in actions and in communications of all types (Fenwick et al, 2000). It seems reasonable to assume that parents who are partners, well informed, and participating in the care are less likely to experience these issues (McGrath, 2005a).

Promoting Parenting in the Neonatal Intensive Care Unit

A major nursing goal in the NICU for care of the family is to optimize parenting skills and discharge an intact family unit. There are different ways to ease parental anxiety during the NICU experience. Open visiting policies, especially 24-hour visiting, provide the parents more opportunities to be with their infant while allowing them to deal with other responsibilities. Restricted visiting may imply that the staff is hiding details of the infant's condition. Unrestricted access to the infant allows the attachment and parenting processes to begin (Franck & Spencer, 2003).

One of the fundamentals of family-centered care is the belief that the family is an active member of the caregiving team right from admission. Members of the caregiving team are not visitors. They are not asked to leave for rounds or procedures. In many NICUs the practice of inviting family members to participate in medical rounds is being explored. Families are part of the decision-making process and as such are given information so that they can decide when they would like to be present and when they feel they would rather not be involved (Tait et al, 2001). They are involved in the assessment of and planning for their child (Simons et al, 2001). Caregiving issues related to scheduling, teaching of medical staff, and confidentiality for families are still unresolved and remain a concern for care providers (Ladd & Mercurio, 2003). However, for the most part, units where these practices are now common have found that the partnership between the family and the medical team is worth the effort required to implement such relationships. Providing for and facilitating the family's role as the constant in the child's life is the best approach for the child's long-term development. Critical pathways also are an excellent means of providing education and anticipatory guidance to parents and families, especially when teaching must be done over a long hospitalization or by several staff members.

Interventions with families must acknowledge the individuality of each of the members and of the family as a unit. Understanding that the needs of the whole are not equal to, greater than, or less than those of the parts is often a difficult concept for the neonatal nurse, who is involved more specifically with the care of the high-risk infant (Beveridge et al, 2001). Researchers repeatedly have found that hospital-based neonatal nurses view caring for families as not within their realm of practice (and certainly not the priority in their practice), but as something extra they do "when there is time." These views are not congruent with family-centered care practices and must be discarded (Saunders et al, 2003; Moore et al, 2003). However, this cannot happen without the support of the institution. Staffing plans that allow health care providers, especially nurses, time in their schedules to spend with families must be a priority if family-centered practices are truly fundamental to the care (Johnson, 2003, 2004).

Parents repeatedly have reported that they felt that health care professionals did not recognize them as the expert caregivers of their child and the constant in their child's life (Beveridge et al, 2001; Cescutti-Butler & Gavin 2003). This perception may lead to mistrust in the developing partnership between the caregivers and the professionals and may intensify the stress for the child and parent during the hospitalization (McGrath, 2001). Acknowledging that parents are the experts and nurses are the consultants to whom parents may come for information or support is a shift that is still difficult for some professionals (Johnson, 2003, 2004). Parents are empowered by nurses when they are respected, involved in the plan of care, provided with complete, unbiased information, and given a sense of control in the health care setting (Johnson, 2003, 2004; McGrath, 2001). Additional interventions that empower and support families include the following:

- Introducing the family to support systems in the form of families with children who are undergoing or have undergone similar experiences
- Providing the family with resources from the community (e.g., spiritual, economic, and social help, as well as information)
- Assisting the family in recognizing and using their strengths and coping skills or facilitating development of new coping strategies
- Encouraging the family to explore positive ways of coping with the situation
- Assisting the family to resolve guilt feelings

Critical pathways and caregiving protocols have been developed to aid in the organization and evaluation of nursing assessments and interventions with children and families. These pathways help promote continuity of care and aid the nurse in prioritizing the needs of the child and family. They are outcome oriented and provide an excellent means of documenting nurses' actions. They can be used to enhance interaction between parents and their preterm infant. The pathway serves as a means to educate parents about the changing needs of their developing preterm infant. Implementation of the pathway increases parents' knowledge and responsiveness to their infant's behavior and helps parents develop independent, cue-based caregiving skills with their infant. Other pathways have been developed with five areas of emphasis: environmental organization, the structure of caring and feeding (all of which relate more to the infant), and family involvement and education (which relate more to the needs of the family). Outcomes for infants include physiologic stability, behavioral organization, and establishing predictable behavioral patterns; outcomes for the family include enhancing social support, increasing knowledge, and increasing involvement in the infant's care while preparing for discharge. Critical pathways also are an excellent means of providing education and anticipatory guidance to parents and families, especially when teaching must be done over a long hospitalization or by several staff members.

Family conferences can be used to evaluate the intervention strategies and how well they were able to meet the family's goals. Collaboration during conferences allows all present the opportunity to examine individual perspectives and goals while negotiating and reevaluating strategies to increase satisfaction with the treatment plan (Partridge et al, 2005). The type of information communicated is also an important consideration. Health care professionals have often provided families with a lot of information about their infant in the here and now; what is sometimes missing is the "so what" of that information. The result of this type of communication is that parents are not always provided with all the information they needed to understand the whole situation for their child now and in the future so that appropriate participation in decision making can occur (McGrath, 2005a; Sudia-Robinson & Freeman, 2000).

The attachment process begins at birth. With a sick or premature infant, this process is delayed until the parents can establish eye contact with and begin touching their infant. Bonding and attachment are enhanced by allowing the parents to touch and hold the infant as soon as the child's condition allows. The preterm neonate's physical appearance, disorganized behavioral responses, and variable physiologic response to touch can cause much anxiety in the parents as they attempt to interact with their infant. However, it is important that the bedside nurse, who is well versed in what the sick or premature infant will tolerate, explain those maturational limitations to the parents. It is vital that parents understand an infant's immaturity and inability to respond or to tolerate eye contact or parental voice cues; otherwise parents may misinterpret cues or detach from their infant. It also is important for the nurse to work with the parents to help them to recognize an infant's distress signals (e.g., hiccups, apnea, cyanosis, bradycardia, or mottling) so that parents can gauge their interactions by their infant's behavior.

A quiet, comforting atmosphere with low lighting helps calm both the infants and their families (Chapter 24). External stimuli in the NICU must be controlled; unnecessary stimuli aggravate these infants' already overwhelmed immature nervous systems, and loud monitor alarms and excessive staff noise can be upsetting and unnerving to parents (McGrath, 2000). Jamsa and Jamsa (1998) found that parents in the NICU felt that the technologic environment was frightening and that it delayed their ability to parent their children. In general, the equipment made the families feel like outsiders. Their discomfort inhibited interaction with their child and delayed their participation in caregiving. These researchers suggested changes in the technology of the NICU, such as use of different kinds of alarm signals with diminished volume; wireless, handheld information terminals; and remote monitoring. Some of this technology already is appearing in the NICU. The technology used in the NICU must be continually reevaluated and designed with a parent- and consumer-based perspective (McGrath, 2000). Achieving a balance between the high-technology environment and the need of parents to touch their infant frequently helps foster parental self-confidence. This balance must be a priority for the neonatal nurse.

Recommendations for single rooms in the NICU and other acute care areas through-out the hospital setting are now included in the 2006 Guidelines for the Design and Construction of Hospital and Healthcare Facilities (http://www.aia.org/aah_gd_hospcons). These guidelines are based on several significant research studies where single rooms throughout the health care setting were found to offer higher occupancy rates, reduced transfer costs, and reduced labor costs, even when the cost of new construction was calculated into the equation. In addition, hospital-acquired infection and medication error were reduced in these settings. Most patients and families also report better communication with health care professionals in single rooms because the provider often spends more time, answers questions more thoroughly, and is more compassionate and caring. Last, patient length of stay has been documented to be shorter in private single rooms, which again adds to the decrease in costs (please see the guidelines for more information about this research). This movement to single rooms in the hospital setting is also important for compliance with the patient and family privacy requirements under the Health Insurance Portability and Accountability Act (HIPAA) of 2003, which includes speech privacy rulings.

So how do these guidelines affect the NICU? There is little research directly related to the effects of neonatal single-room design. Most units across the United States have always been equipped with a few isolation rooms that have been used for infants with highly infectious diseases and, more recently, to isolate extremely-low-birth-weight (ELBW) preterm infants

who appear to be most overstimulated by the big open room environment of the NICU. With new construction, and a greater emphasis on individualized family-centered developmentally supportive care, more units have added more of these single rooms, and some units have chosen to move to an entirely single-room design (McGrath, 2005b). Research to support a less stressful NICU environment with lower lights and less noise and activity has demonstrated shorter lengths of stay, decreased iatrogenic effects, and increased deep sleep and alerting behaviors in the infant, which may provide greater opportunities for more normal cognitive development (Saunders et al, 2003). Moreover, in changing the environment to meet the needs of infants and families, the less stressful environment is often times more positive for caregivers and should have a positive impact on patient outcomes and a decrease in medication errors. The challenge in providing care in these designs is finding a balance between the needs of infants, families, and caregivers in the NICU. This may be best achieved in a single-room design, where areas in the unit can be designed to meet the needs of those who use them most and yet allow others to adjust their individualized areas or rooms to meet their needs (Bowie et al, 2003). Evidence-based design standards for the NICU do exist and should be considered with any remodeling or new construction project (White et al, 2002). These guidelines should be used as a standard, especially when data are needed to support the need to invest upfront in more space, better traffic patterns, multiple kinds of lighting, and noise reduction materials. Paying attention to design is especially important for vulnerable infants who are at risk to develop disabilities. Research data also exist and should be used to support the need to choose colors and textures that increase health and well-being for all who interface in health care settings. For staff to transition to and work with ease in single-room designs, they must have access and become comfortable with central monitoring and communication systems that provide them knowledge about patient status even from remote locations. Work areas for nurses must also be near the private rooms and allow for interaction and teamwork among staff. More research is needed in this area and should be a focus for the future.

Parent participation in the caregiving must begin at admission. Soothing touch, providing containment, gentle infant massage, holding the infant, bathing, and skin-to-skin holding, or "kangaroo care," are just a few of the "high-touch" avenues for promoting parenting in the NICU. Each of these tasks should be provided and reserved for families to implement with their infant. (For more information on environmental factors and how they affect neonatal development, see Chapter 24.) When parents are providing these interventions there are physiologic and behavioral benefits for the infant as well as benefits to parents, including early bonding, increased confidence in parenting skills, and a sense of control; parents begin to have a sense of confidence that their infant is well cared for and may survive (Just, 2005; Prentice & Stainton, 2004).

Staff members may resist including families in these interventions because of the degree of risk to the infant. Nurses must also take into consideration that these short-term physiologic losses for the infant might outweigh the long-term gains for the family and make a decision with the family that is in the best interest of the infant. Established protocols and education of both staff members and parents help with the transition to increased parental participation in the NICU (Just, 2005; Ward, 2001). If the infant is transported from another facility or being transferred to another hospital, parents need time to be with their infant prior to the move and should go on the transport with the infant whenever possible. These brief interactions reduce inaccurate fantasies about the neonate, and promote bonding and attachment behaviors (Evans & Madsen, 2005). Occasionally, the mother's condition is unstable and she or a family member cannot visit the NICU. Instant pictures can be taken and given to the mother as soon as possible.

Throughout the infant's illness, parents need accurate, timely information about their child's condition (Box 25-5). Loo and associates (2003) view parent learning as a process where parents focus on information that is provided when it is timely to the current needs of their infant. If the information provided is not timely and does not anticipate the needs of the parents as related to their relationship with their infant, it may not be helpful and may actually hamper the care (Sudia-Robinson & Freeman, 2000). That information should be direct and honest and should not be contradictory. Parents also appreciate the use of drawings and diagrams when their infant's condition is explained to them, and they appreciate being encouraged by staff members to ask questions. Presenting this information with some optimism allows the family some hope. Ideally, the information should be presented to both parents at the same time. It should be expressed in simple terms with short explanations. The parents are under much stress, and this information may be unfamiliar. Facts may have to be repeated several times before they are absorbed. Parents need a clear understanding of the information provided to make informed decisions about their infant's care. Family-friendly language in understandable terms should be used when delivering care and information. Medical information from a primary caregiver, such as a neonatal nurse practitioner or primary physician, provides consistency, especially when the news is difficult or "bad" (Box 25-6). Families also need information about visiting hours, unit policies, equipment, procedures, and treatments

---

BOX 25-5

Guidelines for Providing Information to Families of Ill Infants

Focus the teaching session so as to build confidence and foster independence in the family.

1. Begin by assessing what the family members already know.
2. Establish a working rapport with the family; work to ease their anxiety and fear and to convey confidence and assurance to family members.
3. Ask family members what they expect to learn from the session and provide information directed toward their concerns.
4. Initially, focus teaching on the diagnosis or current crisis.
5. Use language the family understands; avoid jargon.
6. Include the key characteristics of the plan of care and treatment.
7. Explain the ways in which the illness or medication regimen will affect daily life.
8. Use a variety of teaching materials and styles. All information should be provided orally and reinforced with handouts to be taken home.
9. Keep the information simple and concrete; reinforce oral communication with handouts. Expect to repeat the information and do so readily.
10. Avoid fear tactics but provide information on both benefits and detrimental effects.
11. Use praise to instill confidence.
12. Include anticipatory guidance.

BOX 25-6

Providing Difficult Information

Although difficult information most often is provided by physicians, nurses often are part of the team, especially if the information will be painful to the family. Nurses must know how to support families in these difficult situations.

1. Develop a therapeutic relationship with parents before the need to deliver difficult information and explore what families already know about the status of the infant or diagnosis.
2. Provide unbiased information that is clear, direct, detailed, and understandable; during the discussion, get to the point quickly.
3. Provide the information with compassion and caring in a gentle but confident style; a private, quiet place free of distractions should be used for the discussion.
4. Personalize the information to this baby or child and this family.
5. Allow the family time to express feelings and ask questions, and provide support for those feelings and questions.
6. Provide information about resources and anticipatory guidance. Explain risks in several ways. Provide meaningful statistics or ratios to support the explanations. Draw pictures whenever possible.
7. Arrange an opportunity for the family to meet another family with a child with a similar diagnosis or who has experienced a similar situation or crisis.
8. Be prepared for emotional responses. Allow for tears and outbreaks. If parents need to vent, they should be able to do so in a safe place. If need be, offer to discuss issues at another time.
9. Establish a plan for next actions, including the next interaction with the family; regularly scheduled meetings are helpful.
10. After the interaction, document the exchange, noting what information was imparted, how it was received, what decisions were made or were not made, and the time that you plan to speak again with the family. Engage in self-reflection about your feelings and reactions to the interaction. What could be improved and what needs to be continued? Difficult information is often not the messenger's fault, and fault and blame should be put aside.

Data from McGrath JM (2005). Partnerships with families: a foundation to support them in difficult times. *Journal of perinatal and neonatal nursing* 19(2):94-96.

their infant is receiving. Direct telephone access allows an update from their nurse or physician at all times. After oral communication, written information helps parents remember important facts and a place to refer back to when the information is more relevant to the care of the infant.

Many times the neonatal intensive care hospitalization is the beginning of chronicity for the infant and the family. Parenting a chronically ill child is qualitatively different from parenting a normal child. Nurses must promote the parents' and family's role as the caregiver for the child by determining the family's mode of coping and supporting those strategies while promoting family adaptation to the chronic illness. A major goal of care for these families is to integrate the child back into the family unit rather than making the child with a chronic illness a "special nucleus" that becomes the only priority or focus of family needs.

Family-centered care of an infant or child with any chronic illness is based on the premise that the family is the main source of support and caregiving for the child. Thus family-centered care can be achieved through specific nursing strategies aimed at creating opportunities for families to use their own strengths and abilities to meet their child's and family's needs. Ultimately, family-centered interventions empower families to develop and maintain healthy lifestyles, leading to overall improvement of the family's quality of life.

The number of nursing or medical personnel in nondescript surgical scrub outfits who interact with the parents can be overwhelming. Therefore introductions by name and position are important to families, and personnel should wear name tags to help further identify each staff member. Many institutions have adopted the primary nursing concept. Families often feel more secure knowing that one nurse or team of nurses direct their baby's nursing care throughout the hospitalization, and this allows a trusting, collaborative relationship to be established (Box 25-7). A friendly approach opens communication and demonstrates openness and approachability.

Using language that invites participation also is important (Box 25-8). The primary nurse can act as liaison between the family and the health care team. The liaison ensures that information about the infant's current condition, any changes in condition, and long-term outcomes for the infant are communicated to the family. The liaison role becomes essential if the infant is transported back to a community hospital or to another unit in the same facility (Evans & Madsen, 2005). Parents need to know what to expect in the new unit and to understand how this environment is now actually better suited to meet the changing needs of their infant. Otherwise, parental mistrust may develop (Evans & Madsen, 2005; McGrath, 2001).

Staff members' attitudes are an important part of the development of positive parenting (Box 25-9). Staff behaviors and attitudes can inhibit or encourage parenting skills. Conflict about parenting roles can exist between parents and staff members, and this conflict may escalate into a struggle for control. Parents may view the staff members as acting as the infant's parents or the infant as belonging to the staff because staff members provide most of the care (Cescutti-Butler & Gavin, 2003). The staff members' pet names for the neonate further reinforce parents' fears. Nursing staff can help the family by encouraging them to personalize the infant's care and then following their lead with naming and dressing. Bringing in clothes, toys, and pictures of other family members and

---

BOX 25-7

Principles of Family-Professional Collaboration

Family-professional collaboration accomplishes the following:

- Promotes a relationship in which family members and professionals work together to ensure the best services for the child and family.
- Recognizes and respects the knowledge, skills, and experience that families and professionals bring to the relationship.
- Acknowledges that the development of trust is an integral part of a collaborative relationship.
- Facilitates open communication so that families and professionals feel free to express themselves.
- Creates an atmosphere in which the cultural traditions, values, and diversity of families are acknowledged and honored.
- Recognizes that negotiation is essential in a collaborative relationship.
- Brings to the relationship the mutual commitment of families, professionals, and communities to meet the requirements of children with special health needs and their families.

Modified from Bishop KK et al (1993). *Family-professional collaboration for children with special health care needs and their families.* Burlington, VT: Department of Social Work, University of Vermont.

BOX 25-8

Language That Facilitates Collaboration

"Do you prefer us to call you by your first name or your last name?"

"Here's what I'm thinking, but I'm wondering how this will work for you."

"Tell me, how can I help you?"

"Our institution usually does _____ this way. Would that work for you?"

"These are the things I plan to do for your child today. Would you like to do some of these activities?"

"What goals do you have for your child's care?"

"How does your child look to you today?"

"Do you have any questions or suggestions about your child's care?"

"This sounds important; help me understand your concern."

"Who would you like to have included in discussions about your child's care?"

"Let's talk about how much you want to be consulted."

Modified from Fialka J (1994). You can make a difference in our lives. *Early on Michigan* 3(4):6-7, 11; and Curley MA (1988). Effects of the nursing mutual participation model of care on parental stress in the pediatric intensive care unit. *Heart lung* 17(6):682-688.

---

making cassette tapes of family voices are ways parents contribute to caretaking.

Nurses who care for families need to provide support and promote the family as a unit; however, overinvolvement of nurses can be detrimental to the family unit. Establishing appropriate relationships with families in our care can

---

BOX 25-9

Key Content of Family-Centered Training Programs

- Principles of family-centered care
- Cultural competence
- Child development
- Family systems
- Communication with children and families
- Building of collaborative relationships with families
- Support for and strengthening of families in their caregiving roles
- Impact of hospitalization, illness, and injury on children and families, including the impact of health care costs on family resources
- Support for the developmental and psychosocial needs of children and families through hospital policies and programs
- Function and expertise of each discipline in the medical setting
- Multidisciplinary collaboration and team building
- Ethical issues and decision making
- Community resources for children and families

From the Association for the Care of Children's Health (ACCH), 19 Mantua Road, Mount Royal, NJ 08061; and Johnson BH et al (1992). *Caring for children and families: guidelines for hospitals.* Bethesda, MD: ACCH.

BOX 25-10

Nurse Behaviors That May Become Barriers to Positive Parenting

- Infant "belongs" to the nurse and the NICU rather than to the family; nurse refers to assignments or primaries as "my babies."
- Family is not considered a member of the caregiving team; for example, they are asked to leave for rounds and shift report.
- Family is not asked about the characteristics of their infant or included in discussions related the infant. Families are not seen as the expert about their infant. They are talked about rather than talked with.
- Care is task oriented, and staffing is acuity based rather than based on meeting the needs of families. Families are not invited to participate in the child's care.
- Infant's schedule belongs to the nurse and the NICU rather than to the family, so that feeding and caregiving might occur when the family is unavailable to participate. Scheduling is inflexible.
- Family is seen as an adjunct to the infant and his or her care. They are not the client or patient. Spending time with families is not considered a priority but rather a luxury. Spending time with families is not seen as essential to providing care for the infant.

---

sometimes be difficult. It is necessary to identify inappropriate nursing behaviors and correct them. Educating the nursing staff about the parenting process facilitates identification of inappropriate nursing behaviors (Box 25-10). The education can be initiated during orientation of new staff members and reinforced at intervals with continuing education workshops on the subject. Nurses must provide support while always acknowledging the boundaries of the family. Some families build walls and are so private about family matters that it is difficult to obtain enough information to meet family needs, whereas other families become overly dependent on the nursing staff, needing their support at every moment. Interventions that promote independent family decision making include the following (Johnson, 2003, 2004):

- Respecting the family as a unique unit
- Providing unbiased care to all families
- Providing as much continuity in care provider as possible to promote family strengths
- Allowing the family to determine the implementation of the plan of care

With adequate staffing, nurses can promote parenting in the NICU. Overworked nurses can become frustrated and stressed, overwhelmed by their own anxieties. These feelings may impede their ability to interact calmly and therapeutically with a fragile family unit. Nursing management considerations should include provision for adequate staffing to allow nurses the time and emotional energy to meet the needs of parents in crisis. Patient assignments should be evaluated not only for the technical care an infant requires but also for the psychosocial demands of the family. Institutional policies should be carefully evaluated as to how they meet the needs of families (Figure 25-1).

Caretaking is a normal part of parenting. However, parents of sick or premature infants have been deprived of the time to prepare psychologically and to develop their caretaking skills (Just, 2005). If nurses do not allow the family to become involved in caretaking tasks, parents may feel inadequate or may resent the nurses. Positive reinforcement builds self-confidence in parenting abilities (Figure 25-2). As the nurse prepares the parents for their infant's discharge from the NICU, it is important that the parents feel prepared to care for their infant. Nurses can use several key techniques to prepare parents for working with their infant and the technology in the NICU:

- Give constructive criticism.
- Encourage parents to discuss their concerns and emotions.
- Provide parents with information specific to their infant's care or condition.
- Clarify information that parents have received through other channels.
- Draw the parents' attention to positive points about their infant, including how the child responds to the parents.
- Keep the channels of communication open by remaining nonjudgmental.

Parents can be given one last boost in confidence by allowing them to room in with sick newborns before discharge. Parents feel secure knowing that nurses are close by if they are needed. This process also allows parents the assurance that they can care for their babies adequately.

Parent networking can be a vital tool for promoting parenting. Knowing that other families have survived this crisis can be reassuring. Support groups generally are helpful; however,

Checklist for Family-Centered Care in Neonatal and Pediatric Critical Care Units

This checklist can be used by hospital administrators, care providers, and families to plan or evaluate policies, programs, and practices in critical care settings.

Environment and Design
- Are families' first impressions of the unit positive?
- Do the environment and design say that this is a caring place, a place for children and families?
- Are inappropriate, overwhelming stimuli minimized?
- Are maximum efforts made to control noise?
- Is the lighting comfortable for babies, children, and care providers?
- Does the lighting encourage normal diurnal rhythms?
- Is adequate, accessible work space available around the baby or child to allow staff members to provide care efficiently?
- Is a comfortable space available around the baby or child for families to provide care and nurturing?
- Is private space available for families (for day-to-day interactions, special situations, and meetings with health professionals)?
- Are families encouraged to make their baby's or child's immediate environment as homelike as possible?
- Are telephones, restrooms with diaper changing areas, breast-feeding rooms, water fountains, and food services nearby and easy to find?
- Are secure places available for families to hang coats and store other personal belongings such as purses, boots, and umbrellas?
- Is a comfortable space available near the unit in which the parents can sleep?
- Are space and support available for families to learn and practice new caregiving skills?
- Are there separate corridors for transporting critically ill children?

Patterns of Care
- Is care consistent and predictable?
- Do staffing patterns promote consistency and predictability of care?
- Does each child and family have a single, identified care coordinator?
- Are contributions from different disciplines coordinated and integrated into the care plan?
- Are care procedures and treatments planned to cluster and minimize unpleasant disturbances?
- Are measures taken to reduce the frequency and duration of painful treatments and procedures?
- Are pleasurable experiences routinely integrated into care?
- Are promoting and supporting family-child relationships seen as essential care practices?
- Are procedures in place to ensure smooth transitions from the unit to other settings, including home or home care or community services?

Family-Professional Partnerships
- Do staff members interact respectfully with *all* families?
- Do staff members view all families as having strengths and competencies?
- Are families who have experienced the unit involved in developing and evaluating the unit's policies, programs, and practices?
- Do unit practices promote parent-professional collaboration, beginning at the time of admission?
- Are families supported as full members of the health care team?
- Are all members of the team fully aware and respectful of the role the family has chosen on the team?
- Are the roles of the other team members clear to the family?
- Are families satisfied with the ways in which they are involved in decision making about their infant's or child's care?
- Are disputes between staff members and parents resolved in a positive and supportive manner?
- Is an ethics committee available to families and staff members?

Child and Family Support
- Does the unit define family in an inclusive way that incorporates all those who are most important in the child's life?
- Is the family encouraged to define itself?
- Is affordable temporary housing for families available near the hospital?
- Is financial support available (e.g., for parking, transportation, and lodging) to help families visit the hospital or stay nearby?
- Is the unit welcoming to parents 24 hours a day? To those in the parents' support network?
- Are visiting policies and practices supportive of children and families?
- Is staff or volunteer support available to ensure that visits by brothers and sisters and extended family members are positive experiences?
- Are translators and interpreters available for families who do not speak English or that use sign language?
- Are parents of newborns supported in their nurturing and caregiving roles?
- Are mothers who are hospitalized on another unit or in another hospital fully supported and kept informed about their baby?
- Are fathers and other men in fathering roles specifically supported and encouraged as partners in care?
- Is teaching parents about their baby's uniqueness and development an integral part of care?
- Are families encouraged to see positive physical and developmental progress in their baby or child and to celebrate milestones?
- Are opportunities facilitated for parent groups and for family-to-family support?
- Are a parent group and a family-to-family support group associated with the unit?
- Are referrals to such groups made on a regular basis?
- Is the NICU or PICU linked to a family-to-family support group in the community?
- Are children and families provided information and educational resources on topics of interest to them?
- Are written materials available in a language the family understands?
- Are materials for families written at a reading level no higher than a newspaper (about fifth grade)?
- Are audiovisual and other media available for families who cannot read?
- Are physical, emotional, and spiritual supports available to families to aid them in dealing with the intense feelings associated with having an infant or child in critical care?
- Are developmental specialists and staff members trained in family support regularly included on each child's health care team?

FIGURE **25-1**
Checklist for assessing family-centered care provided in neonatal and pediatric critical care units. From Hanson JT et al (1997). *Family-centered care: changing practice, changing attitudes.* Bethesda, MD: Institute for Family-Centered Care.

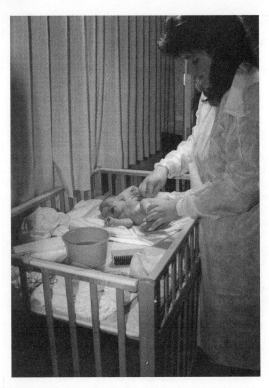

FIGURE **25-2**
Participation in infant care promotes self-confidence and supports the development of parenting skills.

they are not appropriate for every situation (Carvajal, 2002). Some couples need counseling so they can feel more comfortable with decision making and participation in care (Partridge et al, 2005). The primary nurse plays a key role in assessing signs that the family is not coping and needs therapeutic counseling. Support groups or counseling helps families look at problems objectively and learn alternative behavior for adaptive coping. The nurse also can assist parents in identifying additional means of support. Ideally, parents should be permitted to define their "family" as needed to provide support during this crisis, allowing family members to visit as unit policy dictates. Grandparents, extended family, neighbors, and friends may constitute this group.

Grandparents may be a source of support in some instances. They may be forced into an uncomfortable role by seeing their own child in pain without a way to relieve that pain. Grandparents may also relive their own birthing experiences, which may result in associated anxieties and prevent them from providing support for the parents. Extended family members may be more helpful if discord exists between grandparents and the nuclear family.

Friends of the family can be an asset if they are effective listeners. They can offer to provide transportation for the mother and child care for brothers and sisters, or they can take over meal preparation and housekeeping chores to help alleviate family responsibilities. Just having someone to make telephone calls to other friends and family to update them on the infant's condition can be a great relief for the family.

Social workers involved early in the hospital stay provide parents with an objective person and contact with community resources. Families are reluctant to express dissatisfaction with

their child's care to nurses. Social workers can help parents express concerns without fear of retaliation against their child. Clergy provide spiritual support for a family. Families often turn to religion for comfort and support at a time of crisis. It is important to offer parents privacy with the clergy to exercise their religious freedom.

SIBLINGS

Siblings have needs, because they are an important part of the new infant's life. Sibling visits may help relieve anxieties and make the birth a reality. Siblings have a variety of responses to a newborn's arrival in the home, especially after a lengthy hospitalization. Family routines are disrupted by a "normal" birth and are further disturbed by an admission to the NICU and then again at the time of discharge. Siblings may feel displaced while parents are visiting the ill infant. Siblings often are left with baby-sitters when they have rarely had experience with caretakers outside the immediate family. Fathers who may be uncertain about their family role may embrace their familiar work role and spend more time on the job. In these ways routines are disrupted, and parents are less available for their other children. These feelings may result in a variety of acting-out experiences. An example of a family's response to the homecoming of a new brother who had been in the NICU is presented in Box 25-11.

The birth of a new baby precipitates a family upheaval and the need for realignment of relationships and positions within the family constellation. Becoming a sibling is known to be a stressful or "crisis" experience for young children and can have an effect on their mental, emotional, and social development. The birth of a preterm or critically ill neonate who requires intensive care constitutes a further crisis for parents and consequently disrupts the equilibrium of the family system (Munch & Levick, 2001). Parents are reported to experience feelings of anxiety, grief, fear, anger, and guilt in response to the unanticipated events. Siblings are also affected and may experience helplessness, powerlessness, guilt, and anger in addition to the disruption of their daily routines and separation from their parents. The siblings may feel very alone because their worried parents are preoccupied with the newborn baby. Siblings feel like the forgotten family member at the very time they need attention most (Munch & Levick, 2001).

Addressing the needs of families of hospitalized patients has gained acceptance and support among nurses since the advent of the concept of family-centered care (Johnson, 2003, 2004). All members of the family, parents and siblings, may exhaust their coping strategies and feel unsupported by those who are usually available emotionally and physically. The philosophy of family-centered care in the NICU is reported to encourage not only parent participation but also involvement of the well sibling or siblings in the family process. This involvement allows children to see their new sibling and to feel as if they are a part of the family process. Feelings of isolation may engender fantasies about what is taking place in the NICU. At any age, it is easier to cope with reality than with what can be imagined.

Increasing numbers of hospitals are allowing the participation of children at a sibling's birth, sibling contact with the infant at birth, sibling contact with the infant on the postpartum unit, and sibling visiting in intensive care nurseries. For nurses facing these challenges, the philosophy of family-centered care can provide a firm foundation in striving toward

BOX 25-11

Example of a Sibling Response to an Infant's Homecoming

John Jones was born at 33 weeks' gestation. The nurses described him as a typical preemie with respiratory distress syndrome (RDS) and intermittent apnea and bradycardia. He required continuous positive airway pressure (CPAP) for several days and then hood oxygen for a week. After being weaned to room air, he was moved to the transitional nursery, where he stayed for another week until he mastered sucking, swallowing, and breathing. John's mother visited often. Mrs. Jones kept John supplied with breast milk and the latest drawings from his two sisters, Suzie, age 6, and Becky, age 4. John's father visited once in a while on his way home from work but did not take an active role in caretaking. He said that he was afraid to hold John but that he would once John got bigger and stronger. John was a cuddly little guy who had an uneventful recovery and was discharged after 3 weeks in the NICU.

Several days before discharge, John's mother confided in his primary nurse that she was about at the end of her rope because her husband was working longer hours and her daughters were acting up in ways they never had before. Becky had demonstrated regression behaviors of bed-wetting and thumb-sucking. She had also started carrying around her "blankie" again, something she had stopped doing long ago. Becky was particularly close to her mother, and after her mother's daily visit to the NICU, Becky would hit her mother, crying, "I hate you! I wish the baby would go away!" Mrs. Jones said that when she tried to console Becky, the child ran and hid under her bed, crying, "Leave me alone! You only love that baby!" If that weren't bad enough, Suzie had begun waking up with stomachaches and refusing to go to school. Suzie had always loved her teacher and classmates and now was frequently in trouble for misbehaving in class. When Mrs. Jones would make Suzie go to school, the little girl would cry and say, "I hate that baby! I'd like to run over him with Daddy's car!" Mr. Jones had withdrawn from family life and was spending long hours at work. Mrs. Jones was beside herself.

How might the nurse counsel Mrs. Jones? What three strategies could be used to help her deal with her daughters?

her husband? and her own needs? Would a visit to the NICU for the girls be helpful at this time? How might the nurse and Mrs. Jones encourage greater involvement in the care of the children from Mr. Jones? Would a meeting before discharge be helpful to these parents? What should be discussed at this meeting and who should be included? In addition to the support group in the community, would connecting this mother to another mother in the NICU in a similar situation be helpful to this mother? How and why?

The nurse was able to reassure Mrs. Jones that the behaviors of her husband and daughters were typical. Although this reassurance didn't immediately alter the situation, at least Mrs. Jones knew that many families respond to NICU hospitalization in this way and that, given time, the family would reestablish equilibrium. Mrs. Jones was encouraged to take the weekend off from her NICU visiting routine. She was able to spend a couple of special days with her daughters and engage her husband in life outside the worries of the NICU.

However, this did not provide Mrs. Jones with emotional support or help with her feelings of being overwhelmed and depressed. The nurse was able to listen to her concerns and then put her in touch with a parent organization that had been formed to help support families through the transition home. The parent organization offered peer support from parents who had been through the experience. They were also able to help Mrs. Jones place the experience in its proper perspective.

The girls had enjoyed their weekend with their mother and were in a better frame of mind for the homecoming. Peer support helped Mrs. Jones so that she could in turn be available to her family. John was about ready for discharge and had progressed normally. Once John was home, Mrs. Jones included the girls in the baby's routine as much as possible by asking them to get his diapers and having them feed their dollies while she fed John. Suzie brought pictures of John to school for show and tell, and after Mrs. Jones called to speak to the teacher to explain the disruptions at home, Suzie gradually quit misbehaving. Becky continued to have problems with thumb-sucking and bed-wetting for several months while John was incorporated into the family and while a new family routine was established.

---

excellence in the practice of caring for children and families (Ahmann et al, 2003). The development of a sibling-infant bond is vital to establishing and enhancing the relationship within the family unit. Holistic care surrounding childbirth may set up patterns or pathways that dramatically affect subsequent family interactions.

Sibling Visitation to the NICU

Sibling visitation in the hospital after the delivery of a newborn has become common practice. However, limited recent research exists that examines the consequences of permitting and prohibiting sibling visits in the NICU despite the argument that sibling involvement is consistent with the concept of family-centered perinatal care. Early studies of NICU sibling visitation programs provided valuable descriptive data on siblings' responses to the sick neonate. NICU visits provided an opportunity for the older brother or sister to see, touch, and

talk to the newborn. This exposure was reported to help the children integrate the reality of the experience, to prepare for the possible loss of the newborn, and in some cases to reverse regressive behavior that had begun during the newborn's hospitalization. However, the findings of these studies reflected the perceptions of providers and not necessarily those of the parents or siblings. More research is needed in this area. Some NICUs restrict sibling visitation during RSV season, some do not have a strict policy for how visiting might still occur during this time of the year. Again, more research is needed in this area. (Refer to the Evolve website for more on this topic.) *evolve*

Implications for Practice

Nurses have a unique opportunity to support the development of positive sibling relationships in the NICU environment. Evolving models of comprehensive care no longer overlook or delegate the care and needs of the whole family. Research on the families of NICU neonates has demonstrated parents' desire for a family-centered approach to care. Siblings are an integral part of any family, and their adjustment or lack of adjustment to the birth of a newborn greatly affects the well-being of the whole family. Siblings' adjustment to the once-sick infant needs further exploration.

When the birth of a sibling is further complicated by the baby's being ill or at risk, professionals caring for the baby are in a position to reassure parents that siblings will respond to the neonate in various ways based on each child's personality, age, and interests. Professional reassurance can help parents realize that siblings cannot help feeling angry and displaced by the baby. The parents' ability to accept their older children's competitive feelings and yet continue to love them helps those children to integrate ambivalence. Support through this ambivalence facilitates acceptance of the baby and the baby's incorporation into the family.

Increasing parents' knowledge about promoting positive sibling relationships through parent education programs may influence the parents' attitudes, thereby enhancing the future sibling relationship. In response to consumer demand, many hospitals have implemented sibling visitation and educational programs. This preparation can help siblings deal with the realities of the experience. Special attention from the NICU staff also can help siblings feel recognized, supported, and appreciated during this time of stress. Encouraging the sibling to gently touch and talk to the infant and allowing gifts of toys or even a drawing of themselves to be kept with the baby are activities that may foster attachment and growing connection with the newborn.

The death of a sibling usually has profound and lasting effects on surviving children. Surviving siblings, however young, may need some evidence that the baby existed; a visit to see the ill newborn in the incubator, a photograph, or a chance to participate in the funeral. Regardless of the child's age, it seems that the level of care offered to these siblings is crucial to determining the psychologic and life adjustment of the bereaved child. Nurses need to be alert to the range and depth of childhood reactions.

Many of the research findings discussed here can serve as invaluable guides to help NICU nurses promote and facilitate effective sibling interactions and positive involvement between the sick neonate and the siblings. An appropriate environment in which nurses can assist children in coping with the profound changes that affect the sibling bond should also be provided, because such efforts help siblings fully integrate this major event into their young lives.

SUMMARY

The birth of any infant produces tremendous change in the lives of each member of the family. Normal adaptation can be complicated by the birth of a premature, critically ill infant or one with congenital anomalies. If the family does not have adequate coping strategies or resources, this crisis could produce much role stress and strain, which ultimately can weaken or destroy the family unit. The nurse plays an integral role in guiding the family to appropriate resources and support services. By promoting adaptive rather than maladaptive roles, the nurse can ensure an intact family unit after the crisis (Figure 25-3).

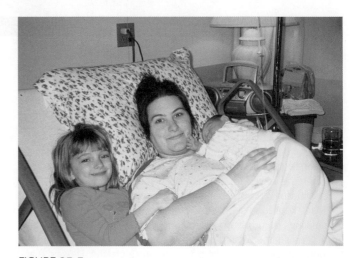

FIGURE **25-3**
The ultimate goal of the nurse is to ensure the integration of the infant into the changing family unit.

REFERENCES

Ahmann E et al (2003). *Changing the concept of families as visitors: supporting the presence and participation of families*. Bethesda, MD: Institute of Family-Centered Care.

Aita M, Snider L (2003). The art of developmental care in the NICU: a concept analysis. *Journal of advanced nursing* 41(3):223-232.

Amankwaa LC (2005). Maternal postpartum collapse as a theory of postpartum depression. *Qualitative report* 10(1):21-38.

Beveridge J et al (2001). Family-centered care in the NICU. *Canadian nurse* 97(3):14-18.

Bowie BH et al (2003). Single-room infant care: future trends in special care nursery planning and design. *Neonatal network* 22(4):27-34.

Brazy JE et al (2001). How parents of premature infants gather information and obtain support. *Neonatal network* 20:41-48.

Bruns DA, McCollum JA (2002). Partnerships between mothers and professionals in the NICU: caregiving, information exchange, and relationships. *Neonatal network* 21:15-23.

Callahan JL, Hynan MT (2002). Identifying mothers at risk for postnatal emotional distress: further evidence for the validity of the perinatal posttraumatic stress disorder questionnaire. *Journal of perinatology* 22: 448-455.

Carter BS (2002). How can we say to neonatal intensive care unit parents amid crisis, "You are not alone." *Pediatrics* 110(6):1245.

Carvajal S (2002). A parent support group in the neonatal intensive care unit. *Central lines* 18(5):4-5.

Cescutti-Butler L, Gavin K (2003). Parents' perceptions of staff competency in a neonatal intensive care unit. *Journal of clinical nursing* 12(5):752-761.

Davis L et al (2003). Mothers' involvement in caring for their premature infants: an historical overview. *Journal of advanced nursing* 42(6):578-586.

Doering LV et al (2000). Correlates of anxiety, hostility, depression and psychosocial adjustment in parents of NICU infants. *Neonatal network* 19(5):15-23.

Doucette J, Pinelli J (2004). The effects of family resources, coping, and strains on family adjustment 18 to 24 months after the NICU experience. *Advances in neonatal care* 4(2):92-104.

Evans R, Madsen B (2005). Culture clash: transitioning from the neonatal intensive care unit to the pediatric intensive care unit. *Newborn and infant nursing reviews* 5(4):188-193.

Fenwick J et al (2000). Interactions in neonatal nurseries: women's perceptions of nurses and nursing. *Journal of neonatal nursing* 6(6):197-203.

Franck LS, Spencer C (2003). Parent visiting and participation in infant caregiving activities in a neonatal unit. *Birth* 30(1):31-35.

Franck LS et al (2005). Measuring neonatal intensive care unit-related parental stress. *Journal of advances in nursing* 49(6):608-615.

Gates L et al (2004). Family issues professional partnerships. In Kenner C, McGrath JM, editors. *Developmental care of newborns and infants: a guide for health professionals* (pp 343-372). St Louis: Mosby.

Hanson SMH, Boyd ST (2001). *Family health care nursing: theory practice and research nursing*, ed 2. Philadelphia: FA Davis.

Heaman DJ (1995). Perceived stressors and coping strategies of parents who have children with developmental disabilities: a comparison of mothers with fathers. *Journal of pediatric nursing: nursing care of children and families* 10(5):311-320.

Hegedus KS (1999). Providers' and consumers' perspectives of nursing caring behaviours. *Journal of advanced nursing* 30(5):1090-1096.

Higgins I, Dullow A (2003). Parental perceptions of having a baby in a neonatal intensive care unit. *Neonatal, pediatric and child health nursing* 6:15-20.

Holditch-Davis D, Miles MS (2000). Mothers' stories about their experiences in the neonatal intensive care unit. *Neonatal network* 19(3):13-21.

Hulac P (2001). Creation and use of "You are Not Alone," a video for parents facing difficult decisions. *Journal of clinical ethics* 12:251-253.

Hynan MT (2005). Supporting fathers during stressful times in the nursery: an evidence-based review. *Newborn and infant nursing reviews* 5(2):87-92.

Institute for Family-Centered Care (Fall 2002). *Advances: changing the concept of families as visitors in the hospital.* Bethesda, MD: Institute of Family-Centered Care.

Jamsa K, Jamsa T (1998). Technology in the neonatal intensive care: a study of parents' experiences. *Technology and healthcare* 6(4):225-230.

Johnson BH (2003). Patient and family-centered care. In *AHA news.* Bethesda, MD: Institute of Family-Centered Care.

Johnson BH (2004). Families are allies for enhancing quality, patient safety. In *AHA news.* Bethesda, MD: Institute of Family-Centered Care.

Just A (2005). Parent participation in care: bridging the gap in the pediatric ICU. *Newborn and infant nursing reviews* 5(4):179-187.

Ladd RE, Mercurio MR (2003). Deciding for neonates: whose authority, whose interest? *Seminars in perinatology* 27(6):488-494.

Lipson JG et al (1996). *Culture and nursing care: a pocket guide.* San Francisco: USCF Nursing Press.

Loo KK et al (2003). Using knowledge to cope with stress in the NICU: how parents integrate learning to read the physiologic and behavioral cues of the infant. *Neonatal network* 22(1):31-37.

Major DA (2003). Utilizing role theory to help employed parents cope with children's chronic illness. *Health education research* 18(1):45-57.

McCubbin HI, Patterson J (1983). The family stress process: the double ABCX model of adjustment and adaptation. In McCubbin HI et al, editors. *Social stress and the family: advances and developments in family stress theory and research* (pp 7-37). New York: Haworth.

McGrath JM (2000). Developmentally supportive caregiving and technology: isolation or merger of intervention strategies? *Journal of perinatal and neonatal nursing* 14(3):78-91.

McGrath JM (2001). Building relationships with families in the NICU: exploring the guarded alliance. *Journal of perinatal and neonatal nursing* 15(4):1-10.

McGrath JM (2005a). Partnerships with families: a foundation to support them in difficult times. *Journal of perinatal and neonatal nursing* 19(2):94-96.

McGrath JM (2005b). Single room design in the NICU: making it work for you. *Journal of perinatal and neonatal nursing* 19(3):210-211.

Miles M, Brunssen SH (2003). Psychometric properties of the parental stressor scale: infant hospitalization. *Advances in neonatal care* 3(4):186-196.

Moore KAC et al (2003). Implementing potentially better practices for improving family-centered care in neonatal intensive care units: successes and challenges. *Pediatrics* 111(4):450-460.

Munch S, Levick J (2001). I'm special too: promoting sibling adjustment in the neonatal intensive care unit. *Health and social work* 26(1):45-49.

O'Shea J, Timmins F (2002). An overview of parents' experiences of neonatal intensive care: do we care for both parents? *Journal of neonatal nursing* 8(6):178-183.

Partridge JC et al (2005). International comparison of care for very low birth weight infants: parents' perceptions of counseling and decision-making. *Pediatrics* 116(2):e263-e271.

Patterson JM (1995). Promoting resilience in families experiencing stress. *Pediatric clinics of North America* 42(1):47-63.

Pinelli J (2000). Effects of family coping and resources on family adjustment and parental stress in the acute phase of the NICU experience. *Neonatal network* 19(6):27-37.

Prentice M, Stainton MC (2004). The effects of developmental care of preterm infants on women's health and family life. *Neonatal, pediatric and child health nursing* 7(3):4-12.

Saunders RP et al (2003). Evaluation and development of potentially better practices for improving family-centered care in the neonatal intensive care unit. *Pediatrics* 111(4):e437-e349.

Simons J et al (2001). Parent involvement in children's pain care: views of parents and nurses. *Journal of advanced nursing* 36(4):591-599.

Spear M et al (2002). Family reactions during infants' hospitalization in the neonatal intensive care unit. *American journal of perinatology* 19(4):205-213.

Sudia-Robinson TM, Freeman SB (2000). Communication patterns and decision-making among parents and health care providers in the neonatal intensive care unit: a case study. *Heart & lung: the journal of acute and critical care* 29(2):143-148.

Sydnor-Greenberg N, Dokken D (2000). Coping and caring in different ways: understanding and meaningful involvement. *Pediatric nursing* 26(2):185-190.

Tait AR et al (2001). Parents preferences for participation in decision-making regarding their child's anesthetic care. *Paediatric anesthesia* 11:283-290.

VandeVusse L (1999). Decision making in analyses of women's birth stories. *Birth* 26(1):43-50.

Ward K (2001). Perceived needs of parent of critically ill infants in the neonatal intensive care unit (NICU). *Pediatric nursing* 27(3):281-286.

Weiss SJ, Chen J (2002). Factors influencing maternal mental health and family functioning during the low birthweight infant's first year of life. *Journal of pediatric nursing* 17:114-125.

White RD et al (2002). *Recommended standards for newborn ICU design: Report of the Fifth Consensus Conference on Newborn ICU Design.* Clearwater Beach, FL: Committee to Establish Recommended Standards for Newborn ICU Design. Available at: http://www.nd.edu/~kkolberg/DesignStandards.htm. Retrieved May 15, 2005.

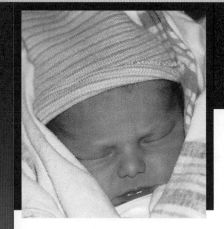

Chapter **26**

Palliative and End-of-Life Care

Carole Kenner • Tanya Sudia-Robinson

In the neonatal intensive care unit (NICU), the assurance that "everything possible is being done" often is interpreted as meaning that the patient is receiving state-of-the-art technologic care. Yet the health care system fails both infants and their families when death occurs. The failure lies not in the infant's death itself, but rather in the neglect to emphasize state-of-the-art palliative care. Until it is evident that all dying infants receive highly skilled palliative care, as well as advanced technologic care, modern medicine cannot say that the best possible care has been provided to these infants and their families. This chapter focuses on the care of infants and their families who are facing life-threatening illnesses or are dying and the urgent need for exemplary neonatal and pediatric hospice and palliative care programs.

ETHICAL OBLIGATION TO PROVIDE OPTIMUM END-OF-LIFE CARE

It can be argued that all members of the health care team have an ethical obligation to plan and implement end-of-life (EOL) care; to provide highly skilled care at all times except at the end of life is to ignore the essence of comprehensive health care. The ethical dimensions of neonatal EOL care include an obligation to provide compassionate care; beneficent and non-maleficent care, especially in regard to infant pain; and recognition of the moral authority of caring, informed parents as surrogate decision makers for their infants.

Compassionate Care at the End of Life

More than a decade ago, Pellegrino and Thomasma (1993) argued that health care professionals have a special responsibility to provide compassionate care at the end of life. They identified compassion and temperance as among the essential virtues of medical practice and cautioned against overuse of high-technology equipment in place of human engagement with patients. They noted that particularly at the end of life, health care professionals can become so focused on technologic processes that they use them as "substitutes for human and compassionate care."

Even today, infants in the NICU frequently die while still intubated and connected to various pieces of equipment. A recent study of childhood deaths in Canadian hospitals found that the acuity of care was high before death and that most of the decisions about EOL issues were made very close to the actual time of death (McCallum et al, 2000). In that study, most of the children were intubated at death (73%), and most died in the intensive care unit (83%). In the United States most pediatric deaths also occur in hospital intensive care units (Kerr, 2001), and there is evidence that children often suffer needlessly before death (Stephenson, 2000; Wolfe et al, 2000). Approximately 54,000 children die annually in the United States, with most of these deaths still occurring in hospitals (Solomon et al, 2002). A random survey of 30 NICUs across the United States indicated that although most of these units had policies regarding postmortem and bereavement care services, none had procedural guidelines for EOL care. Since the late 1990s when this study was done, some progress has been made in the creation of policies and procedures (Carter et al, 2004). Catlin and Carter (2002) developed a palliative care protocol that has assisted many perinatal and neonatal centers in the development of policies to assist with EOL and palliative care issues.

New approaches must be taken to establish compassionate EOL care for all infants in the NICU. This challenge is intensified in a system in which health care professionals are oriented toward active intervention with technologic devices rather than toward an acceptance of death (Jecker & Pagon, 1995; Kenner & McSkimming, 2006). As Jecker and Pagon said, health care professionals are "applauded for acting, intervening, and forestalling death. Once set in motion, these active, goal-directed virtues can easily acquire a momentum of their own." These researchers urge an increased understanding and application of virtues such as patience, cautiousness, and humility in the perinatal setting. Some settings are developing a connection with perinatal hospices when a problem is detected prior to delivery that may result in a stillborn or "born dying" infant. One example of this is "Alexander's House" in Kansas City, MO (Pearce, 2006). Children's Hospital Medical Center, Cincinnati, OH, and their perinatal hospice program called "Star Shine Hospice" is another example of a hospice that is specifically focused on children. (For more information see: http://www.cincinnati-childrens.org/svc/alpha/s/hospice/.)

Wolfe (2000) also serves as an advocate for compassionate care for children at the end of life. She identified the "principle of family" in pediatric EOL care: that is, an obligation to treat the whole family. Wolfe saw the health care staff as having an ethical obligation to "pursue comfort aggressively" and to fully engage the parents in the decision-making process for their child.

Obligation to Provide Beneficent Care

The widely accepted principle of beneficence requires that health care professionals actively provide care that directly benefits their patients. As defined by Beauchamp and Childress (2001), the principle of beneficence encompasses both positive beneficence and actively providing benefit and utility, which requires a balancing of benefits and adverse effects. Professional codes of ethics require that nurses and physicians act in a manner that benefits those entrusted to their care. Health care professionals therefore are obligated to examine their actions with regard to intended beneficial outcomes while simultaneously considering the drawbacks or adverse consequences of their actions.

Obligation of Nonmaleficence

Health care professionals also have a legal and moral obligation to avoid inflicting harm on their patients (Beauchamp & Childress, 2001). Adherence to this principle, known as nonmaleficence, may encompass the provision of life-sustaining treatment, as well as the cessation of such treatment. For example, when a treatment ceases to provide the intended benefit for a patient, it may be considered futile, and the health care professional therefore is no longer obligated to continue that treatment (Beauchamp & Childress, 2001). It also refers to the adequate management of pain and not inflicting undue harm from inadequate management.

Health care professionals who continue to provide futile and burdensome treatments may be viewed as doing more harm than good. The distinction is made by meticulously balancing the benefits and burdens to the patient. For critically ill infants in the NICU, procedures or treatments can be considered inhumane if they inflict pain or discomfort on the infant without actual benefit (Jecker & Pagon, 1995). Jecker and Pagon noted, "Medical interventions provided without benefit rob patients of their very humanity. Inhumanity implies that medical care aimlessly prolongs a patient's pain or suffering, making the use of medical technologies a torture or punishment. Inhumanity suggests a failure to empathize with the sufferings of patients."

Despite these arguments for humane care, burdensome, futile treatments sometimes still are given in the NICU. Weir (1984, 1995) has argued that death should not be considered the worst outcome for some infants, particularly when the chances for survival are remote or when physiologic survival is accompanied by unrelieved pain and suffering. In such cases, health care providers may be merely prolonging dying.

Recognition of Parents' Moral Authority

Parents have both legal and moral authority to serve as surrogate decision makers for their infants. A growing body of literature supports parental decision-making authority, particularly for extremely premature or near-viable infants (Ho, 2003; Jecker & Pagon, 1995; Manning, 2005; Raines, 1996; Pinkerton et al, 1997); however, few studies have examined ways to empower parents to exercise this authority fully. Furthermore, a body of literature written by both parents and health care professionals suggests that parents may not be involved adequately in decisions about prolonged, aggressive treatments for their infants (Stinson & Stinson, 1979; Harrison, 1993; Pinch & Spielman, 1993, 1996; Raines, 1996). It can be argued that parents may not be as fully involved in decisions about their infant's care as they would like and have the authority to be, especially in cases in which aggressive therapies are of uncertain benefit to the infant. As Catlin and Carter (2002) point out, the real need in these instances is clear communication with parents and an understanding of how they wish to be involved in these decisions.

A consensus is growing among ethicists, clinicians, and families that when the benefits of life-sustaining therapies are questionable, parental involvement in treatment decision making is an ethical imperative.* When life-sustaining therapies have proved futile, parents and professionals often are uncertain how to provide end-of-life care. The following quote is from Robert Stinson, father of Andrew, who was born in 1976 at 24 weeks' gestation. At that time Andrew's survival was unprecedented. He underwent intensive care for 6 months, was critically ill throughout this time, and was resuscitated numerous times before his death.

> What they never understood was that one can care deeply enough about a child like Andrew to want his misery ended. Allowing Andrew to die naturally was what we wanted for him, not just to him. I thought often, when I did go in to see him, about his massive pain. He was sometimes crying then; a nearly soundless, aimless cry of pain, undirected and unlistened to except, I sometimes thought, by me. As often as I wanted to gather him into my arms, I wanted him to be allowed to die. What is the name for that? (Stinson & Stinson, 1979).

Although the Stinsons' experience occurred more than 25 years ago, evidence suggests professionals do not always incorporate the parental perspective into care decisions,† particularly with regard to burdensome, futile treatments (Yellin et al, 1998).

Burden of Treatment

The burden of treatment experienced by extremely premature infants in the NICU, especially those with minimal chance for survival, requires further ethical examination. In a national survey of physicians certified in neonatal-perinatal medicine, Yellin and colleagues (1998) found that many neonatologists believe that "there is an ethical or legal obligation to perform treatments that are not in the infant's best interests, regardless of parental preference." Yellin and coworkers concluded that because some neonatologists are unwilling to withdraw treatments, they may be overtreating some infants in

---

*President's Commission for the Study of Ethical Problems in Medicine and Biomedical and Behavioral Research, 1983; Harrison, 1993; Jakobi et al, 1993; Penticuff, 1987, 1988, 1995, 1998).
†Mehren, 1991; King, 1992; Harrison, 1993; Pinch & Spielman, 1996; Raines, 1996.

the NICU. Unfortunately this situation has not changed that much today (Kenner & McSkimming, 2006).

The inordinate medical intervention that occurs for some infants stems from the lack of consensus surrounding the issue of futility (Avery, 1998; Penticuff, 1998). Penticuff (1998) identified harm that ensues for infants, families, the health care team, and society when there is no accepted definition of futility. Such harm includes "needless infant suffering through prolongation of the process of dying" and "psychologic entrapment of the medical team and the family," in which initial aggressive therapies lead inexorably to more aggressive therapies, with only death as the stopping point.

Brody and colleagues (1997) call for compassionate clinical management during the withdrawal of intensive life-sustaining treatment for adult patients using a strategic approach with well-defined goals that dictate the plan of care. Once the goals have been identified, the team examines both the benefits and burdens of the proposed treatment plan with the family. With this approach, any treatment that is more burdensome than beneficial is limited or eliminated. Brody and coworkers identified pain and discomfort as components of treatment burden and said that there is "no sound rationale for withholding adequate analgesia or sedation" during EOL care. This is an area that requires further examination as it relates to critically ill neonates at the end of life.

NEONATAL PAIN MANAGEMENT AT THE END OF LIFE

Research is limited on the provision of analgesia and sedation for infants at the end of life. One study focused on medications administered during life-support (e.g., ventilator) withdrawal. Partridge and Wall (1997) conducted a retrospective chart review to examine the practice of opioid analgesia administration in one NICU at the time of life-support withdrawal. They found that, of infants who had a known painful condition (e.g., acute abdominal or surgical pain) and were receiving analgesia before the decision was made to withhold further life-sustaining treatment, 84% received opioid analgesia during life-support withdrawal. An interesting finding of this study was that the infants who did not receive any analgesia at the time of life-support withdrawal had also not received any pain medication before the decision was made to discontinue life support. These findings suggest that analgesia is not being given to ease the possible suffering associated with withdrawal of life support, but rather to manage specific disease processes. (Additional aspects of neonatal pain management are discussed in Chapter 17.) It is recognized that even the smallest of patients have rights, and these include palliative care. Box 26-1 lists the Core Principles for Care of Patients (Newborns and Infants).

HOSPICE CARE

The use of hospice and palliative care has made a significant difference in EOL care for adults. However, the movement toward hospice care for neonates and young children has been slow to take hold.

Hospice is both a philosophy and a system of compassionate, team-oriented care for individuals at the end of life. According to the National Hospice and Palliative Care Organization (2000), the guiding philosophy of hospice is that "each of us has the right to die pain free and with dignity, and that our families will receive the necessary support to allow us to do so."

BOX 26-1

Core Principles for Care of Patients (Newborns and Infants)

- Respecting the dignity of both child and caregiver.
- Being sensitive to and respectful of the family's wishes.
- Using the most appropriate measures that are consistent with the family's choices.
- Encompassing alleviation of pain and other physical symptoms.
- Assessing and managing psychologic, social, and spiritual/religious problems.
- Ensuring continuity of care (the child should be able to continue to be cared for, if so desired, by his/her primary care and specialist providers).
- Providing access to any therapy that may realistically be expected to improve the child's quality of life, including alternative or nontraditional treatments.
- Providing access to palliative care and hospice care.
- Respecting the right to refuse treatment that may prolong suffering of life.
- Respecting the physician's professional responsibility to discontinue some treatments when appropriate, with consideration for both child and family's preferences.
- Promoting clinical evidence-based research on providing care at the end of life.

From Kenner C, Lott JW (2003). *Neonatal nursing handbook* (pp. 468-469). St Louis: Mosby. Modified from Cassel CK, Foley KM (1999). *Principles of care of patients at the end of life: an emerging consensus among the specialties of medicine.* New York: Milbank Memorial Fund. Available at: http://www.milbank.org/reports/endoflife/.

Hospice care can be provided in select hospitals, in individual hospice facilities, or in a person's home. Although there has been a national movement toward making hospice care available to most adults, there are few examples of hospice centers specifically designed for children and their families.

Pediatric Hospice Care

Although there are few pediatric hospices in the United States, those that exist provide exemplary care for children and their families. One example of a model program is the newly opened Kids Path Hospice and Palliative Care of Greensboro, North Carolina. At Kids Path, care is provided for children with acquired immune deficiency syndrome (AIDS), congenital anomalies, chromosomal disorders, and cancer (Kerr, 2001). It is the only children's hospice facility in North Carolina and among the fewer than 25 such facilities in the United States. Kids Path uses an interdisciplinary care team that includes a pediatric nurse practitioner, registered nurses, medical director, social worker, counselors, and a chaplain. This issue was addressed by the Oklahoma Attorney General's Task Force Report on the State of End-Of-Life Health Care (Edmondson, 2005), where it was recognized that such specialized services are needed.

Barriers to Pediatric Hospice Service

Unfortunately, many barriers obstruct the availability and provision of hospice care to all children and families who could benefit from it. The National Hospice and Palliative

Care Organization (2000) has described psychologic, financial, educational, and regulatory barriers to pediatric palliative care (NHPCO, 2000). One of the psychologic barriers is the association of palliative care with the concept of giving up or going against hope (Kenner & McSkimming, 2006). Families often avoid palliative care, rather than identifying with the life-enhancing benefits it offers. Financial barriers arise because the home-based, multidisciplinary care is often not reimbursed. The educational barriers for care providers are evident in the lack of palliative care training for most physicians and the avoidance of discussing hospice care with parents. Regulatory barriers also exist because the reimbursement system is based on the needs of adults. Ignoring the differences in care needs between children and adults creates barriers to hospice as an option for many families.

PEDIATRIC PALLIATIVE CARE

The American Academy of Pediatrics (AAP) (2000) has issued guidelines for the care of children with life-threatening and terminal conditions. The AAP recommends palliative care for infants when "no treatment has been shown to alter substantially the expected progression toward death." According to the AAP guidelines, palliative care incorporates control of pain, symptom management, and care of the psychologic, social, and spiritual needs of children and their families. The AAP also has established five principles of palliative care: (1) respect for the dignity of patients and families, (2) access to competent and compassionate palliative care, (3) support for the caregivers, (4) improved professional and social support for pediatric palliative care, and (5) continued improvement of pediatric palliative care through research and education.

Respect for the Dignity of Patients and Families

Respect for patients' and families' dignity means that information about palliative care should be provided, and the parents' ability to make their own choice of a program should be respected. Also, the plan of care must incorporate and respect the parents' expressed wishes for their child's care, specifically with regard to testing, monitoring, and treatment (AAP, 2000). This respect should include considerations for religious beliefs and cultural values (Tables 26-1 and 26-2).

Access to Competent and Compassionate Palliative Care

Compassionate palliative care includes alleviation of pain and other symptoms and access to supportive therapies, such as grief counseling and spiritual support. This principle includes provision of adequate respite care for parents (AAP, 2000).

Support for the Caregivers

The AAP recognizes the importance of support for health care professionals involved in the child's care. This support may include paid funeral leave, peer counseling, or remembrance ceremonies (AAP, 2000).

Improved Professional and Social Support for Pediatric Palliative Care

A number of barriers can prevent families from obtaining pediatric palliative care, including the obstacles discussed previously. Health care professionals must help families overcome these obstacles (AAP, 2000).

Continued Improvement of Pediatric Palliative Care Through Research and Education

Health care professionals need continuing education on ways to provide comprehensive palliative care. Also, research is needed that focuses on the effectiveness of palliative care interventions and on models of pediatric palliative care delivery (AAP, 2000). A list of hospice and palliative care resources is provided in Box 26-2.

INCORPORATING PEDIATRIC PALLIATIVE CARE INTO THE NICU

The AAP recommends that palliative care begin at the time of diagnosis of a life-threatening or terminal condition (AAP, 2000). In the NICU, particularly for extremely premature neonates and for neonates with life-threatening anomalies, palliative care should begin at the time of admission. For many health care professionals, this requires a rather dramatic shift from providing intensive high-technology care to providing intensive palliative care. At times, particularly during the early diagnostic phase, palliative care can be provided along with technologic care; this arrangement allows the staff to focus on symptom management and pain control while weighing the benefits and harm of treatment. It also provides for interdisciplinary team members who can provide the support the family needs.

Often, when a neonate is born at the edge of viability, the clinical course shows a downward trend. The neonate's physiologic parameters cause concern as evidence mounts that the organ systems are failing. This scenario represents the inevitable point at which intensive efforts to prolong life merely serve to prolong the infant's dying. In such cases, both infants and their families would benefit from a smooth transition to intensive palliative care. This requires a level of skilled care that is not always present in the NICU. The care providers must be able quickly to recognize the futility of sustained therapies and must be expert at providing palliative care to both infant and family. Unfortunately, as research has indicated, all too often infants and children die while still intubated (McCallum et al, 2000); suffer from pain that is inadequately controlled (Partridge & Wall, 1997; Kenner & McSkimming, 2006); and have not received the benefits of palliative care measures (Byock, 1997; Goldman, 1998; Rushton, 2000; Stephenson, 2000). The National Association of Neonatal Nurses (NANN), the Association of Pediatric Oncology Nurses (APON), and the Society of Pediatric Nurses (SPN) have stated that this area of neonatal care is very important. Under the auspices of the National Leadership Academy on EOL Issues, which is sponsored by Johns Hopkins University (www.son.jhmi.edu/newsandmedia/endoflife.html), these three organizations are adapting the Last Acts Precepts (www.lastacts.org) for neonatal and pediatric patients. The Last Acts organization provides support for health care professionals and families through publications and taking action on EOL issues. It believes that appropriate language must be included to reflect cases such as an infant who is literally born dying, as well as the family's unique needs in such cases. This collaboration is a milestone in efforts to recognize that neonatal and pediatric patients and their families deserve the same level of care that adults have received.

Text continues on p. 520.

TABLE 26-1	Religious Influences			
Religious Sect	**Birth**	**Death**	**Organ Donation/ Transplantation**	**Beliefs Regarding Medical Care**
Baptist	Infant baptism is not practiced. However, many churches present the baby and the parents to the congregation when they attend services for the first time after the birth.	It isn't mandatory that clergy be present at death, but families often desire visits from clergy. Scripture reading and prayer are important.	There is no formal statement regarding this issue. It is considered a matter of personal conscience. It is commonly regarded as positive (an act of love).	Some may regard their illness as punishment resulting from past sins. Those who believe in predestination may not seek aggressive treatment. Fundamentalist and conservative groups see the Bible as the infallible word of God to be taken literally.
Buddhist	Do not practice infant baptism.	Buddhist priest is often involved before and after death. Rituals are observed during and after death. If the family doesn't have a priest, they may request one be contacted.	There is no formal statement regarding organ donation/ transplantation. This is seen as a matter of individual conscience.	Believe that illness can be used as a tool to aid In the development of the soul. May see illness as a result of karmic causes. May avoid treatments or procedures on holy days. Cleanliness is important.
Church Of Jesus Christ of Latter Day Saints (Mormon)	Infant baptism is not performed. Children are given a name and a priesthood blessing sometime after the birth, from a week or two to several months. In the event of a critically ill newborn, this might be done in the hospital at the discretion of the parents. Baptism is performed after the child is 8 years old. Church of Jesus Christ of Latter Day Saints feel that a child is not accountable for sins before 8 years of age.	There are no religious rituals performed related to death.	There is no official statement regarding this issue. Organ donation/ transplantation is left up to the individual or parents.	Administration to the sick involves anointing with consecrated oil and a blessing performed by members of the priesthood. Although the individual or a member of the family usually requests this if the individual is unconscious, and there is no one to represent him or her, it would be appropriate for anyone to contact the Church so that the ordinance may be performed. Refusal of medical treatments would be left up to the individual. There are no restrictions relative to "holy" days.
Episcopal	Infant baptism is practiced. In emergent situations, request for infant baptism should be given high priority and could be performed by any baptized person, clergy or lay. Often in situations of stillbirths or aborted fetuses, special prayers of commendation may be offered.	Pastoral care of the sick may include prayers, laying on of hands, anointing, and/or Holy Communion. At the time of death, various litanies and special prayers may be offered.	Both are permitted.	Respect for the dignity of the whole person is important. These needs include physical, emotional, and spiritual.

TABLE **26-1**	Religious Influences—cont'd			
Religious Sect	**Birth**	**Death**	**Organ Donation/ Transplantation**	**Beliefs Regarding Medical Care**
Friends (Quakers)	Do not practice infant baptism.	Each person has a divine nature, but an encounter and relationship with Jesus Christ is essential.	No formal statement, but generally both are permitted.	No special rites or restrictions. Leaders and elders from the Church may visit and offer support and encouragement. Quakers believe in plain speech.
Islam (Muslim/ Moslem)	At birth, the first words said to the infant in his/her right ear are "Allah-o-Akbar" (Allah is great) and the remainder of the Call for Prayer is recited. An "Aqeeqa" (party) to celebrate the birth of the child is arranged by the parents. Circumcision of the male child is practiced.	In Islam, life is meant to be a test for the preparation for the everlasting life in the hereafter. Therefore, according to Islam, death is simply a transition. Islam teaches that God has prescribed the time of death for everyone and only He knows when, where, or how a person is going to die. Islam encourages making the best use of all of God's gifts including the precious gift of life in this world. At the time of death, there are specific rituals (bathing, wrapping the body in cloth, etc.) that must be done. Before moving and handling the body, it is preferable to contact someone from the person's mosque or Islamic Society to perform these rituals.	Permitted. However, there are some stipulations depending on the type of transplant/donation and its effect on the donor and recipient. It is advisable to contact the individual's mosque or the local Islamic Society for further consultation.	Humans are encouraged in the Qur'an to seek treatment. It is taught that only Allah cures. However, Muslims are taught not to refuse treatment in the belief that Allah will take care of them because even though He cures, He also chooses at times to work through the efforts of humans.
International Society for Krishna Consciousness (a Hindu movement in North America based on devotion to Lord Krishna)	Infant baptism is not performed.	The body should not be touched. The family may desire that a local temple be contacted so representatives may visit and chant over the patient. It is believed that in chanting the names of God, one may gain insight and God consciousness.	There is no formal statement prohibiting this act. It is an individual decision.	Illness or injury is believed to represent sins committed in this or a previous life. They accept modern medical treatment. The body is seen as a temporary vehicle used to transport them through this life. The body belongs to God and members are charged to care for it in the best way possible.

Continued

TABLE 26-1	Religious Influences—cont'd			
Religious Sect	**Birth**	**Death**	**Organ Donation/ Transplantation**	**Beliefs Regarding Medical Care**
Jehovah's Witness	Infant baptism is not practiced.	There are no official "rites" that are performed before or after death; however, the faith community is often involved and supportive of the patient and family.	There is no official statement related to this issue. Organ donation isn't encouraged but it is believed to be an individual decision. According to the Watchtower legal corporation for the denomination, all donated organs and tissue must be drained of blood before transplantation.	Adherents are absolutely opposed to transfusions of whole blood, packed red blood cells, platelets, and fresh or frozen plasma. This includes banking of one's own blood. Many accept use of albumin, globulin, factor replacement (hemophilia), vaccines, hemodilution, and cell salvage. There is no opposition to nonblood plasma expanders.
Judaism (Orthodox and Conservative)	Circumcision of male infants is performed on the eighth day if the infant is healthy. The mohel (ritual circumciser familiar with Jewish law and aseptic technique) performs the ritual.	It is important that the health care professional facilitate the family's need to comfort and be with the patient at the time of death.	Permitted and is considered a mitzvah (good deed).	Only emergency surgical procedures should be performed on the Sabbath, which extends from sundown Friday to sundown Saturday. Elective surgery should be scheduled for days other than the Sabbath. Pregnant women and the seriously ill are exempt from fasting. Serious illness may be grounds for violating dietary laws, but only if it is medically necessary.
Lutheran	Infant baptism is practiced. If the infant's prognosis is poor, the family may request immediate baptism.	Family may desire visitation from clergy. Prayers for the Dying, Commendation of the Dying, and Prayers for the Bereaved may be offered.	There is no formal statement regarding this issue. It is considered a matter of personal conscience.	Illness isn't seen as an act of God; rather it is seen as a condition of mankind's fallen state. Prayers for the Sick may be desired.
Methodist	Infant baptism is practiced but is usually done within the community of the Church after counseling and guidance from clergy. However, in emergency situations, a request for baptism would not be seen as inappropriate.	In the case of perinatal death, there are prayers within the United Methodist Book of Worship that could be said by anyone. Prayer, scripture, and singing are often seen as appropriate and desirable.	Organ donation/ transplantation is supported and encouraged. It is considered a part of good stewardship.	In the Methodist tradition, it is believed that every person has the right to death with dignity and has the right to be involved in all medical decisions. Refusal of aggressive treatment is seen as an appropriate option.
Pentecostal Assembly of God, Church of God, Four Square and many other faith	No rituals like baptism are necessary. Many Pentecostals have a ceremony of "dedication," but it is done in the context	The only way to transcend this life; is the door to heaven (or hell). Questions about "salvation of the soul" are very	Many Pentecostal denominations have no statement concerning this subject, but it is generally seen as positive and well	Pentecostals sometimes labeled as "in denial" due to their theology of healing. Their faith in God for literal healing is

TABLE 26-1	Religious Influences—cont'd			
Religious Sect	**Birth**	**Death**	**Organ Donation/ Transplantation**	**Beliefs Regarding Medical Care**
groups are included under this general heading. Pentecostal is not a denomination, but a theological distinctive (pneumatology).	of the community of faith/believers (Church). Children belong to heaven and only become sinners after the age of accountability, which is not clearly defined.	common and important. Resurrection is the Hope of those who "were saved." Prayer is appropriate; so is singing and scripture reading.	received. Education concerning wholeness of the person and nonliteral aspects such as "heart," "mind," have to be explained. For example, a Pentecostal may have a problem with donating a heart to a "nonbeliever."	generally expressed as intentional unbelief in the prognostic statements. Many Pentecostals do not see sickness as the will of God; thus one must "stand firm" in faith and accept the unseen reality, which many times may mean healing. As difficult as this position may seem, it must be noted that, when death occurs, Pentecostals may leap from miracle expectations to joyful hope and theology of heaven and resurrection without facing issues of anger or frustration due to unfulfilled expectations. Prayer, scriptures, singing, and anointing of the sick (not a sacrament) are appropriate/expected pastoral interventions.
Presbyterian	Baptism is a Sacrament of the Church but is not considered necessary for salvation. However, it is seen as an event to take place, when possible, in the context of a worshipping community.	Family may desire visitation from clergy. Prayers for the Dying, Commendation of the Dying, and Prayers for the Bereaved may be offered.	There is no formal statement regarding this issue.	Communion is a Sacrament of the Church. It is generally celebrated with a patient in the presence of an ordained minister and elder. Presbyterians are free to make their own choices regarding the use of mechanical life-support measures.
Roman Catholic	Infant baptism is practiced. In medical facilities, baptism is usually performed by a Priest or Deacon, as ordinary members of the sacrament. However, under extraordinary, circumstances, baptism	Sacrament of the Sick is the sacrament of healing and forgiveness. It is to be administered by a priest as early in the illness as possible. It is not a last rite to be administered at	Catholics may donate or receive organ transplants.	The Sacrament of Holy Communion sustains Catholics in sickness as in health. When the patient's condition deteriorates, the sacrament is given as Viaticum ("food for the

Continued

TABLE 26-1	Religious Influences—cont'd			
Religious Sect	**Birth**	**Death**	**Organ Donation/ Transplantation**	**Beliefs Regarding Medical Care**
	may be administered by a layperson, provided that the intention is to do as the Church does using the formula, "I baptize you in the name of the Father, the Son, and the Holy Spirit."	the point of death. The Roman Catholic Church makes provisions for Prayers of Commendation of the dying, which may be said by any Priest, Deacon Sacramental Minister, or layperson.		journey"). Like Holy Communion, Viaticum may be administered by a Priest, Deacon, or a Sacramental Minister. The Church makes provisions for Prayers for Commendation of the Dying that may be said by any of those listed above or by a layperson.

From Kenner C, Lott JW (2003). Neonatal nursing handbook (pp 486-492). St Louis: Mosby. From Texas Children's Cancer Center—Texas Children's Hospital. (2000). End-of-life care for children (pp 78-79). Houston, TX: Texas Cancer Council.

TABLE 26-2	Cultural Influences on Health Beliefs and Practices	
Ethnic Group	**Health Belief**	**Practices**
Asian Chinese	1. A healthy body is viewed as a gift from parents and ancestors and must be cared for. 2. Health is one of the results of balances of yin (cold) and yang (hot)—energy forces that rule the world. 3. Illness is caused by imbalance. 4. Blood is source of life and is not regenerated. 5. Chi is innate energy. Lack of chi and blood produces fatigue, poor constitution, and long illness.	1. There is wide use of medicinal herbs procured and applied in prescribed ways. 2. Folk healers are herbalist, spiritual healer, temple healer, and future healer.
Japanese	Health beliefs and practices stem from three major belief systems: 1. Shinto religious influence • Humans are inherently good. • Evil is caused by contact with polluting agents (e.g., blood, corpses, skin disease). 2. Chinese and Korean influence • Health is achieved through harmony and balance between self and society. • Disease is caused by disharmony with society and not caring for body. 3. Portuguese influence • Upholds germ theory of disease: evil is removed by purification.	1. Kampo medicine is use of natural herbs. 2. Care for disabled is viewed as family's responsibility. 3. Take pride in child's good health. 4. Seek preventive care, medical care for illness.
Vietnamese	1. Good health is considered to be balance between yin and yang. 2. Believe person's life has been predisposed toward certain phenomena by cosmic forces. 3. Health is believed to be result of harmony with existing universal order; harmony attained by pleasing good spirits and avoiding evil ones. 4. There is a belief in *am duc,* the amount of good deeds accumulated by ancestors.	1. Many use rituals to prevent illness. 2. Practice some restrictions to prevent incurring wrath of evil spirits. 3. Regard health as family responsibility; outside aid is sought when resources run out.

Continued

TABLE **26-2**	Cultural Influences on Health Beliefs and Practices—cont'd	
Ethnic Group	**Health Belief**	**Practices**
Filipino	1. Believe God's will and supernatural forces govern universe. 2. Illness, accident, and other misfortunes are God's punishment for violations of His will. 3. Widely accept "hot" and "cold" balance and imbalance as cause of health and illness.	1. Some use amulets as a shield for witchcraft or as good luck pieces.

African American	1. Illness classified as:
	  • Natural forces of nature against which there is not adequate protection (e.g., cold air, pollution, food and water).
	  • Unnatural, evil influences (e.g., witchcraft, voodoo, hoodoo, hex fix, root work); symptoms often associated with eating.
	2. Believe serious illness sent by God as punishment (e.g., parents, punished by illness or death of the child).
		1. Self-care and folk medicine is very prevalent.
		2. Attempt home remedies first.
		3. May resist health care because illness is "Will of God."
		4. Prayer is common means for prevention and treatment.

Haitian	1. Illnesses have a supernatural or natural origin.
	2. Supernatural illnesses are caused by angry voodoo spirits, enemies, or the dead, especially deceased ancestors.
	3. Natural illnesses are based on conceptions of natural causation: irregularities of blood volume, flow, purity, viscosity, color, and/or temperature (hot/cold).
	  • Gas (gaz).
	  • Movement and consistency of mother's milk.
	  • "Hot/cold" imbalance in the body.
	  • Bone displacement.
	  • Movement of diseases.
	4. Health is maintained by good dietary and hygienic habits.
	5. Health is a personal responsibility.
	6. Foods have properties of hot/cold and light/heavy and must be in harmony with one's life cycle and bodily states.
		1. Supernatural illness treated by healers: Voodoo priest (houngan) or priestess (mambo), midwife (fam saj), and herbalist or leaf doctor (dokte fey).
		2. Amulets and prayer used to protect against illness due to curses or willed by evil people.

Hispanic/Mexican	1. Health beliefs have strong religious association. 2. Body imbalance between caliente (hot) and frio (cold) or "wet" and "dry" is a cause of illness. Some maintain good health is a result of good luck. 3. Illness prevented by performing properly, through prayer, by wearing religious medals or amulets, and sleeping with relics at home. 4. Illness is a punishment from God for wrongdoing, forces of nature, and the supernatural.	1. Seek help from curandero or curandera, especially in rural areas. Curandero(a) receives his/her position by birth, apprenticeship, or a "calling" via dream or vision. 2. Practice for severe illness—make promises, visit shrines, offer medals and candles, offer prayers. 3. Adhere to "hot" and "cold" food prescriptions and prohibitions for prevention and treatment of illness.
Puerto Rican	1. Subscribe to the "hot and cold" theory of causation of illness. 2. Believe some illness caused by evil spirits and forces.	1. Consult spiritualist medium for mental disorders. 2. Santeria is system and practitioners are called santeros.
Cuban	1. Prevention and good nutrition are related to good health. 2. Diligent users of the medical model.	1. Eclectic health-seeking practices: folk medicine of both religious and nonreligious origins; home remedies; in many instances, seek assistance of santeros and spiritualists to complement medical treatment.

Continued

TABLE **26-2**	Cultural Influences on Health Beliefs and Practices—cont'd	
Ethnic Group	**Health Belief**	**Practices**
Native American	1. Believe health is a state of harmony with nature and universe. 2. Respect bodies through proper management. 3. All disorders believed to have aspects of supernatural. 4. Violation of a restriction or prohibition thought to cause illness. 5. Fear of witchcraft.	1. May carry objects believed to guard against witchcraft. 2. Theology and medicine strongly interwoven.

From Kenner C, Lott JW (2003). Neonatal nursing handbook (pp 497-501). St Louis: Mosby. Adapted from Hockenberry MJ, Wilson D (2007). Wong's nursing care of infants and children, ed 8. St Louis: Mosby. Cited in Texas Children's Cancer Center—Texas Children's Hospital (2000). End-of-life care for children. Houston, TX: Texas Cancer Council.

BOX **26-2**

Pediatric Hospice and Palliative Care Resources

American Academy of Pediatrics (www.aap.org)
141 Northwest Point Boulevard
Elk Grove Village, IL 60007
(847) 434-4000
The American Academy of Pediatrics guidelines for palliative care and care guidelines for terminally ill children can be viewed at this site.

Children's Hospice International (www.chionline.org)
901 North Pitt Street, Suite 230
Alexandria, VA 22314
(800) 242-4453
This site provides information about hospice care for children and has links to related sites for families and care providers.

Children's International Project on Palliative and Hospice Services (www.nhpco.org)
National Hospice and Palliative Care Organization
1700 Diagonal Road, Suite 625
Alexandria, VA 22314
(877) 557-2847
This site discusses the hospice philosophy and provides links to related sites.

Footprints Program (www.footprintsatglennon.org)
Cardinal Glennon Children's Hospital
1465 South Grand Boulevard
St. Louis, MO 63104
(877) 557-2847
This is an interdisciplinary program that coordinates community services, bereavement support, and consultation regarding pain and symptom management.

Innovations in End-of-Life Care (www.edc.org/lastacts)
This is an online international journal and forum for leaders in end-of-life care. Volume 2, issue No. 2, 2000, focuses on pediatric palliative care.

Pediatric Palliative Care Project (www.seattlechildrens.org)
Seattle Children's Hospital
4800 Sand Point Way NE
Seattle, WA 98105
(206) 527-5732
This site provides an example of a statewide pediatric palliative care project.

Worldwide, recognition of the need for neonatal and pediatric palliative care is growing, thanks to funding from the Soros Foundation, the Robert Wood Johnson Foundation, City of Hope, Johns Hopkins University, the Association of American Colleges of Nursing, and other organizations that support educational efforts about EOL and palliative care. Nursing curricula are being revised to include content and competencies on EOL care. Training programs such as the End of Life Nursing Education Consortium (ELNEC) (www.aacn.nche.edu/elnec) are broadening nurses' knowledge in this specialty. A new training program was created by ELNEC that focuses on the pediatric population. This has been presented for the past 2 years in the United States and abroad. Modules that focus specifically on developmental issues regarding the concept of death and dying as well as how to assess for pain in the nonverbal child help health professionals to adapt materials to their settings. Organizations such as the International Association of Hospice and Palliative Care, the NHPCO, and the Hospice and Palliative Care Nurses Association, which traditionally have focused primarily on adult issues, have begun incorporating pediatric palliative care concerns into their initiatives. The inclusion of a chapter (Kenner & McSkimming, 2006) on palliative care in the NICU in Dr. Betty Ferrell's palliative care textbook—the gold standard in palliative care—will increase the awareness of the need for EOL care in this population. All these actions bode well for the integration of EOL care into customary pediatric and neonatal care as a standard that is expected and demanded.

BEREAVEMENT

The grief process is unique to each individual and varies in expression, duration, and meaning. Parents often move through the grief process differently. The infant's mother may express her grief by crying, whereas the father may express his grief by isolating himself.

For many parents, the grief process is lifelong. Significant life events can trigger their grieving, as can such routine childhood milestones as seeing a neighbor's child get on the school bus for her first day of kindergarten or, many years later, receiving a high school graduation announcement for what would have been their child's class.

As parents progress through the first year after their loss, it is important to prepare them for the grief they are likely to experience in the future and to help them develop a plan for themselves. Every family is unique and determines their own milestone days, those days that bring special remembrance of their child. Milestone days may include the child's birthday, the anniversary of the child's death, or holidays. It sometimes is helpful for parents to schedule time off on these milestone days so that they can plan a special activity. Some parents may want to be alone and take a quiet walk together. Others may prefer to be surrounded by relatives or a few close friends. Still others may want to spend the day with another parent who has experienced similar grief.

The nurse should stress three important points to bereaved families: (1) grief is individualized; (2) grief is a process; and (3) family members should not hesitate to seek assistance with their grief, even years after the child's death. (A comprehensive discussion of bereavement can be found on the Evolve website.) **evolve**

SUMMARY

Even when death approaches quickly in the NICU, measures can be taken to ease the infant's transition and adequately assist the family. It is no longer enough to provide quality bereavement and postmortem care to infants and their families. Research into and evaluation of care guidelines are needed so that infants can receive the same quality of EOL care afforded other members of society. Neonatal nurses have been at the forefront of this movement and now have the opportunity to serve as leaders in the design and implementation of exemplary neonatal palliative care programs.

REFERENCES

American Academy of Pediatrics (2000). Palliative care for children. *Pediatrics* 106(2):351-357.

Avery GB (1998). Futility considerations in the neonatal intensive care unit. *Seminars in perinatology* 22(3):216-222.

Beauchamp TL, Childress JF (2001). *Principles of biomedical ethics*, ed 5. New York: Oxford University Press.

Brody H et al (1997). Withdrawing intensive life-sustaining treatment: recommendations for compassionate clinical management. *New England journal of medicine* 336(9):652-657.

Byock I (1997). *Dying well: peace and possibilities at the end of life*. New York: Riverhead Books.

Carter BS et al (2004). Circumstances surrounding the deaths of hospitalized children: opportunities for pediatric palliative care. *Pediatrics* 114(3):e361-e366.

Catlin A, Carter B. (2002). Creation of a neonatal end-of-life palliative care protocol. *Journal of perinatology* 22(3):184-195.

Edmondson WAD (2005). The Oklahoma Attorney General's Task Force report on the state of end-of-life health care 2005. Oklahoma City, OK: The Oklahoma Attorney General's Task Force.

Goldman A (1998). ABC of palliative care: special problems of children. *British medical journal* 316(7124):49-52.

Harrison H (1993). The principles for family-centered neonatal care. *Pediatrics* 92(5):643-650.

Ho LY (2003). Perinatal care at the threshold of viability—from principles to practice. *Annals of the Academy of Medicine of Singapore* 32(3):362-375.

Jakobi P et al (1993). The extremely low birth weight infants: the twenty-first century dilemma. *American journal of perinatology* 10(2):155-159.

Jecker NS, Pagon RA (1995). Medical futility: decision making in the context of probability and uncertainty. In Goldworth A et al, editors. *Ethics and perinatology*. New York: Oxford University Press.

Kenner C, McSkimming S (2006). Palliative care in the neonatal intensive care unit. In Ferrell BR, Coyle N, editors. *Textbook of palliative nursing*, ed 2 (pp 959-973). New York: Oxford University Press.

Kerr E (2001). Kids Path cares for children coping with illness or loss. *MD news Piedmont triad* (5):24-26.

King NMP (1992). Transparency in neonatal intensive care. *Hastings Center report* 22(2):18-25.

Manning D (2005). Proxy consent in neonatal care—goal-directed or procedure-specific? *Health Care Anals* 13(1):1-9.

McCallum DE et al (2000). How children die in hospital. *Journal of pain and symptom management* 20(6):417-423.

Mehren E (1991). *Born too soon*. New York: Doubleday.

National Hospice and Palliative Care Organization (NHPCO) (2000). *Compendium of pediatric palliative care*. New Orleans, LA: NHPCO.

Partridge JC, Wall SN (1997). Analgesia for dying infants whose life support is withdrawn or withheld. *Pediatrics* 99(1):76-79.

Pearce EWJ (2006). Perinatal hospice/supportive care for the dying unborn infant. *Supportive voice*. Available at: http://www.careofdying.org/SV/PUBSART.ASP?ISSUE=SV99SU&ARTICLE=N. Retrieved January 2, 2006.

Pellegrino ED, Thomasma DC (1993). *The virtues in medical practice*. New York: Oxford University Press.

Penticuff JH (1987). Neonatal nursing ethics: toward a consensus. *Neonatal network* 5(6):7-16.

Penticuff JH (1988). Neonatal intensive care: parental prerogatives. *Journal of perinatal and neonatal nursing* 1(3):77-86.

Penticuff JH (1995). Nursing ethics in perinatal care. In Goldworth A et al, editors. *Ethics and perinatology*. New York: Oxford University Press.

Penticuff JH (1998). Defining futility in neonatal intensive care. *Nursing clinics of North America* 33(2):339-352.

Pinch WJ, Spielman ML (1993). Parental perceptions of ethical issues post-NICU discharge. *Western journal of nursing research* 15(4):422-440.

Pinch WJ, Spielman ML (1996). Ethics in the neonatal intensive care unit: parental perceptions at 4 years postdischarge. *Advances in nursing science* 19(1):72-85.

Pinkerton JV et al (1997). Parental rights at the birth of a near-viable infant: conflicting perspectives. *American journal of obstetrics and gynecology* 177(2):283-288.

President's Commission for the Study of Ethical Problems in Medicine and Biomedical and Behavioral Research (1983). *Deciding to forego life-sustaining treatment*. Washington, DC: U.S. Government Printing Office.

Raines DA (1996). Parents' values: a missing link in the neonatal intensive care equation. *Neonatal network* 15(3):7-12.

Rushton CH (2000). Pediatric palliative care: coming of age. *Innovations in end-of-life care* 2(2) (online journal).

Solomon MZ et al (2002). *The initiative for pediatric palliative care (IPPC): background and goals*. Newton, MA: Education Development Center, Inc. Available at: www.ippcweb.org. Retrieved January 2, 2006.

Stephenson J (2000). Palliative and hospice care needed for children with life-threatening conditions. *Journal of the American Medical Association* 284(19):2437-2438.

Stinson R, Stinson P (1979). *The long dying of baby Andrew*. Boston: Little, Brown.

Weir RF (1984). *Selective nontreatment of handicapped newborns*. New York: Oxford University Press.

Weir RF (1995). Withholding and withdrawing therapy and actively hastening death. II. In Goldworth A et al, editors. *Ethics and perinatology*. New York: Oxford University Press.

Wolfe J (2000). Suffering in children at the end of life: recognizing an ethical duty to palliate. *Journal of clinical ethics* 11(2):157-161.

Wolfe J et al (2000). Symptoms and suffering at the end of life in children with cancer. *New England journal of medicine* 342(5):326-333.

Yellin PB et al (1998). Neonatologists' decisions about withholding and withdrawing treatments from critically ill newborns. *Pediatrics* 102(3):757.

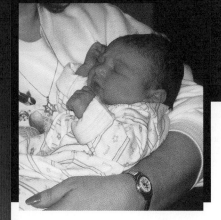

Chapter 27

When a Baby Dies: Caring for Bereaved Families

Karen Kavanaugh • Sara Rich Wheeler

The death of a newborn is a tragic and unexpected outcome of a pregnancy. Instead of experiencing joy with the arrival of a new baby, bereaved parents are faced with unparalleled grief that is often misunderstood by their family or friends. Furthermore, little attention is given to newborn death in popular literature, and the news media focus on births of higher order multiples reinforces the public's impression that smaller, sicker infants survive. This media focus further reinforces the attitude that death is avoidable. Yet, despite drastic reductions in newborn and infant mortality in even the past 20 years (Arias et al, 2003), infant death is still a reality in the neonatal intensive care unit (NICU).

In 2002 there were 27,970 infant deaths in the United States (National Center for Health Statistics, 2005). In that year, the infant mortality rate (IMR), which is the number of deaths in the first year of life, was 7.0 (per 1000 live births) (National Center for Health Statistics, 2005). The neonatal mortality rate (NMR), which is the number of deaths among infants under 28 days of age, was 4.7. These mortality rates remain much higher for African American infants, among whom the IMR is 13.8 and the NMR is 9.9 (National Center for Health Statistics, 2005). The leading causes of death in the neonatal period are disorders related to short gestation, low birth weight, and congenital malformations (National Center for Health Statistics, 2005). The leading causes of infant death in the postneonatal period are sudden infant death syndrome (SIDS) and congenital malformations (National Center for Health Statistics, 2005).

When death occurs in the NICU, the health care professionals should provide expert, compassionate care to the family of the newborn. To do so, they must understand the grief responses of family members and the issues unique to newborn death. This chapter discusses the grief process within the context of theoretic models and a framework for providing care to families.

THEORETIC MODELS

Theoretic models provide a framework for describing responses to loss and developing guidelines for caring for families. A knowledge of grief theory (classic and current), complicated grief, types of loss (sudden or anticipated), and a middle range theory of caring is important both for understanding the responses of families whose newborn has been diagnosed with a life-threatening or terminal illness and for providing care for these families. Selected classic theories of grief are included

to highlight the theorist's contributions to the understanding of grief. However, these theories have been inappropriately applied to the grief of parents after a newborn death; these models have not been adequately tested with parents. Current models of grief are also reviewed, and these provide a fuller understanding of the complex, individual, and continuing nature of grief. These more recent models are based on research with bereaved individuals who have suffered various types of loss, including parental grief. In a recent review of theoretical perspectives of grief, Davies (2004) has also highlighted the relevance of newer models of grief for understanding parental responses.

Classic Theories of Grief

Psychodynamic models of grief were heavily influenced by Freud (1961) and focused on grief as a dilemma resulting from the process of relinquishing a beloved object. Freud differentiated grief from depression and observed somatic distress in grievers, as well as a lack of interest in the outside world, an apparent loss of capacity to love, and painful dejection. Lindemann (1944), who conducted the first empirically, based study of grief on adult survivors of a fire, found that the daily activities of the bereaved changed significantly and that the duration of grief seemed to depend on the person's willingness to mourn. Lindemann coined the term *grief work* to describe the mourning process. He characterized grief work as emancipation from the bondage of the deceased, readjustment to the environment in which the deceased is missing, and the formation of new relationships. Lindemann also described behaviors characterized as "pathologic grief"; however, use of such behaviors as criteria for pathologic grief in parents who have lost an infant has come under criticism (Janssen & Cuisinier, 1996).

Kubler-Ross (1969) studied the emotional responses of terminally ill adult patients as they anticipated their own deaths. In her pioneering work, *Death and Dying,* Kubler-Ross set forth a stage-based model for understanding the task of coping with dying and brought about significant changes in the way people thought about dying. Kubler-Ross reestablished death as a natural part of life and recognized that dying patients and their families want to discuss the impending death. The five-stage model of grief Kubler-Ross developed is her most frequently cited contribution to the literature. The stages she identified are denial, anger, bargaining, depression, and acceptance.

Over the years, many have mistakenly come to view the five-stage model as a predictive, developmental model in which the second stage cannot occur unless the first stage had been completed, and so on. The erroneous belief that the five stages are prescriptive in nature has fostered unrealistic expectations about grief on the part of those dying, the family members, and caregivers. Corr (1993) has identified other limitations with this model. Corr explained that the five stages are really defense mechanisms or ways of coping. Furthermore, these stages do not fully represent all ways of coping and especially do not fully account for the complex experience of dying. Nevertheless, an important lesson from Kubler-Ross's work is that knowledge about dying and grief must come firsthand from those who experience these life events; attentive listening, therefore, is critical to understanding people's responses and needs.

Current Models of Grief

More recently theorists have presented new views of grief, which stand in contrast to the classic view of a process of detaching from the deceased (Klass & Silverman, 1996; Sanders, 1989; Solari-Twadell & Bunkers, 1995; Neimeyer, 2001). Current models of bereavement are based on the meaning of the loss to the person and on attachment theory. Investigators recently demonstrated strong empirical support for these theoretical perspectives for perinatal grief (Uren & Wastell, 2002). Attachment models are rooted in the belief that attachment behavior is instinctive and that attachments are essential to human behavior. The goal of attachment behavior is to maintain effectual bonds; if the bonds are threatened, the individual seeks to preserve them (Bowlby, 1980).

Sanders

Sanders (1989) offers a comprehensive framework for understanding grief as an integrative theory. Her work is based on previous studies by Bowlby (1980), Engel (1961), Freud (1961), and Parks and Brown (1972). Integrative theory focuses on the interrelationship between the bereaved person and environmental factors (internal and external) that will affect the person's grief process. Internal factors include age, gender, personality, physical health, relationship with the deceased, and dependency behaviors. External factors include social support and the type of death (e.g., sudden, anticipated, or the result of long-term illness).

Sanders identified the following phases of bereavement. It is important to remember that the phases coexist, with one or more predominating.

Shock. This phase is the expression of the impossibility of death. Sudden and unexpected loss may generate a greater degree of shock, but even when the death is anticipated, there is still some degree of shock and disbelief. The characteristics of shock are disbelief, confusion, restlessness, and feelings of unreality, regression, helplessness, and a state of alarm. Physical responses to shock may include dry mouth and throat, sighing, loss of strength, crying, uncontrollable trembling, easily startled, upset stomach, loss of appetite, and sleep disturbances. Psychologic responses may be narrowing of the perceptual field, concern for self-needs, preoccupation with thoughts about the baby's death, and psychologic withdrawal. Sanders noted, "Shock can last from a few minutes to many days, but it usually passes into the next phase when the rituals of death are over

and the emotions that have been constricted so tightly begin to release and overflow."

Awareness of Loss. Separation anxiety predominates in this phase of bereavement. On a cognitive level, the bereaved knows the death has occurred, but on another level, the death is not perceived as real. Many environmental cues remind the bereaved of their loss (e.g., the baby's room, a car without a car seat, and other parents with babies). The bereaved may feel physical pain and deep emotions when faced with these cues. There are many emotional struggles during this time. These conflicts are hard to resolve because they usually involve change. Grief takes time and energy that depletes the body's physical and emotional reserves. The immune system becomes impaired because of its response to the stress of grief. The bereaved are more susceptible to infectious diseases. Physical symptoms of this phase include aching arms, a gnawing in the stomach, heart palpitations, and sleep disturbances (e.g., nightmares, waking in the middle of the night thinking that they heard their deceased loved one, and difficulty falling asleep). The psychologic and emotional symptoms are yearning to see the loved one, sensing the presence of the baby, crying, anger, guilt, frustration, shame, oversensitivity, denial, and fear of another loved one's death. Physical and emotional exhaustion are paramount in this phase. This exhaustion motivates the bereaved to withdraw from others in an effort to conserve their strength and energy.

Conservation-Withdrawal. This phase closely resembles clinical depression. The bereaved may feel as if they are "losing their minds." The withdrawal behavior may be reflected in a fatigued feeling and a need for rest. They feel as if they have little strength for everyday activities and need to conserve what energy they do have. Despair prevails because on both a conscious and an unconscious level, the bereaved are aware that the loved one has died and that their life together is over. Life as the bereaved have known it, will never be the same. There is very little support for the bereaved at this time. Extended family members and friends have gone on with their lives and do not realize that the bereaved are still grieving their loss; they think that the bereaved have picked up the pieces and moved on with life. Immediate family members are mustering all their resources to keep themselves going and are unable to help each other. The bereaved may feel very helpless during this phase, especially if the deceased defined the bereaved's role.

Healing. Healing occurs when the person's internal perceptions about himself or herself change from one who is bereaved to one who has experienced and survived the loss of a loved one. In the healing phase, the turning point becomes more defined in the person's thoughts. The bereaved begin to assume control of their lives and to make decisions about the future. This occurs slowly, over time. Men may feel a need to gain better control over their emotions; women may feel a greater need for control over their environment. Decisions about the future include developing a new identity, relinquishing old roles, assuming new roles in life and, for bereaved parents, whether to become pregnant again.

Throughout the grief process, the bereaved have searched for the meaning of their loss. What did the death mean? How will the deceased be remembered? Who will remember the loved one? What did the loved one's death mean to others? This search continues until some conclusion has been reached; this is known as loss integration. As time goes by, the bereaved develop different perspectives on their loss and the events surrounding the death. Kowalski (1991) called this change in how the bereaved remember their loved one and the circumstances of the death "bittersweet grief." Bittersweet grief is the remembering of this experience and their loved one that stimulates a regrief for families. Anniversary dates, life milestones, and special holidays may bring back the grief. Their loved one is not there to take part in the event or is unable to achieve a specific developmental task.

Renewal. This phase of bereavement occurs when the bereaved have dealt with the social consequences of bereavement, experienced an increase in self-esteem, taken charge and responsibility for their lives, and learned to live again. Renewal means new levels of functioning, a new awareness of self. Not all bereaved experience this phase of bereavement. The physical aspects are revitalization, stability in functioning, and the ability to care for one's physical needs. The psychologic aspects include feeling good about oneself again and living life with new vitality.

Klass, Silverman, and Nickman

In their respective research with families experiencing different types of loss (that of a child, spouse, or parent), Klass and colleagues (1996) found that bereaved children and bereaved adults struggle to maintain a connection to the one who has died; they form an inner sense of continuing bond with the deceased. This inner representation provides a connection with the physically absent but emotionally present loved one. Survivors remember the deceased lovingly for a long time, often forever. Remaining connected seems to facilitate the bereaved's ability to cope with the loss and accompanying changes in their lives. The connections provide comfort and support and ease the transition from past to future. This phenomenon cannot be accounted for in the early, classic models of grief.

In explaining parental grief, Klass said that grief involves changing the inner representations of the deceased children in the parent's inner and social worlds. The inner representation of the child is changed in the parent's life when the reality of a child's death and the reality of a parent's continuing bond with the child are made part of the socially shared reality. The end of grief is not breaking the bond with the deceased child; rather, it is integrating the child into the parent's life and into social networks in a different way from when the child was alive. Thus grief is the process by which the bereaved move from the equilibria in their inner and social worlds before a death to new equilibria after a death. Klass reported that it takes 3 to 4 years before the new equilibria seem steady enough to trust. In his work with bereaved parents, he found that, "You do not get over your grief," but it does not stay the same. Also, Klass did not find any prescribed stages of grief.

Cordell and Thomas

Cordell and Thomas (1997) have also expanded our understanding of parental grief. These authors presented their extended concept of parental grief because of the inadequacy of existing theories, particularly the stage models, in accounting for the grief of parents after the death of an infant. According to Cordell and Thomas, parental mourning is an enduring process that, rather than letting go, involves affirming the infant's life and the parent's role. Furthermore, the grief of parents is complex and individual; grief can be severe,

complicated, and enduring and show many variations in emotional state over an extended period. As such, grief is an ongoing process. Parents work through their emotions from day to day and go through a continuous process of reexperiencing emotional reactions. Cordell and Thomas explained that parents are surprised at the intensity of their emotions, that mothers and fathers differ in their response, that this affects communication between them, and that parents perceive that others do not understand what they are going through and expect them to "get over" the death.

Pinwheel Model of Bereavement

Another current model of grief is the pinwheel model described by Solari-Twadell and Bunkers (1995). According to this model, loss and bereavement are unique, individually lived experiences that are based on the personal history of the bereaved (such as who the loved one was and what the person meant to the bereaved). Understanding the history of the bereaved is critical for understanding the individual's loss. Personal history is the context in which other core themes are embedded. These core themes, which characterize the response to loss, include being stopped, pain and hurting, missing, holding, seeking, and valuing. Being stopped describes the interruption in one's life. A cluster of very intense painful emotions characterizes pain and hurting. Missing incorporates the awareness of all that has been lost. Holding is the desire to preserve all from the loved one's existence. Seeking is a search for help, and valuing implies that the loss is cherished by the bereaved.

The individual moves out from these inner experiences through the process of surrender. Surrender occurs when a person begins to reach out to others and rejoin life. Rejoining life can be difficult, because life is different. Acceptance of the fact that life is different allows individuals to include new relationships and events in their lives. According to the pinwheel model, grief is a lifelong experience. It does not last for a specific amount of time, but rather continues indefinitely. Years after the loss, "waves" of feelings occur, even though they may not be as intense or as frequent as the initial period. Bereavement interphases with continuing life experiences, and when this occurs, the loss can be revisited, and the core themes are experienced intensely. Revisiting the loss is a normal part of grief and continues throughout a person's life.

"Pathologic" and Complicated Grief

No firm conclusions can be drawn about "pathologic" or "abnormal" responses to loss in parents after the death of a newborn. In their review of studies on pathologic grief after a perinatal loss, Janssen and Cuisinier (1996) concluded that psychologic and somatic complaints and behavioral changes are common in the first 6 months after a loss; therefore depressive reactions, somatic complaints, and impaired functioning are common for at least the first 6 months. Only about 10% to 15% of mothers of these infants have an extreme response and meet the criteria for a psychiatric mood disorder, and many of these mothers have a history of mental health problems. Uren and Wastell (2002) have recently recommended that for perinatal loss, grief manifestations should be viewed on a continuum rather than dichotomizing them as either normal or pathologic. In the general bereavement literature, complicated grief rather than "pathologic" grief has been described and recently proposed as a distinct psychopathologic diagnostic entity different from other mental health entities, such as depression and posttraumatic stress disorder (Lichtenthal et al, 2004).

Recently, investigators have proposed an explanatory model of health in bereaved parents after a pregnancy loss or infant death (Lang et al, 2004). This model is based on the conceptual model of family stress and focuses on individual and couple strengths as opposed to the negative consequences of loss. In their study of 110 bereaved couples, internal (hardiness) support and external (marital and social) support were the consistent predictors of health over time for both parents. With hardiness, marital satisfaction and social support were predictive of how parents appraised their situation and health status (Lang et al, 2004). The investigators recommend further research to fully understand the variables in this model and ultimately use it to clinical practice. Because of the uniqueness of perinatal loss, others have also recommended further research to more adequately understand the course of perinatal loss, the mental health outcomes associated with this type of a loss, and trials of interventions to determine the best approaches to care (Bennett et al, 2005).

Although there is insufficient evidence to fully understand complicated grief in perinatal loss and identify parents who are at risk for mental health problems after a loss, nurses still need guidelines to determine when a person needs to be referred to a mental health professional. This is critical because it is hard to differentiate between depression and grief: They look similar (Lichtenthal et al, 2004), especially in the first weeks after a loss (Friedrichs et al, 2000). Although it is the responsibility of a qualified mental health professional to distinguish between uncomplicated bereavement and clinical depression, nurses need to be aware of symptoms that may serve as "red flags" to alert the nurse to the need for referral (Box 27-1). Symptoms common to grief and depression include fatigue, sadness, tearfulness, lack of motivation, inability to enjoy oneself, and changes in sleep and appetite. Symptoms specific to depression are acute suicidality (preoccupation with dying, verbalization of purposelessness and a lack of hope, or a plan to hurt or kill oneself), hallucinations or guilt unrelated to the infant, and any one symptom that completely immobilizes a person.

Types of Loss
Sudden Loss
Sudden and unexpected death is very difficult for the family and for the professionals caring for them. There is no time to anticipate the loss, to prepare oneself emotionally, and to mobilize past coping skills. For these reasons, on hearing the bad news many parents and their families find that they cannot comprehend what is being said and are immediately overwhelmed with raw coping and defense mechanisms (avoidance, denial, anger, withdrawal). It may appear as if they have not heard what they were just told. Health care professionals need to be quiet alongside families at this time, not judging what is said or done, but rather creating a safe environment for the expression of emotions of grief and feelings of loss.

Anticipated Loss
Anticipatory grief may develop when a loss is anticipated in the near future. The family who has a critically ill member has the opportunity to entertain the idea that their loved one may die. While the loved one is in intensive care, the pattern of the family's life begins to change from the expected

---

BOX 27-1

Signs That May Indicate a Need for Psychologic Referral

Physical Symptoms

Loss or gain of 15% of the person's body weight

Inability to maintain or initiate basic activities of daily living, including care of surviving children

Abuse of alcohol or mood-altering chemicals

Symptoms of anxiety or depression that interfere with physical health

Worsening of symptoms over time

Emotional Symptoms

Symptoms of anxiety or depression that interfere with functioning at home or work or in social relationships (e.g., social withdrawal, inability to communicate)

Thoughts of suicide that become almost constant, expression of serious suicide intent, or development of a plan for suicide

Emotional responses (e.g., anger, guilt, self-blame) or obsessive thinking that worsens or does not change over time

Social Responses

Feeling of isolation because of inadequate support systems or lack of such systems

Difficulties in relationships with partner, children, family, or friends

Reclusiveness

---

homecoming; instead, they are going home from the hospital without their baby, staying at the hospital instead of being home, and experiencing severe emotional ups and downs with their baby's health. Families begin to learn how to cope with their critically ill baby; they learn the language and special nuances of the unit, where to find information to help them understand what is happening to their baby and, eventually, how to take care of themselves.

Rando (1986) identified family coping tasks for individuals who anticipate the death of a loved one as accepting versus denying the illness, establishing relationships with caregivers, regulating affect, renegotiating family relationships, meeting the needs of the dying, and coping with the postdeath phase. According to Rando, because the loss is anticipated, parents may begin to work through these phases before the death. Some families may even detach from their loved one too soon to protect themselves from the reality of the loved one's death. This may leave the dying baby alone and isolated, which can be frustrating to the health care staff members. During this time, families may be focused on relieving their infant's suffering. A program of hospice care can be an appropriate intervention at this time for all families whose infant is dying.

Middle Range Theory of Caring
A middle range theory of caring (Swanson, 1991, 1993) can be used as a theoretic framework for providing care to bereaved families. Elements of this theory were tested in a caring-based counseling intervention study with women who had miscarriages (Swanson, 1999a). This theory has also been supported in a meta-analysis of caring research (Swanson,

1999b) and in studies of perinatal loss (Kavanaugh, 1997b; Kavanaugh & Hershberger, 2005; Kavanaugh & Robertson, 1999; Lemmer, 1991), and it has been recommended as practice guidelines for perinatal bereavement support (Hutti, 2005; Wheeler & Pike, 1991; Leon, 1992; Hersch & Gensch, 1993). According to Swanson (1993), caring is a "nurturing way of relating to a valued other toward whom one feels a personal sense of commitment and responsibility." For health care professionals, the ultimate goal of caring is to enable patients and their families to achieve well-being.

Caring consists of five therapeutic processes: maintaining belief, knowing, being with, doing for, and enabling. Maintaining belief is sustaining faith in the capacity of families to get through the experience of losing an infant and finding meaning in the experience. Behaviors for this caring process include believing in, offering a hope-filled attitude, going the distance, offering realistic optimism, and helping find meaning. Knowing is striving to understand the experience through the parents' perspective. These behaviors include avoiding assumptions, assessing thoroughly, seeking cues, centering on the other, and engaging the self of both parents. Being with conveys the message of availability and ability to be emotionally and physically present. This includes being there, conveying availability, enduring with, sharing feelings, and not burdening. Doing for is doing for the parents what they would do for themselves and their infant if at all possible by anticipating their needs and preserving both the family's and the infant's dignity. Doing for includes performing skillfully, comforting, anticipating, protecting, and preserving dignity. Finally, enabling is facilitating the parents' passage through the experience by informing, explaining, and helping families to think through important decisions. Enabling includes generating alternatives, informing, validating, supporting, and focusing.

GRIEF RESPONSES OF FAMILIES WHEN AN INFANT DIES

Women's Responses

"My arms still ache to hold our tiny baby."

"I have never been on such an emotional roller coaster; one day you think you're up and are going to make it through all this, and the next moment you're overwhelmed with all of your emotions."

The physical symptoms women report after a stillbirth or newborn death are emptiness, headaches, irritability, nausea, dizziness, backache, chest pains, nervousness, palpitations, muscle tension, aching arms, numbness and tingling, tachypnea, difficulty sleeping, and fatigue (Kavanaugh & Hershberger, 2005; Peppers & Knapp, 1980a, 1980b). The emotional feelings described by these women are disappointment, guilt, failure, embarrassment, emotional cocooning, inadequacy, and anger (Kavanaugh & Hershberger, 2005; Peppers & Knapp, 1980a, 1980b; Hunfeld & Wladimiroff, 1997). Women may want to blame someone or something for the death of their baby, such as God, a member of the medical profession, or themselves, or all of these. Women report feeling cheated and that the death was unfair. Social responses include feeling lonely and ostracized (Cecil, 1994; Rajan, 1994; DeMontigny & Beaudet, 1999; Malacrida, 1999) or experiencing insensitive behaviors or unkind comments (Van & Meleis, 2003). Isolation and lack of social support occur, especially when family and friends had not had the chance to know the infant and therefore minimize

the loss. Other commonly described behaviors include loss of the future, shattered dreams, fears, inability to concentrate, and difficulty being with pregnant women and infants (Kavanaugh, 1997a; Kavanaugh & Hershberger, 2005).

Men's Responses

"Everyone kept telling me I needed to be strong for Jayne; no one ever asked about me."

"I'll tell you what my grief is like. It's like someone rammed their fist down my throat and ripped out my heart."

The physical responses reported by fathers are restlessness, emptiness, sleeping disturbances, nightmares, fatigue, weight gain, high blood pressure, diminished appetite, feelings of exhaustion, and arm pain (Kimble, 1991). The emotional responses of fathers include anger, avoidance of feelings, jealousy, guilt, sadness, unhappiness, crying, disappointment, helplessness, vulnerability, despair, and self-pity (Kimble, 1991; McCreight, 2004; Puddifoot & Johnson, 1997). Some fathers express a feeling of powerlessness over their own lives and emotions (Kavanaugh, 1997a; Kavanaugh & Hershberger, 2005). The father's anger may be directed at God, himself, peers, or unrelated events that make him feel overwhelmed by the things he needs to do (e.g., arranging for the burial, or even carrying out daily tasks) (Kimble, 1991). Social responses include feeling alone and a desire to withdraw from others. Some fathers report that they also feel an overwhelming concern for their spouse's well-being (Kavanaugh, 1997a; Kavanaugh & Hershberger, 2005; McCreight, 2004). Some fathers have felt that their experiences were misunderstood or not acknowledged by family, friends, and coworkers, which left them feeling unsupported by their family and community (McCreight, 2004; Puddifoot & Johnson, 1997; Wagner & Higgins, 1997). Fathers' cognitive responses include difficulty concentrating, disorganized thoughts, and preoccupation with fears for their partner's well-being (Kimble, 1991; Puddifoot & Johnson, 1997).

Couples' Responses

"I really didn't want to go out after Jonathon died, but I would go because Jay would want me to ... so we worked out a signal that I could let him know when I was ready to go home."

"I didn't know what to do ... all she could do was cry, and someone needed to hold it all together or nothing would have gotten done."

Perinatal grief has been associated with marital discord (Wallerstedt & Higgins, 1996). Gilbert (1989) described the effects of perinatal loss on marital relationships. In that study, women appeared to have the additional experience of physically healing after a loss. Many men, however, had the burden not only of dealing with their own responses to the perinatal loss but also of coping with the threat to the wife's health. Couples looked to one another for confirmation of their feelings of loss and for support. Factors that influenced the marital relationship were the couple's ability to share their grief, to accept the differences in each other's grief responses, to be sensitive to each other's needs, to be flexible in role responsibilities, and to spend time together.

Feeley and Gottlieb (2000) found that after a stillbirth, a newborn death, or the death of an infant from SIDS, mothers had a more difficult time communicating their grief, whereas fathers had difficulty expressing their emotions. These fathers also had difficulty coping with the mothers' emotional responses. Peppers and Knapp (1980b) had identified this response as incongruent grief, a term they used to describe the differences in a couple's responses after the death of an infant.

In summary, investigators have found that, compared with fathers, mothers grieve for a longer time and show more intense or a greater number of responses, such as guilt, despair, and crying (Cuisinier et al, 1996; DiMarco et al, 2001; Lin & Lasker, 1996; Theut & Zaslow, 1990). However, investigators have shown that fathers do manifest more intense responses (Conway & Russell, 2000), and in one study, shame proneness in men predicted intensity of grief in men at 13 months after the loss (Barr, 2004). In addition to more intense, more prolonged grieving, mothers reported a longing to hold or to be with the infant and also difficulty being with other infants (Tudehope & Iredell, 1986; Kavanaugh, 1997a; Kavanaugh & Hershberger, 2005). In contrast, fathers described being concerned about their wives and reported feelings of helplessness and a need to be strong (Kavanaugh, 1997a; Kavanaugh & Hershberger, 2005; McCreight, 2004). Several investigators have described different coping mechanisms for mothers and fathers. Mothers coped by talking about the loss (Black, 1991; Rajan, 1994), but fathers coped by returning to work or normalcy (Rajan, 1994) or by engaging in other physical activity (Black, 1991; Kavanaugh, 1997a).

These differences in grief response may be due to the different grieving styles as described by Martin and Doka (2002), with mothers displaying behaviors typical of intuitive grievers and fathers displaying instrumental griever's behaviors. Intuitive grievers experience grief as waves of affect and adapt by finding ways to express their emotions (Martin & Doka, 2002). In contrast, instrumental grievers describe their grief in physical, cognitive, or behavioral manifestations. Thus, expressions and coping strategies tend to be active and cognitive (Martin & Doka, 2002).

Adolescents as Bereaved Parents

The few studies available on adolescent pregnancy loss (miscarriage, stillbirth, or newborn death) suggest that adolescent girls may show a wide range of responses, and many of these girls become pregnant again soon after their loss (Barglow et al, 1973; Stevens-Simon et al, 1996; Wheeler, 1997; Wheeler & Austin, 2001). Barglow and coworkers (1973) found that adolescent girls moved through stages resembling a mourning process. A yearning that was characterized by daydreaming about their infant and a desire to become pregnant again followed initial feelings of shock.

Adolescent parents, both females and males, also experienced guilt, anger, and many somatic complaints. Apathy typically was expressed by a neglect of self-care or by an inability to visualize the future, responses researchers perceived as a way for these young people to cover their pain and despair. Recovery occurred when adolescents became more purposeful in their behavior and began to think about their future.

Adolescent girls who experienced miscarriage, stillbirth, or newborn death had physical disturbances such as exhaustion, change in appetite, aches and pains, dry mouth, and feeling a lump in the throat (Wheeler, 1997; Wheeler & Austin, 2001). Emotional responses included guilt, anger, irritability, fear of failure, crying easily, frequent mood changes, an increase in emotional sensitivity, a desire to scream, and feelings of emptiness or of being barren. Not all adolescents cried at the

time of the loss, and some believed that they could have "done something" to prevent the loss. The social responses of the adolescents included isolating themselves from others and feeling "different." Cognitive responses reflected a disbelief that the loss had occurred, confusion, difficulty concentrating, and preoccupation with thoughts about the baby, the experience itself, and how life would have been different if the pregnancy had continued. Some adolescents viewed the experience as having a positive outcome; they believed that the loss was for the best, that they had a better understanding of the fragility of life, or that they felt more mature. Only a few indicated a desire to die or to be dead.

These studies suggest that miscarriage, stillbirth, or newborn death is a significant life event for most adolescents, and for some it might be followed by grief responses, a bereavement process, and perhaps a rapid repeat pregnancy.

Children's Responses

Little research has been done in the area of children's responses to the death of a newborn sibling. Children's grief responses are influenced by their ability to conceptualize death, their age and vocabulary at the time of the death, their parents' responses to the death, and previous social and cultural experiences with death. Even very young children (i.e., those under the age of 2) can perceive the changes in their family's routines and their parents' feelings and can observe the emotions that accompany the death of an infant. Young children may not understand the concept of death and its irreversibility, but they do understand separation. When children see their parents sad, tense, irritable, and upset, they want to know what made them feel this way. It is very easy for children at any age to interpret their parents' responses to the death of an infant, or even the death itself, as being their fault.

Children cannot cope with the death of a sibling unless their parents can. Parents naturally model behavior for their children. In addition, if parents are withdrawn and remote, the children may suffer a significant secondary loss, the functional loss of their parents (Dowden, 1995). Initially, all children react to the death of their sibling. Therefore, when parents cannot cope with their own loss and that of their surviving children, it is helpful to involve other family members or friends to recognize and acknowledge the surviving child(ren)'s grief (Wilson, 2001). There are common responses among children that can build on each other based on the child's age. Younger children might become more demanding, cling more to their parents, cry or fuss more, express fears of abandonment, have nightmares, or feel guilty. School-age children may become more aggressive at school, withdraw from others, make poorer grades, feel rejected, be angry, or worry more. Adolescents may react similarly to school-age children and may also act confused or stay away from home or become overly involved in taking care of their parents to the exclusion of other friendships. Typically, when children feel that they are not receiving the time and attention they need from their parents, they "act out" in ways that attract the parents' attention.

Both caregivers and parents need to be mindful of the individuality of each child when planning interventions. Parents need to recognize and acknowledge their child's grief, include them in family events, rituals, and practices, and talk about the baby who died (Wilson, 2001; Cote-Arsenault, 2003b). It is important for parents to explain to their children in language and concrete examples that the children will understand. Age-appropriate books can be used to assist with the explanation. It is critical to be honest and not to tell stories that must be changed as the child grows. It is important to answer all questions, even if the answer is "I don't know." Children who have never experienced a death need to be told about death in terms of the body being unable to work any more. Young children understand that toys break, do not work in the same way, and cannot be fixed. Children then will want to know what happens after death. Parents should explain about the rituals they are following in saying goodbye and should include their children if the children want to be included.

One of the most difficult concepts for children to understand is how people get to heaven when they are buried in the ground (if that is the family's spiritual belief) (Schaefer & Lyons, 1993). To explain how souls get to heaven, parents can put a glove, which represents the body, on their hand, and then take the glove off and lay it down, demonstrating staying on earth; they then move the hand that was in the glove in a fluttering motion to show how the soul gets to heaven.

Over time children's grief responses slowly abate. Professional help might be needed if a child is consistently having problems, if the responses worsen instead of improve over time, if the child's responses change suddenly or dramatically, or if the parents feel that they cannot cope.

Grandparents' Responses

A 10-year study by DeFrain (1991) of parents who experienced a stillbirth, newborn death, or SIDS included extended family members, primarily grandparents. Grandparents have a double burden of grief. They see their child suffering from the loss of the baby and are unable to make the situation better for their child. They cannot carry the burden of their own child's grief. They also are grieving for the grandchild who died. They, too, had hopes and dreams of being a grandparent and of whom the baby would resemble and would grow to be like. Grandparents have their own grief process and in their search to determine what happened may inadvertently blame themselves for "bad genes" or their children for not doing all they could during the pregnancy or after birth. DeFrain found that grandparents need information on how they can help their children recover from their loss, how long grief lasts, and the differences between men's and women's grief responses.

NURSING CARE OF BEREAVED FAMILIES

Standardized checklists for caring for families who experience a loss are available (Jansen, 2003) and have been developed at many institutions. These checklists focus on tasks, such as providing infant mementos and encouraging parents to see and hold their infant. However, these checklists should not be used as a standardized approach for all patients without adequately assessing the parent's needs (Hutti, 2005; Leon, 1992). Caring behaviors should be used in conjunction with checklists to guide care to adequately assess and plan for individualized care for bereaved families.

In her study of parents' perceptions of caring after a stillbirth or newborn death, Lemmer (1991) identified two categories of caring: taking care of, which involved providing expert care and information, and caring for or about, which involved providing direct emotional support and individualized, family-centered care; acting as a surrogate parent; facilitating the creation of memories; and respecting the rights of parents.

These caring behaviors are similar to those described in Swanson's middle range theory of caring. Together with the rights of the parents when a baby dies (Box 27-2) and the rights of the deceased infant (Box 27-3), these behaviors can serve as the basis for supportive care of families.

Caring Behaviors
Providing Expert Care

Families expect nurses to be knowledgeable, competent, efficient, and able to anticipate and manage problems in the

---

BOX 27-2

Rights of Parents When a Baby Dies

To be given the opportunity to see, hold, and touch their baby at any time before and after death, within reason

To have photographs of their baby taken and made available to the parents or held in security until the parents wish to see them

To be given as many mementos as possible (e.g., crib card, baby beads, ultrasound and other photographs, lock of hair, footprints and handprints, record of weight and length)

To name their child and bond with him or her

To observe cultural and religious practices

To be cared for by empathetic staff members who will respect their feelings, thoughts, beliefs, and individual requests

To be with each other throughout the hospitalization as much as possible

To be given time alone with their baby, allowing for individual needs

To request an autopsy; in the case of miscarriage, to request to have or not have an autopsy or pathology examination as determined by law

To have information presented in terminology understandable to the parents regarding their baby's status and cause of death, including autopsy and pathology reports and medical records

To plan a farewell ritual, burial, or cremation in compliance with local state regulations and according to their personal beliefs or religious or cultural tradition

To be provided with information on support resources that assist in the healing process (e.g., support groups, counseling, reading material, perinatal loss newsletters)

From SHARE, Pregnancy and Infant Loss Support, Inc., St. Joseph's Health Center, 300 First Capital Drive, St. Charles, MO 63301.

BOX 27-3

Rights of the Deceased Baby

To be recognized as a person who was born and died
To be named
To be seen, touched, and held by the family
To have life-ending acknowledgment
To be put to rest with dignity

From SHARE, Pregnancy and Infant Loss Support, Inc., St. Joseph's Health Center, 300 First Capital Drive, St. Charles, MO 63301.

care of their sick newborn (Kavanaugh, 1997b; Lemmer, 1991; Lundqvist et al, 2002)). The nurse must recognize significant signs and symptoms that reflect a change in the baby and report appropriately to the neonatologist and must be able to identify comfort needs and pain relief for both mother and newborn. Nurses in the NICU should remember that many mothers who have an infant in their unit have recently given birth, and their needs are the same as those of any woman who has given birth (e.g., peri-pads, milk expression or suppression, pain relief, rest, nutrition). Food and fluids for families must be available on the unit or in the parents' lounge to help the mother replenish her physical strength after birth. Beverages should be decaffeinated, to reduce physical stress and promote rest. Comfortable chairs and couches that make up into beds must be available to further ensure adequate rest. Mothers who have experienced a cesarean birth or difficult delivery may have additional physical needs (e.g., pain medication in the NICU, wheelchair access, and outlets for plugging in intravenous pumps).

Families need to be reassured that the nurses and doctors are knowledgeable and technically competent. Many parents have never seen a preterm infant before. Therefore, nurses need to encourage and instill confidence in parents as they become acquainted with their baby (Lundqvist et al, 2002). Parents expect the staff members to talk with each other about the care of their baby so that their child receives consistent care between caregivers, between shifts, and from shift to shift. Parents have been reported to be distressed when they perceive a lack of continuity (Kavanaugh & Hershberger, 2005). When the nurses give special attention to their baby, families appreciate this gesture. Some examples of special attention are notes written on behalf of the baby to the parent or parents, special pictures, remembering holidays celebrated by the family, and unrestricted visitation for siblings, extended family, and friends.

Providing Information

The importance of communicating with parents who experience a perinatal loss has been documented repeatedly in the research literature.[*] Nurses need to remember that when families have an infant in the NICU, they are in crisis. When families perceive themselves as being in crisis, their behavior and understanding of what is being discussed may be different from what the nurses or physicians think it should be or from how they might be under normal circumstances. It is important for nurses to look for cues that tell them the parents or family members have heard what has been said; such cues include eye contact, questions that reflect the information just given, and responses to that information. In most cases the infant's birth has been the only hospital experience the parents have had before the baby's admission to the NICU, and they may not be knowledgeable about the culture of health care (e.g., when their physician will make rounds, how the health care system works, medical terminology, or the purposes of technical equipment and medications). Most parents are either unaware of the questions or are afraid to ask them. Nurses can help

parents determine what questions they need to ask, how to ask them, and when.

Several researchers have offered guidelines for communicating painful medical news.[†] These guidelines include the following:

- Prepare the parents by giving them a warning before actually giving the painful information.
- Have a person who is known to the parents and who knows their baby deliver the news.
- Give the news in person in a private, quiet, comfortable location free of distraction.
- Give the news as soon as possible when problems are suspected.
- Give the news when the parents are with the baby and are together or when other supportive individuals are present.
- Give the news with compassion and caring, paying attention to body position and language.
- Give clear, accurate, information and present it with certainty (or the appropriate degree of certainty); use diagrams and illustrations to include positive characteristics of the baby.
- Give the news at a pace the parents can follow and with an approach that elicits the parents' understanding of the situation.
- Give specific information on referrals, services, and support and a summary of what will be done for the baby.

Nurses and physicians need to communicate with parents at regular intervals; bad news should not come as a surprise at the last minute (Kavanaugh & Paton, 2001). The words used to describe how their baby is doing should be individualized and should convey respect. Nontechnical language should be used, and the infant should be referred to by name, not as "it," "micropremie," or any other abbreviation that leaves the impression the child is less than human (Box 27-4). Expert nurses anticipate the information needs of the parents, offer explanations more than once, and are patient with the process of parents "learning the system." Parents need to be informed of their baby's treatment plan, how it will change with the condition of their infant, possible problems that have a reasonable chance of occurring, and their responsibilities as parents in treatment decisions. They need to be informed about the purposes of the equipment and medication used for their infant. Finally, parents need to know how they can be involved in caring for their infant while in the NICU and after the death.

Providing Direct Emotional Support

Parents consistently describe the benefits of receiving emotional support (DiMarco et al, 2001; Kavanaugh, 1997b; Kavanaugh & Hershberger, 2005; Van & Meleis, 2003). Nonverbal communication of support is shared through eye contact, attentive listening, and concerned facial expressions and, most important, through the nurse's physical presence and willingness to be alongside grieving families. Nurses who wipe their tears, shed a tear for them, check on them often, and used empathetic touch are perceived as caring.

Actualizing the Loss. Some bereaved parents and family members may need help in expressing the experience of their

---

[*]Lemmer, 1991; Covington & Theut, 1993; Calhoun, 1994; Lasker & Toedter, 1994; Crowther, 1995; Kavanaugh, 1997b; Kavanaugh & Hershberger, 2005; Lundqvist et al, 2002; Malacrida, 1997; Radestad & Nordin, 1998.

[†]Fallowfield & Jenkins, 2004; Ptacek & Eberhardt, 1996; Serwint & Rutherford, 2000.

BOX 27-4

What to Say and What Not to Say to Bereaved Parents

What to Say

"I'm sad for you."

"How are you doing with all of this?"

"This must be hard for you."

"What can I do for you?"

"I'm sorry."

"I'm here, and I want to listen."

What Not to Say

"You're young, you can have others."

"You have an angel in heaven."

"This happened for the best."

"Better for this to happen now, before you knew the baby."

"There was something wrong with the baby anyway."

"Fetus" or "it" in referring to the baby

Gundersen Lutheran Medical Foundation; provided by RTS Bereavement Services, 1910 South Avenue, La Crosse, WI 54601.

loss. The nurse should always use the name of their baby or refer to the child as their son or daughter. Open-ended questions or comments that encourage the family to talk about their experience can be helpful, such as the following:

"What has the doctor told you?"

"What have you noticed that's different about Mariah?"

"Whom in your family does Juan look like?"

"I know you were with Laura when she died; what was that like for you?"

"Tell me about your daughter's funeral."

Any statements that minimize the loss, judge the parents, or increase the parent's guilt should be avoided, such as the following:

"Your baby would have been severely damaged. It is better that she only lived an hour."

"Why didn't you go to a specialist during your pregnancy?"

"Didn't you know you were in preterm labor?"

Helping the Survivor Identify and Express Feelings. A grieving family's emotions and expressions of grief can seem overwhelming to nurses. Feelings of anger, guilt, and sadness are heightened in the early moments, days, and months after a death. When a bereaved person expresses feelings of anger, the nurse should identify those feelings by saying, "You look angry" or "What happened to make you feel so angry?" Typically, anger is a surface response for feeling powerless or helpless in their current situation. Once the nurse accepts the feelings of anger and conveys willingness to listen, the anger dissipates, and some problems can be solved.

When an infant dies, families typically have many questions about the loss. "What did I do?" "I did this; did that cause it to happen?" "Do you think I should (could) have done?" These questions represent the phase of bereavement known as awareness of the loss. Parents, family members, and friends all need to find a reason and sometimes a purpose for what happened. This is a major concept of the grief process called loss integration. Part of the grief process is to determine what happened, what the parents' or family's role was, why it happened to them, why it happened to their baby and, ultimately, for some

parents, why God let it happen. The nurse should recognize that the bereaved need to find their own answers to these questions, because that process is a part of their healing. For this reason, instead of just answering the questions, the nurse should encourage the bereaved to talk about their experience more. For example, a mother says, "I hung the wash on the line the day before I went into labor; did that cause the cord to be wrapped around the baby's neck so tight?" The nurse's response should be, "You sound like you are feeling guilty for what happened; I'd be trying to find a reason, too. What else have you thought about?" Only giving the bereaved advice or answering their questions does not help them process their grief. Many times the nurse could pinpoint what physically happened to cause the baby's death and answer the parent's questions; however, the ultimate questions of "why, why me, why my child, why God" remain.

The research of Davidson (1984) reveals that the overpowering emotions that occur with the loss of a child, such as sobbing, crying, and anger, comes in waves that typically last only 15 minutes at a time. However, being with someone who is sobbing, crying, choking on their tears, or angry can be extremely difficult. The initial response is to touch the person who is crying or to hand them a tissue. Although such a response may seem supportive at the time, the expression of emotion may be halted or stifled.

Careful assessment must be made when touch is used as a therapeutic technique to convey empathy. When touch is used appropriately, the bereaved continues to cry, although perhaps not as strongly. Inappropriate touch distracts the bereaved from the expression of emotion and causes the person to stiffen, pull way, startle, freeze, look at the spot that was touched or, more important, stop the expression of emotion. Nurses should quietly support the bereaved by being present, sitting quietly alongside and accepting any expressed emotion, with their hands folded, mouth shut, and body positioned in a mirroring, empathetic manner. This presence leaves the mourners with the feeling of being cared for. Safe means of touching when caring for the bereaved might be placing an arm around the shoulder; clasping an elbow, knee, or hand; or wiping the person's tears when they have stopped crying. In handing a tissue, the nurse needs to watch for signals that the bereaved is ready to wipe away the tears (e.g., the person wipes the eyes or nose, raises the head, looks around, or reaches for a tissue). Telling someone it is all right to cry, handing them a tissue, and patting them on the back does not create an open atmosphere for expressing feelings.

Providing Time to Grieve. On a busy unit it may be hard for the nurse to slow the system down for families to say goodbye to their baby. When an infant dies, parents are no longer aware of shift changes or any needs the hospital system might have. Having a special room or area available to the family is ideal. In less than ideal circumstances, curtains could be drawn, or the family and baby could be moved off the unit. When families are pushed or rushed into making decisions, they typically respond to the health care system's needs, not their own. Nurses must be sensitive to the family's needs at this time. Providing time for them to see and hold their baby in private, for taking pictures, and for making arrangements for their baby to be returned to them helps the family create special memories. Delaying the processing of consent forms for autopsy or removal from the hospital can help the family have more time with their baby, as well as help mobilize support systems. These strategies help further the family's acceptance of the loss and offer the opportunity for a last good-bye before returning to the real world; they also leave the family feeling well cared for.

Interpreting Normal Feelings. Many of the parents whose baby dies in the NICU have never experienced a loss of this magnitude. The physical, emotional, and cognitive grief responses they experience at the time of their loss are so overwhelming they may be afraid of losing control, or they may feel that they are going crazy or losing their mind. Because most parents have never felt this way before, they have little understanding of normal grief responses. It is important for the nurse to remember that the grief responses bereaved parents have after a loss for the most part are new coping mechanisms and that initially any response should be considered normal unless the person has had a previous mental health diagnosis. Some parents may respond to their baby's death with comments or behavior that seems inappropriate to the nurse.

The importance of giving anticipatory guidance about grief has been documented consistently in the literature.[*] Therefore, when the time is right and definitely before the parents leave the hospital, nurses need to reassure and educate them about the grief process, their feelings, the differences between men's and women's grief responses, and how other family members and friends may respond. Reading material on the grief process and on the differences between men's and women's grief, talking with children, accepting the responses of family and friends, and planning a special good-bye can satisfy some of the educational needs of bereaved families. Other strategies for providing parents with information and education can be pursued through follow-up phone calls, by having the parents talk with other parents who have suffered a similar loss, by referring the parents to a perinatal bereavement support group (Box 27-5), and by providing a suggested reading list for the parents or their children.

Allowing for Individual Differences. Grief is very personal, and many families want to keep it private. How a person responds to loss and grief depends on the individual's age, gender, culture, religion, socioeconomic status, and perception of loss, as well as on the expectations of others, previous experiences with loss, and many other factors. Nurses may observe many different types of response in a single family. Men typically want to protect their partners; grandparents want to protect their children from further hurt; and bereaved parents are not sure they can share their grief with their children. Family members' feelings of powerlessness and helplessness may be hidden behind behaviors such as expressing anger, resisting ideas, overcontrolling the situation, or blaming others. Using an individual family member as an example, the nurse can respond to these underlying feelings in the following ways:

1. Position yourself as being on the same side as the resistant person.
   - Recognize how painful this time is for the parent, grandparent, or child.
   - Acknowledge how difficult it must be to feel so responsible for making sure that everything and everyone is taken care of.

- Ask about the individual's personal hopes, dreams, and feeling of loss.
2. Use self-disclosure carefully in terms of your own experience or your experiences in caring for other families in similar situations.
3. Gently confront when necessary. (For example, "I can see how you are struggling to help your ——.")

These techniques can help the nurse guide the resistant person to a position where the individual's needs can be meet. Some families need to be asked more than once (but should not be asked more than three times during the initial phase of grief) when important decisions need to be made. This gives them the opportunity to change their minds, to express their needs to each other, and to make decisions based on their individual needs, as well as the family's needs.

Respecting the Rights of the Parents

Parents must make many decisions after their infant's death. They need to be guided through this process (Figure 27-1), and their rights must be respected so that decisions are made in the best interests of the parents.[†] Families need to be involved in the decision-making process because the decisions made at the time of the loss and over the next few days will provide them with memories for a lifetime. Parents must be given adequate time to make the necessary decisions and must be given an opportunity to change their minds within a time period appropriate to the decision. Many bereaved parents are clueless as to their needs for memories or their rights as parents. It sometimes is difficult for the nurse to create an environment in which information and options are offered to parents without making them feel guilty if they do not choose to exercise those rights or if the parents' choices are not the ones the nurse would make. Finally, whenever a bereaved parent expresses a need, regardless of how unusual the request may sound to the nurse, the nurse must try to meet the request. Unmet needs can lay the groundwork for the development of complicated bereavement, and they leave the parents feeling unimportant and not valued.

Seeing, Holding, and Caring for the Infant. Parents need the opportunity to "parent" their baby after death. For some parents this may be their first opportunity to bathe, diaper, or dress the child. Parents appreciate the opportunity for extended time spent with the infant, and especially appreciate those nurses who allow their infants to remain in the room until the mother's discharge from the hospital (Kavanaugh & Hershberger, 2005). Mothers who are hospitalized on nonmaternity units should also be allowed to see their infant even when the mother is cared for in an intensive care unit. Bereaved parents need to have the option to have time alone with their baby to say and do the things they would have done had their baby been able to go home (Figure 27-2). Asking parents about what they had dreamed of doing for or with their baby after birth can offer insight into arranging for special memories. The following are a few examples of special memories that some families have requested:

- Taking their son to the park with their dogs for the afternoon because they wanted him to feel the sun on his face before he died.

---

[*]Lemmer, 1991; Sexton & Stephen, 1991; Calhoun, 1994; Harper & Wisian, 1994; Lasker & Toedter, 1994; Malacrida, 1997.

[†]Hughes et al, 2002; Lemmer, 1991; Sexton & Stephen, 1991; Calhoun, 1994; Kavanaugh, 1997b; Lundqvist et al, 2002; Malacrida, 1997.

BOX 27-5

Resources and Web Addresses for Perinatal Loss

Center for Loss in Multiple Birth, Inc. (CLIMB)
Jean Kollantai
PO Box 1064
Palmer, AK 99645
(907) 746-6123
www.climb-support.org
CLIMB provides support by and for the parents of twins, triplets, or higher order multiple birth children who have experienced the death of one or more children during pregnancy, at birth, in infancy, or in childhood.

Centering Corporation
Box 3367
Omaha, NE 68103-0367
(402) 553-1200
www.centering.org
The Centering Corporation provides more than 500 caring resources for children and adults, videos, and sympathy cards, including cards for bereaved parents. They will develop needed books and provide caring workshops.

Center for Loss & Life Transition
3735 Broken Bow Road
Fort Collins, CO 80526
(970) 226-6050
www.centerforloss.com
The Center for Loss & Life Transition is a private organization dedicated to helping both the bereaved, by walking with them in their unique life journeys, and bereavement caregivers, by serving as their educational liaison and professional forum.

Ceremonies for Jewish Living: Pregnancy Loss
www.ritualwell.org/rituals/overview.html
This organization is a charity that provides specialized training and support for professionals to enable them to improve their response to the needs of bereaved families.

The Compassionate Friends
PO Box 3696
Oak Brook, IL 60652-3690
(877) 969-0010
Fax: (630) 990-0246
www.compassionatefriends.org
The mission of the Compassionate Friends is to assist families in the positive resolution of grief after the death of a child and to provide information to help others support the bereaved family.

Hygeia Foundation and Institute for Perinatal Loss and
   Bereavement
http://hygeia.org
Hygeia Foundation and Institute for Perinatal Loss and Bereavement is a nonprofit, tax-exempt organization whose mission is to comfort those who grieve the loss of a pregnancy or newborn child (from all causes, e.g., miscarriage, stillbirth, genetic disorders), to address disparities in access to health care services for medically and economically underserved families with respect, dignity, and advocacy, and to provide advocacy and resources for maternal and child health.

Memory Boxes
Memories Unlimited
Martha and Bill Wittgow
9511 Johnson Point Loop NE
Olympia, WA 98516-9529
(360) 491-9819
Fax: (360) 491-9827
www.memoriesunlimited.com
This organization provides memory boxes and pamphlets that support grieving families.

MISS Foundation
www.missfoundation.org
The MISS Foundation is a nonprofit 501 international organization providing immediate and ongoing support to grieving families, helping them to empower themselves by proactive community involvement and volunteerism, and reducing infant and toddler death through research and education.

March of Dimes: Bereavement Kit
www.marchofdimes.com/professionals/2222_2303asp
This kit is designed especially for parents who experience the loss of a child from conception through the first month of life. The kit contains written material on parental grief and a memory envelope for infant mementos.

Perinatal Hospice: A Gift of Time
http://perinatalhospice.org
A site for parents who have received a prenatal diagnosis that indicates their baby will die before or after birth. Contains resources and information on an upcoming book, *A Gift of Time: Continuing Your Pregnancy Following a Terminal Prenatal Diagnosis.*

A Place to Remember
http://aplacetoremember.com
Uplifting support materials and resources for those who have been touched by a crisis in pregnancy or the death of a baby.

The Pregnancy Loss and Infant Death Alliance (PLIDA)
http://www.plida.org/
PLIDA is a nationwide, collective community of parents and health care professionals. PLIDA works together to ensure that all families experiencing the death of a baby during pregnancy, birth, or infancy will receive comprehensive and compassionate care from diagnosis through the reproductive years. Focuses on increasing awareness about the emotional aspects of this bereavement and advocating for the provision of supportive care to parents. Provides support, and education, including the development of position statements on caring for bereaved parents, and networking opportunities to the professionals who work with bereaved families.

BOX 27-5

Resources and Web Addresses for Perinatal Loss—cont'd

RTS Perinatal Bereavement Program (formerly Resolve Through Sharing)
   RTS Bereavement Services
   1910 South Avenue
   La Crosse, WI 54601
   (608) 791-4747
   www.gundluth.org/bereave
RTS is part of Bereavement Services, a professional, interdisciplinary approach to bereavement care across the life span. RTS provides training and support materials to health care professionals working with parents who have lost an infant during pregnancy or shortly after birth.

   SHARE, Pregnancy and Infant Loss Support, Inc.
   St. Joseph's Health Center
   300 First Capital Drive
   St. Charles, MO 63301
   (636) 947-6164
   www.nationalshareoffice.com
The primary purpose of this organization is to provide support to help parents achieve a positive resolution of their grief at the time of or after the death of an infant. The secondary purpose is to provide information, education, and resources on the needs and rights of bereaved parents and siblings.

The UK-Based Child Bereavement Trust
http://www.childbereavement.org.uk

EriChad Grief Support
www.erichad.com
This site is provided as loving support for bereaved parents and is home to a number of other links, including the following:
   PAILS of Hope—Pregnancy/parenting after infertility/loss support cubby at StorkNet with articles, personal stories and message forum
   Pregnancy/Infant Loss Support—Articles, parent tips, memorial garden and message forum at StorkNet, our parent site
   Parents of Multiples of Forever—For parents of multiples who have experienced the death of a twin or some of their multiple birth babies/children
   Waiting with Love—For parents who choose to continue a pregnancy knowing their unborn baby will die before or shortly after birth and for families who learn their newborn will die

---

- Allowing them to spend the night sleeping with their daughter skin to skin.
- Rocking both babies at the same time when a death occurred with a multiple birth.
- Bathing their son, rubbing lotion on him, dressing him, wrapping him in his blanket, and then placing him in his bassinet.
- Reading a "Golden Books" story while rocking her daughter.
- Listening to her son's heartbeat for one last time.
- Having the infant brought back to the unit from the morgue so that her brother could spend special time with his sister.

Visitation with Other Family Members and Friends. Bereaved parents need to be offered the opportunity to include their children (regardless of age), grandparents, extended family members, and friends, allowing them to see and hold their baby (Kavanaugh & Hershberger, 2005; Lundqvist et al, 2002). Such visits afford others the opportunity to become acquainted with their son or daughter, to understand the parents' loss, to offer their support, and to say good-bye. This experience can help parents explain to their surviving children who their brother or sister was and what death means, and it offers the opportunity for siblings to ask questions. Involving extended family and friends enables parents to mobilize their social support system of people who will be with them at the time of the loss and in the future, and it gives the nurse an opportunity to recommend concrete ways that family and friends can help the parents. Nurses should provide specific information on ways family and friends can provide the various types of

social support, including emotional support, practical help, guidance, and possibly financial assistance (Kavanaugh et al, 2004).

Special Memories.   Parents appreciate tangible memories of their baby (Kavanaugh & Hershberger, 2005; Lundqvist et al, 2002; Van & Meleis, 2003), which allow them to actualize the loss. Parents may want to bring in a previously purchased baby book to be completed during their baby's hospitalization. Memory books, cards, and information on grief and mourning are available for purchase by families, hospitals, or clinics through national perinatal bereavement organizations (Box 27-5).

Pictures are often a very treasured memento (Alexander, 2001; Capitulo, 2004; DiMarco et al, 2001; Kavanaugh & Hershberger, 2005; Lasker & Toedter, 1994; Pector, 2004b). Photographs should be taken whenever possible while the infant is alive and after the infant has died. However, cultural practices should be respected. For example, it may be inappropriate to take pictures for some Native American families (Table 27-1). The most important principle regarding cultural and religious practices is that the nurse should determine the cultural and religious practices the family wishes to carry out. The nurse should not assume that all members of a certain religious or cultural group maintain and practice similar beliefs.

Pictures should include close-ups of the infant's face, hands, and feet. The infant should be clothed in a gown and hat and wrapped in a blanket, and pictures should be taken with the parents, siblings, extended family members, and friends (Figure 27-3). Other photographs of the infant unclothed can

Checklist for Assisting Parents Experiencing Stillbirth or Newborn Death

Mother's discharge date: _____

Mother's name: _____

Address: _____

Phone number: (___) _____

Father's name: _____

Address: _____

Phone number: (___) _____

Optimal call time: _____

RTS Counselor: _____

Unit: _____ Ext.: _____

Regular OB MD/midwife: _____

Religion: _____

Age: ____ Gr: ____ Para: ____ L.C.: ____ Due date: ____

Previous loss: _____

Date/time of birth: _____

Date/time of death: _____

Baby's name: _____ Sex: _____

Children's name(s): _____ Age: _____

_____ Age: _____

_____ Age: _____

Support people: _____

Attending MD &/or pediatrician: _____

Date	Time	Follow Protocol in RTS manual Sec. II, p 3-8			Comments	Initials
		Notify/assign RTS counselor:	☐ Yes	☐ No		
		Pastoral Care notified:	☐ Yes	☐ No		
		Communications notified:	☐ Yes	☐ No		
		Saw baby when born and/or after birth:	☐ Mother	☐ Father		
		Touched and/or held baby: ☐ Mother ☐ Father ☐ Siblings ☐ Grandparents ☐ Friends Offered private time with their baby:	☐ Yes	☐ No		
		Baptism offered (use seashell as vessel, give to parents):	☐ Yes	☐ No		
		Remembrance of Blessing offered:	☐ Yes	☐ No		
		Given option to transfer off Maternity Unit:	☐ Yes	☐ No		
		Patient's room tagged with door card:	☐ Yes	☐ No		
		Autopsy: ☐ Yes ☐ No Genetic studies: ☐ Yes ☐ No Genetic associate notified (see note): ☐ Yes ☐ No				
		Regular physician/midwife notified of death: ☐ Yes ☐ No Memo sent to physician/midwife: ☐ Yes ☐ No				
		Section of fetal monitor strip:	☐ Given to parents	☐ On file		
		ID bands/crib cards/tape measure:	☐ Given to parents	☐ On file		
		Footprints/handprints/weight/length recorded on "In Memory Of" sheet: ☐ Given to parents ☐ On file				
		Lock of hair offered:	☐ Yes	☐ No ☐ Given to parents ☐ On file		

A

FIGURE **27-1**

A, Sample checklist for helping parents whose infant was stillborn or whose newborn has died. Gundersen Lutheran Medical Foundation; provided by RTS Bereavement Services, 1910 South Avenue, La Crosse, WI 54601.

Date	Time	Follow Protocol in RTS manual Sec. II, p 3-8			Comments	Initials
		Mementos (clothing, hat, blanket, pacifier, crib cards, basin, thermometer, silk flower): ☐ Given to parents ☐ On file				
		Complimentary birth certificate: ☐ Given to parents ☐ On file				
		Resolve through sharing photographs taken (clothed, unclothed, with props, family photo):				
		Polaroid (3 or more):	☐ Given to parents	☐ On file		
		35 mm (6-12 pictures):	☐ Given to parents	☐ On file		
		Medical photographs:	☐ Yes	☐ No		
		Informed about postponing funeral until mother is able to attend:	☐ Yes	☐ No		
		Services/funeral arrangements, options discussed: ☐ Self-transport ☐ Grave site services ☐ Visitation ☐ Hospital chapel ☐ Cremation ☐ Funeral home ☐ Burial at foot or head of relative's grave ☐ Specific area for babies in cemetery				
		Funeral arrangements made by: Discussed:	☐ Mother ☐ Seeing baby at funeral home ☐ Taking pictures there ☐ Providing outfit or toy for baby ☐ Dressing baby at funeral home	☐ Father		
		Follow protocol in RTS manual (Sec. II, p 3-8)	☐ Mother	☐ Father		
		Grief information packet given to:	☐ Mother	☐ Father		
		Discussed grief process and incongruent grief with:	☐ Mother	☐ Father		
		Discussed grief conference:	☐ Yes	☐ No		
		RTS Parents Support Group brochure given to:	☐ Mother	☐ Father		
		RTS business card given to:	☐ Mother	☐ Father		
		Pregnancy & Infant Loss Card sent to RTS secretary:	☐ Yes	☐ No		
		Follow-up calls: 1 week: _____ 3 weeks: _____ Due date: _____ 6-10 months: _____ Anniversary date: _____				
		Grief conference planned with parents: Date: ____ Time: ____ Place: ____ Letter of confirmation sent:	☐ Yes	☐ No		
		Parent support group, first meeting attended: Date _____ Follow-up meetings attended: Dates: _____				
		Would like another parent to call: Parent contact: _____	☐ Yes ☐ Ask later	☐ No		

B

FIGURE **27-1**

B, Sample checklist for helping parents whose infant was stillborn or whose newborn has died. Gundersen Lutheran Medical Foundation; provided by RTS Bereavement Services, 1910 South Avenue, La Crosse, WI 54601.

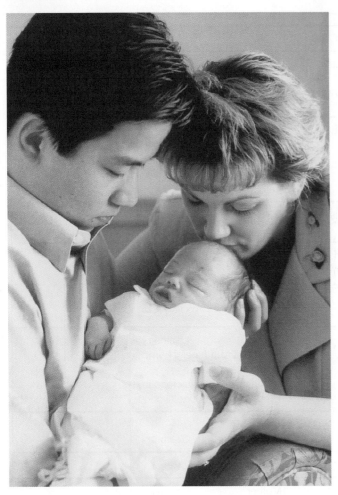

FIGURE **27-2**
Parents with deceased infant.

TABLE **27-1**	Selected Cultural and Religious Aspects of Perinatal Death Practices
Perinatal Death Practice	**Cultural/Religious Practice**
Burial options	Cremation is forbidden, discouraged, or allowed only under unusual circumstances for Baha'is, Jews, and members of the Christian and Missionary Alliance, Church of Jesus Christ of Latter-Day Saints, and Greek Orthodox Church. Cremation is customary for Hindus and Unitarian Universalists.
Embalming	The body is not to be embalmed for Jews and Baha'is unless required by state law.
Pictures	Picture taking may conflict with the beliefs of some cultures, such as those of Native Americans, Eskimos, Amish, Hindus, and Muslims. It is important to offer these families a choice; within the culture as a whole, a photograph may not be acceptable.
Sacraments	Most Protestant denominations and some Roman Catholics perform baptism usually only if the infant is living. Judaism, Hinduism, and Islam have rituals for preparing the body for burial.

be taken at the parents' request. Flowers, blocks, stuffed animals, or toys can be placed in the background to make the picture seem less stark. Black and white film can be used when it would be sensitive to minimize the harshness of colored photographs (e.g., with severe bruising). Keeping a camera nearby and taking pictures when parents are spending special time with their baby can provide families with important memories. Disposable cameras can be purchased so that parents can take numerous photographs of the infant and family. Some families may have their own camera or video equipment and may prefer that the nurse record them parenting their baby as they bathe, dress, or diaper. Asking families what their dreams were for parenting their baby can give the nurse insight into creating a memorable pictorial history of the infant's short life.

The nurse should provide the family with the infant's weight, length, and head circumference. Footprints and handprints can be taken and placed with the other information on a memorial card or in a memory book or baby book. If the footprint or handprint does not turn out, the nurse can trace around the desired body part, or an impression can be made by using a product similar to plaster of Paris called Orthostone (Dentsply International, York, PA). Impressioning is an excellent way to preserve memories for parents (Brown & Kozick, 1994). Any article that comes in contact with the infant during care (e.g., tape measure, blanket, hat, hospital

undershirt, lotion, shampoo, comb, pacifier, identification bands, crib cards) should be saved, placed in a resealable bag, and given to the parents. Articles should not be washed or cleaned beforehand, so that the parents can keep the smell of their baby. A lock of hair may be an important keepsake for the parents' memories. The nurse must ask one or both parents' permission before cutting a lock of hair, which can be removed from the nape of the neck, where it is not noticeable.

Rituals of Remembrance. Many families may have spiritual needs at the time of a loss, and these needs can be an important part of their care, support, and memories. Spiritual needs can be met through various rituals, which are an important component of care surrounding the end of life (Anderson, 2003). Relying on one's own religious and spiritual beliefs may be one of the most important coping strategies for parents, particularly for some ethnic and cultural groups (Kavanaugh & Hershberger, 2005; Van & Meleis, 2003). However, support from the clergy is an option that should be offered to all families. Families may wish to have their own pastor, priest, rabbi, or spiritual leader contacted, or they may wish to see the hospital's chaplain. Nurses can offer the opportunity for the presence of clergy by saying, "It's customary in our hospital when a family is experiencing (a crisis or loss of a loved one) that we notify pastoral care. Can I do this for you?" Members of the clergy may offer families the opportunity for baptism,

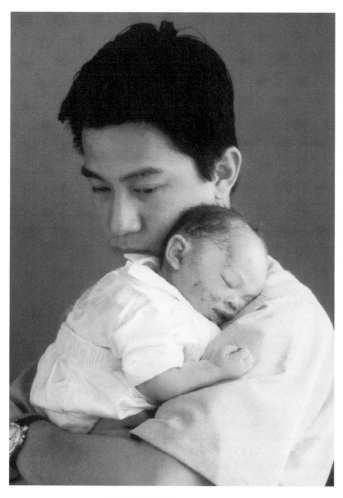

FIGURE **27-3**
Father with deceased infant.

sacrament of the sick, anointing, a naming ceremony, a blessing, special prayers, a memorial service, or other rituals relevant to their spiritual belief. For many families, having the clergy involved in their care can bring a sense of peace in a crisis situation. It is important that the nurse not impose personal religious practices, such as baptism, on the infant without a parent's request or consent.

Autopsy and Organ Donation. The importance of autopsy and burial counseling has been described.[*] Health care professionals must acknowledge to parents that although these decisions are difficult, the consequences become more important as time passes. A good understanding of the differences between a partial and a complete autopsy and of which organs typically are used in infant organ donation is necessary. Health care professionals also should examine their feelings and attitudes concerning autopsies, because these might influence the way in which the consent is obtained (Chiswick, 1995; Khong, 1997). An autopsy can be instrumental in determining the cause of death. For some families this information is helpful for understanding why their loss occurred, for processing their

grief, and perhaps for preventing another loss. Other families may be concerned about the invasive nature of the procedure and may not consent (McHaffie et al, 2001). Some religions prohibit autopsy. These decisions are difficult for families to make, and they will need time to discuss this option.

Organ or tissue donation can be an aid to grieving, an opportunity for the family to see something positive associated with this experience. Before this option is offered to the family, however, the nurse should contact the regional organ bank so that it can be determined whether the infant is a candidate for organ donation. This determination actually should be made before the infant has died. Donation of selected organs may be possible if the infant was born at 36 weeks' gestation or later.

Taking the Infant to the Morgue. Before taking the infant to the morgue, nurses should prepare the child's skin by gently putting cold cream on the eyelids, hands, and face to keep the skin from dehydrating during refrigeration. The infant should be undressed, placed on a large, smooth blanket with the arms at the side (as infants are seen in the nursery), and carefully wrapped with a smooth blanket to prevent impressions from being made on the face.

The nurse should transport the child to the morgue according to hospital protocol, usually by placing the infant in a crib or by carrying the infant in the arms. The infant should be placed face up, with the blanket loose over the face, in the refrigeration unit of the morgue. If the infant is to be placed in a casket, the child should be positioned comfortably. If the infant is too large for the casket, the arms can be positioned on the chest, or the infant can be placed on the abdomen with the head turned and the knees tucked under the chest in the fetal position.

Funeral Arrangements. In making final arrangements for their baby, families may want a special service. They may choose to have a service in the hospital chapel, visitation at a funeral home or their own home, a funeral service, or a graveside service. Families can make any of these services as special, personal, and memorable as they like through music, poems, or readings. Some families may want to buy an outfit for their baby to be buried in, or they may want to use something already purchased. They also may want to bathe and dress their baby again at the funeral home, hold their baby one last time, and place their son or daughter comfortably in the casket. This can be done even if an autopsy has been performed on the infant. However, families need to know what to expect (e.g., the incisions, coolness, and rigidity of the body after embalming). Meaningful mementos chosen by the parents or the baby's siblings can be placed in the casket with the infant. Some parents may want to carry the casket to the vehicle used for transport or to the gravesite. Caskets used for babies typically are made of Styrofoam; therefore the outside can be decorated with magic markers or spray-painted by family members or siblings. Some parents or grandparents may want to build a casket from wood or dig the grave, which would depend on the rules and requirements of the cemetery.

Parents should be given information about choices for the final disposition of their baby, and cultural practices should be respected (Table 27-1). In research with parents who were low-income (Kavanaugh & Hershberger, 2005), contrary to popular belief, parents based their decision for infant burial on what they felt was best for them and their infant, not always on economic factors or the perceived stress of arranging a

---

[*]McHaffie et al, 2001; Sexton & Stephen, 1991; Calhoun, 1994; Harper & Wisian, 1994; Lasker & Toedter, 1994; Crowther, 1995; Primeau & Lamb, 1995; Kavanaugh, 1997b; Khong, 1997; Malacrida, 1997; Limbo & Wheeler, 1998; Radestad & Nordin, 1998.

private service. Therefore, parent decisions should be respected. Final disposition can include burial or cremation. Depending on the cemetery's policies, babies who are placed in a casket or the ashes from babies who are cremated can be buried in a special place designated for babies, at the foot of an already deceased relative, in a separate plot, or in a mausoleum. The remains may also be scattered in a designated area (many states have regulations regarding where ashes can be scattered). A local funeral director or a state's Bureau of Vital Statistics should have information about the state's rules, codes, and regulations regarding live births, death certificates, burial requirements, transportation of the deceased by parents, and cremation. Parents who will bury their baby a distance from where they live or where the infant died may want to transport their baby to the funeral home in the area where the infant is to be buried. Nurses should be knowledgeable about the process of self-transport and the required forms.

Follow-Up Care

Some investigators have recommended follow-up care for parents who experience a perinatal loss (Harper & Wisian, 1994; Kavanaugh & Hershberger, 2005; Malacrida, 1997). Follow-up care is a necessary component of a program of support because of the documented social isolation of the parents after discharge (Rajan, 1994; Kavanaugh & Robertson, 1999; Malacrida, 1999) and the frequent accounts of parents' lack of understanding of the events surrounding the loss (Covington & Theut, 1993; Crowther, 1995; Radestad & Nordin, 1998; Kavanaugh & Robertson, 1999; Kavanaugh & Hershberger, 2005). Some investigators have documented the importance parents ascribe to follow-up contact with a health care professional (Harper & Wisian, 1994; Malacrida, 1997) and the importance of support groups for some parents (DiMarco et al, 2001; Sexton & Stephen, 1991; Calhoun, 1994; Van & Meleis, 2003) or support via the Internet (Capitulo, 2004). Follow-up can also be a time when parents can be given the opportunity to talk about and receive suggestions about ways to honor their babies. Some ways parents hold their babies in memory include creating a family ritual where the name of the baby is mentioned during prayer and using symbols such as planting a shrub in the garden (Cote-Arsenault, 2003b).

Follow-up phone calls or visits (or both) should be made to the family after a newborn death. Phone calls made within 1 week after a loss and again in 1 to 2 weeks, or in conjunction with the mother's postpartum appointment, are critical components of follow-up. Sample questions for the initial telephone call are presented in Box 27-6. During this follow-up contact, the health care professional should clarify information, validate the parents' feelings, and help the parents identify effective ways of coping and sources of support (Friedrichs et al, 2000).

If the parents have consented to an autopsy, the health care professional who has maintained contact with the family should be a part of the autopsy conference. It is helpful for institutions to develop specialized perinatal loss clinics where families, including those who have not consented for an autopsy, meet with an interdisciplinary team of health care professionals (e.g., perinatologist, neonatologist, nurse, mental health professional, and genetic counselor) to have their questions answered and their emotional needs assessed and met. Parents may want to review the previous pregnancy and loss to

---

BOX 27-6

Questions for an Initial Follow-Up Telephone Call After the Death of a Baby

"You might recall that you were told that someone from the hospital would call you in (number) weeks."

"Is this a good time to talk?"

"Are there any issues that you have been thinking about that perhaps I could follow up on for you?"

"Have you been back yet for a postpartum checkup?"

"Some parents have noticed a change in their sleeping or eating habits. Has this been a problem for you?"

"How has (name of other parent) responded to your loss? Sometimes it is hard for both parents to talk about it. How has it been for you?"

"Do you have other family members or friends that you have been able to talk to? What types of things have they been able to do for you?"

"Do you have plans to work outside your home? The first few days at work can be especially difficult. Have you thought about how it might be for you?"

"Did you receive any information on support groups for parents?"

"Are there any other materials you received in the hospital that you have questions about?"

"Are there any other questions that I can answer for you?"

"During the call you stated that …"

"I will call you again on (date)."

Friedrichs J et al (2000). Follow-up of parents who experience a perinatal loss: facilitating grief and assessing for grief complicated by depression. *Illness, crisis and loss* 8(3):302.

---

understand what happened, how it happened, and what they might do differently during a subsequent pregnancy. Also, it is important to remember that even though parents might not bring up the previous loss during a routine follow-up postpartum appointment, the health care professional should not be afraid to discuss the loss with them and ask them if they have any concerns. The health care team must be honest and must not hedge when questions are asked. It is important to instill confidence in the woman and in her body's ability to have a successful pregnancy. This helps create an atmosphere of trust and helps the woman and her partner to be more open.

SPECIAL CONSIDERATIONS
Multiples

"When I have the girls out in the stroller and everyone is remarking how cute our twins are, I just want to scream, 'They're triplets … their brother died!'"

Parents who experience the death of a twin or higher order multiple have special needs because of their unique experiences (Pector & Smith-Levitin, 2002). Being informed about the special needs of these bereaved parents is especially important because technologic advances in perinatal care and reproductive technology have led to a subsequent increase in twin and high-order multiple births (Arias et al, 2003). Since 1980 the number of twin births has increased 59%, and after 2 years of decline the number of triplet and other high-order multiple births rose 3% in 2002 (Arias et al, 2003).

Experiencing the death of an infant who is a multiple is often referred to as "bittersweet" because of the dual emotions of joy and grief that parents experience. Having multiples is a special parenting experience, and with the death of an infant who was a multiple, parents lose the unique opportunity to parent the multiples (Cuisinier et al, 1996; Swanson-Kauffman, 1988). Yet, the results of research with parents of twins have shown that it is critical for parents to be recognized as parents of multiples even after one infant has died (Sychowski, 1998) (Figure 27-4). When parents experience the death of a twin or higher order multiple, they also are parenting the surviving infant (or infants), who often is being cared for in the NICU. Thus parents are undergoing the stress of the NICU experience in addition to their grief, and they may fear that something will happen to their surviving infant. Parents have reported that family and friends expect them to move on with their grief and focus on their surviving infant (Sychowski, 1998). Health care professionals often fail to acknowledge the deceased infant and instead focus on the survivor, especially if the survivor is in the NICU (Pector, 2004a). Thus, it is critical to recognize the special needs of parents of multiples (Pector, 2004b; Pector & Smith-Levitin, 2002; Swanson et al, 2002). Some suggestions include:

- Some parents may find it difficult to be around other multiples in the NICU; consideration should be given to moving the surviving multiple away from other multiples in the nursery if this approach would be supportive to the parents.
- Nurses should ask parents how the remaining multiples should be identified. Nurses must remember that a surviving multiple is still a multiple and should be referred to according to the wishes of the parents.
- Parents should be allowed time to see and hold all multiples together, whether or not they are still alive.
- Similar kinds of infant mementos should be created for all infants as desired by the parent. A variety of pictures should be taken of the infants, including pictures of all multiples together even if one infant has already died. Parents have often superimposed their infants' pictures at a later date when these pictures were not taken in

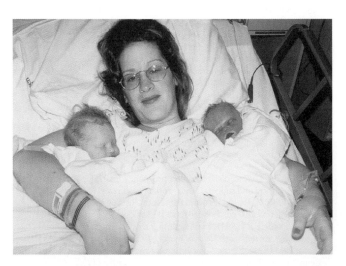

FIGURE **27-4**
Mother with surviving twin and deceased twin.

the hospital or have had artists create a drawing that includes all infants.

- The parents should be given a copy of a newsletter from the Center for Loss in Multiple Birth (Box 27-5).
- Nurses should not be reluctant to talk about the infant who died when the parents visit their surviving multiple in the NICU.

Parents worry about the grief of the surviving multiple as the child grows up (Sychowski, 1998). Also, the surviving multiple serves as a reminder of the other child (Cuisinier et al, 1996; Swanson-Kauffman, 1988; Sychowski, 1998). These concerns are an important part of anticipatory counseling for the parents, especially in regard to the milestone events in the survivor's life.

Subsequent Pregnancy After a Loss

"We wanted to get pregnant right away ... so we had sex every day and sometimes several times a day. I began to feel like a robot ... what used to be special became routine."

"God made a terrible mistake, and he wouldn't do it again."

"I knew when the baby was inside of me, it was safe; it was when he would come out everything could change."

"My body doesn't do pregnancy well. I hated to have to be pregnant again to get what I wanted most."

One of the questions most asked by bereaved parents who have suffered a miscarriage, stillbirth, or SIDS death is when or if they should become pregnant again (DeFrain, 1991). Some parents may be too fearful to attempt a subsequent pregnancy (Kavanaugh & Hershberger, 2005; Van & Meleis, 2003). Yet other parents feel an overwhelming need to become pregnant again (Limbo & Wheeler, 1998). This obsession may occur shortly after the loss and is perpetuated by the feelings of emptiness, aching arms, and dreams of the infant that are part of the physical and emotional grief responses. Some fathers may think that another pregnancy may be something they can do to help their partners feel better. The reasons for getting pregnant again may vary, and it is important to remember that parents take different paths to parenting and how meaning is reconstructed in their lives after an infant dies (Grout & Romanoff, 2000).

Davis and Stewart (1989) studied physicians' recommendations for attempting to conceive after a perinatal loss and found that most physicians recommended a specific waiting period before trying to conceive. However, most parents did not want to be told when to get pregnant again and followed their own ideas about when to conceive. If couples who have experienced a stillbirth or newborn death conceive soon after their loss, they may experience an anniversary of the infant's death and the birthday of their subsequent baby within a relatively short period. Some mothers and fathers experience emotional flashbacks of the previous pregnancy, labor and delivery, and time spent in the NICU. These flashbacks can be frightening and confusing and may cause them to be concerned about their mental health.

Investigators have also consistently documented increased anxiety in mothers during a pregnancy subsequent to a perinatal loss (Capitulo, 2004; Theut & Pedersen, 1988; Davis & Stewart, 1989; Armstrong & Hutti, 1998; Cote-Arsenault, 2003a; Cote-Arsenault & Marshall, 2000; Van & Meleis, 2003). Parents in these studies also were more reserved with social customs during the pregnancy (e.g., announcing the pregnancy, having a baby shower). For these parents, pregnancy was seen as a task with a goal, to produce a healthy baby, rather than as a time of enjoyment. Despite these findings, investigators have also demonstrated that a subsequent pregnancy after a loss diminishes the intensity of the parents' grief response (Zeanah, 1989). Nurses should provide anticipatory counseling to parents who are contemplating a subsequent pregnancy and to their families, so that they are aware of the feelings they may experience (Robertson & Kavanaugh, 1998; Wallerstedt et al, 2003).

CARE FOR THE CAREGIVER

Nurses experience varying degrees of stress in their work. The major source of stress for those who work on a continuing basis with the dying can be organizational, work related, interpersonal, or intrapersonal (Marino, 1998). Working with the dying and the bereaved can touch health care professionals in profound ways (Worden, 1982, 1991). Nurses who have children at home, who are pregnant, or who want to have children can strongly identify with parents when their baby dies. It increases anxiety in terms of their personal relationships and death awareness. Working with the dying can affect nurses' sense of power, mastery, and control (Rando, 1986). Nurses who have not worked through their grief for their professional losses are more vulnerable to unresolved grief. The reasons for not beginning or not completing the grief process often are not addressed in the work place or at home and are difficult for some nurses to articulate. Furthermore, nurses who express their grief might be perceived by their peers or the hospital administration as not being in control of their feelings and emotions; therefore those behaviors would not be supported.

Newborn deaths in an NICU can occur at the same time or serially within a short period. This can lead to bereavement overload, or cumulative grief. Cumulative grief can lead to emotional exhaustion, depression, anxiety, displacement, feelings of decreased professional competency, or a generalized lowering of self-esteem. One of the more serious effects of cumulative grief is denial. As Marino (1998) found, "Distorted or masked grief, which is the grief exhibited in terms of physical illness, substance abuse, or risk-taking behaviors, also can occur."

Learning how to cope with feelings and emotions that occur as a result of infant death is difficult. The loss needs to be dealt with personally, psychologically, socially, and institutionally. Fortinash and Holoday-Worret (2000) have identified personal coping measures and techniques for adapting to stress. Exercise, recreational activities, music therapy, humor, relaxation exercises (e.g., progressive, guided imagery and biofeedback), and yoga all can provide a sense of well-being and of being in control of life events. Psychologic and social supports need to be a blend of both personal and institutional resources.

Nurses generally do not receive adequate preparation for coping with the stress of the work place and of caring for the dying (Feldstein & Gemma, 1995). Adequate education about death and dying, grief theory, feelings associated with loss, and coping strategies help nurses to understand their feelings and the need to develop adaptive coping mechanisms. Health care professionals who care for families who experience a perinatal loss should be well informed about the behaviors and needs of family members. Educational programs on perinatal loss and support of families should be included in employee orientation programs. Health care professionals skilled at caring for families who experience a loss should serve as mentors for their colleagues to ensure the availability of competent health care professionals. Continuing education programs centered on death and grief, including staff feelings about loss, should be offered routinely. Case reviews could be used to provide both novices and experts with the opportunity to learn. This approach would also underscore the importance of meeting the educational and support needs of the professional staff, so that they can provide bereaved families with the best possible care.

Institutions should develop guidelines, policies, and procedures to help the nurse cope when a life can no longer be saved. These processes are aimed at helping the nurse to feel confident and competent in caring for an infant who is dying and at the time of death. Institutions should also formally offer grief support to nurses whose patients have died. This can be done through team debriefing after the death and continuing opportunities to share, offer, and receive support; these measures further enhance nurses' feelings of competency and their sense of mastery and control over their work.

Flexibility in scheduling should allow nurses to attend the funeral, memorial service, or gravesite service for a patient. Nurses should be given time to participate in any institution-sponsored memorial service for infants or other individuals who have died and to take time off to recover or regroup after a stressful period at work. Also, the need for referral for counseling should be assessed if a nurse appears to be experiencing cumulative grief and is unable to cope.

SUMMARY

Because of their continuous presence in the NICU, nurses bear witness to deeply personal experiences with families of infants. When an infant dies, the nurse is in a critical position to provide supportive care to the families. Adequate knowledge of the responses and needs of family members who experience a newborn death can help the nurse provide optimum care and can make a profound difference in how the family experiences this tragic event.

REFERENCES

Alexander KV (2001). The one thing you can never take away. *American journal of maternal child nursing* 26(3):123-127.

Anderson M (2003). *Sacred dying: creating rituals for embracing the end of life.* New York: Marlow & Company.

Arias E et al (2003). Annual summary of vital statistics—2002. *Pediatrics* 112(6):1215-1230.

Armstrong D, Hutti M (1998). Pregnancy after perinatal loss: the relationship between anxiety and prenatal attachment. *Journal of obstetric, gynecologic, and neonatal nursing* 27(2):183-189.

Barglow P et al (1973). Responses of unmarried adolescent mothers to infant or fetal death. *Adolescent psychiatry* 2:285-300.

Barr P (2004). Guilt- and shame-proneness and the grief of perinatal bereavement. *Psychology and psychotherapy: theory, research, and practice* 77:493-510.

Bennett SM et al (2005). The scope and impact of perinatal loss: current status and future directions. *Professional psychology: research and practice* 36(2):180-187.

Black RB (1991). Women's voices after pregnancy loss: couples' patterns of communication and support. *Social work in health care* 16(2):19-36.

Bowlby J (1980). Loss, sadness, and depression. In Bowlby J, editor. *Attachment and loss*, vol 3. New York: Basic Books.

Brown CE, Kozick P (1994). Impressioning: a way to preserve memories. *American journal of maternal child nursing* 19:285-287.

Calhoun LK (1994). Parents' perceptions of nursing support following neonatal loss. *Journal of perinatal and neonatal nursing* 8(2):57-66.

Capitulo KL (2004). Perinatal grief online. *American journal of maternal child nursing* 29(5):305-311.

Cecil R (1994). "I wouldn't have minded a wee one running about" : miscarriage and the family. *Social science and medicine* 38(10):1415-1422.

Chiswick M (1995). Perinatal and infant postmortem examination: difficult to ask for but potentially valuable. *British medical journal* 310(6973):141-142.

Conway K, Russell G (2000). Couples' grief and experience of support in the aftermath of miscarriage. *British journal of medical psychology* 73:531-545.

Cordell AS, Thomas N (1997). Perinatal loss: intensity and duration of emotional recovery. *Omega: journal of death and dying* 35(3):297-308.

Corr CA (1993). Coping with dying: lessons that we should and should not learn from the work of Elisabeth Kubler-Ross. *Death studies* 17:69-83.

Cote-Arsenault D (2003a). The influence of perinatal loss on anxiety in multigravidas. *Journal of obstetric, gynecologic, and neonatal nursing* 32(5):622-629.

Cote-Arsenault D (2003b). Weaving babies lost in pregnancy into the fabric of the family. *Journal of family nursing* 9(1):23-37.

Cote-Arsenault D, Marshall P (2000). One foot in, one foot out. Weathering the storm of pregnancy after perinatal loss. *Research in nursing and health* 23(4):473-485.

Covington SN, Theut SK (1993). Reactions to perinatal loss: a qualitative analysis of the National Maternal and Infant Health Survey. *American journal of orthopsychiatry* 63(2):215-222.

Crowther ME (1995). Communication following a stillbirth or neonatal death: room for improvement. *British journal of obstetrics and gynecology* 102(12):952-956.

Cuisinier M et al (1996). Grief following the loss of a newborn twin compared with a singleton. *Acta paediatrica* 85:339-343.

Davidson GW (1984). *Understanding mourning.* Minneapolis, MN: Augsburg.

Davies R (2004). New understandings of parental grief: literature review. *Journal of advanced nursing* 46(5):506-513.

Davis DL, Stewart M (1989). Postponing pregnancy after perinatal death: perspectives on doctors' advice. *Journal of the American Academy of Child and Adolescent Psychiatry* 28(4):481-487.

DeFrain J (1991). Learning about grief from normal families: SIDS, stillbirth, and miscarriage. *Journal of marital and family therapy* 7(3):215-234.

DeMontigny F, Beaudet L (1999). A baby has died: the impact of perinatal loss on family social networks. *Journal of obstetric, gynecologic, and neonatal nursing* 28(2):151-156.

DiMarco MA et al (2001). Evaluating a support group for perinatal loss. *American journal of maternal/child nursing* 26(3):135-140.

Dowden S (1995). Young children's experience of sibling death. *Journal of pediatric nursing* 10(1):72-79.

Engel GL (1961). Is grief a disease? A challenge for medical research. *Psychosomatic medicine* 23:18-22.

Fallowfield L, Jenkins V (2004). Communicating sad, bad, and difficult news in medicine. *Lancet* 363:312-319.

Feeley N, Gottlieb LN (2000). Nursing approaches for working with family strengths. *Journal of family nursing* 6(1):9-24.

Feldstein MA, Gemma PB (1995). Oncology nurses and chronic compounded grief. *Cancer nursing* 18(3):228-236.

Fortinash KM, Holoday-Worret PA (2000). *Psychiatric mental health nursing,* ed 2. St Louis: Mosby.

Freud S (1961). Mourning and melancholia. In Strachey J, editor. *The standard edition of the complete psychological works of Sigmund Freud,* vol 14. London: Hogarth.

Friedrichs J et al (2000). Follow-up of parents who experience a perinatal loss: facilitating grief and assessing for grief complicated by depression. *Illness, crisis, and loss* 8:296-309.

Gilbert KR (1989). Interactive grief and coping in the marital dyad. *Death studies* 13(6):605-626.

Grout LA, Romanoff BD (2000). The myth of the replacement child: parent stories and practices after a perinatal death. *Death studies* 24:93-113.

Harper MB, Wisian NB (1994). Care for bereaved parents: a study of patient satisfaction. *Journal of reproductive medicine* 39(2):80-86.

Hersch L, Gensch B (1993). *RTS counselor manual,* ed 3. La Crosse, WI: Lutheran Hospital.

Hughes P et al (2002). Assessment of guidelines for good practice in psychosocial care of others after stillbirth: a cohort study. *Lancet* 360:114-118.

Hunfeld JAJ, Wladimiroff JW (1997). The grief of late pregnancy loss. *Patient education and counseling* 31(1):57-64.

Hutti MH (2005). Social and professional support needs of families after perinatal loss. *Journal of obstetric, gynecologic, and neonatal nursing* 34(5):630-638.

Jansen JL (2003). A bereavement model for the intensive care nursery. *Neonatal network* 22(3):17-23.

Janssen HJEM, Cuisinier MCJ (1996). A critical review of the concept of pathological grief following pregnancy loss. *Omega: journal of death and dying* 33(1):21-42.

Kavanaugh K (1997a). Gender differences among parents who experience the death of an infant weighing less than 500 grams at birth. *Omega: journal of death and dying* 35(3):281-296.

Kavanaugh K (1997b). Parents' experience surrounding the death of a newborn infant whose birth is at the margin of viability. *Journal of obstetric, gynecologic, and neonatal nursing* 26(1):43-51.

Kavanaugh K, Hershberger P (2005). Perinatal loss in low-income African American parents. *Journal of obstetric, gynecologic, and neonatal nursing* 34:595-605.

Kavanaugh K, Paton J (2001). Communicating with parents who experience a perinatal loss. *Illness, crisis, and loss* 9:369-380.

Kavanaugh K, Robertson PA (1999). Recurrent perinatal loss: a case study. *Omega: journal of death and dying* 39(2):133-147.

Kavanaugh K et al (2004). Social support following perinatal loss. *Journal of family nursing* 10(1):70-92.

Khong TY (1997). Improving perinatal autopsy rates: who is counseling bereaved parents for autopsy consent? *Birth* 24:55-57.

Kimble DL (1991). Neonatal death: a descriptive study of fathers' experiences. *Neonatal network* 9(81):45-50.

Klass D, Silverman PR (editors) (1996). *Continuing bonds: new understandings of grief.* Washington, DC: Taylor & Francis.

Kowalski K (1991). No happy ending: pregnancy loss and bereavement. *NAACOG critical issues* 2(3):368-380.

Kubler-Ross E (1969). *On death and dying.* New York: Macmillan.

Lang A et al (2004). Explanatory model of health in bereaved parents post-fetal/infant death. *International journal of nursing studies* 41:869-880.

Lasker JN, Toedter L (1994). Satisfaction with hospital care and interventions after pregnancy loss. *Death studies* 18(1):41-64.

Lemmer SCM (1991). Parental perceptions of caring perinatal bereavement. *Western journal of nursing research* 13(4):475-493.

Leon IG (1992). A critique of current hospital practices. *Clinical pediatrics* 31(6):366-374.

Lichtenthal WG et al (2004). A case for establishing complicated grief as a distinct mental disorder in DSM-V. *Clinical psychology review* 24:637-662.

Limbo RK, Wheeler SR (1998). *When a baby dies: a handbook for healing and helping.* La Crosse, WI: Lutheran Hospital.

Lin SX, Lasker JN (1996). Patterns of grief reaction after a pregnancy loss. *American journal of orthopsychiatry* 66(2):262-271.

Lindemann E (1944). Symptomatology and management of acute grief. *American journal of psychiatry* 101:141-149.

Lundqvist A et al (2002). Both empowered and powerless: mothers' experiences of professional care when their newborn dies. *Birth* 29(3):192-199.

Malacrida CA (1997). Perinatal death: helping parents find their way. *Journal of family nursing* 3:130-148.

Malacrida C (1999). Complicating mourning: the social economy of perinatal death. *Qualitative health research* 9:504-519.

Marino PA (1998). The effects of cumulative grief in the nurse. *Journal of intravenous nursing* 21(2):101-104.

Martin TL, Doka KJ (2002). *Men don't cry . . . women do. Transcending gender stereotypes of grief.* Philadelphia: Taylor and Francis.

McCreight BS (2004). A grief ignored: narratives of pregnancy loss from a male perspective. *Sociology of health and illness* 26(3):326-350.

McHaffie HE et al (2001). Consent to autopsy for neonates. *Archives of disease in childhood* 85(1):F4-F7.

National Center for Health Statistics (2005). *Health, United States, 2005. With chartbook on trends in the health of Americans.* Hyattsville, MD: National Center for Health Statistics.

Neimeyer RA (2001). *Meaning reconstruction and the experience of loss.* Washington, DC: American Psychological Association.

Parks CM, Brown RJ (1972). Health after bereavement: a controlled study of young Boston widows and widowers. *Psychosomatic medicine* 34(5):449-461.

Pector EA (2004a). How bereaved multiple birth parents cope with hospitalization, homecoming, disposition for deceased, and attachment to survivors. *Journal of perinatology* 24(11):714-722.

Pector EA (2004b). Views of bereaved multiple-birth parents on life support decisions, the dying process, and discussions around death. *Journal of perinatology* 24:4-10.

Pector EA, Smith-Levitin M (2002). Mourning and psychological issues in multiple birth loss. *Seminars in neonatology* 7:247-256.

Peppers L, Knapp RJ (1980a). *Motherhood and mourning a perinatal death.* New York: Praeger.

Peppers LG, Knapp RJ (1980b). Maternal reactions to involuntary fetal/infant death. *Psychiatry* 43(2):155-159.

Primeau MR, Lamb JM (1995). When a baby dies: rights of the baby and parents. *Journal of obstetric, gynecologic, and neonatal nursing* 24(3): 206-208.

Ptacek JT, Eberhardt TL (1996). Breaking bad news: a review of the literature. *Journal of the American Medical Association* 276(6):496-502.

Puddifoot JE, Johnson MP (1997). The legitimacy of grieving: the partner's experience at miscarriage. *Social science and medicine* 45(6):837.

Radestad I, Nordin C (1998). A comparison of women's memories of care during pregnancy, labour, and delivery after stillbirth or live birth. *Midwifery* 14(2):111-117.

Rajan L (1994). Social isolation and support in pregnancy loss. *Health visitor* 6(33):97-101.

Rando TA (editor) (1986). *Parental loss of a child.* Champaign, IL: Research Press.

Robertson P, Kavanaugh K (1998). Supporting parents during and after a pregnancy subsequent to perinatal loss. *Journal of perinatal and neonatal nursing* 12(2):63-71.

Sanders CM (1989). *Grief: the mourning after—dealing with adult bereavement.* New York: Wiley Interscience.

Schaefer D, Lyons C (1993). *How do we tell the children?* New York: Newmarket.

Serwint JR, Rutherford L (2000). Sharing bad news with parents. *Contemporary pediatrics* 17:45-46, 49-50, 53-54, 56, 59-60, 62, 64, 66.

Sexton PR, Stephen SB (1991). Postpartum mothers' perceptions of nursing interventions for perinatal grief. *Neonatal network* 9:47-51.

Solari-Twadell PA, Bunkers SS (1995). The pinwheel model of bereavement. *Image: journal of nursing scholarship* 27(4):323-326.

Stevens-Simon C et al (1996). Absence of negative attitudes toward childbearing among pregnant teenagers. A risk factor for a rapid repeat pregnancy? *Archives of pediatric and adolescent medicine* 150(10): 1037-1043.

Swanson KM (1991). Empirical development of middle range theory of caring. *Nursing research* 40(3):161-166.

Swanson KM (1993). Nursing as informed caring for the well-being of others. *Image: journal of nursing scholarship* 25(4):352-357.

Swanson KM (1999a). Effects of caring, measurement, and time on miscarriage: impact on women's well-being. *Nursing research* 48(6):288-298.

Swanson KM (1999b). What's known about caring in nursing science: a literary meta-analysis. In AS Hinshaw et al, editors. *Handbook of clinical nursing research* (pp 31-60). Thousand Oaks, CA: Sage.

Swanson PB et al (2002). How mothers cope with the death of a twin or higher multiple. *Twin research* 5(3):156-164.

Swanson-Kauffman K (1988). There should have been two: nursing care of parents experiencing the perinatal death of a twin. *Journal of perinatal and neonatal nursing* 2(2):78-86.

Sychowski SMP (1998). Life and death: in the all at once. *Mother baby journal* 3(1):33-39.

Theut SK, Pedersen FA (1988). Pregnancy subsequent to perinatal loss: parental anxiety and depression. *Journal of the American Academy of Child and Adolescent Psychiatry* 27(3):289-292.

Theut SK, Zaslow MJ (1990). Resolution of parental bereavement after a perinatal loss. *Journal of the American Academy of Child and Adolescent Psychiatry* 29(4):521-525.

Tudehope DI, Iredell J (1986). Neonatal death: grieving families. *Medical journal of Australia* 144(6):290-292.

Uren TH, Wastell CA (2002). Attachment and meaning-making in perinatal bereavement. *Death studies* 26:279-308.

Van P, Meleis AI (2003). Coping with grief after involuntary pregnancy loss: -perspectives of African American women. *Journal of obstetric, gynecologic, and neonatal nursing* 32(1):28-39.

Wagner T, Higgins PG (1997). Perinatal death: how fathers grieve. *Journal of perinatal education* 6(4):9-16.

Wallerstedt C, Higgins PG (1996). Facilitating perinatal grieving between the mother and the father. *Journal of obstetric, gynecologic, and neonatal nursing* 25(5):389-394.

Wallerstedt C et al (2003). Interconceptional counseling after perinatal and infant loss. *Journal of obstetric, gynecologic, and neonatal nursing* 32(4):533-542.

Wheeler SR (1997). Adolescent pregnancy loss. In Woods JR, Woods JL, editors. *Loss during or in the newborn period: principles of care with clinical cases and analyses.* Pitman, NJ: Janetti.

Wheeler SR, Austin J (2001). The impact of early pregnancy loss on adolescents. *American journal of maternal child nursing* 26(3):154-159.

Wheeler SR, Pike M (1991). *Grief resources manual.* Danville, IL: Grief, Ltd.

Wilson RE (2001). Parents' support of their other children after a miscarriage or perinatal death. *Early human development* 61:55-65.

Worden JW (1982). *Grief counseling and grief therapy.* New York: Springer.

Worden JW (1991). *Grief counseling and therapy.* New York: Springer.

Zeanah CH (1989). Adaptation following perinatal loss: a critical review. *Journal of the American Academy of Child and Adolescent Psychiatry* 28(3):467-480.

Chapter 28

Complementary and Integrative Therapies

Nadine Kassity-Krich • Jamieson Jones

The use of complementary and alternative medicine (CAM) is a growing trend in this country and abroad. This topic is included in a neonatal text because little research has been done in the area of CAM in the newborn; yet many of the families we serve use these therapies. In addition some health care professionals are beginning to apply the concepts of holistic care and alternative modalities to this population. This emerging area of medicine has become so widespread that the National Institutes of Health (NIH) created the National Center for Complementary and Alternative Medicine (NCCAM). Monies are now set aside for in-depth research of CAM therapies. Health care professionals must recognize these therapies as well as the gaps in our scientific knowledge regarding CAM. In the neonatal unit, CAM therapies may soften the high-tech environment by adding the more nurturing elements one would expect around newborns. This chapter briefly describes some of the most popular and promising CAM therapies, explores how these options are used in the neonatal intensive care unit (NICU) and other infant populations, and identifies areas for further study.

COMPLEMENTARY AND ALTERNATIVE MEDICINE

The merging of complementary and alternative therapies with mainstream Western medicine is often called integrative medicine. In integrative medicine, health professionals are expanding their view of Western medicine to a more holistic perspective. Two views are now being integrated—one that views disease as having specific causative agents and another that views the mind-body connection as a significant influence on health. In treating disease, practitioners of mind-body medicine look at many factors, including the nature of relationships—such as the relationship between parents and infants and the dynamic between healer and patient. This new integrative, holistic model has thus increasingly challenged our profession to broaden definitions of healing to include all aspects of relationship as part of health and wholeness.

In neonatal care, proponents of complementary therapies believe that the integration of CAM may minimize iatrogenic complications associated with prematurity or interventions to treat prematurity. The high-tech environment may overwhelm the infant with excessive stimulation. Alternatively, these infants may be touch-deprived from weeks in incubators. CAM therapies may provide balance to support the amazing technologic advances we have made.

Alternative medicine, like conventional medicine, has pros and cons, promotes good ideas and bad ones, and promises to hold both benefits and risks. To keep an open, skeptical mind will allow examination of our current medical model with its focus on the "cure" and allow us to broaden our perspective on healing and health. Nursing and nursing care is naturally compatible with CAM, since nursing care is based on a holistic approach. The operative word *care* connotes a friendlier, humanistic value than the word *cure* does. Caring (communication, sensitivity, holistic approach) are some of the hallmarks of our profession. Much of CAM is based on expanding these areas as well as broadening our awareness of many different subtleties in healing.

The complementary categories that were established by the National Center for Complementary and Alternative Medicine (NCCAM) are used for discussion:

- Lifestyle Therapies (Developmental Care)
- Aromatherapy, Music, Light, Kangaroo Care, Cobedding
- Biomechanical Therapies
- Massage, Reflexology, Osteopathy/Cranial-Sacral Therapy
- Bioenergetic Therapies
- Acupuncture, Energy Healing, Healing Touch, Reiki
- Biochemical Therapies
- Herbs and Supplements; Homeopathy

Although some practices could fit in more than one category, the categories are useful for general description. For instance, some view homeopathy as a vibrational medicine because its effect is energetic rather than biochemical. Some also consider techniques that focus on environmental manipulation more alternative in nature. These fall into the realm of either family-focused care (Chapter 25) or the NICU environment (Chapter 24).

LIFESTYLE THERAPIES (DEVELOPMENTAL CARE)

General Developmental Care

Neurodevelopmental care includes any intervention undertaken to improve neurodevelopmental outcome. These include developmentally supportive NICU design (appropriate lighting and use of circadian light/dark cycles; low noise levels in the unit and incubator), nursing care plans (infant positioning and handling, feeding and bathing methods, speaking before handling), and pain management.

Research is needed to assess sensory overstimulation in preterm infants, as well as to demonstrate the efficacy of providing soothing sensory input to ameliorate the NICU experience for infants and their families. One benefit of all of these developmental therapies is they tend to encourage early participation by family members in caregiving, which has been shown to enhance bonding (Chapter 25).

Aromatherapy

The intent of aromatherapy is to alter a person's mood or behavior and to facilitate physical, mental, or emotional well-being through the use of aromatic and essential oils from herbs and flowers. People respond immediately and involuntarily to scents, which may release neurotransmitters in the brain and cause calming, sedating, pain-reducing, stimulating, or euphoric effects. For example, truck drivers are known to use peppermint aromatherapy to keep them awake during long night drives. A month-long Japanese study of aromatherapy found that when the air in an office for keypunch operators was scented with jasmine, error rates dropped 33%; the scent was also found to increase efficiency and relieve stress among employees. Could NICU staff use this anxiety-relief and stress reduction technique as well?

Aromatherapy is the fastest growing of all complementary therapies among the nursing field in the United States. It is only in the past few years that aromatherapy has become recognized by the U.S. State Board of Nursing as a legitimate part of holistic nursing (Buckle, 2001). Lavender, of all the essential oils, has been the most studied by health care providers. Various studies mention the use of lavender on pillows in order to alleviate insomnia, as well as to help ICU patients cope with stress. Questions that arise include: If a newborn is having sleepless nights, might this be mitigated by using olfaction? Could we use lavender rather than sedatives for sleep? Could chamomile help regulate sleep-wake cycles? Could peppermint in incubators as an "olfactory caffeine"—as a stimulant to minimize or eliminate apnea and bradycardia events in preemies? A French study recently published in *Pediatrics* demonstrates a 36% reduction in apnea with the introduction of the odor vanillin (used because of its weak trigeminal activation) when used in the treatment of apneas unresponsive to caffeine and doxapram (Marlier et al, 2005).

There are several recent articles addressing the role of olfaction as a tool in preterm infants. One article assessed the effects of familiar odors (maternal breast milk, amniotic fluid, etc.) used on healthy preterm infants during routine blood draws (heelsticks and venipuncture) noting a decrease in crying and grimacing compared to baseline in infants given various types of odorization (Goubet et al, 2003).

Researchers have reported that newborns have an acute sense of smell. Indeed, the natural odor that emanates from the mother forms part of the complex bonding process. Dr. Hisanobu Sugano, director of the Life Science Institute at Moa Health Science Foundation in Fukuoka, Japan, demonstrated through his numerous studies in subtle energies and aromatherapy that newborns could correctly identify their mothers' milk from nine other specimens. Several other experiments have shown that when used and unused breast pads are placed on either side of the newborn's head, the newborn will turn more often to the side of the used pad. Within a week after birth, the newborn can discern its mother's milk on a breast pad from the milk of other mothers. Surely babies are sensitive to the noxious odors of our

environment from alcohol and Betadine swabs to the newest cousins of our skin cleansers.

The calming or stimulating effects of CAM therapies could be a productive area for research. With the fragrance perception of newborns, is it possible to manipulate the scents to achieve effects from olfactory stimulants, anxiolytics, or enhanced attachment? In some cultures this process is already done. For instance, Filipino families often leave the mother's clothing in the newborn's crib to calm the child in her absence. Some suggestions might be to have the family bring in an article of the parent's clothing and place it in the bed in order to help calm and reassure the infant. Another would be to allow the infant to smell the breast milk container, reinforcing the mother's smell with feedings. Or place a small amount of milk on a pacifier for tube-fed babies. This fosters the formation of the nerve pathways and associations between smell/taste and feeding (McDowell, 2005).

A variety of aromatherapy oils are used for diaper rashes, such as lavender sitz baths, almond oils, and beeswax. Another oil, Brazilian guava, found to have analgesic effects is being investigated for use in babies. Some aromas are recommended for colic. They are believed to reduce infant anxiety as well as parental stress, which many feel plays a role in colic. This is another area that needs further research.

Music Therapy

For several years now, media attention has turned toward what is called the Mozart effect. This focuses on music as an auditory vehicle that can soothe and stimulate developing infants in utero as well as once they are born (Campbell, 1997). Lullabies have been linked with infants throughout history; music therapy carries this tradition over into the NICU. For the past 10 years, music therapy has been used in the NICU to mediate stress and promote positive development. We know that by the 18th week of gestation, the auditory capabilities of the fetus are present. In utero the uterine blood flow provides a soothing musical waterfall and the maternal heart beat a continuous tick-tock chant. Many studies have measured heart rate changes in the fetus when exposed to certain music in utero. The music and the tempo can assist with accelerating the heart rate in terms of bradycardia or decelerating the heart rate to help with stress-induced increases.

Hospital noise differs markedly from in utero acoustics or the sound of soothing music (Ernst, 1996). Ambient noise in the NICU may cause distress, and attempts have been made to cover the noise in the NICU by using sound to negate other sounds. This is called sonic camouflage, or acoustic masking, aimed at sound reduction and minimization of vestibular stimulation.

Music has been shown to promote both neurologic development and language development if words accompany the music (Standley, 2001). Music with or without vocalization has been shown to sooth a crying infant or to decrease a heart rate and increase oxygen saturation levels. In the first meta-analysis of music therapy studies of premature infants, Standley reported that the observed state, heart and respiratory rates, oxygen saturation levels, weight gain, length of stay, feeding rate, and nonnutritive sucking rates were all positively influenced by music therapy (Standley, 2002). Recent literature on the pacifier activated lullaby (PAL) allows the infant to coordinate music and sucking (Marwick, 2000).

Music may even alleviate some of the distress infants sustain with suctioning (Chou et al, 2003) and heelsticks (Butt & Kisilevsky, 2000). It has been theorized that music therapy during performance of nursing interventions may enhance the infant's quality of life.

Based on experience rather than evidence from controlled studies, Standley (2001), a certified music therapist, suggests the following guidelines for music in the NICU:

- Music selection: sounds in the NICU should be soothing, constant, stable, and relatively unchanging to reduce alerting responses.
- Volume level: in the 65 to 70 dB range is recommended.
- Maximum time per day for continuously playing music: 1.5 hours (alternating 45 minutes on and 45 minutes off).
- Approval for auditory stimuli: daily approval of the nurse providing care to the infant should be obtained for provision of music stimulation.[*]

Light Therapy

Research has demonstrated the scientific significance of phototherapy. Aside from the classically recognized effects of diminishing bilirubin and activation of vitamin D, numerous studies have shown this therapy's effect on thyroid stimulation alterations in renal and vascular parameters, increased gut transit times, and a host of other metabolic alterations. Hypothetically, other wavelengths of light may have physiologic effects. This hypothesis is the basis for the field of color and light therapy.

Regulation of ambient lighting in the NICU has been recognized as an important concern. Research in this area falls under the category of NICU design and environment and is discussed in Chapter 24. Constant exposure to light can result in disorganization of the infant's state (Jones et al, 2001). For this reason, procedural lighting and blanket covers are used to shield infants in incubators from direct light. Research is needed to determine whether light therapy—exposing the infant to varying light cycles—alters circadian rhythms or physiologic stability through its effects on endocrine function. Assessing and broadening our current understanding could expand concepts of light, color, or other wavelengths for newborns as well as staff.

Kangaroo Care

Kangaroo care (KC) was first described by Gene Cranston Anderson (1991) about twenty years ago in the mountains of Bogotá, Colombia, yet the practice may be older than recorded history. In this practice, the newborn was placed skin-to-skin, usually on the chest between the mother's breasts to keep the baby warm. The effect of skin-to-skin care on physiologic stability and bonding has been investigated in many studies. Engler and Ludington (1999) conducted a survey of 1133 NICUs in the United States to determine what percentage of those NICUs used KC. They found 82% of the units practiced some form of skin-to-skin care.

To date, studies indicate that KC can positively affect both the mother (or caregiver) and the infant. When a parent holds the infant against his or her skin, the infant's breathing, oxygen saturation, and heart rate become more regular; the flexion and tone improve; and the sleep state becomes less disorganized (Ludington-Hoe et al., 2004). Various body positions also seem to affect gastric emptying and reflux. KC provides a sensory dialogue for the infant and caregiver as well as a method of central nervous system regulation of the autonomic motor and state systems. Mounting evidence in favor of KC to promote physiologic stability has encouraged more studies with very immature, unstable infants (Eichel, 2001).

Cobedding

Cobedding of twins and higher order multiples (HOMs) is a growing practice. The rationale is that during their gestational development, multiple-gestation fetuses lived side by side. Once born, they are normally separated and put in a single bed, partly because of concerns over infection and because of the size of standard infant beds. Studies are underway that examine the effects of the practice of cobedding on physiologic stability, soothing, motoric organization, proprioceptive stimulation, and enhanced growth. One completed study (Altimier & Lutes, 2001) focused on premature twins and higher order multiples admitted to a large Midwestern tertiary center. Twenty-three sets of twins, 4 sets of triplets, and 1 set of quadruplets were included. The control group consisted of 15 sets of twins, 7 sets of triplets, and 2 sets of quadruplets. A randomized control design was used on infants weighing less than 1500 g. The following protocol was indicated:

- Twins and HOMs being cared for in the same NICU were put together when stability was achieved.
- Oxygen requirement was limited to nasal cannula only.
- IVs, gavage feeding, cardiopulmonary monitoring, pulse oximetry, and phototherapy were permitted.
- All equipment, clothing, and chart forms were color-coded to match each twin/multiple. The multiples wore hospital identification bands at all times.
- Positioning of multiples in the womb was replicated, if this was known. Otherwise, siblings were placed side by side, either facing each other, facing the other one's back, or in a head-to-toes position. Repositioning of one or more infants was considered if infant(s) appeared restless.
- One blanket was lightly swaddled around the multiples; hands were free to reach their own face or a sibling to facilitate each other's motor organization.
- Caregiving was clustered to address all infants' needs during the same interaction. (The infant in the most awake state received care first.)
- If one infant demonstrated temperature instability, the temperature probe was placed on that infant, otherwise on the smallest infant. All infants were dressed or undressed depending on their individualized thermoregulatory needs.[†]

The results demonstrated that the cobedded group had a more positive growth rate in weight and in head circumference than the control group. No differences in nosocomial rates or in thermal needs were noted between the two groups (Altimier & Lutes, 2001). Cobedding is considered a developmentally supportive care strategy (Nyqvist & Lutes, 1998). This therapy is being considered as part of some hospitals' quality improvement programs to support family-centered,

---

[*]Used with permission from Standley J (2001). Music therapy for the neonate. *Newborn and infant nursing reviews* 1(4):211-216.

[†]Used with permission from Altimier L, Lutes L (2001). Co-bedding multiples. *Newborn and infant nursing reviews* 1(4):205-206.

developmental care for multiple gestation families (Polizzi et al, 2003). Before this therapy is completely embraced, further research needs to determine the benefits and safety in this population of neonates. Recently concerns have been raised again about the linkage between cobedding and sudden infant death syndrome (SIDS) (Burnett & Adler, 2006). The connection may be the tight swaddling of infants when cobedded. Until further research findings are released this practice should be undertaken with caution if at all.

Infant Massage

Massage develops our first language, the expression of touch. There are many types of massage from gentle stroking, superficial friction, pressure, kneading, containment, vibration, and percussion to the more intense manipulations of Rolfing (Caroll, 2006).

Fields (2000) has conducted infant massage research since the 1970s, much of which focused on the premature infant. Fields reported that massaged infants have a 47% greater weight gain and better organized sleep states; moreover, they are more responsive to social stimulation, have more organized motor development, and are commonly discharged 6 to 10 days earlier from the hospital. This allows the newborn to go home earlier, adding a significant cost savings.

Fields' study (2000) of cocaine-exposed newborns suggested that touch therapy increases vagal activity, which in turn releases the hormones gastrin and insulin, which may explain the weight gain in the premature infant. Massage stimulates the parasympathetic nervous system. If an infant is more attentive, it may follow that more stimulation from the parent is elicited, thus improving the dyad interactions and performance on the infant developmental assessment tools (Fields, 2000).

"Touch promotes bonding and well being and is therefore an essential therapy for the benefit of parents, babies and health care professionals" (Feary, 2002). The efficacy of infant massage depends on respect and consideration for the infant's readiness. Massage should be state dependent; for example, the deep sleep state is not the best time for a massage. A time when the infant is fussy, however, may be the perfect time. Being aware of the baby and his or her receptivity and alertness is important in determining the best time for a massage rather than relying on a predetermined time. The type and amount of massage depends on the infant's gestational age, degree of illness or stability, and ability to engage. Fields (2000) has also suggested many benefits to the "massager"— such as lower stress hormone levels and decreased postnatal depression (Feary, 2002; Glover et al, 2002). Some researchers have focused on massage as a way to reduce stress and to increase bonding and attachment when a parent performs massage. A significant emphasis has been placed on fathers performing massage as a bonding tool, as breastfeeding would be for the mother.

Research on the benefits of massage is increasing. Kirpatrick (2001, personal communication) has found in her NICU experience that massage helps reduce postoperative edema through stimulation of cardiac and lymphatic activity and decreases the need for postoperative narcotics. Physical activity when combined with infant massage seems to stimulate bone growth and mineralization in premature infants. However, with osteopenia, which can be a major course for morbidity in this population, further investigation is warranted (Aly et al, 2004).

Concerns as to whether infant massage can produce overstimulation and therefore adverse effects have been raised. Further research is needed through controlled trials to determine the benefits as well as the risks of this therapy.

Reflexology

Reflexology is an ancient form of healing, somewhat similar to traditional acupuncture. It is a healing method based on the principle that there are reflexes in the hands and feet specific to each organ, gland, function, and part of the human body. The goal of reflexology is to stop or reverse the negative chain reactions that occur within the mind-body and to restore the energy balance. According to the tenets of reflexologists, health problems occur when the flow of life energy (chi) is blocked or disturbed and that it is alleviated when the flow of chi is restored by manipulation of the reflex points. Applying pressure to these points can also bring about stress relief by improving circulation and minimizing pain. This modality can be considered the opposite of the heelstick blood draw; it involves the same area but a reverse technique. However, more research is needed in this area.

The presumed mechanisms in reflexology, from a Western medical perspective, are (1) that the treatment of reflex zones stimulates the body's blood flow; (2) that pressure to these points increases the body's production of endorphins; and (3) that it assists in the elimination of waste materials.

It is the opinion of this author that reflexology may be useful in a neonatal unit to help balance and soothe the patient's bioenergy, which might decrease periods of fussiness or disorganization. Reflexology may also benefit the infant by increasing blood flow to specific organ sites, increasing perfusion to the kidneys, and increasing cardiac output.

Osteopathy/Cranial-Sacral Therapy

Osteopathy medicine is based on the premise that the body has within it an inherent therapeutic potency. The body is its own medicine chest. Most of the biomechanical manipulations in the pediatric osteopathic community fall under the healing category of cranial-sacral therapy. A practitioner of cranial-sacral therapy works with the subtle pressure fluctuations of the cerebral spinal fluid to optimize a patient's health. A practitioner of this discipline may gently realign cranial bones to bring them into the proper relationship.

A basic tenet of osteopathy is that many problems begin at birth. Birth (labor and delivery) is viewed as one of the most traumatic experiences and can cause skeletal strains that can cause problems throughout life. Recognition and treatment of these dysfunctions in the immediate postpartum period is considered an essential preventive measure. In the cranial-sacral system, misalignment of structure that is not corrected can lead to potential alterations in function. The occipital area is believed to sustain most of the trauma during delivery. A study by Frymann (1998) explored the relationship between symptomatology in the newborn and the anatomic physiologic disturbances of the central nervous system (CNS). The study suggested that strains within the unfused fragments of the occipital bones produced problems in the nervous system, that is, vomiting, reflux, hyperactive peristalsis, colic, tremor, hypertonicity, and irritability.

Frymann (1998) reported that compression of the hypoglossal nerve can cause a newborn's failure to grasp the nipple and suck effectively. If left untreated, these newborns may exhibit tongue thrust and may have deviant swallowing patterns, speech problems, and even malocclusion. Problems such as sucking-swallowing difficulties and recurrent reflux after birth are so common that many mothers and doctors consider them to be normal. According to cranial-sacral theory, these can be easily rectified. When the vagus nerve is compressed, for example, recurrent vomiting or reflux can occur. Decompress the condylar parts of the occiput, and the vomiting stops. In temporal bone development, misalignment may cause recurrent otitis media. If the sphenoids are involved, the child may have headaches. Until the structural cause of the problem is recognized and addressed, the underlying pathophysiology will not change. Osteopaths often feel that every child should be structurally evaluated after any type of trauma, especially birth.

This field presents some interesting opportunities for research. What portals of understanding could this field open in the search for intraventricular hemorrhage (IVH)? Could daily CS therapy assist in developing a more womblike analogue for brain and spinal development? Could they palpate and help guide the developmental energies in the CS system by tuning in and tracking the system to retrace its normal developmental pattern, and bringing the memory of health to play? As osteopathy's founder, Dr. Andrew Still, once said, "To find health should be the objective of the doctor. Anyone can find a disease."

BIOENERGETIC THERAPIES

Acupuncture

Acupuncture is part of a complex system known as traditional Chinese medicine (TCM) that has been practiced in China for more than 2000 years. This is an energy-based approach rather than a disease-oriented approach through the conventional diagnostic and treatment model. The main concept behind this philosophy is that of energy in the body. This energy is called chi (immeasurable by current instrumentation in Western science) (Freeman, 2001a), which underlies and supports all aspects of the physical body. This energy circulates throughout the body along specific pathways called meridians. Obstructions in the flow of chi may cause disease. Acupuncturists rebalance the flow of energy by gently placing thin, solid, disposable, metallic needles into the skin along the meridians where chi is blocked. These needles either are briefly left in place or are stimulated with electricity heat, laser, or moxibustion (burning of the moxa herb over the acupuncture point).

Acupuncture has shown promising results in use for anesthesia, postoperative pain, and addiction recovery. In the West, acupuncture has been used since the early 1970s for various forms of addiction and withdrawal in expectant mothers, as well as for infants to help reduce the residual effects of drug exposure in cases of prenatal substance abuse. This therapy is based on research done with acupuncture and withdrawal of drugs and alcohol (Janssen et al, 2005).

Researchers are currently considering whether acupuncture can help treat colic, constipation, diminished postoperative urine output, apnea, and bradycardia as well as the improvement cardiac output and control of postoperative pain. Currently in China, acupuncture is used to treat infants with jaundice (augmenting hepatic chi), skin problems, teething, ear infections, constipation, conjunctivitis, and peripheral nerve injury.

Acupressure, which is similar to acupuncture, appears more popular in pediatric patients because it does not involve the use of needles. Acupressure involves applying pressure at acupuncture points along the 14 major energy meridians to promote the flow of chi. Numerous studies show that acupressure, like acupuncture, stimulates physical reactions in the body, such as changes in brain activity and blood chemistries, in addition to enhancing immune and endocrine functions (Jones & Kassity, 2001).

Healing Touch

Healing touch (HT) is an energy-based therapy developed by Mentgen and the American Holistic Nurses Association in the late 1980s. This therapy is considered experimental and requires parental consent and a certified practitioner. It is another therapy that reaches out to the human desire to be touched. It is a way to further humanize the health care relationship for the nurse as well as the patient. As noted previously, touch promotes healing and the formation of a bond.

During an HT session, infants are not to be disturbed. They usually are scheduled for at least two sessions per week that last from 15 to 40 minutes. HT consists first of a hand scan to assess the infant's condition. This assessment is done by gently and slowly moving a hand from head to toes, often 6 inches or more above the body, to detect changes in the infant's energy field. Once the assessment is completed, a variety of techniques can be used: energy field centering, comfort infusion, energy infusion or modulation, modified magnetic unruffling, spiral healing light, and halo. All of these methods use the hands-on technique or the movement of the hands over the body to balance the energy field of the infant.

Comfort infusion is a technique that parents can be taught. It is believed to relieve pain. Parents place the left palm over the infant, encouraging the pain to move through their palm, up through their body and drain out of their right hand. When parents no longer sense pain, the right hand is placed palm on or over the infant and the left one turned upward to infuse healing energy. This technique empowers parents to actively participate in care of their infants.

In any of these modes, the infant may be observed to calm down (if unsettled before HT), relax, and even fall into a sleep state. The spiral healing light uses a visualized light beam for those infants who are much compromised. A beam of healing light is visualized flowing through the crown chakra "energy center" down the arm and out the first two fingers and thumb as they are held together. Starting at the center of the infant's body, the beam is slowly directed in a clockwise spiral that expands to cover the whole body. The healing light touches every cell of the body and infuses healing energy. When the edges of the body are reached, the spiral is brought back to the center of the body while the practitioner visualizes the healing beam of light, thus giving the infant strength and energy to help the cells release excess fluid, carbon dioxide, bilirubin, or infection. When the center of the body is reached, a clear blue healing light is visualized as flowing through the practitioner's hand and is held over the infant's crown, thus washing away what has been released. Along with traditional medicine, healing touch promotes a calm, restful state and relieves discomfort, which helps support the body, mind, and spirit's natural healing process.

Energy-based healing is growing in popularity in hospitals and medical and nursing school curricula around the country.

Results of healing touch studies support its use in depression, cancer, pain, and many other conditions. It also adds a spiritual dimension to our increasingly high-tech health care system.

Reiki

Reiki, is another form of energy healing, in which energy is transferred from the hands of a practitioner to a patient using a sequence of hand positions above the body. Reiki relaxes and heals by clearing energy meridians and chakras (vortices of energy along the spine), thus restoring balance, relieving pain, and accelerating the healing process. Respiration slows; blood pressure decreases; emotional clearing and calming occur. Blockages are dissolved and the vibrational frequency of the body is thought to increase.

Few studies of Reiki have been done in the United States. In one study from New Hampshire, more than 872 patients underwent a 15-minute Reiki treatment both before and after surgery (Alandydy & Alandydy, 1999). The patients reported an increased sense of relaxation, reduction in stress, and a possible enhancement of the natural healing ability of their bodies. Notably, no infants were included in the study; this is an area in need of further study.

Reiki treatments may be applicable for pregnancy and infancy in many situations. Simply increasing relaxation and improving the body's healing ability could be valuable in many circumstances surrounding pregnancy and birth. Further study is needed regarding the efficacy and safety of these techniques.

BIOCHEMICAL INTERVENTIONS

Homeopathy

The basic idea behind homeopathy is respect of the innate wisdom of the body. The premise is to honor the symptoms of illness that one's body experiences as it responds to defend, heal, or protect itself against stress or infection. The way a homeopath views this process is that the body's internal wisdom will defend and heal itself by choosing a beneficial response. Homeopathy is based on the "like cures like principle": a symptom in a patient is treated with a remedy that causes this same symptom, thus further stimulating the body's current responses (similar in philosophy to a vaccine). Homeopaths explain that when a truly effective therapy is underway, a temporary exacerbation of certain symptoms may appear. This idea contrasts with the suppression theory of conventional medicine, which homeopaths feel works on disease suppression rather than elimination. A homeopath's use of the principle of similars tries to minimize the wisdom of the body rather than suppress its symptoms (Ullman, 1999). Homeopathic remedies are an enigma to those unaware of the concepts of the energetic memory of water and the potentizing successions that enhance the memory of the water, but appear to physical science as a mere series of dilutions.

A review of 89 clinical studies showed that patients who were given a homeopathic medicine were 2.45 times more likely to improve than those who received placebos (Linde et al, 1997). These findings were based on the efficacy of homeopathic remedies in healing and treating a variety of conditions such as asthma, ear infections, postsurgical complications, sprains, rheumatoid arthritis, and those found around childbirth.

Homeopathy can be considered a catalyst to "jump start" the body and its healing process. Professional homeopaths prescribe medicine that is very patient specific and is based on that particular patient's past health history, past medical treatments, genetic inheritance, and the totality of the physical, emotional, and mental or spiritual symptoms. Unfortunately, titrating individualized medicine(s) for everyone, especially newborns, is not always easy. It sometimes takes more than a single visit to a homeopath to find the correct remedy to start the healing process (Linde et al, 1997). Chubby babies require different constitutional remedies from small or low-birth-weight babies, as do babies who sleep through the night compared to those who do not. Some research on homeopathic remedies for pregnant women has been done. One must keep in mind that a mother who receives homeopathic remedies during pregnancy and childbirth will pass its benefits onto the fetus. Postnatal treatment of the mother will also benefit the child if he or she is breastfed (Linde et al, 1997).

Infants who endure traumatic labors with bruising or other injury (i.e., postnatal IV infiltrates) are considered to benefit from a remedy called arnica, which aims to optimize the body's attempts to heal its wounds, both physical and psychologic. In addition to arnica, *Hypericum perforatum* can be used for IV burns for the mother or newborn during hospitalization.

It is hypothesized that homeopathic remedies such as arnica, staphysagria, and calendula can help circumcised newborns heal from the physical and psychologic trauma of circumcision. Chamomilla is the most effective of many remedies suggested for colic and is also the most common remedy for teething pain in older infants. Other remedies for teething pain may include calcarea carbonica, calcarea phosphorica, and silicea. Magnesium phosphorica relieves the symptoms of gas, bloating, and burping. Nux vomica may be used when the woman has ingested alcohol or therapeutic or recreational drugs and the newborn exhibits colicky behavior. Aethusa is used for newborns who are intolerant of milk or who reflux shortly after milk has been ingested. Calendula given externally for diaper rash will soothe the newborn's bottom and help fight infection. In Europe, carbovege is a homeopathic remedy used for apnea and bradycardia in the infant. Homeopathy offers much to learn and information that can be assimilated into care to broaden the current medical understandings.

Herbal Medicine

The use of botanical medicine is ancient. Hippocrates (466–377 BC) integrated herbal medicine into his practice and teaching. The World Health Organization estimates that about 75% of the world population relies on botanical medicines; indeed, 30% of Americans also use botanical remedies, and the practice is growing in popularity (Barrett et al, 1999). It behooves health care professionals to be familiar with the expanding field of herbal medicine. Substances first isolated from plants account for approximately 25% of the Western pharmacopoeia and another 25% is derived from modification of chemicals first found in natural products (Barrett et al, 1999; Freeman, 2001b). Digitalis, the ever-popular echinacea, and caffeine all are herbal and have effects and side effects (Boullata & Nace, 2000).

The bulk of phytomedicinal research has been conducted in Germany, where the medical and social culture is more accepting of herbal medicine. In Germany, millions of prescriptions are written for herbal medicines each year. In the United States herbal medicines are classified as food supplements and are often available without a prescription. They receive minimal regulatory governing from the Food and Drug Administration. Herbal remedies sold in the United States require no proof of efficacy, safety, potency, or standardization and may vary considerably from brand to brand (Gurley et al, 2000; ISMP, 1998; Klepser & Klepser, 1999). For instance, 24% of a sampling of more than 2600 traditional Chinese medicines (herbs) at the Institute for Safe Medicine contained a therapeutic drug adulterant, and more than 50% contained two or more adulterants—including anti-inflammatory, analgesic, and diuretic agents (Huang et al, 1997). Moreover, some Americans mistakenly believe that a natural herb is necessarily a safe herb. On the contrary, some are potent drugs Barrett, 2004). In taking family history, nurses should ask whether any herbal substances are regularly used or were used during pregnancy. Knowing what, if any, herbal remedies nursing mothers use is essential, because the substances can be passed through breast milk to children.

Parents of neonates have been known to ask about aloe vera as a skin protectant or for its use with burns and skin irritations, as it has long been used as a folk remedy. Other creams made from comfrey, plantain, or marigold have been used for treatment of rashes and cradle cap. Calendula is used in Russia for conjunctivitis. Tree tea oil is an antifungal. Dandelion has diuretic properties, and chamomile is an antispasmodic, as are herbs such as valerian, fennel, aniseed, and cardamom. Peppermint stimulates bile flow and lowers loweresophageal spinetic pressure. Milk thistle increases enterohepatic circulation. Tripola increases intestinal peristalsis. Kava can be used to induce oral numbness, which would be helpful with endotracheal tube discomfort. St. John's wort is used for nervous unrest and, more commonly, to treat depression. Immune stimulants such as echinacea and astragalus and all of the herbs in this discussion will surely be studied more extensively in adults before their use is standardized for children and infants. Caffeine is the leading herb therapy in the United States and is used for apnea and bradycardia in infants. Marked expansion can come out of phytomedicines if we remain open-minded to the worldwide wisdom accrued through its extensive use.

RESEARCH

CAM is growing in its use in neonatal care. Unfortunately, for a variety of reasons, little research has been done to support its use. As health care professionals, we can either help gain the evidence to support these practices or watch them be incorporated in possibly unsystematic, unhealthy ways. Currently, many in the medical community condemn these therapies without even making a genuine scientific inquiry into their efficacy. We need to encourage our researchers to conduct the studies necessary to move these modalities safely into the mainstream.

Because of the lack of broad research in these areas, many aspects of how CAM therapies work are not yet fully understood from a Western perspective. Nevertheless, some exciting developments have occurred. Thus far, much of the research on CAM has focused on psychoneuroimmunologic (PNI) effects and has examined how various complementary therapies affect the stress response. For many years bench researchers have studied stress responses in animals and in

humans. We know that two pathways mediate the body's response to a stress. These are the sympathetic-adrenal-medullary (SAM) pathway and the hypothalamic-pituitary-adrenal (HPA) pathway. Each feeds information into the body to put it in "fight-or-flight" or "calm" mode. In the newborn a stressor such as a cool environment within the delivery room activates the stress response pathway. The body responds by releasing cortisol. This, in turn, activates the hypothalamus, which either sends signals down directly to the body via SAM or indirectly through the HPA axis. If SAM is followed, the sympathetic pathway is activated and stimulates the adrenal medulla and then the sympathetic postganglionic neurons. Finally, norepinephrine is released. If the HPA axis is stimulated, the anterior pituitary is stimulated; the adrenal cortex follows; and finally cortisol is released. Often these events are used as outcome measures in CAM research.

Other areas of research are evolving from multisensory interventions (White-Traut, 2004) to kinesthetic stimulation for preventing apnea (Henderson-Smart & Osborn, 2000). Multiple recent articles mention the use of probiotics in decreasing the incidence of necrotizing enterocolitis in very low birth weight infants. Examination of safety and efficacy through larger clinical trials will be needed (Kliegman & Willoughby, 2005).

Another area of CAM focus might be parents—for example, the development of "parent circles" that assist parents in gaining perspective on their situation is a complementary addition to the routines of an NICU (Pearson & Anderson, 2001). Additionally, complementary ideas could be used to meet the often-overlooked needs of siblings. A program that includes this support might be very useful and is worthy of further study (Ballard, 2004).

As research continues, CAM therapies may give us many new insights into the nature of the mind-body system and the overall complexities of health and healing. For instance, if no biochemical mechanisms exist in some CAM therapies, what are the mechanisms of action? If it is subtle energy, what can we do to measure it? Some scientists, for example, have begun to look at the heart rhythms and brain waves of energy healers to detect subtle changes in the overall patterning. In other cases, researchers are turning to double-blind studies to determine whether a CAM therapy is effective, even if the mechanism through which it works is not yet understood. CAM therapies have been traditionally viewed with suspicion by mainstream medicine. However, researchers and practitioners are looking increasingly at these therapies as new areas for scientific inquiry. Attaining reliable risk-benefit analysis and focusing on outcome research should be a long-term goal for practitioners interested in CAM therapies so that they may be used efficiently and without concern.

SUMMARY

CAM may offer important potential for the NICU: some evidence suggests that preterm neonates benefit from the soothing, calming properties of these therapies; these therapies may help the infants conserve energy and improve weight gain, and may augment bonding. CAM may also assist with consolation during painful procedures. It is exciting to observe the complexion of our profession changing so dramatically, from one so technically focused to the rebirth of a nurturant focus. The process can be inspiring as the search for a new sense of care is struggling to be born. The information given in this chapter is merely the tip of the iceberg. Further research to determine the benefits and risks of many of these therapies is needed. Complementary medicine may contribute to increased effectiveness of clinical practice for enhanced patient and family care.

REFERENCES

Alandydy P, Alandydy K (1999). Performance brief: using Reiki to support surgical patients. *Journal of nursing care and quality* 13(4):89-91.

Altimier L, Lutes L (2001). Co-bedding multiples. *Newborn and infant nursing reviews* 1(4):205-206.

Aly H et al (2004). Physical activity combined with massage improves bone mineralization in premature infants: a randomized trial. *Journal of perinatology* 24(5):305-309.

Anderson GC (1991). Current knowledge about skin-to-skin (kangaroo) care for preterm infants. *Journal of perinatology* 11(3):216-226.

Ballard KL (2004). Meeting the needs of siblings of children with cancer. *Pediatric nursing* 30(5):394-401.

Barrett B et al (1999). Assessing the risks and benefits of herbal medicine: an overview of scientific evidence. *Alternative therapies* 5(4):40-49.

Barrett S (2004). The herbal minefield. Available at: http://www.quackwatch.org/01QuackeryRelatedTopics/herbs.html. Retrieved July 19, 2006.

Burnett LB, Adler J (2006). Pediatrics, Sudden Infant Death Syndrome. *Emedicine*. Available at: http://www.emedicine.com/EMERG/topic407.htm. Retrieved July 19, 2006.

Boullata JL, Nace AM (2000). Safety issues with herbal medicine. *Pharmacolotherapy* 20:257-269.

Buckle J (2001). The role of aromatherapy in nursing care. *Nursing clinics of North America* 36(1):57-72.

Butt ML, Kisilevsky BS (2000). Music modulates behaviour of premature infants following heel lance. *Canadian journal of nursing research* 31(4):17-39.

Campbell D (1997). *The Mozart effect*. New York: Avon Press.

Carroll RT (2006). Rolfing. *The Skeptic's Dictionary*. Available at: http://skepdic.com/rolfing.html. Retrieved July 19, 2006.

Chou LL et al (2003). Effects of music therapy on oxygen saturation in premature infants receiving endotracheal suctioning. *Journal of nursing research* 11(3):209-216.

Eichel P (2001). Kangaroo care. *Newborn and infant nursing reviews* 1(4):224-228.

Engler A, Ludington SM (1999). Kangaroo care in the United States: a national survey. *Journal of investigative medicine* 47(2):168A.

Ernst E (1996). *Complementary medicine: an objective appraisal*. Oxford: Butterworth-Heinemann.

Feary AM (2002). Touching the fragile baby: looking at touch in the special care nursery (SCN). *Australian journal of medical herbalism* 9(1):44-48.

Fields TM (2000). *Touch therapy*. St Louis: Churchill Livingstone.

Freeman LW (2001a). Acupuncture. In Freeman LW, Lawlis GF, editors. *Mosby's complementary and alternative medicine: a research-based approach*. St Louis: Mosby.

Freeman LW (2001b). Herbs as medical intervention. In Freeman LW, Lawlis GF, editors. *Mosby's complementary and alternative medicine: a research-based approach*. St Louis: Mosby.

Frymann VM (1998). *The collected papers of Viola M. Frymann, DO: legacy of osteopathy to children*. Ann Arbor, MI: Edward Brothers.

Glover V et al (2002). Benefits of infant massage for mothers with postnatal depression. *Seminars in neonatology* 7(6):495-500.

Goubet N et al (2003). The olfactory experience mediates response to pain in preterm newborns. *Developmental psychobiology* 42:171-180.

Gurley BJ et al (2000). Content versus label claims in ephedra-containing dietary supplements. *American journal of health-systems pharmacy* 57:963-969.

Henderson-Smart DJ, Osborn DA (2000). Kinesthetic stimulation for preventing apnea in preterm infants. *Cochrane database of systematic reviews* 2:CD000373.

Huang WF et al (1997). Adulteration by synthetic therapeutic substances of traditional Chinese medicines in Taiwan. *Journal of clinical pharmacology* 37:344-350.

Institution for Safe Medication Practices (ISMP). (1998). An overview of herbal medicines and adverse events. *ISMP Medication Safety Alert! August 26, 1998*. Available at: http://www.ismp.org. Retrieved July 19, 2006.

Janssen PA et al (2005). Acupuncture for substance abuse treatment in the downtown eastside of Vancouver. *Journal of urban health* 82(2):285-295.

Jones J et al (2001). Complementary care alternatives for the NICU. *Newborn and infant nursing reviews* 1(4):207-210.

Jones J, Kassity N (2001). Varieties of Alternative Experience: Complementary Care in the Neonatal Intensive Care Unit. *Clinical obstetrics & gynecology* 44(4):750-768.

Klepser BT, Klepser ME (1999). Unsafe and potentially safe herbal therapies. *American journal of health-systems pharmacy* 56:125-138.

Kliegman RM, Willoughby RE (2005). Prevention of necrotizing enterocolitis with probiotics. *Pediatrics* 115(1):171-172.

Linde K et al (1997). Are the clinical effects of homeopathy placebo effects? Metaanalysis of placebo-controlled trials. *Lancet* 350(9081):834-843.

Ludington-Hoe SM (2004). Randomized controlled trial of kangaroo care: cardiorespiratory and thermal effects on healthy preterm infants. *Neonatal network* 23(3):39-48.

Marlier L et al (2005). Olfactory stimulation prevents apnea in premature newborns. *Pediatrics* 115(1):83-88.

Marwick C (2000). Music hath charms for care of preemies. *Journal of the American Medical Association* 283(4):468-469.

McDowell BM (2005). Nontraditional therapies for the PICU—part 1. *Journal for specialists in pediatric nursing* 10(1):29-32.

Nyqvist KH, Lutes LM (1998). Co-bedding twins: a developmentally supportive care strategy. *Journal of obstetric, gynecologic, and neonatal nursing* 27(4):450-456.

Pearson J, Anderson K (2001). Evaluation of a program to promote positive parenting in the neonatal intensive care unit. *Neonatal network* 20(4):43-48.

Polizzi J et al (2003). Co-bedding versus traditional bedding of multiple-gestation infants in the NICU. *Journal of healthcare quality* 25(1):5-10.

Standley JM (2001). Music therapy for the neonate. *Newborn and infant nursing reviews* 1(4):211-216.

Standley JM (2002). A meta-analysis of the efficacy of music therapy for premature infants. *Journal of pediatric nursing* 17(2):107-113.

Ullman D (1999). *Homeopathy A-Z*. Carlsbad, CA: Hay House.

White-Traut R (2004). Providing a nurturing environment for infants in adverse situations: multisensory strategies for newborn care. *Pediatric nursing* 30(5):394-401.

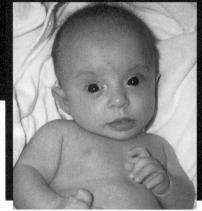

Chapter 29

Postdischarge Care of the Newborn and Infant

Carole Kenner • Susan Ellerbee

In the United States, according to the March of Dimes, 1 of every 8 babies born daily is premature (March of Dimes [MOD], 2005). Approximately 7.8% of all live births were low birth weight (<2500 g) in 2002 (MOD, 2005). Very-low-birth-weight infants—weighing less than 1000 g—comprised about 1.5% (MOD, 2005). Survival rates are at about 90% for very low birth weight and 95% for low birth weight infants thanks to improved technology and better prenatal care (MOD, 2005). Of all infant deaths (deaths in the first year of life), 16% were attributable to prematurity and low birth weight (MOD, 2005).

The multiple neonatal problems that bring an infant to a neonatal intensive care unit (NICU) have been described, in depth, throughout the preceding chapters. The one common factor when caring for these infants is the parent. Parents also require complex care during and following the infant's discharge. This is the focus of this chapter: parents and family.

We believe that parents are not visitors and that they are an integral part of their infant's care during the hospital stay. We also believe that many neonatal nurses are now caring for past NICU graduates through the first year of life; thus the transition to home has extended well beyond the immediate NICU stay. We also recognize that the transition to home may be even more difficult if the infant requires technology in the home. We have included evidence to support what the transition is like for these mothers.

THE NEONATAL INTENSIVE CARE UNIT EXPERIENCE

Try to remember the first time you walked into the NICU. What were your thoughts and feelings? We know what ours were—an overwhelming urge to flee. Time seemed to be running. People were rushing and talking loudly; alarms were buzzing, intercoms were blaring, and doors were slamming. We suddenly felt tense, on edge, and fearful of our ability to survive in such an environment. We were almost immobilized —yet we recognized some of the ventilators, intravenous pumps, and monitors. Surely, with this passing acquaintance, we could learn to work in this environment and actually care for the critically ill infant. Then we walked over to an incubator and peered in at a premature infant—born at 28 weeks' gestation and weighing less than 1000 g—who looked as though she had been through a war. Scratches and cuts were visible. Tape cut into the infant's face to hold an endotracheal tube in place. The right arm was pinned to the bed to hold an intravenous line in place, and her legs were restrained to prevent

dislodgment of an umbilical arterial line that was being used for blood gas sampling. Our hearts sank. We could never be responsible for providing care to this type of infant. We tried to summon the courage to walk—if not run—out of there.

If we, as beginning professionals, could not at first face the unit or the responsibility of care, what must parents feel? They have the additional fear of the death of a family member. For the most part, they lack the knowledge about the medical diagnosis, equipment, treatments, and routines necessary to support neonates. The mothers must, in addition, make a physiologic and psychologic postpartum adjustment. They are also in need of care, yet most express the need to put aside their own time for healing to focus on their infants. For the fathers, the need to run between two units (the postpartum and the NICU) is an added stress even if these units are in the same institution. The parents' concern for their partners and their children often forces them between the two. For the family with other children at home, the stress becomes even greater. Who can take charge of the children? How long will it be necessary for another person to help out with family responsibilities? Is someone who can or will step in to help even available? These are very real family concerns. Along with these concerns comes the assumption of the new parental role. This role adjustment occurs for both first-time and experienced parents. It requires a change from a previous functional pattern to a new one. This change marks a developmental passage or transition.

PARENTAL TRANSITION

Transition involves change—leaving behind the familiar and trying something new. Throughout life, events necessitate change. These life changes are often viewed as turning points. Taking on a new role requires energy, commitment, and most of all a change in the pattern of functioning—thus a transition. A new role requires an adjustment, a setting of new priorities, and an examination of new expectations. This transition can be negative or positive, depending on the perceptions of the person involved in the transition. The role of parent is a good example of the transition process. Once a pregnancy is confirmed, the mother and father begin the task of examining their individual roles. For first-time parents, this means considering what it will be like to be a mother or father to a dependent infant. For parents with other children, the new infant will bring a unique personality and another dimension to the already formed family unit. This infant, too, will require role adjustment on the part of the parents.

Acquisition of the maternal role and maternal identity, as described by Rubin (1984) and Mercer (1995), focused on mothers of healthy, term infants. When the infant is premature or sick and does not fit the image of the desired child, women lose their normal frame of reference for the development of their own role expectations and the expectations of their infants as well. The impact of this change has consequences that may extend beyond the immediate post–hospital discharge period. Some long-term consequences will be discussed, although most are beyond the scope of this chapter.

Attachment

The immediate process of attachment occurs with wanting of the pregnancy, positive maternal feelings, seeing the infant soon after birth, immediate contact with the infant after birth, and being unable to have other children. Delayed attachment occurs with a premature infant, uncertain outcomes, a handicapped child, poor maternal health, prolonged ventilation of the infant, a poor attitude in the partner, a lack of social support, drug dependency, and a taking-one-day-at-a-time attitude. Problematic attachment occurs in some mothers when the infant is born sick or premature. Attachment, which is usually considered dyadic, becomes a triadic relationship in the NICU, in which NICU personnel—especially nurses—can alter the process (Bialoskurski et al, 1999). Nurses can hinder or facilitate a mother's attachment to her infant by encouraging mother-infant touch or by forbidding it. The mother of a premature infant is also a premature mother. Not only are the binding-in and claiming processes affected but the mother herself is a "preemie" as well. Her pregnancy has ended before her own needs are fulfilled. Some or all of the social rituals that socialize mothers into their impending role and prepare them for their new responsibilities—such as baby showers, parenting classes, and birth announcements—may have been forgotten with the birth of a premature or ill infant. Friends and family who would normally be happy to help celebrate the joyous occasion of birth with the exuberant parents may feel uncomfortable and helpless around them. Their support may not be offered, thus leaving the parents more alone and isolated. Thus the transition to a new role becomes more difficult.

For parents of a NICU infant, the transition may have two phases—one associated with becoming parents at the time of birth and the other occurring at the time of discharge. The first phase—becoming parents at the time of the infant's birth—has been discussed in a previous chapter. The second transition is explored in this chapter.

Although the time of NICU discharge is the overriding goal for the health care professional and the family, the actual transition to home can be a time of crisis for the family. The actual assumption of the new parental role can be quite overwhelming. Some researchers and clinicians view this transition as a crisis rather than just a developmental passage to a new functional level.

Transition as a Crisis

The idea that a crisis is a state of disequilibrium is based on the postulate that humans strive for homeostasis by constantly using coping mechanisms to maintain equilibrium. When a situation that upsets the equilibrium arises, a person employs the usual coping mechanisms to solve the problem. When the usual coping methods do not return the person to a state of equilibrium, a crisis evolves. The outcome of a crisis depends on whether resources are available to support the individuals undergoing the crisis. Even when a healthy newborn is brought into a family, a crisis can ensue. For premature or sick infants, however, the meaning to the family usually is viewed as a crisis. A crisis usually lasts 4 to 6 weeks, and crisis intervention is most effective when used during this period. When intervention is applied as close to the time of the crisis as possible, it becomes even more effective. The aim of crisis intervention is not to restructure a person's personality but to help the person deal with the present problem and to rely on history only as it pertains to the present situation. Many things can initiate a crisis in a family. Families see bringing a premature or ill infant who has been in the NICU as a crisis. Contemplating taking home a medically fragile infant or one that is technology-dependent may create a crisis situation for a parent (Scholtes et al, 1994; Jackson et al, 2003).

For neonatal nurses, knowing when a family is in crisis and the causes of the crisis is very important. When an impending or a true crisis is recognized, neonatal nurses can implement interventions that will help prevent or alleviate it. Anticipatory planning for future crises involves reviewing with the family their coping strategies and how they handled the crisis. Coping, then, is the process by which an individual regulates stress. An outcome of coping is usually either control over the stress or being taken over by the stress, as in learned helplessness.

For many parents, the NICU reinforces learned helplessness. Parents express the need to understand their role and what is expected of them in relationship to their infants' care needs; yet they feel "in the way" and unable or incapable of caring for their infants. Thus they learn to be helpless. The picture changes, however, at the time of discharge. The parents are told: "Now it is your turn." It is no wonder that this discharge can be cognitively appraised as being a stress. Nor is it unusual that parents feel helpless and hopeless when it comes to accepting total responsibility for their infants.

When given the opportunity to discuss their concerns, parents are very vocal about their feelings regarding their NICU care and preparation for discharge. Another way to meet the needs of those who are problem-focused copers is to present them with transition programs such as case management or home care (American Academy of Pediatrics, 2004; Hummel & Cronin, 2004; Johnson et al, 2005).

Parental Concerns

Kenner (1988) and Bagwell and associates (1990) found that parents from level II and III units had similar concerns. Their concerns fell into five categories: (1) informational needs; (2) grief; (3) parent-child development; (4) stress and coping; and (5) social support.

Informational Needs

The informational needs of parents include how to provide routine newborn care; how to recognize normal newborn characteristics, both physical and behavioral; how to keep the infant healthy after discharge; their own responsibilities about how to provide care; the equipment used on their infant while in the NICU; and a complete explanation of the medical diagnosis and the expected prognosis (McKim, 1993a).

Parents want to feel that they are important enough to know what is really wrong with their infant (Kenner, 1988; Kenner et al, 1996). One family stated, "The only time that the physicians really asked us our opinion or told us about the baby's condition was when they were obligated to get informed consent for an experimental treatment." Another family said, "We would ask the nurses about the baby's apnea, but they said they had to check with the physicians and they would have to talk to us." Other comments included, "I never understood why nurses just came over and turned off our baby's sounding alarms without seemingly looking at the baby"; "No one told me how difficult it would be to breastfeed a preemie"; "I did not realize how different from my other children the sleep cycle would be for my preemie." These are just a few examples of information that the parents wanted. Parents felt better about their role and the information about their infant's care if they were considered part of the care team.

Grief

The category of grief was first called anticipatory grief (Kenner, 1988)—the rationale being that parents expressed the loss of their expected child once the reality of the neonatal problem shattered their hopes and fantasies. However, as time went on, parents continued to grieve but in the form of anticipating that the infant would eventually die if he or she were sick enough to require special or NICU care. They continued to anticipate this death or at least that the infant would get sick again and require hospitalization after discharge. Their perceptions suggest that the concept seems more appropriately considered grief than anticipatory grief. The process of grief and the period of mourning begin once the infant does not meet the parents' expectations of the fantasy or ideal child. If the parents have other children, they speak of how different this child is from their others or how different the infant is from their expectations. Although the parents anticipate further problems, it is probably not anticipatory grief but rather a continuation of the grief process. Another component of grief seems to be for the loss of the expected parenting role—that is, their normal, familiar role. This feeling may not be different from that of parents of normal, healthy infants, because the homecoming of those infants also requires a role adjustment. This assumption is an area still in need of further research.

Parent-Child Development

This category refers to the parents' and children's role expectations. For anyone making a transition or entering a new level of functioning or a new stage of life, certain expectations about what is to come exist. New parents of healthy infants make adjustments in how they carry out the tasks of daily living once their newborn is at home. Each time a new member is introduced into the family, adjustments are made. When a problem with the infant that requires special care arises, parents may have to set aside their ideal expectations of their roles. The hospitalization may reinforce their roles or may hinder them.

Parents learn a lot about parenting by observing health care professionals. They learn what is valued. When a mother calls the unit for a progress report, she is usually told the infant's weight, amount of feedings, stooling patterns, percentage of oxygen, and how many times apnea occurred. It is not surprising that during home follow-up, parents, particularly mothers, want more information about feeding, formula, breastfeeding, elimination patterns (especially constipation), fear of the infant's losing weight (many say they have been told that if the infant loses weight, rehospitalization may be necessary), and whether the infant's breathing pattern seems normal. Nurses also may

communicate to parents that the parents are not capable of caring for their infants. One family said, "I read all the literature about bonding and knew it was important to hold the baby, but we were not allowed"; "One nurse would say 'maybe in a couple of hours, maybe 4,' but that time would never come"; and "We were in the unit for 3 days before we held the baby, and he was the least sick of any of the infants in the nursery." This family was from a level II unit, and the infant was experiencing some periods of apnea. Thermoregulation was not a concern in this case. The parents felt that they were not needed, not important, and certainly not capable of parenting their infant. These feelings only add to the stress of having a sick infant (Kenner et al, 1996).

Parental responses to their preterm infant vary. The vulnerable child syndrome is one such response. Green and Solnit (1964) hypothesized that, when children are expected to die prematurely, the result is disturbed psychosocial development based on the parent-child relationship. Because the child is seen as "vulnerable," parents make more visits to health care providers for relatively minor illnesses and may discipline the child in a gentler manner. Although some studies (Scheiner et al, 1985; Culley et al, 1989) did not support this premise, more recent studies do. Allen and associates (2004) found a negative association between maternal perception of child vulnerability and adaptive functioning in preterm infants with chronic lung disease at 1-year adjusted age. The mothers who perceived their children as more vulnerable were more anxious, more depressed, and perceived a greater impact of the illness on the family. Greater perceived vulnerability was associated with longer hospitalization, but not gestational age, birth weight, or length of mechanical ventilation. The authors acknowledged that the population of infants with chronic lung disease may limit generalization of the results. Rautava and colleagues (2003) followed 170 Finnish preterm infants and their families for 12 years. At 3 years of age, children in a high-risk group, according to their medical risk at hospital discharge, were reported as having more sleep and behavioral problems than children in a low-risk group. However, all of these differences disappeared by the time the children were 12 years old. The importance of the vulnerable child syndrome for current practice was further explicated in a 1998 commentary (Shonkoff, 1998). With infants being discharged at lower weights, at earlier postconceptional ages, and with more care needs, this concept needs to be considered by those providing posthospital care. The encouraging news is that perception of increased vulnerability tends to disappear as the infant's health status improves.

Stress and Coping

For many families, no warning is available that a problem is pending with the infant's birth or that the infant will be sick. Therefore they are unprepared, and the reality of a sick neonate comes suddenly. The expected feelings of joy and the months of anticipation are replaced by sharply contrasting feelings of fear, shock, and overwhelming sadness. The family experiences disbelief that there could be a problem. Even when a premature or complicated birth is expected or a neonatal problem is diagnosed in utero, many parents still do not believe that a problem will occur. They are usually angry that their infant is sick. Demystification is the understanding of the medical condition—that is, having the informational needs about the prognosis and plan of treatment met. The conditional acceptance is integration of the infant's problem into the family. Even if this is a time-limited condition, the illness must be incorporated into the family's attitude about the unit and the demands that are facing them.

Adaptation coping is necessary for reaching a stage of conditional acceptance. This form of coping comes about through the identification of the family's stresses from their own perspective. It also requires a determination of the resources that are available to the family. These resources might be parent support groups, parent hotlines, extended family members, friends, financial resources, or home care. Adaptation also requires a change of attitude. Information and acknowledgment of feelings before and after discharge both help to ease the transition process to home and into the role of parent. Acknowledging that other parents have been scared about assuming responsibility for their infants' care and introducing them to successful parents decreases stress and increases coping.

Peeples-Kleiger (2000) studied the hospitalization in the neonatal intensive care as a traumatic stressor on parents and their adaptation. She used the definition of *traumatic stressor* that is given in the American Psychiatric Association's *Diagnostic and Statistical Manual of Mental Disorders* (1994): "actual or threatened death or serious injury, or a threat to the physical integrity of self or others." She drew the following conclusions:

- Families who acknowledge the severity of the problem and talk about it cope better than those who do not.
- Parents must learn to manage their feelings in order to adapt.
- Parents must learn that traumatic events will lead to involuntary memories for weeks, months, and years to come.
- Parents must learn that trauma-related symptoms such as lack of sleep and edginess can occur at any point, even after the crisis.
- Parents will feel helpless and may have unchanneled aggression related to the helplessness.
- Parents will need to learn to rebuild their lives and resolve their grief.

Continued stress, feelings of failure, and grieving for the loss of the fantasy child all have the potential for leading to maternal and paternal depression. Parental anxiety and the presence or absence of depressive symptoms should be assessed at regular intervals and be part of routine follow-up care (American Academy of Pediatrics, 2004; Melynk et al, 2002).

Social Support

Parents expressed the feeling that social support had both positive and negative facets. They meant that they saw the NICU nurses as having a lot of power and the potential to explain their infants' progress. They also believed that nurses had the potential to explain why medical treatment plans changed when house staff changes took place in teaching institutions. Nonetheless, parents did not feel that, for the most part, nurses fulfilled their role as advocates. The NICU nurses did not anticipate that the parents might be confused, and the parents readily admitted that they were too confused or intimidated by the health care professionals to ask questions. They assumed that the nurses knew how they felt. They also thought that the nurses were working too many shifts in a row or too many long hours to be bothered with their seemingly trivial concerns. Some parents went so far as to describe the

nurse's role as providing expert infant care but not parent care. Other parents expressed frustration over having to reorient nurses to their infant's condition. They often did not see the same nurse twice, even during a prolonged stay. Although the parents saw the potential for support, they did not feel that the support was always given. Primary nurses for continuity and mother-baby nurses for the level II parents were viewed as helpful for support.

The physician's role was viewed as being for infant care and not for the support of the family. For most families, the physician was the gatekeeper regarding what they were allowed to know about their infant. Physicians even regulated communication to parents via the nursing staff. Even after discharge, parents believed that the physician's permission was necessary to make even the smallest change in the infants' routines that had been established in the hospital. These feelings might be tied to the parents' need for structure and their attempt to continue the safety of the NICU at home. Parents also viewed nurses as gatekeepers of information. The nurses would let parents know when it was not appropriate, for instance, to hold the infant, but only occasionally did they say when parents could hold the infant. Once again, parents did not always see support for their parenting role as readily given. Unfortunately, a side effect of this perception is the parents' sense of a lack of trust that they can provide care or a feeling that the truth about their infants' conditions is being withheld from them.

The positive side of support was also expressed: the caring attitude by some professionals, the friendly hug, and the taking time to talk with the parents, even if it was about something other than their infant's problems. Acknowledgments of the mother's own physical discomfort conveyed a caring and supportive attitude. The availability of a phone number and the potential for a home visit were viewed as positive. Positive social support affects parents' views of their children's care. Van Riper (2001) studied parental well-being in relationship to the family-provider relationship. She found that parents who had positive relationships with the child's caregiver in the NICU and viewed the care as family-centered had more satisfaction with the care. For many parents, the home visit provides a way to vent feelings that otherwise must often be suppressed around family and friends (McKim, 1989, 1993b).

Parents also believed that many times family and friends withdrew their support. For other parents, family and friends were afraid to approach the parents for fear of doing the wrong thing. Still other times, parents felt that their family and friends wanted to tell them what they were doing wrong and how they should parent their infants. For instance, the advice several mothers got included statements such as "Don't breastfeed your preemie; he will get sick. Don't allow visitors; they will only make the baby sick." Positive reaction from family and friends included comments about how well the parents were doing with their infants, how well they were coping, and how normal their feelings of inadequacy are. Social support differs, however, by whether it is professional or personal.

Social support is an important aspect of coping and managing stress. If support is not provided, family functioning and health may suffer. Once social support needs are identified, a plan of action must be implemented. Because there are both positive and negative aspects of social support, it is probably more correct to term this category as social interaction. There is an interaction between at least two people, and whether it is positive or negative, support is determined by the recipient (McKim et al, 1995).

The five categories of parental concerns just discussed may represent a taxonomy for transitional care follow-up. These categories form the basis for transition to home.

INTERVENTION STRATEGIES

Many interventions can alleviate a crisis situation for a family of a premature infant at discharge. The NICU nurse—in the role of primary nurse, clinical nurse specialist, or neonatal nurse practitioner—can advocate for positive parental discharge. Recognizing parents' need for information about their infants and the required at-home care facilitates development of a collaborative, interdisciplinary plan of care, including discharge and follow-up. This type of collaborative plan should include the parents' demonstrating competence and comfort with routine newborn care. Mothers, in particular, need support and reassurance, even after discharge (Bagwell et al, 1990; Kenner, 1988; Scholtes et al, 1994). Swartz (2005) found that five themes emerged when looking at parenting of premature infants studies. These five themes were "adapting to risk, protecting fragility, preserving the family, compensating for the past, and cautiously affirming the future." The nurse therefore needs to make sure the family is included in the "team." These interventions also need to be culturally sensitive (McEvoy et al, 2005; Melynk et al, 2002). The nurse needs to ensure that the parents are completely comfortable with bathing, feeding, and diapering their infant and with administering any special care procedures, such as medication or oxygen therapy. The parents also need to be taught how the NICU infant's temperament differs from that of a normal newborn. Good discharge teaching includes all this as well as developmental information (American Academy of Pediatrics, 2004; Melynk et al, 2002).

Parents also need continuity of care. Many parents express the frustration of trying to build a rapport with medical staff, who change monthly, and with nurses, who change daily. This situation will not necessarily improve, as more nurses work part-time flexible hours or work from agencies that float them between several intensive care units.

Parents also need to be informed and reminded that even though their infant is 6 months old by chronologic age, she or he may be only 3 months old by conceptional age. Thus the infant may act more like a 3-month-old than like a 6-month-old. Tips on helping the infant adapt to home should also be included in the discharge information. Parents of former premature infants have offered such advice as leaving radios and lights on to help the infant adapt to the new environment. This need for increased stimuli may change as NICU infants begin to recognize a developmentally supportive environment (Cicco et al, 1996). Nursing research is needed in this area to determine whether NICU infants require more lights or noise at home.

Parents often report that they feel supported and reassured if a professional in addition to family or friends advise them. Neonatal nurse practitioners (NNPs) are often responsible for follow-up care. Follow-up nurses recognize that failure to use available community resources or follow professional advice may be related to coping difficulties. If this is true, avoidance of these failures may stop the cycle of stress and coping difficulties. Scheduling home visits at frequent intervals is a good strategy for assessing the family's progress.

Parental concerns often center on feeding issues. In the hospital, infants are usually fed on a rigid, every-3-hour schedule with a specified minimum intake at each feeding. The evidence base for this practice, rather than cue-based, or demand feedings, is being challenged. Crosson and Pickler (2004), in an integrative review of the literature on the topic, suggest that demand feedings may be appropriate for most healthy preterm infants. Even with methodologic flaws and inconsistent approaches, studies consistently reported improved behavior state organization, shorter hospital stays, and better weight gain among infants who were demand-fed.

Information given to parents about feeding patterns of preterm infants should include differences and similarities between term and preterm infants. Preterm infants often have shorter periods of sustained sucking, whether receiving feedings from the breast or bottle. Signs of adequate intake are similar for both groups: exhibiting feeding cues on a regular basis, 7 to 10 feeds per 24 hours, and 5 to 6 wet diapers and 2 to 3 stools per 24 hours. Daily weights, routinely done in the hospital, are not practical for home care of most infants, although scales are available if needed. For breastfed infants, the value of weighing before and after feedings to determine actual intake is controversial (Hurst et al, 2004; Hall et al, 2002). For infants being fed artificial baby milk (ABM) (aka, formula), an expected amount of milk to be consumed in a 24-hour period is more realistic than a specific amount per feeding.

Transition to direct breastfeeding should begin as soon as the infant is able to feed orally. Direct breastfeeding for 24 to 48 hours prior to discharge is optimal. If available, an international board-certified lactation consultant (IBCLC) assists the mother as this transition is made. Some preterm infants will require continued supplementation with expressed breast milk (EBM) or ABM for several days or weeks postdischarge. Supplementation can be provided via bottle, cup, or gavage. Mothers should also be instructed to continue pumping four to five times per day to maintain milk supply. This is often needed because the now near-term infant may not yet be able to suckle well enough to stimulate the production of prolactin. Maintaining an adequate milk supply is essential to successfully make the transition to primarily breastfeeding (Wooldridge & Hall, 2003). Continued support of the breastfeeding mother is essential to decrease the risk of early weaning. More longitudinal studies in this area are needed (Callen & Pinelli, 2005).

Regardless of the chosen feeding method, maternal fatigue is often a major issue when the infant comes home. Balancing infant care with other demands is difficult, at best. A cue-based feeding schedule is more likely to help in this area as well as other family issues.

Family Care

The concept of the family as a unit is another point addressed in care-by-parents or transition units (Costello & Chapman, 1998). The father and siblings are often forgotten during discharge preparation. Most fathers want to participate in care and decision making for a healthy or sick/premature newborn (Bolzan et al, 2004). The responses of fathers are sometimes different from those of mothers (Rautava et al, 2003; Allen et al, 2004).

Siblings must also adjust to the infant, who may not seem real to them until they are able to visit the infant in the NICU.

Many units now encourage sibling visits to help ease the infant into the family well before the actual discharge.

Communication

Communication is a key element to successful relationships. It is a new focus for medical care. Nurses are expert communicators. The art of nursing has revolved around the ability to convey care and personal attention to the client. Unfortunately, because of today's health care crisis, nursing shortages have resulted in staff mixes and use of unskilled personnel, coupled with economic constraints resulting in shortened hospital stays; nurses are also falling into the trap of assembly-line health care delivery. However, nurses have the advantage of being able to identify and assess a family's needs and to convey these needs to other health care team members. Being an advocate for the family is an essential part of preparing a family for discharge. Follow-up, in essence, is allowing an open line of communication among health care professionals, the health care delivery system, and the family. It allows a partnership to develop between the health care team and the family. It gives the family back some control. Follow-up moves the family away from the learned helplessness acquired in the hospital to a more participative role. Nurses are often sought out by families who want to vent feelings and concerns—as long as the family feels that the nurses care enough to be concerned. Parents need to be able to openly express their concerns about their infant's appearance and about their feelings of helplessness without fear of being judged as bad parents. Nonverbal cues can get in the way of communication. The nurse's expertise, knowledge, and use of medical terminology without explanations all convey the nurse's need to be in control. Someone has to be in control, but relinquishing some control to the family does not lessen one's credibility as a professional. It conveys to the family that they have a role in their infant's care and that they are important, too.

Another facet to this communication system is the other health care team members. Nurses cannot afford to withhold information that might help the physicians, social workers, and financial counselors who work with the family. Nurses need to convey information and coordinate the assessment data. Application of the nursing process may sound trite, but it is important in terms of not only collecting data but also using the data to identify problems, make nursing diagnoses, and develop a plan of care before and after discharge.

Long-Term Implications for the Family Unit

The breakdown of communication or of family functioning can lead to a less than optimal environment for the infant and child to grow. Studies have documented that the infant of very low birth weight, in particular, is at risk for child abuse, neglect, nonorganic failure to thrive, and developmental and behavioral problems, and that the caregivers of these infants experienced more daily stress than did the average caregiver.

Collaboration among pediatric medical follow-up, parent support or psychosocial assessments at home, and obstetrical follow-up for the mother is essential. Each health care professional has something to contribute to the family's overall well-being. It is essential not to compete but to work with other professionals for the good of the family. This means that turf issues must be settled behind the scenes. It also means that each profession must share information that it receives from the family. It is not unusual during a home visit for the family

to say, "I did not tell the OB [or pediatrician] about my concern over changing from cloth diapers to disposables because I did not want to bother him about that. Yet I am afraid to make even the smallest change in my baby's routine set up by the hospital." These statements demonstrate the need for a discharge protocol for the family.

Miles and Holditch-Davis (1995) and Wereszczak and associates (1997) found in retrospective research studies that the NICU stay has long-lasting effects on mothers of premature infants. When the children are 3 years old, these mothers experience what these researchers term compensatory parenting. This parenting style is overcompensation for feeling sorry for or guilty about having an infant in the NICU. They reported trying to provide special experiences and more stimulation to foster development with these children. At the same time they have shielded their children from other life situations to protect them from further hurt (Miles & Holditch-Davis, 1995).

Quality-of-life issues, which extend beyond the immediate postdischarge period, also need to be addressed (Theunissen et al, 2001; Klassen et al, 2004). NICU graduates have been reported to have behavioral and developmental problems up to the age of 4 (Klassen et al, 2004), although one study (Benzies et al, 1998) found no differences between preterm and term children. Donohue (2002) suggests that quality-of-life measures should be included when assessing the preterm child's health and well-being.

To determine specialized needs, systematic assessments should be done to determine the infant's developmental progress as well as the home environment of the family. Such tools include the Nursing Child Assessment Satellite Training Scales (NCAST; University of Washington, Seattle, WA) developed by Dr. Kathryn Barnard. These are measures that examine sleep-wake organization, feeding, parent-infant interaction, and the home environment. Parts to this assessment include sleep-activity record, Feeding Scale, and Teaching Scale. The Home Observation for Measurement of the Environment (HOME) scale was developed by Dr. Betty Caldwell and colleagues to measure the impact of the home on the infant's development. Out of the NCAST work grew a program called Nursing Systems Toward Effective Parenting—Preterm (NSTEP-P) (University of Washington, Seattle, WA). This program contains protocols for care and teaching guides for the nurses for their home visits and their parent teaching (Johnson-Crowley & Sumner, 1987a,1987b).

Technology-Dependent Infants

In recent years the number of technology-dependent infants discharged home has increased, because of the many early discharge programs available and the survival of extremely-low-birth-weight infants with chronic conditions. Although a fair amount has been written about setting up early discharge programs and the positive financial rewards associated with early discharge, little research is available to look at the effects of having a technology-dependent infant at home.

Spangler-Torok applied the concepts of transition to this unique population. Spangler-Torok (2001) studied mothers receiving and caring for their technology-dependent infants in the home. The experiential descriptions were from eight mothers, aged 17 to 42, who were the primary caretakers of their technology-dependent infants. All of the mothers were interviewed within the first 4 weeks of receiving their infant into the home. Although this was a phenomenologic study, it provides support for the concepts of the Kenner Transition Model.

Information Needs

Mothers in this study understood the need to learn about care and equipment so that the infant could be discharged. Mothers described moving from learning care to making judgments regarding the infant's health. Gathering information is a way of seeking control of the situation. The mothers in this study sought information to make an overwhelming experience more manageable. The mothers described initial fear of caring for the infant at home and their ability to move beyond the fear and do what needed to be done. As more information was gathered, mothers described using their judgment with infant health decisions. When receiving and caring for a technology-dependent infant in the home, more information seems to give mothers more control, confidence, and peace of mind.

Grief

The mothers in this study feared the infant becoming ill and requiring rehospitalization. Several of the mothers voiced concern that the infant might die. Mothers grieved over the loss of the "ideal" pregnancy and infant. Mothers would report that they were managing the home care experience, "but this is not what I planned for." Mothers grieved about the life their infants would have and vowed to give them "as normal a life as possible." Mothers worried about what others would think: "Will they think it was something I did while I was pregnant that caused this to happen to the baby?" Mothers felt the need to "warn" others that the baby was different before they approached the infant.

Parent-Child Role Development

Once they were at home, mothers in this study believed that they were getting to know their infants and that their infants were getting to know them as their mothers. Mothers reported learning things about their infants that they didn't know until they were home, such as when their fussy times were. Mothers believed that as they learned more about infant preferences and health-related behaviors, they were able to make appropriate adjustments to infant care.

Regardless of whether they had other children, the mothers saw a need to adjust the parenting role and expectation to accommodate the premature infant. They realized that this infant was different and required special care—in some instances, more vigilant care. They discussed how the increased needs of this infant took time away from other children and spouses, but acknowledged that being home was easier than extended hospital visits. Most of the mothers in this study quit their jobs or school to care for the infant, which they would not have planned to do if the infant had been healthy. The mothers discussed lifestyle changes since the infant came home from the hospital such as decreased number of outings, staying indoors more, and limiting visitors to the home.

Stress and Coping

Mothers in this study acknowledged that receiving and caring for a technology-dependent infant in the home is a lot of work. One mother stated it is "a ton of work . . . 10 times more work than a normal infant." Mothers report that more time is needed with infant care as well as with supplemental tasks such as dealing with insurance companies, managing supplies, and checking equipment. A lot of time is required to prepare the infant for outings, and time is needed for the infant to readjust to home after outings. Mothers reported problems with infant digestion and temperament when away from home. "She may require 2 or 3 days to recover from an outing to the doctor's office." All of the mothers described the extra work and time the infant required, but most felt it was worth it to have infant home with them. This initial anxiety decreases as the infant's respiratory status improves and the infant becomes less dependent on oxygen therapy (Zanardo & Freato, 2001).

Two mothers described being overwhelmed with infant care in the home and felt they faced too many demands. One mother felt torn between caring for the infant and spending time with her other children. She is "only one person" and can "only be in one place at a time." She appreciates the break the home nurses provide but feels guilty that her infant receives care from others. Another mother describes frustration in dealing with the equipment. She has a "hard time looking" at the feeding tube but is less bothered by the tracheotomy. She gets angry when her husband gravitates towards Holly, the "normal" twin, and leaves all the work for Grace to her. This mother is afraid that her infant will pick up on her frustration with the equipment and feel that she doesn't love her.

Social Interaction

Several mothers in this study attributed their ability to care for this infant at home to the support of family and friends. Mothers stated they could focus on infant care because others were handling household chores and running errands for them. One mother described how strangers who heard of their situation were delivering food to them. The same mother felt that their experience was probably easier than others because "so many people have pitched in to do things." In describing her experience, one mother stated, "We just needed a lot of family." Having people come and help seems to make the experience more manageable for some of the mothers.

One mother described being supported by the home care nurses. "It's wonderful to have the nursing staff here, because when you want to break down and cry, they're there to tell you, rub your hand, or your shoulder and say, 'you're doing a good job, don't think that you're not; you are.'" She is thankful for them and uses the nurses for other things so that she can spend time with the infant.

Although some mothers spoke of the assistance they received, others described the lack of support from family and friends. A mother spoke of being "annoyed" with her husband. She discussed how supportive they were of each other during their infant's hospitalization and that she had assumed that would continue once they were home. She was disappointed by her husband's lack of support and assistance with infant care and home management. "Hey, we have special circumstances here, this isn't just your average baby and you need to help me," she said. Another mother describes a lack of support from husband, children, and friends. She says her husband helps with the cooking, but it takes her three times as long to clean up. Although her 12-year-old daughter is old enough to help, she doesn't. She also wonders why friends have not come to see her. She believes they are afraid to see the baby and therefore do not visit. She sometimes feels alone in her responsibility for the baby.

The experiences of mothers receiving and caring for their technology-dependent infants in the home support the Kenner

Transition Model (1998). Mothers saw the need for information before the infant was discharged and after the infant was home. Mothers grieved for the child they had envisioned during pregnancy and worried what others would think about their infant's special needs. Once they were home, mothers felt they learned more about their infant's likes and dislikes. They also saw the need for an adjustment in roles and responsibilities. Mothers reported increased work and worries when caring for the infant in the home. Two mothers expressed feelings of being overwhelmed. Many mothers reported that the support and assistance of others made the experience more manageable. Two mothers reported lack of support and problems coping with the increased demands. Other studies report similar findings (Zanardo & Freato, 2001; McLean et al, 2000).

HOME CARE

With the shift from acute-care hospitals to providing home care for infants, even technology-dependent infants, the transition to home can be even more traumatic than expected. Some families are expected to set up a "mini" intensive care in the home, even providing ventilators or intravenous medications. There are several types of home care.

Types of Home Care

Home care, for most practical purposes, is classified as short-term, long-term, or hospice care. Other programs involve respite care, day care, and foster care.

Short-Term Care

Short-term care is considered by many health care services to be less than 6 months in duration. Short-term care of an infant at home may include phototherapy for hyperbilirubinemia (Madlon-Kay, 2001), administration of supplemental oxygen to treat respiratory distress, home monitoring for apnea of the premature infant, medication administration for various neonatal conditions, and alternative feeding methods such as gavage for nutritional support (Collins et al, 2005). The primary caregivers in the home usually attend to these treatment modalities. Parents and families are carefully instructed in the use of any equipment placed in the home to administer health care. Extensive teaching before hospital discharge must convey the precise reasons for the therapy, the necessity for close observation of the infant by the caregivers, and the importance of communication and supervision by the primary care physician. In situations of short-term home care, the condition is usually self-limiting, and the home therapy can be discontinued at a predetermined end point.

Long-Term Care

The point at which care becomes long-term is determined by the nature of the health care needs of the individual. The providers of extended care and the insurers paying for the care also arbitrarily set the time frame for long-term care. In general, long-term care indicates that the duration of the condition and the need for care will exceed 6 months. Long-term home care addresses situations for children with disease processes such as bronchopulmonary dysplasia (BPD), short-bowel or short-gut syndrome, congenital heart disease, physical and cosmetic defects, neurologic and metabolic disorders, and numerous other prolonged pathologic conditions.

On discharge, these children may require home care services performed by professional home care agencies or pro-

grams. Families gradually become integrated into the health care routine. The family's responsibility changes as the infant's condition changes. The primary care physician must be closely involved and should be able to rely comfortably on the caregiver's judgment for making assessments and alterations in the home care plan. Long-term home care requires open communication among the family, community physicians, tertiary resources, community health care providers, home medical equipment providers, and financial providers. Many hospital records are now incorporating discharge notes, especially nursing case management notes or orders for the actual discharge and home care follow-up plan. These notes are a good vehicle for communication among the community health care providers and the discharging hospital.

Hospice Care

Congenital anomalies are the leading cause of infant mortality in the United States and are also a major contributor to childhood morbidity, long-term disability, and loss of years of potential life. The proportion of infant deaths attributed to birth defects has remained significantly high. Our human immunodeficiency virus (HIV) epidemic is improving but still takes it toll on the neonatal population. Those infants require specialized home care and in some instances palliative care. In addition, with technologic advances the ability to prolong lives has increased. Infants who are born dying do go home, where they need end-of-life (EOL) or palliative care. When it becomes clear that an infant will no longer benefit from acute intervention, plans for health care should focus on physical and emotional comfort. The transition from acute care to palliative care involves the concept of hospice.

Hospice care is a philosophy of caring when cure is no longer a reasonable expectation. This care is not strictly a kind of terminal care, but rather an effort to maximize current quality of life without giving up all interest in a cure. Hospice provides comfort measures and emphasizes alleviation of symptoms. Whether the infant is terminally or chronically ill, the ultimate goal is to provide an environment that comforts the child and supports the family.

Criteria for Home Care

Some hospitals throughout the country are developing specialized outreach and home care services as an extension of their inpatient services. Regardless of how services are to be provided, the decision to facilitate early discharge from hospital care to home care must be based on standards that are safe and that provide effective ongoing therapy. The infant, the family, the home equipment, and the follow-up health care system must meet criteria for discharge to home care.

Infant Criteria

The infant's home health care needs must be assessed as to technical feasibility and medical requirements. Nutritional support must be evaluated. How does the infant feed and how frequently? How often does the infant require gavage feedings, and which feeding techniques are required? Pharmacologic support assessment must be evaluated. What medication does the infant need and how often? What are the desired and adverse effects of these drugs? Does the infant require supplemental oxygen, respiratory therapy treatments, or chest physical therapy? The assessment of the level of care required must be matched to the ability and skills of the home care providers. It must be determined before discharge that care in the home will be safe and meet the needs of the infant and family.

The specific criteria for discharge of special groups of children—such as those with BPD, short-bowel or short-gut syndrome, neurologic disease, cardiac disease, and other pathologic conditions—are addressed in the preceding chapters.

Family Criteria

The assessment of the family's commitment to home care is perhaps the most critical factor determining the success or failure of home health care. After extensive discharge teaching, skills development, and repeated occasions of caregiving, the family must want the child at home and under their care. They must be willing and able to devote the time and energy required to meet the physical and emotional needs of the child. These factors are essential for the well-being of the family unit.

To prepare families for the discharge of their sick or high-risk infant, NICU personnel must begin teaching them as soon as the neonate is admitted to the unit. Once the family is confident and capable of meeting the needs of the infant, a home assessment should be completed. Basic facilities such as heat, water, telephone, electricity, and transportation must be available. Appropriate support systems must be set up in the home, including the technology necessary for the delivery of care. The operation of phototherapy lights or blankets, oxygen delivery systems, portable suction equipment, respiratory and cardiac monitoring systems, ventilators, and numerous other devices must be thoroughly understood by the caregivers. Clear instructions need to be given to the family members by the providers of the home care technology. Ideally, the parents should bring the equipment to the hospital, or the equipment company can help transport it to the hospital before discharge. The rationale is that the parents can be taught on their own equipment. If a problem arises, it can usually be identified before the infant's discharge. The parents should spend at least 24 hours providing total care before discharge. This time under health professional's supervision helps the family gain confidence in their caregiving abilities. They can also be reassured that they have the proper equipment.

Home Equipment Criteria

The most common equipment needs for neonates are cardiopulmonary monitoring, oxygen, suction, and feeding implements. The family's first decision is how to select a home care equipment company. Most hospital discharge planners or the nurse responsible for the discharge can make recommendations. Burstein (1995) outlined the criteria for selecting a home care pulmonary equipment company. These criteria (Box 29-1) can be used for other types of equipment suppliers as well.

Once the supplier has been selected and the necessary equipment identified, parent education can begin. This education should include neonatal cardiopulmonary resuscitation (CPR). The parents should be given written instructions to take home and a checklist for the CPR procedure that can be clearly posted. If parents cannot read, visual charts outlining the steps should be made available.

A cardiopulmonary monitor is the most common equipment needed in the home. Infants who should be placed on this type of monitoring are those whose sibling died of sudden infant death syndrome (SIDS) or who are at risk for SIDS.

BOX 29-1

Criteria for Selecting a Home Care Pulmonary Equipment Provider Accredited by the Joint Commission on Accreditation of Healthcare Organizations (JCAHO)

Location: within an hour's driving radius of home
Availability of equipment and supplies required for care
Experience with equipment required for care
24-hour on-call service for emergencies
Professional home care clinicians or staff
Record system available to communicate with physician
Availability of backup equipment on site
Experience with similar clinical situations
Acceptance of assignment on insurance benefits
Some areas may require professional services to be contracted. Contracted professionals must be available on 24-hour on-call basis.

From Czervinske MP, Barnhart SL, editors (2002). *Perinatal and pediatric respiratory care*, ed 2. Philadelphia: Saunders.

These infants are usually monitored until age 6 to 12 months (Burstein, 1995). An infant on home oxygen or one who has neurologic impairment is at risk for apneic or bradycardic episodes. Most of these monitors have built-in impedance pneumography capabilities that allow strips to be watched or viewed by home care nurses. In some instances, these can be sent via computer modems. The parents should be told that when an episode of apnea or bradycardia occurs, they must mark on the strip the infant's color, activity, and what they had to do, if anything, to stop the episode (Burstein, 1995). Burstein (1995) made two important points about this type of monitor. For infants on mechanical ventilation, movement is maintained artificially so that a change in heart rate will have to occur before an alarm will sound. Also, for infants who have tracheostomies, the monitoring is to identify episodes in which breathing may stop as a result of mucus plugs or thickened secretions. The survival instinct of the infant to struggle to breathe will not allow the respiratory monitor alarm to sound as movement is detected. It is the cardiac portion of the monitor that at a much later stage detects bradycardia. Parents need to understand these delays and how to respond.

Suctioning equipment is needed for patients with tracheostomies. This equipment requires electricity and running water. One type of suctioning equipment must be portable and battery-powered for trips to and from the clinic and other excursions out of the home. It should have a regulator valve to adjust the amount of suction. If the valve is not present, negative pressure can be very great and cause mucosal trauma to the nasopharyngeal and tracheal tissues. The battery-powered suction machines can be recharged much like portable phones with a direct A/C adapter into a wall outlet or via a cigarette lighter adapter (Burstein, 1995). Most run about 2 hours without recharging. The recharging process takes about 12 hours. The other type of suctioning equipment can be a stationary setup. Parents should be taught clean suctioning technique, which is used as long as no danger of cross-contamination with other infectious agents in the home exists, as may be the case when siblings are ill. Nosocomial infections and cross-contamination are very real possibilities when the infant is hospitalized. The parents should also be taught sterile technique, which should be used only when illness that may put the infant at risk for cross-contamination is present in the home.

Suctioning should be taught according to the physician or practitioner's orders. Usually this is done on an as-needed basis. Signs that indicate the need for suctioning are the same as those used by health professionals in the NICU: restlessness, decreased color, coughing, increased respiratory effort, or sounds of congestion. In general, suctioning is necessary every 2 to 4 hours. Parents should keep a log of the timing of the suctioning and the type of secretions obtained. In addition to the suctioning equipment, parents will need a 50-pound-per-square-inch (PSI) portable air compressor and possibly compressed oxygen with a portable reservoir. Portable or stationary oxygen devices vary in size and the amount of time that they will last. They are classified as sizes AA through K. G, H, and K are large and stationary, whereas the others are portable. The oxygen tanks for these devices differ from those of liquid oxygen in that they can be stored and will not leak if the shutoff valve is left on. They are larger and are filled under high pressure, so they are more difficult to move. A slight danger from pressure occurs if they are accidentally dropped or damaged. The liquid oxygen is more portable and smaller in size. It does not require external electricity or battery-powered sources. The cylinder is small and filled under very little pressure. The liquid oxygen must be moved from the base of the chamber to a portable reservoir. It is more costly than gas pressure oxygen cylinders.

These infants often also need an oxygen concentrator. The concentrator is like the old-fashioned mix-box used in the NICU to mix air and oxygen to achieve the desired oxygen concentration. It separates oxygen from nitrogen in room air and collects oxygen (Burstein, 1995). The concentrations that are possible with these home devices are between 45% and 95% (Burstein, 1995). They cannot deliver very low flow rates such as 0.5 L/min. They are electrically powered. Portable units are needed outside the home. A backup gas oxygen cylinder is necessary for electrical failures and for excursions outside the home. It is beyond the scope of this chapter to detail the exact procedure for the suctioning and care of the tracheostomy tube. The equipment needed for an infant with a tracheostomy is listed in Box 29-2.

Humidification of the airway is necessary for infants with artificial airways, regardless of whether they are on oxygen. If the airway is not humidified, mucous membranes may dry and crack, creating areas that may become infected. Volume jet nebulizers can provide humidification with a 50-PSI portable air compressor. Humidification levels of 35% to 100% can generally be achieved (Burstein, 1995). This compressor should be capable of providing high- or low-pressure aerosol. This capability is important if the infant requires a mist tent at night but during the day is connected to a tracheostomy collar or other airway devices. Some companies suggest use of a heat and moisture exchanger (HME), which can be used for travel and is used by itself and not in conjunction with other humidifying devices. It can be attached to the airway without intermediate equipment (Burstein, 1995).

Mechanical ventilation is another area of home care. Information on home use of ventilators can be obtained from the National Center for Home Mechanical Ventilation. The physician or practitioner orders the specific type of ventilator

---

BOX 29-2

Equipment Supply List for Tracheostomy Patient

Heat and moisture exchangers (1 to 2 boxes per month) for apnea-bradycardia monitor
Electrodes (2 pairs)
Lead wire (2 pairs)
Belts (2 each)
Tracheostomy tubes (same size) (4 per month)
Tracheostomy tubes (one size smaller) 1 each
Velcro tracheostomy ties (2 boxes per month)
Twill tape (1 roll)
Free-standing suction machine (1 each)
Portable suction machine
Suction connecting tubing (4 per month)
Suction catheters (4 cases per month)
DeLee traps (6 each)
50-PSI portable air compressor
Jet nebulizers (4 per month)
Corrugated aerosol tubing (100-ft roll)
Tracheostomy collars (4 per month)
Liquid oxygen with portable reservoir (as needed)
Oxygen connecting tubing (4 each)
Sterile water (2 to 3 cases per month)
Normal saline, 3-ml vials (2 boxes month)
Heat and moisture exchangers (1 to 2 boxes per month)
Scissors (2 pairs)
Nonsterile gloves (2 boxes per month)
Manual resuscitation bags (2 each)
Sterile cotton-tipped applicators (2 boxes per month)
Hydrogen peroxide (2 bottles per month)
Stethoscope

From Czervinske MP, Barnhart SL, editors (2002). *Perinatal and pediatric respiratory care*, ed 2. Philadelphia: Saunders.

---

on the basis of the infant's need. The decision also takes into consideration the family's lifestyle. If the family anticipates movement from home to other areas or other relatives' homes, a portable unit may be best. All portable units must have an internal and external battery. An emergency backup unit must be available—whether it is housed in the home or at immediate dispatch from the equipment company does not matter, as long as it is available for times when equipment failures occur with the portable device. Battery backup is also necessary. Usually a 12-volt battery with 74-amp/hour potential is suggested; such a battery can go about 18 to 20 hours without recharge.

These areas of home care monitoring are the most common. Specific instructions on which equipment is necessary and how to use it in each situation should be obtained from the home health care agency that is to provide care, the hospital equipment vendors, and the home health care equipment vendors. Nurses who are responsible for discharge should be very familiar with the advantages and disadvantages of the equipment that the family will need. The family's lifestyle and capabilities also have to be considered when an infant is sent home on equipment.

Home care equipment and supplies must fit the patient just as it did in the hospital. The nurse responsible for the discharge must make sure that the child's size is considered when ordering equipment. For example, if the infant is now 12 pounds, do you still use a preemie stethoscope? If the child has a tracheostomy, is there a backup of proper size?

Ideally the nurse should make a home visit before the discharge to assess the home environment for safety hazards. For example, is the house/apartment too hot or cold? Either condition can lead to apneic spells. Are there exposed wires in the house? Peeling paint? Open flames used for cooking when oxygen is going to be used in the house? Are there any strong or chemical odors that may be harmful to a child with respiratory compromise? Is there an emergency phone? Have utility companies been notified? Is there a backup plan in case of a power outage? Is there a plan for continued health promotion, such as immunizations? All aspects of the home and the community setting should be considered when discharging the infant and family.

Follow-Up System Criteria

Criteria for home care cannot be complete without accurate assessment of the availability of follow-up after discharge. Environmental conditions and social supports are two of the strongest influences on the ability of the parents to nurture their child in the home.

Hospital-based programs that provide home health services may establish home health visits. Community-funded home health care agencies are often available to provide some home follow-up. The departments of public health and other publicly funded agencies can be of assistance with home care follow-up.

The visiting resource person must be appropriately knowledgeable about the physical and emotional needs of the family. To be effective, the home visitor should be sensitive to cultural and ethnic differences and incorporate knowledge about them into the follow-up plan.

A mandate to provide services for NICU graduates is found in Public Law 99-457 concerning education of the handicapped. These children must be referred to early intervention programs to promote the most positive development possible. Any infant who has a developmental delay, is at risk for a developmental problem, or has a condition with a high probability for developmental problems, such as Down syndrome, is eligible (Stepanek, 1996). Resources for information in early intervention services include the National Early Childhood Technical Assistance System (NECTAS), 137 East Franklin Street, Suite 500, Chapel Hill, NC 27514, 919-962-2001, and the Technical Assistance for Parents Program (TAPP), 95 Berkley Street, Suite 104, Boston, MA 02116, 617-482-2915 (Stepanek, 1996).

SUMMARY

The interventions discussed have been shown to have some effect in decreasing parental anxiety and thus lessening the crisis situation of the transition from the NICU to home. More research is needed to help determine whether a specific way exists to alleviate the crisis situation for a family taking home a premature infant. Existing studies also must be replicated to demonstrate that the interventions are as effective as the original research suggests. A specific research question to be considered is whether all parents of premature infants need interventions as extensive as described, or whether only parents of extremely ill or premature infants need such interventions. None of the existing studies address which groups of

parents are more at risk for crisis problems. The results of such a study might show that all parents, not only the parents of extremely ill or premature infants, need these types of interventions.

REFERENCES

Allen EC et al (2004). Perception of child vulnerability among mothers of former premature infants. *Pediatrics* 113:267-273.

American Academy of Pediatrics (2004). Follow-up care of high-risk infants. *Pediatrics* 114:1377-1397.

American Psychiatric Association (1994). *Diagnostic and statistical manual of mental disorders*, ed 4. Washington, DC: Author.

Bagwell GA et al (1990). *Parent transition from a special care nursery to home: a replicative study.* Unpublished master's thesis. Cincinnati, OH: University of Cincinnati College of Nursing and Health.

Benzies KM et al (1998). Impact of marital quality and parent-infant interaction on preschool behavior problems. *Public health nursing* 15(1):35-45.

Bialoskurski M et al (1999). The nature of attachment in a Neonatal Intensive Care Unit. *Journal of perinatal and neonatal nursing* 13(1):66-77.

Bolzan N et al (2004). Time to father. *Social work health care* 39(1-2):67-88.

Burstein L (1995). Home care. In Barnhart SL, Czervinske MP, editors. *Perinatal and pediatric respiratory care*. Philadelphia: Saunders.

Callen J, Pinelli J (2005). A review of the literature examining the benefits and challenges, incidence and duration, and barriers to breastfeeding in preterm infants. *Advances in neonatal care* 5(2):72-88.

Cicco R et al (January 1996). *Making NICUs more developmentally appropriate for infants: parents and families.* Paper presented at the Physical and Developmental Environment of the High Risk Neonate, University of South Florida College of Medicine, Clearwater Beach, FL.

Collins CT et al (2005). Early discharge with home support of gavage feeding for stable preterm infants who have not established full oral feeds. *Cochrane database of systematic reviews*, 3, ID #CD003743.

Costello A, Chapman J (1998). Mothers' perceptions of the care-by-parent program prior to hospital discharge of their preterm infants. *Neonatal network* 17(7):37-42.

Crosson DD, Pickler RH. (2004). An integrated review of the literature on demand feedings for preterm infants. *Advances in neonatal care* 4(4):216-225.

Culley BS et al (1989). Parental perception of vulnerability of formerly premature infants. *Journal of pediatric health care* 3:237-245.

Donohue PK (2002). Health-related quality of life of preterm children and their caregivers. *Mental retardation and developmental disabilities research reviews* 8(4):293-297.

Green M, Solnit AA (1964). Reactions to the threatened loss of a child: a vulnerable child syndrome. *Pediatrics* 34:58-66.

Hall WA et al (2002). Weighing preterm infants before and after breastfeeding: Does it increase maternal confidence and competence? *American journal of maternal child nursing* 27(6):318-327.

Hummel P, Cronin J (2004). Home care of the high-risk infant. *Advances in neonatal care* 4(6):354-364.

Hurst NM et al (2004) Mothers performing in-home measurement of milk intake during breastfeeding of their preterm infants: maternal reactions and feeding outcomes. *Journal of human lactation* 20(2):178-187.

Jackson K et al (2003). From alienation to familiarity: experiences of mothers and fathers of preterm infants. *Journal of advanced nursing* 43(2):120-129.

Johnson-Crowley N, Sumner GA (1987a). *Concept manual: nursing systems toward effective parenting—preterm*. Seattle, WA: NCAST Publications.

Johnson-Crowley N, Sumner GA (1987b). *Protocol manual: nursing systems toward effective parenting—preterm*. Seattle: NCAST Publications.

Johnson S et al (2005). Randomised trial of parental support for families with very preterm children: outcome at 5 years. *Archives of disease in childhood* 90(9):909-915.

Kenner CA (1988). *Parent transition from the newborn intensive care unit (NICU) to home.* Unpublished doctoral dissertation. Indianapolis, IN: Indiana University.

Kenner C (1995). The transition to parenthood. In Gunderson LP, Kenner C, editors. *Care of the 24-25 week gestational age infant: small baby protocol*, ed 2, Petaluma, CA: NICU Ink.

Kenner C (April 1998). Transition model. Presented at the University of Cincinnati, Cincinnati, OH.

Kenner C et al (1996). Parenting in the NICU. In Zaichkin J, editor. *Newborn intensive care: what every parent needs to know*. Petaluma, CA: NICU Ink.

Klassen AF et al (2004). Health status and health-related quality of life in a population-based sample of neonatal intensive care unit graduates. *Pediatrics* 113:594-600.

Madlon-Kay DJ (2001). Home health nurse clinical assessment of neonatal jaundice: comparison of 3 methods. *Archives of pediatric and adolescent medicine* 155(5):583-586.

March of Dimes (MOD) (2005). Prematurity: the answers can't come soon enough. Available at: http://www.marchofdimes.com/prematurity/prematurity.asp. Retrieved July 25, 2005.

McEvoy M et al (2005). Are there universal parenting concepts among culturally diverse families in an inner-city pediatric clinic? *Journal of pediatric health care* 19(3):142-150.

McKim E (May 1989). *The support needs of mothers of premature infants.* Presented at the Third International Nursing Research Symposium, McGill University School of Nursing, Montreal, Quebec, Canada.

McKim E (1993a). The information and support needs of mothers of premature infants. *Journal of pediatric nursing* 8(4):233-244.

McKim EM (1993b). The difficult first week at home with a premature infant. *Public health nursing* 10(2):89-96.

McKim EM et al (1995). The transition to home for mothers of healthy and initially healthy newborns. *Midwifery* 11:184-194.

McLean A et al (2000). Quality of life of mothers and families caring for preterm infants requiring home oxygen therapy: a brief report. *Journal of paediatrics and child health* 36(5):440-444.

Melynk BM et al (2002). Evidence-based practice. Effectiveness of informational / behavioral interventions with parents of low birth weight (LBW) premature infants: an evidence base to guide clinical practice. *Pediatric nursing* 28(5):511-516.

Mercer RT (1995). *Becoming a mother: research from Rubin to the present.* New York: Springer.

Miles MS, Holditch-Davis D (1995). Compensatory parenting: how mothers describe parenting their 3-year-old, prematurely born children. *Journal of pediatric nursing* 10(4):243-253.

Peeples-Kleiger MJ (2000). Pediatric and neonatal intensive care hospitalization as traumatic stressor: implications for intervention. *Bulletin of the Menninger Clinic* 64(2):257-280.

Rautava P et al (2003). Effect of newborn hospitalization on family and child behavior: a 12-year follow-up study. *Pediatrics* 111:277-283.

Rubin R (1984). *Maternal identity and the maternal experience.* New York: Springer.

Scheiner A et al (1985). The vulnerable child syndrome: fact and theory. *Developmental and behavioral pediatrics* 6(5):298-301.

Scholtes PF et al (1994). Management of medically fragile infants and children. *Physician executive* 20(9):41-43.

Shonkoff JP (1998). Commentary: Reactions to the threatened loss of a child: a vulnerable child syndrome, by Morris Green, MD, and Albert A. Solnit, MD, Pediatrics, 1964;34:58-66. *Pediatrics* 102(1, Part 2):239-241.

Spangler-Torok L (2001). *Maternal perceptions of the technology-dependent infant.* Unpublished dissertation. Cincinnati, OH: University of Cincinnati College of Nursing.

Stepanek JA (1996). Early intervention services for the high-risk infant. In Ahman E, editor. *Home care for the high-risk infant,* ed 2. Gaithersburg, MD: Aspen.

Swartz MK (2005). Parenting preterm infants: a meta-synthesis. *American journal of maternal child nursing* 30(2):115-120.

Theunissen NC et al (2001). Quality of life in preschool children born preterm. *Developmental medicine and child neurology* 43(7):460-465.

Van Riper M (2001). Family-provider relationships and well-being in families with preterm infants in the NICU. *Heart and lung* 30(1):74-84.

Wereszczak J et al (1997). Maternal recall of neonatal intensive care unit. *Neonatal network* 16(4):33-40.

Wooldridge J, Hall WA (2003). Posthospitalization breastfeeding patterns of moderately preterm infants. *Journal of perinatal and neonatal nursing* 17(1):50-64.

Zanardo V, Freato F (2001). Home oxygen therapy in infants with bronchopulmonary dysplasia: assessment of parental anxiety. *Early human development* 65(1):39-46.

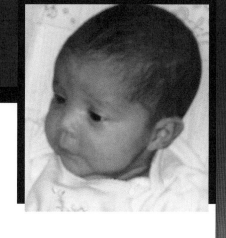

C h a p t e r **30**

Trends in Neonatal Care Delivery

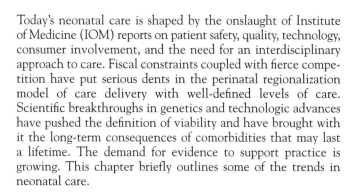

Carole Kenner • Jana L. Pressler

Today's neonatal care is shaped by the onslaught of Institute of Medicine (IOM) reports on patient safety, quality, technology, consumer involvement, and the need for an interdisciplinary approach to care. Fiscal constraints coupled with fierce competition have put serious dents in the perinatal regionalization model of care delivery with well-defined levels of care. Scientific breakthroughs in genetics and technologic advances have pushed the definition of viability and have brought with it the long-term consequences of comorbidities that may last a lifetime. The demand for evidence to support practice is growing. This chapter briefly outlines some of the trends in neonatal care.

LEVELS OF CARE

In the early 1990s the report Toward Improving the Outcome of Pregnancy: The 90s and Beyond (TIOP II) (Committee on Perinatal Health, 1993) illustrated the need for levels of care and a regionalization plan for education and practice. The need to have high-risk perinatal care that also provided educational outreach to the community was embraced. The definitions were incorporated in the work by the American Academy of Pediatrics (AAP) and the American College of Obstetrics and Gynecology (ACOG) in Guidelines for Perinatal Care (AAP/ACOG, 2002). Today this work has been continued by AAP's Committee on Fetus and Newborn (2004a, 2004b) to recognize that as the specialty has become more complex, and as smaller and smaller infants are surviving, the three levels of care are not adequate. Some very highly specialized technologies do not need to be available in every community. Uniformity of care and integration of services are important to the quality and outcome factors today. Box 30-1 reflects the proposed definitions for levels of care.

Another area of concern is high-risk follow-up. As more infants are surviving the relative lack of consistency of how follow-up is conducted or who even receives follow-up is a gap in knowledge. To this end, in June 2002 the National Institute of Child Health and Human Development (NICHD), National Institute of Neurologic Disorders and Stroke (NINDS), and the Centers for Disease Control and Prevention (CDC) convened a workshop to begin to examine this gap. They also

recognized that differences in data collection methods have led to difficulties with comparing outcomes within centers and across centers (NICHD, NINDS, & CDC, 2004). To improve long-term developmental and physical neonatal outcomes, the follow-up care must be clearly defined with levels designated much like NICU levels of care. In the next decade this seminal work will shape the post-NICU experience.

DEVELOPMENTAL CARE

Developmental outcomes have been at the forefront of care for many years, but today the movement is to support individualized family-centered care. This care coincides with the Institute of Medicine's (2001) emphasis on patient-focused care as a method to increase quality. Another aspect of this care supports IOM's initiative in interprofessional or interdisciplinary care, and that is developmentally supportive care. This care incorporates the knowledge of growth and development; factors that interfere with positive growth such as prematurity, environmental noise, and lighting levels; the interface with physiologic responses to stress-inhibited growth factors and increases in cortisol levels; and positioning, just to name a few. Chapter 24 gives more in-depth information on this topic. The NICU environment and its impact on development from a long-term perspective have spawned a growth in the use of Recommended Standards for Newborn ICU Design (White, 2002) throughout the world. (For more information, please see Chapter 24.) These recommendations come from an interdisciplinary group of architects, institutional planners, developmental specialists, nurses, physicians, and parents. The use of such standards to renovate or build new NICUs will increase, as will the overall incorporation of individualized, family-centered, developmental care. One sign of this is the publishing of an interdisciplinary book on this subject, *Developmental Care of Newborns & Infants* by Kenner and McGrath (2004).

NEONATAL STATISTICS

Neonatal statistics are difficult to follow because of the lack of consistent terminology about the age of the fetus, neonate, and infant. To that end the AAP Committee on Fetus and Newborn

BOX 30-1

Proposed Uniform Definitions for Capabilities Associated with the Highest Level of Neonatal Care Within an Institution

Level I Neonatal Care (Basic)

Well-newborn nursery: has the capabilities to:
- Provide neonatal resuscitation at every delivery
- Evaluate and provide postnatal care to healthy newborn infants
- Stabilize and provide care for infants born at 35 to 37 weeks' gestation who remain physiologically stable
- Stabilize newborn infants who are ill and those born at <35 weeks' gestation until transfer to a facility that can provide the appropriate level of neonatal care

Level II Neonatal Care (Specialty)

Special care nursery: level II units are subdivided into two categories on the basis of their ability to provide assisted ventilation including continuous positive airway pressure

Level IIA: has the capabilities to:
- Resuscitate and stabilize preterm or ill infants before transfer to a facility at which newborn intensive care is provided
- Provide care for infants born at >32 weeks' gestation and weighing ≥1500 g (1) who have physiologic immaturity such as apnea of prematurity, inability to maintain body temperature, or inability to take oral feedings or (2) who are moderately ill with problems that are expected to resolve rapidly and are not expected to need subspecialty services on an urgent basis
- Provide care for infants who are convalescing after intensive care

Level IIB: has the capabilities of a level IIA nursery and the additional capability to provide mechanical ventilation

for brief durations (<24 hours) or continuous positive airway pressure

Level III (Subspecialty) NICU

Level III NICUs area subdivided into three categories.

Level IIIA NICU: has capabilities to:
- Provide comprehensive care for infants born at >28 weeks' gestation and weighing >1000 g
- Provide sustained life support limited to conventional mechanical ventilation
- Perform minor surgical procedures such as placement of central venous catheter or inguinal hernia repair

Level IIIB NICU: has the capabilities to provide:
- Comprehensive care for extremely-low-birth-weight infants (≤1000 g and ≤28 weeks' gestation)
- Advanced respiratory support such as high-frequency ventilation and inhaled nitric oxide for as long as required
- Prompt and on-site access to a full range of pediatric medical subspecialists
- Advanced imaging, with interpretation on an urgent basis, including computed tomography, magnetic resonance imaging, and echocardiography
- Pediatric surgical specialists and pediatric anesthesiologists on-site or at a closely related institution to perform major surgery such as ligation of patent ductus arteriosus and repair of abdominal wall defects, necrotizing enterocolitis with bowel perforation, tracheoesophageal fistula or esophageal atresia, and myelomeningocele

Level IIIC NICU: has the capabilities of a level IIIB NICU and also is located within an institution that has the capability to provide extracorporeal membrane oxygenation (ECMO) and surgical repair of complex congenital cardiac malformations that require cardiopulmonary bypass.

From Committee on Fetus and Newborn (2004a). American Academy of Pediatrics (AAP) policy statement: organizational principles to guide and define the child health care system and/or improve the health of all children. *Pediatrics* 114(5):1341-1347.

(2004a, 2004b) developed definitions of gestational, post-menstrual, chronologic, and corrected ages. These definitions are given in Table 30-1.

According to the March of Dimes Birth Defects Foundation, White Plains, NY, one in every eight babies born in the United States is premature. According to the National Center on Health Statistics the U.S. infant mortality rate rose in 2002 to 7 per 1000 live births. This is the first rise in several years; the causes are speculated to be lack of insurance coverage for mothers and babies, with thus little or no prenatal care, and the increasing ability to deliver very immature or sick infants, only to lose them to complications such as gross anomalies incompatible with long-term survival, infections, and prematurity. The incidence of extremely low birth weight infants, those weighing less than 750 g, increased by 500 times over previous years (National Center on Health Statistics, 2005; http://www.cdc.gov/nchs/).

On a global level approximately 130 million infants are born annually. Of these, 4 million die during the neonatal period (first 4 weeks of life) (Horton, 2005). Concern for future generations has resulted in two partnership programs: the Healthy Newborn Partnership, started in 2000 by Save the Children and USA's Saving Newborn Lives initiative, Washington, DC; and Partnership for Safe Motherhood and Newborn Health, a World Health Organization (WHO) initiative. These are both aimed at decreasing maternal and infant morbidity and mortality by examining prenatal interventions and education and neonatal interventions and education, including the use of high technology and low technology such as birth attendants. As might be expected, much of the global infant mortality occurs in the poorest regions such as southeast Asia and sub-Saharan Africa (75% of the mortality globally) (Tinker et al, 2005). The Millennium Development Goal to promote child survival cannot be met

TABLE 30-1	Age Terminology During the Perinatal Period	
Term	**Definition**	**Units of Time**
Gestational age	Time elapsed between the first day of the last menstrual period and the day of delivery	Completed weeks
Chronologic age	Time elapsed since birth	Days, weeks, months, years
Postmenstrual age	Gestational age + chronologic age	Weeks
Corrected age	Chronologic age reduced by the number of weeks born before 40 weeks of gestation	Weeks, months

From Committee on Fetus and Newborn (2004b). American Academy of Pediatrics (AAP) policy statement: organizational principles to guide the child health care system and/or improve the health of all children. Pediatrics 114(5):1362-1364.

unless neonatal mortality is addressed. At present 38% of all child deaths globally occur during the neonatal period (Lawn et al, for the Lancet Neonatal Survival Steering Team, 2005). The Council of International Neonatal Nurses (COINN) (http://www.coinnurses.org/contact.htm) is participating as a partner in the Safe Motherhood and Newborn Health initiative to build capacity in developing countries and support a network of health professionals that will assist in developing standards of professional practice and care. This is one example of the grassroots level of policy that grew out of neonatal nurses coming together at formalized conferences in their own countries (United Kingdom, United States, Australia, and New Zealand—listed in order of formation) to talk about global needs.

MATERNAL/FETAL NEONATAL UNITS

Fetal surgery has been performed for more than a decade. Until recently, fetuses that remained in utero until a viable birth occurred were cared for in a normal NICU. Now there is recognition for the need for more specialized care. Maternal/fetal/neonatal subunits or additions to NICUs have developed. Prototypes of this model are found at Children's Hospital of Philadelphia (CHOP) and Cincinnati Children's Hospital. These units have perinatal/neonatal/pediatric specialists who are familiar with fetal surgery, genetics, pediatric surgery, and the needs of the neonate and family after birth (http://www.fetalcarecenter.org/). These units will continue to flourish as the emphasis on consumer-driven health care models and care coordination continues to grow.

GENETICS

Genetic breakthroughs as a result of the Human Genome Project (HGP) are influencing health and health care. Genomics, the term that refers to the interaction between genetic makeup and the environment, is gradually shaping how health is promoted. The U.S. Surgeon General, along with the work of the National Human Genome Research Institute (NHGRI) (www.genome.gov), advocates the use of the Family History Tool, which incorporates health history in the traditional sense along with genetic history. Use of this tool coupled with knowledge of, say, newborn screening tests will influence how health professionals plan and implement care. One of the newer areas of emphasis by NHGRI is severe combined immunodeficiency syndrome (SCID), which appears to be related to several genetic mutations that may be preventable in the future (http://www.genome.gov/13014325). As another example, if an infant is born to a family with a history of diabetes, then the development of healthy eating habits to avoid obesity and other risk factors for diabetes can start in the neonatal period. The genomics thrust then changes how care is planned and how it needs to be individualized. It also emphasizes the need for individualized family-centered care.

Another aspect of genetics is the controversy over the numbers of tests that a newborn should have to prevent long-term complications of neonatal conditions and to improve quality of life. The March of Dimes (MOD) advocates up to 30 tests, whereas some state newborn screening programs suggest only four. The question becomes: just because the test can be run and is minimally invasive, should it be done? Who decides? What are the ramifications—is there any danger of insurance discrimination? These ethical questions are at the heart of the debate about newborn screening and the intersection with genetic testing. There are websites and organizations dedicated to providing consumer-friendly information for parents on these topics to help them decide a course of action. Two good sources of information are KidsHealth for Parents (http://kidshealth.org/parent/system/medical/genetics.html) and the March of Dimes (http://www.marchofdimes.com/pnhec/298_834.asp).

Another site that focuses on policy and newborn screening is the Genetics & Public Policy Center (http://www.dnapolicy.org/genetics/testing.jhtml). For general information on the Human Genome Project (HGP) and resources for health professionals and families, see http://www.ornl.gov/sci/techresources/Human_Genome/home.shtml. Advances in genetic frontiers will continue to change neonatal care and improve outcomes.

GLOBALIZATION

Recommendations for NICU standards and professional programs such as Neonatal Resuscitation are being used globally. Neonatal care issues are international. This era of globalization is changing the way care practices and outcomes are viewed. Protocols for care are developed so they can be adapted for cultural sensitivity, technology availability, and geographic needs. The push toward evidence-based practice and use of Cochrane Reviews, the Joanna Briggs Institute Collaborative Systematic Reviews, and Vermont Oxford materials all are bringing neonatal care to a level that is supported by scientific findings rather than tradition. This movement is global and is influenced by hospitals seeking Magnet Status, which espouses evidence-based practice guidelines to ensure quality care and more positive outcomes. As this influence continues, there will be shifts in how care is implemented.

Kercsmar (2003) summarized trends to include need for more evidence-based resuscitation strategies, ventilator management, and diagnostic tests such as pulmonary functioning and newer oximetry methods. Other trends include emphasis on long-term problems or complications such as asthma, respiratory syncytial virus, bronchiolitis, croup, and other respiratory-related problems (Kercsmar, 2003). Genetic linkage to the development of chronic conditions will continue, as will techniques to incorporate pharmacogenomics in care to avoid resistant infections and increase knowledge about therapeutic levels. This knowledge will aid in palliative care.

PALLIATIVE AND END-OF-LIFE CARE

There is an increasing awareness of the need for effective pain management. The Joint Commission on Accreditation of Healthcare Organizations (JCAHO) has declared pain as the fifth vital sign across the life span. For neonates, pain management is complicated by the patient's nonverbal status and the need to rely on physiologic parameters to measure pain and pain management responses. There is a need for more evidence to support pain management as seen in Chapter 17. One area that has increased the recognition of this gap in our neonatal care knowledge is palliative and end-of-life care.

Whether we like to acknowledge it or not, some children are born dying. There are infants that we cannot save despite our technology, and others who have life-threatening illnesses and who may survive. Those in the latter group, like all our patients, deserve comfort or palliative care. Chapter 26 reports on this new frontier of neonatal care.

SUMMARY

This chapter has briefly highlighted some of the trends in neonatal care. With all the new breakthroughs in care, it is hard to imagine what the next decade will bring.

REFERENCES

American Academy of Pediatrics (AAP) and American College of Obstetrics and Gynecology (ACOG) (2002). *Guidelines for perinatal care.* Elk Grove Village, IL: Authors.

Committee on Fetus and Newborn (2004a). American Academy of Pediatrics (AAP) policy statement: organizational principles to guide and define the child health care system and/or improve the health of all children. *Pediatrics* 114(5):1341-1347.

Committee on Fetus and Newborn (2004b). American Academy of Pediatrics (AAP) policy statement: organizational principles to guide the child health care system and/or improve the health of all children. *Pediatrics* 114(5):1362-1364.

Committee on Perinatal Health (1993). *Toward improving the outcome of pregnancy: the 90s and beyond.* White Plains, NY: March of Dimes Birth Defects Foundation.

Horton R (2005). Newborn survival: putting children at the centre. *The Lancet: Neonatal survivor series.* Available at: http://www.activemag.co.uk/lancet.htm. Retrieved March 6, 2005.

Institute of Medicine (IOM) (2001). *Crossing the quality chasm: the IOM health care quality initiative.* Washington, DC: National Academies Press.

Kenner C, McGrath JM (2004). *Developmental care of newborns & infants: a guide for health professionals.* St Louis: Mosby.

Kercsmar MC (2003). Current trends in management of pediatric asthma. *Respiratory care* 48(3):194-205; discussion 205-208.

Lawn JE et al, for the Lancet Neonatal Survival Steering Team (2005). Neonatal survival 1:4 million neonatal deaths: When? Where? Why? *The Lancet: Neonatal survivor series.* Available at: http://www.activemag.co.uk/lancet.htm. Retrieved March 6, 2005.

National Center for Health Statistics (2005). *Monitoring the nation's health.* Available at: http://www.cdc.gov/nchs/. Retrieved March 6, 2005.

National Institute of Child Health and Human Development (NICHD), National Institute for Neurologic Disorders and Stroke (NINDS), and the Centers for Disease Control and Prevention (CDC) (2004). Follow-up care of high-risk infants. *Pediatrics* 114(5):1377-1397.

Tinker A et al (2005). A continuum of care to save newborn lives. *The Lancet: Neonatal survivor series.* Available at: http://www.activemag.co.uk/lancet.htm. Retrieved March 6, 2005.

White R (2002). Recommended standards for newborn ICU design: report of the fifth consensus conference on newborn ICU design. Available at: http://www.nd.edu/~kkolberg/DesignStandards.htm. Retrieved October 29, 2005.

Chapter 31

Electronic Medical Records and Technology

Rebecca Lynn Roys Gelrud • Tony C. (Chris) Carnes •
Willa Drummond

Hospitals have used information technology quite successfully for decades to support administrative and financial functions. Recent government mandates such as the Institute of Medicine (IOM) series on quality improvement and other agencies aimed at the improvement of clinical health care have awakened many hospitals' interest in the value of using information technology to support patient care. Effective use of information technologies in NICUs, or any ICU, can greatly improve patient care, patient outcomes, and clinician workload as well as provide hospitalwide cost savings. A recent study conducted at George Washington University Medical Faculty Associates (MFA) hospital revealed that after the implementation of their electronic health records, their first-year savings was $335,900 due solely to a 70% decrease in paper chart pulls. MFA estimates savings of more than $6.3 million over the first 5 years in chart-related staffing expenses alone (Badger et al, 2005). Adoption of computerized technologies holds great promise as computer systems improve each year. Full functionality requires integrating health care systems by adhering to emerging industry standards for computer-to-computer communication, health care data vocabularies, and management quality. This chapter focuses on the current status and near-future advances of NICU computerization, as well as how to evaluate and select an information system for your unit.

BACKGROUND INFORMATION

As health care and computer technology began to blend in the late 1950s, the field of informatics evolved. Informatics was created as a new field with the first computerization of a cardiac catheterization laboratory by Dr. Homer Warner, Sr. Informatics has evolved and expanded quickly as external technologic innovations rapidly diffused throughout the heath care environment. Informatics pioneers were first classified as a subgroup of bioengineering. Many new names for the field appeared: medical computer science, medical information processing, and medical computer technology. Over time, other health care professionals began substituting the term *health* for *medical* because *informatics* is a broad term that pertains to many health care disciplines, not just medicine. In the late 1960s and early 1970s, Russians, English, Germans, and the French all began to use and define variations of the word *informatics*. By the 1980s, the terms *clinical*, *health*, and *nursing* informatics surfaced. The field was searching for a

commonly accepted definition for each new and complex domain of knowledge. Various subgroups attempted to define their "domains" in order to clarify their differences and similarities (Collen, 1995).

After several definitions were created for "generic" medical informatics, a consensus definition was written by the Long-Range Planning Committee of the National Library of Medicine (NLM):

> Medical informatics attempts to provide the theoretical and scientific basis for the application of computer and automated information systems to biomedicine and health affairs. . . . Medical informatics studies biomedical information, data, and knowledge—their storage, retrieval, and optimal use for problem-solving and decision-making. It touches on all basic and applied fields in biomedical science and is closely tied to modern information technology, notably in the areas of computing and communication (Lindberg, 1987).

The consensus definition has not been seriously challenged since.

The field of nursing informatics has evolved rapidly from the predominately physician-populated field of medical informatics. In 1989, Judith Graves and Sheila Corcoran, authors of "The Study of Nursing Informatics" (Graves & Corcoran, 1989), defined nursing informatics as "a combination of computer science, information science, and nursing science designed to assist with the management and processing of data, information, and knowledge to support the practice of nursing and the delivery of nursing care."

Graves and Corcoran's classic definition considers functional components (i.e., "management and processing"), combined with conceptual components (i.e., "data, information, and knowledge"), and then recognizes the "process" where the functional components operate on the conceptual components. In short, Graves and Corcoran believe that nursing informatics should be more concerned with how the data are structured and organized than with the content of the data.

Lindberg and Graves and Corcoran's definitions of informatics hint at the enormous size of this relatively young field of health care. In this infancy stage of development, informatics continues to morph and to grow rapidly. The two strongest influences on the informatics field are evolving health care and advances in technology. Informatics attempts to merge these two dynamic influences to better the delivery of health care.

TYPES OF INFORMATION SYSTEMS

According to Hebda and colleagues (2001), the term *information system* (IS) refers to "a computer system that uses hardware and software to process data into information in order to solve a problem." Others argue that information systems also include those manual data management systems that still exist today. More specifically, clinical information systems are information systems that provide access to and methods for recording and managing clinical data. Some examples include paper and electronic flow sheets, daily notes, physician orders, and pharmaceutical systems.

Flow Sheet Replacement and Monitoring

Critical care bedside clinicians are "hands-on" providers. The care environment is complex and filled with many simultaneous processes that feed medical decision making. Intensive care units are often crowded with both people and devices. Care providers are often summoned from one task to a more urgent one in seconds, making computer use/access/logoff difficult or impossible with existing systems. Clinical data acquisition and integration at most ICU bedsides still depends on pen-and-paper flow-sheet methods. This practice is very time-consuming and creates an "information overload" of poorly organized, often illegible data, which can lead to oversights and potentially avoidable errors (Cole, 1996).

Real-time integration of machine and ancillary data into a user-defined presentation format to support bedside patient care is an unmet dream of most intensive care doctors and practitioners. Past attempts to computerize aspects of ICU bedside physiologic data management have led to sophisticated, free-standing commercial bedside physiologic monitoring and treatment systems (monitors, ventilators, pumps, flowmeters). Each machine relates to a subset of the patient's overall problems (cardiac, respiratory, brain, etc.). Unfortunately, these existing bedside machines have no formal open communication standards with today's computers.

A second challenge for NICU computerization is acquiring and integrating important off-site ancillary data such as those from labs, pharmacy, and radiology. Computer tools to obtain, analyze, and present patient data trends and information important for clinical caregivers in complicated ICU situations are not yet commercially available.

As flow-sheet replacement systems evolve, more complete solutions are being developed to reduce the drawbacks that have prevented the adoption of many of the early electronic flow-sheet systems. The more complete solutions enable real-time temporal integration and storage of clinical patient information derived from many different clinical data sources. They have effective interfaces to analyze and display these data both for immediate patient care and for clinical research and quality assurance initiatives. On some of these new systems, touch-screen interfaces are available that provide a single point of contact for patient data that returning from hospital information systems (HIS) and from laboratory and pharmacy systems, along with data collected from the output of attached bedside machines. This type of automated integration greatly reduces the amount of data that must be re-entered by the bedside nurse. Time-sensitive graphical displays provide a convenient mechanism for caregivers to review current and historical data about the patient so clinicians can quickly grasp a more complete picture of a critical care patient's status. With real-time integrated systems, many critical data points are harder to overlook in situations where multiple simultaneities compete for a caregiver's time, such as crisis situations during transport or in the ICU. The most complete of these automated flow sheet systems improve on current practices by:

1. Integrating important data from the HIS, laboratory, pharmacy, and bedside devices, then displaying the information at the patient bedside or point of care;
2. Capturing and integrating patient parameters (vital signs, labs, etc.) into a daily note system;
3. Enabling remote access to integrated patient data, just as if the clinician were at the point of care;
4. Interfacing patient data collected during transport with the patient electronic record;
5. Providing deidentified or scrubbed patient information to a data warehouse to support a broad range of quality assurance, medical, and pharmaceutical research activities.

Current paper-based flow-sheet standards have appeared to be adequate throughout history. However, it is evident that a properly designed automated flow-sheet system could decrease time spent collecting, communicating, and analyzing patient data. This saved time can then allow clinicians to focus more on treatment and patient care.

Interdisciplinary Notes: Daily Documenting Challenges

Every day, in every ICU, many different notes must be generated that outline the care being provided for the patient by the nurse, the doctor, the respiratory therapist, and others on the care team (pharmacists, social workers, physical therapists, etc.). Generating these notes, from the initial history and physical (H&P), to the daily progress note, to the final discharge note, has often been problematic and is very time consuming.

The information contained in many of these notes is used both for communicating and documenting daily care and eventually for billing. Over the years, attempts to generate a "readable" note have taken on several forms. Traditionally, a clinician would record a few key words when moving from patient to patient or use a preprinted card with check boxes to record appropriate information. Later, in a more private, less chaotic space, the clinician may try to recall everything about the encounter and create a narrative note. The clinician might type the note, but this data entry method has slowed, and often disgruntled, clinicians. More often, the clinician would dictate the encounter narrative to a dictation service. Some number of hours or days later, a complete note would appear for the clinician to sign and place in the chart, as a prerequisite for reimbursement. The dictation is expensive for the hospital. The delay in returning the dictation to the care venue, plus the delay in signing, compounds ongoing operational problems of coordinating daily communication among different caregivers, especially in a cross-disciplinary, teamwork-based NICU.

To try to overcome the delay-related issues, several companies have developed "voice recognition" systems. In some disciplines with "limited" vocabulary and quiet work environments (e.g., radiology), voice recognition systems have achieved some popularity. If voice recognition systems can be made to work well, the daily note is theoretically available as soon as the clinician finishes speaking, and any edits that need to be done can be made immediately. The usual drawback of such systems is that the "vocabulary" to be recognized must be greatly restricted in order for the system to work well. In addition, each clinician using the system must "train" the system to recognize his or her personal speech patterns. Extraneous noise can greatly influence the accuracy of the word recognition, so the dictation must be done in a relatively quite environment, which is difficult to attain in the daily life of many ICUs. To achieve this, the clinician must, once again, be removed from the point of care to record the encounter. This can lead to errors and often requires first written, then verbal narration of facts in hopes to precisely record the encounter. This could potentially cause decreased accuracy and waste precious time duplicating facts, leading to increased frustration and therefore decreased product usage. However, when used in an optimal setting, voice recognition systems often excel.

Types of daily note systems based on templates are gaining popularity. A template is a document, either paper or electronic, that contains commonly used elements in a predefined format. The idea behind these templates is that the format of the template (e.g., daily note) is fairly static for a given patient type (neonate, cardiac, transplant, etc.), with the need to track parameter changes from day to day. One of the more tedious tasks when using this writing system is gathering parameters (such as blood pressure, oxygen saturations, and heart rate from the flow sheet) and retyping them. Another downfall is that the users could begin to rely on only those predefined elements within the template, thereby potentially missing extraneous elements. However, templates that utilize a note system configured to accept bedside data from an automated data acquisition system can greatly reduce the time needed to generate daily notes and often can increase completeness and comprehensibility of the daily note.

Order Entry

The mandate to reduce medical errors has given rise to a new type of electronic information system known as computerized provider order entry (CPOE). The promise of these systems includes a reduction in errors through improved legibility, immediate cross-checking for prescription interactions, and more immediate fulfillment of orders. The jury is still out on the efficacy of the CPOE systems. Currently only about 2% to 5% of hospitals are using CPOE (Briggs, 2003). Many hospitals, after investing millions of dollars, have abandoned CPOE systems because of a revolt by the care provider (Payne et al, 2003). Poor training and system usability seem to be the root causes of these problems (Kuperman & Gibson, 2003). Oftentimes these systems were created by replicating bad paper models and did not have the end users involved in the development process. Although some hospitals have failed in implementing CPOE systems, there are also many hospitals with successful implementations. Among these success stories, studies have indicated that benefits such as a reduction in medical errors, improved quality of patient care, and a positive effect on costs of health care are directly related to CPOE systems (Mekhijan et al, 2002; Saathoff, 2005).

Pharmacy

Several pharmacy-related electronic information systems have been introduced in recent years that have reduced medication errors. Many ICUs have adopted electronic dispensing systems to help ensure that the ordered medicine is given to the correct patient. Bar-code medication administration has also been widely adopted. With such a system, bar codes on the medication are scanned along with an identification band on the patient, ensuring that the selected medication is given to the selected patient without worry of poor drug interactions. These systems require bar codes to be assigned to a patient and to each prescription filled by the pharmacy. For these systems to be most effective, a medication history must be made available to the pharmacy, and someone must be available to enter the historical data.

Other Systems

In addition to the systems outlined, many other IS systems exist within hospital settings providing data regarding a patient's condition. Imaging systems to store and display radiographs, computerized tomographic (CT) scans, and magnetic resonance imaging (MRI) results are widely available. Lab systems that can send information to the HIS or store the results locally are being used by most modern hospitals.

An underlying layer of complexity with all of the mentioned systems is the hardware that is used to display the data. For example, most hospitals' information systems are hardwired, requiring a clinician to view and document patient data at a stationary computer. A rapidly emerging option is to make most interfaces wireless, allowing mobile access to patient information. Wireless solutions include notebook personal computers (PCs), personal digital assistants (PDAs), tablet PCs, smart phones, and mini-PCs. Currently no one solution has emerged as a preferred option in health care (Schuerenberg, 2005).

The problem with having so many different information systems is that ensuring accurate communication between systems is difficult. Such difficulties as code differences among systems, multiple logins, variable security protocols, and reducing data redundancy all point to a more complex integration problem.

INTEGRATING COMPUTER INFORMATION SYSTEMS

Integration issues can be likened to language barriers. Suppose your organization's flow sheet system was in Spanish, your daily notes system in Russian, and your pharmacy system in Chinese. Obviously communication would be difficult unless you spoke all three languages, or had interpreters. In informatics, the "interpreter" that would make these systems communicate is called an interface. Currently interfaces are necessary because each independent system (flow sheet, daily notes, pharmacy, laboratory, etc.) within a hospital needs to communicate patient information with the other systems and with the end users. Although interfaces are currently necessary as a solution, they are not perfect. In intensive care units, optimal clinical care currently depends on clear integration of many different kinds of timely and accurate data. The data needed to support bedside clinical decision making are generated in many departments throughout the hospital. Caregivers such as nurses, respiratory therapists, doctors, social workers, and physical therapists all contribute a specific set of important clinical observations to the clinical data matrix.

Current hospital systems integrate critical clinical information and convey it to the caregiving team in a myriad of ways. Communication efforts currently involve both formal and informal methods, including charting on large paper flow sheets, printed laboratory reports, verbal reports, dictation, and handwritten or typed progress notes. Interestingly some of these methods that are paper based exist within a partially computerized system due to poor integration and virtually no interface between departments. Current practices using paper are notorious for being time consuming, illegible, and laborious. They are also error prone, allow only limited access (only one user can view at any one time), create storage nightmares, and have data redundancy. Furthermore, the problem is complicated because any new computer systems installed oftentimes are not able to integrate with the original, or "legacy" systems, some of which were developed as far back as the 1970s. Future systems would obviously work to correct many of these problems. Costs are another factor to consider. Sharing information data is complicated by the sometimes exorbitant costs associated with the middle-ware or integrator system. Unless these costs are reduced, many health care delivery systems will not be able to afford to share data effectively.

The ideal future method of communication would automate and integrate, in real time, all bedside information, laboratory results, medications, daily notes, and order entry directly into a centralized system. This centralized system would also have a decision support element that notices trends occurring in the patient, alerts the clinician, and recommends possible interventions. Additionally, this type of system provides data to hospital administrators so that decisions can be made regarding staffing, billing, materials management, and quality assurance, to name a few.

To make the leap from current to future systems, hospitals are faced with hundreds of different products from which to choose. Prior to 1996, many of the larger products boasted that they were a "complete system," but did not use standardized communication methods. The companies creating these products were unable to come to an agreement as to a unified common standard, and as a result the government created a law, titled HIPAA, that attempts to mandate development of a common computer communication standard.

Intercommunication Standards and HIPAA

Background of HIPAA
The Health Insurance Portability and Accountability Act of 1996 (HIPAA) (P.L. 104-191, Title II, Subtitle F) is one of the largest pieces of health care legislation in history. According to Friedrich (2001), HIPAA was passed with three main goals: (1) to improve access to health insurance, (2) to reduce fraud and abuse, and (3) to increase the efficiency and effectiveness of the health care system. The initial goal of increasing accessibility is twofold. One aspect is related to making health insurance portable and continuous for those changing employment locations. The second aspect deals with deterring insurance companies from rejecting individuals with pre-existing health conditions. Friedrich also explains that the second goal of HIPAA, related to fraud and abuse, and the third goal, related to increasing the efficiency and effectiveness of health care, fall under the Administrative Simplifications section of HIPAA (2001). The Administrative Simplifications involve the development of both computer communication standards and writing regulations for accessing,

transmitting, and storing medical data. There are two broad types of regulations according to Friedrich (2001). There are standards related to electronic transmission of data and those intended to ensure the security and privacy of patient information.

The HIPAA legislation mandated that specific code sets and computer communication strategies (both called "standards") be decided and implemented by specific dates, now all past. The start dates for use of HIPAA-mandated coding and interconnection strategies were between 2003 and 2005. The foundational work for completing health care computer communication standards is in progress now. No one "standard" was, or is, completely finished. Standards-setting groups meet regularly. These groups are mostly voluntary. Overcoming the proprietary interests of vendors, which have a large vested interest in proprietary (secret) software, communication strategies, and clinical expression codes, did require the federal HIPAA legislation. New systems will be required to be "HIPAA compliant." At the time of this writing (fall 2005), all aspects of HIPAA compliance rules are an enormous "work in progress."

HIPAA Mandates
Codes Set Standards. Before HIPAA, there were no communication standards in place for health care providers and payers to transfer information electronically. More than 400 different formats for electronic transactions had been created for communications between providers and health plans (DHHS, 2000). HIPAA reduced the number to eight clinical code sets and two electronic transaction/computer communication standards for health care administrative and financial communications (U.S. Department of Health and Human Services [DHHS], 2000). Congress made major operational modifications to the original plan in response to comments, problems, and evolving situations in May 2002 (DHHS, 2002).

Codes in HIPAA-defined health care rules are precisely formatted numbers and letters that match some clinical concept, such as a diagnosis, medication, or treatment. Communication standards provide a specific place assignment where programmers insert needed coded information, such as a patient identifier, whether they are writing a lab system, a clinical system, or an administrative system. The HL7 (Health Level 7) and ASC_X12N computer communication standards provide uniform programming structure so different vendors of clinical, lab, or hospital information systems can send medical and administrative information to each other, meaningfully.

A *code set* is any organized system of codes for listing data elements, such as tables of terms, medical diagnosis codes and medical procedure codes (DHHS, 2002). Code sets now defined under the HIPAA legislation are considered code set standards. Examples of these include ICD-9-CM, HCPCS, CPT, CDT, and NDC. ICD-9-CM (International Classification of Diseases, 9th or 10th Edition, Clinical Modification) is used for diagnoses and hospital patient service codes. To report supplies, durable medical equipment, and generic drugs under Medicare plans, HCPCS (Health Care Financing Administration Common Procedural Coding Systems) is employed (DHHS, 2002). CPT (Current Procedural Terminology) is mandated for coding physician services. Dental services are coded under CDT (Current Dental Terminology), and NDC (National

Drug Code) is used only for medications and drug systems for retail pharmacies (DHHS, 2002).

Computer communication standards defined under HIPAA include ASC_X12N and HL7 standard programming structures. ASC_X12N, Version 4010 (Accredited Standards Committee, 2005) is used for health claims, attachments and encounters, payment and remittance advice, claim status, eligibility, referrals, health care enrollment, health plan premium payments, and first report of injury. This communication standard condenses more than 400 transaction formats with one set of specific transaction standards that are formatted in one language (DHHS, 2000). HL7 (Health Level Seven), is an accredited Standards Developing Organization (SDO) that produces standards (sometimes called specifications or protocols) for a particular health care domain such as pharmacy, medical devices, imaging, or insurance (claims processing) transactions. Health Level Seven's domain is clinical and administrative data (HL7, 2005).

As you can see, the elements defining the aforementioned code set standards are independent, not interdependent. Problems therefore quickly arose with initial attempts to apply HIPAA administrative code set standards to computerized clinical medical records. According to Chute (2002), most HIPAA-approved code-set vocabulary standards such as ICD-9 and CPT could lose more than half the underlying, detailed clinical information because these code sets were originally established for billing purposes. Loss of pertinent clinical details needed for bedside care and communication can be detrimental for the patient, the providers, and the institution. Because of the obvious need for standard vocabularies in the clinical setting (medical, nursing, and laboratory), the Office of the National Coordinator for Health Information Technology (ONCHIT) was established in late 2004 to coordinate these efforts (AAP, 2005; DHHS, 2005). The hoped-for outcome of these efforts is rapid development of complete clinical code-set standards for care-based computerized patient records.

Different from the foregoing HIPAA-defined code-set standards, clinical code-set standards either in use or nearly ready for release are SNOMED (Systematized Nomenclature of Medicine), NIC (Nursing Interventions Classification), NOC (Nursing Outcomes Classification), NANDA (North America Nursing Diagnosis Association), and LOINC (Regenstrief Institute, Indianapolis, IN) (Logical Observation Identifiers Names and Codes). The "SNOMED CT (Systematized Nomenclature of Medicine Clinical Terms) core terminology contains over 366,170 health care concepts with unique meanings and formal logic-based definitions organized into hierarchies" (SNOMED, 2005). NIC, NOC, and NANDA are independent code sets used for documentation of nursing diagnoses, treatments, and outcomes. Each of the three have issues such as an inability to combine and link unique concepts as a single concept, poor coding, and an inability to reduce concepts to an anatomic level. A large group of nursing informaticists is currently working in the "Vocabulary Unification Summit" to unify and modernize the three code sets into a single well-designed code set for computerizing nursing processes (Ozbolt et al, 2001). Last is LOINC (Regenstrief Institute, Indianapolis, IN), which facilitates "the exchange and pooling of results, such as blood hemoglobin, serum potassium, or vital signs, for clinical care, outcomes management, and research" (Regenstrief, 2005).

Identifiers. Identifiers are numbers assigned to health care providers (individuals, groups, or organizations) that deliver medical services, other health services, or medical supplies. The final rule for the National Provider Identifier (NPI) was published in January 2004 (Centers for Medicare and Medicaid Services [CMS], 2005). However, the proposed rules for assigning unique identifiers to employers and health plans are not yet fully operational (Gue, 2004). Employee identification numbers (EINs) are under scrutiny because the number to be used was determined by the Internal Revenue Service to be the taxpayer identifying number, also known as the social security number (SSN). This was thought to be a good idea since most employees should already have a social security number assigned before being hired by an organization. However, the use of the SSN has caused controversy because health information and financial information will be directly linked to the same number. National Health Plan Identifiers (NHPIs) are also undetermined at this time (CMS, 2005).

Privacy. Before HIPAA, legal protection of patients' privacy and confidentiality was fragmented across state, federal, and commercial insurance systems, which left many gaps in patient privacy (Hebda et al, 2001; DHHS, 2001). Evolving, implementing, and testing patient privacy rules under HIPAA law is an ongoing process. The effective compliance date was April 14, 2003. Confusion at every level still persists because of various degrees of interpretation of the law (Murray, 2005).

The Privacy Rule was constructed in hopes of protecting verbal, written, or electronic personal health information (PHI) that can be traced to an individual. This PHI refers to any record containing any of the 18 elements defined as personal health data (e.g., name, birth date, social security number, address). The rule protects PHI not only within the walls of the hospital but also while it is in transit to other locations (Friedrich, 2001). The rule applies to health plans, health care clearing houses, and those health care providers who electronically conduct financial and administrative transactions (DHHS, 2001). Consent must be obtained from the patient prior to any release of their private information for treatment, payment, or other health care operations. Patients will have the right to restrict the use and disclosure of their information, and the option to file formal complaints if their privacy has been violated. All shared data must be stripped of PHI information unless sharing is authorized by the patient. In addition, patients must have full access to their medical records (DHHS, 2001).

Security. Security regulations refer to technical protection of computerized PHI that is transmitted electronically within and among provider and payer organizations. Security standards have three categories: (1) administrative security, such as access controls and contingency plans; (2) technical security mechanisms, such as authorizations and audit controls; and (3) physical security, such as limits on physical access to workstations (Hirsch, 2003). Although these three categories are different, the security measures proposed in each category require similar forms of intervention.

For clinical users, HIPAA has created a very tenuous balance between security and usability (Dawes, 2001). For example, many paper-based units have removed all charts from the bedside, including flow sheets, to keep the patient's data more secure. This poses a workflow problem, especially in an ICU, because that information is best served at the bedside. In computerized systems, excess security has become a burden because hospitals are requiring excessive password usage to gain access to EMRs. In an emergency this process tends to delay patient care when it is needed most.

Penalties. According to the U.S. Department of Health and Human Services (DHHS, 2001), there are two types of penalties: civil and federal criminal. For a civil penalty, the minimum fine for failure to comply with a standard is $100 per violation with a maximum of $25,000 for identical violations per year for each requirement violation. Criminal charges start at $50,000 with a maximum of 1 year in prison for wrongful disclosure (DHHS, 2001).

Clearly there are numerous layers of complexity when considering clinical information systems. Various types of information systems are available to consider for all aspects of the delivery of patient care. However, even more important is to consider whether and how these systems communicate or integrate with one another. Whether your NICU is in the process of replacing an entire HIS, or making a smaller change such as an automated flow sheet, it is important to use a formal process to evaluate and select the system that is the best fit for your organization.

INFORMATION SYSTEM EVALUATION, SELECTION, AND IMPLEMENTATION

Bedside caregivers in the NICU need to have an understanding of general guidelines for evaluation, selection, and implementation of information systems into their hospital organization. Bedside caregivers *must* play an integral role in this extensive and elaborate process. The bedside caregivers who interact with the clinical information system on a daily basis are called *end users*. End users help to define the requirements of the system in the early stages of evaluation and to give input during the selection process. End user satisfaction is the key to the successful implementation of a system. We now give a brief overview of these important processes to ensure that modern-era bedside caregivers have an understanding of their roles and expectations during selection and implementation of a NICU information system.

Researching Information System Solutions

Many hospital organizations are initiating the switch from paper-based charting systems to electronic charting systems. This type of project is a massive undertaking for a hospital, both financially and logistically. Therefore, for future purchases, most hospitals are beginning to develop structured planning, purchasing, and implementation processes in an effort to avoid future project failures.

The first stage in the system evaluation and selection process is to identify the problems with the current system. Then it is important to research alternative technologic solutions to the identified problem, or enhancements that might correct it. Often a multidisciplinary (IT, IS, clinical, and administrative representation) approach to these brainstorming sessions yields enough ideas to structure a more substantial search. Initially a Request for Information (RFI) can be directed to vendors that specialize in clinical information systems. The vendor will in turn reply with introductory product information. An RFI is a standard and affordable business process that is used to collect information about the capabilities of various products. The RFI is normally formatted

so it can be used as an initial assessment tool for comparing vendors (Amatayakul, 2004).

Once the vendor list is at a manageable size, a more detailed comparison process begins, using a Request for Proposal (RFP). The main purpose of the RFP is to document the vendor's claims in terms of system functionality, support, training, cost, and implementation approach, including staff education. The hospital's Informatics or Information Systems (IS) department will likely compose this document. However, at this step, input from the end users (practicing clinicians) is vital. An RFP should be created for an individual unit and include its unique workflow issues. When you use an individualized approach, it is harder for the vendor to provide broad, generic answers that may be technically capable, but do not really address your specialized requirements.

One of the most essential sections of the RFP describes the system's functional and technical requirements. Functional requirements are developed using input from bedside caregivers based on the daily workflow needs and data management goals for the specific unit. These detailed requirements are listed by the requesting hospital in a table format. Technical requirements pertain to issues such as network and hardware specifications that are required to make the system run (Amatayakul, 2004). Response columns should be provided for the vendor to reply to each requirement in terms of how their system meets each specification. Each requesting hospital should provide a predetermined response key similar to a scoring system for the vendor to use. The pre-established response key assists the purchasing team in making cross-vendor comparisons.

In addition to the functional and technical requirements, the implementation and maintenance plan for the proposed system should be requested of the vendor. In the RFP response, the vendor should provide, in writing, their plan for implementation, training, and support of their system (Amatayakul, 2004). These components can make or break the success of the system. Finally, the RFP should request a detailed cost matrix of all aspects of the vendor's system and its implementation.

The completed RFP is sent out, and formal proposal replies are expected within weeks. If composed appropriately, the RFP will require the vendors to comb through their systems to verify that they meet the details of the request. Their responses will contain information that will allow a thorough evaluation and selection process.

Evaluation and System Selection

As the vendor proposals return, it is important for the IS or Informatics department to begin the evaluation process. A metric scoring scale can be applied to the objective sections of the submitted proposals. The objective sections include the functional, technical, and financial requirements. The scoring scale allows the hospital to evaluate the vendor's systems objectively and consistently. A numerical weight value will be assigned to each response. For example, a response of "Not available" should receive a weighted score of zero, whereas a response of "Available and already successfully installed in a health care facility" should receive the highest weight on the response key scale. All objective sections of each vendor's proposal can be scored based on their responses. Then a summary table can be created to display the final numeric results and ranking of each vendor.

Financial comparisons evaluate whether the requesting hospital can afford the high-scoring vendors. Typically, the financial department of the hospital assists in this phase. Several financial evaluation tools are commonly used. A cost-benefit analysis (CBA) is traditionally done by comparing the cost of each system to the proposed benefits. However, the CBA is purely an estimation approach and incorporates such concepts as "intangible" benefits that are difficult to quantify for parallel comparisons. A second approach is a cost-effectiveness analysis (CEA), including a Payback Analysis, a Return on Investment (ROI) estimation, and Net Present Value (NPV) assessment. The ROI and Payback Analysis are both methods that determine the time for each system to repay its costs. Once a system pays for itself, cost savings for the hospital will begin. The NPV calculates the value of each system at any given time, and thus determines the profitability in today's dollars (Amatayakul, 2004). Typically, the financial department performs these analyses. End users who are active in the selection process should be familiar with commonly used comparison methods.

Once the objective scoring is complete and the cost analyses are done, vendors should be ranked according to their scored percentages. This ranking acts as a consistent comparison tool to determine which vendor best meets the hospital's desired criteria. This process is important because the purchasing organization must be able to quantify necessary functions for their desired system.

Finalist vendors' products can be further evaluated in many ways. One way to evaluate a finalist is reference checks—using telephone interviews of the specific vendor's clients to get an overall feel of client satisfaction with the vendor's installed system (Amatayakul, 2004). A standard questionnaire is another useful telephone tool that can again compare client feedback on an equal basis. There are several Web-based agencies that conduct and publish results of satisfaction surveys that can be helpful to a buyer.

The next step is to conduct on-site vendor demonstrations. Demonstrations are necessary for end users to test whether their functional requirements can actually be met. A demonstration evaluation tool should be created to assess how each system functions with actual daily workflow for the particular unit. Part of the tool should use case scenarios that are unique to the unit and also taxing to a system. An example of such a scenario might be: "Demonstrate the admission of unnamed triplets where two were born before midnight and one was born after midnight." The demonstration tool should also assess usability and functionality of clinical documentation. For example, "What happens if a nurse is documenting an assessment but gets called away from the bedside before finishing? Is his/her work saved and time-stamped?"

The final step of product evaluation is to conduct site visits at other hospitals. Select similar hospital units that currently use the information system of interest. To obtain a true picture of how the system functions, it is best to conduct these site visits without the vendor present. It also allows the end users to express how they really feel about the system (Amatayakul, 2004). The site visit team should be multidisciplinary for gathering feedback from various perspectives, including different types of end users (i.e., nurses, respiratory therapists, doctors). The site visit team should use the same evaluation tools that were used in the vendor demonstration to observe and evaluate the product function during real-life scenarios

in real time. It is also important for the site visit team to note the physical layout of the unit and how the system fits into the staff's workflow. For example, is there a computer terminal in each patient room, or do the staff share one terminal for several patients? If the computers are mobile, do they easily fit into each patient room, or do the patient's visitors have to leave before the computer can come in? The site visit team can apply the on-site observations to their own NICU. In addition to environment and workflow observations, a site visit questionnaire can be created to gather more structured information from current end users.

As the evaluation process closes, a final decision-making team should review (1) subjective and objective information; (2) reference telephone interviews; (3) demonstration evaluation tool results; and (4) site visit feedback from questionnaires. Hospitals usually select a finalist and a runner-up vendor. The two finalist vendors' supporting information is presented to the project steering committee (i.e., the final decision makers). This committee will likely include representation from high-level executives (CEO), financial personnel (CFO), nursing (CNO), medical (CMO), IS/Informatics (CIO), and so forth. Once the selection is made and contract negotiations are finished, the implementation phase will begin.

Implementation

The key to a successful system conversion (i.e., switching the old system out and bringing the new system in) is a well-thought-out implementation plan. A project implementation team should include end-user representation, IT personnel, and vendor representation. End users who are bedside caregivers are integral to the installation process, because they provide functional knowledge for both the system design team and the training team. IT team members can provide technical services and schedule planning tools to ensure a smooth transition. Team members from the vendor facilitate local customization efforts and training based on their full understanding of their system's inner workings.

The implementation team is responsible for (1) installing hardware and software; (2) educating themselves on 100% of the system's functions; (3) customizing the system; (4) testing the system; (5) creating implementation and user documentation; (6) educating users hospitalwide; (7) overseeing the actual system conversion; and (8) conducting the postimplementation evaluation. The first five steps typically are done by the hospital's implementation team before conversion. These steps make the system mesh with the subtle nuances of the hospital or the particular unit (i.e., the NICU). The last three steps rely heavily on end-user participation. The success of the system conversion is judged based on actual usability by the intended users in the clinical environment.

Before the installation of the hardware (monitors, keyboards, etc.) and software (instructions for the computer), the IT staff on the implementation team should verify the physical layout of the unit and should check and supplement power sources, lighting, noise, and privacy limitations. IT staff should walk through the unit with end-user representatives while they visualize and verbalize issues unique to the unit. This step (a "cognitive walkthrough") helps prevent surprises and delays during the systemwide installation process.

Meanwhile, the vendor representatives of the implementation team should initiate system education and training of the end users within the team. The first end users trained will eventually become the trainers (Amatayakul, 2004). The end user-trainers need to know the operation of the system, its limitations, and backup plans in the event of an unexpected system shutdown.

System customization, the third responsibility of the implementation team, ensures that the system is tailored to meet the unit's workflow needs. For example, the NICU may want to integrate the hospital laboratory list within the new system, so they can view the results of ordered lab tests. It is important for the implementation team to determine that all customization or modification requests are sensible. Sometimes the customization process becomes unrealistic as individual end users' desires expand. For example, one user may want to view vital signs with heart rate as the initial value while another user may prefer the temperature first. Usually an entire NICU must form a consensus of how the standard data are to be represented. Keep in mind that many small modifications to the system usually are needed within the first 6 months of the installation. Expect to give the vendor reasonable time to make those changes.

System testing is a very important responsibility of the implementation team. As customization occurs, it is important to verify that the system is working properly with the new changes. The testing steps should be done by members of the team who are not affiliated with the vendor. Each module of the system should be thoroughly tested for functionality using actual clinical situations. Clinical scenarios should include a sample of the most complex as well as common cases managed on the unit. The flow of data between modules should be verified and validated. System response times should be tested at peak volume of staff using the system simultaneously. All system tests must be fully documented for historical and legal purposes.

As the system is being customized, modified, and thoroughly tested in the NICU, the implementation team begins to create and revise the system's documents. User guides and educational material are created during this phase. Typically, materials supplied by the vendor will need to be updated because of local changes made to the product. The hospital education department should be included at this phase to aid with hospitalwide training.

The hospitalwide end-user education phase should start a few weeks before the "go-live" (conversion) date. The users need to know what to expect of both the system and the rollout process. They should feel prepared for the upcoming change. Choose several "super users" who are computer savvy end users and are eager to help roll out the new system. In terms of system training, a diffusion approach tends to be the most successful. With the diffusion approach, super users, once trained, can train their co-workers with enthusiasm and real-life scenarios. It is best if the initial exposure to the system is in a quiet, comfortable, and well-lit area. Distractions should be kept at a minimum so the training material can be fully absorbed. This session should not exceed 2 hours. If more time is needed, then subsequent sessions should be scheduled. After exposure to the system, move the users to the patient care setting. After go-live (see the following paragraph), trainers should be available in the unit around the clock until the end users are comfortable navigating and using the system.

When the implementation team has completed all planning, testing, documentation, and training steps, it is time for the final conversion or "go-live" step. There are several types of go-live options that have led to successful system conversions: (1) parallel conversion; (2) pilot conversion; (3) phased conversion; and (4) crash conversion. The parallel method involves running both the old and new system at the same time until the users are comfortable with the new system. This approach is time consuming and expensive, but is safe in terms of bridging documentation gaps. The pilot conversion involves changing only one unit at a time. This approach is timely and effective for some organizations. The phased conversion involves installing application modules individually throughout the hospital. This phased conversion takes a considerable amount of time, but may ease the users into the system at a more comfortable rate. The crash approach involves shutting off the old system and turning on the new system. This approach can be quite stressful for the end users and may lead to poor patient care. However, if the staff are adequately trained and are comfortable with the new system, this approach may be optimal, especially if the new system solves many pre-existing problems. Each hospital should carefully weigh the pros and cons of each approach before choosing the best go-live scenario.

A postimplementation evaluation should be made several months after the system conversion. Samples of the people directly involved in the conversion should provide feedback on the go-live process and on the system performance. This feedback may uncover gaps in the system use or performance. Structured feedback may also aid in the redesign of subsequent system conversion approaches. The postimplementation evaluation results should also be analyzed to evaluate operating costs, benefits, and system stability.

The implementation process requires careful planning and much work. Without a solid multidisciplinary implementation team, the system conversion could fail, costing the hospital millions of dollars. The implementation team's stepwise responsibilities are critical to the ultimate success of the system. By following the eight implementation guidelines just outlined, a hospital should be able to avoid pitfalls and complete a successful implementation.

SUMMARY

The intensive care environment has always depended on the most advanced technologies to care for patients. Traditionally these technologies have been limited to bedside devices. It is inevitable that the device-based technology will expand to include information systems. Information systems, such as the electronic medical record, are necessary to capture the data that these devices report throughout the ICU. With the help of advanced computer systems we can view and analyze patient data in ways that traditional paper-based methods cannot permit. As we evolve into the information age in health care, it is important that bedside caregivers have an understanding of the pros and cons of various types of information systems and the importance of an integrated system, as well as the complexities that arise when implementing such a system into their own hospital unit.

REFERENCES

AAP Division of Health Care Finance and Practice (2005). Alphabet soup: making sense of acronyms used by electronic health record organizations. *American Academy of Pediatrics news* 26(6):14.

The Accredited Standards Committee (ASC) X12 (2005). About ASC X12. Available at: http://www.x12.org/x12org/about/index.cfm. Retrieved October 1, 2005.

Amatayakul M (2004). *Electronic health records: a practical guide for professionals and organizations.* Chicago: AHIMA.

Badger S et al (2005). Rapid implementation of an electronic health record in an academic setting. *Journal of health care information management* 19(2):34-40.

Briggs B (2003). CPOE: Order from chaos. Available at: http://www.health datamanagement.com/html/current/PastIssueStory.cfm?PostID=14048&PastMonth=February&PastYear=2003. Retrieved October 20, 2005.

Centers for Medicare and Medicaid Services (CMS) (2005). HIPAA Administrative Simplifications—identifiers. Available at: http://www.cms.hhs.gov/hipaa/hipaa2/regulations/identifiers/default.asp. Retrieved October 20, 2005.

Chute CG (November 2002). Medical concept representation: from classification to understanding. Presented at AMIA Symposium 2002, San Antonio, Texas.

Cole WG (1996). Cognitive integration of data in intensive care and anesthesia. *International journal of clinical monitoring and computing* 13(2):77-79.

Collen MF (1995). *A history of medical informatics in the United States: 1950's to 1990.* Indianapolis, IN: Hartman.

Dawes B (2001). Patient confidentiality takes on a new meaning. *AORN journal* 73(3):596, 598, 600.

Friedrich MJ (2001). Health care practitioners and organizations prepare for approaching HIPAA deadlines. *Journal of the American Medical Association* 286(13):1563-1565.

Graves JR, Corcoran S (1989). The study of nursing informatics. *IMAGE: Journal of nursing scholarship* 21(4):227-231.

Gue DG (2004). HIPAA regs: national identifiers—how they fit into the HIPAA puzzle. *HIPAAdvisory.* Available at: http://www.hipaadvisory.com/regs/natlident.htm. Retrieved October 26, 2005.

Health Level Seven (HL7) (2005). What is HL7? Available at: http://www.hl7.org. Retrieved October 1, 2005.

Hebda T et al (2001). *Handbook of informatics for nurses and health care professionals,* ed 2. Upper Saddle River, NJ: Prentice Hall.

Hirsch R (2003). On HIPAA—the HIPAA Security Rule. *Healthcare informatics* 20(4):56.

Institute of Medicine (IOM) (1999). *To err is human: Building a safer health system.* Washington, DC: National Academies Press.

Institute of Medicine (IOM) (2001). *Crossing the quality chasm: a new health system for the 21st century.* Washington, DC: National Academies Press.

Institute of Medicine (IOM) (2003). *Capabilities of an electronic health record.* Washington, DC: National Academies Press.

Institute of Medicine (IOM) (2003). *Patient safety: achieving a new standard for care.* Washington, DC: National Academies Press.

Institute of Medicine (IOM) (2004). *Quality chasm summit.* Washington, DC: National Academies Press.

Institute of Medicine (IOM) (2004). *Keeping patients safe: transforming the work environment of nurses.* Washington, DC: National Academies Press.

Kuperman GJ, Gibson RF (2003). Computer physician order entry: benefits, costs, and issues. *Annals of internal medicine* 139(1):31-39.

Lindberg DAB (1987). NLM long range plan. Report of the Board of Regents. Bethesda, MD: National Library of Medicine.

Mekhijan HS et al (2002). Immediate benefits realized following implementation of physician order entry at an academic medical center. *Journal of the American Medical Informatics Association* 9(5):529-539.

Murray RBJ (2005). The subpoena and a day in court: guidelines for nurses. *Psychosocial nursing mental health services* 43(3):38-44.

Ozbolt J et al (2001). The nursing terminology summit: collaboration for progress. *Medinfo* 10(part 1):236-240.

Payne TH et al (2003). Preparation and use of preconstructed orders, order sets and order menus in a computerized provider order entry system. *Journal of the American Medical Informatics Association* 10(4):322-329.

Regenstrief Institute (2005). Logical Observation Identifiers Names and Codes (LOINC). Available at: http://www.regenstrief.org/loinc. Retrieved October 20, 2005.

Saathoff A (2005). Human factors considerations relevant to CPOE implementations. *Journal of healthcare information management* 19(4):71-78.

Schuerenberg BK (2005). How does mobile tech measure up? *Health data management* 13(7):42-50.

SNOMED International (2005). SNOMED CT. Available at: http://www.snomed.org/snomedct/index.html. Retrieved October 1, 2005.

U.S. Department of Health and Human Services (DHHS) (2000, last updated). *Frequently asked questions about electronic transaction standards adopted under HIPAA.* Available at: http://aspe.hhs.gov/admnsimp/faqtx.htm#whynational. Retrieved October 1, 2005.

U.S. Department of Health and Human Services (DHHS) (2001, May 9). *Protecting the privacy of patients' health information.* Available at: http://aspe.os.dhhs.gov/admnsimp/final/pvcfact2.htm. Retrieved October 1, 2005.

U.S. Department of Health and Human Services (DHHS) (2002, May 31). *Health insurance reform: modifications to electronic data transaction standards and code sets (45 CFR Part 162).* Available at: http://www.ebglaw.com/article_807.pdf. Retrieved August 23, 2006.

U.S. Department of Health and Human Services (DHHS) (2005). *Office of the National Coordinator for Health Information Technology (ONC).* Available at: http://www.hhs.gov/healthit. Retrieved October 1, 2005.

BIBLIOGRAPHY

Abbott PA (2001). *Implementation of health care information systems* [copyrighted presentation], Baltimore, MD.

Abbott PA (2001). *Standards for identifiers & codes & messages. Unit 8: Nursing terminology models; standards in HIS* [copyrighted presentation], Baltimore, MD.

Abbott PA (2001). *System selection documents* [copyrighted presentation], Baltimore, MD.

Adams K (2004). Hemodynamics assessment; the physiologic basis for turning data info clinical information. *AACN clinical issues* 15(4):534-546.

Adler K (2005). RFID in health care; the right strategies can minimize risk. *Health care informatics* 22(5):24.

Arzt N (2005). The new alphabet soup. *Journal of health care information management* 19(3):17-19.

Atack L, Rankin J (2002). A descriptive study of registered nurses' experiences with Web-based learning. *Journal of advanced nursing* 40(4):457-465.

Bichsel L et al (2003). Request for proposal (RFP) essentials. *Journal of cardiovascular management* 14(3):22-24.

Bishop P (2003). A new assessment tool: fetal oxygen saturation monitoring. *Nursing management* 34(3):37.

Bodenheimer T, Grumbach K (1998). *Understanding health policy a clinical approach,* ed 2. New York: Lange Medical Books/McGraw-Hill.

Briggs B (2004). Diagnostic images flowing among clinicians. *Health data management* 12(11):42-50.

Briggs B (2005). Safety innovators put I.T. on the line; some provider organizations are using technology to try to bring them under control. *Health data management* 13(5):46-54.

Carpenter J (1998). Practice brief. Issue: writing an effective request for proposal (RFP). *Journal of the American Health Information Management Association* 69(7, suppl 2):65.

Clemmer T (2004). Computers in the ICU: where we started and where we are now. *Journal of critical care* 19(4):201-207.

Coyle-Toerner P, Collins L (2003). How the clinical customization of an EMR means good business: a case study of Queen City Physicians. *Journal of medical practice management* 19(1):27-31.

Cross M (2004). Doctors to PDAs: 'Check, please.' *Health data management* 12(11):70-74.

Cross M (2004). Expanding the mobile menu. *Health data management* 12(12):50-54.

Featherly K (2005). Electronic health records. *Health care informatics* 22(2):42-46.

Featherly K (2005). IT and biomedical devices. *Health care informatics* 22(2):54-56.

Forgey D, Vickery J (2005). Informatics; how an emerging field of study benefits HIM. *Journal of AHIMA* 76(6):46-49.

Galt KA et al (2005). Instrument development: physician use of hand-held computers. *AHRQ advances in patient safety* 4:93-108.

Gassert CA (1990). Structured analysis: methodology for developing a model for defining nursing information system requirements. *ANS advances in nursing science* 13(2):53-62.

Gillespie G (2005). Systems integration; the electronic records linchpin. *Health data management* 13(5):34-44.

Gillespie G (2005). Involving physicians in I.T. decisions. *Health data management* 13(7):52-60.

Goedert J (2005). Medical devices meet electronic records. *Health data management* 13(8):38-44.

Hagland M (2005). Bar coding and RFID. *Health care informatics* 22(2):36-37.

Hagland M (2005). Interoperability conundrum; EMR implementation options go beyond core vendor and best of breed. *Health care informatics* 22(5):29-24.

Hagland M (2004). Reshaping radiology; change management and workflow optimization give PACS new punch. *Health care informatics* 21(11):24-28.

Haugh R (2000). Confronting HIPAA. *Hospitals and health networks* 74(3):58-62, 64.

Jossi F (2004). Electronic follow-up; bar coding and RFID both lead to significant goals—efficiency and safety. *Health care informatics* 21(11):31-33.

KLAS Market Intelligent Leaders (2005). *Vendors and firms evaluated.* Available at: http://www.healthcomputing.com/. Retrieved October 26, 2005.

Krohn R (2005). RFID: It's about more than asset tracking. *Journal of health care information management* 19(3):20-23.

Lee T (2004). Nurses' adoption of technology: application of Rogers' Innovation-Diffusion Model. *Applied nursing research* 17(4):231-238.

Lee T et al (2005). Factors affecting the use of nursing information systems in Taiwan. *Journal of advanced nursing* 50(2):170-178.

Makaryus AN, Friedman EA (2005). Patients' misunderstanding of discharge diagnoses and treatment plans. *Mayo Clinic proceedings* 80(8):991-994.

Malone E et al (2005). Developing and implementing a patient-centered IT strategy. *Journal of health care information management* 19(3):47-55.

Marietti C (2005). Regional networks. *Health care informatics* 22(2):62-65.

Mason D, Leavitt J (1998). *Policy and politics in nursing health care*, ed 3. Philadelphia: Saunders.

Matthews P (2000). Maximizing information systems purchases: a primer on system selections. *Nursing administration quarterly* 24(4):36-50.

McCaffree J (2005). The request for proposal: a primer. *Journal of American Dietetic Association* 105(4):522-523.

Meijden MJ et al (2003). Determinants of success of inpatient clinical information systems: a literature review. *Journal of American Medical Informatics Association* 10:235-243. First published online as doi:10.1197/jamia.M1094.

Nash P, editor (2002). Follow these steps for conducting a privacy gap analysis. *Briefings on HIPAA* 2(1):1-2, 7.

O'Connor KJ (2005). Everything you always wanted to know about software escrow agreements—and then some! *Journal of health care informatics* 19(1):10-12.

Poissant L et al (2005). The impact of electronic health records on time efficiency of physicians and nurses: a systematic review. *Journal of American Medical Informatics Association.* Published ahead of print on May 19, 2005, as doi:10.1197/jamia.M1700.

Schuerenberg BK (2005). An Rx for reducing medication errors; seeking to improve patient safety, providers are automating the medication administration process—despite some significant challenges. *Health data management* 13(5):68-76.

Schuerenberg BK (2005). CPOE progress: no guts, no glory. *Health data management* 13(6):28-36.

Smith K et al (2005). Evaluation the impact of computerized clinical documentation. *CIN: computers, informatics, nursing* 23(3):132-138.

Staggers N, Parks PL (1993). Description and initial applications of the Staggers and Parks nurse-computer interaction framework. *Computers in nursing* 11(6):282-290.

Tabar P (2000). Hello HIPAA! *Physician and sports medicine* 28(5 e.MD): 19-22.

Tang P (2000). The HIPAAcratic oath: do no harm to patient data. *Physician executive* 26(3):50-56.

Timmons S (2003). Nursing resisting information technology. *Nursing inquiry* 10(4):257-269.

Wikstrom A (2004). Technology—an actor in the ICU: a study in workplace research tradition. *Journal of clinical nursing* 13:555-561.

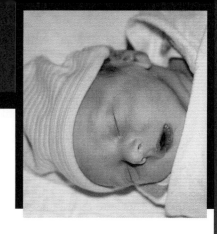

Chapter 32

Impact of Genomics on Neonatal Care

Carole Kenner • Kristie Nix

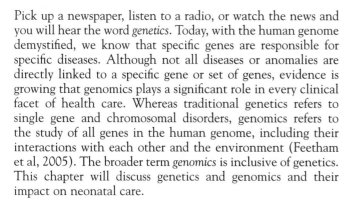

Pick up a newspaper, listen to a radio, or watch the news and you will hear the word *genetics*. Today, with the human genome demystified, we know that specific genes are responsible for specific diseases. Although not all diseases or anomalies are directly linked to a specific gene or set of genes, evidence is growing that genomics plays a significant role in every clinical facet of health care. Whereas traditional genetics refers to single gene and chromosomal disorders, genomics refers to the study of all genes in the human genome, including their interactions with each other and the environment (Feetham et al, 2005). The broader term *genomics* is inclusive of genetics. This chapter will discuss genetics and genomics and their impact on neonatal care.

INCIDENCE OF GENETIC CONDITIONS

Approximately 150,000 infants in the United States have a birth defect (March of Dimes, 2005). These include structural and metabolic disorders, congenital infections, and other environmental causes such as perinatal substance abuse. Thus some newborns have birth defects that have a genetic basis, whereas other newborns suffer from a genetic disease. The distinction is that a genetic disease results from an aberration in the infant's deoxyribonucleic acid (DNA), such as occurs with cystic fibrosis and sickle cell anemia (Scheuerle, 2001).

For many neonatal nurses, genetic mechanisms and the role of genes in disease were not part of basic nursing education. Typically, little information about genomics was included in the curricula beyond the mendelian laws or single gene inheritance. With the exponential increase in genomic information, an expanded genomic knowledge base is required. Families can easily obtain highly technical (and sometimes wrong) information about their infant's condition and the possible genomic basis for that condition. Health professionals must be knowledgeable about genomics and certain that families clearly understand their infant's condition. This chapter briefly discusses the new frontier of genomics as it relates to neonatal and infant care.

HUMAN GENOME PROJECT

The Human Genome Project (HGP) determined that each human comprises approximately 1 billion DNA base pairs that construct the body's protein. Genes make up only about 2% of the human genome, equating to about 20,000 to 25,000 genes (Human Genome Project, 2005).

The genetic code directs the body's cells in how to perform,

what to produce, and even when to die. It carries the "recipes" for the body's proteins, the building blocks of all tissues. When one of these recipes fails or is altered, so is the structure of the body. In some cases this alteration is so subtle that only the cellular level or genetic level is affected. In other cases, however, the mistake results in a disease or structural defect, such as occurs with neurofibromatosis or some forms of cancer.

A genomic map now shows which genes are located on what chromosome, and a region on the chromosome where defective genes are located. Although a condition may be known to be dependent on these defective genes for expression, the genes surrounding the defective ones may or may not be affected. However, the location gives the health professional a starting point to do some detective work about possible health risks.

Through the efforts of the HGP, medical science has gained knowledge of the specific locations of genes on specific chromosomes; this creates the opportunity to design therapies directly targeted to the defective gene. Pharmacogenomics, the science of genomic variation in drug response, will seek to engineer drugs to treat a person's unique genomic makeup (Feetham et al, 2005). Therapy will also take into account the interaction of the environment with an individual's genomic makeup. For example, exposure to second-hand smoke is linked to asthma, but asthma also has a genomic basis. So the interaction of genes with exposure may result in disease—asthma. Such specific knowledge also gives health professionals the opportunity to predict the likelihood that specific family members will develop certain conditions. Prenatal teaching or preconception education becomes more important in light of this new information. True health promotion, and in some cases disease prevention, can be a reality. Dr. Barton Childs (1998) refers to this move away from the disease model to consideration of genetic foundations as using a genetic lens to view health.

With scientific advances in genomics, health professionals have raised many concerns about the ethical dilemmas and legal issues arising from the HGP. The Ethical, Legal, and Social Implications (ELSI) Branch of the HGP has launched studies to analyze situations that pose problems for health professionals and for the children and families they serve. As the National Human Genome Research Institute (NHGRI) has pointed out:

> For some diseases . . . our ability to detect the nonfunctional gene has outpaced our ability to do anything about

the disease it causes. Huntington disease is a case in point. Although a predictive test for high-risk families has been available for years, only a minority of these individuals has decided to be tested. The reason? There is no way to cure or prevent Huntington disease, and some individuals would rather live with the uncertainty than with the knowledge they will be struck, sometime in midlife, with a fatal disease. And what might happen if a health insurance company or a potential employer learns that an individual is destined to develop Huntington disease; might that person be denied coverage or a job? (National Human Genome Research Institute [NHGRI], 2001).

Similar issues are being raised by advances in newborn screening and testing. Most screening is also genetic testing, as many of the conditions have a genetic underpinning. Tandem mass spectrometry (MS/MS) permits testing for more than 30 disorders. The ethical dilemma becomes: Should testing be done for conditions that have a poor prognosis or no effective treatment (Kenner & Moran, 2005)? Among the concerns to emerge were whether the tests should be mandatory or remain voluntary, and who would have access to the information. Discrimination in insurance coverage when a genetic problem is found is also a major ethical issue (Kenner & Moran, 2005). Only time, debate, negotiations, and perhaps legislation will determine the outcome of these ethical issues. However, when headlines in the popular press and the health professional literature proclaim linkages between sleep apnea, sudden infant death syndrome (SIDS), and genetics, it is difficult to view the negatives; if this linkage between a missing enzyme and SIDS is true, much good could be derived from this testing (Gaultier & Gallego, 2005).

Nurses must continue to advocate for infants and families; to do this, they must have a solid grounding in genomic knowledge, including foundational genetics starting at the molecular level. Knowledge of the molecular level starts with the structure of the DNA molecule and includes the coding pattern for a protein.

Deoxyribonucleic Acid

DNA is composed of two very long chains (strands) of interlocking nucleotides (Figure 32-1). Each nucleotide is composed of a molecule of any one of the following four bases: adenine (A), guanine (G), thymine (T), and cytosine (C). Adenine and guanine are purine bases; thymine and cytosine are pyrimidine bases. These bases are attached to a five-carbon sugar (a pentose arrangement called a ribose), which is connected to a phosphate group. The phosphate groups actually provide the linkage between the individual bases, forming the long strands. The phosphate connections therefore are the actual "backbone" of the DNA strand.

In human beings, DNA does not exist as a single strand; rather, the DNA is double stranded in an antiparallel arrangement. The two strands are not directly physically connected; instead, a number of relatively weak ionic forces hold the two strands in proximity. These ionic forces are different for the two groups of bases, and these differences are responsible for adenine always pairing with thymine (and vice versa) and guanine always pairing with cytosine (and vice versa). Thus the two strands of DNA are lined up together and are composed of interacting bases that form base pairs. Because the bases are specific in their attractions, the two

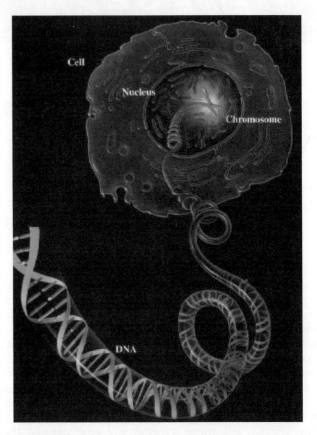

FIGURE **32-1**
DNA is composed of two very long chains (strands) of interlocking nucleotides. Courtesy National Human Genome Research Institute, Bethesda, MD.

strands of DNA are complementary in terms of their nucleotide sequence. If the sequence of one DNA strand is known, the sequence of the complementary DNA strand can be accurately predicted.

In its native state during the reproductive resting state of the cell (G0), the double-stranded DNA has a loosely coiled helical (double strand) arrangement. At various times in the cell cycle, the DNA becomes more tightly packed together by further coiling at well-regulated intervals around protein substances called histones; this gives the DNA the appearance of beads on a string. The complex of DNA wound around each histone is called a nucleosome. In addition to the histone proteins that come into contact with the DNA at specific points in the strand and at certain times in the cell cycle, nonhistone proteins are associated with the DNA. During cell division, the DNA must become even more tightly packed together to form dense structures called chromosomes. Each chromosome is composed of a relatively large section of DNA containing many genes.

The basic structure of chromosomes is presented in Figure 32-2. Most of the nomenclature currently used to describe specific areas or features of chromosomes is derived from the 1971 Paris Conference of the International Human Genetics Congress.

Chromatids are the two long structures that make up the two longitudinal halves of the chromosome, present during metaphase of cell division. Chromatids on the same chromosome are called sister chromatids. The point at which the two sister chromatids are joined is called the centromere.

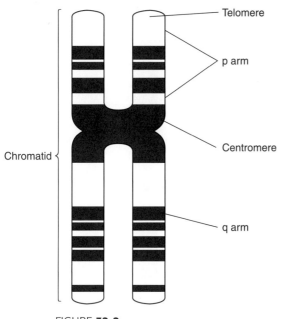

FIGURE **32-2**
The basic structure of chromosomes.

Many chromosome features are described in relation to the centromere. The portions of the chromatids above the centromere are shorter than those below the centromere and are called the p arms (or "short" arms). The portions of the chromatids below the centromere are called the q arms (or "long" arms). The distal ends of the chromosome are called the telomeres or the terminals.

Normally, human beings have 46 chromosomes (23 different pairs) in all cells except mature red blood cells and the mature sex cells (sperm and ova). This number, called the diploid number (2N) of chromosomes for human beings, constitutes the genome, or the complete set of human genes. Of the 23 pairs, 22 pairs are autosomal chromosomes (autosomes), which code for and regulate somatic cell development and function. One pair of chromosomes constitutes the sex chromosomes, which code for and regulate sexual development and function. Mature red blood cells have no nucleus and therefore have no chromosomes. Mature sex cells (gametes) have only 23 chromosomes (half of each pair). This number is known as the haploid number (1N) of chromosomes for human beings.

Genetic Testing
The constitutional chromosomes of an individual can be studied through a process called chromosome analysis (karyotyping), which can be performed only on dividing cells. This process involves obtaining a sample of sterile, living tissue that is capable of relatively rapid cell division. Blood lymphocytes or skin fibroblasts are most often used for this purpose. The tissue is incubated with nutrient fluids at 37° C for several hours to several days to encourage more cells to enter the reproductive cycle and proceed to the mitotic phase. The dividing cells are artificially trapped in the metaphase stage of mitosis, fixed with preservative, placed on microscope slides, stained, and evaluated under the microscope.

Chromosome analysis then is carried out through examination of karyotypes. Microscopic photographs of metaphase chromosomes are made, and from these photographs the chromosomes are karyotyped; that is, grouped in sequences of pairs according to the size of the chromosome pairs and the positions of the centromeres. Each group begins with the largest pair of chromosomes that has the centromeres most centrally located. Subsequent chromosome pairs are ordered according to descending size and more distally located centromeres. Analysis of the photographed karyotype can determine numeric chromosome aberrations. However, this method of chromosome analysis is haphazard because specific individual chromosomes cannot be identified precisely. There are approximately 1000 genes on each chromosome, but only about 100 genes in each band (i.e., the light and dark areas of the chromosome that appear using laboratory techniques) (Scheuerle, 2001).

A more sophisticated chromosome analysis is obtained when standard cytogenetic techniques are combined with the process of banding. Giemsa banding (G-banding) is the banding technique most often used for chromosome analysis. In G-banding, the fixed slides are exposed to a proteolytic enzyme (usually trypsin), which selectively digests areas of the chromosome, and the slide is then stained with Giemsa stain. The areas in which protein has been digested do not take up the stain, which leaves a white space (negative band) on the chromosome. The areas in which protein was not digested do take up the stain, leaving a dark area (positive band) on the chromosome. As a result of this process, each chromosome pair has a unique banded or striped appearance, which permits absolute identification of specific chromosomes (Figure 32-3).

Chromosome analysis that uses banding techniques can identify structural chromosomal abnormalities within individual chromosomes, as well as numeric chromosome abnormalities. However, even this technique has severe limitations, because the smallest chromosome area that can be observed under standard light microscopy has at least 10,000 base pairs. Many genetic disorders are known to involve deletions or rearrangements of genes much smaller than 10,000 base pairs.

Molecular testing is also used to determine whether an aberration is present; this technique involves examining the DNA directly. Another form of testing involves examining the gene directly; this test requires a knowledge of which gene alteration results in a specific disease process. A mutation that results in sickle cell anemia, for example, can be detected by this method of analysis, which uses allele-specific oligonucleotide (ASO) techniques (Scheuerle, 2001). The direct mutation technique depends on knowledge of the sequence of base pairs that is altered in a suspected disease. This technique can detect fragile X or a breakable area of a chromosome (Scheuerle, 2001). Linkage testing is used when one or more family members have a known genetic problem and the health professional wants to determine if the condition exists in the infant. The results of linkage testing are not considered diagnostic in the first person affected, but rather only after a second possibly affected family member has been identified. This testing is useful for diseases such as cystic fibrosis and Duchenne's muscular dystrophy.

Blood tests for DNA analysis are also used. These have been popularized for paternity issues and for use in criminal cases. The test is considered diagnostic. Protein tests performed on blood examine the structure of the protein. The test helps when a suspected protein structural defect is believed to be involved in the defect or disease, such as Ehlers-Danlos

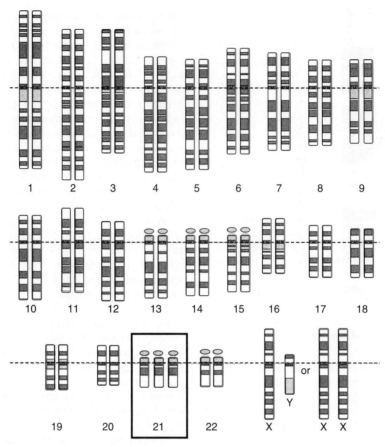

FIGURE **32-3**
Each chromosome pair has a unique banded or striped appearance, which permits absolute identification of specific chromosomes. Courtesy National Human Genome Research Institute, Bethesda, MD.

syndrome, osteogenesis imperfecta, and Marfan syndrome. Each of these conditions is a connective tissue or protein abnormality (Scheuerle, 2001).

Biochemical screening is used when a defect in the metabolic enzymes is suspected. Measurement of amino or organic acids results in identification of an abnormality. The technique is considered a screening test and must be followed by direct measurement of the enzymes for diagnostic purposes.

Cellular Division

For human beings, development begins when one haploid egg is fertilized by a single haploid sperm. The result of this union is a single cell containing the entire human genome, 23 pairs of chromosomes, half of each pair from the maternal gamete (egg or ovum) and half from the paternal gamete (sperm). For the one-celled organism to develop successfully into a complete human being, cell division by duplication is necessary. Duplication divisions occur through the process of mitosis.

Mitosis

Mitosis permits duplication division of one cell to form two daughter cells, which are identical to each other and to the original cell. The complete process of cellular reproduction, including actual mitosis, involves four phases, which collectively are called the cell cycle (Figure 32-4). The primary purpose of the processes involved in mitosis is to ensure that

each daughter cell precisely inherits the exact human genome. Although the process of mitosis usually results in an equal division of all cellular structures and contents for the two daughter cells, it is absolutely essential for function that the genetic material inherited by each daughter cell be identical to that of the original cell. The DNA synthesis phase, therefore, is a critical stage of cell division.

The cell cycle is actually a model depicting various activities that cells must accomplish for successful cell division that results in high-fidelity duplication. It is important to remember that the cell cycle refers only to the reproductive cycle of a cell; it does not take into consideration the cell's total life cycle. After development is complete, most cell types do not spend much time in the actual reproductive cycle. Rather, they exist as functional cell citizens that are performing all their specific and appropriate duties except reproduction. This nonreproductive state is called G0. Normal cells leave this state and enter the reproductive cycle only if (1) they are a specific cell type that is capable of cell division (some cells, such as neurons, skeletal muscle cells, and cardiac muscle cells, do not divide after development is complete); and (2) the particular cell type is needed for normal growth or replacement of dead or damaged cells.

G1 Phase

On entering the G1 phase of the cell cycle, the cell is committed to divide; this is an irreversible step for normal cells. At this time the cell takes on added nutrients to form

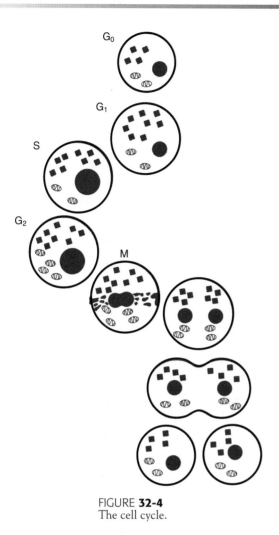

FIGURE **32-4**
The cell cycle.

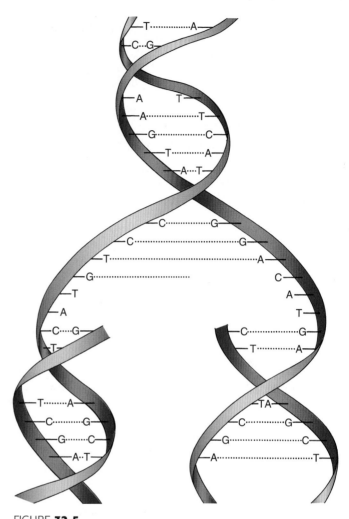

FIGURE **32-5**
The loosened strands separate into two single strands so that each single strand can be used as a template for the new DNA.

energy substances needed for the strenuous processes involved in actual cell division. In addition, the cell increases the fluid and membrane content to accommodate the needs of two cells.

S Phase

For each daughter cell to inherit the proper human genome, the DNA content of the original cell must first duplicate itself. The process of making more DNA to form a new cell is called DNA synthesis (S phase of the cell cycle), and it occurs entirely within the nucleus. The original strands of DNA temporarily loosen from the tight helical arrangement. The loosened strands separate into two single strands so that each single strand can be used as a template for the new DNA (Figure 32-5). A series of enzymes is required for this process.

To achieve duplication, the DNA strands relax; the strands unwind from the histones; and the helix straightens out slightly. An additional enzyme enters the straightened area and separates the two strands over a limited area. Another enzyme enters and prevents the two strands from rejoining. A different enzyme attaches itself to one strand, travels down it, "reads" the base sequence of this strand, and forms a new strand of DNA that is complementary to the one being read. This process is called the semiconservative mode of DNA synthesis because it results in two identical double helices, each containing one original strand of DNA and one newly created strand of DNA.

After the strands of DNA have been duplicated (replicated), they return to supercoiled chromosomes and line up so that they are ready to be pulled apart (split) during the M phase of the cell cycle. This splitting permits the two sets of DNA to become part of two new cells instead of just one cell.

G2 Phase

The G2 phase of the cell cycle is characterized by intense protein synthesis. The cell synthesizes all the enzymes and other complexes necessary to carry out the actual division of the cell, as well as the proteins needed for the regular "housekeeping" duties of the cell. Increased numbers of various organelles also are synthesized to meet the needs of two future cells.

M Phase

The actual part of the cell cycle in which two new cells are formed from the original cell is called mitosis, and it is the only time when the DNA is organized into chromosomes. This phase is further divided into subphases.

From the time the cell's DNA is duplicated in the S phase through the G2 phase, the cell's nucleus is said to be in interphase. During interphase the DNA is loosely coiled into nucleosomes and is widely dispersed throughout the nucleus. Only the nucleolus and two centrioles are distinguishable under standard light microscopy. At this time the two centrioles each begin to form a daughter centriole. As the cell leaves the G2 phase and begins the M phase, the DNA begins to condense. In early prophase, long spaghetti-like strands of newly formed chromosomes are discernible. Throughout prophase, the DNA continues to condense until recognizable chromosomes are present. Later in prophase, the centrioles move to opposite poles of the cell and begin to synthesize spindle fibers. During prometaphase, these spindle fibers attach to the kinetochores of chromosomes on or near the centromeres, and the nuclear membrane begins to disintegrate. During metaphase of mitosis, the chromosomes are in the most compact and readily visible structural forms. The chromosomes line up in the middle of the cell along the equatorial plane. At this point the cell enters anaphase of mitosis, during which the two sister chromatids of each chromosome are pulled apart toward the pole to which each is attached. This process is called nucleokinesis, indicating that the nucleus has moved and separated into two nuclei within the one cell. Under normal conditions, the chromosomes separate in such a way that the two daughter cells receive genetic components that are identical to each other and identical to those of the originating cell. The spindle fibers continue their pulling motion, and the cell begins cytokinesis, or the separation of the single cell body into two separate cell bodies, each with one nucleus. Cytokinesis is completed during telophase of mitosis, and at this time the DNA begins to loosen from the compacted chromatids. When the nuclear material is completely dispersed throughout the nucleus with only the centrioles and nucleolus discernible, the two new daughter cells are in interphase.

During early embryonic development, the initial fertilized egg with 46 chromosomes undergoes many duplication divisions, resulting in a large, hollow ball of cells (blastocyte), each with the same amount and organization of genetic material in its nucleus and exactly the same appearance and function. Although individual genes can undergo mutations after conception that result in altered gene expression, the actual genetic fate of this future human being, determined at the time of conception, is irreversible and cannot be changed.

At this point, these early embryonic cells are called undifferentiated because none of these cells has yet taken on the specific appearance (morphologic characteristics) and function or functions of the mature cell type it eventually will become. Obviously, something has to change during the course of development, because normal human infants are not born as large balls of undifferentiated cells.

Between 8 and 10 days after conception, the human embryonic cells initiate the steps that lead to differentiation. In response to an unknown signal or signals, each cell commits itself to a specific maturational outcome. At the time of commitment, the cell has not taken on any differentiated features or functions, but it now positions itself within a group that eventually will take on specific morphologic characteristics and functional behavior. The process of commitment involves turning off specific genes that regulated and directed the early rapid growth and turning on other specific genes that control the expression of particular differentiated functions. The uncommitted, pluripotent cell is

referred to as the stem cell. Stem cell transplants are used to treat leukemia and other forms of autoimmune suppression. Stem cell research has sparked considerable controversy over the use of fetal tissue in such experimental situations. Time, debate, negotiation, and perhaps legislation will surround these complex issues.

It is critical to remember that all differentiated somatic cells (body cells, not including sex cells) retain all the genes in the human genome. At one time the differences in appearance and function between cell types were explained by the theory that different cells actually "lost" the genes they did not need and retained only those required to reproduce and to perform special functions. We now know that this is not the way differentiation occurs and is maintained. Instead, all cells (excluding the sex cells) retain all genes. However, genes are selectively expressed or repressed in different cell types. For example, the gene for insulin is present in all cells; however, only in the beta cells of the pancreas is the insulin gene expressed, or "turned on," to meet the body's need for insulin production. There is nothing wrong with the insulin genes in other cell types (e.g., in skin cells or skeletal muscle cells); simply put, because the special functions of these other cells do not include the production of insulin, the insulin gene in these cells is maintained in a repressed, or "turned-off," state. This turning off of early embryonic genes appears to be accomplished through the activity of special repressor genes that function solely to repress the activity of the early embryonic genes so that they can no longer be freely expressed. This knowledge offers potential for future genetic treatment for many diseases.

Meiosis

The process by which early embryonic cells destined to become mature sex cells achieve maturation is somewhat different from that for somatic cells. Early in development, the committed sex cells continue to undergo mitotic cell division to increase their overall numbers. The cells resulting from these mitotic divisions continue to be diploid. Before the sex cells can completely mature, however, they must reduce their chromosome complement to the haploid rather than the diploid number through meiotic cell division.

Meiosis is the form of cell division that reduces the genetic complement of the cells by half, an actual reduction division that is different from the duplication division of mitosis. The result of meiosis is the production of new daughter cells that are identical to each other (in terms of their autosomes) but different from the originating cell. This process is necessary for gametogenesis, the final formation of sex cells. To accomplish this, the entire process of meiosis involves two completely separate series of cell divisions, one stage of which closely resembles a mitotic cell division. As a result of meiosis, four haploid cells are formed from a single diploid precursor sex cell.

As the precursor gametes (sex cells) prepare to become haploid gametes, each diploid precursor undergoes one round of DNA replication (synthesis), just as mitotic cells do in the S phase of mitosis. At this point in the process, the diploid precursor cell is now tetraploid (4N), with twice the normal number of chromosomes (92).

The cell now enters prophase of the first meiotic division. Each chromosome has two sister chromatids joined only at the centromere. Early in prophase, or meiosis I, the chromosomes condense and coil up, and the homologous pairs of chromosomes form a synapse. During synapse the homologous pairs of chromosomes associate with each other, lying side by side to form a tetrad with four chromatids. Because they are so close and because they are not yet compacted completely, some "crossing over" of genetic material occurs, both from the chromatids on the same chromosome (sister chromatids) and from the chromatids on the homologous pair (nonsister chromatids). Many genes are located on each chromatid. This crossing over of genetic material from nonsister chromatids has the effect of randomly "reshuffling" the maternally and paternally derived genes within the chromatids of homologous pairs, producing a wide variety of new combinations.

All the autosomes undergo this reshuffling process during synapse. The sex chromosomes have only a few limited exchanges at the telomeres. This limitation of exchanges is necessary because the chromatids of the X and Y chromosomes are different, each with unique areas. By not exchanging unique areas, the integrity of the sex chromosomes is maintained. In this way, the species continues with only two genders.

After synapse the two centrioles in the cell move to opposite poles on the nucleus and begin to form spindles. The synaptic pairs of chromosomes further condense and move to the equatorial plane of the nucleus, where metaphase of meiosis I begins; this stage is similar to metaphase in mitosis. The newly created spindles attach to the centromeres of the chromosomes. Contraction of the spindles causes whole chromosomes to be separated from chromosome pairs, but the newly reorganized chromatids of each chromosome remain together (anaphase I). At this point, disjunction occurs as the chromosomes form dyads or pairs of sister chromosomes, and the cell completes cytokinesis so that two new cells with 46 chromosomes each are formed. However, because of the crossing over that occurred during synapse and because the new chromosomes randomly assort into pairs, the two newly created cells do not contain the identical gene complement of the precursor sex cell that began the process of meiosis. The new combination of chromosomes cannot be equally separated by maternal and paternal origin. Although the two new cells each contain 22 pairs of autosomes and one pair of sex chromosomes, some of the pairs may be composed wholly of maternally derived chromosomes; others may be composed wholly of paternal chromosomes; and still others may be composed of varying combinations of maternal and paternal genetic material.

These two cells, which contain 46 chromosomes each (two copies of each chromatid), now spend some time in interphase before completing meiosis. The amount of time spent in interphase varies, with secondary oocytes remaining considerably longer in interphase (years) than secondary spermatocytes. No further duplication or synthesis of DNA occurs in these cells.

Meiosis is completed after the second meiotic division. In meiosis II, the two new interphase diploid cells created in meiosis I enter prophase and begin condensing their DNA so that chromatids are formed. The centrioles in each of the two nuclei separate to opposite poles and form spindles that attach to the centromere of each chromosome. The cells now enter metaphase as the nuclear membrane begins to disintegrate.

The chromosomes in each of the two cells move to the equatorial plane and line up. The spindles separate the chromatids. Each pair of chromosomes has four chromatids.

When these chromatids separate, one chromatid from each chromosome is segregated to each new daughter cell; each daughter cell therefore receives two chromatids from each pair of chromosomes. However, because the four chromatids segregate independently to the two daughter cells, there is no guarantee that each daughter cell will receive a chromatid from each chromosome of the chromosome pair. It is highly likely that for some chromosome pairs, the daughter cell will inherit two chromatids from one chromosome of a pair and none from the other chromosome.

The result of the entire process of meiosis is the formation of four haploid gamete cells from one diploid precursor sex cell. The crossing over of genetic material from homologous pairs of chromosomes during synapse with random assortment of chromatids in meiosis I, followed by independent segregation of chromatids in meiosis II, has some intriguing consequences. Even though all gametes are descended from the same clone of precursor sex cells and have identical genetic constitutions, the reshuffling of paternal and maternal whole genes and alleles (recessive as well as dominant) can result in hundreds or even thousands of possible minor variations in the genetic makeup of the gametes. Given this range of possibilities, the astounding fact is not that brothers and sisters sometimes do not resemble each other, but rather that they ever do.

PROTEIN SYNTHESIS

All cells that make protein have in their DNA the code for that protein, the actual gene for that protein. The unique DNA pattern (gene) for a specific protein is first converted into a piece of ribonucleic acid (RNA). RNA is similar to DNA, but instead of containing thymine (T), RNA contains uracil (U).

Proteins are formed by the linkage of individual nitrogen units, called amino acids, into a linear strand. There are 22 different amino acids; each has a unique three-base code sequence, called a codon, that identifies the DNA and RNA recipe specific for that amino acid. Some amino acids have only one codon, whereas others have as many as four different but closely related codons:

Amino Acid	RNA Codon
Methionine	AUG
Alanine	GCU, GCC
Valine	GUU, GUC, GUA, GUG
Phenylalanine	UUU, UUC

The total number of amino acids in a specific protein and the exact order in which they are connected determine the nature and activity of the protein. The making of protein, or protein synthesis, is similar to some of the steps in DNA synthesis, although carried out on a smaller scale.

The cell must loosen the area of DNA that contains the amino acid code (gene) for a specific protein such as insulin. The DNA in the region of the gene to be read loosens and unwinds slightly from the histones, using enzymes that are similar to those involved in DNA synthesis. Once the appropriate area of DNA has unwound and the two strands are separated and held open, a special RNA enzyme binds to the gene area of the DNA and reads it. When the enzyme recognizes a "start" signal, it moves along the strand and synthesizes a new strand of RNA complementary to the gene area of the DNA. When the enzyme reaches the end of the gene sequence, a "stop" signal tells the enzyme to stop making new RNA. The newly created RNA strand moves away from the gene. The DNA closes back together and recoils into the normal helical formation. The new piece of RNA is called messenger RNA (mRNA or sometimes just the "message") because it contains the special coded pattern sequence (the message) for building the specific protein (in this case, insulin).

After the mRNA has been transcribed from the gene, the mRNA interacts with two other types of RNA. Individual amino acids are present inside the cytoplasm, waiting to be properly aligned to form a protein, in a process called translation. Substances called ribosomes, which are made up of special bunches of ribosomal RNA, also are present, along with yet another type of RNA called transfer RNA (tRNA).

Transfer RNAs are adapter molecules that assist in bringing the correct amino acid into the lineup at the proper time. Each tRNA can carry or hold only one amino acid at a time, and the tRNA has an anticodon that is complementary to that specific amino acid's codon. Therefore, because each tRNA can bind to only one of the 22 different amino acids, there must be at least 22 different types of tRNA.

In the cytoplasm, the ribosome attaches to the mRNA strand and begins the reading process along the strand. When a three-base code is read and interpreted by the ribosome as a specific codon for a specific amino acid, the ribosome allows the tRNAs to come in and attempt to match their anticodons to the codon. When the correct tRNA matches up with the codon on the mRNA, that tRNA releases its amino acid and allows the amino acid to bind to the growing protein strand. This process is repeated all the way down the mRNA until all the correct amino acids are aligned in the right order to make the specific protein.

PATTERNS OF INHERITANCE

Gregor Mendel and others established general rules or concepts concerning the inheritance of specific traits governed by single genes. Much of the preliminary information was obtained through observation and manipulation of many generations of plant reproduction; however, these concepts proved to be generally accurate and applicable for the transmission of some human traits.

Mendelian Laws of Gene Expression

Mendel's work explained the concept of dominant and recessive traits. Through his observations of different types of garden peas, Mendel determined that specific varieties of peas had unique traits. For example, one variety of peas always produced wrinkled seeds when fertilized with pollen from the same pea type, whereas another variety of peas always produced smooth seeds when fertilized with pollen from its same pea type. Modeling out this information yielded the following table, in which P1 indicates the original parent generation; F1 indicates the first-generation offspring or progeny; F2 indicates the second-generation offspring or progeny; F3 indicates the third-generation offspring or progeny; and so forth for succeeding generations. Each generation of progeny was fertilized with pollen from the same generation.

Generation	Smooth Seeds	Wrinkled Seeds
P1	Smooth × smooth	Wrinkled × wrinkled
	↓	↓
F1	All smooth seeds	All wrinkled seeds
	↓Self-pollination	↓Self-pollination
F2	All smooth seeds	All wrinkled seeds
	↓Self-pollination	↓Self-pollination
F3	All smooth seeds	All wrinkled seeds
	↓Self-pollination	↓Self-pollination
F4	All smooth seeds	All wrinkled seeds

When Mendel experimented with cross-pollination (cross-breeding) of pea varieties, the inheritance of the traits came out differently than expected. The following model depicts Mendel's results when he fertilized a smooth pea variety with the pollen of a wrinkled pea variety.

P1 Smooth × wrinkled
F1 All smooth seeds
  Self-pollination
F2 Smooth and wrinkled seeds
  (3:1 ratio of smooth to wrinkled)

Mendel's explanation for this observation was that the trait for seed texture was determined by the inheritance of a pair of hereditary elements, now known as gene alleles (an allele is any possible alternative form of a gene), and that the relative "strength" of these two alleles varied. This variation in strength resulted in variable expression of the trait when the pair of hereditary elements was mixed (heterogeneous). When both parent seeds had the same hereditary element or genotypes (homogeneous), all the offspring in succeeding generations had the same appearance, or phenotype, of the expression of that element. For homogeneous pairs, the phenotypes and the genotypes were identical. When the parent seeds were heterogeneous for a particular hereditary element, the first-generation offspring expressed only the stronger or dominant element, even though both elements were present in all offspring. In this situation, the phenotype was different from the genotype; that is, the appearance of the peas in the F1 generation was smooth even though the hereditary elements for texture of these peas was heterozygous and consisted of one gene allele for smooth texture and one gene allele for wrinkled texture.

The mixed appearance of the peas in the second self-fertilized generation led Mendel to determine that the hereditary element (gene allele) for smooth texture was dominant and the hereditary element for wrinkled texture was recessive. Dominant traits could be expressed in the phenotype when the genotype for that trait was either homogeneous or heterogeneous, but recessive traits could be expressed in the phenotype only when the genotype for that trait was homogeneous.

Further experimentation with cross-pollination of plants led to the finding of codominance or incomplete dominance.

In cross-pollinating red roses with white roses in the parental generation, Mendel predicted that only the dominant color trait would be expressed in the F1 generation, with both colors being expressed in the F2 generation (in a 3:1 ratio). Because red was a stronger, bolder color, Mendel expected that the first-generation flowers from this cross-pollination would all be red. Instead, the roses in the first-generation progeny were all pink, indicating that the gene for red and the gene for white were equally dominant. Roses in the second generation of this cross-pollination were red, pink, and white in a 1:2:1 ratio. Therefore in codominance, the phenotype accurately expresses the genotype. Red roses must have two red gene alleles (homogeneous), pink roses must have one red gene allele and one white gene allele (heterogeneous), and white roses must have two white gene alleles (homogeneous).

The mendelian rules for patterns of inheritance apply only to traits or characteristics regulated by a single gene with multiple possible alleles.

Patterns of Traits Inherited by Single-Gene Transmission

A single gene, whether dominant or recessive, may control a trait. The locations of many genes have been specifically identified, or mapped, on human chromosomes. Even without establishing a gene's chromosomal location, it is possible to determine genetic transmission through multiple generations of a family, as specific patterns that indicate whether the gene is dominant, recessive, located on an autosomal chromosome, or located on one of the sex chromosomes. This information can be elucidated without identifying the specific gene through the use of family pedigree analysis. Determination of inheritance patterns for a specific trait allows more accurate prediction of the risk of trait transmission.

A pedigree graphically represents a person's medical and biologic history (Olsen et al, 2004). It is a schematic drawing of a family history (Figure 32-6), which allows a pictorial representation of patterns of inheritance over many generations. Construction of a pedigree involves the use of symbols denoting standardized pedigree nomenclature (Bennett et al,

1995). The pedigree usually is started with the proband (also known as the prepositus), the individual who draws medical (genetic) attention to the family. The proband usually is indicated with an arrow.

In analyzing a pedigree, the answers to the following specific questions are noted:

1. Is any pattern of inheritance present, or does the trait appear sporadic?
2. Is the trait transmitted equally or unequally to males and females?
3. Is the trait present in every generation, or does it skip a generation?
4. Do only affected individuals have children affected with the trait, or can unaffected individuals also have children who express the trait?

Construction of a pedigree as part of history taking:

- Facilitates note taking, increasing the accuracy of the history and serving as a means to organize collected information.
- Serves as a means of communication, allowing information collected by one health team member to be shared with other professionals working with the individual or family so that information is not repeated.
- Provides a means for professionals working with an individual or family to visualize and validate the relationships of affected individuals within a family scope. Creating a visual image of relationships may assist family members in clarifying who is or is not a blood relative of an affected individual.
- Facilitates the emergence of patterns of inheritance for a specific trait in a specific family.
- Enhances analysis of gene expression and transmission of more than one trait through linkage studies.
- Helps to identify individuals at risk within a kinship more accurately (these individuals then can undergo examination or receive counseling).

The four types of inheritance patterns associated with traits controlled by a single gene are autosomal dominant, autosomal recessive, sex-linked dominant, and sex-linked recessive.

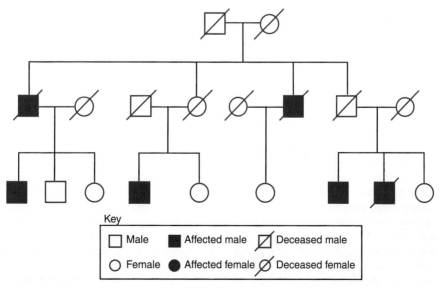

Key

| | Male | ■ | Affected male | ⊠ | Deceased male |
| ○ | Female | ● | Affected female | ⊘ | Deceased female |

FIGURE **32-6**
A pedigree. Courtesy National Human Genome Research Institute, Bethesda, MD.

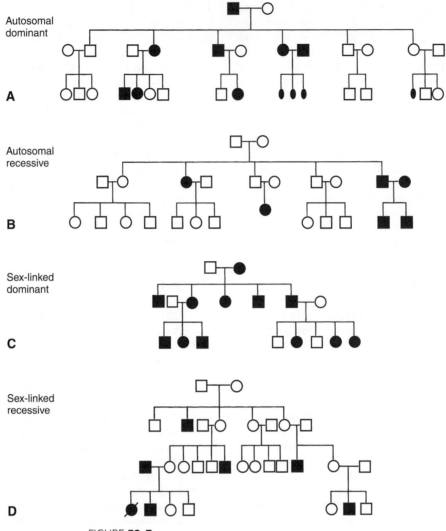

FIGURE **32-7**
Variety of typical pedigrees for a number of inherited traits.

Figure 32-7 shows a variety of typical pedigrees for a number of inherited traits. Each of these inheritance patterns is defined by specific criteria.

Traits with an Autosomal Dominant Pattern of Inheritance

Autosomal dominant single-gene traits require that the gene controlling the trait be located on an autosomal (nonsex) chromosome, and the trait usually is expressed even when the gene is present on only one chromosome of a chromosome pair. A typical autosomal dominant pattern of inheritance that meets all the defining criteria would be:

1. The trait appears in every generation with no skipping. When the trait is a result of a new mutation (de novo), this criterion is demonstrated only in the branch of the pedigree stemming from the person who first exhibited the new mutation.
2. The risk for affected individuals to have affected children is 50% with each pregnancy.
3. Unaffected individuals do not have affected children; therefore their risk is 0%.
4. The trait is found equally in males and females.

Autosomal dominant patterns of inheritance are associated with many normal variations in body structure, such as brown eye color, widow's peak hairline, and curly hair. In addition, this pattern of inheritance has been demonstrated in a variety of genetically transmitted problems, including achondroplasia, familial hypercholesterolemia, Huntington's disease, dentinogenesis imperfecta, brachydactyly, allergic hypersensitivity, Marfan syndrome, and familial hypercalcemia.

Traits with an Autosomal Recessive Pattern of Inheritance

Autosomal recessive single-gene traits require that the gene controlling the trait be located on an autosomal chromosome, and the trait can be expressed only when the gene is present on both chromosomes of a chromosome pair. A typical autosomal recessive pattern of inheritance that meets all the defining criteria would be:

1. The trait appears in alternate generations of any one branch of a kinship.
2. The trait or characteristic usually first appears only in siblings (progeny of unaffected parents) rather than in the parents themselves.

3. Approximately 25% of a kinship is affected and expresses the trait.
4. The children of an affected father and an affected mother are always affected (risk is 100% for each pregnancy). Two affected individuals cannot have an unaffected child.
5. Unaffected individuals who are carriers (have the gene on only one chromosome of a chromosome pair) and do not express the trait themselves can transmit the trait to their offspring if their mate either is a carrier or is affected. The risk of a carrier having a child who expresses the trait is 25% with each pregnancy when the carrier is married to another carrier, 50% with each pregnancy when the carrier is married to an affected individual, and 0% with each pregnancy when the carrier is married to a noncarrier. The risk of the unaffected carrier having a child who is a carrier for the trait is 50% with each pregnancy.
6. The trait is found equally in males and females.

Autosomal recessive patterns of inheritance are associated with many normal characteristics and variations in body structure and function, such as blue eye color, straight hair, and the Rh-negative blood type. In addition, this pattern of inheritance has been demonstrated in a variety of genetically transmitted conditions, including albinism, sickle cell anemia, cystic fibrosis, phenylketonuria, Tay-Sachs disease, Hurler's syndrome, Bloom syndrome, Fanconi's anemia, galactosemia, and hyperextensible thumb.

For some of these diseases, the carrier has no symptom of the trait, and in other conditions the carrier does not express the full-blown condition but may express a milder form when predisposing environmental or personal events are present. For example, carriers of sickle cell disease (SCD) may have some sickling of their red blood cells under conditions of extreme hypoxia, although the sickling is never as severe or widespread as it is in the person who is homozygous for SCD. For the most part SCD is not a single gene mutation. Research has identified many versions of SCD that involve modifier genes such as those responsible for beta-globin genotype, fetal hemoglobin (HbF), beta S gene cluster haplotype, and alpha-thalassemia, as well as interaction with the environment in order to produce the disease (Kenner et al, 2005).

Sex-Linked Patterns of Inheritance

Some genes are present only on the sex chromosomes. The Y chromosome appears to have few genes that are not also present on the X chromosome. However, the X chromosome has many single genes that do not appear to be present elsewhere in the human genome. For all intents and purposes, then, the discussion of sex-linked patterns of inheritance is really a discussion of X-linked patterns of inheritance.

Because X chromosomes are distributed unequally between males and females (1:2 ratio, respectively), the X-linked chromosome genes likewise are distributed unequally between the two genders. Males have only one X chromosome and are said to be hemizygous for any gene on the X chromosome. As a result, X-linked recessive genes have a dominant expressive pattern of inheritance in males and a recessive expressive pattern in females. This difference in expression occurs because males do not have a second X chromosome to balance the expression of any recessive gene on the first X chromosome.

Dominant Patterns

For a sex-linked (X-linked) dominant single-gene trait to be expressed, the gene controlling the trait must be located on only one of the X chromosomes. A typical sex-linked dominant pattern of inheritance meets certain criteria that are obvious in the pedigree. The defining criteria are:
1. There is no carrier status; all individuals with the gene are affected.
2. Female children of affected males are all affected (risk is 100%), whereas male children of affected males are unaffected (risk is 0%). Therefore the overall risk of an affected male having affected children is 50% for each pregnancy, since the probability of having a female is also 50%. It is the inheritance of the trait by female offspring of affected males that defines the problem as X-linked dominant, because the inheritance pattern among the offspring of affected females is identical to an autosomal dominant pattern.
3. The trait appears in every generation.
4. For homozygous females, the risk of having an affected child is 100% with each pregnancy, and offspring of both genders are affected equally. For heterozygous females, the risk of having an affected child is 50% with each pregnancy, and children of both genders are equally at risk.
5. In the general population, X-linked dominant problems affect twice as many females as males, but heterozygous females usually express a milder form of the problem than do hemizygous males.

Common X-linked dominant problems include fragile X and hypophosphatemia.

Recessive Patterns

X-linked recessive single-gene traits are among the best-defined inherited health problems. This pattern of inheritance requires that the gene controlling the trait be present on both X chromosomes for the trait to be fully expressed in females (females must be homozygous for the trait) and on only one of the X chromosomes for the trait to be expressed in males (males must be hemizygous). A typical sex-linked recessive pattern of inheritance meets all the following defining criteria:
1. Expression, or incidence, of the trait is much higher among males in a kinship (and in the general population) than among females.
2. The trait cannot be transmitted from father to son because the father contributes only the Y chromosome to his son's sex chromosome pair.
3. Transmission of the trait occurs from father to all daughters (who are all carriers but either do not express any of the trait or express it in a very mild form).
4. Female carriers have a 50% risk (with each pregnancy) of transmitting the gene to their offspring. Female offspring who inherit the trait are carriers, and male offspring who inherit the trait are affected.

Sex-linked recessive inheritance patterns may be responsible for normal variation of some secondary female sex characteristics. This pattern of inheritance also has been associated with a variety of disorders, including hemophilia (A and B), Duchenne's muscular dystrophy, ichthyosis, Lesch-Nyhan syndrome, and color blindness. For some of these disorders, females who are heterozygous for the gene express no overt symptoms (such as color blindness). For other disorders, female heterozygotes express some mild aberrations (e.g., increased bleeding tendency in carriers of hemophilia). Few females who express homozygosity have been found; it may be that homozygosity related to sex-linked recessive diseases leads to such a severe disorder that it is lethal in embryonic or early fetal life.

Multifactorial Inheritance

The use of the term *multifactorial* refers to the new understanding of the interaction of the genome with the environment. As genetic knowledge increases it is recognized that few conditions are really single gene conditions, as described above with SCD.

Gene Variation and Nontraditional Inheritance

In addition to variation in the expression of single genes, a single gene may be responsible for the expression of many effects that appear unrelated. This concept, known as pleiotropy, probably involves changes or aberrations in regulatory genes rather than in structural genes. One example of pleiotropy is Marfan syndrome. This syndrome is transmitted as an autosomal dominant trait, but its expression involves a variety of aberrations in unrelated tissue types. These aberrations include excessive growth of long bones, the presence of or predisposition to development of an aortic aneurysm, and severe nearsightedness.

Some heritable problems are associated with more than one gene. For example, congenital deafness or Usher's syndrome is an outcome associated with a variety of abnormal genes, although not all of the genes have to be abnormal for deafness to result (Kenner et al, 2005). When more than one gene is responsible for a specific characteristic or trait, the trait is controlled through polygenic expression. Cleft palate and neural tube defects are other examples of developing tissues that require polygenic expression for normal development and that can develop abnormally if any of the required genes is not normal.

Mitochondrial Disorders

Mitochondria, intracellular organelles involved in energy production, have their own DNA (mtDNA) distinct from nuclear DNA (nDNA), discussed earlier in this chapter. A unique finding about mtDNA is that it is inherited exclusively through the maternal line. Each cell has numerous mtDNA molecules, so a single cell with an mtDNA mutation may also have other mtDNA without the mutation, a condition termed heteroplasmy. This heterogeneity in DNA composition contributes to variable expression in mitochondrial diseases. Conditions attributed to mtDNA mutations include Leber hereditary optic neuropathy (LHON), Kearns-Sayre disease, deafness, and Alzheimer's disease.

CHROMOSOMAL ABERRATIONS

As discussed previously, chromosomes are formed during the metaphase of mitosis from tightly packed, supercoiled DNA. Each chromosome contains hundreds of genes; detectable aberrations of any chromosome can result in aberration in the structure or expression of one or more genes.

Numeric Aberrations

The normal diploid number of human chromosomes at metaphase of mitosis is 46: that is, 23 pairs. Some individuals have missing or extra whole chromosomes. This type of aberration usually is the result of abnormal or delayed disjunction (nondisjunction) in gamete formation during meiosis I or meiosis II. Instead of all gametes having 23 chromosomes each, some gametes have 24, some have 22, and some have the normal 23. When a 24-chromosome gamete is united with a 23-chromosome gamete of the opposite sex during fertilization, the resulting individual has 47 chromosomes. One chromosome set contains three copies of a chromosome instead of the normal two copies; this situation is called a trisomy. When a 22-chromosome gamete from one parent is united with a 23-chromosome gamete of the other parent during fertilization, the resulting individual has 45 chromosomes. One chromosome set contains only one copy of a chromosome instead of the normal two copies; this is called a monosomy. Whenever the individual has more or fewer chromosomes than normal, some malformations and abnormal developmental processes are expressed. Nondisjunction is most commonly associated with advanced maternal age at the time of conception, presumably as a result of primary oocytes spending years in prophase of meiosis I. It is important to note, however, that nondisjunction can occur at any age.

In theory, nondisjunction can occur within any chromosome pair. However, nondisjunction of some chromosome pairs leads to embryolethal consequences. The most common chromosomal aberration found among all conceptuses is a missing X chromosome, or Turner syndrome (45,XO). Most conceptuses with a chromosome constitution of 45,XO do not survive beyond the embryonic period. The most common chromosomal aberration observed among newborns is trisomy 21 (Down syndrome) (47,XX or XY, 21). Other syndromes of trisomy that can be observed among newborns are trisomy 13, trisomy 15, trisomy 18, and sex chromosome trisomies (47,XXX; 47,XXY; 47,XYY). Trisomy 16 has been identified in embryonic and early fetal wastage, but this abnormality does not usually lead to a fully developed newborn. Autosomal monosomes may be conceived but rarely survive to the stage of birth, although monosomy 21 has been reported among newborns.

All individuals with autosomal trisomies experience some degree of mental retardation. In addition, each trisomy is associated with a specific set of abnormalities, malformations, and unique developmental patterns. This is why individuals with trisomy may share heritable characteristics with their normal family members (e.g., hair color and texture, skin tone, eye color), but many of their structural features tend to resemble those of unrelated individuals who have the same trisomy.

Individuals with missing or extra whole sex chromosomes tend to be intellectually normal and have fewer recognizable physical malformations compared with individuals with autosomal numeric aberrations. Somewhat controversial is the finding that these individuals have behavioral patterns that are not completely normal, such as attention deficit problems and other learning disorders.

Structural Aberrations

Structural aberrations can occur in one of two ways: (1) parts of chromosomes can break off and either become lost or attach themselves to other chromosomes, resulting in translocation of chromosomal material from one chromosome to another; or (2) one whole chromosome can become joined to another whole chromosome, a translocation of chromosomes called robertsonian translocation.

When chromosomes are broken and translocated to other chromosomes, the total amount of chromosomal material may be balanced (normal) or unbalanced (abnormal). If the total amount of chromosomal material present in the individual's cells is balanced, even though it is not located in the usual positions, the individual phenotypically is normal. Problems do not arise until this individual reproduces. Because some of this individual's gametes are not normal (i.e., not balanced) as a result of random assortment and independent segregation of chromatids during gametogenesis, the person is at risk for having chromosomally unbalanced and abnormal offspring. This individual should be referred for genetic counseling. The same situation is true for individuals with robertsonian translocations. As long as the normal amount of chromosomal material is present in all the individual's cells, the individual is phenotypically normal, even though the chromosomes' locations might be abnormal.

PRENATAL TESTING AND SCREENING

For an increasing number of heritable conditions, prenatal screening is available for determining if a fetus is affected. The issue of prenatal diagnosis is complex. Many of the tests are expensive, carry some degree of risk to the pregnancy, and cannot always provide conclusive results. Tests may be performed directly on fetal cells or indirectly on products synthesized by the fetus, or by imaging. Some tests are even done before implantation.

Preimplantation Genetic Diagnosis

Preimplantation genetic diagnosis (PGD) is used with in vitro fertilization (IVF), oftentimes to determine if the zygote has any readily detectable genetic abnormalities. The cells from the zygote are biopsied and analyzed using a polymerase chain reaction (which consists of a series of events or reactions that occur as a substance moves down the strands of DNA) or fluorescence in situ hybridization (FISH) (see explanation later in this chapter). The FISH test can detect conditions such as Duchenne's muscular dystrophy, cystic fibrosis, and severe combined immunodeficiency (SCID) (Harris & Verp, 2001). More commonly, tests are performed on fetal cells or enzymes.

Fetal Ultrasonography

Fetal ultrasonography involves the use of high-frequency sound waves that are reflected differently in various media and in tissues of different densities. With computer enhancement, ultrasonography can provide a relatively detailed image of the embryo and fetus. Interpretation of the images produced has been refined to such a degree that even minor structural aberrations can be detected. Ultrasonography often is used to locate the placenta, cord, embryo or fetus, amniotic fluid pockets, and other associated structures before more invasive diagnostic procedures are performed. Fetal ultrasonography can provide information about fetal age, the amount of amniotic fluid present, and a variety of structural abnormalities (Hata et al, 1998), including the following:

- Neural tube defects (spina bifida, encephaloceles, microcephaly, anencephaly, hydrocephaly)
- Skeletal dysplasia (fractures, disproportions, bowing)
- Gastrointestinal anomalies (gastroschisis, atresias, tracheoesophageal fistulas)
- Congenital heart disease (coarctation of the aorta,

transposition of the great vessels); echocardiograms can be performed in conjunction with ultrasonography to determine chamber and valvular abnormalities, hypoplastic ventricles, and septal defects
- Genitourinary problems (horseshoe kidneys, polycystic kidneys, exstrophy of the bladder, Potter's syndrome or sequence)
- Cystic hygromas

Tests on Fetally Derived Cells

A wide variety of tests can be performed directly on fetal cells. The most common methods of obtaining fetal cells are through amniocentesis and chorionic villus sampling.

Chromosome Analysis by Amniocentesis

Amniocentesis is an invasive procedure in which the amniotic cavity is accessed under sterile conditions through the abdominal wall of the mother. This procedure usually is performed in conjunction with fetal ultrasonography to minimize the risk of puncturing vital fetal structures with the relatively large-bore amniocentesis needle. The ideal gestational age for safe amniocentesis is 16 weeks after conception has occurred. At this time considerable amniotic fluid is present, and the fetus is capable of shedding many viable cells. Once the needle is in place, approximately 20 ml of amniotic fluid is withdrawn. Some viable fetal cells will be present in the fluid. This test sometimes is referred to as midtrimester testing, because it is used from 15 to 20 weeks' gestation.

Early amniocentesis, which is performed before 14 weeks' gestation, also is used. Usually, not enough fetal cells are obtained to ensure an adequate sample size for most tests, so cells are cultivated in tissue culture, then tested. The tests most often performed include chromosome analysis, enzyme analysis, tests for the presence or absence of a specific biochemical product, and examination of genes using molecular probes.

Chromosome Analysis by Chorionic Villus Sampling

Chromosome analysis can also be performed on fetal tissue obtained through chorionic villus sampling (CVS). This technique involves removing a piece of tissue from the growing placenta after its location has been identified through ultrasonography. The needle can be inserted either through the cervical os (more common method) or by transabdominal puncture. This procedure can be performed during the first trimester, as early as 9 to 10 weeks' gestation.

Enzyme Analysis

Some genetic metabolic diseases are caused by a deficiency of a specific enzyme in the fetus. Often these children are normal at birth because maternal enzymes crossed the placenta and performed the specific function in the fetus. However, after birth, maternal enzymes can no longer be used. The pathway affected by the missing or inactive enzyme malfunctions, and the body begins to demonstrate abnormal buildup of products or abnormal metabolism.

Fetal cells cultured for several weeks without the influence of maternal enzymes can express the same metabolic abnormalities that the child would show after birth. Enzyme analysis of the cells or culture fluid (or both) can determine whether a specific enzyme is present at all or whether it is present in normal concentrations. Some genetic metabolic problems that can be identified through enzyme analysis of fetal cells are Tay-Sachs disease, Hurler's syndrome, metachromatic leukodystrophy, galactosemia, and homocystinuria.

Alpha-Fetoprotein

Alpha-fetoprotein (AFP) is normally synthesized in measurable quantities only during embryonic and fetal life. In the early embryo, the yolk sac synthesizes AFP; later the fetal liver and gastrointestinal cells assume this function. AFP is present in fetal blood and in some extracellular fluids, and it serves the same function that albumin does in human blood after birth. Because the fetal and maternal circulations are integrated, substances made by the fetus that are small enough move down their concentration gradients into maternal serum. AFP also is present in fetal urine and therefore in amniotic fluid. The synthesis of AFP is well regulated, and the pattern of normal amniotic fluid levels specific to gestational age is known. Variation from this normal pattern is associated with developmental problems.

AFP can be measured in the amniotic fluid (requiring amniocentesis) or in maternal serum. The maternal serum alpha-fetoprotein (MSAFP) test is one of the more commonly used prenatal screening tests. The accuracy of both the amniotic fluid and MSAFP measurements requires exact identification of gestational age at the time the fluid or serum is obtained. An AFP value is considered elevated if it is at least twice the mean for that specific gestational age. The most common problem associated with elevated AFP is an open neural tube defect (the open tube provides a means for extra AFP to leak into the amniotic fluid). A lower than normal AFP value also has been associated with fetal developmental problems, although this phenomenon shows more variability. The most common condition consistently associated with low AFP is Down syndrome, although the phenomenon is not consistent enough to be used as the only screening test for Down syndrome. Other conditions associated with low AFP are gestational diabetes and spontaneous abortion.

Multiple Marker Screen

The multiple marker screen, or quad screen, is more sensitive for aneuploidy than is AFP by itself. This screen can detect changes in the maternal AFP, human chorionic gonadotropin (hCG), unconjugated estriol (uE3), and dimeric inhibin-A (DIA). These biologic markers are particularly useful in detecting conditions such as trisomies. The same factors that can affect AFP levels, of course, can cause inaccurate results in the multiple screen including wrongly estimated dates of confinement and multiple gestations (twins).

The multiple marker screen is performed between 15 and 20 weeks' gestation. If an abnormality is found, ultrasonography should be used to confirm the problem. The exact mechanism involved in the alteration marker levels when a chromosomal problem exists is unknown, although it probably relates to a problem with the fetal liver (Harris & Verp, 2001).

Percutaneous Umbilical Blood Sampling (PUBS)

PUBS is another test that can be useful from 18 weeks' gestation. It requires use of ultrasonography to visualize the positioning of the catheter into the umbilical cord. Blood is withdrawn and tested for genetic abnormalities. PUBS is an invasive procedure through which fetal blood can be obtained for karyotyping, but FISH is replacing PUBS in many perinatal centers.

Fluorescence in Situ Hybridization (FISH)

FISH uses DNA probes that resemble chromosomal sequences or regions. These probes are fluorescent, and when they bind with areas in or on the chromosome, they are visible. FISH probes were first developed for several of the most common numerical chromosome abnormalities (i.e., 13, 18, 21, and X and Y) (Harris & Verp, 2001). The conditions for which they are used include Prader-Willi syndrome and aneuploidy (Harris & Verp, 2001).

Other Molecular or DNA Probes

In some cases the actual gene associated with a specific problem has been identified, and molecular probes complementary to the gene have been made. These probes can be used to determine whether the gene is present in fetal cells. Use of molecular probes does not require dividing fetal cells, although a sufficient volume of cells is necessary. In some cases, enough fetal cells can be obtained through amniocentesis or CVS so that the test can be performed directly on the DNA of the tissue. At other times, a greater volume of fetal cells is required, and the fetal cells must be grown in culture before the DNA can be extracted and probed.

Many molecular probes are commercially available, which makes testing more accessible and less costly. Genetic metabolic diseases for which molecular probes are commercially available include cystic fibrosis, hemophilia B, Huntington's disease, retinoblastoma, sickle cell disease, and thalassemia. Testing for genetic metabolic diseases for which probes are not commercially available can be performed in genetic research centers.

NEWBORN TESTING AND SCREENING

Advances in genetic technology have resulted in increased testing capability for numerous disorders, including infections, genetic disease, and metabolic disorders with a single blood spot (ACOG, 2003; Banta-Wright & Steiner, 2004). Individual state statutes vary widely in the number of tests mandated, from as few as four to as many as 30 (U.S. National Newborn Screening and Resource Center, 2006). Although many tests are currently available for newborn screening, for some of the identified diseases there are no effective treatments. Nationwide universal testing for 29 "core panel" conditions has been recommended (ACMG, 2005), along with 25 "secondary targets," conditions that are part of the differential diagnosis of a core panel condition (table available: http://www.mchb.hrsa.gov/screening/). Twenty-three of the 29 core conditions can be tested with a single blood spot using tandem mass spectrometry (MS/MS) (ACMG, 2005). However, debate continues about tests in the screening panel because most states are not prepared with a system of notification for follow-up and treatment when infants have positive test results. Unfortunately, molecular technology has eclipsed health care provider preparation in genomic knowledge. Nursing must respond to this gap in order to provide quality care in response to parental questions about testing, results, risk interpretation, and follow-up. In addition, nurses must be educated in order to contribute knowledgably to the many ethical and legal issues that have been raised about newborn testing, such as storing blood spots for future testing, cost effectiveness of universal testing, parental consent for testing, and privacy protection.

FAMILY HISTORY TOOL AND NURSING

Today there is recognition that a three-generation family history is essential for good health. To focus attention on the importance of family health history, U.S. Surgeon General Richard H. Carmona launched a national public health campaign in 2004 to encourage all American families to learn more about and record their family health history using Centers for Disease Control and Prevention's (CDC) Family History Tool (Yoon et al, 2002) or the U.S. Department of Health and Human Services "My Family Health Portrait" (U.S. Department of Health and Human Services, 2005). Recognition of the significance of accurate health history is a byproduct of the HGP. Nurses are often the professionals involved in taking a health history that could result in a pedigree. Typical information obtained for the three-generation family history and pedigree includes age and year of birth; age and cause of death for those deceased; ethnic background of each grandparent; relevant health information; illnesses and age at diagnosis; information regarding prior genetic testing; information regarding pregnancies including infertility, spontaneous abortions, stillbirths, and pregnancy complications; and consanguinity issues (Bennett, 1999). Together, history and pedigree have the capacity to demonstrate linkages between current health and future health risks. For example, sickle cell disease (SCD) and its alterations at the cellular level may put the infant at risk as a teenager or adult for stroke. Understanding this risk, nurses can plan efforts for health promotion.

SUMMARY

Neonatal nurses must keep abreast of new genomic knowledge and prenatal/neonatal testing that can be done to impact long term health (Williams et al, 2004). Many health problems have genetic aspects for perinatal and neonatal nursing, such as prenatal screening and diagnosis, assistance with infertility testing and intervention, diagnosis of congenital syndromes and associations and metabolic disease, identification of reproductive hazards in the workplace and the surrounding environment both for health professionals and for the public, identification of congenital problems that occur secondary to substance abuse, and fetal therapy and surgery and the neonatal implications of such procedures (Feetham et al, 2005; Jenkins et al, 2005; Loescher & Merkle, 2005; Olsen et al, 2003).

All health professionals at every level of education must have a knowledge of genomics. In 2001 the National Coalition of Health Professional Education in Genetics (NCHPEG) published a list of core competencies, which are considered necessary for all health professionals in all disciplines (Jenkins, 2001). The nursing profession led this movement, recognizing the importance of genomics to all areas of nursing practice. A list of the genetics core competences is available (http://www.nchpeg.org).

A nurse with a subspecialty in genomics may act as a genetic counselor, informing families of their genetic risks, providing information, and giving support during the initial diagnosis and through follow-up. However, the holistic nature of nursing, which takes in biopsychosocial needs, extends beyond just counseling measures as they often are defined; it includes a broader perspective of care. The six roles of the professional nurse—advocate, practitioner, collaborator, investigator, educator, and leader—are all essential in working with patients and families with genetic and congenital disorders.

The nurse can also act as an advocate for the family and refer them to community resources such as genetics clinics, family support groups, or specialized home health care services. Access to care is an important aspect of advocacy for these families. The neonatal nurse involved in community-based follow-up care has a special need for updated genomic information. Prenatal and newborn screening and early identification of genetic, congenital, or familial problems often occurs in this practice setting. This nurse is also involved in the treatment of the actual disease, such as phenylketonuria or cystic fibrosis, and must help educate the family about the need for complying with treatment and for continuing follow-up care. The nurse should also be aware of community resources, for both the public and the professional, that provide treatment, support, and education for such medical-genetic disorders. A list of available Web-based resources is provided in Table 32-1. The National Coalition for Health Professions Education in Genetics (NCHPEG) developed interprofessional core competencies (http://www.nchpeg.org). Currently a nursing group led by Dr. Jean Jenkins and colleagues are adapting these to reflect the nursing profession and care.

TABLE **32-1**	Websites for Genomic Resources and Professional Organizations	
Name	**Website**	**Description**
American College of Medical Genetics (ACMG)	http://www.acmg.net/	Education and resources for professionals in medical genetics
American Medical Association (AMA)	http://www.ama-assn.org/ama/ pub/category/4646.html	Information about genetics and genetic resources; professional organization for medical doctors
American Nurses Association	http:www.nursingworld.org	Registered nurses professional organization; continuing education; genetic articles; ethical issues; standards of practice

Continued

TABLE 32-1	Websites for Genomic Resources and Professional Organizations—cont'd	
Name	**Website**	**Description**
American Society of Human Genetics (ASHG)	http://www.ashg.org/	Professional organization of human geneticists; genetics professional information and research
Association of Women's Health, Obstetric and Neonatal Nurses	http://www.awhonn.org	Clinical position statement
Center for Disease Control (CDC) Office of Genomics and Disease Prevention (OGDP)	http://www.cdc.gov/genomics	Genetics information and research; tool for family history; public health priorities; common questions
Cincinnati Children's Hospital Genetics Education Program for Nurses (GEPN)	http://www.cincinnatichildrens.org/ ed/clinical/gpnf/	Offers modularized learning online for those practicing nurses or faculty who want to gain more genetic knowledge
Dolan DNA Learning Center	http://www.dnalc.org/	Educational resources for children, parents, professionals
Ethical, Legal and Social Implications (ELSI) Research Institute	http://www.genome.gov/10001618	Federal program to fund research related to ethical, legal, and social implications of genomic research
Gene Tests	http://www.genetests.org/	Free genetics information, disease reviews, international directory of laboratories and clinics
Genetics	http://ghr.nlm.nih.gov/	National Library of Medicine website for consumer information about genetics
Genetic Alliance	http://www.geneticalliance.org/	Coalition for genetic advocacy
Genetics and Public Policy Center	http://www.dnapolicy.org/	Genetic technology and public policy information
Genetic and Rare Diseases (GARD) Information Center	http://rarediseases.info.nih.gov	Provides information specialists to answer consumer questions about rare diseases
Genetics Education Center, University of Kansas	http://www.kumc.edu/gec/	Genetics education; links to large number of Internet resources
Genetic Resources on the Web (GROW)	http://www.nih.gov/sigs/bioethics/ grow.html	Forum for organizations/professionals who desire high-quality information availability on the Internet
Genetic Education Materials (GEM) Database	http://www.gemdatabase.org/ GEMDatabase/index.asp	Searchable listing of public health genetics policy documents and clinical genetics educational materials
Health Resources and Services Administration (HRSA)	http://www.hrsa.gov	Federal resource for research funding, policy development
Harvard Medical School, Department of Continuing Education	http://cme.med.Harvard.edu	Professional online continuing education
International Society of Nurses in Genetics (ISONG)	http://www.isong.org	Nursing organization devoted to genetics; genetics education, practice, and resources
International Council of Nurses (ICN)	http://www.icn.ch/matters_genetics. htm	International nursing organization; genetics policy statements
March of Dimes	http://www.marchofdimes.com	Professional and consumer education about genetics, newborn screening, prevention of birth defects
National Coalition in Health Professional Education in Genetics (NCHPEG)	http://www.nchpeg.org	Multiprofessional organization supporting core education in genetics. Core competencies in higher education of professionals
National Guideline Clearinghouse	http://www.guideline.gov	Searchable site for guidelines relating to genetics
National Human Genome Research Institute (NHGRI)	http://www.genome.gov	Research and news about genomics
National Newborn Screening and Genetics Resource Center (NNSGRC)	http://genes-r-us.uthscsa.edu/	Information on newborn screening by state; genetic resources
National Society of Genetics Counselors (NSGC)	http://www.nsgc.org	Professional organization of genetics counselors; genetic information; tools for collecting family history

TABLE 32-1	Websites for Genomic Resources and Professional Organizations—cont'd	
Name	**Website**	**Description**
Online Mendelian Inheritance in Man (OMIM)	http://www.ncbi.nlm.nih.gov/entrez/query.fcgi?db=OMIM	Database of human genes and genetic disorders
Secretary's Advisory Committee on Genetics, Health and Society (SACGHS)	http://www4.od.nih.gov/oba/SACGHS.HTM	Committee of professionals and interested individuals representing public stakeholders in genetics issues
Summer Genetics Institute (SGI), National Institute of Nursing Research (NINR)	http://ninr.nih.gov/research/summer_institutes/summer_genetics_institute/	Eight-week graduate-level competitive nursing program to provide foundation for molecular genetics education and research
World Health Organization (WHO) Genetics Resource Centre	http://www.who.int/genomics/en/	Worldwide genomics progress
US Department of Energy Office of Science Genome Programs	http://www.doegenomes.org	Federal programs related to genomics

REFERENCES

American College of Medical Genetics (ACMG) (2005). Newborn screening: toward a uniform screening panel and system. Available at: http://www.mchb.hrsa.gov/screening/. Retrieved September 29, 2005.

American College of Obstetricians and Gynecologists (ACOG) (2003). ACOG committee opinion number 287, October 2003: newborn screening. *Obstetrics and gynecology* 102(4):887-889.

Banta-Wright SA, Steiner RD (2004). Tandem mass spectrometry in newborn screening: a primer for neonatal and perinatal nurses. *Journal of perinatal and neonatal nursing* 18(1):41-60.

Bennett RL (1999). *The practical guide to the genetic family history.* New York: Wiley-Liss.

Bennett RL et al (1995). Recommendations for standardized human pedigree nomenclature. Pedigree Standardization Task Force of the National Society of Genetic Counselors. *American journal of human genetics* 56(3):745-752.

Childs B (1998). Medicine through a genetic lens. In Hager M, editor. *The implications of genetics for health professional education.* New York: Josiah Macy, Jr. Foundation.

Feetham S et al (2005). Nursing leadership in genomics for health and society. *Journal of nursing scholarship: an official publication of Sigma Theta Tau International Honor Society of Nursing* 37(2):102.

Gaultier C, Gallego J (2005). Development of respiratory control: evolving concepts and perspectives. *Respiratory physiology and neurobiology* 149(1-3):3-15.

Harris CM, Verp MS (2001). Prenatal testing and interventions. In Mahowald MB et al, editors. *Genetics in the clinics: clinical, ethical, and social implications for primary care.* St Louis: Mosby.

Hata T et al (1998). Three-dimensional ultrasonographic assessments of fetal development. *Obstetrics and gynecology* 91(2):218-223.

Human Genome Project (2005). The science behind the human genome project: basic genetics, genome draft sequence, and post-genome science. Available at: http://www.ornl.gov/sci/techresources/Human_Genome/project/info.shtml. Retrieved July 25, 2005.

Jenkins J (2001). *Core competencies in genetics essential for all health care professionals.* Rockville, MD: National Coalition for Health Professional Education in Genetics (NCHPEG).

Jenkins J et al (2005). Nurses and the genomic revolution. *Journal of nursing scholarship* 37(2):98-101.

Kenner C, Moran M (2005). Newborn screening and genetic testing. *Journal of midwifery and women's health* 50(3):219-226.

Kenner C et al (2005). Promoting children's health through understanding of genetics and genomics. *Journal of nursing scholarship* 37(4):308-314.

Loescher LJ, Merkle CJ (2005). The interface of genomic technologies and nursing. *Journal of nursing scholarship* 37:111-119.

March of Dimes (2005). Birth defects. Available at: http://www.marchofdimes.com/pnhec/4439_1206.asp. Retrieved July 25, 2005.

National Human Genome Research Institute (NHGRI) (2001). *About the human genome project. The Human Genome Research Project: from maps to medicine.* Available at: http://www.genome.gov/12011238. Retrieved July 18, 2006.

Olsen S et al (2004). Case for blending pedigrees, genograms, and ecomaps: nursing's contribution to the "big picture." *Nursing and health sciences* 6(4):295.

Olsen SJ et al (2003). Creating a nursing vision for leadership in genetics. *MEDSURG nursing* 12(3):177-183.

Scheuerle AE (2001). Diagnosis of genetic disease. In Mahowald MB et al, editors. *Genetics in the clinics: clinical, ethical, and social implications for primary care.* St Louis: Mosby.

Secretary's Advisory Committee on Genetic Testing (SACGT) (2001). *What's new: TGAC [The Genome Action Coalition] Hotline, 2000.* Available at: http://www4.od.nih.gov/oba/SACGHS.htm. Retrieved July 18, 2006.

U.S. Department of Health and Human Services (2005). *U.S. Surgeon General's family history initiative.* Available at: http://www.hhs.gov/familyhistory/. Retrieved July 25, 2005.

U.S. National Screening Status Report (2006). Washington, DC: National Newborn Screening and Genetics Resource Center. Available at: http://genes-r-us.uthscsa.edu/nbsdisorders.pdf. Retrieved July 18, 2006.

Williams JK et al (2004). Advancing genetic nursing knowledge. *Nursing outlook* 52:73-79.

Yoon PW et al (2002). Can family history be used as a tool for public health and preventive medicine? *Genetics in medicine* 4(4):304-310.

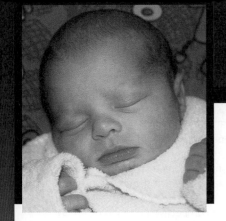

Chapter 33

Neonatal Research and Evidence-Based Practice

Kathleen R. Stevens • Lynda Harrison

Knowledge guides every clinical decision and action taken by a nurse. The underlying rationale for a nursing intervention may come from past experiences, trial and error, authority, a nursing procedure manual, a textbook, or science produced through systematic inquiry (research). Nursing care policies often represent a source of knowledge known as authority. Multiple sources of knowledge may underlie a policy—the policy maker's own clinical experience, tradition ("we have always done it this way"), internal or external benchmarks, and textbooks. Whatever the knowledge base for the action, it carries with it a likelihood that an intervention will produce the desired health outcome for the patient or the accuracy with which the diagnostic approach will assess the patient's health status. The focus of this chapter is on linking neonatal nursing practice and research in such a way that the strongest knowledge—that derived from research—is put into practice. The chapter presents the basis of evidence-based practice, models of evidence-based quality improvement, various research roles for neonatal nurses, identification of clinical problems amenable to research, and current trends in neonatal nursing research.

EVIDENCE-BASED NEONATAL NURSING PRACTICE

Not all sources of knowledge are highly reliable, nor does care based on various sources consistently produce the desired patient outcome. Experience and trial and error are good teachers; however, the knowledge gained through these approaches contains bias. That is, the results may be due to something other than the intervention, something that is outside of the nurse's awareness, or the results from one situation may not be applicable to another situation or client. Clinical decisions drawn on experience and trial and error are not the most effective at producing desired patient outcome because these sources do not expose the full truth or validity of the broader reality. These sources do not represent the underlying science for nursing care.

Quality of care and resulting patient outcomes improve when research results guide that care. The primary concept of evidence-based practice (EBP) is that research studies produce the most reliable source of knowledge on which to base clinical decisions. Today, the measure of "best practice" is that interventions are based on "best evidence," that is, scientific findings. The new social mandate for evidence-based quality improvement provides ample impetus for implementing

evidence-based practice (Stevens & Staley, 2006). However, putting research into practice can be hampered by obstacles. The work within the EBP paradigm has removed a number of the obstacles in applying research results in practice. EBP has produced a new way of applying research evidence in clinical decision making to ensure the best outcome that science knows how to produce. Individual clinician decisions about care as well as agency policies about care standards should reflect the best evidence produced to date. The end result of applying state-of-the-science patient care is that health care status goals are effectively and efficiently met within the context of preferences of the patient and health care provider (Sackett et al, 2000). This rapidly advancing movement of EBP embodies new methods and represents a new paradigm of research application in clinical care. The care environment in neonatal nursing will exhibit many aspects of EBP in which the entire health care team is engaged.

WHAT IS EVIDENCE-BASED PRACTICE?

Evidence-based practice is a process through which scientific evidence is identified, appraised, converted, and applied in health care interventions (Stevens, 2004). A commonly used definition of evidence-based practice is the conscientious, explicit, and judicious use of current best evidence in making decisions about the care of individual patients; EBP is the integration of best research evidence with clinical expertise and patient preference (Sackett et al, 2000). The objective of evidence-based practice is application of the best available evidence in clinical care in order to increase the likelihood that the desired patient outcome is achieved.

Although evidence and knowledge can be drawn from a variety of sources, the best evidence is specifically identified as that evidence drawn from scientific investigation, or research (Guyatt & Rennie, 2002). Using research evidence as the basis for care is best because it allows the nurse to gauge the certainty and predictability that the care will produce the outcome. Implementation of evidence-based practices generates more accurate diagnosis, maximally effective and efficient intervention, and most favorable patient outcomes. These ends can be accomplished through newly developed evidence-based practice methods, processes, and models.

A MODEL OF EVIDENCE-BASED NURSING

Evidence-based nursing can be described as a process of establishing research-based practice by transforming the evidence through a full cycle, into practice and patient outcomes. Nurse scientists developed the ACE Star Model of Knowledge Transformation (Figure 33-1) to emphasize the steps necessary to reduce volume and complexity of research knowledge, convert one form of knowledge to the next, and incorporate a broad range of sources of knowledge throughout the evidence-based practice process (Stevens, 2004). The Star Model provides a framework in which to consider how research knowledge must be converted into a form that has utility in clinical decision making. Knowledge Transformation is depicted as a five-point process (Box 33-1). The steps in this process are primary research, evidence summary, translation, integration, and evaluation (Stevens, 2004).

Primary research is the research approach with which we are familiar—individual reports of research studies. Over the past 3 decades, nurse researchers have produced literally thousands of research studies on a wide variety of nursing clinical topics. The cluster of primary research studies on any given topic may include both strong and weak study designs, small and large samples, and conflicting or converging results, leaving the clinician to wonder which study is the best reflection of cause and effect in selecting effective interventions. In addition, research studies on a given clinical topic may number in the hundreds and thus are not useful in the clinical setting. Historically, nurses focused on primary research studies in research utilization that detailed ways to move a single research study into practice. EBP experience has now taught us how this leads to errors in care.

Using this approach, two hurdles emerged: the form of the knowledge and the volume and complexity of research literature. These hurdles are addressed by new approaches used in EBP. The EBP solution to the form of knowledge is the transformation of knowledge through various stages into a clinically useful form (Stevens, 2004). The EBP solution to the complexity and volume of literature is an evidence summary. In the

second stage of knowledge transformation, the evidence summary, teams gather together all primary research on a given clinical topic and summarize it into a single statement about the state of our knowledge on the topic. This summary step is the main feature that distinguishes evidence-based practice from simple research application and research utilization in clinical practice. Systematic reviews (SRs) transform research knowledge in a number of notable ways and offer distinct

---

BOX 33-1

The Five Points of the Star Model and the Competencies for Nurses

Star Point	Competency
1—Original Research	"Recognize ratings of strength of evidence when reading literature including web resources"
2—Evidence Summary	"List advantages of SRs as strong evidential foundation for clinical decision making"
3—Translation	"Using specified databases, access CPGs on various clinical topics"
4—Integration	"Assist in integrating practice change based on EB CPGs"
5—Evaluation	"Participate in EB quality improvement processes to evaluate outcomes of practice changes"

From Stevens KR (2005). *Essential competencies for evidence-based practice in nursing.* San Antonio, TX: ACE-University of Texas Health Science Center. Reprinted with express permission. SR, Systematic review; CPG, clinical practice guideline; EB, evidence-based.

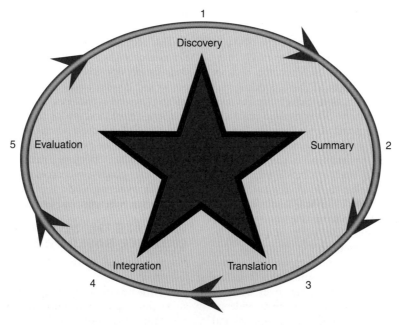

FIGURE **33-1**
ACE Star Model of Knowledge Transformation. Reprinted with express permission from Stevens KR (2004). *ACE star model of knowledge transformation.* San Antonio, TX: Academic Center for Evidence-based Practice, The University of Texas Health Science Center at San Antonio. Available at: http://www.acestar.uthscsa.edu. Retrieved August 5, 2006.

BOX 33-2

Advantages of Systematic Reviews

A systematic review accomplishes the following:
- Reduces large quantities of information into a manageable form
- Integrates existing information for decisions about clinical care, economic decisions, future research design, and policy formation
- Increases efficiency in time between research and clinical implementation
- Establishes generalizability across participants, across settings, and treatment variations and different study designs
- Assesses consistency and explains inconsistencies of relationships across studies
- Increases power in suggesting the cause and effect relationship
- Reduces bias from random and systematic error, improving true reflection of reality
- Provides better continuous updates of new evidence

Adapted from Mulrow C (1994). Rationale for systematic reviews. *British medical journal* 309:597-599.

advantages, as is summarized in Box 33-2. Evidence summaries are also called evidence synthesis, systematic reviews, integrative reviews, and reviews of literature. The most widely used methods in rigorous evidence summary produce a systematic review that reflects the methods established in the mid 1990's (Alderson et al, 2003). A systematic review is a type of evidence summary that uses a rigorous scientific approach to combine results from a body of original research studies into a clinically meaningful whole and therefore produces new knowledge through synthesis and typically uses the statistical procedure meta-analysis to combine findings across multiple studies. In this way, evidence summaries remove the obstacle of voluminous and rapidly expanding bodies of research literature. Evidence summaries in the form of systematic reviews are a significant advancement through EBP—overriding the previous paradigm of research utilization. Systematic reviews have been identified as the "heart of evidence-based practice" because they provide a new form of knowledge to guide clinical decision making (Stevens, 2001). Evidence summaries communicate the latest scientific findings in a palatable and accessible form for the clinical nurse to readily apply the research in clinical decisions—that is, evidence summaries form the basis on which we build evidence-based practices. When developing an evidence summary, one must keep in mind that nonsignificant findings can be as important to practice as positive results. However, nonsignificant findings tend not to be published and so are underrepresented in the literature. Developing sound evidence summaries requires scientific skill and extensive resources—often over a year's worth of scientific work. If done to rigorous standards, evidence summaries will review research across all relevant disciplines and across the globe, screen studies for relevance and quality of design, use multiple reviewers to abstract findings, and analyze the results to combine findings and examine the extent of bias in the set of research studies. For this reason, evidence summaries

are often conducted by scientific and clinical teams that are specifically prepared in the methodology.

In the third stage of EBP, translation, experts are called on to consider the evidence summary, fill in gaps with consensus expert opinion, and merge research knowledge with expertise to produce clinical practice guidelines. This process translates the research evidence into clinical recommendations. Clinical practice guidelines are commonly produced and sponsored by a clinical specialty organization. For example, the International Lactation Consultant Association developed an excellent example of a clinical practice guideline (National Guideline Clearinghouse [NGC], 2005). The association combined research evidence and clinical expertise to produce evidence-based multidisciplinary breastfeeding management strategies for the first 14 postpartum days to prevent premature weaning (NGC, 2005). Such guidelines are present throughout all organized health care—in the form of clinical pathways, nursing care standards, and unit policies. Well-developed clinical practice guidelines, nursing care standards, and such share several characteristics: A specified process is followed during guideline development; the guideline identifies the evidence based on which each recommendation is made, whether it is research or expert opinion; and the evidence is rated using a strength-of-evidence rating scale.

Once guidelines are produced, integration is accomplished through change at both the individual clinician and organizational level. Planned change approaches often are used to overcome resistance and move the individual and organization to a higher standard of practice based on evidence. Guidance for planned change is provided by several principles and theories: because quality is a system property, systems must be changed with EBP; adoption of new practices can be amplified using principles from theories such as Rogers' theory of diffusion of innovation (Rogers, 1995). In neonatal nursing, as advances emerge, it is essential that all members of the health care team be actively involved in making quality improvement changes. Nurses will be leaders and followers in contributing to such improvement at their individual level of care as well as the system level of care.

The fifth stage in knowledge transformation is evaluation. Practice changes are followed by evaluation of the impact on a wide variety of outcomes, including effectiveness of the care in producing desired patient outcome; patient outcomes; population outcomes; efficiency and cost factors in the care (short- and long-term), and satisfaction of providers and patients alike. Evaluation of specific outcomes has risen to a high level of public interest given our new awareness that American health care is neither safe nor effective (Institute of Medicine [IOM], 2000). As a result, quality indicators have been established for health care improvement and for public reporting (e.g., Agency for Healthcare Research and Quality [AHRQ], 2005).

WHAT ARE THE MAJOR FEATURES OF EVIDENCE-BASED PRACTICE?

Major features of evidence-based practice include the following:
- It is heavily interdisciplinary.
- Development of clinical practice is based on evidence summary of the topic.
- Translation of evidence into clinical practice guidelines repackages the evidence for use by the clinician.
- Individual provider and organizational factors guide integration and rate of adoption.

- Evaluation includes determining effectiveness and efficiency in terms of patient outcomes and economy (Stevens, 2001).

Barriers to implementing research-based practice, when they exist, are removed by using evidence synthesis. Systematic reviews "efficiently integrate valid information and provide a basis for rational decision making" in clinical care (Mulrow, 1994). Only in rare instances will a single research study offer highly reliable answers to a clinical question. A systematic review provides stronger conclusions about the cause and effect (intervention and outcome) than a single study; therefore interventions based on systematic reviews are more likely to produce the desired health outcome. Because conducting evidence syntheses is a new, resource-intensive, and rigorous process, it is beyond the capacity of the typical clinician. For this reason, awareness of existing sources of synthesized evidence is critical for the clinician. Box 33-3 presents examples of evidence summaries from credible sources. In addition, Table 33-1 describes the most credible sources for evidence summaries to date. In some cases, conclusions from the evidence summary support current practice and increase confidence that the nursing care will produce the desired outcome. In other cases, the evidence points to a needed change in practice. In either case, examining current practice in light of the state of the science is becoming an expectation for health care.

SOURCES OF EVIDENCE FOR PRACTICE

Synthesis work is conducted by several organized agencies such as the Agency for Healthcare Research and Quality (AHRQ) and the Cochrane Collaboration. Because the conduct of a systematic review requires specialized scientific methods and significant resources, it is usually a sponsored activity conducted by groups of scientists. The prime sponsors are the Cochrane Collaboration (a global collaborative headquartered in the United Kingdom) and the Agency for Healthcare Research and Quality (a federally funded agency in the United States). Another source is the Joanna Briggs Institute, headquartered in Adelaide, South Australia, that has centers for EBP and conducts systematic reviews around the world. In turn, these agencies disseminate the evidence summaries for use by clinicians, health policy makers, and consumers of health care.

SKILLS ESSENTIAL IN EMPLOYING EVIDENCE-BASED PRACTICE

Each form of knowledge requires a different approach and process to increase its utility in clinical practice. For example, summarizing research requires that the scientific methodology for systematic review be implemented. Therefore, different tasks are required at the various stages of knowledge transformation and employment of EBP. The wide variety of tasks requires an EBP team so that sufficient skills, time, and other resources are applied to the task at hand. The EBP team will likely include clinical staff (all involved disciplines), advanced practice nurses, physician directors, other health professions, librarians, quality assurance leaders, informatics services, health care scientists, and administrators. The collective skills of the members of the group will enable them to accomplish the "knowledge work" necessary to convert knowledge around points of the Star Model into clinically useful recommendations that are enacted in care. Consensus from across the nation about essential competencies for evidence-based practice in nursing has been established (Stevens, 2005). Box 33-1 provides examples of these competencies for the staff nurse level, organized by the five points of the Star Model.

HOW TO EMPLOY EVIDENCE-BASED PRACTICE

With new insights into effective clinical decision making that EBP has provided, the question becomes, "How is EBP employed?" Although a number of methods are being developed, tested, and adopted, several guiding principles are apparent.

In clinical settings, often the administrative and managerial teams come to a conclusion that the agency will adopt an initiative: to employ EBP throughout their health care. The commitment requires time, persuasion, and resources, so several planning stages are helpful in making the initiative a success. These are described next.

The plan for employing EBP may initially include announcements, persuasion for buy-in from all vested interests, and identification and mobilization of resources. Of the many resources needed, time in the clinician's workday is a key resource. Other resources can be drawn from existing departments such as the quality assurance department, the medical librarian, and academicians from collaborating universities.

TABLE 33-1	Sources of Systematic Reviews on the Internet
Systematic Review Source	**Address**
Agency for Healthcare Research and Quality	http://www.ahrq.gov (AHRQ)
Cochrane Collaboration	View introductory information at http://www.cochrane.org/cochrane/cc-broch.htm#CC *Cochrane Reviewer's Handbook* at http://www.update-software.com/ccweb/cochrane/hbook.htm
Cochrane Library	Subscription service, free browsing of abstract reviews, and alphabetical listing of all titles in the Cochrane Library available at http://www.update-software.com/cochrane/cochrane-frame.html
Joanna Briggs Institute	Agency for Healthcare Research and Quality (AHRQ)
Sigma Theta Tau International's Worldviews on Evidence-Based Nursing	http://www.blackwellpublishing.com/journal.asp?ref=1545-102X
U.S. Preventive Services Task Force	http://www.ahrq.gov/clinic/uspsfact.htm

Adapted from Stevens KR, Pugh JA (1999). Evidence-based practice and perioperative nursing. *Seminars in perioperative nursing 8(3):155-159.*

BOX 33-3

Examples of Evidence Summaries on Neonatal Care from Cochrane Database of Systematic Reviews

Anderson GC et al (2003). Early skin-to-skin contact for mothers and their healthy newborn infants. *Cochrane database of systematic reviews,* issue 2.

Balaguer A et al (2003). Infant position in neonates receiving mechanical ventilation. *Cochrane database of systematic reviews,* issue 2.

Bellù R et al (2005). Opioids for neonates receiving mechanical ventilation. *Cochrane database of systematic reviews,* issue 1.

Brady-Fryer B et al (2004). Pain relief for neonatal circumcision. *Cochrane database of systematic reviews,* issue 3.

Brocklehurst P (2002). Interventions for reducing the risk of mother-to-child transmission of HIV infection. *Cochrane database of systematic reviews,* issue 1.

Brown S et al (2002). Early postnatal discharge from hospital for healthy mothers and term infants. *Cochrane database of systematic reviews,* issue 3.

Collins CT et al (2003). Early discharge with home support of gavage feeding for stable preterm infants who have not established full oral feeds. *Cochrane database of systematic reviews,* issue 4.

Craft AP et al (2000). Vancomycin for prophylaxis against sepsis in preterm neonates. *Cochrane library (Oxford),* issue 3.

Darlow BA, Graham PJ (2000). Vitamin A supplementation for preventing morbidity and mortality in very low birth weight infants. *Cochrane database of systematic reviews,* issue 3.

Flenady VJ, Gray PH (2002). Chest physiotherapy for preventing morbidity in babies being extubated from mechanical ventilation. *Cochrane database of systematic reviews,* issue 2.

Flint A et al (2005). Continuous infusion versus intermittent flushing to prevent loss of function of peripheral intravenous catheters used for drug administration in newborn infants. *Cochrane database of systematic reviews,* issue 4.

Gray PH, Flenady V (2001). Cot-nursing versus incubator care for preterm infants. *Cochrane database of systematic reviews,* issue 2.

Henderson G et al (2001). Formula milk versus preterm human milk for feeding preterm or low birth weight infants. *Cochrane database of systematic reviews,* issue 3.

Henderson G et al (2005). Calorie and protein-enriched formula versus standard term formula for improving growth and development in preterm or low birth weight infants

following hospital discharge. *Cochrane database of systematic reviews,* issue 2.

Henderson-Smart DJ, Osborn DA (2002). Kinesthetic stimulation for preventing apnea in preterm infants. *Cochrane database of systematic reviews,* issue 2.

Lemyre B et al (2000). Nasal intermittent positive pressure ventilation (NIPPV) versus nasal continuous positive airway pressure (NCPAP) for apnea of prematurity. *Cochrane database of systematic reviews,* issue 3.

McCall EM et al (2005). Interventions to prevent hypothermia at birth in preterm and/or low birthweight babies. *Cochrane database of systematic reviews,* issue 1.

Osborn DA, Henderson-Smart DJ (1999). Kinesthetic stimulation for treating apnea in preterm infants. *Cochrane database of systematic reviews,* issue 1.

Premji S, Chessell L (2002). Continuous nasogastric milk feeding versus intermittent bolus milk feeding for premature infants less than 1500 grams. *Cochrane database of systematic reviews,* issue 4.

Shah V, Ohlsson A (2000). Venepuncture versus heel lance for blood sampling in term neonates. *Cochrane database of systematic reviews,* issue 3.

Shah P, Shah V (2005). Continuous heparin infusion to prevent thrombosis and catheter occlusion in neonates with peripherally placed percutaneous central venous catheters. *Cochrane database of systematic reviews,* issue 3.

Sinclair JC (2000). Servo-control for maintaining abdominal skin temperature at 36° C in low birth weight infants. *Cochrane database of systematic reviews,* issue 3.

Soll RF (2000). Synthetic surfactant for respiratory distress syndrome in preterm infants. *Cochrane database of systematic reviews,* issue 3.

Symington A, Pinelli J (2003). Developmental care for promoting development and preventing morbidity in preterm infants. *Cochrane database of systematic reviews,* issue 4.

Vickers A et al (2004). Massage for promoting growth and development of preterm and/or low birth-weight infants. *Cochrane database of systematic reviews,* issue 2.

Webster J, Pritchard MA (2003). Gowning by attendants and visitors in newborn nurseries for prevention of neonatal morbidity and mortality. *Cochrane database of systematic reviews,* issue 2.

Wells DA et al (2005). Positioning for acute respiratory distress in hospitalised infants and children. *Cochrane database of systematic reviews,* issue 2.

Zupan J, Garner P (2000). Topical umbilical cord care at birth. *Cochrane database of systematic reviews,* issue 3.

To focus the EBP effort, clinical priority topics are identified and set out as the first targets for evidence-based quality improvement. To be successful, the organization and health care team are involved. The criteria useful for selecting priority topics may be those established by the IOM to identify national priorities for health care improvement (IOM, 2003). These are (1) impact in terms of burden on patient, family, health care system, and society; (2) evidence that already exists for improvability but is not yet used in standard care; and

(3) inclusiveness, reflecting applicability to patients across the life span and settings.

After identifying clinical priority topics, the evidence must be located. A comprehensive search is essential and professional information management skills are valuable. Beginning with a search for evidence summaries is often productive in locating reviews that have already been completed. Locating other forms of knowledge, such as primary research and clinical practice guidelines are also important in this step.

Critical appraisal of the evidence can be accomplished by an evidence team. Using existing checklists, the validity and strength of the evidence are rated.

An evidence-base clinical practice guideline (CPG) may be adapted from an existing one or developed by the team. This CPG development process should be standardized to ensure that evidence is explicated and rated in all CPGs that are introduced into practice.

Quality indicators are selected and baseline assessments are made.

A comprehensive plan for change, adoption of innovation, and integration into practice is developed and implemented.

The targeted quality indicators are measured once again and compared to baseline assessment. These outcome measures should include patient outcomes, satisfaction, health status (population) indicators, and cost impact. The impact on the care process is also measured to determine if clinical practice has been true to the prescribed CPG. Feedback from quality audits is effective in stabilizing the change to the new standard of care.

USING THE EBP MODEL TO CHANGE NEONATAL NURSING PRACTICE

Neonatal nurses can use findings from research as well as other evidence to improve and change neonatal nursing practice. The first step in developing an EBP protocol or procedure is the identification of a clinical problem to be addressed. Nurses might identify a problem of concern in their individual clinical setting, or specialty organizations might identify priorities for research utilization projects. For example, in 1990 the Association of Women's Health, Obstetric, and Neonatal Nurses (AWHONN) convened a panel of nurse experts to identify areas with sufficient research to develop research-based protocols that could be tested in multiple settings. Gennaro (1994) described the following neonatal topics that were identified by the AWHONN panel:

1. Use of comfort measures such as nonnutritive sucking during or in anticipation of stressful procedures
2. Removal of barriers to successful breastfeeding and improving breastfeeding success in preterm infants
3. Improving skin integrity of low-birth-weight premature infants
4. Improving thermoregulation of infants
5. Reducing physiologic sequelae of infant suctioning
6. Using findings that indicate that infants do feel pain
7. Using telephone follow-up services for high-risk infants and families

Members of the AWHONN Research Committee recommended that the organization fund an EBP project to evaluate the best method for transition of preterm infants to open cribs and appointed a group of six neonatal nurse researchers to conduct the project (Meier, 1994). After reviewing the literature on the topic, the group held a series of meetings and ultimately developed a weaning protocol that was subsequently tested with 270 infants from 10 different hospitals (Medoff-Cooper, 1994). The evidence of this project suggested that preterm infants could be moved to an open crib at lower weights than had been suggested by results of previous studies.

The AWHONN project is an excellent example of the contributions that clinical professional associations can make to the development of EBP guidelines. This project illustrates several points in the ACE Star Model: evaluation of original research related to thermoregulation, developing a practice guideline based on a review and synthesis of the existing research, and evaluating the outcome of the EBP guideline.

Another example of an EBP project that was developed by professional associations was a collaborative project developed by AWHONN and the National Association of Neonatal Nurses (NANN) using research findings to develop a protocol for neonatal skin care (Lund et al, 2001). As in the transition to open crib project, a group of researchers reviewed extant literature to develop a clinical practice guideline and data collection tools. Site recruitment resulted in participation of 65 coordinators from 60 clinical sites across 27 states. A total of 51 sites completed all phases of the project, which involved 2820 infants in all levels of care. Results of the study indicated that the use of the clinical guideline resulted in improved skin condition of neonates in intensive, secondary, and well-baby nurseries. Nurses also were better able to identify risk factors for impaired skin integrity in neonates.

Another initiative that focuses on enhancing awareness of nurses and consumers of evidence in order to enhance health care is the Near Term Initiative launched in April 2005 by AWHONN. The association first convened an expert panel that identified several gaps in research, education, and clinical practice resources for nurses and families caring for near-term infants. The focus of this initiative will be to enhance awareness of the special needs of the near-term infant among health care providers and consumers, and promote universal adoption of a practice guideline for care of these infants. For more information on this initiative, readers can go to the AWHONN website at http://www.awhonn.org/.

Many professional organizations have developed practice guidelines based on current available evidence. For example, the AWHONN website has links to practice guidelines related to continence for women, nursing management of the second stage of labor, breastfeeding support, and nursing care of the woman receiving regional analgesia/anesthesia in labor (www.awhonn.org/). Similarly, the National Association of Neonatal Nurses (NANN) has published position statements on various practice issues on its website, such as cup and finger feeding of breast milk, pain management, cobedding, and prevention of bilirubin encephalopathy and kernicterus (www.nann.org).

Rogers' (1995) model of diffusion of innovations is widely used in integrating evidence-based CPGs into practice. This model includes five stages: knowledge, persuasion, decision, implementation, and confirmation.

During the evidence summary phase of knowledge transformation, existing research related to the clinical problem is reviewed, evaluated for scientific merit and relevance for the particular clinical setting, and summarized into a single statement. To be most helpful to clinical decision making, strength of evidence included in the summary should be rated—that is, the strength of the conclusion is rated reflecting the likelihood that the intervention causes the outcome. Most rating systems are based on the *research design* and the resulting strength of causality attributed to the design. For example, a descriptive design does not produce evidence of cause and effect between intervention and outcome. However, a true experiment (also called *randomized control trial* [RCT]) does provide evidence of the likelihood that the intervention will produce the targeted outcome. It is widely agreed that a systematic review produces the strongest evidence for clinical decision making.

A number of hierarchies of strength of evidence have been developed and evaluated (AHRQ, 2002). Based on several of the most widely used ratings, the following hierarchy assists nurses in rating the strength of evidence in determining cause and effect:

1-A	Systematic Reviews
1-B	Randomized Control Trials, True Experiments
2-A	Individual Cohort Studies
2-B	Outcomes Research Studies
3	Case-Control Studies
4	Case Series Studies
5	Expert Opinion, Theory, Bench Research Studies

There are a number of resources to help clinicians evaluate the strength of evidence, and there is a variety of appraisal criteria for different types of evidence. Cullum (2000) identified criteria that nurses can use to evaluate the validity of studies of treatment or prevention interventions.

Primary questions to evaluate validity of the study are:

- Was the assignment of patients to treatments randomized, and was the randomization concealed?
- Was follow-up sufficiently long and complete?
- Were patients analyzed in the groups to which they were initially randomized?

Secondary questions to evaluate validity of the study are:

- Were patients, clinicians, outcome assessors, and data analysts unaware of (blinded to or masked from) patient allocation?
- Were participants in each group treated equally, except for the intervention being evaluated?
- Were the groups similar at the start of the trial?
- What were the results?

Questions to consider in evaluating the results include:

- How large was the effect of the treatment? (Another way to say this is "how different were the outcomes for the experimental and control groups?")
- Are the effects "clinically" as well as "statistically" significant?
- Was the sample large enough so that the results can be generalized?
- Will the results help me in caring for my patients?

Two questions to consider when answering this last question are:

1. Are the patients in the study similar to my patients?
2. Are there any risks to my patients in applying the results from this study? (pp 100-102)

Even though descriptive and qualitative studies are ranked as lower levels of evidence than systematic reviews or experimental RCTs, findings from these studies can also provide important evidence for practice. Russell and Gregory (2003) provided guidelines for evaluating qualitative studies

Questions to evaluate validity of a qualitative study are:

- Is the research clear and adequately substantiated?
- Is the design appropriate for the research question?
- Is the sampling method appropriate for the research question and design?
- Were data collected and managed systematically?
- Were data analyzed appropriately?
- What were the results?

Questions to consider in evaluating the results of a qualitative study include:

- Is the description of findings thorough?
- Will the results help me in caring for my patients?

Questions to consider when answering this latter question are:

- What meaning and relevance does the study have for my practice?
- Does the study help me understand the context of my practice?
- Does the study enhance my knowledge about my practice? (pp 36-40)

During the persuasion stage of EBP integration, changes at all levels must be addressed. Vested interest groups from across the agency and across the services and disciplines must be persuaded to consider the practice change. Factors such as cost, potential benefits to the patient and to the institution, and the complexity of the change that is proposed will all influence the willingness of others to adopt the evidence-based change.

The decision to implement an EBP change requires system change. At an agency level, leaders must be persuaded to rewrite practice standards and policies. Melnyk et al (2000) outlined guidelines for implementing EBP and suggested that the practice environment must value EBP, and nursing evaluations should reflect the nurse's provision of evidence-based care. Nurses should work in interdisciplinary EBP teams and use change theory to implement new policies and practices based on best available evidence.

Implementation of the change might be done at the individual nurse, the unit, or the institutional level. A final and critical stage of the research utilization process is to confirm or evaluate the results of implementing the research-based change. This stage requires considerable planning before implementation and commitment to collect the data needed for evaluation.

CONDUCTING RESEARCH IN NEONATAL NURSING

Scientific substantiation of effectiveness of neonatal nursing and neonatal care requires collaboration with other nurses and health professionals. The clinical nurse is often the first to recognize and identify trends in newborn and infant care problems for which there is no apparent evidential base. With the guidance and assistance of other nurses, nurse specialists, and physicians, a collaborative investigation may be used to explore the problem. The combination of expertise from multiple disciplines can make a highly effective research team.

Research is a formal, systematic inquiry or examination of a given problem. The outcome or goal of research is to discover new information or relationships or to verify existing knowledge. Other less formal definitions of research focus on the understanding an event by logically relating it to other events. Some types of research are designed to predict events by relating them empirically to antecedents in time. Still other types of research attempt to control or manipulate an event or procedure to determine its impact on other phenomena.

WHY DO RESEARCH?

Using the research process to discover new information or to confirm empirical knowledge allows for the growth and evolution of nursing practice. Without research, nursing care would be based simply on tradition. The practice of nursing would change slowly and grow little because things would be done the way they have always been done. The failure to conduct research regarding neonatal care has taught us some sobering lessons. Judgments of efficacy based on observation of small numbers of infants or of treatments based on the principle "if a little is good, more is better" have resulted in significant morbidity and mortality for neonates. Misuses of oxygen therapy, chloramphenicol, and vitamin E are examples (Jain & Vidyasagar, 1989). From these experiences, the use of clinical research trials to evaluate new therapies scientifically before widespread application has become more common in neonatal care.

The research process also provides a vehicle for challenging accepted routines and theories. Nurses caring for neonates often identify issues for which adequate scientific information on which to base clinical judgments does not exist.

The investigative role of the nurse is integrated throughout many clinical career ladders and performance competencies. A number of professional nursing organizations also define research within the role of the nurse. The American Nurses Association (ANA) asserts that all nurses are responsible for assuming various research activities and roles as appropriate to their education. In addition, the ANA has issued a position statement specifying that basic-level nurses (associate degree and baccalaureate degree) use research findings in clinical practice and implement nursing research findings (ANA, 1994).

RESEARCH ROLES FOR NEONATAL NURSES

The many different research roles for neonatal nurses include research consumer, participant, facilitator/coordinator, and investigator (Harrison, 2001). All neonatal nurses should be knowledgeable consumers of research, should read reports of research, and should ensure that their practice is research- or evidence-based. To be a knowledgeable research consumer, the nurse must be a critical reader of research articles. A rigorous critique of research should also be carried out before one tries to use the findings in a practice situation. Unfortunately, research findings are sometimes used as a basis for practice without critical review (Perez-Woods & Tse, 1990).

Melnyk et al (2004) identified a number of individual barriers to research utilization of EBP by clinicians that have been identified in prior studies. These barriers include lack of time and heavy patient loads, lack of appreciation for the value of research, difficulty searching for and retrieving studies, difficulty reading, understanding, and evaluating research reports, institutional barriers, and limited autonomy or control over one's own practice. Institutional barriers include inadequate staffing and failure to reward nurses who initiate change based on findings from research. Funk et al (1995) noted that additional barriers to using research include problems with the research and with the presentation of the research. Barriers related to the research itself include lack of replication of the research, uncertainty about the credibility of the research results, and methodologic inadequacies of the research. Barriers related to the way the research was presented include problems with understanding the statistical analysis, failure to identify the implications of the study, and failure to report the research clearly.

In a recent survey of 160 nurses (Melnyk et al, 2004), only 46% of these nurses identified that their current practices were evidence-based. Factors associated with increased evidence-based care were nurses' beliefs about the importance of EBP, knowledge of EBP, length of practice as an advanced practice nurse, use of the Cochrane Database of Scientific Reviews or the National Guideline Clearinghouse, and having a mentor to model EBP. These findings can be used to plan changes for improving the use of EBP in clinical settings.

A key research role for every neonatal nurse is to serve as an advocate for infants and families who are research participants to ensure their rights are protected and their safety is maintained. Thomas (2005) reviewed safety and ethical issues related to research with vulnerable infants and their families, and suggested that neonatal nurses may serve an important role by reporting any safety concerns to the Institutional Review Board (or ethics committee) that originally approved the study.

Neonatal nurses can participate in research in a variety of ways. One effective method to gain knowledge about the research process is to become involved in a colleague's project as a research participant. Nurses can also participate in research as data collectors. Some neonatal nurses work as clinical research coordinators (CRCs) or clinical research associates (CRAs) and assume primary responsibility for implementing clinical studies and protocols (McKinney & Vermuelen, 2000). The Association for Clinical Research Practitioners (ACRP) has a certification program for CRCs as well as for CRAs. (For information, see the ACRP website at http://www.acrpnet.org.)

Another method of participating in the research process is to perform secondary analyses on data that were collected to answer another research question. Often answers to other research questions can be extracted from a single database without having to collect new data. Caution, however, must be used in the design of secondary analysis studies to minimize threats to validity and reliability that are inherent in the method.

Neonatal nurses prepared at the master's or doctoral level might also serve as research facilitators (McGee, 1996). Clinical Nurse Specialists (CNSs) may promote research by coordinating research committees, promoting research utilization, coordinating research activities in the NICU, and providing educational programs to help nurses understand and use findings from research. According to the American Nurses' Association 1994 paper titled "Education for Participation in Nursing Research," preparation of nurse scientists for principal investigator roles begins at the masters' level and is the focus of doctoral preparation. Nurses prepared at these levels assume primary responsibility as principal investigators in research (ANA, 1994).

OBSTACLES TO INVOLVEMENT IN RESEARCH

The reluctance of nurses to become involved in research generally stems from two basic obstacles: lack of knowledge and lack of resources. Both of these obstacles can be overcome. To address these issues effectively, nurses must receive education regarding the research process, have the opportunity to participate in research projects (in data collection or as research participants), and participate with colleagues in sessions to stimulate the formulation of questions from their clinical experience. One can begin by asking the question "why?" of every NICU nursing practice.

Lack of resources—including time, money, and consultation—can be more difficult to address. In many institutions, the conduct of nursing research is still viewed as a frill and not central to the delivery of patient care. In such a setting, nurses who wish to conduct research may initially need to invest their own time and even money. However, once the research process has demonstrated clinical relevance, additional resources are often made available. Collaboration with colleagues within the institution, schools and universities, and industry can enhance resources. Writing grants with colleagues for the purposes of obtaining funds to support research is often the only way that clinical research can be conducted (Kenner & Walden, 2001).

IDENTIFYING THE RESEARCH PROBLEM OR QUESTION

Nurses in the clinical setting are often in the best position to identify and articulate research questions and to carry out research studies that improve the delivery of nursing care. The types of questions posed by clinical researchers include questions about basic physiologic mechanisms, efficacy of different caregiving techniques, and identification and description of new phenomena. Box 33-4 lists topics of current research interest for neonatal nurses.

Many of these research questions are derived from the concern about the prevention of iatrogenic complications of treatments. Others emerge from systematic observation of clinical phenomena or from frustration with current practices.

BOX **33-4**

Some Current Neonatal Nursing Research Questions

Skin Care

How can epidermal damage from tape removal be reduced?

Can the permeable skin of preterm infants be used to deliver medication?

How can the barrier properties of the skin be improved to prevent infection and water loss?

Which cleansing agent and bathing techniques are best for preterm and full-term infants?

Do emollients prevent transepidermal water loss and dermatitis in premature infants?

What is the reliability and validity of the neonatal skin condition score?

Nutrition

How can breastfeeding practices be promoted among mothers of premature infants?

What are the most effective methods of delivering formula (e.g., continuous vs intermittent) to ill infants?

Does providing cheek and jaw support promote sucking patterns of preterm infants during feeding?

What are the effects of kangaroo care on breast milk production?

Is weight gain improved with demand vs scheduled feeding?

How can intravenous access be improved and complications minimized?

What is the effect of nonnutritive sucking on neonatal weight gain?

What is the effect of protein supplementation of breast milk on the weight gain of preterm infants?

How can nurses assess infants' feeding skills and feeding readiness?

What is the best method to verify feeding tube placement in the preterm infant?

Instruments and Procedures

What is the best method for collecting urine?

Which scale provides the most accurate weight?

What is the influence of equipment weights on neonatal daily weight measurements?

Which device provides the most accurate measure of temperature?

What is the effect of routine care tasks, such as bathing or suctioning, on cerebral blood flow velocity?

Which pulse oximeters are most effective in reducing the effects of motion artifact?

What is the efficacy of saline vs heparin locks for peripheral IV flushes in neonates?

Do temperature probe covers contribute to nosocomial infections by providing an environment for skin microbe colonization?

What is the effect of draw-up volume on the accuracy of electrolyte measurements from neonatal arterial lines?

What are the different effects of tub and sponge bathing on preterm infants?

Effect of the Environment and Supplemental Stimulation

What is the impact of light, noise, and handling on infants in the NICU?

What is the appropriate level of stimulation for preterm infants?

What is the effect of supplemental massage and gentle touch on preterm infants?

What are the effects of music therapy on preterm infants?

What is the effect of cycled lighting on preterm infants?

What is the most appropriate method of positioning preterm infants to promote neuromuscular development?

What is the effect of swaddling preterm infants during painful procedures?

Extracorporeal Membrane Oxygenation (ECMO)

Is the initial training and ongoing education of ECMO specialists sufficient to maintain emergency management skills?

What are the long-term effects of ECMO's use?

What are the neurodevelopmental outcomes of infants who were treated with ECMO?

Endotracheal Tube Stabilization and Maintenance

How can slippage of the endotracheal tube within the trachea be measured?

How can movement of the endotracheal tube be minimized?

Is there a difference in the incidence of nosocomial infections, bronchopulmonary dysplasia, or frequency of suction when using closed vs open tracheal suctioning in neonates?

Management of Pain

How can neonatal pain be assessed?

When is pharmacologic treatment appropriate?

What factors influence preterm infants' responses to painful procedures?

Are there long-term consequences of unrelieved pain experienced in the neonatal period?

What is the most effective method for weaning the infant from analgesics?

Does the use of premedication prior to intubation result in fewer signs of physiologic distress during intubation compared to intubation without premedication?

What are effective nonpharmacologic pain-management techniques for use with neonates?

What are the analgesic effects of oral sucrose and pacifier use on preterm infants during painful procedures?

BOX 33-4

Some Current Neonatal Nursing Research Questions—cont'd

Thermoregulation

Which techniques are most effective in minimizing insensible water loss and maintaining thermoregulation in the extremely premature infant?

What are the optimal procedures for maintaining thermoregulation when transferring infants from incubators or warmers to open cribs?

What are the effects of skin-to-skin holding (kangaroo care) on thermoregulation of preterm infants?

Positioning and Holding

Which positions are most effective in promoting optimal oxygenation and in minimizing postural deformities?

What are the effects of skin-to-skin holding of high-risk infants?

What are the effects of containment and swaddling of preterm infants?

How often should infants' positions be changed?

Under what conditions is the prone position linked to sudden infant death syndrome?

What factors influence parents' decisions about sleep positions of their infants?

Developmental Care

What are the outcomes of developmental care?

What are the effects of developmental care training programs on the care delivered by NICU staff?

What are valid and reliable measures of stress in preterm infants?

Is measurement of heart rate variability or vagal tone a reliable means for assessing stability or stress in preterm infants?

Effects of Cocaine

How is the behavior of a cocaine-exposed infant different from that of the nonexposed infant?

What is the appropriate level of environmental stimulation for these infants?

What types of intervention programs are effective for families of cocaine-exposed infants following hospital discharge?

Effective Parent Teaching Techniques

What are the most effective teaching methods for instructing parents in the care of their newborns?

Is computer-assisted instruction effective?

What type of posthospital follow-up is most helpful to parents of infants who are released from the NICU?

Are postdischarge telephone follow-up programs effective in promoting breastfeeding of preterm infants discharged from the NICU?

What are parents' perceptions of a parental care-by-parent program before NICU discharge of their infants?

Family Issues

What nursing interventions help to reduce stressors experienced by families who have infants in the NICU?

What is the incidence of depression among parents of preterm infants?

What interventions help grieving parents?

What interventions help to promote attachment and adaptive parenting between parents and preterm infants and between parents and infants with serious health problems?

What are the outcomes associated with participation in a parent support group for parents of preterm infants?

What are parents' perceptions of the NICU follow-up clinic?

Staff Education

What is the most effective method of orientation of new NICU nurses?

How should formal classroom teaching and clinical preceptorship be integrated?

Are self-paced learning modules an effective teaching methodology for neonatal nurses?

Can neonatal nurses use expert systems to support decision making?

Delivery of Nursing Care

What is the most effective model for delivery of nursing care in the NICU?

Can nonprofessional staff be used in the NICU to support the professional nurse?

Does the use of critical pathways facilitate "costing out" nursing services?

What is the effect of a structured neonatal resuscitation program on delivery room resuscitation practices?

Retention of Nurses in the Critical Care Setting

What are the factors that increase job satisfaction for nurses working in the NICU?

How do NICU nurses cope with stress?

What factors increase the likelihood that nursing jobs will be retained?

Do neonatal nurses perceive technology in the NICU as sources of stress?

Ideas for research come from many different sources, including an individual nurse's experience, the nursing or health literature, discussions of social or health issues, or theory (Burns & Grove, 2001). Quality assurance and quality improvement activities often lead to the design and conduct of research. Nurses are often introduced to issues related to objective data collection through quality assurance audits. Issues of clinical consequence that are identified through quality assurance screening can lead to the articulation of research questions. Research principles can also be used in the evaluation of new procedures, protocols, and products. Evaluation is often an integral part of NICU nursing, but it is performed subjectively. Using research methodology to perform evaluation promotes scientific objectivity. Researchers and professional organizations sometimes conduct surveys or convene expert panels to identify research priorities. These priorities can also help researchers identify researchable problems. For example, the National Institute of Nursing Research (NINR) has identified the following areas of research opportunity for 2006:

- Research in a Multicultural Society: Focus on Preventing and Intervening in HIV and AIDS
- Increasing Health Promotion through Studies on Parenting Capacities
- Biobehavioral Methods to Improve Outcomes Research
- Improving Cognitive Function in Quality of Life in CNS Disorders

- Providing End-of-Life and Palliative Care in Rural and Frontier Areas

(See the NINR website at http://www.nih.gov/ninr.)

CURRENT TRENDS IN NEONATAL NURSING RESEARCH

Over the past 20 years there has been a tremendous increase in the quantity and quality of descriptive as well as experimental and quasiexperimental studies focused on preterm or other high-risk infants and their families. Holditch-Davis and Black (2003) reviewed nursing research on the care of the preterm infant and identified 17 nurse researchers who had developed programs of neonatal research, meaning that the researcher had at least five publications since 1990 and was the first author on at least three of these publications. These programs of research had four themes: infant responses to the NICU environment, pain management, infant stimulation, and infant behavior and development. Holditch-Davis and Black suggested that these research programs had many strengths, including interdisciplinary focus and clinical relevance, but recommended that more studies should focus on the clinically ill infant, and that more studies should be based on a developmental science perspective.

An important source of funding for nursing research is the National Institute of Nursing Research (NINR), an institute within the U.S. Department of Health and Human Service's (DHHS) National Institutes of Health (NIH). There are many different mechanisms for funding of experienced as well as new investigators. Abstracts of research funded by the NIH can be searched and retrieved in the Computer Information on Retrieval of Information on Scientific Projects (CRISP) database (http://crisp.cit.nih.gov/crisp/). A query using the key-words "preterm infant" resulted in a listing of 124 abstracts of research funded by the NINR and other NIH institutes.

In 2004 and 2005, the NINR published an annotated bibliography of recent findings related to the management of high-risk pregnancies and neonatal care. These bibliographies are excellent resources and are published by the NINR in an effort to enhance nurses' awareness of research findings and support EBP. Box 33-5 lists the areas of research interest for 2004 and 2005 that were identified by the NINR.

Another trend in neonatal research is the publication of reports of EBP projects in the NICU. For example, Pollock and Franklin (2004) described an ongoing project to implement developmentally sensitive care in the NICU. Smith (2005) described the process of developing, implementing, and evaluating a feeding guideline for very low birth weight infants. There are many opportunities for neonatal nurses to implement EBP projects to improve the quality of care for patients and families. Sharing experiences by presentations at professional meetings or publication in the professional literature will contribute to the growing body of information about EBP and the implementation of evidence-based neonatal nursing practice.

SUMMARY

With more and more hospitals and health care organizations seeking to be recognized for effective care and identifying the need for the inclusion of evidence-based clinical guidelines for care in these institutions, interest in research and EBP will continue to grow. This chapter has highlighted some of the ways in which neonatal nursing and care is being affected by research and EBP.

BOX **33-5**

Areas of Research Included in the 2004-2005 Annotated Bibliography

2004*
Identifying maternal risk factors
Prenatal care and preventive measures
Pregnancy and HIV/AIDS
Preterm infant growth and development
Parental issues and attachment
NICU care (cycled lighting, individualized vs standard monitoring criteria, feeding, thermal stability, sleep state)
Parenting issues
Follow-up interventions
Long-term outcomes

2005†
Nursing and medical staff in intensive care
Handwashing in the NICU
Issues of genetic testing
Prenatal issues
Care of the preterm infant (thermoregulation, feeding, kangaroo care, sleeping/waking behaviors)
Parental and family issues
Development and early infancy (tactile stimulation, multimodal stimulation, infant colic)

*From National Institute of Nursing Research Division of Extramural Activities (2004). Recent findings from the National Institute of Nursing Research related to neonatal care. *Neonatal network* 23(1):57-63.
†From National Institute of Nursing Research Division of Extramural Activities (2005). Recent findings from the National Institute of Nursing Research related to neonatal care. *Neonatal network* 24(1):65-70.

REFERENCES

Agency for Healthcare Research and Quality (AHRQ) (March 2002). *Systems to rate the strength of scientific evidence.* Summary, Evidence Report/Technology Assessment, No. 47. AHRQ Publication No. 02-E015. Rockville, MD: Agency for Healthcare Research and Quality. Available at: http://www.ahrq.gov/clinic/epcsums/strengthsum.htm. Retrieved September 15, 2006.

Agency for Healthcare Research and Quality (AHRQ) (2005). *National healthcare quality report.* Available at: http://www.ahrq.gov/qual/nhqr05/nhqr05.pdf. Retrieved July 21, 2006.

Alderson P et al, editors (2003). *Cochrane reviewers' handbook 4.2.2* (updated December 2003). Available at: http://www.cochrane.org/resources/handbook/hbook.htm. Retrieved September 30, 2005.

American Nurses Association (ANA) (1994). *ANA position statement: education for participation in nursing research.* Available at: http://www.nursingworld.org/readroom/position/research/rseducat.htm. Retrieved October 15, 2005.

Burns N, Grove SK (2001). *The practice of nursing research: conduct, critique, and utilization,* ed 4. Philadelphia: Saunders.

Cullum N (2000). *Evaluation of studies of treatment or prevention interventions. Evidence-based nursing* 3:100-102.

Funk SG et al (1995). Barriers and facilitators of research utilization: an integrative review. *Nursing clinics of North America* 30(3):395-407.

Gennaro S (1994). Research utilization: an overview. *Journal of obstetric, gynecologic, and neonatal nursing* 23(4):313-319.

Guyatt G, Rennie D (2002). *Users' guides to the medical literature: essentials of evidence-based clinical practice.* Chicago: American Medical Association.

Harrison L (2001). Research roles for neonatal nurses. *Central lines* 17(1):18-20.

Holditch-Davis D, Black BP (2003). Care of preterm infants: programs of research and their relationship to developmental science. *Annual review of nursing research* 21:23-60.

Institute of Medicine (IOM) (2000). *To err is human: building a safer health system*. Washington, DC: National Academy Press.

Institute of Medicine (IOM) (2003). *Priority areas for national action: transforming health care quality*. Washington, DC: National Academies Press.

Jain L, Vidyasagar D (1989). Iatrogenic disorders in modern neonatology. *Clinics in perinatology* 16(1):255-273.

Kenner C, Walden M (2001). *Grant writing tips for nurses and other health professionals*. Washington, DC: American Nurses Foundation/American Nurses Publishing.

Lund CH et al (2001). Neonatal skin care: clinical outcomes of the AWHONN/NANN evidence-based clinical practice guideline. *Journal of obstetric, gynecologic, and neonatal nursing* 30(1):41-51.

McGee P (1996). The research role of the advanced nurse practitioner. *British journal of nursing* 5:290-292.

McKinney J, Vermuelen W (2000). Research nurses play a vital role in clinical trials. *Oncology nursing forum* 27:28.

Medoff-Cooper B (1994). Transition of the preterm infant to an open crib. *Journal of obstetric, gynecologic, and neonatal nursing* 23(4):329-335.

Meier PF (1994). Transition of the preterm infant to an open crib: process of the project group. *Journal of obstetric, gynecologic, and neonatal nursing* 23(4):321-326.

Melnyk BM et al (2000). Evidence-based practice: the past, present, and recommendations for the millennium. *Pediatric nursing* 26(1):77-81.

Melnyk BM et al (2004). Nurses' perceived knowledge, beliefs, skills and needs regarding evidence-based practice: implications for accelerating the paradigm shift. *Worldviews on evidence-based nursing* 1(3):185-193.

Mulrow C (1994). Rationale for systematic reviews. *British medical journal* 309:597-599.

National Guideline Clearinghouse (NGC) (2005). *Management of breastfeeding for healthy full-term infants*. Available at: http://www.guideline.gov. Retrieved August 9, 2006.

National Institute of Nursing Research Division of Extramural Activities (2004). Recent findings from the National Institute of Nursing Research related to neonatal care. *Neonatal network* 23(1):57-63.

National Institute of Nursing Research Division of Extramural Activities (2005). Recent findings from the National Institute of Nursing Research related to neonatal care. *Neonatal network* 24(1):65-70.

Perez-Woods R, Tse AM (1990). Research attitudes, activities, competencies, and interest of NANN members. *Neonatal network* 8(5):57-59.

Pollock TR, Franklin C (2004). Use of evidence-based practice in the neonatal intensive care unit. *Critical care clinics of North America* 16(2):243-248.

Rogers EM (1995). *Diffusion of innovations*, ed 4. New York: Free Press.

Russell CK, Gregory DM (2003). Evaluation of qualitative research studies. *Evidence-based nursing* 6:36-40.

Sackett DL et al (2000). *Evidence-based medicine: how to practice and teach EBM*. Edinburgh: Churchill Livingstone.

Smith JR (2005). Early enteral feeding for the very low birth weight infant: the development and impact of a research-based guideline. *Neonatal network—journal of neonatal nursing* 24(4):9-19.

Stevens KR (2001). An introduction to evidence-based practice. *Newborn and infant nursing reviews* 1(1):6-10.

Stevens KR (2001). Systematic reviews: the heart of evidence-based practice. *AACN clinical issues: advanced practice in acute and critical care* 12(4):529-538.

Stevens KR (2004). *ACE star model of knowledge transformation*. Available at: http://www.acestar.uthscsa.edu. Retrieved August 5, 2006.

Stevens KR (2005). *Essential competencies for evidence-based practice in nursing*. San Antonio, TX: Academic Center for Evidence-Based Practice, The University of Texas Health Science Center.

Stevens KR, Pugh JA (1999). Evidence-based practice and perioperative nursing. *Seminars in perioperative nursing* 8(3):155-159.

Stevens KR, Staley J (2006). The Quality Chasm reports, evidence-based practice, and nursing's response to improve healthcare. *Nursing outlook* 54(2):94-101.

Thomas K (2005). Safety: when infants and parents are research subjects. *Journal of perinatal and neonatal nursing* 19(1):52-58.

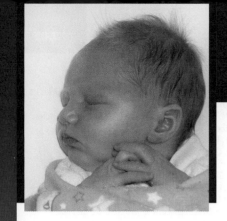

Chapter 34

Legal and Ethical Issues of Neonatal Care

Pamela Holtzclaw Williams • Tanya Sudia-Robinson

Legal and ethical issues in neonatal care challenge the use of critical thinking, negotiating, and decision-making skills and are becoming more commonplace as the age of viability has decreased and technologic advances have increased. These issues often arise when divergent legal, ethical, or moral perspectives exist. The neonatal nurse advocates for the infant and family within an environment of local, state, and federal laws, professional standards of care, and institutional guidelines. Advocacy, therefore, for the neonate requires nurses to exercise navigation skills at various levels, ranging from individual patient care to global concerns. The responsible neonatal nurse incorporates the elements of the formal legal and ethical frameworks into the care. If this is done it can prevent civil liability, criminal charges, or threats to nursing licensure while protecting the infant and family. The framework of rules, laws, codes, and standards is dynamic.

The neonatal nurse can function as a change catalyst in the legal and ethical environmental framework, regardless of the setting. Whether in academic, administration, research, or clinical settings, neonatal nurses can advocate for legal and ethical causes. Nurses create change through individual and collective efforts.

Individual nurses caring for the individual newborn perform the advocacy role at the most direct level while addressing immediate needs of the infant. The nurse providing direct neonatal care must be prepared to meet ethical and legal issues that directly affect relationships with patients, parents, and family, the interdisciplinary team, and the institution. The advent of technology in the neonatal unit has compounded the challenge. Genetic testing, cord blood banking, and the ability to mechanically sustain life in the extremely premature infant are examples of fertile ground from which ethical dilemmas grow.

Collective neonatal nursing organizations function as watchdogs for ethical standard enforcement for neonatal populations. (For the NANN position statement on Code of Ethics, go to: http://www.nann.org/i4a/pages/index.cfm?pageid=1012.) Collectively, nurses also lobby and advocate policy agendas related to ethical issues related to neonatal care. For example, the Childbirth Nurses Interest Group, as part of the Registered Nurses of Ontario website (http://www.rnao.org/), describes itself as an advocate group. In addition, nurse organizations advocate by establishing professional ethical standards. The American Nurses Association created a code of ethics for nurses that is used as a template for specialty organizations

to adapt and can be viewed at http://www.nursingworld.org/ethics/ecode.htm.

This chapter is designed to prepare neonatal nurses to address the myriad of ethical and legal issues related to newborn care. Provided is a methodical approach model for nurse advocates. The intent is to encourage nurses to exercise the role of neonate advocate to the fullest capacity (Peter et al, 2004). Text boxes present examples of legal and ethical issues currently encountered by neonatal nurses. This chapter demonstrates analytical consideration of legal and ethical issues currently encountered by identifying critical elements that nurses navigate in advocacy, critical decision-making and finding dilemma resolutions, and illustrating navigation and resolution strategies for legal and ethical issues existing in neonatal nursing.

ELEMENTS OF LEGAL AND ETHICAL ISSUES IN NEONATAL NURSING

The Ethical Dilemma: An Element of Legal and Ethical Neonatal Nursing Issues

Ethical issues become ethical dilemmas when people of differing perspectives take or propose to take disparate action. Dilemmas are characteristically situations where there are two or more legitimate alternatives for action with different outcomes (Monterosso et al, 2005).

The dilemma may arise when the nurse takes issue with an action that has occurred in the recent past. For example, a physician orders minimal pain medication based on an outdated medical opinion, whereas the nurse's current evidence-based opinion is contrary.

The dilemma may also arise when an action is contemplated for the near future. For example, the family and health care team cannot reach consensus whether an extremely premature infant should continue on mechanical ventilation for life support.

Dilemmas also occur where actions are ongoing and repetitive in newborn patients. Moral distress can occur where the neonatal nurse is required by state law to participate in comprehensive genetic neonatal screening, yet there is no requirement for parental consent and no training in genetic counseling, nor is there sufficient time to provide follow-up for the impact of disclosure of positive or false positive test results. Here the conflicting ethical perspectives are the legislated mandate's determination that screening is a neonatal care priority, balanced against the nurse's professional ethics

Example of an Ethical Dilemma

Legal Perspective vs Health Care Perspective vs Maternal Substance Abuse

Infants are born with substance addiction as a result of maternal substance abuse during pregnancy. In addition to addiction, infants are born at alarming rates with permanent disabilities such as fetal alcohol syndrome. The health care and legal perspectives are not always in consensus as to what is in the best interest of the infant in these situations. The neonatal nurse can be caught in the crossfire of this ethical dilemma.

Health care has consistently maintained that the best interest of the newborn is served by working with, not against, the interests of the mother. (See position statements of various health care organizations.) When feasible, prenatal substance abuse treatment is advocated. Nursing advocates that, where addiction or disability of the newborn is detected, the mother should be supported with substance abuse treatment, not incarceration or legal jeopardy (Kenner et al, 2000).

However, in many states there are legislated policies by lawmakers or law enforcement that the health care provider must report the mother when a child is born addicted or with health impairment due to substance abuse. Criminal charges have been brought against mothers delivering drug-addicted newborns (Foley, 2002).

Neonatal nurses are caught in the crossfire. Such regulations challenge ethical standards of confidentiality and loyalty to the patient. Nurses can ask their institutions for support on protocol in these situations. Ethics committees should be prepared to advise the nurse on how to proceed.

Ethical Issues Providing Potential for Ethical Dilemma

Cord Blood Banking

Technology and genetic knowledge development have combined to create a new option for prospective parents. Blood can be extracted from the umbilical cord after birth and stored. The blood is valued for its stem cells. The blood has potential future use for the newborn, a blood relative, research, or an unrelated donee. Stem cells are currently used for transplanting to treat childhood hematologic cancers. To date, more than 45 disorders can be treated with stem cells from umbilical cord blood. On the horizon are uses for immunodeficiencies or gene therapies.

In an effort to obtain informed consent to store, the issue is what to inform the parent regarding its future use. For now, the most appropriate rationale has been described as a "possibility in the future" or a "just in case." The recommendation now is to obtain informed consent during pregnancy and again after the sample is obtained.

Another issue is the identification of ownership and rights: Can the parent decide to use it as he or she pleases? Who will have access—can donations occur for research or other recipients? These questions have been characterized as a work in progress (Pinch, 2001).

The March of Dimes has deemed the potential ethical issues to merit discussion at their website. The site explains there are many ethical issues in connection with umbilical cord blood banking that have yet to be resolved. Beyond who owns the cord blood sample and how informed consent is obtained, there are more questions. How should the obligation to notify parents and donor children of the results of medical testing for infectious diseases and genetic information be handled? How are privacy and confidentiality to be maintained? How will services for the harvesting of and access to umbilical cord blood be provided fairly? (March of Dimes, 2006).

Where there are ethical questions that can be answered in more than one fashion, there is room for ethical issues to become ethical dilemmas. Can you think of a hypothetical situation where some of these issues could become a dilemma for the parent or the nurse?

focused on parental informed consent, continuity, and competency of care.

Box 34-1 shows an example of an ethical dilemma involving legal perspective vs health care perspective vs maternal substance abuse.

An ethical dilemma has recently been proposed as a NANDA nursing diagnosis. The proposal defines the phenomenon as a perceived conflict of ethical/moral values, principles, and duties/rules underlying thought and/or action (Kopala & Burkhart, 2005).

As the 20th century closed, a study was conducted where nurses identified the ethical dilemmas that were most disturbing. Ethical issues arose most frequently from questions of adequate respect of informed consent, advance directives, accuracy of information about a treatment, and quality of life being adequately balanced against extension of life with technology (Riley & Fry, 2000).

Neonates do not have advance directives. Therefore there is a required surrogate decision making that confounds questions regarding resuscitation or heroic measures to prolong life. Informing parents about the complex technologic interventions and being asked to predict the quality of life for the very premature infant is becoming a frequent area of neonatal nurse responsibility. Therefore, a significant concentration of ethical dilemmas in neonatal nursing for the 21st century is apparent.

Box 34-2 shows an example of clinical issues that may result in ethical dilemmas involving cord blood banking.

The Nurse: Individually and Collectively
Elements of Neonatal Legal and Ethical Issues

At the individual level, the neonatal nurse has relationships with the neonate and family, other interdisciplinary team members, the employing institution, co-worker peers, and him- or herself. Each relationship can develop divergent ethical or legal positions on the right course of action for neonates individually or collectively.

The neonatal nurse must avoid a paternalistic attitude in the relationship with both the neonate and family, while advocating for what is in the best interest of their patient. The nurse as the neonate's advocate must also avoid temptation to be judgmental regarding parents' decisions.

Avoiding unprofessional pitfalls does not equate to passively responding to ethical issues. Nurses can enable themselves to efficiently advocate by assessing and exercising action using their unique personal strengths such as courage, honesty, confidence, assertiveness, unconventionality, diplomacy, communication, and argumentation skills. Experience in advocacy creates greater comfort in the role (Peter et al, 2004).

Institutional support of nursing advocacy is fundamental to the role. This support provides a balance of power in institutional policy. Institutional support reinforces self-efficacy and confidence in the nursing advocacy role. Nurses should be represented on institutional ethics committees to ensure peer review of nursing actions.

Nursing culture can reverse assumptions that it is passive and accepting of being excluded from participation in the resolution of legal and ethical issues. These assumptions are to the detriment of both the nurse and the neonate. The nurse who spends consecutive hours with the patient and family is better positioned than other health care team members to develop decisions on what is in the best interest of the neonate (Peter et al, 2004; Turkoski, 2001).

While performing the advocacy role, the newborn's nurse may encounter obstacles in the environmental framework that prevent the recognized ethical action from being taken. Examples of these are lack of supervisory support, the medical power structure, and institutional policy. The nurse experiences what has been referred to as "painful psychologic disequilibrium." The phenomenon has been described as moral distress. The nurse can face an internal ethical dilemma whether to stay in such an employment environment to suffer or stay loyal to co-workers and most of all, the neonate patients. Efforts are being made to establish measurement tools for nurses facing moral distress (Corley et al, 2001).

Recently NANDA proposed moral distress as a nursing diagnosis for nurses, patients, or family. It is defined as the inability to carry out one's chosen ethical or moral decision or action (Kopala & Burkhart, 2005).

Nursing research recently has developed a reliable and valid tool that could be used to identify ethical issues experienced by neonatal nurses and the frequencies of their occurrence, the Ethical Issues Scale (Fry & Duffy, 2001). Identification and quantification can lead to further development of effective interventions to resolve ethical issues confronted by neonatal nurses.

An example of an ethical issue involving neonatal pain management and professional opinion vs professional opinion is shown in Box 34-3.

The Neonate and Family as an Element of Legal and Ethical Issues in Neonatal Nursing

Newborns present unique factors for decision making and ethical conflict resolution. The neonate is limited in communication and ability to actively participate in decision making. Prenatal care typically omits preparing the family for ethical dilemmas, unless abnormalities have been prenatally detected. Adult patient populations' illness trajectory allows family members to prepare for decision making, and the familial role is ancillary to the patient's decisions. In contrast, the neonatal nurse is typically caring for a family with no advance preparation while being the primary decision maker. This situation invokes the educator and advocacy roles of the neonatal nurse.

BOX 34-3

Example of an Ethical Issue of Neonatal Pain Management

Professional Opinion vs Professional Opinion

The last 20 years have produced many studies regarding neonatal pain. The physiologic ability of the neonate to perceive pain has been established. However, the gap between research and clinical practice has not closed. This creates a foundation for nurses to challenge the ethics of undertreatment of neonates for pain. Except for a small number of advanced practice nurses who have prescriptive authority, physicians hold the power for pharmacologic pain management. The disparity between adults and infants in use of pharmacologic pain management for painful procedures such as arterial line placement and endotracheal intubation has been measured in nursing research.

Nurses are responding in research and clinical practice by development of scientific objective neonatal pain assessment scales. This work is ongoing.

Advanced practice nurses such as neonatal nurse practitioners or clinical nurse specialists with prescriptive authority can directly improve neonatal pain management with appropriate pain management orders (Rouzan, 2001). All nurses can use the best evidence to guide pain assessment and relief, which now is in the form of research and policy statements from professional organizations (Byers & Thornley, 2004).

Parents hold the key decision-making position in all neonatal care (Penticuff & Arheart, 2005). They should be able to expect that the nurse will not advise them of the right decision, but instead will enable them to make decisions by gaining understanding of the relevant factors and foreseeable consequences of alternative options (Penticuff & Arheart, 2005).

Parents exercise their decision making by giving informed consent for care. Informed consent is not simply reading a form and getting a signature. Informed consent is a process.

Parents reach informed decisions in their infant's best interest when the neonatal nurse ensures access to appropriate, understandable information about their infant's condition. This includes potential risks and benefits to the infant of various options for treatment and nontreatment. This information allows the parents to weigh risks and benefits of proposed options and come to a reasoned decision (National Association of Neonatal Nurses [NANN], 2005).

In the rare instance in which the decision of the parent is not consistent with the best interest of the newborn, the nurse may need to advocate intervention. Nursing organizations committed to neonatal interests advocate that "a system of bioethical consultation should be available as well as a system for legal intervention in rare events where parental decisions and infant's rights conflict. Except in extraordinary circumstances the parents' wishes should be honored" (NANN, 2005).

Box 34-4 gives an example of an ethical dilemma involving a parent's decision to opt for heroic measures vs palliative care measures.

BOX 34-4

Example of an Ethical Dilemma

Parent Decides Heroic Measures vs Palliative Care Measures

The beginning of the 21st century witnessed an unexpected increase in the U.S. infant mortality rate. Shortened gestation and low birth weight together lead the causes of death (MacDorman et al, 2005). Technology responded, and now sicker and smaller infants survive premature or catastrophic birth defects with technologic support. In some circumstances technology usage provokes the question whether its use prolongs suffering and deprives the neonate of a dignified death instead of sustaining a life that can realistically experience any notion of quality (Caniano, 2004). The inability to realistically predict whether a proposed technologic application will result in an acceptable future quality of life for the neonate compounds the challenge of decision making for parents and health care providers. The role of the neonatal nurse in these situations becomes further compounded by the shortage of evidence-based standards of advocacy for this issue in neonatal nursing (Monterosso et al, 2005).

The degree of nurses' participation in NICU decision making regarding the use or termination of technologic support varies by setting. One variable is the degree of meaningful collaborative relationships with the doctors on the interdisciplinary care team. A barrier to participation in the NICU decision making regarding the ethical issue of life support termination is the lack of interdisciplinary decision-making models for NICU nurses (Monterosso et al, 2005).

Dilemmas of whether the neonatal nursing care should be palliative in anticipation of death or heroic rescue with technology will increase as technology advances. Both nursing research and clinicians focused on neonatal care can participate in advocacy on this issue by developing theoretical models of decision making on the issues of heroic measures vs palliative care. This would provide an evidence base for the clinical nurse participating in the catastrophic decision making on this very sensitive ethical issue. Interventions described under strategies for resolution of ethical issues are suitable for use in these dilemmas.

The Ethical Framework as an Element of Legal and Ethical Issues in Neonatal Nursing

The ethical framework of nurses has evolved over time with the evolution of the nursing role. The role of the nurse changed from being a physician's assistant, to being a member of an independent profession with its own ethical perspective. Codes of ethics became established for many specialties, including neonatal care (Fry, 2002).

Advocacy has become part of the nursing role. The advocacy construct was reviewed by concept analysis under protocols established in peer-reviewed nursing literature. The analysis concludes that clinical practitioners combine valuing, apprising, and interceding functions in the course of advocacy. Patient advocacy as a nursing concept is an element of addressing legal and ethical issues. It is the method of navigation that relies on the nurse's skills of critical thinking and negotiation.

It is a more ambiguous method than is found in legal advocacy. Nurses exercising patient advocacy have none of the formal rules of engagement or the official forum for resolution that exists in a lawyer's framework (Baldwin, 2003).

The ethical framework for neonatal nurses varies from state to state. The authority to determine much of what controls the institutional environment is at the state level. For example, each state can legislate its own mandatory genetic screening for newborns (Kenner & Moran, 2005), regulations concerning reprisal for professional whistleblowing (Little, 2002), and competency demonstration for licensing advanced nursing specialties. In contrast, ethical codes, professional standards, and position statements are more pervasive in application. They apply to all members of the organizations, regardless of geographical location.

Genetic screening of newborns vs traditional ethics of care is shown in Box 34-5.

Strategies for Ethical Issue Resolution and Risk Management

Strategies for ethical issue resolution are essential for reasons beyond the paramount best interest of the neonate. They also function as risk management strategies to prevent malpractice claims. Neonatal nurses assume a degree of expertise and corresponding responsibility in patient care. In all nursing expertise, levels of responsibility correspond to levels of liability exposure. Because neonatal nurse expertise brings autonomous decision making, there is potential liability separate from that of the physician. Expertise level results in a professional expectation to question, act, intervene, and advocate. Failure to perform these duties creates potential liability (Greenwald & Mondor, 2003). Risk management should not be the responsibility of any one professional on the neonate's health care team. The controversial and significant decisions should be made through the process of parental consent and informed decision making. By incorporating these two processes into the resolution of all ethical dilemmas, the best interest of the neonate is served and liability risk is minimized (Hurst, 2005a). Neonatal nurses are in logistically pivotal positions on health care teams. Endeavors to empower parental decision making from these positions are supported by the professional guidelines of the American Nurses Association (ANA), the Association of Women's Health Obstetric and Neonatal Nurses (AWHONN), the National Association of Neonatal Nurses (NANN), the American Academy of Pediatrics (AAP), and the Principles of Family-Centered Neonatal Care (Hurst, 2005b).

Strategies, based on review of nursing literature, for further support of nurses to increase self-efficacy in advocacy functions include adequate educational preparation. Proposed education goes beyond comprehension of general principles. Ethics education must have a component of strategy or plan of action, so that nurses can be motivated to participate (Peter et al, 2004). The next section provides a three-step strategy.

Three-Step Strategy for Ethical Dilemma Resolution

Step 1: Identification. Identification of any dilemma's existence or recognition of existing precipitating factors (e.g., a neonate born extremely premature) is the first intentional step toward a plan of action to prevent or resolve an ethical dilemma. Stakeholders in the dilemma are included in this identification stage (Wueste, 2005).

BOX **34-5**

Genetic Screening of Newborns vs Traditional Ethics of Care

A fundamental requirement in meeting ethical standards in neonatal care is the informed consent process. Neonatal nurses function to put the educational information in the consent process.

Nurses are also taught to administer care within their scope of expertise, not beyond that scope. Nurses advocate continuity of care and believe that part of competent neonatal care is to adequately prepare the family for foreseeable problems once the patient is discharged. Regardless of these well-established standards of care, many states have passed legislation that requires mandatory genetic screening of newborns. Informed parental consent is required in only a minority of states (Kenner & Moran, 2005). Nurses are expected to participate in the testing without having adequate training in genetics, genetic counseling, or genetic test interpretation. The neonate is usually discharged before there can be any meaningful assessment of the impact of positive or false positive test result disclosure on the family. The technology available to make genetic determinations evolved faster than the readiness of nurses to measure the phenomenon of genetic knowledge impact of families of newborns (American College of Obstetricians and Gynecologists, 2003).

Most disciplines agree that this technology used to predict genetic conditions for intervention purposes benefits newborns. However, the 50 states have not agreed on how to proceed in administering the benefit. Each state has the authority to legislate policy determinations as to which conditions will be screened. The states also establish the protocol regarding consent requirements. The states vary on these issues. For a full explanation, see Figure 34-1.

Nurses participating in screening can address at the individual level some ethical issues raised by genetic screening. Nurses can ensure their competency to provide information regarding particular screening methods and the meaning of test results by self-education. Continuing education courses, professional meetings, and literature reviews will increase the nurse's competency in the genetic screening portion of neonatal care. This approach assists the nurse in practicing within the scope of her knowledge and expertise, an ethical standard of practice.

Nursing research can lead in the development of knowledge regarding the impact of disclosing positive screening results (Bennett Johnson et al, 2004). Advocacy of any position is most persuasive when it relies on scientific evidence. Consequences of deviation from informed consent principles should be studied. Outcomes for infants receiving genetic screening should be measured (Baughcum et al, 2005). Once knowledge is established, professional organizations can rely on evidence to advocate through position statements and political action groups regarding issues of informed consent departure and screening disclosure impact.

Reactions from a base emotion run a risk of jeopardizing not only the nurse's rationale for the particular dilemma, but also the nurse's credibility for future considerations. Patience is part of any strategy for dilemma resolution. Even if the nurse is not substantively persuasive in resolving the initial dilemmas confronted, demonstration to peers and other health care team members of a logical critical thinking method develops future credibility and persuasive authority.

Step 2: Analysis. The second step of the strategy is the analysis task. Dilemmas can be analyzed by different methods. One analytical method is to evaluate the consequences of alternative options. This method evaluates the potential harm and benefit of each option, determining which has the greater potential for benefit with least risk of harm to the neonate (Turkoski, 2001; Wueste, 2005).

Another method of analysis is to examine the nature of the rights and responsibilities of the respective stakeholders. If the rights and responsibilities of each stakeholder are identified and honored, theoretically the correct course of action can reveal itself (Turkoski, 2001; Wueste, 2005).

Step 3: Take Action. The analysis step has provided the rationale and support for the action; now take it. Some suggestions follow.

Intervention for Moral Distress and Ethical Dilemma: Infant Progress Chart (IPC) and Care Planning Meetings (CPMs)

This intervention, published in 2005, was designed to facilitate parent-professional collaboration. This is necessary to the process of informed consent and adequate decision making. The intervention is appropriate for situations where the moral distress or ethical dilemma diagnoses are made.

The IPC increases parental understanding of the infant's condition by reporting the status of all significant health indicators in a chart format. It provides a comprehensive perspective, outlining major foreseeable complications of premature birth such as chronic lung disease, sepsis, and intracranial hemorrhage.

CPMs are held at intervals, at 0 to 3, 9 to 12, and 25 to 28 days of the neonate's life. The parent and a member of the neonate's health care team meet. The intent of the meeting is to facilitate development of parent-professional relationships, open communication, shared decision authority, and trust.

The combination of the IPC and CPMs has proven to be effective. These collaboration strategies offer nurses and other members of the health care team a means to help families understand their infant's care and health status and be more satisfied with the process of decision making (Penticuff & Arheart, 2005).

Other Interventions for Ethical Dilemma and Moral Distress Diagnoses

Three additional interventions are available to respond to ethical dilemmas. In the Nursing Interventions Classification (NIC), the "values clarification" intervention suggests how the nurse may directly assist the patient in evaluation of the situation. The intervention "multidisciplinary care conference" may facilitate communication for foundation of

Text continues on p. 614.

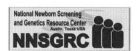

National Newborn Screening Status Report

Updated 09/25/06

The U.S. National Screening Status Report lists the status of newborn screening in the United States.

Dot "●" indicates that screening for the condition is universally required by Law or Rule and fully implemented

A = universally offered but not yet required, **B** = offered to select populations, or by request, **C** = testing required but not yet implemented

D = likely to be detected (and reported) as a by-product of MRM screening (MS/MS) targeted by Law or Rule

STATE	Hearing	Endocrine		Hemoglobin			Other			Additional Conditions Included in Screening Panel (universally required unless otherwise indicated)
	HEAR	CH	CAH	Hb S/S	Hb S/A	Hb S/C	BIO	GALT	CF	
Alabama	A	●	●	●	●	●	●	●	●	G6PD, TOXO, 5-OXO, HHH, NKH, PRO, OTC
Alaska	●	●	●	●	●	●	●	●		
Arizona	A	●	●	●	●	●	●	●	C	
Arkansas	●	●		●	●	●		●		
California	B	●	●	●	●	●	C	●	C	HHH; PRO; EMA
Colorado	●	●	●	●	●	●	●	●	●	
Connecticut	●	●	●	●	●	●	●	●	B	HHH; HIV[2]; NKH
D.C.	●	●	●	●	●	●	●	●	●	G6PD
Delaware	●	●	●	●	●	●	●	●	●	
Florida	●	●	●	●	●	●	●	●	C	
Georgia	A	●	●	●	●	●	●	●		
Hawaii	●	●	●	●	●	●	●	●		
Idaho	A	●	●	●	●	●	●	●		
Illinois	●	●	●	●	●	●	●	●		5-OXO, HIV[2]
Indiana	●	●	●	●	●	●	●	●		
Iowa	●	●		●	●	●	●	●	●	HHH; NKH
Kansas	●	●		●	●	●		●		
Kentucky	A	●	●	●	●	●	●	●	●	
Louisiana	●	●	●	●	●	●	●	●		
Maine	A	●	●	●	●	●	●	●		HHH; CPS (D)
Maryland	●	●	●	●	●	●	●	●	●	
Massachusetts	●	●	●	●	●	●	●	●	A	TOXO; HHH (A); CPS (D)
Michigan	A	●	●	●	●	●	●	●		
Minnesota	A	●	●	●	●	●	●	●	●	
Mississippi	●	●	●	●	●	●	●	●	●	5-OXO; CPS; HHH
Missouri	●	●	●	●	●	●	C	●	C	
Montana	A	●	B	●	●	●	B	●	B	
Nebraska	A	●	●	●	●	●	●	●	●	5-OXO; HHH; NKH (A)
Nevada	A	●	●	●	●	●	●	●		
New Hampshire	A	●	●	●	●	●	●	●	●	TOXO
New Jersey	●	●	●	●	●	●	●	●	●	
New Mexico	●	●	●	●	●	●	●	●	C	
New York	●	●	●	●	●	●	●	●	●	HIV; HHH; Krabbe Disease
North Carolina	●	●	●	●	●	●	●	●		
North Dakota	A	●	●	●	●	●	●	●	●	HHH; NKH
Ohio	●	●	●	●	●	●	●	●	●	
Oklahoma	●	●	●	●	●	●		●	●	
Oregon	A	●	●	●	●	●	●	●		
Pennsylvania	●	●	●	●	●	●	B	●	B	5-OXO; CPS; G6PD; HHH; NKH (B)
Rhode Island	●	●	●	●	●	●	●	●	●	
South Carolina	A	●	●	●	●	●	●	●		
South Dakota	A	●	●	●	●	●	●	●	A	5-OXO; EMA; HHH; NKH
Tennessee	A	●	●	●	●	●	●	●		5-OXO; HHH; NKH
Texas	B	●	●	●	●	●	C	●		
Utah	●	●	●	●	●	●	●	●		
Vermont	●	●	●	●	●	●	●	●		CPS
Virginia	●	●	●	●	●	●	●	●	●	
Washington	A	●	●	●	●	●	●	●		
West Virginia	●	●		●	●	●		●		
Wisconsin	A	●	●	●	●	●	●	●	●	
Wyoming	●	●	●	●	●	●	●	●	●	

[1]Terminology consistent with ACMG report - Newborn Screening: Towards a Uniform Screening Panel and System. Genet Med. 2006; 8(5) Suppl: S12-S252
Newborn screened for HIV only if mother was not screened during pregnancy

Additional Conditions/Abbreviations and Names

BIO	Biotinidase	**CF**	Cystic fibrosis	**GALT**	Transferase deficient galactosemia (Classical)	**HB S/C**	Sickle – C disease	**HEAR**	Hearing screening
CAH	Congenital adrenal hyperplasia	**CH**	Congenital hypothyroidism	**HB S/S**	Sickle cell disease	**HB S/A**	S-βeta thalassemia		

Other Disorders

5-OXO	5-oxoprolinuria (pyroglutamic aciduria)	**G6PD**	Glucose 6 phosphate dehydrogenase	**NKH**	Nonketotic hyperglycinemia
CPS	Carbamoylphosphate synthetase	**HHH**	Hyperammonemia/ornithinemia/ citrullinemia (Ornithine transporter defect)	**PRO**	Prolinemia
EMA	Ethylmalonic encephalopathy	**HIV**	Human immunodeficiency virus	**TOXO**	Toxoplasmosis

FIGURE **34-1**
National Newborn Screening Status Report. From National Newborn Screening and Genetics Resource Center (September 25, 2006). *National newborn screening status report.* Austin, TX: The Author.

Continued

STATE	Core[1] Conditions - Metabolic																			
	Fatty Acid Disorders					Organic Acid Disorders									Amino Acid Disorders					
	CUD	LCHAD	MCAD	TFP	VLCAD	GA-1	HMG	IVA	3-MCC	Cbl-A,B	BKT	MUT	PROP	MCD	ASA	CIT	HCY	MSUD	PKU	TYR-1
Alabama	•	•	•	•	•	•	•	•	•	•	•	•	•	•	•	•	•	•	•	•
Alaska	•	•	•	•	•	•	•	•	•	•	•	•	•	•	•	•	•	•	•	•
Arizona	•	•	•	•	•	•	•	•	•	•	•	•	•	•	•	•	•	•	•	•
Arkansas																			•	
California	•	•	•	•	•	•	•	•	•	•	•	•	•	•	•	•	•	•	•	•
Colorado	•	•	•	•	•	•	•	•	•	•	•	•	•	•	•	•	•	•	•	•
Connecticut	•	•	•	•	•	•	•	•	•	•	•	•	•	•	•	•	•	•	•	•
D. of Columbia	•	•	•	•	•	•	•	•	•	•	•	•	•	•	•	•	•	•	•	•
Delaware		•	•	•	•	•	•	•	•	•	•	•	•	•	•	•	•	•	•	•
Florida	•	•	•	•	•	•	•	•	•	•	•	•	•	•	•	•	•	•	•	•
Georgia			•														•	•	•	•
Hawaii	•	•	•	•	•	•	•	•	•	•	•	•	•	•	•	•	•	•	•	•
Idaho	•	•	•	•	•	•	•	•	•	•	•	•	•	•	•	•	•	•	•	•
Illinois	D	•	•	•	•	•	•	•	•	•	•	•	•	•	•	•	•	•	•	•
Indiana	•	•	•	•	•	•	•	•	•	•	•	•	•	•	•	•	•	•	•	•
Iowa	•	•	•	•	•	•	•	•	•	•	•	•	•	•	•	•	•	•	•	•
Kansas																			•	
Kentucky	•	•	•	•	•	•	•	•	•	•	•	•	•	•	•	•	•	•	•	•
Louisiana	•	•	•	•	•	•	•	•	•	•	•	•	•	•	•	•	•	•	•	•
Maine	D	•	•	D	•	•	•	•	•	•	•	•	•	D	•	•	•	•	•	•
Maryland	•	•	•	•	•	•	•	•	•	•	•	•	•	•	•	•	•	•	•	•
Massachusetts	D	A	•	D	A	A	A	A	A	A	A	A	A	D	A	A	•	•	•	A
Michigan	A	A	A	A	A	A	A	A	A	A	A	A	A	A	A	A	A	A	•	A
Minnesota	•	•	•	•	•	•	•	•	•	•	•	•	•	•	•	•	•	•	•	•
Mississippi	•	•	•	•	•	•	•	•	•	•	•	•	•	•	•	•	•	•	•	•
Missouri	•	•	•	•	•	•	•	•	•	•	•	•	•	•	•	•	•	•	•	•
Montana	B	B	B	B	B	B	B	B	B	B	B	B	B	B	B	B	B	B	•	B
Nebraska		A	•	A	A	A	A	A	A	A	A	A	A	A	A	A	A	A	•	A
Nevada	•	•	•	•	•	•	•	•	•	•	•	•	•	•	•	•	•	•	•	•
New Hampshire			•															•	•	
New Jersey	•	•	•	•	•	•	•	•	•	•	•	•	•	•	•	•	•	•	•	•
New Mexico	C	C	C	C	C	C	C	C	C	C	C	C	C	C	C	C	C	C	•	C
New York	•	•	•	•	•	•	•	•	•	•	•	•	•	•	•	•	•	•	•	
North Carolina		•	•	•	•	•	•	•	•	•	•	•	•	•	•	•	•	•	•	
North Dakota	•	•	•	•	•	•	•	•	•	•	•	•	•	•	•	•	•	•	•	•
Ohio	•	•	•	•	•	•	•	•	•	•	•	•	•	•	•	•	•	•	•	
Oklahoma			•																•	
Oregon	D	•	•	D	•	•	•	•	•	D	D	•	•	D	•	•	•	•	•	•
Pennsylvania	B	B	B	B	B	B	B	B	B	B	B	B	B	B	B	B	B	B	•	B
Rhode Island	•	•	•	•	•	•	•	•	•	•	•	•	•	•	•	•	•	•	•	•
South Carolina	•	•	•	•	•	•	•	•	•	•	•	•	•	•	•	•	•	•	•	•
South Dakota	•	•	•	•	•	•	•	•	•	•	•	•	•	•	•	•	•	•	•	•
Tennessee	•	•	•	•	•	•	•	•	•	•	•	•	•	•	•	•	•	•	•	•
Texas	C	C	C	C	C	C	C	C	C	C	C	C	C	C	C	C	C	C	•	C
Utah	•	•	•	•	•	•	•	•	•	•	•	•	•	•	•	•	•	•	•	•
Vermont	•	•	•	•	•	•	•	•	•	•	•	•	•	•	•	•	•	•	•	•
Virginia	•	•	•	•	•	•	•	•	•	•	•	•	•	•	•	•	•	•	•	•
Washington			•														•	•	•	
West Virginia																			•	
Wisconsin	•	•	•	•	•	•	•	•	•	•	•	•	•	•	•	•	•	•	•	•
Wyoming	•	•	•	•	•	•	•	•	•	•	•	•	•	•	•	•	•	•	•	•

[1]Terminology consistent with ACMG report - Newborn Screening: Towards a Uniform Screening Panel and System. Genet Med. 2006; 8(5) Suppl: S12-S252

Deficiency/Disorder Abbreviations and Names (optional nomenclature)

3-MCC	3-Methylcrotonyl-CoA carboxylase	CUD	Carnitine uptake defect (Carnitine transport defect)	LCHAD	Long-chain L-3- hydroxyacyl-CoA dehydrogenase	PKU	Phenylketonuria/ hyperphenylalaninemia
ASA	Argininosuccinate acidemia	GA-1	Glutaric acidemia type 1	MCAD	Medium-chain acyl-CoA dehydrogenase	PROP	Propionic acidemia (Propionyl-CoA carboxylase)
BKT	Beta ketothiolase (mitochondrial acetoacetyl-CoA thiolase ; short-chain ketoacyl thiolase; T2)	HCY	Homocystinuria (cystathionine beta synthase)	MCD	Multiple carboxylase (Holocarboxylase synthetase)	TFP	Trifunctional protein deficiency
CBL A,B	Methylmalonic acidemia (Vitamin B12 Disorders)	HMG	3-Hydroxy 3 - methylglutaric aciduria (3-Hydroxy 3-methylglutaryl-CoA lyase)	MSUD	Maple syrup urine disease (branched-chain ketoacid dehydrogenase)	TYR-1	Tyrosinemia Type 1
CIT I	Citrullinemia type I (Argininosuccinate synthetase)	IVA	Isovaleric acidemia (Isovaleryl-CoA dehydrogenase)	MUT	Methylmalonic Acidemia (methylmalonyl-CoA mutase)	VLCAD	Very long-chain acyl-CoA dehydrogenase

FIGURE **34-1, cont'd**
National Newborn Screening Status Report. From National Newborn Screening and Genetics Resource Center (September 25, 2006). *National newborn screening status report.* Austin, TX: The Author.

STATE	Fatty Acid Disorders								Organic Acid Disorders						Amino Acid Disorders								Other Metabolic		Hbg
	CACT	CPT-Ia	CPT-II	DE-RED.	GA-II	MCKAT	M/SCHAD	SCAD	2M3HBA	2MBG	3MGA	Cbl-C,D	IBG	MAL	ARG	BIOPT-BS	BIOPT-RG	CIT-II	H-PHE	MET	TYR-II	TYR-III	GALE	GALK	Variant Hbg's
Alabama	•	•	•	•	•		•		•	•	•	•	•	•	•	D	D	•	•	•	•	•			•
Alaska	•	•	•		•			•	•	•	•	•	•	•	•	B	B	•	•	•	•		B	B	•
Arizona	•	•	•		•				•			•	•					D	•		D	D			•
Arkansas																									A
California	•	•	•		•				•	•	•	•	•	•	•			•	•	•	•	•			•
Colorado	•	•	•	•	•				•	•	•	•	•	•	•			•	•	•	•	•			•
Connecticut	•	•	•		•			•				•			•			•	•	•			•	•	•
D. of Columbia	•	•	•	•	•	•	•	•	•	•	•	•	•	•	•	A	A	•	•	•	•	•	•	•	•
Delaware	•		•		•	A			A		A		•		•	A	A	•	•	•	•	•	•	•	•
Florida	•	•	•					•											•		•				•
Georgia																B	B		•				•	•	•
Hawaii	•	•	•		•			•	•	•	•	•	•	•	•	D	D	•	•	•	•	•	B	B	•
Idaho	•	•	•		•			•	•	•	•	•	•	•	•	B	B	•	•	•	•	•	B	B	•
Illinois	•	D	•	D	•	D	•	•	D	•	•	•	•	•	•			D	•	•	•	•	•		•
Indiana	•	•	•	•	•	•	•	•	•	•	•	•	•	•	•			•	•	•	•	•	•		•
Iowa	•	•	•	•	•	•	•	•	•	•	•	•	•	•	•			•	•	•	•	•			•
Kansas																				•					•
Kentucky			A		A			•							A	B	B	•	•	A					•
Louisiana																				•					•
Maine	D	D	•		•			•		D	D	•	D		•			•	•	D	•	D			•
Maryland	•								•							B	B		•	•			•	•	•
Massachusetts	D	D	A		A			A		D	D	A	D		A	D	D	A	•	D	A	D	•	•	•
Michigan	A	A	A	A	A	A	A	A	A	A	A	A	A	A	A	•	•	A	•	A			•		•
Minnesota	•	•	•	•	•	•	•	•	•	•	•	•	•	•	•			•	•	•	•	•			•
Mississippi	•	•	•	A	•	A	•	•	A	•	•	•	•	•	•	A	A	•	•	•	•	•	A	•	•
Missouri	•	D	•	D	•	D	D	•	D	D	D	D	D	D	D	D	D	D	•	•	•	•	D		•
Montana	B		B	B	B	B	B	B	B	B	B	B	B	B		B	B	B	•	B	B	B			•
Nebraska	A		A		A			A		A		A	A	A	A			A	A	A	A				•
Nevada	•	•	•		•			•	•	•	•	•	•	•	•	B	B	•	•	•	•	•	B	B	A
New Hampshire																		•	•	D			•	•	•
New Jersey	•	B	•		•			A	B					A	A			•	•	•			•	•	•
New Mexico																				•					•
New York	•	•	•		•	•	•	•	•	•	•	•	•	•	•			•	•	•	•	•			•
North Carolina	•	•	•		•			•	•	•	•	•	•	•	•			•	•	•	•	•			•
North Dakota	•	•	•		•	•	•	•	•	•	•	•	•	•	•			•	•	•	•	•			•
Ohio	•	•	•		•			•							•			•	•	•					•
Oklahoma																				•					•
Oregon	•	D	•		•			•	D	D	•	•	D	D	D	B	B	•	•	•	•	•	D	B	B
Pennsylvania	B	B	B	B	B	B		B		B	B	B	B	B	B	B	B	B	•	B	B	B			•
Rhode Island			D																•				•	•	•
South Carolina	•		•		•	•		•	•		•	•	•	•	•			•	•	•					•
South Dakota	•	•	•		•			•	•	•	•	•	•	•	•			•	•	•	•	•			•
Tennessee	•	•	•		•			•	•	•	•	•	•	•	•			•	•	•	•	•			•
Texas																				•					•
Utah	•	•	•		•	D		•	•	•	•	D	•	•	D	•	•	•	•	•	•	•	•		•
Vermont	D	D	D		D					D	D				D			•	•	•	D	D	D	•	•
Virginia																				•					•
Washington																				•					•
West Virginia																				•				•	•
Wisconsin	•		•	•	•	•	•	•	•	•	•	•	•	•			•	•	•	•	•	•	•	•	•
Wyoming	A	A	A	A	A	A	A	A	A	A	A	A	A	A	A			A	•	A	A	B			•

[1] Terminology consistent with ACMG report - Newborn Screening: Towards a Uniform Screening Panel and System. Genet Med. 2006; 8(5) Suppl: S12-S252

Deficiency/Disorder Abbreviations and Names (optional nomenclature)

2M3HBA	2-Methyl-3-hydroxy butyric aciduria	**CACT**	Carnitine acylcarnitine translocase	**GA-II**	Glutaric acidemia Type II	**MAL**	Malonic acidemia (Malonyl-CoA decarboxylase)
2MBG	2-Methylbutyryl-CoA dehydrogenase	**CBL-C,D**	Methylmalonic acidemia (Cbl C,D)	**GALE**	Galactose epimerase	**MCKAT**	Medium-chain ketoacyl-CoA thiolase
3MGA	3-Methylglutaconic aciduria	**CIT-II**	Citrullinemia type II	**GALK**	Galactokinase	**MET**	Hypermethioninemia
ARG	Arginemia (Arginase deficiency)	**CPT-Ia**	Carnitine palmitoyltransferase I	**H-PHE**	Benign hyperphenylalaninemia	**SCAD**	Short-chain acyl-CoA dehydrogenase
BIOPT-BS	Defects of biopterin cofactor biosynthesis	**CPT-II**	Carnitine palmitoyltransferase II	**IBG**	Isobutyryl-CoA dehydrogenase	**TYR-II**	Tyrosinemia type II
BIOPT-REG	Defects of biopterin cofactor regeneration	**De-Red**	Dienoyl-CoA reductase	**M/SCHAD**	Medium/Short chain L-3-hydroxy acyl-CoA dehydrogenase	**TYR-III**	Tyrosinemia type III

FIGURE **34-1, cont'd**
National Newborn Screening Status Report. From National Newborn Screening and Genetics Resource Center (September 25, 2006). *National newborn screening status report.* Austin, TX: The Author.

Continued

informed parental consent (Dochterman & Bulechek, 2004; Kopala & Burkhart, 2005).

Ethical committees should be considered as potential intervention tools (Kopala & Burkhart, 2005).

Interventions to Improve Interdisciplinary Communication

Sometimes the conflict is between members of the health care team. Interventions that could improve interdisciplinary communication and ethical decision-making processes in the neonatal setting include (1) participation in case conferences, (2) unitwide education on controversial issues such as pain medication, and (3) consultation with senior medical or nursing staff (Monterosso et al, 2005).

Intervention or Last Resort?

Whistleblowing is a form of addressing observed ethical issues when the nurse has not been officially or informally invited to speak. It is defined as a report by a health team member to the public about a serious wrongdoing or danger created where the whistleblower works (Little, 2002). This form of advocacy does not come without stressful consequences. Interestingly, a recent study evaluated stress-induced physical health problems in nurses as a consequence of whistleblowing or electing not to whistleblow. The findings suggest that stress from whistleblowing situations may cause physical and emotional health problems regardless of whether one blows the whistle or not (McDonald & Ahern, 2002).

Some states have provisions in place safeguarding the employment of nurses who elect to whistleblow (Brownsey, 2001). Other strategies to improve personal protection from reprisals related to whistleblowing include obtaining legal counsel, developing a support system of colleagues and getting consensus, relying on facts, and leaving anger or emotion out of it. Document everything, and be prepared for lack of public support by those who support privately (Little, 2002).

SUMMARY

Choosing to care for neonates can bring professional satisfaction from caring for people during one of a family's most significant events. Unfortunately, some newborns enter the world with incredible uphill challenges. Some meet the world in good health, but find that technology immediately wants to screen for future challenges. Well-meaning health care providers and parents will not always agree on how to respond to infants' challenges. Each new ethical dilemma that arises has its own set of facts.

Nursing is spending research, academic, political, and clinical energy addressing the ethical issues and dilemmas in care of newborns. New sets of issues accompany technologic and scientific advancement. This century promises the development of many new issues due to genetic knowledge and technologic progress. Concentrating on the development of successful navigation strategies that are transferable from issue to issue will yield an enduring legacy for future infants and their health care providers.

REFERENCES

American College of Obstetricians and Gynecologists (ACOG) (2003). ACOG committee opinion number 287, October 2003: newborn screening. *Obstetrics and gynecology* 102(4):887-889.

Baldwin MA (2003). Patient advocacy: a concept analysis [Review]. *Nursing standard* 17(21):33-39.

Baughcum AE et al (2005). Maternal efforts to prevent type 1 diabetes in at-risk children. *Diabetes care* 28(4):916-921.

Bennett Johnson S et al (2004). Maternal anxiety associated with newborn genetic screening for type 1 diabetes. *Diabetes care* 27(2):392-397.

Brownsey D (2001). Nurses and their right to whistle blow. *AORN journal* 73(3):693-697.

Byers JF, Thornley K (2004). Cueing into infant pain [see comment]. *American journal of maternal child nursing* 29(2):84-89; quiz 90-91.

Caniano DA (2004). Ethical issues in the management of neonatal surgical anomalies [Review]. *Seminars in perinatology* 28(3):240-245.

Corley MC et al (2001). Development and evaluation of a moral distress scale. *Journal of advanced nursing* 33(2):250-256.

Dochterman J, Bulechek G (2004). *The nursing interventions classification.* St Louis: Mosby.

Foley EM (2002). Drug screening and criminal prosecution of pregnant women [Review]. *Journal of obstetric, gynecologic, and neonatal nursing* 31(2):133-137.

Fry ST (2002). Defining nurses' ethical practices in the 21st century. *International nursing review* 49(1):1-3.

Fry ST, Duffy ME (2001). The development and psychometric evaluation of the Ethical Issues Scale. *Journal of nursing scholarship* 33(3):273-277.

Greenwald LM, Mondor M (2003). Malpractice and the perinatal nurse [Review]. *Journal of perinatal and neonatal nursing* 17(2):101-109.

Hurst I (2005a). The legal landscape at the threshold of viability for extremely premature infants: a nursing perspective, part I. *Journal of perinatal and neonatal nursing* 19(2):155-166; quiz 167-168.

Hurst I (2005b). The legal landscape at the threshold of viability for extremely premature infants: a nursing perspective, part II. *Journal of perinatal and neonatal nursing* 19(3):253-262.

Kenner C, Moran M (2005). Newborn screening and genetic testing. *Journal of midwifery and women's health* 50(3):219-226.

Kenner C et al (2000). Identification and care of substance-dependent neonates. *Journal of intravenous nursing* 23(2):105-111.

Kopala B, Burkhart L (2005). Ethical dilemma and moral distress: proposed new NANDA diagnoses. *International journal of nursing terminologies and classifications* 16(1):3-13.

Little M (2002). Advocating safety. "Whistle-blowing" in the U.S. and Canada. *AWHONN lifelines* 6(1):18-20.

MacDorman MF et al (2005). Explaining the 2001–02 infant mortality increase: data from the Linked Birth/Infant Death Data Set. *National vital statistics reports* 53(12):1-22.

March of Dimes (MOD) (2006). Umbilical cord blood. Available at: http://www.marchofdimes.com/professionals/681_1160.asp. Retrieved August 24, 2006.

McDonald S, Ahern K (2002). Physical and emotional effects of whistleblowing. *Journal of psychosocial nursing and mental health services* 40(1):14-27.

Monterosso L et al (2005). The role of the neonatal intensive care nurse in decision-making: advocacy, involvement in ethical decisions and communication. *International journal of nursing practice* 11(3):108-117.

National Association of Neonatal Nurses (NANN) (2005). NICU nurse involvement in ethical decisions, position statement #3015. Available at: http://www.nann.org/i4a/pages/index.cfm?pageid=790. Retrieved October 7, 2005.

Penticuff JH, Arheart KL (2005). Effectiveness of an intervention to improve parent-professional collaboration in neonatal intensive care. *Journal of perinatal and neonatal nursing* 19(2):187-202.

Peter E et al (2004). Nursing resistance as ethical action: literature review. *Journal of advanced nursing* 46(4):403-416.

Pinch WJ (2001). Cord blood banking: ethical implications [Review]. *American journal of nursing* 101(10):55-59.

Riley JM, Fry ST (2000). Troubled advocacy: nurses report widespread ethical conflicts. *Reflections on nursing leadership* 26(2):35-36.

Rouzan IA (2001). An analysis of research and clinical practice in neonatal pain management [Review]. *Journal of the American Academy of nurse practitioners* 13(2):57-60.

Turkoski BB (2001). Ethics in the absence of truth. *Home healthcare nurse* 19(4):218-223.

Wueste DE (2005). A philosophical yet user-friendly framework for ethical decision making in critical care nursing [see comment]. *Dimensions of critical care nursing* 24(2):70-79.

Chapter 35

Competency-Based Education in Neonatal Nursing

Frances Strodtbeck • Carole Kenner

As health care moves into the 21st century, the issue of developing, maintaining, and ensuring the competence of neonatal nurses remains at the forefront for many institutions and agencies concerned with the quality of neonatal health care. Although the emphasis on competence is not new, the topic gained prominence during the period of health care reform in the 1980s. As the American health care delivery system reorganized under the umbrella of health care reform, societal concerns about the quality of care received and the providers delivering that care increased (Whittaker et al, 2000). Responding to the escalating concern, credentialing agencies such as the Joint Commission on Accreditation of Healthcare Organizations (JCAHO) issued standards requiring documentation of the clinical competency of all nursing staff (JCAHO, 1999).

Hospitals now were faced with the need to develop systems for assessing both the initial competence of newly hired nurses and the ongoing competence of the existing nursing staff. Unfortunately, this regulatory push for documentation hit hospitals at a time when many were losing their unit-based educators or clinical nurse specialists (or both) as a result of downsizing. This loss was particularly hard for critical care units, such as the neonatal intensive care unit (NICU), that were short staffed and had high turnover rates for nurses at all educational levels. As this movement toward documentation of minimal competencies for hospital nurses was developing, educational institutions were looking at terminal program objectives and the ways in which these might translate into minimal competency statements for graduates. A strategy that gained acceptance during this period of upheaval was competency-based education (CBE). It offered a bridge between the academic center and the hospital or community health care center. The hope was that CBE offered a way to shorten orientation time while improving quality control for nurses' performance. The assumption was, if the academic centers could demonstrate that their graduates' competencies were closely tied to the minimal competencies expected by employers, the orientation could focus on the specialty content and needs in the area where the nurse eventually would work (Avery, 2005; Hodges & Hansen, 1999; Marrone, 1999).

This chapter traces the development of the competency movement in health care, discusses the advantages and disadvantages of competency-based education, and describes the impact of competency evaluation on neonatal nursing practice and education.

HISTORY OF THE COMPETENCY MOVEMENT

The first voice to link improvement in hospital care to the competence of its providers was Florence Nightingale's. In her books, *Notes on Nursing* (1860) and *Notes on Hospitals* (1859), she laid the foundation for changes that revolutionized nursing education and practice. The hospital-based education system that evolved from her teachings became the predominant model for nursing education in the United States. Hospital-based or diploma programs that used an apprentice model to integrate classroom learning and clinical performance dominated the American educational system for nurses until the late 1960s and early 1970s (Chapman, 1999). Subsequently, the growing importance of higher education shifted nursing education from the hospital-based school to the academic school or university and transferred responsibility for the competence of the new graduate nurse from the hospital or employer to the university and its educators (Bechtel et al, 1999). University-based nursing education gained in popularity, and the hospital-based programs began to disappear.

As the new paradigm of nursing education evolved, a gap appeared between the expectations in the practice arena (the hospitals and clinical agencies) and the expectations in the education arena; this gap persists as a major issue in nursing education today. According to Lenburg (1999a), "Employers are experiencing a widening gulf between the competencies required for practice and those new graduates learned in their education programs." This gap in competency adds to the cost of health care, because employers must spend more money on human resource time and expertise in orienting new nurses.

The landmark book *On Competence: A Critical Analysis of Competence-Based Reforms in Higher Education* paved the way for recommendations to reform the education of professionals in American universities and colleges (Grant, 1979). Although published more than 25 years ago, Grant's thoughts on competence are still relevant:

Today, in fact, belief in one's own competence is no longer enough, and a demand for demonstrated competence now motivates much of education. This demand underlies much of the insistence on continuing education and even relicensure in the major professions, and it aims both to uncover cases of self-delusion about one's competence and to prevent apathetic resignation about maintaining one's competence. There is more to know in general; there is more to know about the specialty on which one focuses; and there is more continuous production of new knowledge that requires sifting, even if much of it must be discarded as unproven or redundant.

Eventually government became concerned about the issue of education and competency. In 1986 the National Governors' Association tackled the tough issues of accreditation of institutions of higher learning and their accountability to the public for the competency of graduates (Lenburg, 1999b). As the pressure to become accountable for the competency of university graduates grew, academia responded. The journal of the American Association of Higher Education, *Change*, devoted the entire September/October issue in 1990 to addressing the problems of competence and higher education (Lenburg, 1999a, 1999b, 1999c). Over the next decade, academia imported total quality management concepts and strategies from the business world (Lenburg, 1999b, 1999c). Academic accreditation agencies such as the National League for Nursing Accreditation Corporation (NLN) and the Commission for Collegiate Nursing Education (CCNE) incorporated competency language into their accreditation criteria (NLNAC, 1997; CCNE, 1998). State boards of nursing addressed the issue of ensuring competence and competency validation at the state regulatory level (National Council of State Boards of Nursing, 1998).

Multidisciplinary and consumer organizations concerned about the quality of health care also pushed for reforms to assure the public of the competency of those entering the health care professions and of those already in practice. In 1996 the Citizens Advocacy Center (CAC), an organization of public members of health care regulatory and governing boards, held a 2-day conference titled, "Continuing Professional Competence: Can We Assure It?" The proceedings of the conference, published in 1997, called for stronger measures to assure the public of the continued competence of health care workers and to remove workers who may not be competent (CAC, 1997).

The Pew Health Professions Commission released several documents in the late 1990s calling for education reform and validation of the competency of existing practitioners (Pew Health Professions Commission, 1995, 1998). The first report called for states to "require each board to develop, implement, and evaluate continuing competency requirements to assure the continuing competence of regulated health care professionals" (Pew Health Professions Commission, 1995). A subsequent report called for states to require that health care professionals "demonstrate their competence in the knowledge, judgment, technical skills, and interpersonal skills relevant to their jobs throughout their careers" (Pew Health Professions Commission, 1998). These reports proposed periodic reviews of professional competence at intervals not to exceed 7 years. In addition to mandatory continuing education, the commission advocated repeat testing of professionals using the initial licensing examination or a new examination in the specialty or practice area, chart or peer review (or both), and acceptance of professional credentialing such as certification and recertification.

Despite the differences in the issues of concern to employers, regulators, and politicians, academia, especially health care educators, clearly has been put on notice to shape up and provide society with a competent graduate. The key question for the nursing profession is, how should the nursing educational system be changed to meet this challenge, given the complexities of today's health care environment? The situation is well summarized by Lenburg (1999a): "Substantive reforms in academic and continuing education and in credentialing requirements are needed to accommodate consumer protection, technological innovations, sociodemographic and market forces, and the rising incidence of litigation related to health care."

A seemingly obvious solution would be to return to some variation of the apprentice model used in diploma nursing education; however, the logistics of implementing such a solution in a manner that would preserve the gains made by moving nursing education to institutions of higher learning would be insurmountable. Another obvious solution would be to narrow the gap between nursing education and nursing service. Bargagliotti and colleagues (1999) stressed the need to consider the stakeholders when considering competencies. They suggested that practice and education must work together to determine competencies. As Lenburg (1999b) observed:

> Nurse educators, whether responsible for classroom or clinical learning, are most effective when they engage in some form of clinical practice through which they adapt past skills to current circumstances and learn new ones now required in complex health care environments. Those who practice little, or not at all, are ill equipped to promote competence among students in the ever-changing contemporary work force.

Although a variety of models for integrating education and service have been tried across the country, most nursing academic programs remain separate from institutions that provide nursing services.

Other possible solutions offered have focused on changing the education model for entry into the nursing profession (i.e., requiring the professional doctorate) and on switching from the traditional pedagogy of lectures to alternative models, such as competency-based education and problem-based learning.

Proponents of the professional doctorate model cite the knowledge explosion, the proliferation of medical technology, the complexity of health care delivery systems, and the increasing need for nursing professionals to deal with sophisticated biomedical ethical situations as reasons for moving toward a longer basic nursing educational program (Carter, 1988; Fitzpatrick, 1988; Watson, 1988). The suggested curriculum would parallel the curriculum design for medicine and law; that is, the professional nursing education would be built on a foundation of study for the bachelor's degree in liberal arts or science and prescribed prenursing courses. Individuals interested in nursing careers then would apply for admission to a nursing school. On acceptance, the individual would complete a 3- to 4-year nursing curriculum, and graduates would be awarded a doctor of nursing (ND) degree. With the new movement toward the Doctor of Nursing Practice (DNP), the ND programs have gone away. Although this model had many advantages, as may the DNP, the reality is that the nursing profession is still arguing over the baccalaureate model for entry into practice.

As the competency movement gains strength, the need to prepare competent graduates becomes a de facto obligation for nursing schools. Changing from the traditional model of classroom teaching and learning to alternative models is both realistic and possible. Competency-based education and other similar models are growing in popularity in nursing academia and continuing education.

COMPETENCE AND COMPETENCY

What is competence? What is competency? What is the difference between the two? How is practice competence measured? These are some of the questions nursing educators and managers are asking.

Alspach (1992) defines competence as "the possession of knowledge, skills, and abilities necessary to perform the job" and competency as "the employee's ability to actually perform in the (work) environment in accordance with the role and standards of the institution." The National Institutes of Health (1995) defines competency as "a general statement that describes the knowledge, skills, and abilities necessary for safe nursing practice in a specific area." Competency, according to Benner (1984), is "the ability to perform the task with desirable outcomes under the varied circumstances of the real world." Jeffrey (2000) defines competency as a written statement established by expert opinion that identifies specific standards and direction for the professional's decision making in health care.

In 1994 the American Nurses Association (ANA) defined competency as "the demonstration of knowledge and skills in meeting professional role expectations." More recently, an ANA Expert Panel (2000) published the following definitions of competence:

- Continuing competence: Ongoing professional nursing competence according to the level of expertise, responsibility, and domains of practice.
- Professional nursing competence: Behavior based on beliefs, attitudes, and knowledge matched to and in the context of a set of expected outcomes as defined by nursing scope of practice, policy, [the ANA] Code for Nurses, standards, guidelines, and benchmarks that assure safe performance of professional activities.
- Continuing professional nursing competence: Ongoing professional nursing competence according to level of expertise, responsibility, and domains of practice as evidenced by behavior based on beliefs, attitudes, and knowledge matched to and in the context of a set of expected outcomes as defined by nursing scope of practice, policy, Code of Ethics, standards, guidelines, and benchmarks that assure safe performance of professional activities.

Clearly, competence and competency are related but different. Competence refers to the skills and abilities of the individual; competency is the ability of the individual to demonstrate those skills and abilities in a work setting. Competence and competency are the two sides of one coin, and both are of concern to nursing educators and employers of new nurses.

Traditionally, individual competence is assessed during the interview and hiring process. This assessment usually consists of checking letters of recommendation; verifying educational and state recognition for practice as a registered nurse (RN); evaluating the applicant's self-reported information (e.g., résumé and job application); and conducting a personal interview. Advanced practice nurses (APNs), especially nurse practitioners, often undergo an additional review of their skills and abilities during the credentialing process. The advanced practice skills and abilities are subjected to a peer-review process that often includes verification of previous employment, specialty certification, and state recognition of APN status, in addition to investigations for involvement in malpractice claims and disciplinary actions against the applicant's professional credentials.

Competency, on the other hand, is seen as an ongoing process, one that begins with employment and continues at periodic intervals for the duration of employment. Competency therefore is the issue of concern to employers, regulatory agencies, insurance companies, professional organizations, and society at large (Whittaker et al, 2000), whereas educators are concerned with preparing competent individuals.

Like many other practice disciplines, the profession of nursing has two dimensions, science and art. The science of nursing is imparted in formal educational programs and continuing education. The art of nursing is more elusive and is learned over time. The process of mastering both dimensions is essential. Benner (1984) details this process in her important book, *From Novice to Expert: Excellence and Power in Clinical Nursing Practice*, which is widely recognized within the profession. According to Benner, individuals go through five stages in the development of nursing expertise: novice, advanced beginner, competent, proficient, and expert.

It is noteworthy that competent is the third stage, not the final one. Two stages (proficient and expert) come after the development of competence. The new graduate nurse or the experienced nurse who is changing practice areas cannot reasonably be expected to be competent at the onset of employment in a new area such as the NICU; both will require some type of orientation before they can become contributing members of the NICU staff. It is reasonable to expect that both will acquire initial competency within a reasonable period of time as defined by the unit and the institution.

COMPETENCY-BASED EDUCATION

Understanding competency-based education (CBE) requires an understanding of what a competency is. A competency has three components: the knowledge that forms the basis of nursing practice; the performance skills (psychomotor and problem solving) to apply that knowledge to a clinical situation; and an affective response (Dunn et al, 2000).

Nursing competencies are often divided into levels. Fey and Miltner (2000) describe three levels: core, specialty, and patient care management competencies. Core competencies are the skills and knowledge required for the minimum safe level of nursing performance. Specialty competencies are the skills and knowledge required for the minimum safe level of nursing care for a specific patient population. Specialty competencies are often unit specific. Patient care management competencies demonstrate the integration of core and specialty competencies in the provision of safe patient care.

Competencies are often written in two parts: a statement that describes the performance standard and a list of performance criteria (Luttrell et al, 1999). The differences in the levels of competencies are illustrated in Table 35-1. Special attention should be paid to the progression from the broad (core) to the specific (patient care in a specific population).

Although some competencies are mandated by accreditation agencies such as JCAHO, most nursing competencies are derived from standards of practice developed by professional nursing organizations (Weinstein, 2000). Nursing

TABLE 35-1	Competency Levels Applied to Neonatal Nursing		
	Core Competency	**Specialty Competency**	**Patient Care Management Competency**
Performance standard	The nurse assesses the patient's level of pain.	The nurse recognizes the signs and symptoms of pain in neonates.	The nurse provides care for neonates in the immediate postoperative period.
Performance criteria	The nurse routinely assesses each patient's level of pain.	The nurse assesses the neonates for signs and symptoms of pain every hour.	The nurse cares for a neonate after gastrointestinal surgery for an abdominal wall defect.
	The nurse implements a plan of care to provide pain relief.	The nurse initiates nonpharmacologic pain interventions per unit protocol.	The nurse cares for the preterm neonate after surgery for a patent ductus ligation.

Modified from Fey MK, Miltner RS (2000). A competency-based orientation program for new graduate nurses. Journal of nursing administration 30(3):126-132.

standards of practice define the essential content competencies that form the foundation for CBE (Dozier, 1998). The National Organization of Nurse Practitioner Faculties (NONPF) has developed standardized general nursing competencies for advance practice nurses. These general competencies can be adapted to fit specialties within nursing. Specialty nursing organizations, such as the National Association of Neonatal Nurses (NANN), have a multifaceted role in the development of neonatal nursing competencies. Specialty organizations are responsible for developing the specific standards and clinical guidelines on which professional nursing practice is based (Whittaker et al, 2000). They also are responsible for monitoring issues that affect the practice of nursing, such as the development of an appropriate health care policy, and for supporting research to link nursing interventions to patient outcomes. Finally, nursing organizations support individual competence by providing educational opportunities for nurses to maintain their skills and knowledge, by influencing changes in state nurse practice acts, and by participating in the credentialing process as appropriate (Weinstein, 2000; Whittaker et al, 2000).

Ensuring the competency of a nursing staff requires an organized approach to orientation to the unit and a system of verification and validation of the skills and knowledge applied. Because nurses have a variety of educational and experiential backgrounds, the traditional orientation involving lectures and procedural manuals is no longer an efficient and effective strategy (Dunn et al, 2000). Competency-based orientation (CBO) is one form of CBE and is the preferred model in many institutions because it allows for the variation in nurses' backgrounds. CBO is "the simultaneous integration of the knowledge, skills, and attitudes that are required for performance in a designated role and setting" (Alspach, 1984). Ideally, this type of orientation would be an extension of a generic, competency-based curriculum followed by the academic institutions, adapted to fit the clinical or practice setting.

Competency-based orientation has many advantages and few disadvantages. A major advantage is the shortened orientation for experienced nurses (Stewart & Vitello-Cicciu, 1989; O'Grady & O'Brien, 1992; Marrone, 1999). In the current economic environment, this can result in significant savings for the unit and the institution. Other advantages are (1) measurable performance standards; (2) increased quality control (because performance standards are consistent); (3) elimination of repetitive classroom lectures and presentations; (4) adapt-

ability of the length of orientation to the needs of the new graduate or the experienced nurse; (5) personal accountability on the part of orientees for their own learning (or lack of it); and (6) treatment of orientees as adult learners (Alspach, 1984; O'Grady & O'Brien, 1992; Chaisson, 1995; Marrone, 1999; Mikos-Schild, 1999; Smith et al, 1996). The educator becomes the facilitator of the process rather than the master teacher and gatekeeper of learning (Mikos-Schild, 1999). As unit resources, preceptors serve as expert role models and facilitate the learning of the orientee.

Competency-based education has been criticized as emphasizing the science of nursing while paying little or no attention to the art of nursing. Communication skills, ethics, creative problem solving, and role development skills inherent in the art of nursing are difficult to quantify and to translate into objective, measurable competency statements (Mikos-Schild, 1999). Several authors have argued that the emphasis on skills and the technical aspects of nursing performance does not promote critical thinking and problem-solving skills (Mikos-Schild, 1999). Because of the subjective nature of evaluation and problems in measurability, measuring competency is difficult (Neary, 2001). Competencies often include a laundry list of skills and knowledge that must be attained. This application of competencies, more or less as tasks to be performed, may prolong orientation for the individual who is unable to set priorities or who is not motivated to complete the process (Mikos-Schild, 1999). Despite these disadvantages, CBE is widely used for orientation programs and some academic nursing programs. CBE is well suited to adult learners (Knowles, 1980).

One of the best-known approaches to CBE is the Competency Outcomes and Performance Assessment (COPA) model developed by Lenburg for the New York Regents College Nursing Program (Lenburg, 1999c). In the COPA model, traditional educational objectives are replaced with outcomes that are practice based, realistic, and measurable. The process of switching from the objective model to a competency-based model is governed by four key questions: What are the performance-based competency outcomes required for practice? What are the measurable indicators of competence for each outcome? What are the most effective learning strategies for achieving the outcomes? What are the most effective methods for assessing achievement of outcomes?

According to Lenburg, there are eight core practice competencies, each having subset skills (Table 35-2). The traditional learning objectives focused on the learning process (e.g., the student would be asked to discuss the role of the

TABLE **35-2**	Lenburg's Core Practice Competencies and Examples of Subset Skills
Core Competency	**Subset Skill Examples**
Assessment and intervention skills	Assessment
	Monitoring
	Therapeutic treatments
Communication skills	Oral
	Written
	Computer (information systems)
Critical thinking skills	Problem solving
	Evaluation
	Prioritizing
	Diagnostic reasoning
Human caring and relationship skills	Respect for cultural diversity
	Ethics
	Interpersonal relationships with patients, colleagues, and family
	Patient advocacy
Management skills	Delegation and supervision
	Materials resource management
	Accountability
	Quality improvement
Leadership skills	Professional accountability
	Role behaviors
	Risk taking
	Collaboration
Teaching skills	Health promotion
	Health restoration
	Group teaching
	Individual teaching
Knowledge integration skills	Nursing and related disciplines
	Liberal arts
	Natural and social sciences

Modified from Lenburg CB (1999c). COPA model. Online journal of issues in nursing. Available at: http://www.nursingworld.org/mods/mod110/copafull.htm.

TABLE **35-3**	Psychometric Concepts Used with Competency Performance Assessments
Concept	**Definition**
Critical elements	Statements that collectively define competence for a particular skill; these are single, discrete, observable behaviors that are mandatory to demonstrate competence for the skill.
Objectivity	A procedure that minimizes subjectivity on the part of the assessor (evaluator); two components are used: (1) a written statement of what is expected (e.g., the content of a particular skill or critical element) and (2) the consensual agreement of all directly involved in any aspects of the testing process.
Sampling	The process of selecting the most frequently encountered or most essential skills for the test.
Acceptability	The determination of what percentage of skills will be considered passing (i.e., 85% must be achieved for acceptable performance).
Comparability	The development of procedures to ensure that each test episode is essentially the same with regard to extent and difficulty.
Consistency	The development of procedures to ensure that the testing process is the same regardless of who administers the examination.
Flexibility	The ability to adapt when the performance examination is given in an actual clinical environment rather than as a simulation.
Systematized conditions	The development of procedures for determining the actions to be taken in the event of unanticipated situations in the clinical environment so that evaluators (faculty) respond in a manner that is objective, comparable, and consistent.

Modified from Lenburg CB (1999b). COPA model. Online journal of issues in nursing. Available at: http://www.nursingworld.org/mods/mod110/copafull.htm.

nurse in the NICU). Competency statements focus on the outcomes the institution desires in its graduates or employees. These statements are measurable performance outcomes that lend themselves to criterion-referenced performance evaluations. Objective evaluations based on psychometric concepts are developed to document learner competence for the core practice competencies. The psychometric concepts include critical elements, objectivity, sampling, acceptability, comparability, consistency, flexibility, and systematized conditions (Table 35-3).

Objective evaluations are developed for didactic and clinical learning. Didactic evaluations are called competency performance assessments (CPAs); clinical evaluations are called competency performance examinations (CPEs) (Luttrell et al, 1999). CPAs are used to evaluate didactic learning and classroom projects, such as poster presentations and written papers. CPEs are used in the clinical setting. They often are more exacting because the professional, legal, and ethical aspects of care all must be taken into account. An example of a CPE for newborn assessment is provided in

Figure 35-1. Another example is what Ringerman, Flint, and Huges (2006) present as peer competency validation to demonstrate and measure continuing competency in a cost-saving manner.

An element critical to the success of the COPA model of education is periodic program evaluation to determine the effectiveness of the learning plan in achieving the desired learning outcomes. This periodic review also allows for routine updates as practice or unit procedures change.

Competency Performance Assessment for Newborn Physical Examination

Name: _____ Date: _____ Examiner: _____

Start time: _____ Stop time: _____ Length of examination: _____

General Criteria
1. The student will maintain appropriate asepsis at all times during the examination.
2. The student will maintain patient safety at all times, including temperature control.
3. Skills marked with an asterisk (*) are required and must be performed to pass the performance examination.
4. The student will complete the examination within 30 minutes.

Competency	**Met**	**Unmet**
I. Vital Signs and Measurements		
A. Temperature	_____	_____
B. Heart rate	_____	_____
C. Respiratory rate	_____	_____
D. Weight	_____	_____
E. Length	_____	_____
F. Head circumference	_____	_____
II. General Appearance *(Inspection)*		
*A. Level of alertness/infant state	_____	_____
*B. Posture	_____	_____
*C. General proportions	_____	_____
*D. Symmetry	_____	_____
*E. Hydration/nutritional status	_____	_____
III. Integument *(Inspection, palpation)*		
*A. Skin (temperature, color, lesions)	_____	_____
*B. Hair (distribution, texture, patterns)	_____	_____
*C. Nails (presence, length)	_____	_____
IV. Head, Ears, Eyes, Nose, and Throat (HEENT) *(Inspection, palpation, auscultation)*		
*A. Head (size, shape)	_____	_____
1. Skull and scalp		
*2. Sutures (movement)		
*3. Fontanelles (number, size, position, bruits)		
*B. Face (features, symmetry)		
*C. Eyes (shape, position, measurements, movements, red reflex, discharge, pupil response)	_____	_____
*D. Ears (shape, position, auditory canal, hearing)	_____	_____
*E. Throat (general appearance, color, lesions)	_____	_____

FIGURE **35-1**
Example of a competency performance examination (CPE) for newborn assessment.

A major concern of academics is the measurability and standardization of their clinical evaluation tools. According to the COPA model, the criterion-referenced outcomes used as performance indicators would give faculty and clinic-based educators more confidence in their evaluations. Another advantage of the COPA model is that students could be moved through curricula as they demonstrate competencies, rather than on the basis of "seat time" amassed in a particular course. This means that it would not matter if it took 2 weeks or 20 weeks to master content and perform in a competent manner; passing the course would depend on mastery of the selected competencies (Kenner & Fernandes, 2001). Ideally, this arrangement would allow faculty members to spend more time with students having difficulty and would not hold back those with a solid grasp of the course content. Faculty members could hold back struggling students without feeling obligated to pass them on because the semester is ending. However, some problems arise with application of this model to that extent. Most of these problems center on faculty resources and on satisfying regulatory requirements for a certain number of hours spent in class or a clinical setting. These are hurdles that can be worked out with a

little nursing creativity. Only time will tell if more academic settings will use these strategies to address the nursing shortage and the need to ensure the quality of their graduates.

Some programs are using competency statements to guide their neonatal nurse practitioner (NNP) protocols. This is done not to the extent of moving students through more quickly, but rather to address the need to demonstrate competencies in graduates. One such program is Arizona State University's NNP program. The terminal competencies identified for NNP graduates in the master's of science program are listed in Box 35-1.

IMPLICATIONS FOR NEONATAL NURSING
Orientation to the NICU
Because neonatal nursing is a specialty area of practice, most graduate nurses complete their basic nursing education with very little clinical experience in the NICU. This places the burden of developing practice competence on the unit and the hospital. As a result of the projected nursing shortage, many NICUs will be employing new graduate nurses at a time when the supply of seasoned neonatal nurses may be diminished.

BOX **35-1**

Terminal Competencies for Neonatal Nurse Practitioner Graduates, Master of Science Program, Arizona State University College of Nursing

- Gathers pertinent information systematically and skillfully from all sources: perinatal history, diagnostic tests, and comprehensive physical examination with behavioral and developmental assessments and provides comprehensive health history and physical assessment.
- Differentiates normal and abnormal variations for all body systems.
- Accurately interprets diagnostic tests.
- Analyzes data from multiple sources in making clinical judgments and in determining the effectiveness of a plan of care.
- Develops problem lists with associated differential diagnoses.
- Provides holistic neonatal nursing care to high-risk infants in high-technology tertiary settings.
- Assesses family adaptation, coping skills, and the need for crisis and other interventions.
- Identifies educational needs of the family and assists with teaching.
- Ensures routine opportunities for neonate and parent relationships to emerge with development of bonding and attachment.
- Assists family to restructure daily living activities in ways that meet the needs of the infant and those of other family members.
- Evaluates infant physiologic and behavioral responses to interventions for revision of management plan.
- Communicates with family members regarding the changing health care needs of the infant.
- Initiates and performs measures necessary to resuscitate and stabilize a compromised infant.
- Accurately and appropriately performs routine diagnostic and therapeutic techniques according to established protocol and current standards for practice by neonatal nurse practitioners.
- Plans and implements appropriate pharmacologic therapies.
- Identifies ethical dilemmas in the evaluation and management of the high-risk infant.
- Develops therapeutic nurse-patient relationship.
- Demonstrates management of acute and chronic health alterations across the neonatal care continuum.
- Demonstrates health promotion and health maintenance strategies.
- Prioritizes and initiates pertinent diagnostic tests.
- Determines nursing and medical diagnoses and develops a prioritized comprehensive problem list.
- Establishes appropriate priorities of care.
- Collects patient data on an ongoing basis, prioritized according to immediate conditions or needs.
- In collaboration with the family, physician, staff nurse, and other members of the multidisciplinary health care team, formulates a plan of care that incorporates health care maintenance, discharge, and follow-up care.
- Demonstrates management of complex, rapidly changing clinical situations.
- Evaluates the patient's progress toward attainment of expected outcomes.
- Systemically evaluates and ensures quality and effectiveness of care.
- Demonstrates multidisciplinary consultation and collaboration.
- Initiates referrals based on the infant's and family's needs.
- Seeks appropriate consultation based on the infant's health care needs.
- Facilitates use of organizational resources in caring for the patient.
- Evaluates his or her clinical practice in relation to professional and ethical standards, relevant laws, statutes, and regulations.
- Identifies the legal components of advanced neonatal nursing practice.
- Critiques theories and research and participates in research activities for the evaluation, modification, and enhancement of existing practice.
- Helps provide in-service education programs and functions as a neonatal clinical resource person within the institution.
- Assists in developing unit policies and procedures for nursing care of the high-risk infant and participates in quality assurance measures in the NICU.
- Develops and implements strategies that have a positive effect on the political and regulatory processes related to health care systems and the role of the neonatal nurse practitioner.
- Demonstrates commitment to the role of neonatal nurse practitioner and identifies mechanisms to determine the future direction of the profession.
- Demonstrates cultural sensitivity and cultural competence.

Modified from McGrath J, director, Neonatal Nurse Practitioner Program, Arizona State University, Tempe, Arizona. Personal communication, 2001.

The traditional orientation approach of classroom learning followed by a period of joint clinical practice with an assigned preceptor may not be possible. As the competition for new graduate nurses intensifies, many hospitals are developing internship or externship programs.

Internships and externships for the new graduate nurse are a viable option for NICUs. Most newly graduated nurses recognize the paucity of their knowledge and skills for intensive care units and want some type of formalized educational program to become staff nurses in these areas. Depending on the availability of staff development instructors and seasoned nurses willing to assume preceptor responsibilities, many internship and externship programs offer a mix of traditional classroom teaching and competency-based education. To maximize resources, hospitals often combine nurse interns and externs for the classroom work. For example, a large tertiary hospital may offer a maternal-child nursing option, whereas a children's hospital may offer a critical care option. In the former case, the interns and externs may take classes together on maternity and pediatric nursing. In the latter case, the interns may be in class for the critical care core content.

CBE is also well suited to orientation for new graduate nurses and for experienced nurses who are changing their focus area. For the seasoned staff nurse who switches from adult intensive care, the orientation can focus on the neonatal-specific aspects of critical care. The orientation program for this nurse can be individualized to allow credit for knowledge and skills previously learned. An experienced staff nurse who switches from the well-baby nursery to the NICU needs to focus on the critical care aspects of newborns, because this individual already has a knowledge base about well infants and about concerns common to well babies and those in the NICU, such as thermoregulation and hypoglycemia.

Ongoing Staff Development

The individual employee must pursue the necessary ongoing education, although unit managers are responsible for documenting competency (i.e., validating skills and knowledge). This can be done through continuing education programs offered by professional organizations and by staff development programs offered by the institution. Maintaining individual competence is a professional obligation of every neonatal nurse. This obligation is spelled out clearly in the ANA's Code for Nurses (ANA, 1985):

> The profession of nursing is obligated to provide adequate and competent nursing care. Therefore, it is the responsibility of each nurse to maintain competency in practice. The nurse must be aware of the need for continued professional learning and must assume personal responsibility for currency of knowledge and skills.

Voluntary certification is an excellent mechanism for staff nurses to document their ongoing competence in neonatal nursing. In addition to measuring specialty knowledge, national certification examinations require documentation of ongoing education to maintain the certified nurse's expertise. The National Certification Corporation for the Obstetric, Gynecologic, and Neonatal Nursing Specialties (NCC) offers several examinations for neonatal nurses. These include an examination for neonatal intensive care and low-risk newborn care. Subspecialty areas, such as lactation nursing, are also available to certified nurses (NCC, 2001). An examination in neonatal critical care is available from the American Association of Critical-Care Nurses (AACN) Certification Corporation (AACN, 2006). The findings of a recent study of 19,000 certified nurses indicated that certified nurses make fewer errors in patient care, have fewer adverse events, are more effective in interpersonal skills, and have more confidence in their ability to identify patient complications (Trossman, 2000).

Graduate Programs to Prepare Neonatal Nurse Practitioners

Ensuring the competence of neonatal nurse practitioners is a joint responsibility of the specialty organization that establishes the criteria for NNP programs, the academic institutions that provide this education, and the credentialing agencies that measure entry into practice knowledge. Currently, no specific education standards exist for NNP education programs. Nurse practitioner programs are evaluated against accreditation criteria developed for graduate nursing education. Under the leadership of the National Organization of Nurse Practitioner Faculties, a variety of nursing organizations concerned with nurse practitioner education standards and credentialing worked together to produce a document titled *Criteria for Evaluation of Nurse Practitioner Programs* (NONPF, 1997). Although this document sets forth criteria for nurse practitioner programs, it does not address specialty-specific content, such as that required by a neonatal nurse practitioner. Although the National Association of Neonatal Nurses published guidelines for curriculum development for NNP programs, they are out of date (NANN, 1995). A NANN task force developed educational standards for NNP programs, and these are being used by most of the U.S.-based neonatal programs (NANN, 2002). A critical step in this process is the identification of NNP core competencies. The core competencies will define the practice of the NNP and serve as the foundation for a quality educational program (Williams & Kelley, 1998).

Currently, the competence of new graduate neonatal nurse practitioners is a function of the individual's background in neonatal nursing and the quality of the NNP program attended. The quality of NNP programs varies and depends on a number of factors, including the experience and expertise of the program's faculty, the entrance requirements for students, and the amount of didactic and clinical experience obtained through the program.

Although the trend in academia is to reduce the amount of staff nursing experience required before graduate school, a recent survey of NNP program directors revealed that practice experience is considered essential for NNP education (NANN NNP Education Standards Task Force, 2000). Much work must be done before NNP competency can be ensured.

COMPETENCY VALIDATION

Hospitals are required to document initial competency and the ongoing competence of their nursing staff. Validation is essential to ensure both that the nurse continues to maintain the level of expertise necessary to provide safe care and that the nurse has the knowledge needed to provide the best possible care for the particular problems of patients (Gunn, 1999). Responsibility for validation often falls on the shoulders of the intensive care nursery's unit manager.

The frequency of validation may vary according to the specific skill. The interval for validation of such skills as neonatal resuscitation is determined by the national standard, as set by the Neonatal Resuscitation Program (Bloom, Cropley, American Heart Association and American Academy of Pediatrics [AHA/AAP] Neonatal Resuscitation Steering Committee, 2006). Other skills usually are validated annually or as required by accreditation criteria set forth by JCAHO.

Competency validation can be achieved through a variety of mechanisms, including self-assessment, direct observation of performance, objective examination, and documentation of the number of technical skills or procedures performed in a given time (Miller et al, 1998). For many skills, a combination of methods is used; for example, validation of neonatal resuscitation skills includes objective examinations and performance evaluations.

SUMMARY

Maintaining and ensuring the competence of neonatal nurses are major concerns of hospitals, regulators, insurance companies, and society at large. Changes in the health care industry as a result of managed care, mergers of provider institutions such as hospitals, and significant reorganization within the delivery system have placed new demands on the nursing profession to ensure the ongoing competence of its members. Individually and collectively, nurses are challenged by the need to keep current in the midst of a knowledge and technology explosion, by the demand from payers for greater productivity and efficiency in health care, and by consumers' growing sophistication about the consequences brought about by incompetent providers. Standards of nursing practice and accreditation criteria from agencies such as JCAHO are used to develop the nursing competencies.

Competency-based education provides a mechanism for contemporary nursing to provide a cost-effective, quality approach to nursing orientation. It also allows units and institutions to individualize the orientation program to meet the differing needs of nurses who have significantly different backgrounds and levels of experience. Competency-based education shifts the focus of learning from the traditional model of objectives and classroom teaching to a new model based on competencies and outcomes.

The final aspect of ensuring competency of the nursing staff is the development of a mechanism for validating competencies. A variety of methods currently are used to validate nursing knowledge and skills, including skills checklists, performance appraisals, and formal testing (e.g., posttests).

Ultimately, the individual nurse is responsible for maintaining professional knowledge and skills through continuing education and other educational activities. Educational institutions provide the nurse with the basic nursing education. Passing the registered nurse licensing examination is only the beginning of documentation of competence as a professional nurse. Ongoing competence requires each nurse to become accountable for his or her own practice.

REFERENCES

Alspach JG (1984). Designing a competency-based orientation for critical care nurses. *Heart lung* 13(6):655-662.

Alspach JG (1992). Concern and confusion over competence. *Critical care nurse* 12(4):9-11.

American Association of Critical Care Nurses (AACN) Certification Corporation (2001). *CCRN: certification for adult, pediatric, and neonatal critical care nurses.* Available at: http://www.certcorp.org/certcorp/certcorp.nsf/edcfc72ba47aaa708825666b0064bdcf/373c091694efeaaa88256 6d4007dfa50?OpenDocument. Retrieved August 18, 2006.

American Nurses Association (ANA) (1985). *Code for nurses with interpretive statements.* Washington, DC: Author.

American Nurses Association (ANA) (1994). *Standards of nursing professional development: continuing education, and staff development.* Washington, DC: Author.

American Nurses Association Expert Panel (2000). *Continuing competence: nursing's agenda for the twenty-first century.* Washington, DC: Author.

Avery MD (2005). The history and evolution of the core competencies for basic midwifery practice. *Journal of midwifery and women's health* 50(2):102-107.

Bargagliotti T et al (1999). Reducing the threats to the implementation of a competency-performance assessment system. *Online journal of issues in nursing.* Available at: http://www.nursingworld.org/ojin/topic10/tpc10_5.htm. Retrieved August 18, 2006.

Bechtel GA et al (1999). Problem-based learning in a competency-based world. *Nurse education today* 19(3):182-187.

Benner P (1984). *From novice to expert: excellence and power in clinical nursing practice.* Menlo Park, CA: Addison-Wesley.

Bloom RS, Cropley C, AHA/AAP Neonatal Resuscitation Steering Committee (2006). *Textbook of neonatal resuscitation,* ed 5. Elk Grove Village, IL: American Academy of Pediatrics/American Heart Association.

Carter MA (1988). The professional doctorate as an entry into clinical practice (pp 49-52). *Perspectives in nursing 1987-89: based on the presentations at the Eighteenth NLN Biennial Convention.* National League for Nursing (NLN) Publication #41-2199.

Chaisson SF (1995). Role of the CNS in developing a competency-based orientation program. *Clinical nurse specialist* 9(1):32-37.

Chapman H (1999). Some important limitations of competency-based education with respect to nurse education: an Australian perspective. *Nurse education today* 19(2):129-135.

Citizens Advocacy Center (CAC) (1997). *Continuing professional competence: can we assure it? Proceedings of a citizens advocacy center conference, December 13-17, 1996.* Washington, DC: Author.

Commission for Collegiate Nursing Education (CCNE) (1998). *Standards for accreditation of baccalaureate and graduate nursing education programs.* Washington, DC: Author.

Dozier AM (1998). Professional standards: linking care, competence, and quality. *Journal of nursing care quality* 12(4):22-29.

Dunn SV et al (2000). The development of competency standards for specialist critical care nurses. *Journal of advanced nursing* 31(2):339-346.

Fey MK, Miltner RS (2000). A competency-based orientation program for new graduate nurses. *Journal of nursing administration* 30(3):126-132.

Fitzpatrick JJ (1988). The professional doctorate as an entry into clinical practice (pp 53-56). *Perspectives in nursing 1987-89: based on the presentations at the Eighteenth NLN Biennial Convention.* National League for Nursing (NLN) Publication #41-2199.

Grant G (1979). *On competence: a critical analysis of competence-based reforms in higher education.* San Francisco: Jossey-Bass.

Gunn IP (1999). Regulation of health care professionals. Part 2. Validation of continued competence. *CRNA: clinical forum for nurse anesthetists* 10(3):135-141.

Hodges J, Hansen L (1999). Restructuring a competency-based orientation for registered nurses. *Journal for nurses in staff development* 15(4):152-158.

Jeffrey Y (2000). Using competencies to promote a learning environment in intensive care. *Nursing in critical care* 5(4):194-198.

Joint Commission on Accreditation of Healthcare Organizations (JCAHO) (1999). *Comprehensive accreditation manual for hospitals: the official handbook.* Oakbrook Terrace, IL: JCAHO.

Kenner C, Fernandes JH (2001). Knowledge management and advanced nursing education. *Newborn and infant nursing reviews* 1(3):192-198.

Knowles MS (1980). *The modern practice of adult education: from pedagogy to andragogy.* Chicago: Follet.

Lenburg CB (1999a). Redesigning expectations for initial and continuing competence for contemporary nursing practice. *Online journal of issues in nursing.* Available at: http://www.nursingworld.org/ojin/topic10/tpc10_1.htm. Retrieved August 18, 2006.

Lenburg CB (1999b). The framework, concepts, and methods of the competency outcomes and performance assessment (COPA) model. *Online journal of issues in nursing.* Available at: http://www.nursingworld.org/ojin/topic10/tpc10_2.htm. Retrieved August 18, 2006.

Lenburg CB (1999c). COPA model. *Online journal of issues in nursing.* Available at: http://www.nursingworld.org/mods/archive/mod110/copa2.htm. Retrieved August 18, 2006.

Luttrell MF et al (1999). Competency outcomes for learning and performance assessment. *Nursing and health care perspectives* 20(3):134-141.

Marrone SR (1999). Designing a competency-based nursing practice model in a multicultural setting. *Journal for nurses in staff development* 15(2):535-562.

Mikos-Schild S (1999). Competency-based orientation. *Today's surgery nurse* 21(3):3-17.

Miller E et al (1998). Assessing, developing, and maintaining staff's competency in times of restructuring. *Journal of nursing care quality* 12(6):9-17.

National Association of Neonatal Nurses (NANN) (1995). *Program guidelines for NNP educational preparation*. Petaluma, CA: Author.

National Association of Neonatal Nurses (NANN) NNP Education Standards Task Force. (2000). *Survey of NNP programs*. Unpublished data. Glenview, IL: NANN.

National Association of Neonatal Nurses (NANN) (2002). *Education standards for neonatal nurse practitioner programs*. Glenview, IL: Author.

National Certification Corporation for the Obstetric, Gynecologic, and Neonatal Nursing Specialties (NCC) (2001). *NCC examinations*. Available at: www.necnet.org/ certification.examdesc.htm. Retrieved November 15, 2001.

National Council of State Boards of Nursing (NCSBN) (1998). *Assuring competence: a regulatory responsibility*. Chicago: Author.

National Institutes of Health (NIH) Clinical Center Nursing Department (1995). *Nursing standards*. Rockville, MD: NIH.

National League for Nursing Accreditation Commission (NLNAC) (1997). *Accreditation manual and interpretive guidelines*. NLNAC: New York.

National Organization of Nurse Practitioner Faculties (NONPF) (1997). *Criteria for evaluation of nurse practitioner programs*. Washington, DC: NONPF.

Neary M (2001). Responsive assessment: assessing student nurses' clinical competence. *Nurse education today* 21(1):3-17.

O'Grady TP, O'Brien A (1992). A guide to competency-based orientation: develop your own program. *Journal of nursing staff development* 8(3):128-133.

Pew Health Professions Commission (1995). *Reforming health care work force regulation: policy considerations for the twenty-first century*. San Francisco: Author.

Pew Health Professions Commission (1998). *Strengthening consumer protection: priorities for health care work force regulation: report of the Pew Health Professions Commission*. San Francisco: Author.

Ringerman E et al (2006). An innovative education program: the peer competency validator model. *Journal of nurses staff development* 22(3):114-121, quiz 122-123.

Smith S et al (1996). Examining competency-based orientation implementation. *Journal of nursing staff development* 12(3):139-143.

Stewart SL, Vitello-Cicciu KM (1989). Designing a competency-based orientation program for the care of cardiac surgery patients. *Journal of cardiovascular nursing* 3(3):34-41.

Trossman S (2000). Certified nurses report fewer adverse events: survey links certification with improved health care. *American nurse* 1:9.

Watson J (1988). The professional doctorate as an entry into clinical practice (pp 41-47). *Perspectives in nursing 1987-89: based on the presentations at the Eighteenth NLN biennial convention*. National League for Nursing (NLN) Publication #41-2199.

Weinstein SM (2000). Certification and credentialing to define competency-based practice. *Journal of intravenous nursing* 23(1):21-28.

Whittaker S et al (2000). Assuring continued competence. *Online journal of issues in nursing*. Available at: http://www.nursingworld.org/ojin/topic10/tpc10_4.htm. Retrieved August 18, 2006.

Williams DR, Kelley MA (1998). Core competency-based education, certification, and practice: the nurse-midwifery model. *Advanced practice nursing quarterly* 4(3):63-71.

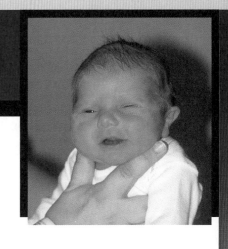

Chapter **36**

Fetal Development: Environmental Influences and Critical Periods

Judy Wright Lott

In this chapter, the major events of prenatal development are described, and critical development periods for the major organ systems are identified. A brief review of the events beginning with fertilization is included, but the reader is referred to an embryology text for a more thorough account. Human genetics is discussed in Chapter 32.

EARLY FETAL DEVELOPMENT

The process of human development begins with the fertilization of an ovum (female gamete) by a spermatocyte (male gamete). The fusion of the ovum and sperm initiates a sequence of events that causes the single-celled zygote to develop into a new human being. During the 38 to 42 weeks of gestation, dramatic growth and development occurs that is unequaled during any other period of life.

Fertilization

Large numbers of spermatozoa are necessary to increase the chances for conception because the spermatozoa must traverse the cervical canal, the uterus, and the uterine (fallopian) tubes to reach the ovum; approximately 200 to 500 million sperm are deposited in the posterior fornix of the vagina during ejaculation. The usual site of fertilization is in the ampulla, the widest portion of the uterine tubes, located near the ovaries. Sperm are propelled by the movement of the tails, aided by muscular contractions of the uterus. The spermatozoa undergo two physiologic changes in order to penetrate the corona radiata and zona pellucida, the barriers around the secondary oocyte. The first change is capacitation, an enzymatic reaction that removes the glycoprotein coating from the spermatozoa and plasma proteins from the seminal fluid. Capacitation generally occurs in the uterus or uterine tubes and takes about 7 hours. The second change, the acrosome reaction, occurs when a capacitated sperm passes through the corona radiata, causing structural changes that result in the fusion of the

plasma membranes of the sperm and the oocyte. Progesterone released from the follicle at ovulation stimulates the acrosome reaction. Three enzymes are released from the acrosome to facilitate entry of the sperm into the ovum. Hyaluronidase allows the sperm to penetrate the corona radiata; whereas trypsin-like enzymes and zona lysin digest a pathway across the zona pellucida (Jirasek et al, 2001; Larsen, 2001; Sadler, 2003).

Only about 300 to 500 spermatozoa actually reach the ovum. When a spermatozoon comes into contact with the ovum, the zona pellucida and the plasma membrane fuse, preventing entry by other sperm. After penetration by a single sperm, the oocyte completes the second meiotic cell division, resulting in the haploid number of chromosomes (22,X) and the second polar body. The chromosomes are arranged to form the female pronucleus (Jirasek et al, 2001; Larsen, 2001; Sadler, 2003).

As the spermatozoon moves close to the female pronucleus, the tail detaches and the nucleus enlarges to form the male pronucleus. The male and female pronuclei fuse forming a diploid cell called the *zygote*. The zygote contains 23 autosomes and one sex chromosome from each parent (46,XX or 46,XY). The genetic sex of the new individual is determined at fertilization by the contribution of the father. The male parent (XY) may contribute either an X or a Y chromosome. If the spermatozoon contains an X chromosome, the offspring is female (46,XX). If the spermatozoon receives one Y chromosome, the offspring is male (46,XY). Individual variation is the result of random or independent assortment of the autosomal chromosomes (Jirasek et al, 2001; Larsen, 2001; Sadler, 2003).

Cleavage

Mitotic cell division occurs after fertilization as the zygote passes down the uterine tube, resulting in the formation of two blastomeres (Figure 36-1). The cells continue to divide, increasing in number, although decreasing in size. The term

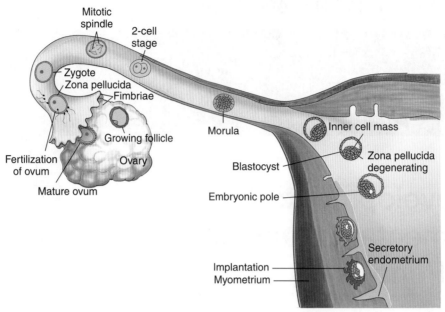

FIGURE **36-1**

Fantastic voyage: from fertilization to implantation. The journey through the fallopian tubes takes approximately 4 days. During this time, mitotic cell division occurs. Implantation occurs on about day 9 through day 12.

cleavage is used to describe the mitotic cell division of the zygote (Figure 36-2). When the number of cells reaches approximately 16 (usually on the third day), the zygote is called a *morula*, because of its resemblance to a mulberry. The zygote reaches the morula stage about the time it enters the uterus. The morula consists of groups of centrally located cells called the *inner cell mass* and an outer cell layer. At this stage the individual cells are called blastomeres. The outer cell layer forms the trophoblast, from which the placenta develops. The inner cell mass, called the *embryoblast*, gives rise to the embryo (Jirasek et al, 2001; Larsen, 2001; Sadler, 2003).

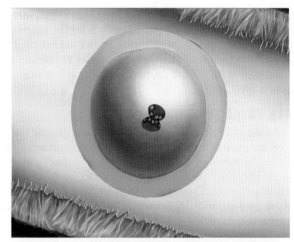

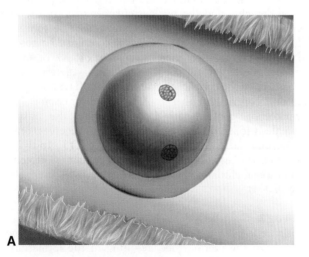

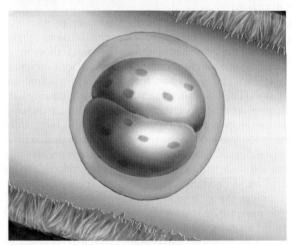

FIGURE **36-2**

Stages of cell division: cleavage. **A,** Zygote. **B,** Zygote undergoing first cleavage. **C,** Two-cell blastomere state.

After the morula penetrates the uterine cavity, fluid enters through the zona pellucida into the intercellular spaces of the inner cell mass. About the fourth day after fertilization, the fluid-filled spaces fuse, forming a large cavity known as the blastocyst cavity. The morula is now called the *blastocyst*. The trophoblast forms the wall of the blastocyst, and the embryoblast projects from the wall of the blastocyst into the blastocyst cavity. The uterine secretions nourish the blastocyst until implantation occurs (Jirasek et al, 2001; Larsen, 2001; Sadler, 2003).

Implantation

Degeneration of the zona pellucida occurs on about the fifth day after fertilization, allowing the blastocyst to attach to the endothelium of the endometrium on about the sixth day. The trophoblasts then secrete proteolytic enzymes that destroy the endometrial endothelium and invade the endometrium. Two layers of trophoblasts develop; the inner layer is made up of cytotrophoblasts, and the outer layer is composed of syncytiotrophoblasts. The syncytiotrophoblast has finger-like projections that produce enzymes capable of further eroding the endometrial tissues. By the end of the seventh day, the blastocyst is superficially implanted (Figure 36-3) (Jirasek et al, 2001; Larsen, 2001; Sadler, 2003).

Formation of the Bilaminar Disk

Implantation is completed during the second week. The syncytiotrophoblast continues to invade the endometrium and becomes embedded. Spaces in the syncytiotrophoblast called *lacunae* fill with blood from ruptured maternal capillaries and secretions from eroded endometrial glands. This fluid nourishes the embryoblast by diffusion. The lacunae give rise to the uteroplacental circulation. The lacunae fuse to form a network that then becomes the intervillous spaces of the placenta. The endometrial capillaries near the implanted embryoblast become dilated and eroded by the syncytiotrophoblast. Maternal blood enters the lacunar network and provides circulation and nutrients to the embryo. Maternal-embryonic blood circulation provides the developing embryo with nutrition and oxygenation and removes waste products before the development of the placenta. Finger-like projections, primary chorionic villi, of the chorion develop into the chorionic villi of the placenta at about the same time (Jirasek et al, 2001; Larsen, 2001; Sadler, 2003).

The inner cell mass differentiates into two layers: the hypoblast (endoderm), a layer of small cuboidal cells, and the epiblast (ectoderm), a layer of high columnar cells. The two layers form a flattened, circular bilaminar embryonic disk. The amniotic cavity is derived from spaces within the epiblast. As the amniotic cavity enlarges, a thin layer of epithelial cells covers the amniotic cavity. During the development of the amniotic cavity, other trophoblastic cells form a thin extracoelomic membrane, which encloses the primitive yolk sac. The yolk sac produces fetal red blood cells. Other trophoblastic cells form a layer of mesenchymal tissue, called the *extraembryonic mesoderm*, around the amnion and primitive yolk sac. Isolated coelomic spaces in the extraembryonic mesoderm fuse to form a single, large, fluid-filled cavity surrounding the amnion and yolk sac, with the exception of the area where the amnion is attached to the chorion by the connecting stalk. The primitive yolk sac decreases in size, creating a smaller secondary yolk sac (Jirasek et al, 2001; Larsen, 2001; Sadler, 2003).

Two layers of extraembryonic mesoderm result from the formation of the extraembryonic cavity. The extraembryonic somatic mesoderm lines the trophoblast and covers the

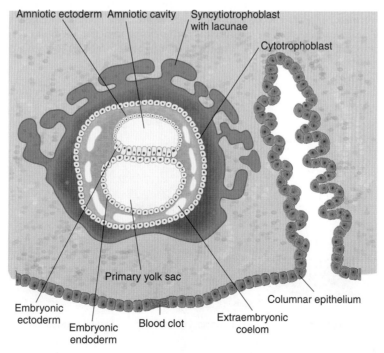

Amniotic ectoderm   Amniotic cavity   Syncytiotrophoblast with lacunae

Cytotrophoblast

Primary yolk sac

Embryonic ectoderm

Embryonic endoderm

Blood clot

Extraembryonic coelom

Columnar epithelium

FIGURE **36-3**
Cross section of a blastocyst at 11 days. Two germ layers are present. The trophoblast has differentiated into the syncytiotrophoblast and the cytotrophoblast.

amnion, and the extraembryonic splanchnic mesoderm covers the yolk sac. The chorion is made up of the extraembryonic somatic mesoderm, the cytotrophoblast, and the syncytiotrophoblast. The chorion forms the chorionic sac, in which the embryo and the amniotic and yolk sacs are located. By the end of the second week, there is a slightly thickened area near the cephalic region of the hypoblastic disk, known as the prochordal plate, which marks the location of the mouth.

Formation of the Trilaminar Embryonic Disk: The Third Week of Development

The third week of development is marked by rapid growth, the formation of the *primitive streak*, and the differentiation of the three germ layers, from which all fetal tissue and organs are derived (Jirasek et al, 2001; Larsen, 2001; Sadler, 2003) (Figure 36-4).

Gastrulation

Gastrulation is the process through which the bilaminar disk develops into a trilaminar embryonic disk. Gastrulation is the most important event of early fetal formation; it affects all of the rest of embryologic development. During the third week, epiblast cells separate from their original location and migrate inward, forming the mesoblast, which spreads cranially and laterally to form a layer between the ectoderm and the endoderm called the *intraembryonic mesoderm*. Other mesoblastic cells invade the endoderm, displacing the endodermal cells laterally, forming a new layer, the embryonic ectoderm. Thus, the hypoblastic ectoderm produces the embryonic ectoderm, embryonic mesoderm, and the majority of the embryonic endoderm. These three germ layers are the source of the tissue and organs of the embryo (Jirasek et al, 2001; Larsen, 2001; Sadler, 2003).

Primitive Streak

Over days 14 to 15, a groove and thickening of the ectoderm (epiblast), called the *primitive streak*, appears caudally in the center of the dorsum of the embryonic disk. The primitive streak results from the migration of ectodermal cells toward the midline in the posterior portion of the embryonic disk. The primitive groove develops in the primitive streak. When the primitive streak begins to produce mesoblastic cells that become intraembryonic mesoderm, the epiblast is referred to as the *embryonic ectoderm* and the hypoblast is referred to as the *embryonic mesoderm* (Jirasek et al, 2001; Larsen, 2001; Sadler, 2003).

Notochordal Process

Cells from the primitive knot migrate cranially and form the midline cellular *notochordal process*. This process grows cranially between the ectoderm and the endoderm until it reaches the prochordal plate, which is attached to the overlying ectoderm, thus forming the oropharyngeal membrane. The cloacal membrane, caudal to the primitive streak, develops into the anus.

The primitive streak produces mesenchyme (mesoblasts) until the end of the fourth week. The primitive streak does not grow as rapidly as the other cells, making it relatively insignificant in size when compared with the other structures that continue to grow. Persistence of the primitive streak or remnants is the cause of sacrococcygeal teratomas (Jirasek et al, 2001; Larsen, 2001; Sadler, 2003).

The *notochord* is a cellular rod that develops from the notochordal process. The notochord is the structure around which the vertebral column is formed. It forms the nucleus pulposus of the intervertebral bodies of the spinal column (Figure 36-5) (Jirasek et al, 2001; Larsen, 2001; Sadler, 2003).

Neurulation

Neurulation is the process through which the neural plate, neural folds, and neural tube are formed. The developing notochord stimulates the embryonic ectoderm to thicken, forming the neural plate. The neuroectoderm of the neural plate gives rise to the central nervous system. The neural plate develops cranial to the primitive knot. As the neural plate elongates, the neural plate gets wider and extends cranially to the oropharyngeal membrane. The neural plate invaginates along the central axis to form a neural groove with neural folds

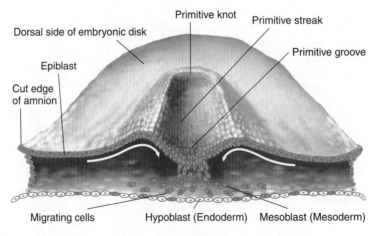

FIGURE **36-4**
Formation of the trilaminar embryonic disk: gastrulation. During gastrulation, the bilaminar embryonic disk is changed to a trilaminar embryonic disk, consisting of the epiblast (ectoderm), hypoblast (endoderm), and mesoblast (mesoderm).

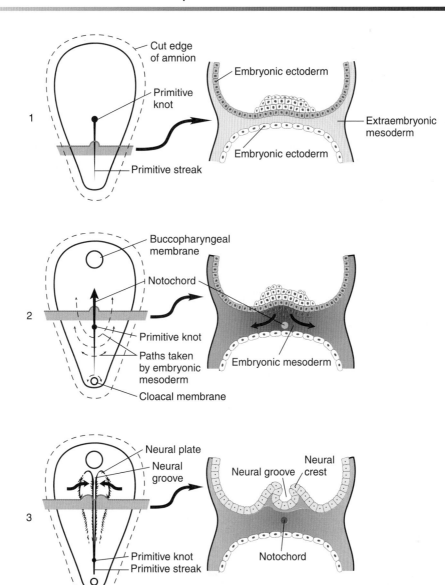

FIGURE **36-5**
Formation of primitive streak, primitive knot, notochord, and neural groove.

on each side. The neural folds move together and fuse, forming the neural tube (Figure 36-6). The neural tube detaches from the surface ectoderm, and the free edges of the ectoderm fuse, covering the posterior portion of the embryo. With formation of the neural tube, nearby ectodermal cells lying along the crest of each neural fold migrate inward, invading the mesoblast on each side of the neural tube. These irregular, flattened masses are called the *neural crest*. This structure's cells give rise to the spinal ganglia, the ganglia of the autonomic nervous system, and a portion of the cranial nerves. Neural crest cells also form the meningeal covering of the brain and spinal cord and the sheaves that protect nerves. The neural crest cells contribute to the formation of pigment-producing cells, the adrenal medulla, and skeletal and muscular development in the head (Jirasek et al, 2001; Larsen, 2001; Sadler, 2003).

Development of Somites

Another important event of the third week is the development of somites, which give rise to most of the skeleton and associated musculature and much of the dermis of the skin. During formation of the neural tube, the intraembryonic mesoderm on each side thickens, forming longitudinal columns of paraxial mesoderm. At about 20 days, the paraxial mesoderm begins to divide into paired into cuboidal bodies known as somites. In all, 42 to 44 somites develop, in a craniocaudal sequence, although only 38 develop during the "somite" period. These somite pairs can be counted and give an estimate of fetal age before a crown-rump measurement is possible (Jirasek et al, 2001; Larsen, 2001; Sadler, 2003).

Intraembryonic Cavity

Another significant process is the formation of the intraembryonic cavity. This structure first appears as a number of small spaces within the lateral mesoderm and the cardiogenic mesoderm. These spaces combine to form the intraembryonic cavity; it is horseshoe-shaped and lined with flattened epithelial cells that eventually line the peritoneal cavity. The intraembryonic cavity divides the lateral mesoderm into the

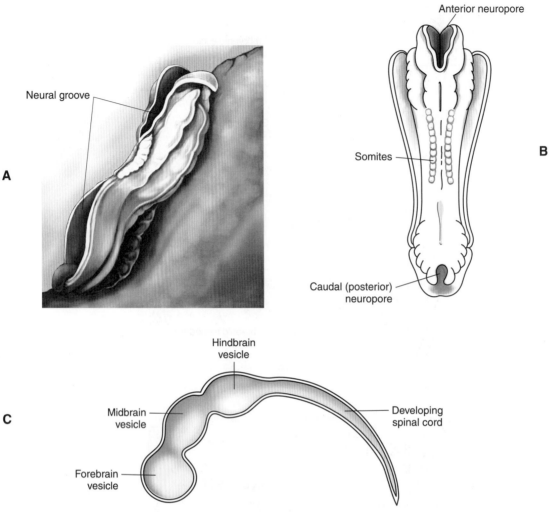

FIGURE **36-6**
Formation of the neural tube. **A,** Neural groove. **B,** Closure of the neural tube almost completed. **C,** Dilation of the neural tube forms the forebrain, midbrain, and hindbrain.

parietal (somatic) and visceral (splanchnic) layers. It gives rise to the pericardial cavity, the pleural cavity, and the peritoneal cavity (Jirasek et al, 2001; Larsen, 2001; Sadler, 2003).

PLACENTAL DEVELOPMENT AND FUNCTION

The rudimentary maternal-fetal circulation is intact by the fourth week of gestation. Growth of the trophoblast results in numerous primary and secondary chorionic villi, covering the surface of the chorionic sac until about the eighth week of gestation. At about the eighth week, the villi overlying the conceptus (decidua capsularis) degenerate, leaving a smooth area (smooth chorion). The villi underlying the conceptus (decidua basalis) remain and increase in size, producing the chorion frondosum, or fetal side of the placenta. The maternal side of the placenta is made up of the chorion and the chorionic villi. On implantation of the conceptus, maternal capillaries of the decidua basalis rupture, causing maternal blood to circulate through the developing fetal placenta (chorion frondosum). As growth and differentiation progress, extensions from the cytotrophoblast invade the syncytial layer and form a cytotrophoblastic shell, surrounding the conceptus

and chorionic villi. This shell is continuous but has communications between maternal blood vessels in the decidua basalis and the intervillous spaces of the chorion frondosum. The latter is attached to the maternal side of the placenta (decidua basalis) by the cytotrophoblastic shell and anchoring villi. The placenta is mature and completely functional by 16 weeks of development (Figure 36-7). If the corpus luteum begins to regress prior to the 16th week and fails to produce enough progesterone (the hormone responsible for readying the uterine cavity for the pregnancy), the pregnancy is aborted because the placenta is not capable of supporting the pregnancy on its own until about this time (Jirasek et al, 2001; Larsen, 2001; Sadler, 2003).

Placental-Fetal Circulation

A simple ebb-and-flow circulation is present in the embryo, yolk sac, connecting stalk, and chorion by 21 days of gestation. By 28 days, unidirectional circulation is established. Deoxygenated fetal blood leaves the fetus via the umbilical arteries and enters the capillaries in the chorionic villi where gaseous and nutrient exchange takes place. Oxygenated blood

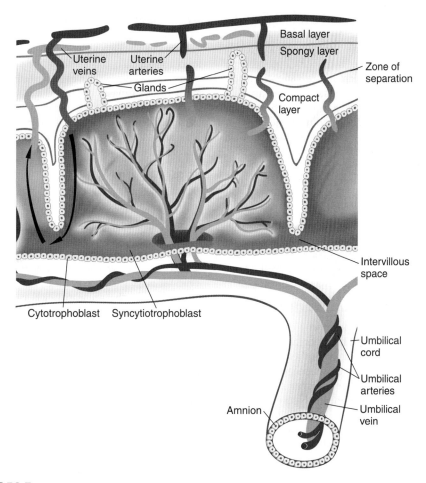

FIGURE **36-7**
Formation of the placenta. The fetal and maternal sides of the placenta. Separation of the placenta from the uterus occurs at the site indicated by the black line labeled *Zone of separation.*

returns to the fetus through the umbilical veins. At first there are two arteries and two veins, but one vein gradually degenerates, leaving two arteries and one vein. If only one artery is present, a congenital anomaly, especially a renal one, should be suspected (Jirasek et al, 2001; Larsen, 2001; Sadler, 2003).

Placental Function
Normal growth and development of the embryo depend on adequate placental function. The placenta is responsible for oxygenation, nutrition, elimination of wastes, production of hormones essential for maintenance of the pregnancy, and transport of substances. In addition, the placenta synthesizes glycogen, cholesterol, and fatty acids, which provide nutrients and energy for early fetal development. Transport across the placental membrane occurs primarily through simple and facilitated diffusion, active transport, and pinocytosis. Oxygen, carbon dioxide, and carbon monoxide cross the placenta through simple diffusion. The fetus is dependent on a continuous supply of oxygenated blood flowing from the placenta (Jirasek et al, 2001; Larsen, 2001; Sadler, 2003).

Water and electrolytes cross the placenta freely in both directions. Glucose is converted to glycogen in the placenta as a carbohydrate source for the fetus. Amino acids move readily across the placental membranes for protein synthesis in the fetus. Free fatty acids are transferred across the placenta by pinocytosis. There is limited or no transfer of maternal cholesterol, triglycerides, and phospholipids. Water- and fat-soluble vitamins cross the placenta and are essential for normal development (Moore & Persaud, 2002a).

The placenta produces and transports hormones that maintain the pregnancy and promote growth and development of the fetus. Chorionic gonadotropin, a protein hormone produced by the syncytiotrophoblast, is excreted in maternal serum and urine. The presence of human chorionic gonadotropin is used as a test for pregnancy. Human placental lactogen, also a protein hormone produced by the placenta, acts as a fetal growth-promoting hormone by giving the fetus priority for receiving maternal glucose (Jirasek et al, 2001; Larsen, 2001; Sadler, 2003).

The placenta also produces steroid hormones. Progesterone, produced by the placenta throughout gestation, is responsible for maintaining the pregnancy. Estrogen production by the placenta is dependent on stimulation by the fetal adrenal cortex and liver. Placental transport of maternal antibodies provides the fetus with passive immunity to certain viruses. IgG antibodies are actively transported across the placental barrier, providing humoral immunity for the fetus. IgA and

IgM antibodies do not cross the placental barrier, placing the neonate at risk for neonatal sepsis. However, failure of IgM antibodies to cross the placental membrane explains the lower incidence of a severe hemolytic process in ABO blood type incompatibilities when compared with Rh incompatibilities. The latter result when an Rh-negative mother has an Rh-positive fetus. If the mother is sensitized to the Rh-positive fetal blood cells, the mother produces IgG antibodies. IgG is transferred from the maternal to fetal circulation, and hemolysis of fetal red blood cells occurs (Jirasek et al, 2001; Larsen, 2001; Sadler, 2003).

The placenta is selective in the transfer of substances across the placenta; however, this selectivity does not screen out all potentially harmful substances. Viral, bacterial, and protozoal organisms can be transferred to the fetus through the placenta. Toxic substances such as drugs and alcohol can also be transferred to the fetus. The effects of these substances depend on the stage of gestation and type and duration of exposure, as well as the interaction of these and other factors, such as nutrition.

EMBRYONIC PERIOD: WEEKS 4 THROUGH 8

The embryonic period lasts from the beginning of gestational week 4 through the end of week 8. All major organ systems are formed during this period. The shape of the embryo changes as the organs develop, taking a more human shape by the end of the eighth week. The major events of the embryonic period are the folding of the embryo and organogenesis (Figure 36-8).

Folding of the Embryo

In the trilaminar embryonic disk, the growth rate of the central region exceeds that of the periphery so that the slower growing areas fold under the faster growing areas, forming body folds. The head fold appears first, as a result of craniocaudal elongation of the notochord and growth of the brain, which projects into the amniotic cavity. The folding downward of the cranial end of the embryo forces the septum transversum (primitive heart), the pericardial cavity, and the oropharyngeal membrane to turn under onto the ventral surface. After the embryo has folded, the mass of mesoderm cranial to the pericardial cavity, the septum transversum, lies caudal to the heart. The septum transversum later develops into a portion of the diaphragm. Part of the yolk sac is incorporated as the foregut, lying between the heart and the brain. The foregut ends blindly at the oropharyngeal membrane, which separates the foregut from the primitive mouth cavity (stomodeum) (Jirasek et al, 2001; Larsen, 2001; Sadler, 2003).

The tail fold occurs after the head fold as a result of craniocaudal growth progression. Growth of the embryo causes the caudal area to project over the cloacal membrane. During the tail folding, part of the yolk sac is incorporated into the embryo as the hindgut. After completion of the head and tail folding, the connecting stalk is attached to the ventral surface of the embryo, forming the umbilical cord. Folding also occurs laterally, producing right and left lateral folds. The lateral body wall on each side folds toward the median plane, causing the embryo to assume a cylindrical shape. During the lateral body folding, a portion of the yolk sac is incorporated as the midgut. The attachment of the midgut to the yolk sac is minimal after this fold develops. After folding, the amnion is attached to the embryo in a narrow area in which the umbilical cord attaches to the ventral surface (Jirasek et al, 2001; Larsen, 2001; Sadler, 2003).

Organogenesis: Germ Cell Derivatives

The three germ cell layers (ectoderm, mesoderm, and endoderm) give rise to all tissues and organs of the embryo. The germ cells follow specific patterns during the process of *organogenesis*. The main germ cell derivatives are listed in Box 36-1. The development of each major organ system is discussed separately. **The embryonic period is the most critical period of development because of the formation of internal and external structures.** The critical periods of development for the organs are also discussed in the section on specific organ development.

FETAL PERIOD: WEEK 9 THROUGH BIRTH

The *fetal period* begins at the start of the ninth week of gestation and extends through the duration of the pregnancy. It is characterized by further growth and development of the fetus and the organs formed during the embryonic period. Other changes that occur include the appearance of vernix caseosa, lanugo, and scalp hair. The eyelids open at about 24 to 26 weeks' gestation. The fetus has the potential for survival at approximately 24 weeks, but the preterm newborn experiences many difficult physiologic adjustments for intact survival. Closer to term, subcutaneous fat is deposited, giving the skin a smooth, firm,

Text continues on p. 637.

BOX 36-1

Germ Cell Derivatives

Ectoderm
Central nervous system (brain, spinal cord)
Peripheral nervous system
Sensory epithelia of eye, ear, and nose
Epidermis and its appendages (hair and nails)
Mammary glands
Subcutaneous glands
Teeth enamel
Neural crest cells
Spinal, cranial, and autonomic ganglia cells
Nerve sheaths of peripheral nervous system
Pigment cells
Muscle, connective tissue, and bone of branchial arch origin
Adrenal medulla
Meninges

Mesoderm
Cartilage
Bone
Connective tissue
Striated and smooth muscle
Heart, blood, and lymph vessels and cells
Gonads
Genital ducts
Pericardial, pleural, and peritoneal lining
Spleen
Cortex of adrenal gland

Endoderm
Epithelial lining of respiratory and gastrointestinal tracts
Parenchyma of tonsils, thyroid, parathyroid, liver, thymus, and pancreas
Epithelial lining of bladder and urethra
Epithelial lining of tympanic cavity, tympanic antrum, and auditory tube

TIMETABLE OF HUMAN PRENATAL DEVELOPMENT
1 TO 6 WEEKS

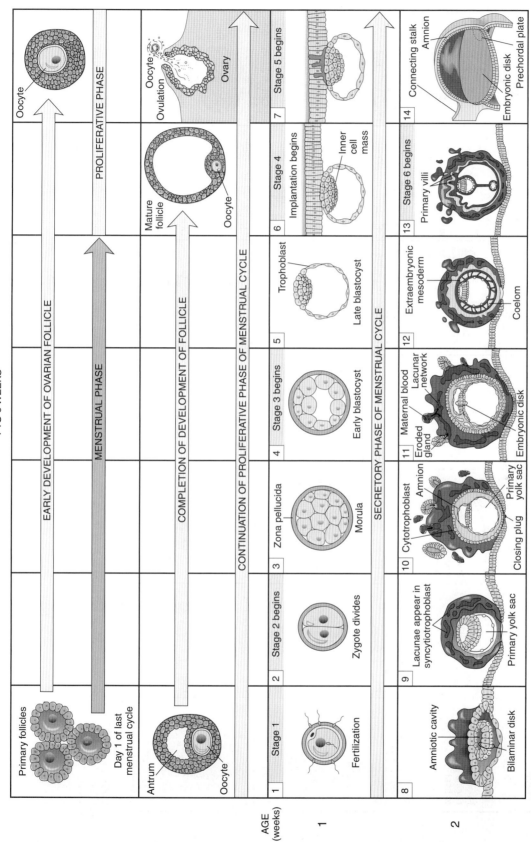

FIGURE **36-8**

Critical periods of development. From Moore KL et al (2003). *Before we are born: essentials of embryology and birth defects,* ed 6. Philadelphia: Saunders. Reprinted with permission.

Continued

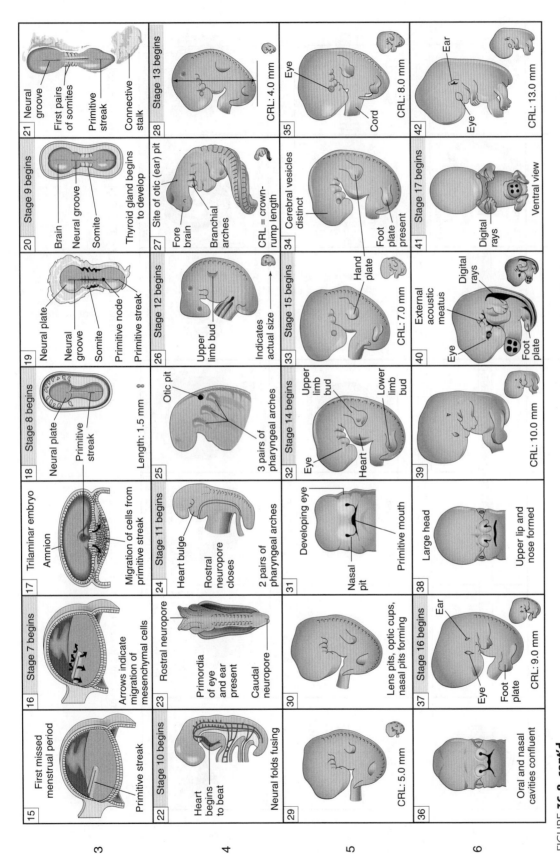

FIGURE **36-8, cont'd**
Critical periods of development. From Moore KL et al (2003). *Before we are born: essentials of embryology and birth defects,* ed 6. Philadelphia: Saunders. Reprinted with permission.

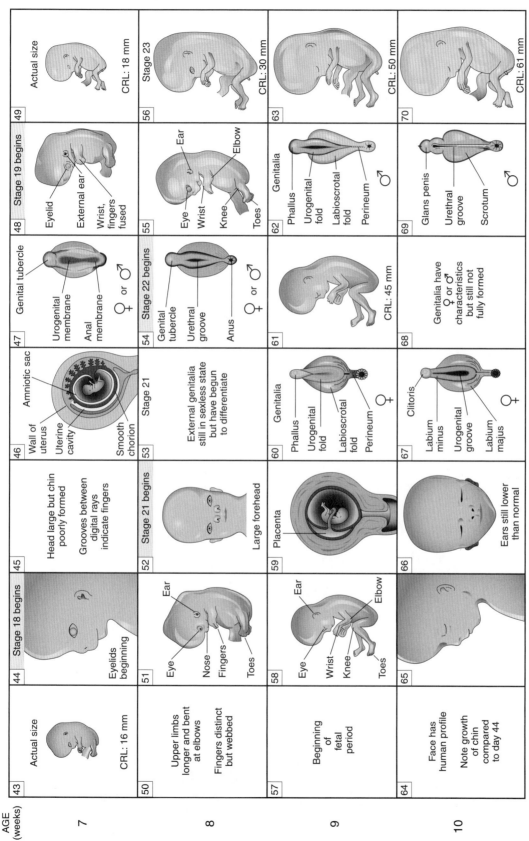

TIMETABLE OF HUMAN PRENATAL DEVELOPMENT
7 to 38 weeks

FIGURE **36-8, cont'd**
Critical periods of development. From Moore KL et al (2003). *Before we are born: essentials of embryology and birth defects*, ed 6. Philadelphia: Saunders. Reprinted with permission.

Continued

Eleventh Week to Full Term

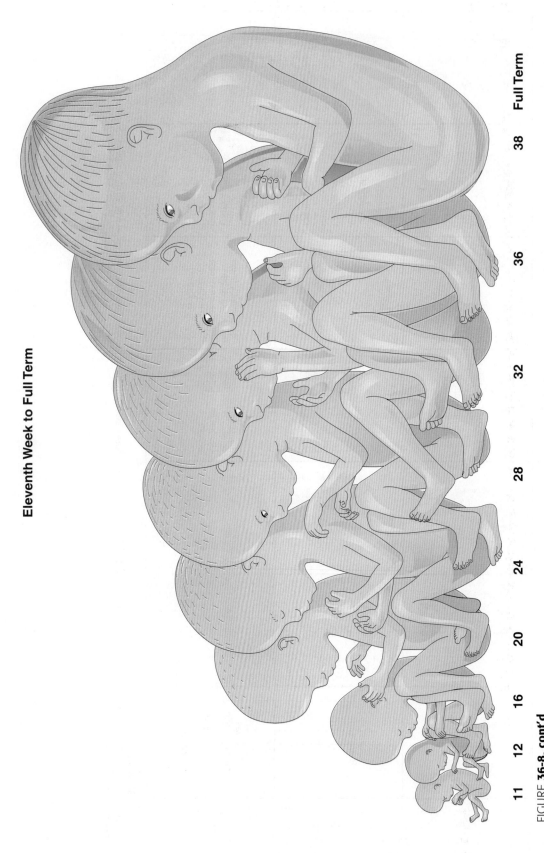

11   12   16   20   24   28   32   36   38   **Full Term**

FIGURE **36-8, cont'd**
Critical periods of development. From Moore KL et al (2003). *Before we are born: essentials of embryology and birth defects*, ed 6. Philadelphia: Saunders. Reprinted with permission.

Three Periods of Fetal Development

Embryonic Period
Extends from the fertilization of the ovum

Period 1: Pre-embryonic Period
Extends from the fertilization of the ovum to the formation of the embryonic disk with three germ layers—week 1 through week 3.

Period 2: Embryonic Period
Period of rapid growth and differentiation; formation of major organ systems occurs—week 4 through week 8.

Period 3: Fetal Period
Further growth and development of organ systems—extends from week 9 to week 40 (term).

Data from Moore KL et al (2003). The developing human: clinically oriented embryology, ed 7. Philadelphia: Saunders.

plump appearance and texture. The last part of the fetal period provides preparation for transition to the extrauterine environment (Jirasek et al, 2001; Larsen, 2001; Sadler, 2003).

The fetus is at less risk for structural defects caused by teratogenic factors than is the embryo; however, there is still a risk for functional impairment of existing structures. This risk is addressed in the section on environmental factors. Changes in specific organs or organ systems during the fetal period are discussed in the section on the development of specific organs. For a summary of prenatal development, see Box 36-2.

DEVELOPMENT OF SPECIFIC ORGANS AND STRUCTURES

Nervous System
The origin of the nervous system is the neural plate, which arises as a thickening of the ectodermal tissue about the middle of the third week of gestation. The neural plate further differentiates into the neural tube and the neural crest. The neural tube gives rise to the central nervous system. The neural crest cells give rise to the peripheral nervous system (Figure 36-9).

The cranial end of the neural tube forms the three divisions of the brain: the forebrain, the midbrain, and the hindbrain. The cerebral hemispheres and diencephalon arise from the forebrain; the pons, cerebellum, and medulla oblongata arise from the hindbrain. The midbrain makes up the adult midbrain (Jirasek et al, 2001; Larsen, 2001; Sadler, 2003).

The cavity of the neural tube develops into the ventricles of the brain and the central canal of the spinal column. The neuroepithelial cells lining the neural tube give rise to nerves and glial cells of the central nervous system. The peripheral nervous system consists of the cranial, spinal, and visceral nerves and the ganglia. The somatic and visceral sensory cells of the peripheral nervous system arise from neural crest cells. Cells that form the myelin sheaths of the axons, called *Schwann cells*, also arise from the neural crest cells (Jirasek et al, 2001; Larsen, 2001; Sadler, 2003).

Cardiovascular System
The fetal cardiac system appears at about 18 to 19 days of gestation, and circulation is present by about 21 days. The cardiovascular system is the *first* organ system to function in utero. The heart and blood develop from the middle layer (mesoderm) of the trilaminar embryonic disk. Tissue from the lateral mesoderm migrates up the sides of the embryonic disk, forming a horseshoe-shaped structure that arches and meets above the oropharyngeal membrane. With further development, paired heart tubes form, which then fuse into a single heart tube (Figure 36-10). The vessels that make up the vascular system throughout the body develop from mesodermal cells that connect to each other, with the developing heart tube and the placenta. Thus, by the end of the third week of gestation, there is a functional cardiovascular system (Jirasek et al, 2001; Larsen, 2001; Sadler, 2003).

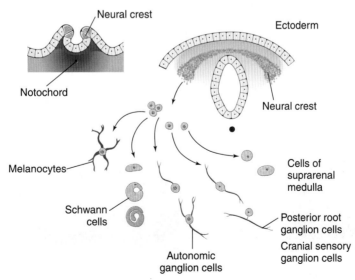

FIGURE **36-9**
Differentiation of the nervous system. The cells of the neural crest differentiate into the cells of the ganglia, Schwann cells, and the cells of the suprarenal medulla and melanocytes.

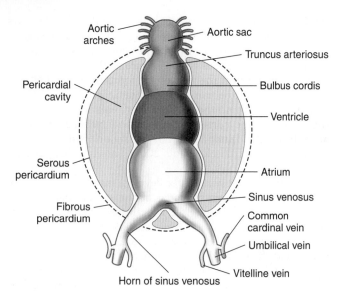

FIGURE **36-10**
Formation of the single heart tube. The appearance of the single heart tube inside the pericardial cavity. Note that the atrium and sinus venosus are outside the pericardial cavity.

As the heart tube grows, the folding of the embryonic disk results in the movement of the heart tube into the chest cavity. The heart tube differentiates into three layers: the endocardial layer, which becomes the endothelium; the cardiac jelly, which

is a loose tissue layer; and the myoepicardial mantle, which becomes the myocardium and pericardium. The single heart tube is attached at its cephalic end by the aortic arches and at the caudal end by the septum transversum. The attachments limit the length of the heart tube. Continued growth results in dilated areas and bulges, which become specific components of the heart. The atrium, ventricle, and bulbus cordis can be identified first, followed by the sinus venosus and truncus arteriosus. To accommodate continued growth, two separate bends in the heart occur. It first bends to the right to form a U shape, and the next bend results in an S-shaped heart. The bending of the heart is responsible for the typical location of cardiac structures (Figure 36-11) (Jirasek et al, 2001; Larsen, 2001; Sadler, 2003).

Initially, the heart is a single chamber; partitioning of the heart into four chambers occurs from the fourth to sixth weeks of gestation. The changes that cause the partitioning of the heart occur simultaneously. The atrium is separated from the ventricle by endocardial cushions, which are thickened areas of endothelium that develop on the dorsal and ventral walls of the open area between the atrium and ventricle. The endocardial cushions fuse with each other to divide the atrioventricular canals into right and left atrioventricular canals. Partitioning of the atrium occurs through invagination of tissue toward the endocardial cushions, forming the septum primum. As the septum primum grows toward the endocardial cushions, it becomes very thin and perforates, becoming the foramen ovale. The septum primum does not fuse completely with the endocardial cushions; it has a lower portion that lies

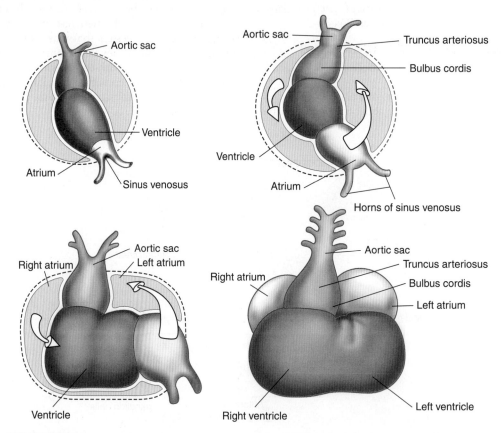

FIGURE **36-11**
Bending of the heart tube inside the pericardial cavity. The bending of the heart tube brings the atrium into the pericardial cavity. The sinus venosus is taken into the right atrium and the coronary sinus.

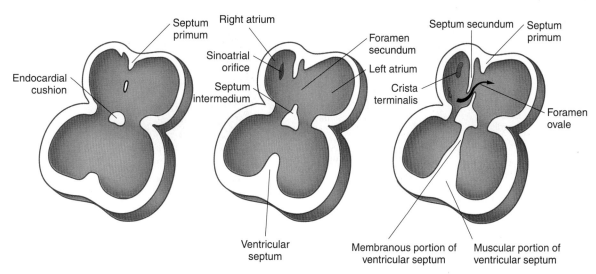

FIGURE **36-12**
Partitioning of the atrium. The partitioning of the atrium into the right and left atria through septation.

beside the endocardial cushions. Overlapping of the septum primum and the septum secundum forms a wall if the pressure in both atria is equal. In utero, the pressure on the right side is increased, allowing blood to flow across the foramen ovale from the right side of the heart to the left side (Figure 36-12) (Breier, 2000; Jirasek et al, 2001; Larsen, 2001; Sadler, 2003).

The ventricle is also partitioned by a membranous and muscular septum. The muscular portion of the septum develops from the fold of the floor of the ventricle. With blood flowing through the atrioventricular canal, ventricular dilation occurs on either side of the fold or ridge, causing it to become a septum. The membranous septum arises from ridges inside the bulbus cordis. These ridges, continuous into the bulbus cordis, form the wall that divides the bulbus cordis into the pulmonary artery and the aorta. The bulbar ridges fuse with the endocardial cushions to form the membranous septum. The membranous and muscular septa fuse to close the intraventricular foramen, resulting in two parallel circuits of blood flow. The pulmonary artery is continuous with the right ventricle, and the aorta is continuous with the left ventricle (Figure 36-13).

The blood flowing through the bulbus cordis and truncus arteriosus in a spiral causes the formation of ridges. The ridges fuse to form two separate vessels that twist around each other once. Thus, the pulmonary artery exits the right side of the heart and is in the left upper chest; the aorta exits the left side of the heart and is located close to the sternum (Jirasek et al, 2001; Larsen, 2001; Sadler, 2003).

The pulmonary veins grow from the lungs to a cardinal vein plexus. Concurrently, a vessel develops from the smooth wall of the left atrium. As the atrium grows, the pulmonary vein is incorporated into the atrial wall. The atrium and its branches give rise to four pulmonary veins that enter the left atrium. These pulmonary vessels, connected to the plexus of the cardinal vein, provide a continuous circulation from lung to heart. The pulmonary and aortic valves (semilunar valves) develop from dilations within the pulmonary artery and aorta. The ebb-and-flow circulation through these structures causes them to hollow out to form the cusps of the valves. The tricuspid and mitral valves develop from tissue around the atrioventricular

canals that thicken and then thin out on the ventricular sides, forming the valves (Figure 36-14) (Jirasek et al, 2001; Larsen, 2001; Sadler, 2003).

Respiratory System

The development of the respiratory system is linked to the development of the face and the digestive system. The respiratory system is composed of the nasal cavities, nasopharynx, oropharynx, larynx, trachea, bronchi, and lungs (Figure 36-15). Development of the lungs occurs in four overlapping stages, which extend from the fifth week of gestation until about 8 years of life. The stages are listed in Table 36-1. At term birth, the normal respiratory system functions immediately. For adequate functioning of the respiratory system, there must be a sufficient number of alveoli, adequate capillary blood flow, and an adequate amount of surfactant produced by the secretory epithelial cells or the type II pneumatocytes. It is the surfactant that prevents alveolar collapse and aids in respiratory gas exchange. In addition, work to identify the role of epidermal growth factor (EGF) in the development of the fetal respiratory system have determined that EGF indirectly promotes branching morphogenesis of the lung epithelium through a direct effect on the mesenchyme (Gresik et al, 1998; Jirasek et al, 2001; Larsen, 2001; Sadler, 2003).

Recent advances in genetics have led researchers to recognize that airway pressure plays a role by altering effector cells (epithelial, mesenchymal, or both). Signal conduction pathways turn "on" or "off" the regulatory genes that play key roles in regulating lung development through induction of transcription factors, growth factors, and other regulatory proteins (Ciley et al, 2000). Further knowledge of genetics may provide solutions to promote lung maturity in preterm infants.

Muscular System

The muscular system develops from mesodermal cells called myoblasts. Striated skeletal muscles are derived from myotomal mesoderm (myotomes) of the somites. The majority of striated skeletal muscle fibers develop in utero. Almost all striated skeletal muscles are formed by 1 year of age. Growth is

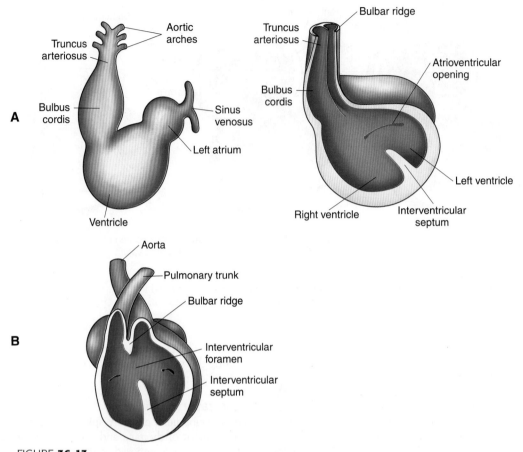

FIGURE **36-13**
Partitioning of the ventricles. **A,** Five chambers are present in the heart at 5 weeks' gestation. **B,** At 6 weeks the bulbus cordis has been taken into the ventricles and the interventricular septum has partitioned the ventricles into right and left sides.

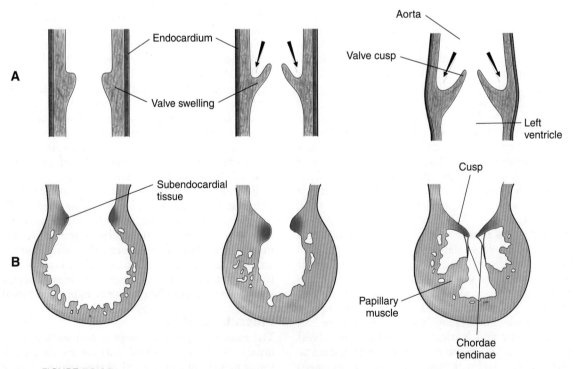

FIGURE **36-14**
Formation of the heart valve. **A,** Formation of the semilunar valves of the aorta and the pulmonary artery. **B,** Formation of the cusps of the atrioventricular valves.

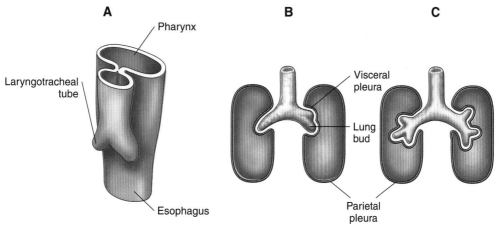

FIGURE **36-15**
Development of the pulmonary system. **A,** The laryngotracheal groove and tube have formed; the margins of the laryngotracheal groove fuse, forming the laryngotracheal tube. **B,** Invagination of the lung buds into the intraembryonic cavity. **C,** Division of the lung buds into the right and left mainstem bronchi.

TABLE **36-1**	Stages of Lung Development
Stage	**Critical Events**
Stage 1: Pseudoglandular period Weeks 5 to 7	Development of the conducting airway
Stage 2: Canalicular period Weeks 13 to 25	Enlargement of the bronchial lumina and terminal bronchioles
	Vascularization of lung tissue
	Development of respiratory bronchioles and alveolar ducts
	Development of a limited number of primitive alveoli
Stage 3: Terminal sac period Week 24 to birth	Development of primitive pulmonary alveoli from alveolar ducts
	Increased vascularity
	Type II pneumatocytes begin to produce surfactant by about 24 weeks
Stage 4: Alveolar period Late fetal period until about 8 years of age	Pulmonary alveoli formed by thinning of terminal air sac lining
	One eighth to one sixth of adult number of alveoli present at term birth
	Number of alveoli increase until age 8 years

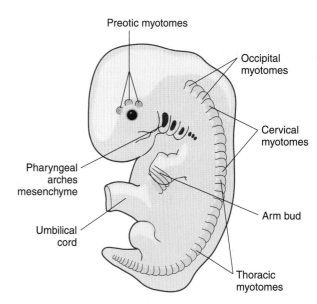

FIGURE **36-16**
Origin of the muscles of the head and neck.

achieved by an increase in the diameter of the muscle fibers, rather than the growth of new muscle tissue. Smooth muscle fibers arise from the splanchnic mesenchyme surrounding the endoderm of the primitive gut. Smooth muscles lining vessel walls of blood and lymphatic systems arise from somatic mesoderm. As smooth muscle cells differentiate, contractile filaments develop in the cytoplasm, and the external surface is covered by an external lamina. As the smooth muscle fibers develop into sheets or bundles, the muscle cells synthesize and release collagenous, elastic, or reticular fibers (Figure 36-16) (Jirasek et al, 2001; Larsen, 2001; Sadler, 2003).

Cardiac muscle develops from splanchnic mesenchyme from the outside of the endocardial heart tube. Cells from the myoepicardial mantle differentiate into the myocardium. Cardiac muscle fibers develop from differentiation and growth of single cells rather than fusion of cells. Cardiac muscle growth occurs through the formation of new filaments. The Purkinje fibers develop late in the embryonic period. These fibers are larger and have fewer myofibrils than do other cardiac muscle cells. The Purkinje fibers function in the electrical conduction system of the heart (Jirasek et al, 2001; Larsen, 2001; Sadler, 2003).

Skeletal System

The skeletal system develops from mesenchymal cells. In the long bones, condensed mesenchyme forms hyaline cartilage models of bones. By the end of the embryonic period, ossification centers appear, and these bones ossify by endochondral ossification. Other bones, such as the skull bones, are ossified by membranous ossification in which the mesenchyme cells become osteoblasts (Figure 36-17).

The vertebral column and the ribs arise from the sclerotome compartments of the somites. The spinal column is formed by the fusion of a condensation of the cranial half of one pair of sclerotomes with the caudal half of the next pair of sclerotomes. The skull can be divided into the neurocranium and the viscerocranium. The neurocranium forms the protective covering around the brain. The viscerocranium forms the skeleton of the face. The neurocranium is made up of the flat bones that surround the brain and the cartilaginous structure, or chondrocranium, that forms the bones of the base of the skull. The neurocranium (chondrocranium) is made up of a number of separate cartilages, which fuse and ossify by endochondral ossification to form the base of the skull (Jirasek et al, 2001; Larsen, 2001; Sadler, 2003).

Gastrointestinal System

The gastrointestinal system is primarily derived from the lining of the roof of the yolk sac. The primitive gut, consisting of the foregut, midgut, and hindgut, is formed during the fourth gestational week (Figure 36-18). The structures that arise from the foregut include the pharynx, esophagus, stomach, liver, pancreas, gallbladder, and part of the duodenum. The esophagus and trachea have a common origin, the laryngotracheal diverticulum. A septum, formed by the growing tracheoesophageal folds, divides the cranial part of the foregut into the laryngotracheal tube and the esophagus. Smooth muscle develops from the splanchnic mesenchyme that surrounds the esophagus. The epithelial lining of the esophagus, derived from the endoderm, proliferates, partially obliterating the esophageal lumen. The esophagus undergoes recanalization by the end of the embryonic period (Jirasek et al, 2001; Larsen, 2001; Sadler, 2003).

The stomach originates as a dilation of the caudal portion of the foregut. The characteristic greater curvature of the stomach develops because the dorsal border grows faster than the ventral border. As the stomach develops further, it rotates in a clockwise direction around the longitudinal axis. The duodenum is derived from the caudal and cranial portions of the foregut and the cranial portion of the midgut. The junction of the foregut and midgut portions of the duodenum is normally distal to the common bile duct (Jirasek et al, 2001; Larsen, 2001; Sadler, 2003).

The liver, gallbladder, and biliary ducts originate as a bud from the caudal end of the foregut. The liver is formed by growth of the hepatic diverticulum, which grows between the layers of the ventral mesentery, forming two parts. The liver forms from the largest, cranial portion. Hepatic cells originate from the hepatic diverticulum. Hematopoietic tissue and Kupffer cells are derived from the splanchnic mesenchyme of the septum transversum. The liver develops rapidly and fills the abdominal cavity. The liver begins its hematopoietic function by the sixth gestational week. Primitive erythropoiesis is characterized by large, nucleated erythrocytes that contain embryonic hemoglobin and are not dependent on erythropoietin (Dame & Juul, 2000).

The smaller portion of the hepatic diverticulum forms the gallbladder. The common bile duct is formed from the stalk connecting the hepatic and cystic ducts to the duodenum. The pancreas is derived from the pancreatic buds that arise from the caudal part of the foregut (Jirasek et al, 2001; Larsen, 2001; Sadler, 2003).

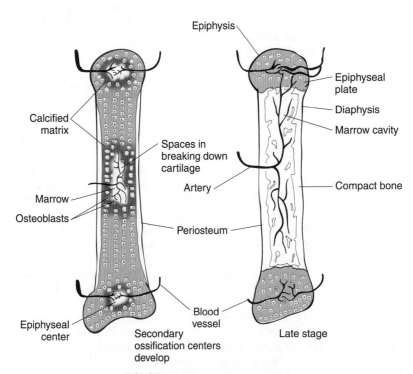

FIGURE **36-17**
Endochondral ossification of bones.

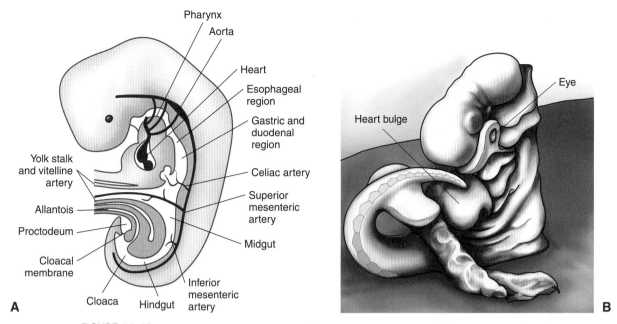

FIGURE **36-18**
A and **B**, The primitive gut. The early gastrointestinal system present in an embryo at about 4 weeks' gestation.

The structures that are derived from the midgut include the remainder of the duodenum, the cecum, the appendix, the ascending colon, and the majority of the transverse colon.

The intestines undergo extensive growth during the first weeks of development. The liver and kidneys occupy the abdominal cavity, restricting the space available for intestinal growth. The growth of the intestines is accommodated through a migration out of the abdominal cavity via the umbilical cord. A series of rotations occurs before the intestines return to the abdomen. The first rotation is counterclockwise, around the axis of the superior mesenteric artery. At about the tenth week, the intestines return to the abdomen, undergoing further rotation. When the colon returns to the abdomen, the cecal end rotates to the right side, entering the lower right quadrant of the abdomen. The cecum and appendix arise from the cecal diverticulum, a pouch that appears in the fifth week of gestation on the caudal limb of the midgut loop (Figure 36-19) (Jirasek et al, 2001; Larsen, 2001; Sadler, 2003).

The hindgut is that portion of the intestines from the midgut to the cloacal membrane. The latter structure consists of the endoderm of the cloaca and the ectoderm of the anal pit. The cloaca is divided by the urorectal septum. As the septum grows toward the cloacal membrane, folds from the lateral walls of the cloaca grow together, dividing the cloaca into the rectum and upper anal canal dorsally and the urogenital sinus ventrally. By the end of the sixth week, the urorectal septum fuses with the cloacal membrane, forming a dorsal anal membrane and a larger ventral urogenital membrane. At about the end of the seventh gestational week, these two membranes rupture, forming the anal canal (Jirasek et al, 2001; Larsen, 2001; Sadler, 2003).

Urogenital System

The development of the urinary and genital systems is closely related. The urogenital system develops from the intermediate mesoderm, which extends along the dorsal body wall of the embryo. During embryonic folding in the horizontal plane, the intermediate mesoderm is moved forward and is no longer connected to the somites. This mesoderm forms the urogenital ridge on each side of the primitive aorta. Both the urinary and genital systems arise from this urogenital ridge. The area from which the urinary system is derived is called the *nephrogenic cord*. The genital ridge is the area from which the reproductive system is derived (Jirasek et al, 2001; Larsen, 2001; Sadler, 2003).

There are three stages of development of the kidney: the pronephros, the mesonephros, and the metanephros. The pronephros, a nonfunctional organ, appears in the first month of gestation and then degenerates, contributing only a duct system for the next developmental stage. The mesonephros uses the duct of the pronephros and develops caudally to the pronephros (Figure 36-20). The mesonephros begins to produce urine during development of the metanephros. The mesonephros degenerates by the end of the embryonic period. Remnants of the mesonephros persist as genital ducts in males or vestigial structures in females. The metanephros appears in the fifth week of gestation and becomes the permanent kidney. The metanephros begins to produce urine by about the 11th week of gestation. The urinary bladder and the urethra arise from the urogenital sinus and the splanchnic mesenchyme. The caudal portion of the mesonephric ducts is incorporated into the bladder, giving rise to the ureters (Jirasek et al, 2001; Larsen, 2001; Sadler, 2003).

Although the genetic sex of the embryo is determined at conception, the early development of the genital system is indistinguishable until the seventh week of gestation. Beginning in the seventh week, the gonads begin to be differentiated. The ovaries and the testes are derived from the coelomic epithelium, the mesenchyme, and the primordial germ cells. Development of female sexual organs occurs in the absence of hormonal stimulation precipitated by the H-Y antigen gene carried on the Y chromosome. If the Y chromosome is present, testes develop; otherwise, ovaries develop (Jirasek et al, 2001; Larsen, 2001; Sadler, 2003).

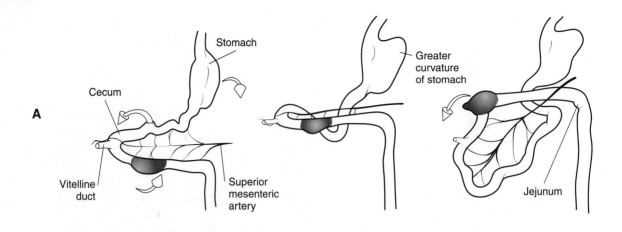

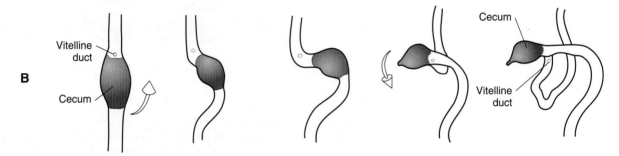

FIGURE **36-19**
Migration and rotation of the midgut. **A,** Counterclockwise 90-degree rotation of midgut loop and "herniation" into extraembryonic cavity. **B,** Counterclockwise 180-degree rotation of midgut loop on return to the abdominal cavity.

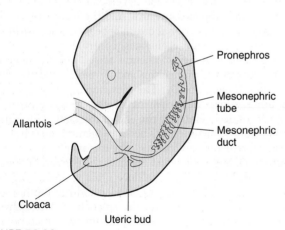

FIGURE **36-20**
Development of the kidney. The locations of the pronephros and mesonephros.

CONGENITAL DEFECTS

Congenital defects or anomalies are structural or anatomic abnormalities present at birth. Congenital defects vary in severity and location, ranging from minor insignificant defects to major organ system defects. Congenital defects are attributed to genetic or chromosomal abnormalities or to maternal or environmental factors. Most congenital defects result from an interaction between genetic and environmental factors, or multifactorial inheritance. The generally reported incidence of congenital

defects is about 2% to 3%. The actual incidence is higher because some defects are not apparent at birth. Close to 12% of birth defects are not discovered until after the newborn period (Felix et al, 2000). The incidence of all defects (including both minor and major defects) is approximately 14%. Almost 20% of all perinatal deaths are caused by congenital defects. Congenital defects caused by single-gene disorders and chromosomal abnormalities are discussed in Chapter 32, "Impact of Genomics on Neonatal Care." The influence of the environment on embryonic development is discussed in this section.

Moore and Persaud (2002a) listed six mechanisms that can cause congenital defects: (1) too little growth, (2) too little resorption, (3) too much resorption, (4) resorption in the wrong location, (5) normal growth in an abnormal position, and (6) overgrowth of a tissue or structure. Embryonic organs are most sensitive to noxious agents during a period of rapid cell growth and differentiation. Damage to the primitive streak at about 15 days of gestation could cause severe congenital malformations of the embryo because of its role in the production of intraembryonic mesoderm, from which all connective tissue is formed. Biochemical differentiation occurs before morphologic differentiation, so organs or structures are sensitive to the action of teratogens before they can be identified.

Critical Periods of Human Development

Environmental influences during the first 2 weeks after conception may prevent successful implantation of the blastocyst and cause abortion of the embryo. The most sensitive period for the embryo is the period of organogenesis, especially from day 15 to day 60. Each organ has a critical period during which its development is most likely to be adversely affected by the presence of teratogenic agents (see Figure 36-8 for critical periods for each major organ system).

Teratogens

Teratogens are agents that may adversely affect embryonic development. About 7% of all congenital defects are caused by exposure to teratogenic agents. Known teratogenic agents include drugs or other chemicals, radiation, and infectious organisms. Very few agents have been proved teratogenic, primarily because risks to humans make scientific study difficult. Some agents have been tested on animal models; however, caution must be used when extrapolating these findings to humans. Some agents have been identified as teratogenic after exposure to the agent resulted in an increased incidence of defects. Limited knowledge about safety of all substances makes it prudent for women to avoid all potential teratogens prior to conception and during pregnancy.

Drugs and Chemicals

Drugs and chemicals account for about 2% to 3% of congenital defects. Few drugs are known to be teratogenic; however, no drug can be considered completely safe. Therefore, all drugs should be avoided unless the benefit of taking the drug outweighs potential risks. Drugs of various classifications have been identified as being teratogenic.

Alcohol has been associated with congenital defects, which include craniofacial abnormalities, limb deformities, and cardiovascular defects. Associated abnormalities include growth deficiency and mental retardation. The term *fetal alcohol syndrome* is used to describe the cluster of defects characteristic of maternal ingestion of alcohol. There is no level of alcohol consumption that can be considered safe; therefore, it is recommended that alcohol be avoided throughout the perinatal period (Baraitser & Winter, 1996).

Certain antibiotics have been identified as teratogens. Tetracycline is deposited in the embryo's bones and teeth, leading to a brown discoloration to the teeth and diminished growth of the long bones. Antituberculosis agents, such as streptomycin and dihydrostreptomycin, have been associated with hearing deficits and damage to cranial nerve VIII. Sulfonamides have been associated with an increased incidence of kernicterus in the newborn. Currently, the safest antibiotic for use in pregnant women appears to be penicillin. This drug has not been associated with an increased incidence of congenital defects (Sanders et al, 2002).

Several anticonvulsant drugs have been implicated in the presence of congenital defects (Sanders et al, 2002). The use of phenytoin may cause craniofacial defects, nail and digital hypoplasia, intrauterine growth retardation, microcephaly, and mental retardation. Other anticonvulsant drugs that have been identified as teratogens include trimethadione (Tridione) and paramethadione (Paradione). The defects include fetal facial dysmorphia, cardiac defects, cleft palate, and intrauterine growth restriction.

Warfarin, an anticoagulant, can cause craniofacial abnormalities, optic atrophy, microcephaly, and mental retardation. Other anticoagulants, although not specifically teratogenic, cross the placental barrier and may lead to hemorrhage in the fetus. Heparin does not cross the placental barrier and is used for anticoagulation in pregnant women.

Antineoplastic agents are particularly teratogenic. Aminopterin and methotrexate have both been associated with major congenital malformations, especially central nervous system defects. Antineoplastic drugs may be harmful to health care workers exposed to them during routine nursing interventions. Women who are pregnant or trying to conceive should not administer antineoplastic agents (Sanders et al, 2002).

Antipsychotic and antianxiety agents are also suspected teratogenic agents. Phenothiazine and lithium have been linked to congenital defects. Diazepam (Valium), meprobamate, and chlordiazepoxide may cause congenital defects. Diazepam is associated with an increased incidence of cleft lip with or without cleft palate.

Hormonal agents are also implicated in the incidence of congenital defects. Androgenic agents (progestins) may cause masculinization of female fetuses. Diethylstilbestrol (DES), a synthetic estrogen used to prevent abortion in the 1940s and 1950s, has been found to cause an increased incidence of vaginal and cervical cancer in female children exposed to the drug in utero. Additionally, there are associated abnormalities of the reproductive system, often causing reproductive dysfunction (Sadler, 2003). Cortisone has been shown to cause cleft palate in animal models but has not been implicated as a factor in cleft palate in human newborns.

Social or recreational drugs are highly suspected of contributing to congenital defects. Drugs such as lysergic acid diethylamide (LSD) have been associated with limb abnormalities and central nervous system abnormalities. Other drugs that may be teratogenic include phencyclidine and marijuana. "Crack" cocaine, a relative newcomer to the social drug inventory, has been associated with congenital abnormalities. The tendency of drug abusers to use multiple drugs, combined with their poor nutritional habits and lack of prenatal care, makes it difficult to establish the effects of the drugs individually.

Miscellaneous drugs from other categories that are suspected of leading to congenital defects include propylthiouracil and potassium iodide, which are associated with neonatal goiter and mental retardation. Amphetamines are associated with oral clefts and heart defects. Salicylates (aspirin), the most commonly used medication during pregnancy, may be harmful to the fetus if taken in large amounts. Retinoic acid (vitamin A) is teratogenic in high doses in humans. Isotretinoin, a drug used to treat acne, causes craniofacial abnormalities, cleft palate, thymic aplasia defects, and neural tube defects (Sadler, 2003).

Environmental chemicals such as pollutants, fungicides, food additives, and defoliants have been suspected of causing congenital defects. There is the most support for the claim that mercury produces neurologic manifestations similar to those seen in cerebral palsy, blindness, and mental retardation (Sadler, 2003). Although there is little evidence to prove that other environmental agents are teratogenic, no data prove that environmental chemicals are not dangerous. Therefore, pregnant women should avoid exposure to potentially toxic chemicals. Unfortunately, because of their many uses it is difficult to recognize exposure to potentially hazardous products (Sadler, 2003).

Radiation

Exposure to high levels of ionizing radiation can result in microcephaly, skull defects, spina bifida, blindness, and cleft palate. Studies of the outcomes of women who were pregnant during the atomic bombing of Hiroshima and Nagasaki showed that 28% had abortions, 25% had liveborns who died within 1 year, and 25% of the survivors gave birth to children with central nervous system disorders (Sadler, 2003). There is no established "safe" level for radiation. The severity of the radiation-induced defects depends on the duration and timing of exposure. There is no evidence that the small amount of radiation required for modern radiographic studies is harmful; however, caution is used to minimize the exposure to the fetus because of the potential for cumulative effects of radiation exposure throughout the life span.

Infectious Agents

Three viral agents have been positively identified as teratogenic to the developing fetus: rubella, cytomegalovirus (CMV), and herpes simplex. There is a 15% to 20% incidence of congenital malformations in newborns of women who have had rubella in the first trimester of pregnancy. The typical malformations include heart defects, deafness, and cataracts. CMV is thought to be the most commonly occurring viral infection of the human fetus. CMV in early embryonic development probably results in spontaneous abortion. CMV infection during the second or third trimester may cause microcephaly and microphthalmia. Herpes simplex infection of the fetus primarily occurs late in the pregnancy, commonly during delivery. Congenital abnormalities in fetuses infected prior to delivery include microcephaly, microphthalmia, retinal dysplasia, and mental retardation.

Maternal infection with *Toxoplasma gondii*, a protozoal parasite, can cause hydrocephalus, cerebral calcification, microphthalmia, and ocular defects. *T. gondii* can be contracted from undercooked meat, by handling feces of infected cats, or from the soil. Untreated primary maternal infections of *Treponema pallidum*, the microorganism that causes syphilis, result in serious fetal infection, but adequate treatment kills the organism, preventing serious defects. Untreated syphilis can lead to congenital deafness and mental retardation. Other viral agents have been implicated as causes of congenital malformations. Such malformations have been reported following maternal infection with mumps, varicella, echovirus, coxsackievirus, and influenza virus. The incidence of congenital malformations following these infections is unknown, but is suspected to be low (Sadler, 2003). (For further information on viral agents, see Chapter 9.)

Another teratogenic factor is hyperthermia. It may be the causative factor in congenital defects associated with viral agents, because of the fever produced by the agents. Hyperthermia can also be caused by maternal use of hot tubs or saunas.

Maternal Substances

The effects of substances present in pregnant women inappropriate amounts (high or low) may contribute to congenital defects in the fetus. There is evidence that high maternal levels of certain physiologic compounds may have a deleterious effect on fetal development. High maternal levels of phenylalanine during pregnancy can result in neurologic damage resembling untreated phenylketonuria (PKU), despite the fetus not having the genotypic PKU. Thyroid deficiency during the last two trimesters of pregnancy and first months after birth can result in mental retardation or other neurologic deficits. Thus, untreated maternal hypothyroidism can also adversely affect the developing fetus (Utiger, 1999). Researchers have postulated that high maternal levels of trans-fatty acids may adversely affect fetal development, although more research is needed before specific recommendations can be made (Carlson et al, 1997).

Good nutrition has long been considered essential for proper growth and development of the fetus. However, with the exception of folic acid, where which there is evidence that deficiencies are causally related to defects of the neural tube, there is little evidence of the role of the micronutrients on fetal development. Supplementation of vitamins and minerals must occur within the appropriate critical period of development to be effective or may be harmful. Environmental factors that have yet to be identified may exert influence on the development of the fetus. It is essential to consider the environment of the fetus in terms of the uterine environment and the environment of the mother in assessment of the influences on fetal development (McArdle & Ashworth, 1999).

SUMMARY

This chapter has provided an overview of embryologic and fetal development, outlined the critical periods of development, and described the more common congenital defects. Knowledge of embryologic and fetal development is essential as a foundation for understanding the role of environment, genetics, physical, or other factors that may have an impact upon anatomy, physiology, or pathophysiology of the organism. The future health of the individual is in large part dependent upon the numerous events that take place during gestation. As knowledge of genetics, development, and human pathophysiology improve, better health care technologies may emerge that can significantly reduce morbidity and mortality and improve quality of life. Box 36-3 contains websites that provide further information about factors that influence fetal development.

BOX 36-3

Websites

Basic Embryology Review Program (BERP) of the University of Pennsylvania Health System: http://www.med.upenn.edu/meded/public/berp/. This Web page follows development from fertilization through birth. This site has been selected in two well-known "best of the Web" reviews.

University of New South Wales (UNSW) Embryology, Faculty of Medicine, School of Anatomy: http://anatomy.med.unsw.edu.au/cbl/embryo/embryo.htm#start. Includes movies of developmental processes, lecture notes, photographs, notes on individual systems development, and much, much more. Website created and maintained by Dr. Mark A. Hill, Lecturer in the School of Anatomy, University of New South Wales and Head of the Cell Biology Laboratory (1995–).

The Human Embryology Website: http://www.med.uc.edu/embryology/. Designed to support the current editions of *Human Embryology and Essentials of Human Embryology* by W. J. Larsen (Churchill Livingstone) and to assist students and teachers of human embryology.

Embryology: http://www.rchc.rush.edu/rmawebfiles/Embryology.htm. Created by Ra-id Abdulla, MD, of Rush University.

The Teratology Society: http://teratology.org/. This multidisciplinary scientific society was founded in 1960. Members study the causes and biologic processes leading to abnormal development and birth defects at the fundamental and clinical levels, as well as appropriate measures for prevention.

Organization of Teratology Information Services: http://www.otispregnancy.org/. Website is designed to assist in the location of teratology information services in all geographic areas of the United States.

Clinical Teratology Web: http://depts.washington.edu/~terisweb/. Designed to serve as a resource guide for health care professionals.

Fetal Development: http://www.w-cpc.org/fetal.html. Site contains information, QuickTime movies, and great photographs of fetal development.

REFERENCES

Baraitser M, Winter RM (1996). *Color atlas of congenital malformation syndromes*. St Louis: Mosby.

Breier G (2000). Angiogenesis in embryonic development—a review. *Placenta* 21(Suppl A, Trophoblast Research,14):S11-S15.

Carlson SE et al (1997). *trans*-Fatty acids: infant and fetal development. Report of an expert panel on *trans*-fatty acids and early development. *American journal of clinical nutrition* 66(3):715S-736S.

Ciley RE et al (2000). Fetal lung development; air way pressure enhances expression of developmental genes. *Journal of pediatric surgery* 35(1):113-119.

Dame C, Juul SE (2000). The switch from fetal to adult erythropoiesis. *Clinics in perinatology* 27(3):507-526.

Felix JF et al (2000). Birth defects in children with newborn encephalopathy. *Developmental medicine and child neurology* 42(12):803-808.

Gresik EW et al (1998). The EGF system in fetal development. *European journal of morphology* 36(Suppl):92-97.

Jirasek JE et al (2001). *An atlas of the human embryo and fetus: a photographic review of human prenatal development* (The encyclopedia of visual medicine series). New York: Parthenon Publishing.

Larsen WJ et al (2001). *Human embryology*. Philadelphia: Churchill.

Moore KL, Persaud TVN (2002a). *The developing human: clinically oriented embryology*, ed 7. Philadelphia: Saunders.

Moore KL, Persaud TVN (2002b). *Before we are born: essentials of embryology and birth defects*, ed 6. Philadelphia: Saunders.

McArdle HJ, Ashworth CJ (1999). Micronutrients in fetal growth and development. *BMJ* 55(3):499-510.

Sadler TW (2003). *Langman's medical embryology*, ed 9. Baltimore: Lippincott Williams & Wilkins.

Sanders RC et al, editors (2002). *Structural fetal abnormalities: the total picture*, ed 2. St Louis: Mosby.

Utiger RD (1999). Maternal hypothyroidism and fetal development. *New England journal of medicine* 341(8):601-602.

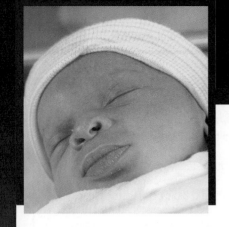

Chapter 37

Prenatal, Antenatal, and Postpartal Risk Factors

Beverly Bowers

Advances in perinatal medicine and technology make it possible for women with high-risk medical conditions to get pregnant, for infertile couples to conceive, for expectant parents to see ultrasound images of the fetus, and for neonates to survive at lower gestational ages than ever before. Despite these advances, adverse outcomes continue to persist such as preterm delivery, low birth weight, congenital anomalies, and other factors that lead to increased neonatal morbidity and mortality. Pregnant women continue to be exposed to harmful physical, psychosocial, behavioral, or environmental conditions that make their pregnancies high risk. There is growing evidence of the genetic influence on some perinatal risk factors and of a link between exposure to environmental triggers and perinatal outcomes. Perinatal care providers must engage in continuous systematic assessment of potential maternal risk factors from preconception through the postpartum period in order to optimize perinatal outcomes. Patient education and assistance with lifestyle alterations necessary for healthy pregnancy are key components of prenatal care. This chapter will present an overview of high-risk factors that contribute to adverse outcomes in the prenatal, intrapartum, and postpartum periods.

PERINATAL OUTCOMES

Some of the adverse perinatal outcomes that are of concern related to maternal risk factors include low birth weight (LBW), intrauterine growth restriction (IUGR), preterm delivery, and perinatal death. These terms will be further defined. LBW is defined as a weight of less than 2500 g or less than 5 pounds 8 ounces at birth. LBW is further broken down into very low birth weight (VLBW) or extremely low birth weight (ELBW). VLBW is defined as a birth weight less than 1500 g or less than 3 pounds 4 ounces, and ELBW is defined as a birth weight less than 1000 g. LBW infants are at higher risk for neonatal and postnatal morbidity and mortality (see Table 37-1).

Low birth weight is one of the most important determinants of the infant's future health and has been linked to obesity, hypertension, diabetes mellitus, and decreased fertility later in adult life (Okah et al, 2005).

Gestational age is estimated through evaluation of neonatal physical and neuromuscular characteristics using a scale such as the Ballard Maturational Assessment of Gestational Age. The neonate's birth weight, frontal occipital head circumference, and length are plotted on graphs by gestational age. The infant is categorized as appropriate for gestational age

(AGA) if birth weight falls between the 10th and 90th percentile for the infant's gestational age; small for gestational age (SGA) if birth weight falls into the lower 10th percentile for weight based on gestational age; or large for gestational age (LGA) if birth weight is greater than 90th percentile for weight based on gestational age. SGA infants might be genetically small, but as many as 10% to 15% of SGA fetuses are actually IUGR fetuses (Mari, 2005). Some authors believe that the incidence of IUGR is underestimated by limiting the definition of IUGR to less than the 10th percentile. IUGR is commonly caused by changes in the maternal vasculature or the placenta due to conditions such as pre-eclampsia, history of smoking or taking drugs, low prepregnancy weight, low weight gain in pregnancy, or inadequate prenatal care (Steward & Moser, 2004). Many of these conditions cause progressive uteroplacental insufficiency that limits the normal exchange of oxygen and nutrients to the fetus. Lack of adequate nutrients interferes with normal growth potential. IUGR can also be caused by maternal genetic factors, fetal chromosomal problems, congenital infection, intrauterine crowding, cord pathology, Rh isoimmunization, or twin-to-twin transfusion (Harper et al, 2005).

There are two types of IUGR, symmetric and asymmetric. Symmetric growth restriction occurs early in pregnancy. The factors that restrict fetal growth are similar to a chronic condition. In this type of IUGR, the head, long bones, abdomen, and soft tissue growth are restricted. Symmetric IUGR is associated with a decreased number of fetal cells. Infants are born with fewer brain cells and tend to have poorer long-term outcomes. They tend to grow more slowly after they are born and their growth seldom catches up to other infants during the first year of life. In contrast, fetuses with asymmetric IUGR have normal fetal head and long bone growth; however, soft tissue and abdominal growth are restricted. The infant usually has a small liver. Infants with symmetric IUGR tend to catch up on the growth charts during the first year of life (Harper et al, 2005). IUGR is best detected prenatally with serial fundal height measurements or serial ultrasound that tracks when fetal growth is not progressing as expected. Severe uteroplacental insufficiency restricts blood flow to the fetus and affects fetal growth and oxygenation. It is a cause of fetal demise; therefore fetuses with IUGR must be identified and closely monitored with nonstress testing, biophysical profiles, or contraction stress tests. Early delivery is indicated if signs of fetal stress or distress are present. After birth, infants with

TABLE 37-1 Live Births by Birth Weight and Percentage of Very Low and Low Birth Weight, by Period of Gestation and Race and Hispanic Origin of Mother: United States, 2003

Birth Weight[1] and Race and Hispanic Origin of Mother	All Births	Preterm					Total 37 to 41 Weeks	Term			Postterm	Not Stated
		Total Under 37 Weeks	Under 28 Weeks	28 to 31 Weeks	32 to 35 Weeks	36 Weeks		37 to 39 Weeks	40 Weeks	41 Weeks	42 Weeks and Over	
Number												
All races[3]	4,089,950	499,008	30,061	49,545	234,074	185,328	3,288,548	2,097,771	807,157	383,620	258,552	43,842
Less than 500 g	6,307	6,132	5,857	247	23	5	6	2	3	1	1	168
500-999 g	22,980	22,319	16,587	5,172	528	32	183	133	35	15	19	459
1,000-1,499 g	29,930	27,759	3,905	16,085	7,179	590	1,508	1,080	297	131	213	450
1,500-1,999 g	63,791	53,171	957	12,259	34,790	5,165	8,984	7,419	1,095	470	794	842
2,000-2,499 g	201,056	105,163	612	4,193	68,175	32,183	88,377	73,882	9,883	4,612	5,175	2,341
2,500-2,999 g	711,003	133,242	908	4,162	60,025	68,147	537,339	412,555	87,702	37,082	32,922	7,500
3,000-3,499 g	1,557,864	100,835	—	4,827	41,100	54,908	1,340,828	888,504	314,513	137,811	99,990	16,211
3,500-3,999 g	1,131,577	39,471	—	2,461	17,514	19,496	993,872	559,499	290,910	143,463	86,878	11,356
4,000-4,499 g	309,721	7,721	—	—	3,805	3,916	271,493	132,782	88,291	50,420	27,172	3,335
4,500-4,999 g	46,690	1,243	—	—	577	666	40,228	18,893	12,804	8,531	4,720	499
5,000 g or more	5,431	211	—	—	98	113	4,577	2,324	1,306	947	566	77
Not stated	3,600	1,741	1,235	139	260	107	1,153	698	318	137	102	604
Percent												
Very low birth weight[4]	1.4	11.3	91.4	43.5	3.3	0.3	0.1	0.1	0.0	0.0	0.1	2.5
Low birth weight[5]	7.9	43.1	96.9	76.8	47.3	20.5	3.0	3.9	1.4	1.4	2.4	9.9

From National Vital Statistics Report, Vol 54, No 2, September 8, 2005, p 87. Available at: http://www.cdc.gov/nchs/data/nvsr/nvsr54/nvsr54_02.pdf.
—, Quantity zero; 0.0, quantity more than zero but less than 0.05.
[1] *Equivalents of the gram weights in pounds and ounces are shown in the "Technical Notes" in original document.*
[2] *Expressed in completed weeks.*
[3] *Includes races other than white and black and origin not stated.*
[4] *Birthweight of less than 1500 g (3 lb 4 oz).*
[5] *Birthweight of less than 2500 g (5 lb 8 oz).*

IUGR often have problems with thermoregulation due to a lack of subcutaneous fat. They also are at increased risk for necrotizing enterocolitis, thrombocytopenia, and renal failure because during fetal development, blood was shunted away from the gastrointestinal and renal system to the brain, heart, and other vital organs as a protective mechanism. As adults, those who were born with IUGR are more at risk to develop a metabolic syndrome with type 2 diabetes, obesity, hypertension, hypercholesterolemia, and heart disease (Harper et al, 2005).

Preterm infants require intensive medical and nursing care. The high cost of providing neonatal intensive care for these vulnerable infants adds a huge financial burden to the health care system. In 2003, the cost of caring for the estimated 4 million infants who were born in the United States was over $10 billion. Over half of that amount was spent on the 12.3% of infants who were born prematurely (delivery at <37 weeks' gestational age). As infant birth weight decreases, the costs of the initial hospitalization increase (Cuevas et al, 2005). Preterm infants account for most neonatal deaths, and if they do survive, they have increased risks for morbidity. Prematurity and LBW places infants at an increased risk for disability, neonatal death, or the development of lifetime chronic health problems. More ELBW infants have survived over the past decade, with a corresponding increased risk for neuro-developmental impairment (Wilson-Costello et al, 2005). Preterm infants are also more at risk for hospital readmission within 6 weeks of birth, adding to the financial burden (Martens et al, 2004). Prevention of preterm birth and LBW has the potential to save lives, to prevent long-term health problems associated with prematurity, and to provide significant savings of health care dollars.

The rate of preterm birth has remained basically unchanged over the past decade, although there was a slight rise from the 1990s (MacDorman et al, 2005). Preterm delivery accounts for 60% of all perinatal deaths (Tekesin et al, 2005). Multiple variables have been associated with increased risks for preterm delivery. Gene-gene interactions or gene-environment interactions might trigger the process of preterm birth. Recently researchers found a significant relationship between the tumor necrosis factor alpha gene (TNF) and preterm labor in mothers who also had presence of bacterial vaginosis (BV) as a postulated environmental trigger (Macones et al, 2004). The search for possible genetic causes of preterm labor is an exciting field for future investigations.

In 2002, infant mortality in the United States increased for the first time in over 40 years to 7.0 per 1000 deaths. Black infants had 2 to 3 times the rates of white infants in all categories of perinatal and infant death (National Center for Health Statistics, 2005). The top 10 causes of infant death during the first year of life were congenital anomalies, LBW, sudden infant death syndrome (SIDS), maternal complications of pregnancy, cord and placental complications, unintentional injuries, respiratory distress, bacterial sepsis, circulatory diseases, intrauterine hypoxia, and asphyxia (see Figure 37-1). The largest increase was in neonatal deaths reported from 0 to 28 days of life, with most of them occurring in the first 7 days of life (Kochanek et al, 2004). In 2002, the infant mortality rate per 1000 births was significantly higher for LBW (59.5) and VLBW (250.8) infants than for infants who weighed over 2500 g (2.4). Singleton births accounted for about 75% of the increase and multiple births contributed about 25% of the increase (MacDorman et al, 2005).

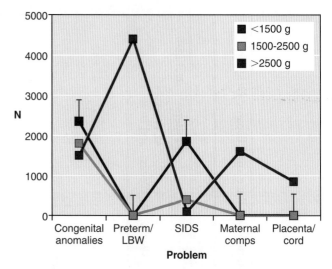

FIGURE **37-1**
The five leading causes of neonatal death by birth weight.

Evaluation of maternal risk factors can help anticipate many of the neonates who will be at increased risk for problems at birth. However, there is no way to accurately predict every neonate who will be at risk, because a cause-and-effect relationship between high-risk maternal characteristics or behaviors and poor outcomes is not always clearly defined. For example, there have been cases of identical twins where one twin was born healthy and the other one was born compromised and required admission to the neonatal intensive care unit (NICU). In such cases, both babies had similar genetic makeup, were exposed to the same environment while in utero, and had the same gestational age, but only one of them had problems.

One of the most essential ways to decrease problems of prematurity, LBW, and perinatal death is to promote optimal pregnancy health. The ideal state is for all women considering pregnancy to seek preconceptual counseling prior to conception. During the preconceptual visit, the woman can learn about risk factors that could potentially cause birth defects or problems with pregnancy. Risk factors may be either modifiable or nonmodifiable. Examples of modifiable risk factors that can be changed include diet, smoking, alcohol use, or substance abuse. Nonmodifiable risk factors are intrinsic factors that cannot be changed such as maternal age, ethnicity, genetic inheritance, or pre-existing health problems. Risk factors usually do not occur in isolation. The presence of one risk factor may lead to other risk factors, causing an additive effect. For example, a pregnant woman who lacks financial resources might also have a poor obstetric history, an inadequate nutritional intake, and increased stress, and she might smoke cigarettes. Some maternal risk factors can be modified through patient education, counseling, lifestyle changes, and support. The purpose of preconceptual care is to help the woman who is contemplating pregnancy get into optimal physical condition prior to conception. Unfortunately, preconceptual counseling is not the norm. Therefore, all women of childbearing age must be encouraged to live healthy lifestyles and to seek early prenatal care in the first trimester of pregnancy. Even the first trimester of pregnancy is not too late to implement interventions or modify lifestyle risk factors that will maximize positive pregnancy outcomes.

PRENATAL MATERNAL RISK FACTORS

Maternal risk factors consist of demographic, behavioral, and psychosocial factors, as well as maternal medical conditions and pregnancy-related conditions. Demographic risk factors include personal characteristics of mothers such as age or previous obstetric history that are associated with high-risk pregnancy or the delivery of a high-risk newborn. Behavioral risk factors include risky behaviors the mother has either prior to or during pregnancy that can harm the fetus, such as smoking or taking drugs. Psychosocial risk factors are variables that relate to the types of social interactions and support that the mother has during pregnancy. Maternal medical conditions include pre-existing or emergent medical conditions that can potentially be harmful to the fetus such as diabetes or pregnancy-induced hypertension (PIH). Pregnancy-related conditions are those conditions that only happen during pregnancy such as multiple gestation, pregnancy-induced hypertension, or gestational diabetes.

A variety of demographic factors are related to neonatal outcomes. A complete maternal history done at the first prenatal visit will help identify important demographic and medical risk factors that might influence the outcomes of the pregnancy. The presence of risk factors should serve as a warning. Many women with identifiable high-risk factors will give birth to healthy infants without problems. The potential influence of demographic risk factors of age, ethnicity, obstetric history, and the health compromising behaviors of nutrition, smoking, alcohol and drug use on pregnancy are further discussed in the following sections.

Maternal Age

The maternal childbearing age range has widened over the past decade, partially because of advances in assisted reproductive technology that have made it possible for women to achieve pregnancy, even into the fifth or sixth decade of life, if desired. Maternal age is considered to be a risk factor at either end of the childbearing age spectrum for poor perinatal outcomes (see Table 37-2).

Young adolescent and teenage mothers are considered high risk because they are biologically immature and their growing body is competing with the fetus for nutrient resources. They have not had the chance to complete their own physical growth and development. Many teenagers do not eat an adequate diet, even when they are not pregnant. If the young immature mother does not consume enough nutrients to maintain her own growth, then she is more at risk to have an LBW infant as compared to an older mother. If teens become pregnant within 2 years of menarche, they are considered reproductively immature (Fraser et al, 1995). Since the young mother's reproductive organs are more immature, she is more likely to have a fetal loss, preterm birth, or infant death. Younger mothers have an infant mortality rate (15.4 in 2002) 2 to 3 times higher than that for women between the ages of 20 and 44 (Menacker et al, 2004). After birth, infants of younger mothers (<19 years of age) had an increased risk for readmission to the hospital within the first 6 weeks after newborn discharge (Martens et al, 2004).

The birth rate for all teenagers declined in 2003 for most ethnic groups. The birth rate for adolescents between the ages of 10 and 14 reached a new low in 2003 at 0.6 per 1000, even despite the fact that this age group had an increase in growth during this time (Martin et al, 2005). Most births to young

teens occurred in girls between the ages of 13 and 14. Girls of this age were also in the group that was least likely to seek early prenatal care. Only 47.1% of young teens sought prenatal care in the first trimester as compared with 78% of other age groups of women (Menacker et al, 2004). Teen mothers have fewer years of formal education. Education is known to be a factor related to promotion of positive pregnancy behaviors. Many teen mothers find it difficult to return to school full time once they assume the parenting role. Dropping out of school can destine them to a lifetime of working in low-paid menial jobs unless they have the parental support necessary to complete their education. Teen mothers are less likely to be married, and they need more financial support for the pregnancy from parents or social agencies. Teen mothers are also more likely to have a repeat teen pregnancy.

Advanced maternal age refers to childbearing by women who are over the age of 35 at estimated date of delivery. Advanced maternal age poses increased risks for decreased fertility, chromosomal abnormalities in the infant, spontaneous abortion, ectopic pregnancy, or stillbirth (Andersen et al, 2000; Cleary-Goldman et al, 2005; Heffner, 2004). Older pregnant women are at an increased risk for medical problems associated with aging such as diabetes or PIH. Diabetes increases the risk for delivery of a macrosomic infant. Advanced maternal age also increases the risks for placenta previa, preterm delivery, or delivery of an LBW infant (Aliyu et al, 2005; Ananth et al, 1996). Women over age 40 tend to gain less weight during pregnancy, a factor that could contribute to the increased risk of LBW (Menacker et al, 2004).

Advanced maternal age creates genetic risks because as the woman gets older, the genetic material contained within her ova ages. All females are born with all of the eggs that they will ever have, which contain the genetic material that each woman will pass on to her progeny. According to maternal aging theory, as the woman chronologically ages, her eggs and all of the genetic material they contain age, too. The genetic material within the aging ovum of a woman over age 35 has a higher chance of being defective because it is older. Aging genetic material is more likely to have errors occur during cell division during meiosis that can result in either a lack of or an excess of chromosomal material (Maternal Age Risks, 2001). This phenomenon most likely accounts for decreased fertility rates as women age and the increased risk of chromosomal abnormalities in their offspring (Heffner, 2004). Trisomy 21 (Down syndrome) and trisomies 18 and 13 are examples of genetic problems resulting from errors in cell division. Down syndrome is the most common chromosomal problem that is linked to advanced maternal age. Normally, a fetus has 23 pairs of chromosomes with half of each pair inherited from each parent. However, with Down syndrome the fetus has an extra chromosome located on chromosome 21 (i.e., three chromosomes instead of two; hence the name trisomy 21). The risk for having an infant with Down syndrome increases with advanced maternal age. For example, a 30-year-old woman's risk to have an infant with Down syndrome is 1 in 885, at age 35 the risk is 1 in 365, and at age 40 the risk is 1 in 109 (Hook & Lindsjo, 1978).

Late fetal and early perinatal death rates are higher for pregnant women between ages 45 and 54 than for any other age groups. Pregnant women over the age of 45 have a rate of spontaneous abortion that is nine times higher than that of pregnant women between the ages of 20 and 24 (Andersen et

| TABLE **37-2** | Selected Abnormal Conditions of the Newborn and Rates by Age and Race of Mother: Total of 48 States and the District of Columbia, 2003 |

Abnormal Condition and Race of Mother	All Births[1]	Abnormal Condition Reported	Age of Mother							Not Stated[2]
			All Ages	Under 20 Years	20-24 Years	25-29 Years	30-34 Years	35-39 Years	40-54 Years	
			All races[3]							
Anemia	3,863,502	3,604	0.9	1.0	0.9	0.9	0.9	1.0	1.2	22,046
Birth injury[4]	3,460,109	9,774	2.8	3.1	3.0	2.8	2.9	2.4	2.5	21,979
Fetal alcohol syndrome[5]	3,793,462	132	0.0	*	0.0	0.0	0.0	0.0	*	21,963
Hyaline membrane disease/RDS	3,863,502	23,214	6.0	6.6	6.3	5.8	5.7	6.1	6.9	22,046
Meconium aspiration syndrome	3,863,502	4,788	1.2	1.5	1.4	1.2	1.1	1.2	1.5	22,046
Assisted ventilation less than 30 minutes[6]	3,743,733	79,727	21.4	21.6	20.3	20.8	22.2	23.1	24.1	21,364
Assisted ventilation 30 minutes or longer[6]	3,743,733	34,699	9.3	10.8	9.2	8.6	8.9	10.1	12.0	21,364
Seizures[6]	3,863,502	1,755	0.5	0.5	0.5	0.4	0.4	0.4	0.6	22,046

Excerpted from National Vital Statistics Report, Vol 54, No 2, September 8, 2005, p 95. Available at: http://www.cdc.gov/nchs/data/nvsr54/nvsr54_02.pdf.
Rates are number of live births with specified abnormal condition per 1000 live births in specified group.
0.0, Quantity more than zero but less than 0.05.
*Figure does not meet standards of reliability or precision; based on fewer than 20 births in the numerator.
[1]Total number of births to residents of areas reporting specified abnormal condition.
[2]No response reported for the abnormal condition item.
[3]Includes races other than white and black.
[4]Nebraska and Texas do not report this condition.
[5]Wisconsin does not report this condition.
[6]New York City does not report this condition.
NOTES: Excludes data for Pennsylvania and Washington, which implemented the 2003 Revision to the U.S. Standard Certificate of Live Birth for data year 2003. This change has resulted in a lack of compatibility between data based on the 2003 Revision and data based on the 1989 Revision to the U.S. Certificate of Live Birth. See "Technical Notes" in original document. Race and Hispanic Origin are reported separately on birth certificates. Race categories are consistent with the 1977 Office of Management and Budget Standards. In this table all women (including Hispanic women) are classified only according to their race: see "Technical Notes" in original document.

al, 2000). Women over age 40 are at increased risk for placental abruption and perinatal mortality (Cleary-Goldman et al, 2005). Although fertility tends to decline with advanced maternal age, women between the ages of 35 and 39 actually have an increased risk of conceiving twins without the assistance of fertility treatments, another factor that increases their risk status (Andersen et al, 2000).

Advanced paternal age has been associated with increased risk of miscarriage, especially if the man is over age 40 or if both partners are of advanced age (de la Rochebrochard & Thonneau, 2002). Advanced paternal age should also be considered when evaluating prenatal risks, as it is associated with rare congenital anomalies in offspring due to dominant mutations such as neural tube defects, congenital cataracts, upper limb reduction defects, and Down syndrome (MacIntosh et al, 1995). Older fathers are more likely to have offspring with such autosomal dominant genetic conditions as Marfan syndrome, achondroplasia, Huntington's chorea, and von Willebrand's disease (Heffner, 2004). A careful assessment of family history of both parents will help alert the health care provider to these potential risks.

Ethnicity

Even though birth outcomes have dramatically improved over the past 25 years for all ethnic groups, serious ethnic disparities continue to exist. Black mothers are 2 to 3 times more likely to die from pregnancy-related causes, have a fetus or infant who dies, have preterm labor, have an LBW infant, or have an infant with congenital anomalies than mothers of other ethnic groups. Black women are more likely to have a spontaneous abortion, an ectopic pregnancy, or a cesarean section than white women (Gennaro, 2005; Hogue & Bremner, 2005; Rich-Edwards et al, 2003). Although black mothers are more likely to be socially disadvantaged and live in poor neighborhoods with higher levels of poverty (Rich-Edwards et al, 2003), even infants of college-educated black women who seek first-trimester prenatal care are at increased risk to die as a result of prematurity or VLBW.

Black and white interracial couples also have an increased risk for stillbirth, SGA, and neonatal mortality. Preterm and SGA births are more common in pregnancies with mixed white mother–black father (WB) or black mother–black father (BB) parent combinations than for white mother–white father (WW) parent combinations. WW parents have more LGA infants. Infant death rate is higher for infants of WB parents (6.0), black mother–white father (BW) parents (5.9), and BB parents (7.6) than for those of WW parents (3.9). There are differences in socioeconomic factors, with more teen parents, unmarried women, and failure to seek prenatal care in the BW, WB, and BB groups. Paternal genetic factors might influence some of these outcomes; this needs further study (Getahun et al, 2005).

Weathering and Stress Age

Racial disparities in birth outcomes cannot be totally explained by the presence of maternal risk factors. Even special programs developed in attempts to address ethnic disparities in birth outcomes have not been able to make much of a difference. The effects of lifetime stress were proposed as a possible reason for continued ethnic disparities in birth outcomes for black infants. Geronimus (1992) noted that infants of teenaged African American women had a survival

advantage over infants of older African American women. Maternal "weathering" was proposed as a possible explanation for these disparities. Weathering is a term for premature aging that is caused by stress. The weathering hypothesis proposes that socioeconomic disadvantage contributes to an earlier decline in the health of African-American women (Geronimus, 1996). This early decline affects the entire body, including the reproductive system. Theoretically, the reproductive system functions most optimally during the time of a woman's life that would maximize her chances to reproduce a healthy child. If women delay childbearing past this optimal time, then their aging reproductive systems do not function as efficiently (Geronimus, 1996). Furthermore, prepregnancy chronic stress might lead to accelerated physiologic aging of the female reproductive system and thus to poor pregnancy outcomes. Therefore, women who are under stress have increased risks for delivery of preterm or LBW infants because of the decreased efficiency of their reproductive systems. Maternal age is a marker for how long the woman has endured exposure to stressful hardships (Rich-Edwards et al, 2003).

According to the theory of stress age, a term synonymous with weathering, the cumulative effects of lifetime exposure to acute stress and experiences of chronic day-to-day stress increase the risk of stress-related disease during pregnancy (Hogue & Bremner, 2005). Additional stress experienced during pregnancy can add to the mother's cumulative lifetime stress, therefore elevating her risk for preterm labor or an LBW infant. Many African American women experience more than the usual level of lifetime stressors because of their encounters with racial and gender discrimination and violence throughout their lifetimes. Racial discrimination can be a source of chronic stress and can alter the individual's stress reactivity (Patrick & Bryan, 2005). Because of increased lifetime stress, women may experience increased stress age that could influence pregnancy outcomes that are stress sensitive. Researchers have established links between some pregnancy-related diseases and later chronic illness; for example, women with gestational diabetes have an increased risk for type 2 diabetes later in life. A possible explanation is that poor pregnancy outcomes represent initial signs of aging of the endocrine, immune, and reproductive systems (Rich-Edwards & Grizzard, 2005). Hardiness, resilience, and social support might act as stress buffers in some women, lessening the impact of stress (Patrick & Bryan, 2005). The "weathering hypothesis" offers an interesting explanation for the increased incidence of preterm delivery and LBW infants for older childbearing women or women who are under stress.

Hogue and Bremner (2005) proposed an epidemiologic model demonstrating some of the possible mediators and moderators of stress age (Figure 37-2). Stress age is affected by lifetime exposure to acute or chronic personal stressors (such as violence or racism). The social, cultural, and physical environment, such as underlying health problems, anemia, hypertension, lifestyle choices, and exercise, add additional stressors that influence acute and personal stressors. Stress is mediated as it enters the host organism through mechanisms that help provide immunity to the effects of incoming stress. Stress mediators include (1) blame reflection (i.e., how much the host attributes the stressor to external or internal causes); (2) stress reducers (actions the host takes to reduce stress such as exercise or diet); (3) spiritual strength (use of prayer or faith); (4) social resources (support network available); (5) economic

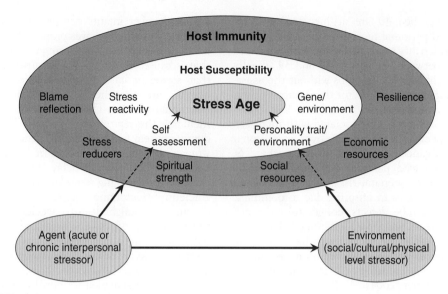

FIGURE **37-2**
Hypothesized effect of stress on stress-aging, with the use of the agent/host/environment model. From Hogue CR, Bremner JD (2005). Stress model for research into preterm delivery among black women. *American journal of obstetrics and gynecology* 192:S47-55.

resources (availability of resources to provide for needs such as prenatal care, food, or medication); and (6)resilience. The host is susceptible to the effects of stress through the influence of the following factors: (1) stress reactivity (how the host reacts to stress); (2) self-assessment (the host's perception of stress); (3) personality or trait environment of the host (including a tendency toward anxiety or anger); and (4) the genetic environment that could influence susceptibility to stress. Exposure to high levels of stress compromises the host's ability to withstand stress and increases susceptibility to stress-related diseases such as hypertension, as well as increasing the likelihood of infections. Maternal stress can affect immune, endocrine, and vascular function; any one of these factors may trigger preterm labor or cause LBW.

The exact mechanism by which maternal stress causes preterm labor is not fully understood, but it is thought to occur by one of two mechanisms. Corticotropin-releasing hormone (CRH) released as a byproduct of maternal stress could stimulate neuroendocrine pathways within the maternal-fetal-placental unit that trigger labor; or maternal stress could cause increased maternal and fetal susceptibility to inflammation and infection, triggering labor through an immune-inflammatory pathway (Hogue & Bremner, 2005; Rich-Edwards & Grizzard, 2005). Although more research is needed to test the stress age theory, it does offer a promising new direction to explain ethnic disparities related to preterm birth and LBW.

Differences in LBW and preterm delivery are not totally explained by race or sociodemographic factors. Mexican women who immigrate to the United States have demographic and socioeconomic factors such as high rates of teen pregnancy, less educated mothers, and higher rates of no prenatal care or late prenatal care in the third trimester that put them at high risk for poor perinatal outcomes. On the other hand, Asian Indian women who immigrate to the United States have demographic and socioeconomic risk factors similar to those of white women that put them at low risk. Asian Indian women have higher education levels with more college graduates,

have less teenaged pregnancy, and are more likely to get adequate prenatal care. However, an "epidemiologic paradox" occurs, and outcomes do not occur as predicted. African American women have the highest incidence of LBW, SGA, and fetal and neonatal deaths in the United States at rates almost twice that of white women. Foreign-born Mexican women with demographic and socioeconomic risk factors comparable to those of African American women have better perinatal outcomes than expected, including less LBW and fewer neonatal deaths than white women. Asian Indian women have higher incidences of prematurity, LBW, SGA, and fetal death than white women. This "epidemiologic paradox" suggests that there are other factors that give foreign-born women either a perinatal advantage or disadvantage, such as environmental factors, diet or lifestyle factors, or genetic factors (Gould et al, 2003). It is possible that ethnic differences in LBW might be a factor of ethnically determined differences in weight by gestational age. For example, based on a given gestational age, white infants will generally weigh more than Hispanic infants, and Hispanic infants will weigh more than black infants (Chung et al, 2003).

Obstetric Factors

Obstetric history is a good indicator of the presence of maternal risk factors. Women with previous obstetric complications are more at risk for problems with the current pregnancy. History of infertility, previous stillbirth, preterm infant, infant with IUGR, infant with genetic problems, complications during pregnancy or birth, or other poor outcomes are clues indicating that the pregnancy must be closely monitored. Prepregnancy health status is another factor associated with the risk of preterm delivery. Women who are in poor physical condition prior to conception (i.e., underweight, having poor pre-pregnancy physical function, chronic hypertension, or smoking before pregnancy) have an increased risk for preterm delivery (Haas et al, 2005). Important obstetric factors that can compound pregnancy risk are the adequacy of prenatal care, the number of previous pregnancies, interpregnancy level, the use of assisted reproductive technology, and postterm pregnancy.

Prenatal Care

Prenatal care that begins in the first trimester of pregnancy and continues until birth helps promote good birth outcomes. Most women seek prenatal care during the first trimester of pregnancy. Only a small percentage of women start prenatal care during the last trimester or have no prenatal care. Native American/Alaskan Native, non-Hispanic black, and women of Mexican origin have higher rates of late or no prenatal care. The decision to seek prenatal care is influenced by the woman's attitudes toward pregnancy, cultural preference, or lifestyle factors. Inadequate prenatal care increases the risk for LBW, preterm birth, and perinatal death (Fraser et al, 1995; Vintzileos et al, 2002). Higher postneonatal death rates seen in infants of women who did not have prenatal care might be associated with lack of access to care providers or lack of use of pediatric medical care (Vintzileos et al, 2002).

Parity

Parity, or number of previous deliveries, is another perinatal risk factor to consider. The risk for having an LBW infant, a preterm delivery, abruptio placentae, or placenta previa increases as parity increases (Aliyu et al, 2005). Women with five or more previous births are more likely to have inadequate prenatal care and are at an increased risk for having a macrosomic infant. Women with high parity are usually older and are more likely to have aging-associated diseases such as diabetes or hypertension that can affect pregnancy outcomes.

Interpregnancy Level

Interpregnancy level is defined as the amount of time between delivery of a baby and the subsequent conception of another child. A short interpregnancy level of less than 6 months increases the risk for maternal complications including third-trimester bleeding, premature rupture of membranes, puerperal endometritis, anemia, and maternal death. Women with longer interpregnancy levels have the highest risk for pre-eclampsia, eclampsia, and gestational diabetes, again probably related to older maternal age. The risk for prematurity is increased when the interpregnancy level is 18 months or less or greater than 59 months (Fuentes-Afflick & Hessol, 2000).

Assistive Reproductive Technology

Assistive reproductive technology (ART) is any procedure or medical treatment used to assist a woman in achieving pregnancy. ART is an option for many couples who have a history of infertility. ART methods include use of medications to stimulate ovulation and release of eggs, or procedures where eggs and sperm are removed and mixed outside of the body to achieve fertilization. Some techniques require that the fertilized egg remain outside the body for a few days before being implanted back into the woman's body. In some cases the eggs, sperm, or embryos might be frozen for later use or manipulated with instrumentation during the earliest stages of cell formation.

ART increases the risk for a multiple pregnancy, prematurity, and LBW. Most ART procedures result in high rates of multiple pregnancies since couples may choose to have multiple embryos implanted to maximize their chances for success. A multiple pregnancy naturally increases risks for preterm labor, cesarean delivery, and LBW and provides one explanation for the increase in number of LBW and preterm infants over the past few years. The risk for congenital anomalies doubles for infants conceived with ART, including sex and autosomal chromosomal anomalies such as Beckwith-Wiedemann and Angelman's syndromes. Infants conceived by ART have a fourfold to sevenfold increased risk for retinoblastoma (Green, 2004).

Couples who electively conceive through ART with a large number of embryos may have to make tough ethical decisions, including options for selective reduction later in the pregnancy, in order to protect the health of compromised fetuses. The risk for prematurity and LBW increases as the number of fetuses increases, increasing risks of poor outcomes for the infants. The decision to maintain a pregnancy with a large number of fetuses can be economically and emotionally catastrophic for the family. Outcomes for the babies who survive depend in part on the number of fetuses and gestational age at delivery. Some countries have set mandatory limits on the numbers of embryos that can be implanted during ART procedures to help address some of these issues (Green, 2004).

Postterm Pregnancy

Postterm pregnancy is defined as a pregnancy that continues past 42 weeks (294 days) or 14 days past the estimated due date (ACOG Committee on Practice Bulletins [ACOG], 2004). Incidence is in about 7% of all pregnancies. The cause of postterm pregnancy is not known, but it occurs more often with male fetuses and may have a genetic basis. Some cases of postterm pregnancy can be attributed to inaccurate dates used to calculate the estimated date of confinement. Ultrasound dating of pregnancy is considered to be accurate if done during the first trimester; however ultrasound dating of pregnancy has a margin of error.

Postterm infants are more likely to have macrosomia, with increased risks for prolonged labor or cephalopelvic disproportion (CPD). Macrosomia increases the risk for cesarean section or shoulder dystocia that leads to increased risks of possible musculoskeletal injury (i.e., fractured clavicle or brachial plexus injury). Postmaturity also predisposes to uteroplacental insufficiency in about 20% of cases. Postmature infants who have been exposed to uteroplacental insufficiency present with chronic IUGR and are more at risk for cord compression due to oligohydramnios or presence of thick meconium (Morantz & Torrey, 2004). Adverse outcomes are more likely in the presence of oligohydramnios (ACOG, 2004). Postterm pregnancy has also been related to lower umbilical artery pH levels and lower Apgar scores (Caughey et al, 2005). ACOG recommends surveillance of postterm pregnancies between 41 and 42 weeks because of increased risks of fetal complications as gestational age advances. Postterm fetuses should be evaluated by nonstress testing or biophysical profiles. Delivery is not indicated as long as the results of these tests are reassuring (ACOG, 2004). When the amniotic membranes rupture and if meconium is present, measures must be taken to prevent meconium aspiration at birth. Meconium aspiration increases the risk of death for postterm infants. At birth the nose, mouth, and hypopharynx must be suctioned thoroughly prior to delivery of the shoulders and the cords should be visualized and suctioned of any meconium prior to initiation of the first breath. If the infant with meconium is breathing spontaneously, then intubation is not necessary for cord visualization.

After delivery postterm neonates will need careful assessment for possible birth injuries. Infants with meconium aspiration will need intensive treatment for respiratory complications. All postterm infants should be monitored for possible hypoglycemia and temperature instability.

Environmental Influences

Every individual is conceived with a unique genetic makeup called a genotype. The phenotype, or the person's ultimate physiologic and psychologic makeup, is determined during the postconceptual period until after birth. The expression of the genetic inheritance (i.e., actual physiologic and psychologic makeup of the person) is the result of complex gene-gene interactions and environmental influences on genes that occur at the molecular level. Exposure to environmental toxicants during pregnancy can precipitate gene-environment interactions that can alter these molecular interactions, especially if the exposure to the harmful substance occurs at critical periods of fetal development. Two critical periods when gene-environmental interactions can be most harmful are during organogenesis (when fetal organs are being formed during the first trimester of pregnancy), and during the fetal period (after the eighth week of pregnancy) when there is rapid growth of all systems. Spina bifida is an example of a gene-environment interaction. At conception a fertilized egg might inherit the genes to have an intact neural tube. Neural tube defects occur when there is a lack of adequate folic acid at a critical stage of development while in utero. Exposure to teratogens, substances that are known to cause birth defects, during these times can result in birth defects or other adverse outcomes. Two pregnant women could be exposed to the same toxicants at the same point during pregnancy and could have infants with different outcomes. For example, two infants could inherit the genetic trait for sickle cell disease, yet when they are born they could have different expressions of the disease based on other complex molecular interactions that happen within genes and that could be influenced by the environment. The study of epigenetics is an evolving science that looks at factors such as genetic inheritance, imprinting, or nutritional factors that are hypothesized to mediate genetic interactions at the molecular level and that may one day provide more insight into these complex processes.

Environmental hazards are found in air, water, and food. These seemingly innocuous substances can contain high levels of contaminants such as pesticides, heavy metals, and solvents (Silbergeld & Patrick, 2005). Maternal exposure to air pollutants during the first trimester of pregnancy has been associated with decreased fetal birth weight (Gouveia et al, 2004). Poor or socially disadvantaged women, especially women of color, are more often exposed to environmental hazards because they tend to live in older sections of town or work in areas with high exposure. Their homes are usually older, increasing the risk for lead paint exposure. Poor parts of town are often located close to factories where pregnant women are exposed to incinerator emissions or other sources of air pollution. The poor are more likely to be exposed to agricultural pesticides or chemicals as they are more likely to work on farms or as migrant workers. In fact, fetal congenital anomalies and death were noted in the offspring of male agricultural workers who worked where pesticides were used.

More fetuses died in seasons when pesticide usage was highest (Regidor et al, 2004). The disadvantaged might be more likely to reside on land that once served as a hazardous waste dumpsite (Silbergeld & Patrick, 2005). Cultural practices such as pica place some pregnant women at increased risk for exposure to environmental pollutants including heavy metals.

Health-Compromising Behaviors

Health-compromising behaviors (HCBs) such as smoking and drug or alcohol use can affect overall maternal health during pregnancy and can negatively influence fetal well-being. Prepregnancy maternal health status and health behaviors may play a role in preterm labor risk. Babies born to mothers who smoke, drink alcohol, or take drugs weigh less than babies of mothers who do not smoke, drink, or take drugs (Okah et al, 2005; Reichman & Teitler, 2003).

Cigarette smoking is a major predictor of LBW, possibly because of impaired oxygen delivery (hypoxia) and nutrient delivery from the mother to fetus (Chiriboga, 2003). Infants of mothers who smoke have an increased risk of spontaneous abortion, late fetal death, preterm delivery, and neonatal mortality. Women who smoke are more likely to use alcohol or illicit drugs during pregnancy than those who do not smoke.

Substance abuse is a concern for childbearing women of all ages. More teenagers are experimenting with drugs, alcohol, and smoking cigarettes and marijuana than in the past (AAP, 2001a). Marijuana smoking results in carbon monoxide levels five times higher than those from cigarette smoking, another factor that limits fetal growth and oxygenation (Chiriboga, 2003). Women under the influence of mind-altering substances are more likely to make poor choices and increase the risk of engaging in promiscuous behavior resulting in an unplanned pregnancy.

Maternal alcohol ingestion during pregnancy can result in fetal alcohol syndrome (FAS). Incidence of FAS may be related to both environmental exposure and genetic susceptibility. Alcohol is believed to have a direct teratogenic effect that limits fetal growth and brain growth. The fetal effects of drinking are most pronounced if the fetus is exposed during the first trimester of pregnancy. The minimum amount of alcohol that is harmful to the fetal brain is not known. It is known that binge drinking (ingestion of more than five drinks at one occasion) leads to higher levels of blood alcohol. Binge drinking is a special concern in early pregnancy when the fetal brain is developing and women may not yet even realize that they are pregnant (Maier & West, 2001; Okah et al, 2005).

Pregnant women who abuse illicit drugs such as cocaine have higher levels of LBW and IUGR infants than women who do not use cocaine and are less likely to seek or receive adequate prenatal care (Brady et al, 2003). Individual health-compromising behaviors such as smoking, alcohol, and drug abuse are discussed elsewhere in this text. The influence of nutrition, illicit drug consumption, and environmental factors are further discussed here as health-compromising behaviors.

Nutrition

Adequate nutrition prior to conception and during pregnancy is important for maternal and fetal health. The pregnant woman needs to consume enough calories and nutrients to meet her own physiologic needs as well as those of the developing fetus. Nutritional risks to consider include inadequate or excessive weight gain, medical conditions that complicate pregnancy such as hyperemesis gravidarum, dental conditions that compromise the ability to take in food, or inadequate resources to access food. Lack of adequate nutrients prior to or during early pregnancy can lead to birth defects. It has been well established that it is important for all women of childbearing age (between 15 and 45) to consume at least 400 mcg of folic acid daily to help prevent neural tube defects. The Centers for Disease Control and Prevention (CDC) estimates that 50% to 70% of all birth defects could be prevented by this simple measure! Another important nutritional consideration is prevention of maternal anemia during pregnancy. Maternal anemia during the first half of pregnancy has been associated with an increased risk for preterm labor at less than 37 weeks' gestation (Scholl & Reilly, 2000).

Maternal eating disorders prior to or during pregnancy increase the risk for LBW or SGA infants. These infants are more likely to have a smaller head circumference with a reduced brain size. A decreased food intake with less availability of nutrients to the fetus is the most likely cause of LBW; decreased head circumference is attributed to increased maternal stress level (Kouba et al, 2005). Prolonged periods of time without food can lead to increased maternal corticotropin-releasing hormone and can subsequently increase the risk for preterm delivery (Gennaro, 2005). Women living on low incomes do not get adequate nutrition during pregnancy. Nutritional support during pregnancy including basic and specialized nutrition education, and participation in the Special Supplemental Nutrition Program for Women, Infants, and Children (WIC) have been demonstrated to increase the mean birth weight and reduce the odds for LBW for infants of poor women on Medicaid. WIC is an important part of prenatal programs for poor or at-risk women (Reichman & Teitler, 2003).

Maternal obesity is another nutritional concern. Infants of obese women (defined as body mass index [BMI] >30.0 kg/m^2) have more than twice the risk for stillbirth and neonatal death after adjusting for other factors including smoking, alcohol, maternal age, parity, hypertension, and diabetes (Kristensen et al, 2005).

The increased use of bariatric surgery to correct obesity in the United States creates a new maternal risk factor with implications for pregnancy. There are two types of bariatric surgery: restrictive and malabsorptive (Edwards, 2005). The complications for the fetus and neonate appear to be secondary to maternal and fetal malnutrition, particularly deficiencies in vitamin B$_{12}$. Infants are more likely to be SGA. Breastfed infants may have continued nutritional deficiencies such as organic failure to thrive or megaloblastic anemia; however, breastfeeding should not be discouraged in these mothers (Edwards, 2005). Most experts recommend that women wait at least 18 months to get pregnant following either type of bariatric procedure. Infants need to receive good follow-up care focusing on nutritional needs, weight gain, and growth patterns.

Maternal food-borne illness or ingestion of toxic substances during pregnancy can be harmful to the fetus. *Listeria monocytogenes* is a special concern in pregnancy, because about one third of all cases occur in pregnant women. Women who ingest food contaminated with *Listeria* do not usually feel ill; however, the fetus can be significantly affected. Eating food contaminated by microorganisms such as *Listeria* or substances

such as heavy metals can cause abortion, stillbirth, preterm delivery, neonatal infections, fetal brain or kidney problems, or even maternal death. The "Food Safety for Moms-to-Be" program from the U.S. Food and Drug Administration (2005) educates pregnant women about prevention of food-borne illness. Teach pregnant women simple basic precautions such as handwashing, separating meats from other foods during storage, cooking food to proper temperatures, and placing food in the refrigerator to help prevent food-borne illness during pregnancy.

Pica is an interesting dietary practice seen more often in African American women during pregnancy. Women ingest substances such as starch, ice, clay, or dirt. Ingestion of these substances might be an attempt to increase iron or calcium in the diet and is not generally harmful to the fetus. Women who practice pica tend be more underweight at the start of their pregnancy, have lower hematocrit levels, and smoke less than other women (Corbett et al, 2003). One concern is if the mother eats dirt that is contaminated with lead or other heavy metals. These heavy metals could be harmful and possibly cause anemia or lead poisoning (Silbergeld & Patrick, 2005).

Cultural dietary practices cannot be ignored as possible risk factors and must be assessed. Asian women who ingest betel nuts, which contain arecoline, are at higher risk for spontaneous abortion, LBW, preterm birth, and placental changes, and their infants are at risk for neonatal substance withdrawal (Garcia-Algar et al, 2005). The health care practitioner must become familiar with the food and complementary medicine cultural practices of local ethnic groups as they may affect pregnancy outcomes.

Over-the-Counter and Complementary Drugs

Drugs taken during pregnancy can have harmful effects on the fetus whether they are controlled substances or over-the-counter medications. Despite warnings not to take any medications without consulting with their heath care provider, many pregnant women take over-the-counter or nonprescribed medications during pregnancy, including complementary therapies that they might not consider as harmful. About 44% of women of childbearing age between the ages of 18 and 34 report taking at least one prescription drug within the past month and 10% report taking three or more drugs in past month (National Center for Health Statistics, 2005). Many women regularly take over-the-counter drugs such as cold remedies, aspirin, nonsteroidal anti-inflammatory drugs (NSAIDs), or herbal teas. In some cases women might take medications that could be harmful to the fetus before they know that they are pregnant. Even vitamins and dietary supplements taken in excessive dosages can be harmful to the fetus. Pregnant women with pre-existing medical problems such as asthma, arthritis, heart problems, diabetes, or epilepsy will usually have to continue to take their prescribed medications. In some cases, the prescribed medication will need to be changed to one that is less harmful to the fetus.

Health care providers must be cognizant of Food and Drug Administration (FDA) pregnancy categories and drugs that must be used with caution or that are contraindicated in pregnancy (Table 37-3). One concern is that thalidomide received FDA approval for treatment of leprosy in 1998 and is currently being evaluated in clinical trials for renal cell cancer, AIDS, and tuberculosis. Thalidomide was withdrawn from the market in the 1960s after it was linked to fetal limb-shortening birth

TABLE 37-3	Drug Safety Pregnancy Categories	
Pregnancy Category	**What Category Means**	**Examples of Drugs in This Category**
A	Tested and were found to be safe during pregnancy	Thyroid, vitamin B_6, and folic acid
B	Used by many women during pregnancy and do not appear to have risks	Some antibiotics, acetaminophen, aspartame, famotidine, prednisone, insulin, metformin, Arcabose, and ibuprofen (do not take in last trimester of pregnancy)
C	No human studies to show that they are harmful to the fetus although there might be animal studies, or no animal studies conducted. May be used if the benefits outweigh the risks	Ciprofloxacin, fluconazole, pseudoephedrine, prochlorperazine, and some antidepressants. ACE inhibitors and ARBs are category C in first trimester, then category D thereafter—discontinue before pregnancy.
D	Have evidence of harmful fetal effects from studies done after the drug was approved for use in pregnant women, but they can be used if there is a favorable benefit-to-risk ratio	Lithium, phenytoin, and most chemotherapy drugs
X	Contraindicated during pregnancy because they have known teratogenic effects	Accutane, diethylstilbestrol (DES), thalidomide, and drugs for psoriasis such as Tegison (no longer marketed in the United States) or Soriatane, statins used for treatment of diabetes (discontinue before conception).

defects when it was used during pregnancy. Now there are stringent educational requirements, warnings about risks in pregnancy, and mandatory contraception for both men and women who use thalidomide. It is possible that pregnancy could occur despite these measures.

MATERNAL MEDICAL AND OBSTETRIC CONDITIONS

Diabetes, hypertension, and bleeding disorders are some of the most common maternal complications of pregnancy. These complications can lead to preterm delivery or perinatal death, or can influence fetal morbidity. Rates of maternal complications increase with maternal age (Salihu et al, 2003).

Diabetes

About 0.3% to 0.5% of all pregnancies in the United States are complicated by pregestational diabetes (Bernasko, 2004). Women with pregestational diabetes should seek preconceptual care prior to getting pregnant. The preconceptual visit should include a complete physical examination with evaluation of blood glucose levels, cardiovascular and renal health, gastrointestinal system, an eye exam to check for diabetic retinopathy, and evaluation of the presence of neuropathy. A team approach with a diabetes nurse educator and dietician can teach the woman how to implement the dietary and lifestyle changes needed for a healthy pregnancy. Oral hypoglycemics should be changed to human insulin prior to pregnancy. Ideally the woman with diabetes should maintain euglycemia for several months prior to pregnancy and during pregnancy. This is sometimes difficult since insulin needs change with each trimester. Women with pregestational diabetes have increased risks for having a miscarriage, a stillbirth, or an infant with a congenital birth defect if blood glucose levels during pregnancy are not controlled. Glycosylated hemoglobin levels (HbA1c) should be maintained as close to the normal range as possible during pregnancy, especially during the period of fetal organogenesis (American Diabetes Association [ADA], 2005).

Universal blood glucose screening of all pregnant women with a 1-hour glucose tolerance test between 24 and 28 weeks' gestation is recommended to identify women with gestational diabetes. About 5% of pregnancies are complicated by gestational diabetes (ADA, 2005). Identification and treatment of women with gestational diabetes is the key to promoting positive neonatal outcomes. The most important principle of diabetes management for all pregnant women with diabetes is to maintain tight glycemic control. Poor glycemic control increases the risks for miscarriage or stillbirth, and increases the infant's risk for birth defects (i.e., cardiovascular, musculoskeletal, and central nervous system anomalies), hypoglycemia, hyperbilirubinemia, erythrocytosis, respiratory complications, and shoulder dystocia (Langer et al, 2005; March of Dimes, 2005a; Schaefer-Graf et al, 2000). Risks for birth defects are similar in gestational diabetics as compared with women with type 1 diabetes (Schaefer-Graf et al, 2000).

Diabetes during pregnancy is frequently accompanied by maternal vascular changes that can compromise uteroplacental circulation; therefore fetal nonstress testing is recommended during the last trimester. If early delivery is indicated, amniocentesis can be done to determine fetal lung maturity; however, results of tests of the lecithin/sphingomyelin (L/S) ratio are often inaccurate for infants of mothers with diabetes. Infants of diabetic mothers generally have macrosomia. These large babies have increased risks for birth injuries due to shoulder dystocia, including fractured clavicles or nerve palsies. Large infants are more likely to be delivered by cesarean section. Infants of diabetic mothers should be closely monitored for hypoglycemia in the immediate postbirth period and until feeding is well established.

Hypertension in Pregnancy

Approximately 5% to 10% of pregnancies are complicated by hypertensive disorders. The National High Blood Pressure Education Working Group (NHBPWEG) Report on High Blood Pressure in Pregnancy (2000) recently updated the classification of hypertensive disorders in pregnancy (Table 37-4). Chronic hypertension exists when there is a history of hypertension prior to the pregnancy, but it can also be diagnosed during pregnancy for the first time. About 20% of women with pre-existing hypertension develop superimposed pre-eclampsia during their pregnancy (Seely & Solomon, 2003). Women with chronic hypertension who develop proteinuria are at increased risks for fetal complications, especially if serum creatinine levels are above 1.4 mg/dl at conception. They are also at increased risk for placental abruption. Gestational hypertension is diagnosed during pregnancy and usually disappears within 12 weeks after delivery. Pre-eclampsia is a pregnancy-specific disease that usually occurs after 20 weeks of pregnancy. It is characterized by hypertension and proteinuria. As the condition progressively worsens, maternal lab work indicates elevations in liver enzymes and low platelets.

PIH causes vasoconstriction with subsequent poor maternal circulatory and placental perfusion. Decreased uteroplacental circulation compromises the fetus; therefore it is more likely to be growth restricted, SGA, or at increased risk for stillbirth. Women with PIH are also at increased risk for abruptio placentae. Delivery is the definitive treatment for PIH; however, it might not be appropriate if the fetus is immature. Early delivery will be based on stability of the mother and outcomes of fetal testing. A serious risk for the pre-eclamptic mother is eclamptic seizures due to cerebral edema and central nervous system excitability. Seizures increase the risk for a placental abruption. Therefore, if the mother's condition worsens, early delivery will be elected as the definitive treatment. However, the ability of the fetus to survive must be considered. Corticosteroid administration is advised at 33 to 34 weeks' gestational age and may be beneficial for promotion of fetal lung maturity (NHBPWEG, 2000). Patients with pre-eclampsia tend to have infants with lower gestational ages at delivery and lower birth weights than do patients with gestational hypertension alone (Barton et al, 2001). Women with severe gestational hypertension (defined as BP >160/110) without proteinuria tend to have higher rates of preterm delivery and are more likely to have a baby who is SGA as compared to mothers who are normotensive or have mild gestational hypertension or mild pre-eclampsia (Buchbinder et al, 2002). The earlier that hypertensive disease occurs in pregnancy, the more likely it is that proteinuria will develop. The development of proteinuria in women with gestational hypertension increases the chances for adverse maternal and neonatal outcomes (Barton et al, 2001).

If pre-eclampsia worsens, the pregnant woman is admitted to the hospital for stabilization and delivery. If the woman has a seizure, oxygen should be provided during and immediately following the seizure and the fetus should be monitored for signs of distress. Magnesium sulfate is the drug of choice to prevent central nervous system excitability from cerebral edema. Infants rarely have harmful effects from in utero exposure to magnesium sulfate prior to delivery, but should be monitored for signs of respiratory depression or hypotonia.

Ethnic differences in the progression of hypertensive disorders in pregnancy have been noted. African American women were hospitalized earlier in the pregnancy for treatment of PIH. Their babies had lower gestational age and birth weight. African American women also had a higher incidence of abruptio placentae, stillbirths, and neonatal deaths than

TABLE **37-4**	Classification of Hypertension in Pregnancy		
Type	**BP Parameters**	**Proteinuria**	**Other Manifestations**
Chronic hypertension	140 mm Hg systolic 90 mm Hg diastolic	Not present	Hypertension that is present before pregnancy or within first 20 weeks of gestation. Hypertension that is diagnosed for the first time during pregnancy and does not resolve after delivery.
Gestational hypertension	>140 mm Hg systolic; >90 mm Hg diastolic in a woman who was previously normotensive	Not present	BP returns to normal within 12 weeks of delivery.
Pre-eclampsia	>140 mm Hg systolic; >90 mm Hg diastolic	>0.3 g in 24 hours	Headache, blurred vision, abdominal pain Low platelet count Hemolysis Elevated liver function tests Eclamptic seizures Disseminated intravascular coagulation
Pre-eclampsia superimposed on chronic hypertension	>140 mm Hg systolic >90 mm Hg diastolic *or* a sudden increase in BP that has been previously well controlled	New-onset proteinuria >0.3 g during 24 hours	Platelet count <100,000/mm^3 Increase of alanine aminotransferase (ALT) or aspartate aminotransferase (AST) to abnormal levels

From National Heart Lung and Blood Institute (2000). National high blood pressure education program: working group report on high blood pressure in pregnancy. *Rockville, MD: National Guideline Clearinghouse, Agency for Healthcare Research and Quality.*

other ethnic groups. More Hispanic women developed proteinuria during pregnancy, and their disease was more likely to progress to severe pre-eclampsia (Barton et al, 2002).

Premature Rupture of Membranes

Premature rupture of membranes (PROM) is a cause of preterm delivery and occurs in about 3% of all births. Once the membranes rupture, the fetus is at high risk for problems related to oligohydramnios, cord compression, chorioamnionitis, and abruptio placentae. Women with PROM may report that they are leaking fluid from the vagina or may have experienced a gush of fluid. Sterile speculum exam, nitrazene testing, and microscopic examination of fluid for ferning are methods to evaluate if membranes have ruptured. The decision of whether to deliver or to use expectant management must weigh the advantage of postponing delivery until gestational age increases against the risk for maternal or fetal sepsis. About 13% of pregnancies complicated with PROM develop chorioamnionitis (Ramsey et al, 2005). Signs of intrauterine infection include fever greater than 100.4° F (38.0° C), uterine tenderness, and maternal or fetal tachycardia. Results of the white blood cell count tests should be used judiciously as indicator of infection, especially if steroids have been given within the previous 5 to 7 days.

Fetal outcomes after PROM are related to gestational age at time of membrane rupture and whether the infant is delivered without complications of infection or asphyxia from cord compression or prolapse. Prior to 23 weeks' gestation, if the fetus is delivered after PROM it will not survive. As gestational age increases from 23 to 32 weeks' gestation, outcomes after PROM improve. Preterm PROM near term occurs between 32 to 36 weeks' gestation, and infants who are delivered at this time are more likely to survive if they do not have other complications. Sometimes in the absence of other indications, a wait-and-see approach might be taken where delivery is not expedited. Maternal monitoring for signs of infection (i.e., fever, uterine tenderness, maternal and fetal tachycardia) and initiation of antibiotics have been shown to prolong the interval from PROM to delivery and improve fetal outcomes. A single course of corticosteroids should be administered to the mother to promote fetal lung maturity if PROM occurs prior to 32 weeks or up to 34 weeks if fetal immaturity is suspected (Mercer, 2003). If PROM occurs at earlier gestational ages, the risk for chorioamnionitis increases. At delivery, infants of women with chorioamnionitis tend to be of younger gestational age and to weigh less than infants of women who do not have chorioamnionitis. Neonatal morbidity is increased when chorioamnionitis occurs as a complication of PROM. The use of prophylactic antibiotics given to the mother when chorioamnionitis is present does not prevent poor neonatal outcomes (Ramsey et al, 2005). However, antibiotic therapy has been demonstrated to lower the number of infants with respiratory distress syndrome, death, early sepsis, severe intraventricular hemorrhage, and severe necrotizing enterocolitis. Antibiotics also reduced the incidence of group B streptococcus sepsis, amnionitis, and pneumonia (Mercer, 2003).

Maternal Infections

Maternal infections can be transmitted to the infant in utero, during the birth process, or even during the postpartum period. Fetal infections can cause congenital anomalies, LBW,

respiratory illness after birth, or even death. Infectious agents include protozoal infections, helminthic infections, sexually transmitted infections, viruses, and bacterial organisms. Hepatitis and HIV/AIDS can be passed to the fetus during pregnancy, during the birth process, or during breastfeeding. In the United States about 280 to 370 infants a year still contract HIV from their mothers (March of Dimes, 2005b). In 2002 the CDC made the recommendation that all pregnant women be offered universal screening for HIV/AIDS because of the effectiveness of the antiretroviral medications in prevention of vertical transmission from mother to baby. A protocol that includes preconceptual HIV/AIDS testing, initiation of zidovudine (ZDV) as early as 14 weeks' gestation and throughout pregnancy, and continued administration of ZDV to the newborn for 6 weeks after birth decreases the risk of transmission to the infant by 66%. In cases where the pregnant woman in labor has not been treated during pregnancy, giving a combination of ZDV and nevirapine has been demonstrated to help reduce the risk to the baby. Delivery by cesarean section prior to rupture of membranes is recommended as another way to decrease transmission risks.

Every pregnant woman must be screened for risk factors for infection. Early identification and treatment of women with STDs or blood-borne infections will improve neonatal outcomes. Infectious conditions are discussed elsewhere in this book.

Abruptio Placentae

Abruptio placentae, or premature separation of the placenta prior to delivery, is a leading cause of stillbirth and neonatal mortality. Placental separation is thought to be due to changes in placental vasculature, thrombosis, and reduced placental perfusion. It has been speculated that there is a genetic basis for abruptio placentae that causes these changes. Placental separation occurs in several ways. In marginal separation, the edges of the placenta separate and bright red bleeding is present. Occult or hidden abruptio placentae occurs when the edges of the placenta are intact but the central part of the placenta detaches from the uterus, allowing blood loss to accumulate behind the placenta without any outward signs of bleeding. Complete abruptio placentae occurs when the placenta totally detaches, a situation that is incompatible with fetal survival. Over half of neonatal deaths complicated by abruptio placentae are because the infant was born prematurely. Infants of mothers with abruptio placentae who survive must be closely monitored for signs of blood loss and shock.

Risk factors for abruptio placentae include smoking, multiple pregnancy, and maternal age greater than 50. Increased risk in older women could be related to increased rates of chronic hypertensive disorders or aging of the uterine blood vessels. Although the risk of abruptio placentae increases with a multiple pregnancy as the number of fetuses increases from singleton to triplet pregnancies, perinatal death from abruptio placentae is higher for singletons than for multiples. IUGR might play a factor in this finding, because singleton infants delivered in abruptio placentae cases weigh less than other infants of the same gestational age, indicating IUGR. The increased stillbirth rate in singletons might be related to chronic fetal compromise, LBW, or blood loss from the abruption, whereas in multiples a different etiology could be a factor (Salihu et al, 2005).

POSTPARTUM RISK FACTORS

After birth the five leading causes of infant death are complications of congenital anomalies, complications of prematurity and LBW, SIDS, result of maternal complications, and placental-cord complications. Congenital anomalies account for most neonatal deaths in the first month of life. Infants who are LBW are more likely to die from complications of prematurity (respiratory distress, infections, or anemia), maternal complications in pregnancy, or placenta or cord conditions. In addition to these leading causes of death, other risk factors could affect the health of the neonate or cause injury such as maternal smoking or drug usage. Providing information and anticipatory guidance to the parents to increase awareness of some of these factors might be enough to protect the infant and to promote positive outcomes.

Drugs Excreted in Maternal Milk

Maternal medications taken while lactating are a concern as they may alter the milk supply or cross to the infant through the milk supply. Although many medications have been demonstrated to be safe, there are still others that have not been reported about in the literature. Psychotropic drugs pose a special concern since there has been an increase in their use. These drugs and their metabolites have long half-lives and are detectable in infant tissues and the developing brain. The long-term consequences of this exposure have not been thoroughly studied. As new drugs are placed on the market, their safety for the infant must be evaluated. Some untoward effects on the infant from use of prescribed maternal drugs include possible immune suppression; neutropenia; skin rash; central nervous system changes including irritability, restlessness, sleepiness, lethargy, or convulsions; or gastrointestinal effects such as feeding problems, vomiting, diarrhea, slow weight gain, blood in stool, jaundice, or dark urine. A comprehensive list of drugs, foods, and environmental agents that are excreted in human milk and that could be potentially harmful to neonates is available from the American Academy of Pediatrics (AAP).

The AAP Committee on Drugs (2001b) recommends that whenever drugs are prescribed for lactating women, the following factors be considered. When a medication is absolutely necessary, the baby's pediatrician and mother's physician should consult together to select the most appropriate drug for the mother with minimal effects on lactation and minimal transfer to the infant. Select the safest drug when there are several to choose from. Consider measuring the infant's blood concentration of the drug if there are potential risks from the drug for the infant. Advise the nursing mother to take the medication immediately after breastfeeding the infant or after a feeding that will be followed by an expected infant sleep period, to minimize infant drug exposure (AAP, 2001b).

Sudden Infant Death Syndrome (SIDS)

SIDS is the leading cause of death in infants after the neonatal period despite dramatic reductions in the SIDS death rate since 1992. That was the year when the American Academy of Pediatrics implemented the "Back to Sleep" campaign. Parents were encouraged to place their infants on their backs instead of prone for sleeping. This change in practice lowered the SIDS death rate by 50%, from 1.2 per 1000 live births in 1992 to 0.56 per 1000 live births in 2001 (AAP, 2005b).

Although this decrease has been a dramatic improvement, SIDS still is one of the leading causes of infant death. More than 70 causes of SIDS have been proposed. SIDS has been blamed on environmental factors such as soft bedding, overheating, entanglement in blankets, immunizations, smoke exposure, or bed sharing with parents. Genetic factors have also been blamed for findings. Prolonged QT interval has been found in up to 30% to 35% of SIDS cases. The diminished arousal response that precedes death in infants with SIDS might be explained by possible structural defects in the brain that control cardiac and respiratory function. SIDS is not always sudden; some infants have evidence of chronic hypoxia on autopsy (Burnett & Adler, 2004). In reality the cause of SIDS is most likely multifactorial. The triple risk theory proposes that multiple complex factors (including genetics, prenatal risk factors, and environmental risk factors) might make some babies more vulnerable to environmental triggering events and unable to respond to these events through usual homeostatic mechanisms (AAP, 2005b; Burnett & Adler, 2004).

Infants at risk for SIDS have many of the same risk factors seen with prematurity and LBW. Preterm or LBW infants and infants with a history of apnea are at increased risk for SIDS. The peak age at death from SIDS is between 2 to 4 months. SIDS is unusual after the age of 6 months. Ethnic disparities exist with SIDS. It is more common in African Americans and Native Americans, with death rates in black infants 2.5 times that of white infants. Maternal risk factors include young, single mothers with a history of prenatal smoking or substance abuse. Environmental risk factors for SIDS include maternal smoking, soft bedding or sleeping surfaces, thermal stress or overheating, and bed sharing with parents or siblings, especially if a bed partner consumes alcohol (AAP, 2005b; Hunt, 2005). Term infants who have had apparent life-threatening events with apnea, cyanosis, choking and gagging are at increased risk for SIDS (Burnett & Adler, 2004). No definitive link between SIDS and immunizations has been established.

Sleeping in the prone position has been highly associated with SIDS and is one reason the "Back to Sleep" campaign has been so successful in reducing SIDS death rates. The rate of SIDS increases for preterm infants who are placed in the prone position. Many parents of premature infants place their infant to sleep on their stomachs or sides once at home. It is possible that new parents are learning the practice of putting their baby in either the prone position or side-lying position by watching caregivers in the NICU. Neonatal care practices that place preterm infants in the prone or side-lying positions are providing poor role models for parents. Every time parents see their baby in a prone or side-lying position while in the hospital, they are getting reinforcement of a poor practice about how to provide care to their baby at home. Infants become habituated to the prone position for sleeping, especially if they have had a prolonged hospitalization, which makes it more difficult for parents to change the baby's sleeping position to the back-lying position (Burnett & Adler, 2004). Another concern is that about 20% of SIDS deaths occur while the infant is in the home of a child-care provider. Placing the infant in an unaccustomed prone position for sleep increases the risk for SIDS. Many child-care providers are not knowledgeable of newer recommendations for supine sleep positions. Nurses need to educate parents to share information with their childcare providers about placing the baby on the back to sleep (AAP, 2005b). Neonatal nurses must continue to educate each parent about the risk factors for SIDS and remind parents that the safest place for a baby is in its own crib in the parents' room for the first 6 months.

Child Abuse

Child abuse in infants is sometimes difficult to identify. Parents of an injured infant arrive for emergency treatment and are severely distraught and worried about their child's injuries. They often offer reasonable explanations for the injury that must be ruled out with medical tests. The victims, the babies, cannot speak for themselves to describe what happened. New parents are subject to many stressors that could trigger child abuse, such as lack of sleep, financial strain, and dealing with inconsolable infants. Health care providers have a legal and ethical duty to report cases of suspected child abuse to child protective services (Smith, 2003). Two forms of child abuse are discussed further: shaken baby syndrome and Munchausen syndrome by proxy.

Shaken baby syndrome (SBS) describes a serious form of head trauma caused by abusive shaking of an infant causing a whiplash-type injury. When the infant is shaken, the head flops back and forth, causing rapid acceleration, deceleration, and/or rotational forces of the brain within the skull, stretching, shearing, and tearing the blood vessels of the brain. Infants are more at risk for severe injury from SBS because of their weak neck muscles, proportionately large head size with soft skull and open fontanelles, and immaturity of brain development (King et al, 2003).

Several types of injuries occur with SBS. Intracranial injuries cause direct brain injury and damage to the axons. Shearing forces exerted on the veins that bridge from the dura to the brain cause intracranial bleeding. During shaking there is a lack of oxygen to the brain that is further compounded by chemical processes that occur in the damaged cells. These injuries lead to swelling of the brain and increased intracranial pressure that further compromises brain oxygenation. At least half of all SBS children also have retinal hemorrhages (Reece & Kirschner, 2005). Whereas external signs of injury to the face or head are uncommon, injuries or bruising of the long bones, thorax, or abdomen may occur as a result of firmly grasping the infant during the shaking episode (Reece, 2005).

SBS most often results when a parent becomes frustrated with an infant who is crying and inconsolable. Parents who are stressed with the parenting role, parents of premature infants, those who are sleep deprived, or parents who do not have support or help to care for their baby's needs may have low tolerance of infant crying. In frustration they may pick up the baby and shake it to try to quiet the baby. Newborns are more susceptible to the forces of shaking and may sustain injury even if not shaken as roughly as an older child. Once a parent shakes the child and gets a response, the parent might shake the child again over time, causing the infant to be injured repeatedly. Because the intracranial bleeding can be slow initially, the child might not manifest symptoms until 48 to 72 hours after the injury.

When parents seek medical attention for the infant, the history of events that preceded the infant's symptoms is often vague. The father or boyfriend is more likely to be the person responsible for the injury, and the mother may be unaware that the shaking incident occurred (King et al, 2003). Signs of SBS vary based on extent of the injury and are sometimes subtle, such as feeding difficulties, vomiting, lethargy, hypothermia, failure to thrive, and increased somnolence. More life-threatening signs include seizures, bulging fontanelle, apnea, coma, bradycardia, or complete cardiovascular collapse. Outcomes are poor for children who present with coma; approximately 60% will die. Sequelae for survivors of coma include severe neuromotor impairment, visual impairment, and developmental delay. They may require shunting for hydrocephalus. Long-term occupational therapy, physical therapy, and speech therapy will be needed to help the child achieve his or her maximum potential (Wallis & Goodman, 2000). Approximately 20% of infants might die as a result of the shaking abuse. A small percentage of children will have no outward ill effects from the shaking. The remaining children have long-term sequelae including ongoing neurologic injuries and visual impairment. A delay of 12 to 18 months might occur before symptoms are evident (King et al, 2003).

New parents need to be taught not to shake their infant at any time. Prior to discharge, time should be spent exploring parents' concerns about taking a newborn home, their sources of support, and their coping strategies under stress. Referral for stress management techniques, anger management, and provision of a parenting hotline number might help prevent this devastating injury.

Munchausen Syndrome by Proxy

Munchausen syndrome by proxy (MSBP) is a form of child abuse where a parent, usually a mother, fabricates illness in a dependent child in order to draw attention to herself as the parent of a sick child. Four criteria are required for a diagnosis: (1) A parent or guardian fabricates illness in the child; (2) the child is presented for medical care; (3) the perpetrator denies knowledge of the cause of the child's illness; and (4) the signs and symptoms subside if the child is separated from the perpetrator (Barber & Davis, 2002). The diagnosis of MSBP includes two diagnoses, one for the child and one for the parent. The parent response might range from exaggerating symptoms of the sick child to actually inducing the symptoms in the child by attempts to suffocate or poison the child. About 1200 new cases of MSBP occur each year (Schreier, 2002). Some of the most common types of fabrications include gastrointestinal (diarrhea), neurologic (seizures), infections (fevers), dermatologic (strange rashes), and cardiopulmonary (acute life-threatening events). Some children will die as a result of the parent's abuse or ministrations. Unwittingly, physicians or health care workers can be drawn into the situation, attempting to help the child based on the parent's descriptions of what is occurring. Health care professionals might prescribe unnecessary diagnostic tests or treatments for the child (Yonge & Haase, 2004). Health care professionals need increased awareness of MSBP and should question cases where children are seen constantly for parentally reported conditions not witnessed by anyone else. Cases where children who are not gaining weight begin to gain during hospitalization are also suspect. The child may need to be placed into a protective environment if the parent is approached and refuses to get psychologic help, or if the child has been subjected to a major illness because of the parent. MSBP has long-term psychologic implications for the child, and when older, the child is at risk to develop MSBP (Barber & Davis, 2002).

PERINATAL CARE IN DEVELOPING NATIONS

Pregnant women in developing nations have many of the same risk factors for prematurity and LBW as women in the United States such as poor prepregnancy physical condition, inadequate spacing between pregnancies, inadequate nutrition, low weight gain during pregnancy, maternal anemia, and lack of access for perinatal care. They also have to contend with other risk factors not even seen in the United States, such as malaria (Tucker & McGuire, 2004). Poverty and lack of education about pregnancy health are sometimes compounded by lack of skilled care providers, lack of transportation to health care centers, problems of war, civil unrest, and low status of women (USAID, 2005).

Maternal and neonatal death rates in developing nations are much higher than in the United States. Countries in sub-Saharan Africa and Asia have some of the highest rates of maternal death and neonatal death. The U.S. maternal death rate ranged from 8 to 12 per 100,000. In the same year in Africa it was 1000 per 100,000. According to the World Health Organization (WHO, 2005), each year more than 500,000 mothers worldwide die during pregnancy, and 4 million babies will die during the first 3 weeks of life; most of these are from developing nations (Mavalankar & Rosenfield, 2005). Each day 11,000 infants under the age of 4 weeks of age dies and another 11,000 are stillborn (USAID, 2005). The primary causes of neonatal death globally are estimated to be prematurity (28%), severe infection (26%), and asphyxia (23%) (Lawn et al, 2005). Many more die because of the unavailability of basic obstetric and pediatric care services.

Many neonates worldwide die from preventable conditions. Some congenital anomalies could have been prevented with maternal folic acid supplementation. Death from birth asphyxia might have been prevented with timely neonatal resuscitation at delivery. Deaths from prematurity could have been prevented with adequate prenatal care or a system of neonatal care for premature infants. Death from infections could have been prevented with immunizations, antibiotics, patient teaching about cord care, or maternal treatment for HIV during pregnancy.

Infections kill more women and babies in developing nations because basic immunization practices that are taken for granted in the United States, such as tetanus or rubella vaccination, may be unavailable to women or infants in developing countries. Tetanus, a disease that can be easily prevented, accounts for about 7% of neonatal deaths in developing nations. Tetanus develops in newborns because of unclean cord handling practices, including instrumentation and use of traditional cord salves that can cause infection. Once infected, the infant loses the ability to suck within a few days of exposure and progresses through stiffness, seizures and death (Lawn et al, 2005). Malaria is still a concern in developing nations and kills about 10,000 pregnant women and 200,000 infants each year. About 100,000 babies are born each year with congenital rubella (WHO, 2005).

Four interventions are recommended to improve birth outcomes and decrease neonatal loss in developing nations. These perinatal programs can be tailored to meet the specific needs of each country. First, antenatal care should be implemented on a local level, not only for screening for possible problems but also to educate women about how to promote a healthy pregnancy. Promoting adequate nutrition prior to pregnancy is key in many settings. Anemia is a serious problem affecting about half of pregnant women worldwide. It is more prevalent in nonindustrialized nations because of poor nutrition, iron-deficient diets, presence of parasitic disease, and incidence of HIV/AIDS. Women who are anemic are less likely to withstand blood loss during delivery and have increased risks of perinatal death, LBW, stillbirths, and prematurity (WHO, 2005). Optimal timing and spacing of pregnancy is another important part of prenatal care to promote mothers who are in the best physical condition prior to conception. Prevention and control of infection are also important during the prenatal period. Proper medical treatment of women who are infected with sexually transmitted diseases or HIV/AIDS during pregnancy will increase the infant's chances of healthy survival.

Antenatal screening alone cannot predict or prevent most problems during pregnancy or delivery; therefore the second intervention is that all pregnant women should be considered high risk and must have access to skilled birth attendants and timely emergency obstetric care. Nations with the highest rates of neonatal and maternal mortality are those that have the lowest number of births attended by a skilled birth attendant. In some countries access to medical care is difficult because of living in remote village locations, a lack of basic transportation, or poor infrastructure making it difficult to transport women or infants with problems to specialized centers. Sometime the policies of developing nations interfere with the provision of safe obstetric care. For example, some countries limit the type of health care providers who can perform cesarean sections or administer anesthesia, thereby limiting access to these services (Mavalankar & Rosenfield, 2005).

Third, basic training and equipment for infant resuscitation at birth will help prevent some of the poor birth outcomes related to birth asphyxia. Many facilities in developing nations are working with antiquated equipment as they attempt to provide care for neonates. Textbooks are often outdated or are not written in the native language of the health care provider. The American Academy of Pediatrics (AAP) Neonatal Resuscitation Program (NRP) has been demonstrated to be an effective method to provide immediate resuscitative care to neonates. This program has been translated into at least 20 languages and is being taught in other countries through formally organized courses through the AAP or by independent efforts of NRP instructors (AAP, 2005a). Countless infant lives can be saved worldwide through implementation of the neonatal resuscitation guidelines (Contributors and Reviewers, 2000). Neonatal mortality is lower when the mother has received professional care during the antenatal period and during childbirth.

The fourth recommendation is to provide postpartum care that includes parent teaching about infant care and family planning services to help prevent close interpregnancy levels. Strategies for successful breastfeeding, proper cord care, recognition of signs of illness, and promotion of psychosocial well-being are all skills that parents need to have in order to promote optimal newborn health. Women of childbearing age need to learn the importance of being in optimal physical condition prior to and during pregnancy. Family planning services will help women become empowered to make choices about when to have children and will help prevent unnecessary abortions.

There have been some inroads made to improve maternal and child health internationally. There are still many barriers for many nations, including creation of the infrastructure needed to support the WHO recommendations and training of adequate health care professionals to provide care. Some countries are beginning to see successes in reducing their maternal and infant mortality. A sustained worldwide effort is needed to continue to improve these outcomes.

SUMMARY

This chapter has presented an overview of prenatal, intrapartal, and postpartal risk factors that influence neonatal health. The perinatal nurse must be aware of potential risk factors in order to screen pregnant women and provide counseling and support. Presence of risk factors can point to an increased chance that a baby will be born with problems; however, many more babies will be born without problems even though they have mothers with risk factors. Prediction of which neonates will be at risk helps ensure that adequate personnel and equipment are available at birth to manage problems, should they occur. Patient education about modifiable risk factors and support for altering health-compromising behaviors during pregnancy can help prevent some adverse neonatal outcomes.

REFERENCES

Aliyu MH et al (2005). High parity and fetal morbidity outcomes. *Obstetrics and gynecology* 105(5):1045-1051.

American Academy of Pediatrics (AAP), Committee on Child Health Financing and Committee on Substance Abuse (2001a). Improving substance abuse prevention, assessment, and treatment financing for children and adolescents. *Pediatrics* 108(4):1025-1029.

American Academy of Pediatrics (AAP), Committee on Drugs (2001b). The transfer of drugs and other chemicals into human milk. *Pediatrics* 108:776-789.

American Academy of Pediatrics, Neonatal Resuscitation Program (2005a). *International activities: NRP Abroad.* Available at: http://www.aap.org/nrp/intl/intl_abroad.html. Retrieved November 20, 2005.

American Academy of Pediatrics (AAP), Task Force on Sudden Infant Death Syndrome (2005b). The changing concept of sudden infant death syndrome: diagnostic coding shifts, controversies regarding the sleeping environment, and new variables to consider in reducing risk. *Pediatrics* 116(5):1245-1255.

American College of Obstetricians and Gynecologists (ACOG) Committee on Practice (2004). Management of postterm pregnancy. ACOG practice bulletin: Clinical management guidelines for obstetrician-gynecologists. No. 55. *Obstetrics and gynecology* 104(3):639-646.

American Diabetes Association (ADA) (2005). Standards of medical care. *Diabetes care* 28:S4-S36.

Ananth C et al (1996). Effect of maternal age and parity on the risk of uteroplacental bleeding disorders in pregnancy. *Obstetrics and gynecology* 88(4 part 1):511-516.

Andersen A et al (2000). Maternal age and fetal loss: population based register linkage study. *British medical journal* 320(7251):1708-1712.

Barber M, Davis P (2002). Fits, faints, or fatal fantasy? Fabricated seizures and child abuse. *Archives of disease in childhood* 86:230-233.

Barton C et al (2002). Mild gestational hypertension: differences in ethnicity are associated with altered outcomes in women who undergo outpatient treatment. *American journal of obstetrics and gynecology* 186(5):896-898.

Barton J et al (2001). Mild gestational hypertension remote from term: progression and outcome. *American journal of obstetrics and gynecology* 184(5):979-983.

Bernasko J (2004). Contemporary management of type 1 diabetes mellitus in pregnancy. *Obstetrical and gynecological survey* 59(8):628-636.

Brady T et al (2003). Maternal drug use and the timing of prenatal care. *Journal of health care for the poor and underserved* 14(4):588-607.

Buchbinder A et al (2002). Adverse perinatal outcomes are significantly higher in severe gestational hypertension than in mild preeclampsia. *American journal of obstetrics and gynecology* 186(1):66-71.

Burnett L, Adler J (2004). *Pediatrics: sudden infant death syndrome.* E-Medicine. Available at: http://www.emedicine.com/emerg/topic407.htm#section~author_information. Retrieved October 24, 2005.

Caughey A et al (2005). Neonatal complications of term pregnancy: rates by gestational age increase in a continuous not threshold fashion. *American journal of obstetrics and gynecology* 192:185-190.

Chiriboga C (2003). Fetal alcohol and drug effects. *Neurologist* 9(6):267-279.

Chung J et al (2003). Ethnic differences in birth weight by gestational age: at least a partial explanation for the Hispanic epidemiologic paradox? *American journal of obstetrics and gynecology* 189(4):1058-1062.

Cleary-Goldman J et al (2005). Impact of maternal age on obstetric outcome. *Obstetrics and gynecology* 105(5):983-990.

Contributors and Reviewers for the Neonatal Resuscitation Guidelines (2000). International guidelines for neonatal resuscitation: an excerpt from the guidelines 2000 for cardiopulmonary resuscitation and emergency cardiovascular care: international consensus on science. *Pediatrics* 106(3):e29. Available at: http://pediatrics.aappublications.org/cgi/content/full/106/3/e29. Retrieved November 20, 2005.

Corbett RW et al (2003). Pica in pregnancy: does it affect pregnancy outcomes? *MCN: American journal of maternal child nursing* 28(3):183-191.

Cuevas K et al (2005). The cost of prematurity: hospital charges at birth and frequency of rehospitalizations and acute care visits over the first year of life: a comparison by gestational age and birth weight. *American journal of nursing* 105(7):56-64.

de la Rochebrochard E, Thonneau P (2002). Paternal age and maternal age are risk factors for miscarriage; results of a multicentre European study. *Human reproduction* 17(6):1649-1656.

Edwards JE (2005). Pregnancy after bariatric surgery. *Lifelines* 9(5):388-393.

Fraser AM et al (1995). Association of young maternal age with adverse reproductive outcomes. *New England journal of medicine* 332(17):1113-1118.

Fuentes-Afflick E, Hessol NA (2000). Interpregnancy interval and the risk of premature infants. *Obstetrics and gynecology* 95(3):383-390.

Garcia-Algar O et al (2005). Prenatal exposure to arecoline (areca nut alkaloid) and birth outcomes. *Archives of disease in childhood: fetal and neonatal edition* 90(3):F276-F277.

Gennaro S (2005). Overview of current state of research on pregnancy outcomes in minority populations. *American journal of obstetrics and gynecology* 192(5 Suppl):S3-S10.

Geronimus A (1992). The weathering hypothesis and the health of African-American women and infants: evidence and speculations. *Ethnicity and disease* 2(3):207-221.

Geronimus A (1996). Black/White differences in the relationship of maternal age to birthweight: a population-based test of the weathering hypothesis. *Social science and medicine* 43(4):589-597.

Getahun D et al (2005). Adverse perinatal outcomes among interracial couples in the United States. *Obstetrics and gynecology* 106(1):81-88.

Gould J et al (2003). Perinatal outcomes in two dissimilar immigrant populations in the United States: a dual epidemiologic paradox. *Pediatrics* 111(6):676-682.

Gouveia N et al (2004). Association between ambient air pollution and birth weight in São Paulo, Brazil. *Journal of epidemiology and community health* 58(1):11-17.

Green N (2004). Risks of birth defects and other adverse outcomes associated with assisted reproductive technology. *Pediatrics* 114(1):256-259.

Haas J et al (2005). Prepregnancy health status and the risk of preterm delivery. *Archives of pediatric and adolescent medicine* 159(1):58-63.

Harper T et al (2005). Fetal growth restriction. E-Medicine. Available at: http://www.emedicine.com/med/topic3247.htm. Retrieved October 5, 2005.

Heffner LJ (2004). Advanced maternal age—how old is too old? *New England journal of medicine* 351(19):1927-1929.

Hogue CR, Bremner JD (2005). Stress model for research into preterm delivery among black women. *American journal of obstetrics and gynecology* 192(5 suppl):S47-S55.

Hook E, Lindsjo A (1978). Down syndrome in live births by single year maternal age interval in a Swedish study: comparison with results from a New York State study. *American journal of human genetics* 30(1):19-27.

Hunt CE (2005). Gene-environment interactions: implications for sudden unexpected deaths in infancy. *Archives of disease in childhood* 90(1):48-53.

King W et al (2003). Shaken baby syndrome in Canada: clinical characteristics and outcomes of hospital cases. *Canadian Medical Association journal* 168(2):155-159.

Kochanek K et al (October 2004). *National vital statistics reports, deaths: final data for 2002.* CDC. Available at: http://www.cdc.gov/nchs/data/nvsr/nvsr53/nvsr53_05.pdf. Retrieved October 7, 2005.

Kouba S et al (2005). Pregnancy and neonatal outcomes in women with eating disorders. *Obstetrics and gynecology* 105(2):255-260.

Kristensen J et al (2005). Pre-pregnancy weight and the risk of stillbirth and neonatal death. *BJOG: international journal of obstetrics and gynaecology* 112(4):403-408.

Langer O et al (2005). Gestational diabetes: the consequences of not treating. *American journal of obstetrics and gynecology* 192(4):989-997.

Lawn J et al (2005). 4 million neonatal deaths: when? where? why? *Lancet* 365(9474):1845.

MacDorman M et al (2005). Explaining the 2001–2002 infant mortality increase: data from the linked birth/infant death data set. *National vital statistics reports* 53(12). Hyattsville, MD: National Center for Health Statistics.

MacIntosh G et al (1995). Paternal age and the risk of birth defects in offspring. *Epidemiology* 6(6):640-641.

Macones G et al (2004). A polymorphism in the promoter region of TNF and bacterial vaginosis: preliminary evidence of gene-environment interaction in the etiology of spontaneous preterm birth. *American journal of obstetrics and gynecology* 190(6):1504-1508.

Maier S, West J (2001). Patterns and alcohol-related birth defects. *Alcohol research and health* 25(3) [Electronic version]. Available at: http://www.niaaa.nih.gov/publications/arh25-3/168-174.htm. Retrieved September 23, 2005.

March of Dimes (2005a). *Diabetes in pregnancy: professionals and researchers.* Available at: http://www.marchofdimes.com/professionals/681_1197.asp. Retrieved October 18, 2005.

March of Dimes (2005b). *HIV and AIDS in pregnancy: professionals and researchers.* Available at: http://www.marchofdimes.com/professionals/681_1223.asp. Retrieved October 1, 2005.

Mari G (2005). *Intrauterine growth retardation.* Vol 1, No 8. Hygeia Foundation. Available at: http://www.hygeia.org/poems8.htm. Retrieved September 22, 2005.

Martens P et al (2004). Predictors of hospital readmission of Manitoba newborns within six weeks postbirth discharge: a population-based study. *Pediatrics* 114(3):708-713.

Martin J et al (2005). Births: final data for 2003. *National Vital Statistics Reports* 54(2):1-116.

Maternal age risks (2001). Emory University School of Medicine. Department of Human Genetics, Division of Genetics. Available at: xhttp://www.genetics.emory.edu/pdf/Emory_Human_Genetics_Maternal_Age_Risks.PDF. Retrieved August 28, 2005.

Mavalankar DV, Rosenfield A (2005). Maternal mortality in resource-poor settings: policy barriers to care. *American journal of public health* 95(2):200-203.

Menacker F et al (November 15, 2004). Births to 10–14 year old mothers, 1990–2002: trends and health outcomes. *National Vital Statistics Reports* 53(7). CDC, Center for Vital Statistics. Available at: http://www.cdc.gov/nchs/data/nvsr/nvsr53/nvsr 53_07.pdf. Retrieved September 3, 2005.

Mercer B (2003). Preterm premature rupture of the membranes. *Obstetrics and gynecology* 101(1):178-193.

Morantz C, Torrey B (2004). Practice guideline briefs: management of postterm pregnancy. *American family physician* 70(9) [electronic version]. Available at: http://www.aafp.org/afp/20041101/practice.html. Retrieved November 22, 2005.

National Center for Health Statistics—National Vital Statistics System (2005). *Chartbook on trends in the health of Americans: fetal deaths.* U.S. Department of Health and Human Services. Available at: http://www.cdc.gov/nchs/about/major/fetaldth/abfetal.htm. Retrieved October 25, 2005.

National Heart Lung and Blood Institute (2000). *National high blood pressure education program: working group report on high blood pressure in pregnancy.* National Guideline Clearinghouse. Available at: http://www.guideline.gov/summary/summary.aspx?doc_id=1478. Retrieved on October 30, 2005.

Okah F et al (2005). Term-gestation low birth weight and health-compromising behaviors during pregnancy. *Obstetrics and gynecology* 105(3):543-550.

Patrick T, Bryan T (2005). Research strategies for optimizing pregnancy outcomes in minority populations. *American journal of obstetrics and gynecology* 192:S64-S70.

Ramsey P et al (2005). Chorioamnionitis increases neonatal morbidity in pregnancies complicated by preterm premature rupture of membranes. *American journal of obstetrics and gynecology* 192:1162-1166.

Reece R (2005). *What the literature tells us about rib fractures in infancy.* National Center on Shaken Baby Syndrome. Available at: http://www.dontshake.com. Retrieved October 7, 2005.

Reece R, Kirschner R (2005). *Shaken baby syndrome/shaken impact syndrome.* National Center on Shaken Baby Syndrome. Available at: http://www.dontshake.com/Audience.aspx?categoryID=8&PageName=SBS_SIS.htm. Retrieved October 7, 2005.

Regidor E et al (2004). Paternal exposure to agricultural pesticides and cause specific fetal death. *Occupational and environmental medicine* 61(4):334-339.

Reichman N, Teitler J (2003). Effects of psychosocial risk factors and prenatal interventions on birthweight: evidence from New Jersey's HealthStart program. *Perspectives on sexual and reproductive health* 35(3):130-137.

Rich-Edwards JW, Grizzard TA (2005). Psychosocial stress and neuroendocrine mechanisms in preterm delivery. *American journal of obstetrics and gynecology* 192(5 suppl):S30-S35.

Rich-Edwards JW et al (2003). Diverging associations of maternal age with low birthweight for black and white mothers. *International journal of epidemiology* 32(1):83-90.

Salihu H et al (2003). Childbearing beyond maternal age 50 and fetal outcomes in the United States. *Obstetrics and gynecology* 102:1006-1014.

Salihu H et al (2005). Perinatal mortality associated with abruptio placenta in singletons and multiples. *American journal of obstetrics and gynecology* 193(1):198-203.

Schaefer-Graf U et al (2000). Patterns of congenital anomalies and relationship to initial maternal fasting glucose levels in pregnancies complicated by type 2 and gestational diabetes. *American journal of obstetrics and gynecology* 182(2):313-320.

Scholl TO, Reilly T (2000). Anemia, iron and pregnancy outcome. *Journal of nutrition* 130:S443-S447.

Schreier H (2002). Munchausen by proxy defined. *Pediatrics* 110(5):985-988.

Seely E, Solomon C (2003). Insulin resistance and its potential role in pregnancy-induced hypertension. *Journal of clinical endocrinology and metabolism* 88(6):2393-2398.

Silbergeld E, Patrick T (2005). Environmental exposures, toxicologic mechanisms, and adverse pregnancy outcomes. *American journal of obstetrics and gynecology* 192(5 suppl):S11-S21.

Smith J (2003). Shaken baby syndrome. *Orthopaedic nursing* 22(3):196-203.

Steward D, Moser D (2004). Intrauterine growth retardation in full-term newborn infants with birth weights greater than 2,500 g. *Research in nursing and health* 27(6):403-412.

Tekesin I et al (2005). Assessment of rapid fetal fibronectin in predicting preterm delivery. *Obstetrics and gynecology* 105(2):280-284.

Tucker J, McGuire W (2004). Epidemiology of preterm birth. *British medical journal* 329(7467):675-678.

US Food and Drug Administration (2005). Food safety for moms-to-be. Available at: http://www.cfsan.fda.gov/~pregnant/pregnant.html. Retrieved November 1, 2006.

USAID (2005). *Saving the lives of women and children.* Maternal and Child Health. Available at: http://www.usaid.gov/our_work/global_health/mch/mh/index.html. Retrieved October 15, 2005.

Vintzileos A et al (2002). The impact of prenatal care on postneonatal deaths in the presence and absence of antenatal high-risk conditions. *American journal of obstetrics and gynecology* 187(5):1258-1262.

Wallis W, Goodman G (2000). Neurotrauma in infants: shaken impact syndrome (inflicted head injury). *Critical care nursing clinics of North America* 12(4):489-498.

Wilson-Costello D et al (2005). Improved survival rates with increased neurodevelopmental disability for extremely low birth weight infants in the 1990s. *Pediatrics* 115(4):997-1003.

World Health Organization (WHO) (2005). *The world health report 2005—make every mother and child count.* Available at: http://www.who.int/whr/2005/whr2005_en.pdf. Retrieved October 20, 2005.

Yonge O, Haase M (2004). Munchausen syndrome and Munchausen syndrome by proxy in a student nurse. *Nurse educator* 29(4):166-169.

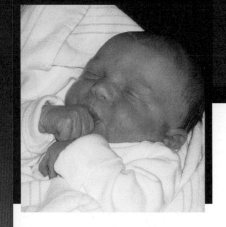

Chapter 38

Resuscitation and Stabilization of the Newborn and Infant

Gail A. Bagwell

The vulnerable and sick infant requires the health professional to quickly assess and take action when signs of cardiac or respiratory depression are present. This chapter begins with a discussion of risk factors that predispose the newborn to cardiorespiratory depression. The remainder of the content describes the actions taken to avoid this depression or to alleviate the symptoms and reverse a downward spiral.

CAUSES OF CARDIORESPIRATORY DEPRESSION IN THE NEWBORN

The combined effects of numerous maternal, fetal, and intrauterine factors determine the condition of an infant at birth (some of these factors are listed in Table 38-1). Although some of these factors emerge only during labor and delivery (e.g., cord prolapse), most arise during gestation (e.g., placenta previa) or even before conception (e.g., maternal diabetes). Regardless of the site or time of origin, the influence of each of these problems can become manifest as cardiorespiratory depression in the newborn.

To provide effective care, the nurse must be able not only to recognize potential risk factors but also to understand the ways in which they disrupt cardiorespiratory function. Ideally, the health professional determines that cardiorespiratory depression may occur and is thoroughly prepared to intervene. Although many risk factors come into play, the underlying pathogenic processes can be divided into six major categories. The mnemonic TAMMSS can be used as a simple but effective means of remembering these etiologic groups:

- **T** Trauma
- **A** Asphyxia (intrauterine)
- **M** Medication
- **M** Malformation
- **S** Sepsis
- **S** Shock (hypovolemia)

Trauma

Traumatic injury to the central or peripheral nervous system is an uncommon occurrence that can result in immediate or delayed respiratory depression. Because the skull is incompletely mineralized and has open sutures, it can undergo considerable distortion without fracture. However, the underlying membranes and vessels are much less resilient and are easily stretched or torn if overly compressed, particularly if the pressure is abruptly applied. Similarly, forced traction or torsion of the neck during delivery may damage the spinal cord or the phrenic nerve, with con-sequent paralysis of the diaphragm. An unusually long and difficult labor, a precipitous delivery, multiple gestation, abnormal presentation (especially breech), cephalopelvic disproportion (secondary to macrosomia or a small or contracted pelvis), shoulder dystocia, or rapid extraction by forceps (as may be required for fetal distress) frequently is involved. Despite their generally low birth weight, premature infants also may be at risk because of the unusual compliance of their skulls.

Asphyxia (Intrauterine)

The most common cause of cardiorespiratory depression at birth is fetal hypoxia and asphyxia. Any condition that reduces oxygen delivery to the fetus may be the cause. Such conditions include maternal hypoxia (from hypoventilation or hyperventilation, respiratory or heart disease, anemia, postural hypotension); maternal vascular disease that results in placental insufficiency (from pre-existing or pregnancy-induced diabetes, primary or pregnancy-induced hypertension); and accidents involving the umbilical cord (compression, entanglement, or prolapse). Postterm pregnancies also are at risk, perhaps because of placental aging and progressive placental insufficiency. An asphyxial episode occasionally may trigger the passage and aspiration of meconium in utero.

Medication

Pharmacologic agents given to the mother during labor and delivery as well as any medications or herbs taken by the mother prior to the delivery of the neonate may affect the fetus both directly and indirectly. Indirectly, these agents may cause maternal hypoventilation and hypotension or adversely affect placental perfusion. Hypnotic, analgesic, or anesthetic drugs may depress maternal respirations, resulting in reduced oxygen intake and delivery to the tissues and organs, including the uterus and placenta. Anesthetic agents, because of their effect on the sympathetic nervous system, may also cause peripheral vasodilatation, diminished cardiac output, and hypotension with decreased placental perfusion. Narcotic analgesics, which rapidly cross the placenta, may directly depress neonatal respiratory drive. Oxytocin (Pitocin), on the other hand, may cause uterine hyperstimulation and shorten placental perfusion time. Each of these conditions places the fetus at greater risk of fetal hypoxia and asphyxia. In addition, medications and herbs that the mother may take prior to delivery may also affect the fetus. Many street drugs, especially opiate derivatives, are known to cause infants to be depressed on delivery.

TABLE 38-1	Conditions Associated with Asphyxiation of Newborns
Source of Problem	**Conditions**
Maternal	Amnionitis, anemia, diabetes mellitus, pregnancy-induced hypertension, heart disease, hypotension, respiratory disease, maternal genetic cause, drugs, infection, maternal deformities
Uterine	Preterm labor, prolonged labor, multiple pregnancies, abnormal fetal presentation
Placental	Placenta previa, abruptio placentae, placental insufficiency, postterm pregnancy
Umbilical	Cord prolapse, entanglement, or compression
Fetal	Cephalopelvic disproportion, congenital abnormalities, erythroblastosis fetalis, intrauterine infection Iatrogenic causes: Mechanical (difficult forceps delivery) Drugs

Malformation

Infants may have any of a vast array of congenital anomalies, but the ones that cause the most concern during the first few minutes of life are those with associated facial or upper airway deformities and conditions that lead to pulmonary hypoplasia. Many of these conditions can be diagnosed through antenatal ultrasonographic examinations and other screening techniques, but suspicion also should be raised if oligohydramnios or polyhydramnios is reported.

Oligohydramnios is seen with prolonged rupture or leakage of membranes and in infants with renal agenesis or dysplasia or urethral obstruction. If fluid is lost or diminished, the developing fetal structures may be compressed, leading to characteristic Potter facies (including micrognathia) or pulmonary hypoplasia. Polyhydramnios is seen in infants with impaired swallowing ability (as in anencephaly and neuromuscular disorders); in those with real or functional obstruction high in the gastrointestinal tract (as with esophageal atresia); and in those with profuse leakage of cerebrospinal fluid (as in neural tube defects), which contributes to the volume of amniotic fluid. Polyhydramnios is also noted with diaphragmatic hernia and hydrops fetalis.

Sepsis

The fetus may acquire bacterial or viral agents from infected amniotic fluid, from maternal blood crossing the placenta, or by direct contact on passage through the birth canal. An infant is especially susceptible to infection if born prematurely (because these infants are relatively immunocompromised) or if born to a mother who had a premature rupture of membranes or a history of infection or chorioamnionitis. If infection is acquired in utero, the lungs tend to be heavily involved, and the alveoli may be filled with exudate. The infant may be apneic at birth, may be slow to establish a spontaneous and regular breathing pattern, or may show frank signs of respiratory distress.

Shock (Hypovolemia)

Most of the blood lost during delivery is from the maternal side of the placenta and therefore is of no consequence to the newborn. However, blood loss from the fetal side of the placenta as a result of abruptio placentae or placenta previa can lead to acute hypovolemia and cardiovascular collapse. Normally the umbilical cord is unusually strong, but ruptures are possible if cord tension increases suddenly, as in a precipitous delivery, or if the vessels are superficially implanted in the placenta (velamentous insertions). In rare cases acute hypovolemia may occur without frank hemorrhage. With severe cord compression, for example, blood flow to the fetus is impeded. The umbilical arteries, however, are much more resistant to compression and continue to pump blood back to the placenta. In this case, the effects of hypovolemia and asphyxia may be superimposed. Infants with chronic blood loss (as in fetal-to-maternal hemorrhage or twin-to-twin transfusions) generally are asymptomatic immediately after delivery.

PREPARATION FOR DELIVERY

The success of resuscitative efforts depends on three factors: (1) anticipation of the need, (2) the presence of trained personnel, and (3) ready availability of necessary equipment and supplies. The most competent personnel and the finest equipment are useless if they are not present in the delivery room. Frantic calls for assistance or a scavenger hunt for equipment should never occur; they needlessly delay intervention and can compromise the patient's outcome.

Anticipation

The antepartum and intrapartum history of each pregnant woman must be carefully reviewed to identify those at risk of delivering a depressed infant. Especially worrisome is a fetus that clinically demonstrates the effects of asphyxia (i.e., a nonreassuring fetal heart rate pattern, particularly bradycardia and loss of beat-to-beat variability; acidosis, as determined by fetal scalp blood sampling; or meconium-stained amniotic fluid).

Personnel

Although most risk factors can be identified at some time during the pregnancy, many may not become apparent until birth. Delivery through meconium-stained amniotic fluid and unexpected diaphragmatic hernia are just two cases in point. Consequently, at least one person competent in neonatal resuscitation should be present at every delivery. Obviously, additional personnel should be made available if a depressed newborn is expected (Bloom & Cropley, 1994; Kattwinkel, 2006).

When a team is required, the role each member is to play in the resuscitative effort should be predetermined. The head of the team generally is the person who will establish and maintain the airway, the one responsible for ventilation and intubation. A second person is responsible for monitoring the heart rate and for initiating chest compressions if needed. If intravenous (IV) medications are required, two additional individuals are needed, one to catheterize the umbilical cord and administer the drugs and the other to pass equipment and prepare the medications. The person who passes equipment and prepares the medications may also be responsible for documenting the resuscitation process, but a fifth person is preferable for this because minute-to-minute notations must be made. The individual delivering the baby is not considered part of this resuscitative team.

Equipment and Supplies

A newly born infant is predisposed to heat loss (particularly evaporative and radiant losses) and, if unprotected, can quickly become cold stressed. The consequences of such stress include hypoxemia, metabolic acidosis, and rapid depletion of glycogen stores with hypoglycemia. All are conditions that may exacerbate asphyxia and thus complicate resuscitation. Clearly, measures to prevent hypothermia must be part of any resuscitative effort. The delivery room should be kept warm, and the radiant bed should be preheated if possible. Prewarming of linens, towels, and caps or other head coverings also is helpful. For extremely premature babies less than 28 weeks' gestation, the use of a food-grade polyethylene bag has been found to be helpful in maintaining the infant's body temperature in the delivery room (Kattwinkel, 2006).

Possible exposure to blood and body fluids is of particular concern in the delivery room. Gloves, gowns, masks, and protective eyewear should be worn during procedures that are likely to generate droplets or splashes of blood or other body fluids (Kattwinkel, 2006).

The additional equipment and supplies needed to carry out a full resuscitation (Box 38-1) should be checked as a part of the daily routine. Small supplies should be organized according to frequency of use and may be displayed on a wall board kept in the radiant warmer (if there is sufficient drawer space) or stored in a cart or specially designed tackle box. Breakaway security clips may be used to safeguard materials when they are not in use, but foolproof or locking closures that require a key are not appropriate in delivery rooms, birthing rooms, or nurseries. A bedside table or flat surface (other than the bed) should be within reach to provide space for catheter trays and medication preparation.

As the delivery nears, the team should double-check all supplies and make sure the equipment is in working order. Hospital infection control policies dictate how far in advance packaged supplies can be opened, connected to tubing, and otherwise prepared. A backup or duplicate set of materials should be maintained in case of equipment failure, contamination, or multiple births. All items used should be restocked as soon as possible after resuscitation.

GENERAL CONSIDERATIONS

The two goals of resuscitation are (1) to remove or ameliorate the underlying cause of asphyxia and (2) to reverse or correct

---

BOX 38-1

Equipment and Supplies Needed for Full Resuscitation

Suction Equipment
Bulb syringe
Mechanical suction device and tubing
Suction catheters (5 or 6 French, 8 French, 10 French, or 12 French)
8 French feeding tube and 20-ml syringe
Meconium aspirator

Bag and Mask Equipment
Self-inflating bag *or* flow-inflating bag with pressure manometer and oxygen source
Face masks, newborn and premature sizes (cushioned rim masks preferred)
Oxygen with flowmeter (flow rate up to 10 L/min) and tubing

Intubation Equipment
Laryngoscope with fresh batteries and functioning light source
Straight blades—No. 0 (preterm) and No. 1 (term)
Extra bulbs and batteries for laryngoscope
Endotracheal tubes—2.5, 3, 3.5, and 4 mm internal diameter
Stylet (optional)
Scissors
Tape or securing device for endotracheal tube
Alcohol sponges
CO_2 detector

Medications
Epinephrine 1:10,000 (3-ml or 10-ml ampules)
Isotonic crystalloid (normal saline or Ringer's lactate) for volume expansion

Sodium bicarbonate 4.2% (5 mEq/10 ml, 10-ml ampules)
Naloxone hydrochloride (0.4 mg/ml, 1-ml ampules; or 1 mg/ml, 2-ml ampules)
Dextrose 10% (250 ml)
Normal saline (for flushes)
Feeding tube, 5 French (optional)

Umbilical Vessel Catheterization Supplies
Sterile gloves
Scalpel or scissors
Povidone-iodine solution
Umbilical tape
Umbilical catheters—3.5 French, 5 French
Three-way stopcock
Syringes—1, 3, 5, 10, 20, 50 ml
Needles—25, 21, 18 gauge—or puncture device for needleless system
Tape or method to secure catheter
Paper tape measure (optional)

Miscellaneous
Gloves and appropriate personal protection
Radiant warmer or other heat source
Firm, padded resuscitation surface
Shoulder roll
Clock with second hand (timer optional)
Warmed linens
Stethoscope (neonatal head preferred)
Cardiac monitor and electrodes or pulse oximeter and probe (optional for delivery room)
Oropharyngeal airways—0, 00, 000 sizes or 30, 40, and 50 mm lengths

---

Adapted from Kattwinkel J, editor (2006). *Textbook of neonatal resuscitation*, ed 5 (Lesson 5: Endotracheal Intubation). Elk Grove Village, IL: American Academy of Pediatrics and American Heart Association.

the associated chain of events (hypoxia, hypercarbia, acidosis, bradycardia, and hypotension). To achieve these ends, resuscitation management should be centered on attempts to expand, ventilate, and oxygenate the lungs, with cardiac assistance provided as necessary. However, intervention must be specific to each infant in extent and form and must be determined by appropriate assessment.

The Apgar score provides a shorthand description of the infant's condition at specific intervals after birth and may be useful as a rough prognostic indicator of long-term outcome; however, it does have limitations. Although it is a quantitative tool, the scoring often is subjectively or retrospectively applied. It often is poorly correlated with other indicators of well-being, such as cord pH. Its usefulness is suspect with extremely preterm infants who may have poor respiratory drive and who may be relatively hyporeflexive and hypotonic because of immaturity rather than distress. Finally, waiting until the first Apgar score is assigned at 1 minute of age causes unnecessary delay in care. For these reasons, the Apgar score should not be used to determine the need for or course of resuscitation (Bloom & Cropley, 1994; Kattwinkel, 2006).

The initiation and progression of resuscitation are based on three signs: respiratory effort, heart rate, and color. As soon as the infant has been positioned under a radiant warmer, thoroughly dried, and suctioned, these signs are assessed at 30-second intervals and interventions are carried out as needed.

The basics of neonatal resuscitation are as easy as ABC: airway, breathing, and circulation. These are the critical elements of any resuscitative effort.

Airway Control
Positioning
Airway control is a fundamental prerequisite for effective oxygenation and ventilation. To achieve this, the infant should be placed in a flat supine position. The practice of placing the infant in a slight head-down tilt (Trendelenburg position) has been abandoned. This maneuver historically was used under the presumption that fluids from the lower extremities would be redistributed to the intrathoracic compartment. Studies with healthy adults in the Trendelenburg position have demonstrated improvement, albeit transient (lasting <10 minutes), in the stroke volume of the heart, but they have also indicated that a tilt as slight as 10 degrees may cause blood to pool in the dependent cerebrovascular bed. Infants have only a limited ability to increase stroke volume but are at greater risk than older children or adults for intraventricular hemorrhage secondary to rupture of the vulnerable microvessels of the germinal matrix; consequently, the potential benefit, if any, of the head-down tilt position is not believed to be worth the risk.

Once the infant is in the supine position, the neck is placed in a neutral or slightly extended "sniff" position (Bloom & Cropley, 1994; Kattwinkel, 2006). Compared with the adult tongue, an infant's tongue is relatively large in proportion to the mouth, and this slight extension moves the tongue and epiglottis away from the posterior pharyngeal wall and opens the airway. Care must be taken to avoid full extension, however, which reduces the circumference of the airway and increases airway resistance. The reasonably safe extension posture appears to be no more than 15 to 30 degrees from neutral (Reiterer et al, 1994). An oral airway should be placed if the tongue is unusually large (as in Beckwith-Wiedemann syndrome) or if the chin is unusually small, causing posterior dis-

placement of the tongue (as in Pierre Robin sequence or Potter association). Because newborns also have a relatively large head in comparison with the chest and tend naturally to fall into a flexed position, a shoulder roll, $\frac{3}{4}$ to 1 inch thick, may be used to raise the chest and align the cervical vertebrae. This roll may be particularly helpful if the occiput is exaggerated in size by molding or edema. If these procedures fail to provide an unobstructed airway, intubation is indicated (Bloom & Cropley, 1994).

Suctioning
If time permits, the mouth, nose, and posterior pharynx should be suctioned while the head is on the perineum before the thorax has been delivered. After delivery the infant is placed on the warming bed and quickly dried and positioned, and the airway is more thoroughly cleared with a bulb syringe. Because suctioning may cause inadvertent stimulation and gasping, the mouth should always be suctioned before the nose. Mechanical suction often is mentioned as an alternative to the bulb syringe, but it generally should not be used immediately after delivery. If infants are suctioned vigorously within the first 5 minutes of life, apnea or arrhythmias may follow. These symptoms probably are due to vagal stimulation, with reflex bradycardia. If a bulb syringe can be used instead of a suction catheter, this situation usually can be avoided. If mechanical suction is required (i.e., for meconium removal), it should be applied for no longer than 5 seconds at a time with an 8 or 10 French suction catheter and with the equipment set to produce no more than 100 mm Hg (136 cm H_2O) negative pressure (Bloom & Cropley, 1994).

If meconium is present in the amniotic fluid, the first step is to suction the nasohypopharynx with a bulb syringe or a 10 or 12 French suction catheter as soon as the head is delivered and before the shoulders appear. Endotracheal (ET) suctioning may be needed for the most thorough clearing of the airway if the infant is depressed or not vigorous (Niermeyer & Keenan, 2001). This suctioning is performed before the infant is dried or otherwise stimulated and is conducted under laryngoscopy with suction directly applied to the trachea, with the ET tube used as a suction catheter. There is some controversy over the benefit of ET suctioning if the infant is vigorous and the meconium is thin; however, suctioning generally is recommended if the infant is depressed (heart rate below 100 beats/min and the infant is not vigorous) or the meconium is thick or particulate. The suction is applied as the ET tube is slowly withdrawn, and the procedure is repeated as needed until the meconium has been cleared. Techniques involving mouth suction should not be used because of the risk of exposure of personnel to blood and other body fluids. Also, passing a suction catheter through the ET tube or directly intubating the trachea with a suction catheter is an inadequate substitute for the ET tube, because the small bore of these catheters is easily clogged with the thick, tenacious meconium (Bloom & Cropley, 1994).

Tactile Stimulation
In a mildly depressed infant, drying and suctioning generally produce enough stimulation to induce effective respirations. If the respiratory rate and depth are nevertheless diminished, rubbing the spine or flicking or slapping the soles of the feet can briefly stimulate the infant. If the infant's reflexes are intact, 10 to 15 seconds of stimulation should be sufficient to

elicit a response. Longer and more vigorous methods of stimulation should be avoided (Bloom & Cropley, 1994).

OXYGENATION AND VENTILATION

Oxygenation and ventilation are the mainstays of neonatal resuscitation. In fact, most infants who require resuscitation can be revived with oxygen and ventilation alone. Even when more aggressive therapies are required, they ultimately are undertaken to support oxygen delivery to the tissues, either by optimizing the airway (i.e., intubation) or by supporting the "pump" that "pushes" oxygen to the periphery (i.e., chest compressions, medications). Early administration of 100% oxygen is critical and may be accomplished by several techniques. The risks associated with oxygen excess should not be a concern during the brief period required for resuscitation.

Free-Flow Administration of Oxygen

An infant who is breathing spontaneously, but fails to become pink in room air, needs supplemental oxygen. The oxygen can be provided directly from the end of the oxygen tube held in a cupped hand, by a funnel or face mask attached to the tubing, or by a flow-inflating ventilation bag. The flow should be set to deliver at least 5 L/min, and the tubing, funnel, or mask should be held close to the infant's face to maximize the inhaled concentration (Bloom & Cropley, 1994).

Ventilation

If the infant fails to become pink with free-flow oxygen or shows other signs of cardiorespiratory decompensation (apnea or gasping respirations or a heart rate below 100 beats/min), positive-pressure ventilation should be instituted. The initial breaths generally require pressures of 30 to 40 cm H_2O to inflate the lungs. Pressures for succeeding breaths vary with the infant's condition. A ventilation rate of 40 to 60 breaths/min should be used.

Ventilation Bags

Two types of ventilation bags are available for neonatal use, the self-inflating bag and the flow-inflating bag. Self-inflating bags do not require gas flow but do require a reservoir to deliver high concentrations of oxygen. Traditionally these bags have been fitted with a pressure-release "popoff" valve preset at 30 to 40 cm H_2O to prevent overinflation of the lungs and the risk of pneumothorax. Most self-inflating bags must be squeezed to move gas through the circuit and may not be capable of passive, free-flow oxygen delivery.

Flow-inflating bags, on the other hand, are closed systems and therefore must be connected to a compressed gas source. Although self-inflating bags have the advantages of being both easy to operate and gas flow independent, flow-inflating bags provide more reliable oxygen concentrations (particularly at low flow rates), better control of inspiratory times, and a greater range of peak inspiratory pressures, as well as providing free-flow oxygen.

Both types of bags can be used to provide ventilation by mask or ET tube as well as be equipped with a manometer to monitor airway pressure. Though a manometer is important, visualization of the chest is equally if not more important. The degree of chest rise should simulate that seen when a normal newborn takes an easy breath. Excessive chest rise reflects overzealous delivery of tidal volume; if there is no movement, delivery is inadequate. A self-inflating or flow-inflating bag

that has a regulatory valve with a maximum volume of 750 ml should be more than sufficient to deliver the normal tidal volume of 20 to 30 ml for the average newborn (Bloom & Cropley, 1994; Niermeyer & Keenan, 2001).

Methods of Ventilation

For mask ventilation, a face mask is used to provide an oxygen-enriched "microenvironment." An anatomically shaped mask with a cushioned rim is preferred for this purpose. Because masks are available in a variety of sizes, care must be taken to select one that covers the tip of the chin, the mouth, and the nose but not the eyes. Mask ventilation is a simple, noninvasive method of oxygen delivery that can be initiated without delay, but use of a mask has disadvantages. First, it may be difficult to obtain and maintain a good seal between the mask and the infant's face, particularly around the nose. Any leakage of air results in underventilation, which is aggravated if low lung compliance or high airway resistance is a factor. The seal should be "airtight" without excessive pressure applied. Second, the mask itself has a considerable amount of dead space. Consequently, a sufficient tidal volume must be delivered to prevent accumulation and rebreathing of carbon dioxide. Masks used for neonatal resuscitation ideally should have a dead space of less than 5 ml. Finally, prolonged bag and mask ventilation may produce gastric distention from swallowed gas, which in turn impedes diaphragmatic excursions and places the infant at risk of regurgitation and aspiration. However, this problem can be easily avoided by inserting an 8 French orogastric tube if mask ventilation continues beyond 2 minutes. The gastric contents should be suctioned and the tube left in place as a vent as long as mask ventilation is provided (Bloom & Cropley, 1994).

Mask ventilation suffices for most infants, but if it proves ineffective (as evidenced by poor chest rise or continuing bradycardia) or if prolonged ventilation is expected, an ET tube should be inserted. Premature infants (certainly those weighing <1000 g) who have diminished lung compliance, immature respiratory musculature, and decreased respiratory drive may also benefit from early intubation (Bloom & Cropley, 1994). In research comparing outcomes for very low birth weight infants (those weighing <1500 g) who were selectively intubated at delivery or given a trial of spontaneous ventilation, the results showed that the infants who were immediately intubated had higher 5-minute Apgar scores, less acidosis, less hypoglycemia, and fewer pneumothoraces and required slower ventilatory rates.

Infants suspected of having a diaphragmatic hernia, hydrops fetalis, or certain airway or gastrointestinal abnormalities also benefit from immediate intubation. Uncuffed ET tubes with a uniform internal diameter should be used. The proper tube size and depth of insertion are determined by the infant's size by weight (Table 38-2). Most neonatal ET tubes have a black line (vocal cord guide) near the tip of the tube that serves as a guide for insertion. When this guide is placed at the level of the vocal cords, the tube should be properly positioned with its tip in the midtrachea. As an alternative, the distance from the midtrachea (tube tip) to the infant's upper lip may be estimated using the simple tip-to-lip formula:

$$\text{Weight (kg)} + 6 = \text{Tip-to-lip distance}$$

When the tube is properly situated, the centimeter marking on the side of the tube at the level of the upper lip should

TABLE **38-2**	Endotracheal Tube Size and Placement	
Infant's Weight (kg)	**Tube Size (mm)**	**Insertion Depth (cm)**
<1	2.5	<7
1 to 2	3	7 to 8
2 to 3	3.5	8 to 9
>3	3.5 to 4	>9

Data from the American Heart Association Emergency Cardiac Care Committee and Subcommittees (1992). Guidelines for cardiopulmonary resuscitation and emergency cardiac care. VII. Neonatal resuscitation. Journal of the American Medical Association 268:2276-2281; and Kattwinkel J, editor (2006). Textbook of neonatal resuscitation, ed 5. Elk Grove Village, IL: American Academy of Pediatrics and American Heart Association.

be at or near the tip-to-lip distance. For example, infants weighing 1 kg are intubated to a depth of 7 cm (1 + 6 = 7); those weighing 2 kg to a depth of 8 cm (2 + 6 = 8), and so on. Tubes with metallic markers or fiber-optic illumination at the tip may make it possible to determine the depth of the tube transdermally (i.e., by observing a circle of light on the skin or by hearing an audible signal from a transcutaneous locator instrument), but these modifications do not allow differentiation between ET intubation and esophageal intubation and therefore offer no advantage in an emergency situation (Heller & Heller, 1994). Similarly, capnometers used during resuscitation to measure end-tidal carbon dioxide and thus confirm tube placement in the trachea may be inaccurate when pulmonary blood flow is poor or absent (Bhende & Thompson, 1995).

Correct placement is best demonstrated by the tried and true methods: improved clinical signs (heart rate, color, and activity), symmetric chest rise, bilateral and equal breath sounds (as auscultated in the axillae), and fogging of the tube on exhalation. Air should not be heard entering the stomach, and the abdomen should not be distended. If any doubts exist, tube placement can be checked by repeated laryngoscopy; the tube should be clearly seen passing through the glottic opening (Bloom & Cropley, 1994).

ET intubation is the definitive technique for airway management and ventilation. However, agility and accuracy in placement require continual practice. Also, many hospital personnel are restricted by policy or statute from learning or using this skill. The laryngeal mask airway (LMA), which was approved by the U.S. Food and Drug Administration in 1991, has been enthusiastically accepted in some settings as an alternative that offers most of the advantages of intubation but does not require laryngoscopy for placement.

The LMA (Figure 38-1) is a relatively long tube with a bag connector and an inflation port at one end and an inflatable soft cuff at the other. The tube is blindly passed into the hypopharynx so that the tip of the cuff lodges in the esophageal opening. Inflated, the cuff creates a seal around the larynx. The tube then is connected to a bag that delivers oxygen by ventilation through the central aperture of the laryngeal mask.

Little research has been done comparing the LMA with ET intubation, particularly in neonates. However, it appears that for ventilation purposes, the LMA, under controlled circumstances, can be as effective as, but never more effective than, intubation. Also, placement of the LMA is not necessarily

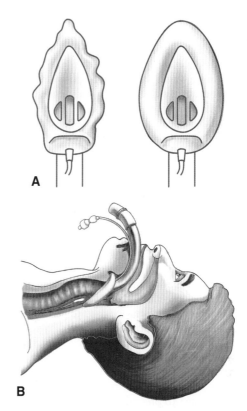

FIGURE **38-1**
A, Laryngeal mask airway deflated for insertion *(left)* and with cuff inflated *(right)*. **B,** Laryngeal mask airway in position with cuff inflated around laryngeal inlet. From Efrat R et al (1994). The laryngeal mask airway in pediatric anesthesia: experience with 120 patients undergoing elective groin surgery. *Journal of pediatric surgery* 29(1):23-41; 29(2):206-208.

easier than intubation. Studies have indicated wide variability in successful placement of the LMA on the first attempt (68% to 100% for those with expertise in airway management), whereas reported success rates for intubation generally are always about 90% to 95%. Even with successful placement, nearly a quarter of infants with a laryngeal mask airway subsequently develop airway obstruction, probably because of displacement during patient movement. The cuff provides only a low-pressure seal around the larynx, which limits the airway pressures that can be achieved during ventilation. The risks of gastric insufflation and regurgitation of gastric contents are reduced but not eliminated. Because of its size, the LMA currently is restricted to term infants, although there have been anecdotal reports of successful use in very small infants (1 to 1.5 kg). The LMA does not provide access to the lower airway and therefore is not suitable for meconium removal or drug administration, nor does it preserve the airway during laryngospasm. Its usefulness in neonates who require chest compressions and in those with oropharyngeal disease or diaphragmatic hernia has yet to be assessed (Brimacombe, 1994, 1995; Efrat et al, 1994; Paterson et al, 1994; Brimacombe & Berry, 1995; Brimacombe & Gandini, 1995; Williams, 1995).

CHEST COMPRESSIONS

Chest compressions rarely are required for resuscitation in the delivery room. They are performed in only 1 of every 1000 deliveries but probably are avoidable even in most of these cases. According to some authorities, approximately one third of the infants who received chest compressions have showed biochemical evidence of asphyxia (acidemia), but the remaining two thirds were found to have a malpositioned ET tube or inadequate ventilatory support (i.e., insufficient rate or pressure). Clearly, the airway should be reassessed and respiratory support should be optimized before chest compressions are initiated (Perlman & Risser, 1995). Assuming that these components are satisfactory, chest compressions are begun if the heart rate drops below 60 beats/min (Kattwinkel, 2006).

Chest compressions provide temporary support for circulation and oxygen delivery. Pressing on the sternum has two effects: it compresses the heart against the vertebral column, and it increases intrathoracic pressure. Both effects cause blood to be pushed out of the heart into the arterial circulation. When the sternal pressure is released, the ventricles return to their original shape; intrathoracic pressure falls toward zero; and venous blood is pulled into the heart by a suction effect (Bloom & Cropley, 1994; Elliott, 1994).

Either of two techniques may be used to perform chest compressions, but the thumb method is preferred by the American Academy of Pediatrics Neonatal Resuscitation Program. For the thumb method, both hands encircle the chest; the fingers support the back, and the thumbs (pointing cephalad either side by side or one on top of the other, depending on the infant's size) are used to press the sternum downward. For the two-finger method, one hand supports the back from below while two fingers of the free hand are held perpendicular to the chest and the fingertips are used to apply downward pressure on the sternum. Comparative studies have shown that higher systolic blood pressure, higher diastolic blood pressure, higher mean arterial pressure, and higher coronary perfusion pressure are generated with less external compression force when the thumb method is used. This method also has had fewer reports of trauma to the liver and other abdominal organs. Moreover, the thumb method is perhaps easier and certainly less tiring to perform. The thumb method therefore is preferred, but the two-finger method may be necessary if the nurse's hands are too small to encircle the chest properly or if access to the umbilicus is needed to facilitate placement of an umbilical venous catheter (UVC) for administration of emergency drugs (Bloom & Cropley, 1994; Elliott, 1994).

For both methods, the pressure is applied to the lower third of the sternum (just below the nipple line but above the xiphoid process) where the right ventricle lies closest to the sternum. Just enough force is used to depress the sternum ½ to ¾ of an inch (Bloom & Cropley, 1994). Research indicates that myocardial and cerebral blood flows are optimal when the downward stroke and release phases of the compression are equal in time (Niermeyer & Keenan, 2001). This equalization is best accomplished with a smooth stroke and release rhythm.

Positive-pressure ventilation with 100% oxygen must be continued while chest compressions are performed. The most recent guidelines recommend interposing chest compressions with ventilations at a 3:1 ratio. Every fourth compression is dropped to allow delivery of a single, effective breath. During the course of a full minute, 90 compressions and 30 ventilations are given (Bloom & Cropley, 1994). Faster rates were recommended in the past, but they only increase the chance of administering simultaneous compressions and ventilations (Bloom & Cropley, 1994; Trautman, 1995). Most research

indicates that simultaneous delivery increases the intrathoracic pressure to a level at which ventilation is impeded and coronary perfusion is reduced. Whether there is any effect on cerebral blood flow is equivocal, but there have been other reports of lower survival rates when simultaneous compression and ventilation was used.

Experimental techniques, such as external circulatory assist devices (e.g., mechanical "thumpers," pneumatic vests, and abdominal binders), counterpoint abdominal compressions (e.g., cough cardiopulmonary resuscitation), and active decompression (e.g., plumber's plunger), have shown promise in animal studies. However, few large-scale clinical trials have been done, and most of those used adults. Consequently, these methods cannot be advocated for neonatal resuscitation at this time.

MEDICATIONS
Epinephrine

Epinephrine is a direct-acting catecholamine with both alpha-adrenergic and beta-adrenergic effects. These effects lead to peripheral vasoconstriction, acceleration of the heart rate, and an increase in the forcefulness of cardiac contractions. The net effect is a sharp rise in blood pressure (pressor effect) and an increase in cardiac output. The marked pressor effect combined with the increased aortic diastolic pressure increases the cerebral and myocardial perfusion pressures, maintaining blood flow to these critical organs during resuscitation. Epinephrine therefore is considered the drug of choice with asystole or persistent bradycardia (heart rate <60 beats/min) despite adequate ventilation with 100% oxygen and chest compressions. For newborns the recommended dosage is 0.1 to 0.3 ml/kg of 1:10,000 solution (0.01 to 0.03 mg/kg) intravenously (Kattwinkel, 2006). The drug is rapidly inactivated by an enzymatically driven process known as sulfoconjugation, in which the active compound is bound to (conjugated with) sulfate (Schwab & von Stockhausen, 1994). The half-life of infused epinephrine is approximately 3 minutes. Consequently, the dose may be repeated every 3 to 5 minutes as clinically indicated.

Epinephrine ideally should be administered the IV/UVC route. Because IV/UVC placement may be difficult and time-consuming during resuscitation, initial doses tend to be given by ET tube. Unfortunately, absorption into the circulation from the pulmonary capillary bed may be highly variable because of the low-blood-flow state associated with resuscitation. In addition, much of the ET-instilled drug remains along the walls of the ET tube and in the conducting airways, with a relatively small amount finding its way into the deep absorptive surfaces of the alveoli. If epinephrine is given by the ET tube, a higher dose of 0.3 to 1 ml/kg of 1:10,000 solution (0.03 to 0.1 mg/kg) should be given (Kattwinkel, 2006).

A number of steps can be taken to aid delivery when the ET route is necessary. First, to optimize blood flow to the lungs, every effort must be made to ensure that chest compressions are performed effectively. Second, epinephrine may be dispersed more quickly to deeper pulmonary tissues by diluting the drug and following the instillation with a few forceful ventilations or a small amount of flush. When diluted, the medication should be mixed with a sufficient amount of normal saline to produce a final volume of 1 to 2 ml (Bloom & Cropley, 1994). As an alternative, some individuals prefer to administer the drug through a 5 French feeding tube positioned through the ET tube. Theoretically, the smaller lumen feeding tube would have less surface area to which the drug could cling, but the actual clinical significance, if any, is unknown. In view of this erratic absorption, subsequent doses should be given by the IV/UVC route as soon as access is achieved. In a study done by Rehan and colleagues (2004) on epinephrine delivery methods, they were able to show that the direct endotracheal tube method was more effective and less cumbersome than the catheter-inserted method for administering epinephrine during resuscitation. In the rare cases in which line placement is unattainable and the infant has failed to respond to standard doses given by the ET route, higher dosages of 1 to 2 ml/kg (0.1 to 0.2 mg/kg) may be considered (Bloom & Cropley, 1994).

Although higher doses of epinephrine administered by the ET route may have a role in exceptional situations, routine IV/UVC administration of high-dose epinephrine is not recommended in newborns. Studies with adults and older children have shown a dose-response relationship, with higher doses bringing about greater improvements in coronary and cerebral blood flow; in neonates, however, the efficacy and safety of high-dose IV/UVC epinephrine have not been adequately evaluated. Most of these studies have been done with patients with a history of coronary artery disease who demonstrate ventricular fibrillation. Neonates, however, more commonly have bradycardia caused by hypoxia. These pathophysiologic differences prevent extrapolation of findings. Furthermore, administration of high doses generally has been followed by a prolonged period of hypertension. Because the newborn, particularly the prematurely born, has a vascular germinal matrix, the risk may be greater for intraventricular hemorrhage. In fact, this area of the brain is most susceptible to hemorrhage when hypertension is preceded by hypotension, which is the case with resuscitation. For this reason, only the standard dose of epinephrine (0.1 to 0.3 ml/kg) should be given by the IV/UVC route.

Volume Expanders

Volume expanders are indicated with evidence or suspicion of acute blood loss with signs of hypovolemia. These signs include pallor despite oxygen therapy, hypotension with weak pulses despite a normal heart rate, and failure to respond to resuscitation (Bloom & Cropley, 1994). Low hematocrit and hemoglobin concentrations are diagnostic of blood loss, but the levels may be misleadingly normal immediately after acute loss. In general, it takes about 3 hours for a sufficient amount of fluid to shift from the interstitial to the intravascular space to produce the degree of compensatory hemodilution reflected by a fall in laboratory values.

The basic requirement for any replacement solution is that the electrolyte and protein composition be roughly equivalent to that which was lost. Otherwise, an osmotic pressure gradient is created, and fluids are driven out of the capillaries into the interstitial tissue. The expansion of circulatory volume is only transient, and the infant is put at risk for secondary problems, particularly pulmonary edema. Clearly, whole blood is the fluid of choice for volume replacement, and it offers the added benefit of oxygen-carrying capacity. Fresh O-negative blood cross-matched against the mother should be used. When blood is not readily available, isotonic fluids (normal saline or Ringer's lactate) may also be used (Bloom & Cropley, 1994). Glucose-containing fluids (e.g., D5W or D10W) should not be given by bolus because of the risk of profound hyperglycemia. Hyper-

glycemia with untreated asphyxia may aggravate metabolic acidosis.

For emergency treatment of hypovolemia, 10 ml/kg of volume expander is given slowly over 5 to 10 minutes by the IV/UVC route (Bloom & Cropley, 1994). Rapid infusion must be avoided, because abrupt changes in vascular pressure in the vulnerable matrix capillaries place the infant (especially a preterm infant) at greater risk of intraventricular hemorrhage. The response usually is dramatic, with a prompt improvement in blood pressure, pulses, and color. If the signs of hypovolemia continue, however, a second volume replacement may be given. Persistent failure beyond this point probably indicates some degree of "pump failure," and further improvement is not likely until cardiac function is improved. In fact, excessive volume administration may so engorge the heart and overstretch the cardiac muscle fibers that the strength of contractions is actually diminished. In such cases, administration of sodium bicarbonate (to correct metabolic acidosis) or an inotropic agent (such as dopamine) should be considered (Bloom & Cropley, 1994).

Dopamine

Dopamine may be used when vascular volume has been restored but hypotension continues to exist because of myocardial decompensation (pump failure). Dopamine increases cardiac output, blood pressure, and peripheral and organ perfusion. A precursor of norepinephrine, dopamine is a naturally occurring catecholamine with alpha-adrenergic, beta-adrenergic, and dopaminergic effects. The beta effects are elicited both directly (by direct interaction with the receptors) and indirectly (by releasing norepinephrine, which interacts with receptors). The effects of dopamine are complex and dose related. In general, low doses (<2 mcg/kg/min) primarily stimulate dopaminergic receptors. Moderate doses (2 to 10 mcg/kg/min) activate dopaminergic receptors. High doses (over 15 to 20 mcg/kg/min) activate all three adrenergic receptors, but alpha stimulation negates the effect of beta stimulation (Young & Mangum, 2005).

Dopamine is metabolized rapidly, having a serum half-life of 2 to 5 minutes. The duration of action is less than 10 minutes. Consequently, the drug must be given by continuous IV infusion. When used after a prolonged resuscitation, dopamine is infused at an initial dosage of 5 mcg/kg/min and titrated in increments of 3 to 5 mcg/kg/min to a maximum of 20 mcg/kg/min until blood pressure and perfusion improve. Heart rate and rhythm and blood pressure must be monitored continuously. Like all catecholamines, dopamine is inactivated by an alkaline solution and therefore should not be mixed with sodium bicarbonate (Bloom & Cropley, 1994; Young & Mangum, 2005).

Sodium Bicarbonate

Of the biochemical events that arise from asphyxia, the most significant is the conversion from aerobic to anaerobic metabolism with the production of lactic acid. As this strong acid accumulates, metabolic acidosis develops, myocardial contractility declines, hypotension worsens, and the cardiac response to catecholamines weakens (Leuthner et al, 1994). In such cases, the best treatment for acidosis is directed at its cause, hypoxemia. Immediate therapy includes ventilation with 100% oxygen and cardiac compressions to restore blood flow and tissue oxygenation. However, if the resuscitation is prolonged and the infant remains unresponsive, alkali therapy may be helpful (Bloom & Cropley, 1994). Sodium bicarbonate is the most frequently used alkalinizing agent, but its use remains controversial; therefore, it should be used only when no improvement is seen (Niermeyer & Keenan, 2001).

Sodium bicarbonate ($NaHCO_3$) is a physiologic buffer. When it is added to a solution of strong acid, such as hydrochloric acid (HCl), the bicarbonate anion (HCO_3^-) combines with the hydrogen ion (H^+) from the acid to form the weaker carbonic acid (H_2CO_3) and a neutral salt, such as sodium chloride (NaCl):

$$HCl + NaHCO_3 \rightarrow H_2CO_3 \; NaCl$$

The carbonic acid rapidly dissociates into water (H_2O) and carbon dioxide (CO_2), and the blood transports the dissolved carbon dioxide to the lungs, where it is eliminated:

$$H_2CO_3 \rightarrow H_2O + CO_2$$

Although sodium bicarbonate historically was considered a pharmacologic mainstay of neonatal resuscitation, a growing body of research suggests that sodium bicarbonate administration may actually be counterproductive and possibly injurious. First and foremost, effective removal of carbon dioxide by the lungs depends on both ventilation and pulmonary blood flow. If either is inadequate (which frequently is the case during resuscitation), CO_2 accumulates, with a shift from metabolic to respiratory acidosis without any real resolution of acid-base imbalance (Leuthner et al, 1994). Second, CO_2 diffuses across cell membranes much more rapidly and easily than does bicarbonate. That is, CO_2 quickly moves out of the capillaries into cells, whereas bicarbonate lags behind in the intravascular space. The blood pH rises, but intracellular pH transiently falls. Therefore, when the cells of the heart are involved, intramyocardial acidosis worsens and cardiac performance declines further (Leuthner et al, 1994). Other possible consequences of sodium bicarbonate administration are intraventricular hemorrhage (as a result of rapid infusion of hypertonic solution) and hypernatremia.

Administration of sodium bicarbonate should not be undertaken lightly and is in fact discouraged for brief resuscitation or episodes of bradycardia. It should be reserved for prolonged arrest unresponsive to other therapy and then used only after effective ventilation and compressions have been established. The dosage currently recommended is 4 ml/kg of 4.2% solution (2 mEq/kg) by the IV/UVC route. This hypertonic solution contains 0.5 mEq/ml and therefore should be given slowly over at least 2 minutes (1 mEq/kg/min) (Bloom & Cropley, 1994). At the first opportunity, samples for blood gas analysis should be drawn from whatever site is available to confirm metabolic acidosis.

Naloxone

For the mother, narcotic analgesics are an effective means of pain control during labor. Unfortunately, these lipid-soluble drugs rapidly cross the placenta and can cause neonatal respiratory depression. Peak fetal narcotic levels occur 30 minutes to 2 hours after administration to the mother. The degree and duration of depression shown by the newborn depend on the dose, the route, and how soon before delivery the drug is given. Affected infants show decreased respiratory effort and muscle tone but typically have a good heart rate and perfusion. If these signs are noted and the mother was given a narcotic within

4 hours of delivery, the infant should be given a narcotic antagonist (Bloom & Cropley, 1994; Wimmer, 1994).

Naloxone hydrochloride is a synthetic narcotic antagonist designed to reverse narcotic-induced respiratory depression. It acts by competing with narcotics for receptor sites in the central nervous system. As a pure competitive antagonist, it binds with but does not activate receptors. Consequently, in the absence of narcotics, naloxone exhibits essentially no pharmacologic activity. As always, ventilatory support is still the first defense against respiratory depression (Niermeyer & Keenan, 2001).

Naloxone is available in a variety of concentrations; however, the American Academy of Pediatrics Committee on Drugs (1990) currently recommends use of either the 0.4 mg/ml preparation or the 1 mg/ml preparation. Neonatal naloxone (0.02 mg/ml) should not be used because of the fluid volume that would be given. The dosage is 0.1 mg/kg, which may be repeated every 2 to 3 minutes as needed. Administration by the IV/UVC is preferred, but the drug also can be given intramuscularly (IM), because affected newborns generally have good perfusion. The IV/UVC route provides the quickest onset of action (generally apparent within 2 minutes), but IM injection produces a more prolonged effect. Adequate ventilatory assistance must be provided until reversal is complete. Close monitoring should continue for 4 to 6 hours after administration. Because the liver rapidly metabolizes naloxone, its duration of effect may be shorter than that of some narcotics, and respiratory depression may recur. If signs reappear, additional doses of naloxone should be given (Bloom & Cropley, 1994; Kattwinkel, 2006; Wimmer, 1994). Although naloxone has no known short-term toxic effects, it is contraindicated in infants born to narcotic-dependent mothers. Because abrupt and complete reversal of narcotic effect may precipitate seizures (withdrawal reaction), assisted ventilation is provided in this circumstance until the respiratory drive is adequate (Bloom & Cropley, 1994).

Because several studies have suggested that hypoxia and acidosis stimulate the release of endogenous opiates (endorphins), it has been theorized that these endorphins might accentuate the depressing effect of hypoxemia on the cardiorespiratory system. However, clinical trials of naloxone administration to infants with 1-minute Apgar scores of 6 or lower have shown no effect on spontaneous respiratory frequency or heart rate.

Other Drugs

Calcium ions play a critical role in the depolarization of cardiac pacemaker cells in the sinoatrial and atrioventricular nodes, and the movement of calcium into and within the cells of the cardiac and vascular smooth muscle accelerates and maintains the chemical reactions necessary for muscle contraction. As a result, administration of calcium salt (e.g., calcium gluconate, calcium chloride) has been widely recommended in the past to increase heart rate, improve myocardial contractility, and raise blood pressure during resuscitation (Proano et al, 1995). Although these effects are theoretically plausible, several studies have failed to show the anticipated improvement in cardiovascular function. However, adverse side effects have been reported even at standard doses. Although preterm and sick newborns may develop hypocalcemia in the first week of life from a variety of causes, low calcium levels are rarely if ever a factor at birth because calcium is actively transported across the placenta from mother to fetus. Administration of calcium in the first few minutes of life therefore may produce dangerously high serum calcium levels. Pacemaker blockade, bradycardia, and even arrest may result from fatigue after excessive and sustained stimulation. Moreover, high intracellular free calcium levels have been implicated in the activation of aberrant enzyme systems, intracellular release of free fatty acids, generation of oxidative free radicals, and cerebral arterial spasm, which may trigger many of the undesirable consequences of asphyxia. In summary, no data currently are available to support the use of calcium, but a considerable amount of evidence indicates that it may actually be deleterious. Although calcium administration may be appropriate under other circumstances as therapy for documented hypocalcemia or to antagonize the adverse effects of hyperkalemia or hypermagnesemia, calcium should not be used for neonatal resuscitation in the delivery room (Bloom & Cropley, 1994; Keenan, 1994).

Another drug that has fallen out of use in neonatal resuscitation is atropine. Atropine is an anticholinergic drug that blocks the action of acetylcholine at cholinergic receptor sites. Parasympathetic (vagal) stimulation of the heart normally inhibits and decelerates cardiac function (Table 38-3). If this stimulation is blocked, cardiac tone and activity returns to normal. Although atropine may be useful for reversing bradycardia of vagal origin (as from airway manipulation during intubation), infants who require resuscitation in the delivery room are typically bradycardic because of hypoxia. Administration of atropine in this situation has a transient effect at best, and bradycardia will return if the hypoxia persists (Burchfield, 1994).

SPECIAL CIRCUMSTANCES

For some infants, changes in or variations of the usual resuscitative measures are needed. Most of these infants have congenital anomalies, structural defects, or conditions that compromise the cardiovascular system, such as neural tube

defects, abdominal wall defects, diaphragmatic hernias, hydrops fetalis, esophageal atresia, pneumothorax, choanal atresia, and laryngeal anomalies. Resuscitative measures with these disorders are discussed in greater detail elsewhere in this text.

Termination of Resuscitation

The law and its underlying ethical principles require that treatment be provided and continued as long as it is judged to be effective in ameliorating or correcting an underlying pathophysiologic process. Unfortunately, the data are insufficient to allow a general recommendation for how long resuscitation should be performed before continuation can be deemed futile and efforts are terminated. Evidence indicates that neonates with a birth weight below 750 g who require cardiac compressions in the delivery room do not survive to discharge. Survival also is unlikely at any birth weight if the Apgar score remains zero after 10 minutes of aggressive resuscitation.

Although many hospitals have guidelines for withholding full resuscitation for extremely low birth weight infants and those with lethal anomalies, early and well-documented discussion with parents is recommended when such events are anticipated prenatally. If the event was not anticipated, great attention should be given to postmortem evaluation. Blood for chromosome examination and other pertinent laboratory work, radiographs, and an autopsy are important both for family counseling and for evaluation of the resuscitation process.

Postresuscitation Stabilization

A successfully resuscitated neonate requires special consideration during stabilization. The goal of care after resuscitation is to reverse the causes of cell death and tissue injury (hypoxia, ischemia, and acidosis) and avoid or treat any exacerbating conditions (hypothermia, hypoglycemia, respiratory failure, infection). The mnemonic S.T.A.B.L.E.™ can aid the nurse in remembering the basic components of the stabilization process (Karlsen, 2006):

TABLE 38-3	Effects of Stimulation of the Autonomic Nervous System			
	Adrenergic (Sympathetic) Effects			**Predominant Parasympathetic (Cholinergic) Effects**
Site	**Alpha Receptors**	**Beta Receptors**	**Dopaminergic Receptors**	
HEART				
SA node	—	↑ Heart rate	—	↓ Heart rate
AV node	—	↑ Conduction velocity	—	↓ Conduction velocity
Cardiac muscle	—	↑ Contractility	—	↓ Contractility
LUNGS				
Bronchial muscle	Constrict	Relax	—	Constrict
ARTERIES				
Coronary	Constrict	Dilate	Dilate	Constrict
Pulmonary	Constrict	Dilate	?	—
Cerebral	Constrict	—	Dilate	Dilate
Renal	Constrict	Dilate	Dilate	
VEINS	Constrict	Dilate	Constrict	

Data from Zaritsky A, Chernow B (1984). Use of catecholamines in pediatrics. Journal of pediatrics 105:341-350.
AV, Atrioventricular; SA, sinoatrial.

S—Safe care and Sugar
T—Temperature
A—Airway
B—Blood pressure
L—Laboratory work
E—Emotional support for the family

Documentation

No resuscitative event can go unrecorded. Unfortunately, the circumstances surrounding resuscitation are fraught with medicolegal hazards. Assessment of the infant generally is limited to the most basic measurements (respiratory rate, heart rate, and color). Immediate response may be affected by many factors unrelated to professional competence. Furthermore, the ultimate outcome may not become apparent for years. Even the best, most appropriate care can look "bad" in retrospect if documentation is incomplete or inaccurate. Yet no area of the hospital is perhaps less conducive to quality documentation than the delivery room, where a variety of professionals (nurses, physicians, and respiratory therapists) from different clinical areas (obstetrics, neonatology, anesthesiology), each with a unique perspective on the situation, are brought together in an emergency. Notes are jotted on bed linen, scrub clothes, paper towels, or anything at hand. More often than not, these brief notes are so hastily written that they are little more than a list of the medications given. When transcribed, the events may be documented in two totally separate charts, one for the mother, and another for the infant. Great care must be taken with record keeping so that events and actions can be accurately reconstructed many years in the future (Thigpen, 1995).

Descriptive charting is most appropriate in this situation. The record should include the pertinent perinatal factors, the physical findings, the activities performed, and the infant's response, but definitive diagnoses should not be offered. It is particularly important that information concerning the pregnancy, labor, and delivery be based on fact and not hearsay. Terms such as "fetal distress" and "asphyxia" tend to take on a life of their own once they have been committed to paper, even if they are not supported by clinical evidence. It is best to record factual data, such as vital signs and blood gas determinations, without adding an interpretation. Ventilation, chest compressions, and administration of medications are essential items for documentation, but the basics should not be dismissed. It is just as important to note that attempts were made to keep the infant dry and warm.

Accurate timing of notes can be critical, because actions are judged by the minute-to-minute changes noted in the chart. A preprinted recording form not only helps in this regard but also can provide a structure for evaluation and decision making. Any form used should be printed in triplicate: one copy (the original) is retained for the medical record; the second copy is sent to the pharmacy so that medications can be quickly restocked; and the third copy is used for quality assessment (Thigpen, 1995).

SUMMARY

Although most depressed infants respond to drying, warming, positioning, suctioning, and tactile stimulation, every obstetric and neonatal unit should be adequately equipped and well prepared to handle neonatal emergencies. To provide neonatal care effectively, nurses must understand the cardiorespiratory transition and must be able to identify factors that may interfere with successful transition, comprehend the principles of resuscitation, and intervene based on assessment of respirations, heart rate, and color.

REFERENCES

American Academy of Pediatrics Committee on Drugs (1990). Naloxone dosage and route of administration for infants and children: addendum to emergency drug doses for infants and children. *Pediatrics* 86:484-485.

American Heart Association Emergency Cardiac Care Committee and Subcommittees (1992). Guidelines for cardiopulmonary resuscitation and emergency cardiac care. VII. Neonatal resuscitation. *Journal of the American Medical Association* 268:2276-2281.

Bhende MS, Thompson AE (1995). Evaluation of an end-tidal CO_2 detector during pediatric cardiopulmonary resuscitation. *Pediatrics* 95:395-399.

Bloom RS, Cropley C (1994). *Textbook of neonatal resuscitation.* Elk Grove Village, IL: American Academy of Pediatrics and American Heart Association.

Brimacombe J (1994). The laryngeal mask airway for neonatal resuscitation [letter]. *Pediatrics* 93:874.

Brimacombe J (1995). Laryngeal mask airway for emergency medicine. *American journal of emergency medicine* 13:111-112.

Brimacombe J, Berry A (1995). The laryngeal mask airway: a consideration for the Neonatal Resuscitation Programme guidelines? *Canadian journal of anaesthesia* 42:88-89.

Brimacombe J, Gandini D (1995). Resuscitation of neonates with the laryngeal mask airway: a caution. *Pediatrics* 95:453-454.

Burchfield DJ (1994). Why *not* use atropine in neonatal resuscitation? *NRP news intermountain West* 1:1.

Efrat R et al (1994). The laryngeal mask airway in pediatric anesthesia: experience with 120 patients undergoing elective groin surgery. *Journal of pediatric surgery* 29:206-208.

Elliott RD (1994). Neonatal resuscitation: the NRP guidelines. *Canadian journal of anaesthesia* 41:742-753.

Heller RM, Heller TW (1994). Experience with the illuminated endotracheal tube in the prevention of unsafe intubations in the premature and full-term newborn. *Pediatrics* 93:389-391.

Karlsen KA (2006). *The S.T.A.B.L.E. Program Learner manual,* ed 5. Salt Lake City, UT: S.T.A.B.L.E.

Kattwinkel J, editor (2006). *Textbook of neonatal resuscitation,* ed 5. Elk Grove Village, IL: American Academy of Pediatrics and American Heart Association.

Keenan B (1994). Calcium use for neonatal resuscitation. *NRP news intermountain West* 1:1-2.

Leuthner SR et al (1994). Cardiopulmonary resuscitation of the newborn: an update. *Pediatric clinics of North America* 41:893-907.

Niermeyer S, Keenan W (2001). Resuscitation of the newborn infant. In Klaus MG, Fanaroff AA, editors. *Care of the high-risk neonate,* ed 5. Philadelphia: Saunders.

Paterson SJ et al (1994). Neonatal resuscitation using the laryngeal mask airway. *Anesthesiology* 80:1248-1253.

Perlman JM, Risser R (1995). Cardiopulmonary resuscitation in the delivery room: associated clinical events. *Archives of pediatric and adolescent medicine* 149:20-25.

Proano L et al (1995). Calcium channel blocker overdose. *American journal of emergency medicine* 13:444-450.

Rehan VK et al (2004). Epinephrine delivery during neonatal resuscitation: comparison of direct endotracheal tube vs. catheter inserted into endotracheal tube administration. *Journal of perinatology* 24:686-690.

Reiterer F et al (1994). Influence of head-neck posture on airflow and pulmonary mechanics in preterm neonates. *Pediatric pulmonology* 17:149-154.

Schwab KO, von Stockhausen HB (1994). Plasma catecholamines after endotracheal administration of adrenaline during postnatal resuscitation. *Archives of disease in childhood* 70:F213-F217.

Thigpen J (1995). Neonatal resuscitation record. *Neonatal network* 14:57-58.

Trautman MS (1995). Neonatal resuscitation: be prepared. *Contemporary pediatrics* 12:101-110, 113.

Williams RK (1995). Resuscitation of neonates with the laryngeal mask airway: a caution. *Pediatrics* 95:454.

Wimmer JE (1994). Neonatal resuscitation. *Pediatrics in review* 15:255-265.

Young TE, Mangum OB (2005). *Neofax: a manual of drugs used in neonatal care,* ed 18. Raleigh, NC: Acorn.

Assessment of the Newborn and Infant

Debra A. Sansoucie • Terri A. Cavaliere

Assessment is a continuous process of evaluation throughout the course of routine care of the neonate and infant. However, periodically a more formalized, comprehensive examination must be undertaken to determine wellness or to evaluate a specific problem. The results of the comprehensive physical assessment serve as the database on which clinical judgments about diagnosis and treatment are based.

A comprehensive physical assessment is performed for various reasons. The assessment may be the initial examination at birth, assessment of extrauterine transition, determination of gestational age, comprehensive assessment after transition, discharge examination, well-baby outpatient examination, or evaluation of an illness or injury. Although these assessments have many commonalities, each has a somewhat different purpose. This chapter discusses various aspects of a comprehensive physical assessment.

FIRST NEONATAL ASSESSMENT AND THE APGAR SCORE

The initial neonatal assessment occurs immediately after delivery with the assignment of Apgar scores. These scores were devised in 1952 by Virginia Apgar as a means of assessing the clinical status of infants immediately after delivery (Apgar, 1953). The Apgar score consists of five components—heart rate, respiratory effort, muscle tone, reflex irritability, and color—and each component is given a score of zero, one, or two; the scores are then added to obtain a total score (Table 39-1). Although the total score originally was assigned at 1 minute after birth, the current recommendation is that it be assigned at 1 and 5 minutes. If the total score is below 7 at 5 minutes, the assessment is repeated every 5 minutes for 20 minutes or until a score above 7 has been achieved twice consecutively.

The value of the Apgar score has been challenged because of its misuse in the identification of birth asphyxia and prediction of neurologic outcome. It is important to recognize that elements of the Apgar score may be influenced by a variety of factors besides birth asphyxia, including, among others, preterm birth, administration of drugs to the mother, and congenital anomalies. A low 1-minute Apgar score does not correlate with the newborn's future outcome. The 5-minute Apgar score, especially the change in the score between 1 and 5 minutes, is a useful indicator of the effectiveness of resuscitation efforts. However, even a 5-minute score of 0 to 3, although possibly a result of hypoxia, is limited as an indicator of the severity of the problem and in and of itself correlates

poorly with future neurologic outcome (Stanley, 1994). Apgar scores are still useful for assessing the condition of the newborn at birth; however, as recognized by the American Academy of Pediatrics (AAP) Committee on the Fetus and Newborn and the American College of Obstetricians and Gynecologists Committee on Obstetrics (1996), additional information is required to properly interpret the scores of infants who require immediate resuscitation.

The value of the Apgar score for the evaluation of extremely premature infants has also been questioned. Several components of the Apgar score, such as reflex irritability, muscle tone, and respiratory effort, are affected by the maturity of the infant; therefore, premature infants are unsurprisingly assigned lower Apgar scores than infants born at term.

OTHER CONSIDERATIONS FOR THE INITIAL NEONATAL ASSESSMENT

A brief physical examination should be performed before the infant leaves the delivery area. Considerations for this assessment include inspection for birth injuries and major congenital anomalies and evaluation of pulmonary and cardiovascular adjustment to extrauterine life. Evaluation of early transition to extrauterine life includes observation of color for adequacy of perfusion and oxygenation, appraisal of respiratory effort, auscultation of breath sounds and heart sounds, and inspection of the amount, color, and consistency of secretions. The infant's tone, activity, and appropriateness of state should also be noted at this time. A cursory inspection of all external areas should be performed before the infant leaves the delivery area, including a general inspection of the external genitalia and, in males, palpation for testes in the scrotum. The entire examination should be performed under a radiant heat source to prevent significant heat loss from the infant.

EVALUATION OF TRANSITION

Adaptation to both intrapartum and neonatal events is reflected in the transition from a fetal to an extrauterine environment. These events result in sympathetic activity that affects the infant's color, respiration, heart rate, behavioral state, gastrointestinal function, and temperature (D'Harlingue & Durand, 2001). It is important to remember that the physiologic and biochemical changes peculiar to the period of transition to extrauterine life affect the physical findings of early examinations. The examination performed during transition is described separately because characteristics that

TABLE 39-1	Apgar Scoring System			
		Assigned Points		
Sign	**0**	**1**	**2**	
Heart rate	Absent	Slow (<100 beats/min)	100 beats/min	
Respirations	Absent	Weak cry; hypoventilation	Good, strong cry	
Muscle tone	Limp	Some flexion	Active motion	
Reflex irritability (response to brisk slap on soles of feet)	No response	Grimace	Cough or sneeze	
Color	Blue or pale	Body pink; extremities blue	Completely pink	

Used with permission of American Academy of Pediatrics Committee on the Fetus and Newborn and the American College of Obstetricians and Gynecologists Committee on Obstetrics (1996). Use and abuse of the Apgar score. Pediatrics 98:141-142.

are normal during transition may be abnormal if they appear at other times.

As the neonate's circulation converts from the fetal route, there may be a period in which pulmonary vascular resistance remains greater than systemic vascular resistance, resulting in a right to left shunt across the ductus arteriosus. Higher preductal oxygen saturation causes the neonate's face and upper body to appear pink while the lower body and legs appear pale or blue; this creates a visible demarcation across the chest. As the fetal circulation successfully converts to the neonatal pathway, this transitional differential cyanosis disappears (D'Harlingue & Durand, 2001).

Acrocyanosis is common during this period. To evaluate babies with deeper skin pigmentation, the nurse should observe the color of the mucous membranes. When the neonate is stimulated, the skin may appear blushed or bright red; this change in color is called erythema neonatorum, or generalized hyperemia, which develops a few hours after birth. It generally resolves within several minutes to an hour and rarely appears with the same intensity. According to Fletcher (1998), "This event of total blushing is noteworthy in that it likely signals the successful completion of fetal to neonatal transition in the cardiopulmonary system and provides some reassurance of health in that infant." Erythema neonatorum is not synonymous with erythema toxicum neonatorum.

The neonatal heart rate may range from 160 to 180 beats/min in the first 15 minutes of life; it slowly falls to a baseline rate of 100 to 120 beats/min by 30 minutes of life. The heart rate is labile, and brief periods of asymptomatic, irregular heart rates are not pathologic. Murmurs are common, because the ductus arteriosus may still be patent. Respirations are also irregular during the first 15 minutes, with rates ranging from 60 to 100 breaths/min. Grunting, flaring, retractions, and brief periods of apnea may also be seen in the neonate. Crackles may be present on auscultation (D'Harlingue & Durand, 2001).

Despite the changes in the heart and respiratory rates during the initial 15 to 30 minutes of life, healthy term infants are awake and alert. They may rest quietly, cry periodically, startle spontaneously, and breastfeed during this period. Full-term babies often show flexed posture with good muscle tone; preterm newborns, in comparison, have less flexion and tone (Sansoucie & Cavaliere, 2002). Temperature is decreased, and gastrointestinal activity includes the establishment of bowel sounds and the production of saliva. This first period of

reactivity may be prolonged in infants who have experienced difficult labor and delivery, in sick term infants, and in well premature infants (D'Harlingue & Durand, 2001).

After the first period of reactivity, the infant is relatively unresponsive or sleeping, and the heart rate drops to a baseline of 100 to 120 beats/min. This interval, which lasts approximately 60 to 100 minutes, is followed by a second period of reactivity, which lasts anywhere from 10 minutes to several hours. During this time the infant may show rapid color changes, intermittent tachypnea and tachycardia, and changes in tone. Healthy infants may have periods during which the respiratory rate is considerably higher than 60 breaths/min; however, the infant does not appear distressed and can slow this rate enough to nipple feed successfully. Meconium often is passed during this period (D'Harlingue & Durand, 2001). The chart in Figure 39-1 summarizes some of the physical changes seen during the transition period.

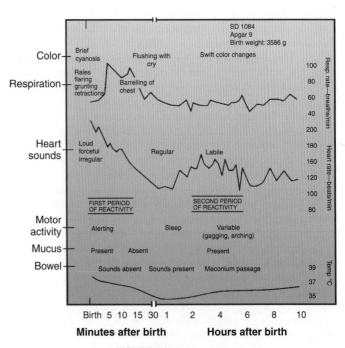

FIGURE **39-1**
Normal transition period.

NEWBORN EXAMINATION

The comprehensive newborn examination generally is performed within the first 12 to 18 hours of life, after transition has been completed successfully. The examination should be initiated when the infant is quiet and should progress from assessments that are least likely to bother the infant to those that are most irritating. An examination sequence based on the infant's state is outlined in Table 39-2.

DISCHARGE EXAMINATION

The purpose of the discharge examination is to assess the infant's ability to be cared for outside the controlled environ-ment of the hospital. The focus of the assessment depends primarily on how long the infant has been hospitalized and for what reasons. The needs of a healthy, full-term infant being discharged home with the mother are different from those of a growing, preterm infant who has been hospitalized for weeks or months and who has significant sequelae. Evaluating the caretaker's capability to care for and observe changes in the infant is an important aspect of the discharge assessment and follow-up plan. Anticipatory guidance regarding feedings, sleeping position and environment, skin care, safety practices, and recognition of signs and symptoms of illness should be provided at this time.

TABLE 39-2	Examination Sequence Based on Infant's State		
Assessment Technique	**Required State**	**Arousing Maneuver**	**Equipment**
Observe general appearance			
Observe color			
Observe resting posture	Quiet		
Observe spontaneous activity	Active		
Count respirations	Quiet		Clock
Count heartbeats	Quiet		Clock
Inspect facies at rest	Quiet		
Auscultate heart sounds	Quiet		Stethoscope
Auscultate breath sounds	Quiet		Stethoscope
Measure blood pressure	Quiet		Blood pressure cuff
Inspect head and neck region			
Stimulate response to sound	Quiet		Calibrated noise maker
Inspect trunk anteriorly			
Palpate abdomen, cardiac impulse	Quiet		
Feel pulses			
Examine genitalia			Lubricant for rectal examination
Inspect trunk posteriorly			
Inspect arms and hands			
Inspect legs and feet			
Assess passive tone			
Assess active tone	Active	X	
Elicit primitive reflexes	Active	X	
Assess muscle strength	Active	X	
Assess gestational age			
Test range in major joints		X	
Manipulate hips		X	
Measure temperature			Thermometer
Examine ears			Otoscope
Determine pupil response			Bright light
Examine fundi	Quiet	X	
Elicit tendon reflexes		X	Percussion hammer
Stimulate response to pain		X	
Weigh infant	Quiet	X	Scales, growth chart
Measure head circumference			Tape measure, growth chart
Measure chest and abdomen circumferences		X	Tape measure
Measure length			Tape measure, growth chart
Transilluminate head		X	High-intensity light
Percuss abdomen	Quiet		
Percuss lungs	Quiet		

Data from Fletcher MA (1998). Physical diagnosis in neonatology. Philadelphia: Lippincott-Raven.

OUTPATIENT EXAMINATION

The focus of the first outpatient examination is the infant's adaptation to the home environment. This examination includes assessment of any issues highlighted at discharge. Some factors to be considered in the infant are temperature stability, ability and success at feeding and elimination, sleep patterns, normal color, drying of the umbilical cord, reassessment of hip stability, and normal state and behavior. Any areas that may have been relatively inaccessible during earlier examinations should be included, such as the eyes, ear canals, and eardrums (Fletcher, 1998).

The birth history, including the birth weight, gestational age, and any problems, should be reviewed. As part of the complete physical examination, height, weight, and head circumference should be plotted and developmental progress observed. The results of newborn metabolic screening and the infant's immunization status should be reviewed. For sick infants, general assessment assists in the establishment of priorities. For example, if a child is experiencing pronounced respiratory problems, assessment of this area is a priority. Anticipatory guidance issues include nutrition, elimination, sleep patterns, development and behavior, social and family relationships, and injury prevention (AAP, 2002). A more detailed description of health maintenance for high-risk infants during the first year of life is presented later in this chapter.

ENVIRONMENT

The routine neonatal assessment should take place in a quiet, warm environment. The room should be lighted well enough for appropriate observation, but the light should not be so strong that the infant is deterred from opening the eyes. Prevention of heat loss is critical to the infant's comfort and to the maintenance of thermal neutrality and glucose homeostasis. Most healthy term infants can tolerate being undressed in a reasonably warm room for the 5 to 10 minutes required to perform the physical assessment. If the environment is cool or drafty or if the infant is sick or preterm, an external heat source should be provided, such as a radiant warmer or heat lamps. If heat lamps are used, the infant's eyes should be shielded to prevent adverse effects from prolonged exposure of the infant's eyes to the bright light of the lamps. The examiner should warm the hands and examination equipment before beginning the assessment. This practice not only prevents heat loss but also avoids upsetting an otherwise quiet and cooperative infant.

The examination should be conducted in a quiet environment with a calm infant. A placid infant provides the best opportunity for gathering meaningful data. Extraneous environmental noise hampers auscultation and assessment of bodily sounds and may overwhelm a sick or immature infant, causing changes in state and cardiovascular status (Fletcher, 1998). Handling the infant gently and speaking in a soothing voice may allow the examiner to complete most of the assessment without distressing the infant. Disturbing components of the examination, such as deep palpation of the abdomen and assessment of the hips, should be performed last.

Having one or both parents present during the routine neonatal assessment offers the opportunity to assess their competence in caregiving and to educate them about the unique physical traits, behavior, and coping skills of their infant. The examiner may also use this time to build rapport and trust with the parents, to listen to their concerns, and to offer pertinent information. Some issues may require privacy for discussion; therefore, confidentiality should be considered when conversing with parents in the presence of others.

COMPONENTS OF A COMPREHENSIVE HISTORY

The neonatal history is very similar to that for an older child or adult, including information about the past medical history, the current condition, and the family. For a newly delivered infant, the initial neonatal assessment probably will be conducted before the nurse speaks to the parents. Basic information about the pregnancy and delivery should be available in the maternal records, but a complete history lays the foundation for the comprehensive newborn examination and should be elicited directly from the parents. Without a complete history, the examiner may lack adequate information to formulate an accurate impression.

The components of a complete history are the identifying data; chief complaint; interim neonatal history or history of presenting problem or illness; antepartum history; obstetric history; intrapartum history; and the maternal medical, family medical, and social histories (Table 39-3). After data collected from the complete history and physical assessment are organized and all expected and unexpected findings have been reviewed, areas of concern are identified and prioritized for further evaluation and attention. This forms the framework for the clinical diagnosis and plan of care.

Interviewing the Parents

The interview with the parents is a vital component of the health assessment of a newborn or an infant. This interview offers the nurse an excellent opportunity to develop a therapeutic partnership with the parents in the care of their baby. Ideally, the interview is conducted in a quiet, comfortable setting; if it takes place at the bedside in a busy intensive care unit, the parents may be distracted and overwhelmed by the sounds and sights customary to this environment. If the ideal setting is not possible, the nurse can provide a focal point of warmth and attention by using a conversational tone of voice, maintaining eye contact, and concentrating fully on the parents. However, this can be done only with a discipline that dispels both personal and professional distractions.

It is important that nurses introduce themselves and clearly state their names and roles in the baby's care. Nurses should make sure they understand the parents' names and should pronounce them correctly. They should ask the baby's name and use it often during the conversation. During this session, the purposes of the health interview and physical assessment should be clarified. Cooperation and sharing are more likely if the parents understand that the questions lead to better care for their infant.

The use of silence and listening, as well as allowing ample time for response to questions, is crucial to reassuring parents that what they say is worthwhile. Also, the parents can easily be shown that the interview is important and will not be rushed. Nurses should fix their attention on the parents and listen and should not interrupt unless necessary. They also should avoid asking the next questions before listening to the complete answer to the current question. They should indicate that they understand the responses and should request clarification if necessary. Nurses should take care to avoid overly

TABLE **39-3**	Components of a Comprehensive Neonatal History
Component	**Data Required**
Identifying data	Infant's name, parents' names, parents' telephone numbers (home and work), infant's date of birth, gender, and race; source of referral (obstetric or pediatric provider) if any.
Chief complaint	Statement of initial known status (age, gender, birth and current weights, gestational age by dates and examination) and problems infant might have; for a newborn or well-baby examination, the statement simply reflects the current health status (e.g., "Full-term male infant, now 1 week of age, for well-baby follow-up").
Interim history/history of presenting problem	Chronologic record of newborn's history from time of delivery to present or, if older infant, chronologic narrative of chief complaint. Narrative should answer questions related to where (location), what (quality, factors that aggravate or relieve symptoms), when (onset, duration, frequency), and how much (intensity, severity).
Antepartum history	Historical data about the pregnancy, including maternal age, gravidity, parity, last menstrual period, and estimated date of delivery. Date and gestational age at which prenatal care began, provider of care, and number of visits should be recorded here. Mother's health during pregnancy, infections, medications taken, use of illicit drugs or alcohol, abnormal bleeding, and results of prenatal screening tests also should be included.
Obstetric history	Significant history regarding previous pregnancies; neonatal problems or subsequent major medical problems of previous children and current age and health status of living children should be noted.
Intrapartum history	Duration of labor, whether it was spontaneous or induced, duration of rupture of membranes, type of delivery, complications; infant's birth weight, presentation at delivery, and Apgar scores; resuscitative measures if required and response to those measures.
Past medical history	Significant maternal history of chronic health problems or diseases treated in the past or during the pregnancy, including surgical procedures and hospitalizations before or during the pregnancy. For older infants, also obtain information about infant's history, including feeding, development, illness, and immunizations.
Family medical history	Significant family medical history of chronic disorders, disabilities, known hereditary diseases, or consanguinity.
Social history	Parents' marital status, paternal involvement, parents' occupations and educational level; sources of financial support, housing accommodations, and insurance status must be noted, as well as any support agencies involved. Family unit should be defined and religious and cultural affiliations noted, along with number of individuals living in the home. Plans for child care should be elicited, as well as any current family stressors (e.g., moving, death in the family).

technical language, medical jargon, and the tendency to inundate the parents with information. They should attempt to verify that the parents understand what has happened and what they have been told and that they seem to be coping. Nurses should always discuss and explain what the parents can expect to happen next; methods of keeping in touch, pertinent telephone numbers, and the visitation policy, if appropriate.

It is often difficult to approach parents about sensitive matters, such as drug or alcohol use or concerns about the death of their infant. The following suggestions may assist in the discussion of sensitive issues (Seidel et al, 2003). Nurses should:

- Respect the individual's privacy
- Avoid discussing sensitive topics where the conversation might be overheard
- Begin the discussion with open-ended questions and ask the least threatening questions first
- Do not be patronizing, but use language that is straightforward and understandable
- Take a direct and firm approach
- Avoid apologizing for asking a question (the nurse is doing nothing wrong)
- Avoid lecturing (the nurse is not there to pass judgment)

- Understand that defensive behavior might be the individual's way of coping
- Proceed slowly and take care not to demean the individual's behavior
- Offer feedback to ensure that the individual agrees that your interpretation is appropriate
- Provide an opportunity for the individual to ask relevant questions

It is vital that, in communicating with parents from diverse cultures, nurses appreciate and respect differences in communication patterns and in childbearing and health practices. A knowledge of cultural variations in family and health practices assists nurses in developing sensitivity to differences; however, the family must be observed carefully for cues to family practices and relationships with children and one another.

Physical Assessment Techniques

The techniques used for physical assessment are inspection, palpation, percussion, and auscultation. Learning these skills requires patience and practice, and the inability of the newborn to provide verbal cues presents an additional challenge. With experience, the practitioner learns to process a multitude

TABLE 39-4	Percussion Sounds				
Type of Sound	**Intensity**	**Pitch**	**Duration**	**Quality**	**Common Locations**
Tympany	Loud	High	Moderate	Drumlike	Gastric bubble; air-filled intestine (simulate by tapping puffed out cheeks)
Resonance	Moderate to loud	Low	Long	Hollow	Lungs
Hyperresonance	Very loud	Very low	Long	Booming	Lungs with trapped air; lungs of a young child
Dullness	Soft to moderate	High	Moderate	Thudlike	Liver, fluid-filled space (e.g., stomach)
Flatness	Soft	High	Short	Flat	Muscle

Data from Engel J (2002). Pocket guide to pediatric assessment, ed 4. St Louis: Mosby.

of observations while assessing individual systems and then to use these data to form a clinical impression and plan of care.

Inspection

Inspection is a crucial skill in the physical assessment of neonates, but it also is a difficult one to master. Inspection is the simple yet intricate use of the auditory and visual senses to evaluate an infant's state, color, respiratory effort, posture, and activity, as well as the shape and symmetry of various body regions. The sense of smell may be used to note unusual odors. The impression obtained from methodical observation establishes priorities for the remainder of the systematic assessment. In the physical examination, thoughtful observation, rather than simple looking, is the most efficient means of detecting changes. Inspection should be used throughout the physical assessment and should continue as long as the infant remains in the nurse's care.

Auscultation

Auscultation is the process of listening for sounds made by the body. The bell of the stethoscope is used for low-pitched sounds (e.g., cardiovascular sounds) and the diaphragm for higher pitched sounds (e.g., lung and bowel sounds). The stethoscope should be placed lightly but firmly against the wall of the body part being assessed. A calm infant and quiet environment facilitate auscultation. Practice in recognizing normal body sounds is required before abnormal sounds can be identified accurately.

Palpation

With palpation, the examiner uses the sense of touch to determine hydration, texture, tension, pulsation, vibration, amplitude, and tenderness, as well as the depth, size, shape, and location of deep structures. The touch used for palpation must be gentle and is performed with the flats of the finger pads rather than the fingertips (Fletcher, 1998). To gather the most accurate information, the infant should be calm at the onset of the abdominal examination. Relaxing the abdominal musculature by flexing the infant's knees and hips with one hand facilitates palpation of the liver and spleen. Gentle pressure must be emphasized during palpation of sensitive organs (e.g., liver, spleen, and skin) that are at greater risk for injury and bleeding in neonates, particular preterm infants or those that have hepatomegaly. Warming of the examiner's hands, use of a pacifier, and progression from superficial to deep

palpation help maintain the infant's comfort throughout most of the examination. Tender areas should always be palpated last.

Percussion

Percussion is the use of tapping to produce sound waves that may be assessed according to intensity, pitch, duration, and quality (Table 39-4). Percussion may be direct or indirect. For direct percussion, the examiner directly strikes the body part to be assessed with the tip of the middle right finger. For indirect percussion, the examiner places the middle finger of the non-dominant hand against the skin of the body part to be assessed and strikes the distal joint with the tip of the middle finger of the dominant hand. The wrist must make a snapping motion, creating a brisk thump with the tip of the right middle finger against the left middle finger's distal joint. Vibrations are transmitted from the bones of the finger joint touching the infant's body to the underlying tissue (Figure 39-2). Although percussion is rarely used in neonatal assessment, it may be a useful technique for examining the older infant or child.

Assessment of Size and Growth

Well-being in the fetal and neonatal periods is reflected by a normal growth pattern. Fetal and neonatal growth rates are predictable and can be measured by various methods. To determine if an individual infant's growth is adequate, an appropriate standard must be used with which the child's measurements can be compared. The growth curves used must

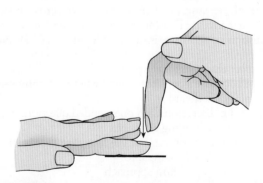

FIGURE **39-2**
Percussion. Note the position of the fingers. From Engel J (2002). *Pocket guide to pediatric assessment*, ed 4. St Louis: Mosby.

match the patient as closely as possible in gender, race, gestational age, genetic potential, and environmental factors, such as altitude. A discussion of the techniques used to estimate and assess fetal growth is beyond the scope of this chapter and can be found elsewhere in this text. Two methods of evaluating adequacy of growth in the newborn are the gestational age assessment and the clinical assessment of nutritional status (CANSCORE).

ASSESSMENT OF GESTATIONAL AGE

A determination of gestational age (GA) is part of the physical examination of every newborn. Classification of newborns by gestational age enables the health care provider to determine the neonatal mortality risk (Figure 39-3) and to identify possible disorders (Figure 39-4) and initiate intervention or screening (Gardner et al, 2002). Figure 39-5 shows the classification of newborns by intrauterine growth and gestational age. Table 39-5 presents terms used in GA assessment and in determining the adequacy of in utero growth.

As was previously mentioned, morbidity and mortality can be predicted from the GA assessment (see Figures 39-3 and 39-4). Neonates with the lowest risk of problems associated with morbidity and mortality are term infants who developmentally are appropriate for gestational age (AGA). Risks associated with categories of gestational age and intrauterine growth restriction are shown in Table 39-6.

After birth, gestational age is determined by the evaluation of physical, neurologic, and neuromuscular characteristics. A number of methods have been developed to assess gestational

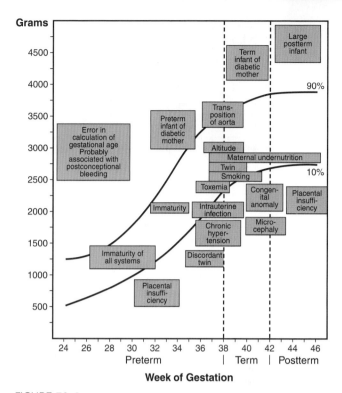

FIGURE 39-4
Deviations of intrauterine growth: neonatal morbidity by birth weight and gestational age. From Lubchenco LO (1967). *The high risk infant.* Philadelphia: Saunders; as adapted from Lubchenco LO et al (1968). In Jonxis JHP et al, editors. *Aspects of prematurity and dysmaturity.* Springfield, IL: Charles C Thomas.

age in newborns. Currently, the New Ballard score (NBS) is the most widely used assessment tool (Figure 39-6). Its advantages over the other scoring systems are its wide range (20 to 44 weeks) and its accuracy (within 1 week) of GA measurement (Southgate & Pittard, 2001). Performing the examination as soon as possible in the first 12 hours of life enhances its accuracy.

Although GA assessment is discussed separately, the components of the assessment should be performed as part of the infant's general physical examination. Table 39-7 presents the essentials of the NBS; each component is scored as shown in Figure 39-6. The total score is calculated, and the resulting GA is plotted on a graph (see Figure 39-5).

CLINICAL ASSESSMENT OF NUTRITIONAL STATUS (CANSCORE)

GA assessment does not identify all infants with intrauterine malnutrition. Although the terms small for gestational age (SGA) and intrauterine growth retardation/restriction (IUGR) are related, they are not synonymous. IUGR represents a reduction in the expected fetal growth pattern, whereas SGA refers to an infant whose birth weight is less than population norms. Not all IUGR infants are SGA, and not all SGA infants are IUGR (Kliegman, 2006; Trotter, 2003).

Many but not all infants who are either SGA or IUGR are malnourished in utero. However, malnutrition can occur in neonates of any birth weight. Because malnutrition alters body composition and can prevent adequate brain growth, it is important to identify infants who have been affected in utero.

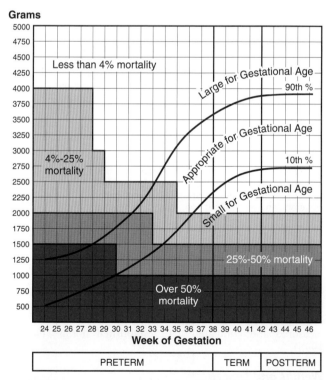

FIGURE 39-3
University of Colorado Medical Center classification of newborns by birth weight and gestational age and by neonatal mortality risk. From Battaglia FC, Lubchenco LO (1967). A practical classification of newborn infants by weight and gestational age. *Journal of pediatrics* 71:159-163.

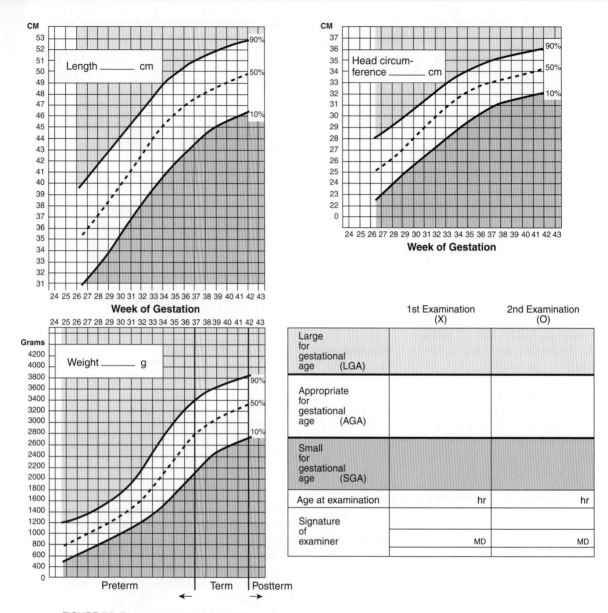

FIGURE **39-5**
Estimating gestational age: newborn classification based on maturity and intrauterine growth. From Lowdermilk DL et al (2007). *Maternity & women's health care*, ed 9. St Louis: Mosby. Modified from Lubchenco L et al (1966). Intrauterine growth in length and head circumference as estimated from live births at gestational ages from 26 to 42 weeks. *Journal of pediatrics* 37:403; Battaglia F, Lubchenco L (1967): A practical classification of newborn infants by weight and gestational age. *Journal of pediatrics* 71:159.

These infants may be at risk for problems associated with aberrant growth (Fletcher, 1998).

McLean and Usher (1970) described physical findings that are suggestive of weight loss or poor nutrition. These physical characteristics form the basis of the CANSCORE used in the clinical evaluation of nutritional status in newborns at term (Figure 39-7).

Measurement Techniques

For most infants the parameters of weight, length, and occipitofrontal circumference (OFC) are adequate for the basic physical assessment. These measurements are compared against standard growth curves. If the infant has any abnormalities in the size of a body component or if the infant shows disproportionate growth, the involved areas should be measured and compared with established norms (Fletcher, 1998).

Weight and Length

The infant should be weighed while unclothed and quiet. Weight can be falsely increased by a significant amount of infant motion (Fletcher, 1998). The weight of the average full-term that is AGA is 3.5 kg, with a range of 2700 to 4000 g (Grover, 2000a; Tappero, 2003). Generally African American,

TABLE **39-5**	Terms and Abbreviations Used in Assessment of Gestational Age and Adequacy of Intrauterine Growth
Term and Abbreviation	**Description**
Low birth weight (LBW)	Infant weighing <2500 g*
Very low birth weight (VLBW)	Infant weighing <1500 g*
Extremely low birth weight (ELBW)	Infant weighing <1000 g*
Appropriate for gestational age (AGA)	Parameter (weight) within the 10th to 90th percentile for gestational age
Large for gestational age (LGA)	Parameter above the 90th percentile for gestational age
Small for gestational age (SGA)	Parameter below the 10th percentile for gestational age
Intrauterine growth restriction (IUGR)	Slowing of intrauterine growth documented by ultrasound; a neonate may be IUGR without being SGA
Symmetric IUGR	Measurements for weight, length, and head circumference all within the same growth curve even if neonate is AGA, LGA, or SGA
Asymmetric IUGR	Measurements for weight, length, and head circumference in different growth curves
Term gestation	Neonate born between 37 and 42 weeks' gestation
Preterm gestation	Neonate delivered before completion of week 37 of gestation
Postterm gestation	Neonate delivered after completion of week 42 of gestation

Regardless of length of gestation.

TABLE **39-6**	Risks Associated with Gestational Age and Intrauterine Growth Restriction
Category	**Risks**
Small for gestational age (SGA), large for gestational age (LGA), intrauterine growth retardation/restriction (IUGR)	Perinatal and long-term problems
Preterm SGA	Problems associated with immaturity of body systems and placental insufficiency
Preterm	Problems associated with immaturity of body systems
Postterm	Problems associated with placental insufficiency
Term LGA	Risks are greatest in perinatal period, but long-term problems can develop

Hawaiian, and Asian neonates weigh less than Caucasian infants (Tappero, 2003).

The crown-to-heel length can be obtained using a measurement board or a standard tape measure. With the infant supine and legs extended, the nurse draws a line on the bed at the baby's head and another at the heels and then measures the distance between these two points (Figure 39-8). The average full-term newborn is 50 cm long with a range of 48 to 53 cm (Tappero, 2003). Other measurement techniques are described in the appropriate sections.

Physical Examination of the Neonate

The following sections describe the newborn examination beyond the transition period.

Vital Signs

Once transition is complete, the neonate has a respiratory rate between 40 and 60 breaths/min, and the rate may be irregular. Respirations are easy and unlabored; breath sounds should be clear on auscultation. The heart rate varies from 100 to 160 beats/min, depending on the infant's state and gestational age (Vargo, 2003). Premature neonates have a higher baseline heart rate. The resting heart rate is the most representative for any baby.

Normal blood pressure ranges depend on gestational and chronologic ages and the methods used. Blood pressure in premature babies is proportional to size; therefore normal values are lower than for term babies (Hegyi et al, 1994). Figures 39-9 and 39-10 and Tables 39-8, 39-9, and 39-10 show normal blood pressure values over various time frames and gestational ages.

Temperature is determined by axillary measurement; acceptable values range from 35.5° to 37.5° C (Blake & Murray, 2002; Southgate & Pittard, 2001).

Cardiovascular Values

The heart is assessed for rate, rhythm, character of heart sounds, and presence of murmurs. During infancy the position of the heart changes and the point of maximal impulse (PMI) shifts (Fletcher, 1998). In the first few days of life the PMI is located at the fourth intercostal space at or to the left of the midclavicular line (Vargo, 2003). Auscultation should be performed at the second and fourth intercostal spaces, cardiac apex, and axilla (D'Harlingue & Durand, 2001). Murmurs are commonly heard before the ductus arteriosus closes completely. However, murmurs that are persistent may not be normal and require evaluation. Brief asymptomatic irregularities in rate and rhythm are not uncommon, especially in the preterm baby. The most common benign dysrhythmias are sinus bradycardia or tachycardia and premature atrial or ventricular contractions (Vargo, 2003). An electrocardiogram (ECG) or heart monitor is needed to properly identify the abnormality. Exact identification of the abnormality cannot be made solely by auscultation.

Neuromuscular Maturity

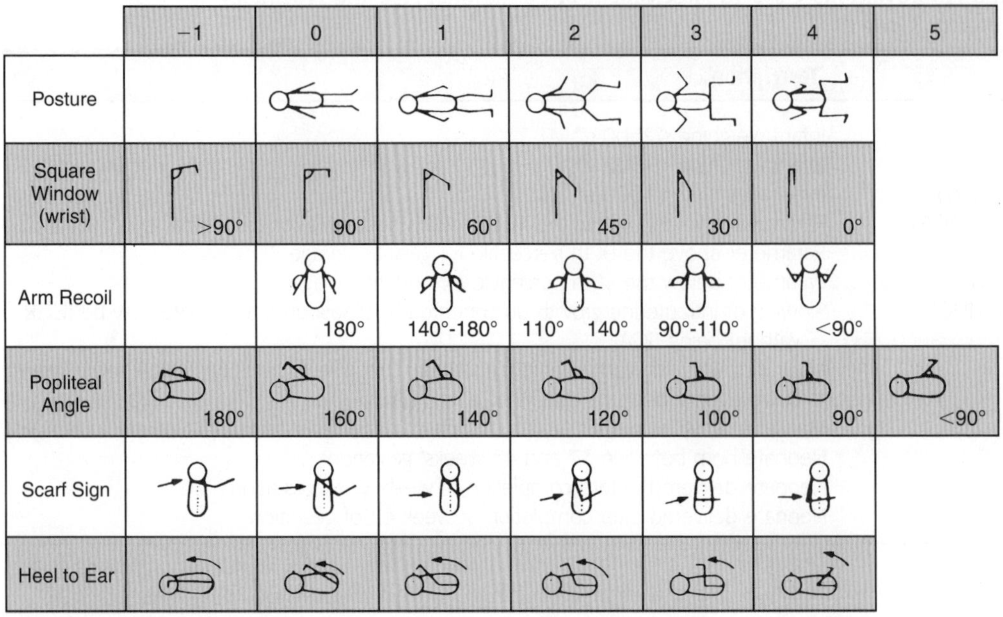

	−1	0	1	2	3	4	5
Posture							
Square Window (wrist)	>90°	90°	60°	45°	30°	0°	
Arm Recoil		180°	140°-180°	110° 140°	90°-110°	<90°	
Popliteal Angle	180°	160°	140°	120°	100°	90°	<90°
Scarf Sign							
Heel to Ear							

Physical Maturity

Skin	sticky friable transparent	gelatinous red, translucent	smooth pink, visible veins	superficial peeling &/or rash few veins	cracking pale areas rare veins	parchment deep cracking no vessels	leathery cracked wrinkled
Lanugo	none	sparse	abundant	thinning	bald areas	mostly bald	
Plantar Surface	heel-toe 40-50 mm: −1 <40 mm: −2	>50 mm no crease	faint red marks	anterior transverse crease only	creases ant. 2/3	creases over entire sole	
Breast	imperceptible	barely perceptible	flat areola no bud	stippled areola 1-2 mm bud	raised areola 3-4 mm bud	full areola 5-10 mm bud	
Eye/Ear	lids fused loosely: −1 tightly: −2	lids open pinna flat stays folded	sl. curved pinna; soft; slow recoil	well-curved pinna; soft but ready recoil	formed & firm instant recoil	thick cartilage ear stiff	
Genitals (male)	scrotum flat, smooth	scrotum empty faint rugae	testes in upper canal rare rugae	testes descending few rugae	testes down good rugae	testes pendulous deep rugae	
Genitals (female)	clitoris prominent labia flat	prominent clitoris small labia minora	prominent clitoris enlarging minora	majora & minora equally prominent	majora large minora small	majora cover clitoris & minora	

Maturity Rating

score	weeks
−10	20
−5	22
0	24
5	26
10	28
15	30
20	32
25	34
30	36
35	38
40	40
45	42
50	44

FIGURE **39-6**
Maturational assessment of gestational age: New Ballard scoring system. From Ballard JL et al (1991). New Ballard Score, expanded to include extremely premature infants. *Journal of pediatrics* 119:417-423.

A precordial impulse may be visible along the left sternal border during the first 6 hours (Fletcher, 1998; Southgate & Pittard, 2001). In premature neonates, because of their thin skin and absence of subcutaneous fat, the precordial impulse may be visible for a longer period.

Pulses are palpated for rate, strength, and synchrony. Figure 39-11 shows the location of pulses in the neonate (Vargo, 2003). Radial or brachial pulses are compared for timing and intensity, and the same is then done for bilateral femoral pulses. Finally, the preductal and postductal pulses are examined.

The adequacy of the infant's perfusion is determined by checking the capillary refill. This is assessed by depressing the skin over the abdomen or on an extremity until the area blanches. The capillary refill time is the number of seconds that elapse until the color returns to the area. This should be less than 3 seconds.

TABLE 39-7	New Ballard Scoring System		
Component	**Assessment Technique**	**Effect of Maturity**	**Comments**
NEUROMUSCULAR MATURITY			
Posture	Observe infant while baby is unrestrained and supine; note amount of flexion and extension of extremities.	Extensor tone is replaced by flexor tone in a cephalocaudal progression.	Knees may be hyperextended in a frank breech delivery.
Square window	Flex wrist; measure minimum angle formed by ventral surface of forearm and palm.	Angle decreases; at term no space exists between palm and forearm.	Response depends on muscle tone and intrauterine position.
Arm recoil	Place infant in supine position with head in midline. Flex elbow and hold forearm against arm for 5 seconds; fully extend elbow, then release; note time required for infant to resume flexed position.	Angle decreases and recoil becomes more rapid.	
Popliteal angle	Flex hips, placing thighs on abdomen; keeping hips on surface of bed, extend knee as far as possible until resistance is met; estimate popliteal angle.	Popliteal angle decreases.	Amount of extension can be overestimated if knee is extended beyond point where resistance is first met; this assessment also is affected by intrauterine position and hip dislocation.
Scarf sign	With head in midline, pull hand across chest to encircle neck; note position of elbow relative to midline.	Increased resistance to crossing the midline.	Reflects muscle tone; response is altered by obesity, hydrops, or fractured clavicle.
Heel to ear	Keep infant supine with pelvis on mattress; press feet as far as possible toward head, allowing knees to be positioned beside abdomen; estimate angle created by arc from back of heel to mattress.	Angle decreases; hip flexion decreases toward term.	Reflects muscle tone.
PHYSICAL MATURITY			
Skin	Observe translucency of skin over abdominal wall.	Skin becomes thicker and ultimately dry and peeling; pigmentation increases.	Skin becomes drier hours after birth; phototherapy or sunlight enhances pigmentation.
Lanugo	Assess for presence and length of hair over back.	Lanugo emerges at 19 to 20 weeks and is most prominent at 27 to 28 weeks; it then gradually disappears, first from the lower back and then from at least half of the back.	The degree of pigmentation and quantity of hair are related to race, gender, and nutritional status.
Plantar surface	Measure length of foot; determine presence or absence of true deep creases (not merely wrinkles).	Early in gestation, foot length correlates with fetal growth; creases develop from toes to heel, and absence of creases correlates with immaturity.	Plantar creases also reflect intrauterine fetal activity; accelerated creasing is seen with oligohydramnios; diminished creasing suggests lack of activity in a mature fetus.
Breast	Estimate diameter of breast bud; assess color and stippling of areola.	Definition and stippling of areola and pigmentation are evident near term; bud size increases because of maternal hormones and fat accumulation.	With intrauterine growth restriction, breast tissue may be diminished, but development of areola proceeds regardless of malnutrition.

Continued

TABLE 39-7	New Ballard Scoring System—cont'd		
Component	**Assessment Technique**	**Effect of Maturity**	**Comments**
PHYSICAL MATURITY—cont'd			
Ear cartilage	Fold top of auricle; observe speed of recoil.	Cartilage becomes stiff, and auricle thickens.	Compression in utero and absence or dysfunction of auricular muscles diminishes firmness.
Eyelid opening	Without attempting to separate eyelids, evaluate degree of fusion.	Opening begins at 22 weeks; lids are completely unfused by 28 weeks.	Fused eyelids should not be considered a sign of nonviability; lids may be fused at term with anophthalmia.
EXTERNAL GENITALIA			
Male	Palpate scrotum to assess degree of descent of testes; observe rugae and suspension of scrotum.	At 27 to 28 weeks, testes begin to descend into scrotum; rugae formation begins at about 28 weeks; by term rugae are well defined, and scrotum is pendulous.	Rugae are decreased with scrotal edema; testes may be absent (cryptorchidism).
Female	Assess size of labia minora and labia majora.	Labia minora increase in size before labia majora; at term labia majora cover labia minora completely.	Size of labia majora depends on amount of body fat; with malnutrition, size may be diminished; edema may increase size of labia majora.

Data from Fletcher MA (1998). Physical diagnosis in neonatology. Philadelphia: Lippincott-Raven; and Southgate WM, Pittard WB (2001). Classification and physical examination of the newborn infant. In Klaus MH, Fanaroff AA, editors. Care of the high risk neonate, ed 5. Philadelphia: Saunders.

General Appearance

The infant's general appearance is indicative of nutritional status, maturity, and overall well-being. Term neonates normally are well formed and rounded and have stores of subcutaneous fat. They assume the fetal position at rest. Premature babies may display less flexion than those born at term. Movement should be spontaneous and tremulous. Neonates range in mood from quiet to alert; they are consolable when crying. The cry is strong and sustained (Sansoucie & Cavaliere, 2002).

Skin

The skin is assessed for maturity, consistency, and color. Discolored areas, variations, or abnormalities are noted for size and location. The skin of a full-term newborn contains subcutaneous fat that provides insulation against heat loss. It is smooth, pink, and wrinkle free. Premature infants lack subcutaneous fat; their skin is thinner than that of term babies and has visible blood vessels over the chest and abdomen. Extremely immature babies often have a gelatinous appearance with transparent skin. They commonly have a red, ruddy color caused by underdevelopment of the stratum corneum. Subcutaneous fat also is lacking in neonates who are IUGR. This group of babies may have loose skin folds, particularly around the knees.

Vernix is the greasy yellow or white substance found on fetal skin, particularly in the axillary, nuchal, and inguinal folds. Composed of sebaceous gland secretions, lanugo, and desquamated epithelial cells, it protects against fluid loss and bacterial invasion (Fletcher, 1998). Vernix is most abundant during the third trimester and decreases in amount as the fetus approaches 40 weeks.

Lanugo is fine, downy hair that first appears on the fetus at 19 to 20 weeks' gestation and becomes most prominent at 27 to 28 weeks. It begins to disappear from the lower back and usually is not present at term.

Head

The head is inspected for shape, symmetry, bruises, and lesions. Neonates delivered by cesarean section generally have a rounded head. Infants born vaginally in vertex position can have overriding sutures; this results in an irregularly shaped head that persists only for a few days in full-term neonates but may be evident for several weeks in premature babies (Sansoucie & Cavaliere, 2002). The head circumference is measured in the occipitofrontal plane and is the largest diameter around the head. It is obtained with the tape measure placed snugly above the ears, the eyebrow ridges, and the occiput of the head. The average OFC in a full-term neonate is 35 cm, with a normal range of 31 to 38 cm (Sansoucie & Cavaliere, 2002). The major bones of the head, as well as sutures and fontanelles, are shown in Figure 39-12.

The head should be palpated to assess the firmness of bone and the size and configuration of fontanelles and sutures and also to detect swelling, masses, or bony defects. The amount of overlap of sutures may vary, depending on the extent of molding. Normally the sutures should move freely when gentle pressure is applied to the bones on opposite sides of the suture lines (Furdon & Clark, 2003). Directly after birth it may be difficult to determine if the sutures are fused or merely

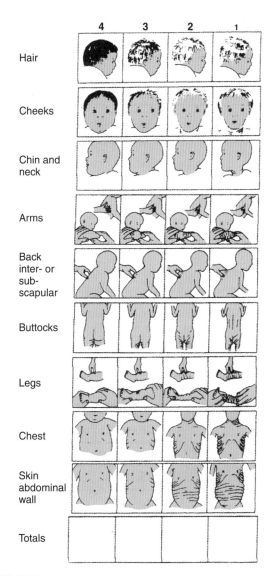

FIGURE **39-7**
Clinical assessment of nutritional status at birth (CANSCORE system). Nine signs are used to assess the nutritional status of newborn term infants. Each sign is rated from 4 (best) to 1 (worst). The CANSCORE is the sum of the nine signs. *Hair:* Large amount, smooth, silky, easily groomed (4 points); thinner, some straight "starring" hair (3 points); still thinner, more straight, with depigmented stripe (flag sign). *Cheeks:* Progression from full buccal pads and round face (4 points) to significantly reduced buccal fat with narrow, flat face (1 point). *Chin and neck:* Double or triple chin fat folds, neck not evident (4 points) to thin chin, no fat folds, neck with loose, wrinkled skin very evident (1 point). *Arms:* Full, round, cannot elicit accordion folds or lift folds of skin from elbow or triceps area (4 points) to striking accordion folding of lower arm (to elicit this sign, the examiner uses the thumb and fingers of the left hand to grasp the infant's arm just below the elbow, and the thumb and fingers of the right hand to encircle the infant's wrist, and then moves the two hands toward each other); skin loose, easy to grasp and pull away from the elbow (1 point). *Back:* Skin in interscapular area difficult to grasp and lift (4 points) to skin in interscapular area loose, easily lifted in a thin fold (1 point). *Buttocks:* Full, round gluteal fat pads (4 points) to virtually no evident gluteal fat, skin of buttocks and upper, posterior thigh loose and deeply wrinkled (1 point). *Legs:* Same as for arms. *Chest:* Full and round, ribs not seen (4 points) to progressive prominence of ribs with obvious loss of intercostal tissue (1 point). *Abdomen:* Full, round, no loose skin (4 points) to distended or scaphoid but with very loose, easily lifted, wrinkled skin with accordion folds demonstrable (1 point). From Metcoff J (1994). Clinical assessment of nutritional status at birth, *Pediatric clinics of North America* 41:875-891.

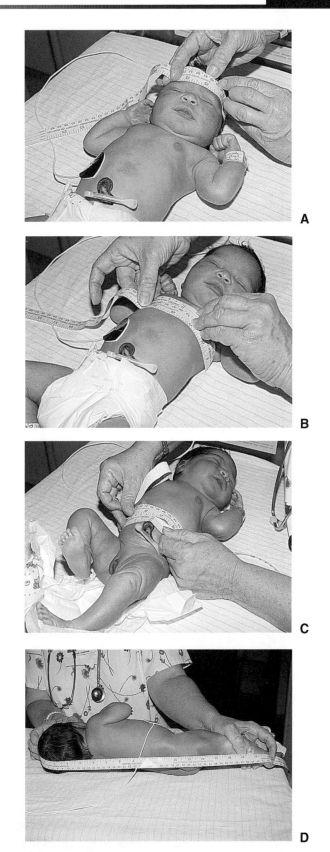

FIGURE **39-8**
Newborn measurements. **A,** Circumference of head. **B,** Circumference of chest. **C,** Circumference of abdomen. **D,** Length, crown to rump. (Total length includes the length of the legs.) If the measurements are taken before the infant's first bath, the nurse must wear gloves. From Lowdermilk DL et al (2000). *Maternity and women's health care,* ed 7. St Louis: Mosby. Courtesy Marjorie Pyle, RNC, Lifecircle, Costa Mesa, CA.

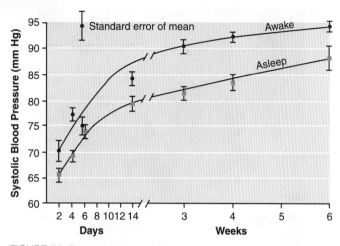

FIGURE **39-9**

Increase in systolic blood pressure between ages 2 days and 6 weeks in infants awake and asleep (values obtained by cuff measurement). From Early A et al (1980). Blood pressure in the first six weeks of life. *Archives of disease in childhood* 55:755-757.

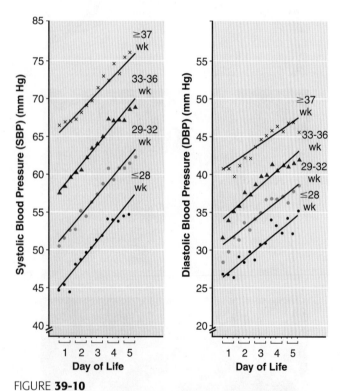

FIGURE **39-10**

Systolic and diastolic blood pressures plotted for the first 5 days of life, with each day subdivided into 8-hour periods. Infants are categorized by gestational age into four groups: 28 weeks or younger (*n* = 33), 29 to 32 weeks (*n* = 73), 33 to 36 weeks (*n* = 100), and 37 weeks or older (*n* = 110). From Zubrow AB et al (1995). Determinants of blood pressure in infants admitted to neonatal intensive care units: a prospective multicenter study. Philadelphia Neonatal Blood Pressure Study Group. *Journal of perinatology* 15:470.

TABLE **39-8**	Blood Pressure Values According to Site and Age		
	Blood Pressure (mm Hg)		
Site and Age	**Systolic**	**Diastolic**	**Mean**
Right Arm			
Less than 36 hours old	62.6 ± 6.9	38.9 ± 5.7	48 ± 6.2
Over 36 hours old	68.4 ± 8.8*	43.5 ± 6.2*	53 ± 7.3
Total	64.7 ± 8.1	40.6 ± 6.2	49.8 ± 7
Calf			
Less than 36 hours old	61.9 ± 7	39.6 ± 5.3	47.6 ± 6
Over 36 hours old	66.8 ± 10.1*	42.5 ± 7.3*	51.5 ± 9*
Total	63.6 ± 8.6	40.6 ± 6.3	49 ± 7.5

Values were obtained by blood pressure cuff measurement in 219 healthy term infants, 140 less than 36 hours old and 79 over 36 hours old. Values are given as means ± standard deviation.
**Significantly different from values in infants less than 36 hours old ($p < 0.05$).*

TABLE **39-9**	Blood Pressure Ranges in Different Weight Groups of Premature Newborns	
	Blood Pressure (mm Hg)	
Birth Weight (g)	**Systolic**	**Diastolic**
501-750 (*n* = 18)	50-62	26-36
751-1000 (*n* = 39)	48-59	23-36
1001-1250 (*n* = 30)	49-61	26-35
1251-1500 (*n* = 45)	46-56	23-33
1501-1750 (*n* = 51)	46-58	23-33
1751-2000 (*n* = 61)	48-61	24-35

From Hegyi T et al (1994). Blood pressure ranges in premature infants. The first hours of life. Journal of pediatrics 124:627-633.
Measurements were obtained by blood pressure cuff or umbilical artery transducer in the first 3 to 6 hours of life.

TABLE **39-10**	Oscillometric Measurements: Mean Arterial Blood Pressure		
	Mean Arterial Pressure ± Standard Deviation		
Birth Weight (g)	**Day 3**	**Day 17**	**Day 31**
501-750	38 ± 8	44 ± 8	46 ± 11
751-1000	43 ± 8	45 ± 7	47 ± 9
1001-1250	43 ± 8	46 ± 9	48 ± 8
1251-1500	45 ± 8	47 ± 8	47 ± 9

From Fanaroff AA, Wright E (1990). Profiles of mean arterial blood pressure (MAP) for infants weighing 50 to 1500 grams. Pediatric research 27:205A.

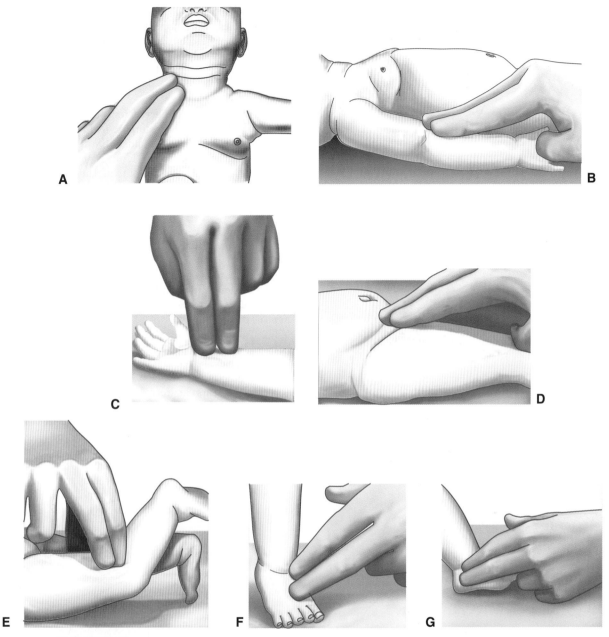

FIGURE **39-11**
Palpation of arterial pulses. **A,** Carotid. **B,** Brachial. **C,** Radial. **D,** Femoral. **E,** Popliteal. **F,** Dorsalis pedis.
G, Posterior tibial.

overlapping. Re-evaluation when molding and overlap have resolved may yield more reliable information about the presence of craniosynostosis (Fletcher, 1998).

The anterior fontanelle is 2 to 3 cm wide, 3 to 4 cm long, and diamond shaped (see Figure 39-12). It should be flat and soft; tense, bulging fontanelles may be reflective of intracranial pressure while a sunken fontanelle can signify dehydration (Johnson, 2003). The posterior fontanelle is 1 to 2 cm wide and triangular. It may be difficult to palpate the fontanelles directly after birth because of cranial molding (Sansoucie & Cavaliere, 2002). Tension in the fontanelle should be assessed with the infant both recumbent and upright. Serial measurements of the width of the anterior fontanelle are more helpful

than a single measurement because of wide variations in size and differences in measurement techniques (Fletcher, 1998).

Hair is evaluated for color, length, continuity, texture, quantity, position and number of hair whorls, and hairlines. Term newborns have fine hair with identifiable individual strands. Hair may appear disheveled for the first several weeks to months (Fletcher, 1998). In premature neonates the hair is more widely dispersed and is described as "fuzzy." Normally, hair color is fairly uniform, although some neonates have a blend of light and dark hair (Furdon & Clark, 2003). Sporadic patches of white hair may be a familial trait and is a benign finding, but a white forelock and other pigmentation defects in the eyes or skin may be associated with deafness or mental

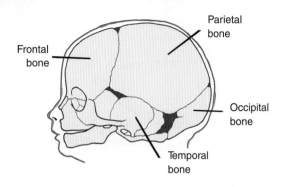

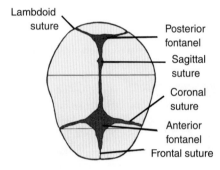

FIGURE **39-12**

Major bones of the head in the newborn with sutures and fontanelles. From Lowdermilk DL et al (2000). *Maternity and women's health care,* ed 7. St Louis: Mosby.

retardation (Fletcher, 1998; Waardenburg, 1951). The anterior hairline varies, with normal growth of pigmented hair onto the forehead of hirsute babies. The posterior hairline ends at the neck crease. Usually one off-center hair whorl is present in the parietal region (Fletcher, 1998; Furdon & Clark, 2003).

Face and Neck

The face should be inspected for shape, symmetry, and the presence of bruising or dysmorphic features. The overall facial configuration should be evaluated; the features should be proportional and symmetric. Unusual facial features may be familial or pathognomonic of a malformation syndrome. Gag, sucking, and rooting reflexes should be evaluated.

The newborn has a relatively short neck that should be palpated or observed for symmetry, appearance of the skin, range of motion, masses, and fistulous openings. The neck should be symmetric with the head, demonstrating full range of motion (Sansoucie & Cavaliere, 2002). In utero positioning can cause asymmetry of the neck. Redundant skin or webbing may be evident (Sneiderman & Taeusch, 2005). The clavicles can be palpated at this time; they should be intact and without crepitus or swelling.

Ears

The ears are evaluated and compared for shape, configuration, position, amount of cartilage, and signs of trauma. The position of the ears at term should be similar bilaterally; approximately 30% of the pinna should lie above a line from the inner and outer canthi of the eye toward the occiput. The rotation of the ears should also be assessed; the long axis of the pinna should lie approximately 15 degrees posterior to the true vertical axis of the head (Fletcher, 1998) (Figure 39-13). Abnormalities of the external ear may be associated with syndromes, but often they represent minor structural variations and may be within the normal range (Johnson, 2003).

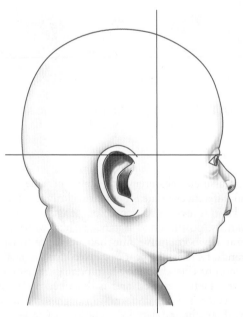

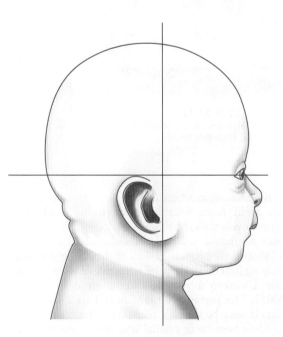

Normal ear location   Low-seated ear

FIGURE **39-13**
Ear position.

The presence and patency of the auditory canal can be documented by inspection. Otoscopic examination is not usually part of the examination in the newborn period because the ear canals are filled with vernix, amniotic debris, and blood. This condition clears in approximately 60% of term infants by 1 week of age but may persist for weeks. Less debris is seen in preterm babies, whose canals may clear more quickly.

Because infants frequently remain hospitalized beyond the neonatal period and because evaluation of the middle ear is part of a health maintenance examination, it is appropriate to include otoscopic examination in this section. The otoscope is used differently in young infants than in adults. In a neonate the ear lobe is pulled toward the chin, and the speculum is directed toward the face. The ear canals of preterm babies are prone to collapse because they are more pliable. Positive pressure applied through the pneumatic otoscope prevents the cartilaginous ear canal from obscuring the view (Fletcher, 1998). The neonatal tympanic membrane is thicker, grayer, and more vascular than that of an adult or older child (Figure 39-14).

Infants should also be assessed for behavioral response to noise stimuli. However, routine formal audiologic testing is becoming more common in the newborn period.

Eyes

The eyes should show spontaneous range of motion and conjugate movements. The lids should be symmetric in both horizontal and vertical placement, and the lashes should be directed outward in an orderly fashion. The eyes should be clear and should have an evenly colored iris, which may be dark gray, blue, or brown, depending on race. Pigmentation should be similar between the two eyes. Permanent eye color is not established for several months, but darker races may show permanent pigmentation in the first week of life. The surface of the conjunctiva should be smooth. During the first few days of life, the cornea may appear slightly hazy as a result of corneal edema, but thereafter the cornea should be clear and shiny. The sclerae normally are white, but a bluish coloration may be noted in premature and other small infants because their sclerae are thinner (Fletcher, 1998; Gupta et al, 2006).

An ophthalmoscope is used to assess the pupillary and red reflexes. The light should be directed on the pupils from a distance of approximately 6 inches. The pupils should be round and equal in diameter and should constrict equally in response to light (pupils equal and reactive to light, or PERL) (Johnson, 2003). The beam of light illuminating the retina causes the red reflex. The retina (fundus) appears as a yellowish-white/gray or red background, depending on the amount of melanin in the pigment epithelium. The pigment varies with the complexion of the baby; in dark-skinned infants the reflex will be pale or cloudy (Honeyfield, 2003; Wright, 1999).

Nose

The nose should be evaluated for shape and symmetry, patency of nares, skin lesions, or signs of trauma. The nasal mucosa should be pink and slightly moist; secretions should be thin, clear, and usually scanty (Fletcher, 1998). The nose should be midline. Immediately after birth the nose may be misshapen as a result of compression in utero, but this should correct spontaneously in a few days (Fletcher, 1998; Sansoucie & Cavaliere, 2002). Obstructions and deformities may denote anatomic malformations or congenital syndromes. The patency of the nares can be demonstrated by alternate occlusion of each naris using gentle pressure (Fletcher, 1998). Nasal flaring may be indicative of respiratory distress but "the use of ali nasi activation in otherwise healthy premature infants varies with activity and sleep states, so by itself cannot be used as a sign of respiratory distress" (Fletcher, 1998).

Mouth

The mouth is inspected for size, shape, color, and presence of abnormal structures and masses. It should be evaluated both at rest and while the infant is crying. The speed of response and intensity of neonatal reflexes, such as rooting, gag, and suck, are also assessed. The mouth is a midline structure, symmetric in shape and movement. The mouth, chin, and tongue should be in proportion, with the lips fully formed (Sansoucie & Cavaliere, 2002).

The mucous membranes should be pink and moist, and oral secretions should be thin and clear. Excessive secretions or drooling suggests inability to swallow or esophageal or pharyngeal obstruction. Both the hard and soft palates should be inspected and palpated to rule out clefts. A high-arched palate may be seen in malformation syndromes, but it generally is insignificant if it appears as an isolated characteristic (Lissauer, 2006).

The tongue should be smooth on all surfaces; the lingual frenulum may be short but not so short as to restrict tongue movement. Limitation of movement would be obvious on crying, when the tip of the tongue would form an inverted V (Fletcher, 1998).

Thorax

The chest is evaluated for size, symmetry, musculature, bony structure, number and location of nipples, and ease of respiration (Southgate & Pittard, 2001). It should be symmetric in shape and movements. Because the anteroposterior diameter is approximately equal to the transverse diameter, the chest

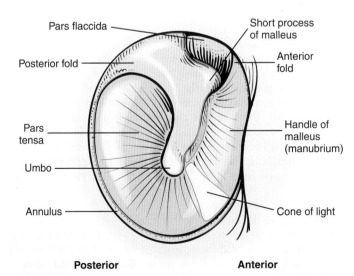

Posterior   **Anterior**

Pars flaccida
Posterior fold
Pars tensa
Umbo
Annulus
Short process of malleus
Anterior fold
Handle of malleus (manubrium)
Cone of light

FIGURE **39-14**
Normal landmarks of the right tympanic membrane as seen through an otoscope. From Lewis SM et al (2000). *Medical-surgical nursing: assessment and management of clinical problems*, ed 5. St Louis: Mosby.

appears round. The chest circumference of a term infant should be about 2 cm smaller than the head circumference (Askin, 2003). At all gestational ages, the chest measurement normally is smaller than the OFC (Fletcher, 1998).

Occasional mild subcostal retractions may be seen in healthy newborns because of decreased compliance of the ribs. A paradoxical breathing pattern is typical of newborns, especially during sleep. On inspiration the chest wall is drawn in and the abdomen protrudes; the reverse occurs on expiration (Fletcher, 1998).

The amount of breast tissue depends on the gestational age and birth weight, whereas areolar development reflects only gestational age. Two nipples should be present in equal alignment. The internipple distance varies by gestational age and chest circumference, but the ratio of internipple distance to chest circumference should be less that 0.28 (Fletcher, 1998). Widely spaced nipples are associated with a variety of congenital syndromes.

Newborn breast tissue may hypertrophy as a result of the influence of maternal hormones. A milky substance (witches' milk) may appear toward the end of the first week of life, and this discharge may persist for a few weeks to several months (Askin, 2003; Fletcher, 1998).

Abdomen

The abdomen is inspected for contour and size, symmetry, character of skin, and umbilical cord location and anatomy. Palpation yields information about muscle mass and tone of the abdominal wall, location and size of viscera, tenderness, and masses (Fletcher, 1998). Bowel sounds are detected on auscultation; they are relatively quiet in newborns until feedings are established. Compared with term babies, preterm neonates have less active bowel sounds. Evaluating changes in bowel sounds from the infant's baseline is more clinically useful than an isolated assessment (Fletcher, 1998).

The normal abdomen in an infant is round and soft and protrudes slightly. The umbilical cord should be bluish white, shiny, and moist and should have two arteries and one vein. To facilitate palpation, the knees and legs should be flexed toward the hips, which allows the abdominal muscles to relax. The edge of the liver can be palpated 1 to 2 cm below the right costal margin at the midclavicular line; this edge should be smooth, firm, and well defined (Goodwin, 2003). The tip of the spleen can be felt below the left costal margin in newborn infants. The size of the spleen depends on variables such as circulating blood volume, day of life, method of delivery, and type of therapy, which must be considered when interpreting the significance of mild enlargement (Fletcher, 1998).

The kidneys are located in the flanks. The lower pole of both kidneys should be palpable because of the reduced tone of neonatal abdominal muscles (Vogt et al, 2006). The kidneys should be smooth and firm to the touch. Enlarged kidneys are somewhat easy to detect, but normal-size neonatal kidneys may be somewhat more difficult to find. The presence of renal tissue is confirmed when voiding has occurred (Cavaliere, 2003).

Anogenital Area

The anogenital area should be examined with the infant supine. Gestational age affects the appearance of the external genitalia. Maturational changes are described in Figure 39-6 and Table 39-7. The genitalia should be readily identifiable as male or female.

- Males: The normal length of the penis at term is 3.5 cm (plus or minus 0.7 cm) (Fletcher, 1998). Gentle traction is applied on the foreskin to visualize the urethral meatus; the opening should be at the central tip of the glans. Physiologic phimosis, a nonretractable foreskin, normally is seen in newborns. The opening in the prepuce should be large enough to allow urination. The urine stream should be forceful and straight. The inguinal area and scrotum should be palpated for masses, swelling, and the presence of testes. The testes should be firm, smooth, and comparatively equal in size. Testicular descent begins at approximately 27 weeks' gestation. At term both testes should be in the scrotum, which should be fully rugated. The scrotum should be more deeply pigmented than the surrounding skin (Cavaliere, 2003).
- Females: The labial, inguinal, and suprapubic areas are inspected and palpated to detect masses, swelling, or bulges. The clitoris should be located superior to the vaginal opening. Hymenal tags and mucous/bloody vaginal discharges are benign, transient findings.

Edema of the genitalia is common in both sexes in breech deliveries. It may also be due to the effects of transplacentally acquired maternal hormones. The perineum should be smooth and should have no dimpling, fistulae, or discharges (Cavaliere, 2003; Gardner et al, 2002).

The anus is evaluated for patency and tone. Patency can be documented by gentle insertion of a soft rubber catheter. The passage of meconium does not confirm a patent anus, because meconium may be passed through a fistulous tract (Fletcher, 1998). Gentle stroking of the anal area should produce constriction of the sphincter, known as the anal wink (Sansoucie & Cavaliere, 2002).

Back

The infant should be placed in the supine position while the back is examined for curvature, patency, and presence of structural abnormalities. Vertebrae are palpated for enlargement and pain. Symmetry should be seen on both sides of the back and between the two scapulae. The spine should be straight and flexible and should have no visible defects, such as pits, hair tufts, or dimples (Sansoucie & Cavaliere, 2002).

Extremities and Hips

The extremities are observed for symmetry, degree of flexion, and presence of defects and fractures. Full range of motion should be present, and the extremities should move symmetrically. Although symmetry of gluteal skin folds suggests normal hips, the Ortolani and Barlow maneuvers should be performed to confirm the stability of the hips (Figure 39-15). The Ortolani maneuver reduces a dislocated femoral head into the acetabulum, and the Barlow maneuver reflects the ability of the femoral head to be dislocated (Fletcher, 1998; Tappero, 2003).

The limbs should be equal in length, and they should be in proportion to the body; they also should be straight and should have no edema or crepitus. Palpation or movement of the limbs should not produce a painful response. The digits should be equally spaced and have no webbing. The nails should extend to the end of the nail beds.

Reflexes

The most common neonatal reflexes are presented in Table 39-11.

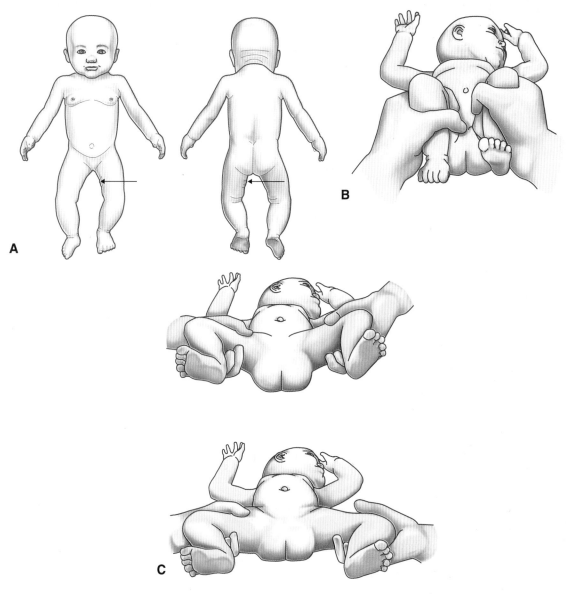

FIGURE **39-15**
Signs of congenital dislocation of hip. **A,** Asymmetry of gluteal and thigh folds. **B,** Barlow maneuver.
C, Ortolani maneuver. Redrawn from Wong DL (2003). *Wong's nursing care of infants and children,* ed 7.
St Louis: Mosby.

Variations and Abnormal Findings on Physical Examination

Minor variations and abnormal findings of the physical examination are presented in Table 39-12.

HEALTH MAINTENANCE IN THE FIRST YEAR OF LIFE

The goal of health maintenance, or primary care, is to provide consistent preventive health care for the infant and education for the parents. In addition to the basic surveillance provided for all infants, high-risk infants have other needs that must be addressed. Primary care for these infants often requires a multidisciplinary approach, and the health care provider is responsible for coordinating medical, developmental, and social services. Because high-risk infants face the possibility of developmental delays, neurologic sequelae, and nutritional deficits, follow-up must include formal developmental, neurologic, and nutritional assessments in addition to routine screening tests. The health care provider may need to schedule longer and more frequent visits to evaluate the infant adequately and to assess the family's adjustment to caring for the child. The health care provider also is responsible for giving the parents comprehensive anticipatory guidance (AAP, 2002; Sifuentes, 2000).

The American Academy of Pediatrics (AAP) has published guidelines for health supervision (AAP, 2002). These guidelines indicate the elements that can be included in office visits for patients from birth to 21 years of age. The guidelines are intended to be used in the care of infants, children, and adolescents whose "health and adaptation are thought to be within the normal range" (AAP, 2002). However, the approach has been designed to be flexible and can easily be

Text continues on p. 708.

TABLE 39-11	Assessment of Neonatal Reflexes		
Reflex	**Technique**	**Response**	**Comments**
Asymmetric tonic neck	With infant supine and in light sleep or quiet awake state, turn head to right until jaw is over shoulder; hold for 15 seconds, then release.	Occipital flexion and mental extension; right arm and leg are extended; left arm and leg are flexed. Premature neonates may lie at rest in this position for extended periods.	Reflex appears at 35 weeks' gestationand disappears by 6 to 7 months of age.
Babinski	Using thumbnail, scratch sole of foot at lateral side from toes to heel.	Dorsal flexion of great toe with extension of other toes.	Care must be taken not to elicit plantar grasp by stimulating sole of foot. Reflex appears at 34 to 36 weeks' gestation, is well established at 38 weeks, and disappears at 12 months of age.
Doll's eyes	Rotate head from side to side, observing eye movement.	As head is moved to right or left, eyes move in opposite direction.	Lack of eye movement with head rotation or movement of eyes in same direction as head may indicate brainstem or oculomotor nerve dysfunction. Reflex is well established and may even be exaggerated at 24 to 25 weeks' gestation.
Galant (truncal incurvation)	Place infant prone, either lying on flat surface or in suspension; lightly stroke along either side of spinal column from shoulder to buttocks.	Normal response is strong incurvation of whole vertebral column toward stimulated side.	Reflex is first seen at 28 weeks' gestation.
Glabellar	Hold head firmly and tap forehead just above nose.	Normal response is tighter closure of both eyes and wrinkling of brow.	Asymmetry, absent or exceptionally strong response (closure longer than1 second), or generalized startle is abnormal.
Moro	Hold infant suspended over mattress, supporting head with one hand and body with other hand; rapidly lower both hands 10 to 20 cm without flexing neck, but do not allow baby to drop back to mattress.	Symmetric abduction of arms and extension at elbows with hands open completely, followed by adduction of arms and flexion at elbows with curling of fingers; infant cries or grimaces at conclusion.	Response attenuates and ultimately disappears with repetition as habituation occurs. No response is seen at <26 weeks' gestation; extension only at 30 weeks; variable adduction at 34 weeks; complete response at 38 weeks. Reflex disappears at 6 months of age.
Palmar grasp	Stimulate palmar surface of hand with a finger.	Neonate grasps finger; grasp tightens with attempt to remove finger.	Reflex appears at 28 weeks' gestation, is well established after 32 weeks, and disappears at 2 months of age.
Pupillary	Elicit in darkened environment by presenting bright, sharply focused light from periphery.	Pupils constrict equally.	Reflex is sluggish but present between 28 and 32 weeks' gestation in healthy neonates; it is fully present after 34 weeks.
Rooting	Stroke cheek and corner of mouth.	Mouth opens and head turns toward stimulus.	Reflex appears at 28 weeks' gestation, followed by long latency period beginning at 30 weeks; it is well established at 32 to 34 weeks and disappears by 3 to 4 months of age.
Stepping	Hold neonate upright and allow feet to touch flat surface.	Alternating stepping movements.	Reflex appears at 35 to 36 weeks' gestation, is well established at 37 weeks, and disappears at 3 to 4 months of age.
Sucking	Touch or stroke lips.	Mouth opens, and neonate begins to suck.	Reflex appears at 28 weeks' gestation, is well established by 32 to 34 weeks, and disappears at 12 months of age.

Data from Carey B (2003). Neurologic assessment. In Tappero EP, Honeyfield ME, editors. Physical assessment of the newborn, ed 3. Petaluma, CA: NICU Ink; Fletcher MA (1998). Physical diagnosis in neonatology. Philadelphia: Lippincott-Raven; and Vannucci RC, Yaeger JY (2002). Newborn neurologic assessment. In Fanaroff AA, Martin RM, editors (2002). Neonatal-perinatal medicine: diseases of the fetus and infant, ed 7. St Louis: Mosby.

TABLE **39-12**	Abnormalities and Variations Found on Physical Examination of Newborns and Infants

Finding	Definition/Description	Comments
SKIN		
Color	Acrocyanosis (blue discoloration of the hands, feet, and perioral area), commonly seen in the first 6 to 24 hours of life.	Occurs when blood flow to an area is sluggish and all available oxygen has been extracted (Fletcher, 1998); exacerbated by cooling and diminished by warming; normal variation but abnormal if persists beyond the first 24 hours of life.
	Cutis marmorata (mottling of the skin in response to cold or other stressful stimuli); caused by dilation of capillaries, usually greatest on the extremities but may be seen on the trunk.	May be suggestive of other conditions (e.g., cardiovascular hypertension, hypothyroidism) if mottling is extensive, shows no improvement with warming, or persists beyond first few months (Fletcher, 1998).
	Cyanosis (blue discoloration of the skin, tongue, and mucous membranes).	Caused by excess of desaturated hemoglobin in the blood (cardiopulmonary disease) or a structural defect in the hemoglobin molecule (methemoglobin); always an abnormal finding.
	Jaundice (yellow coloring of the skin, mucous membranes, and sclerae).	Caused by deposition of bilirubin; may be physiologic.
	Pallor (absence of color or paleness of the skin).	Caused by a decrease in cardiac output, subcutaneous edema, anemia, or asphyxia (Lissauer, 2006).
	Plethora (ruddy skin coloration in the newborn).	Caused by high circulating red blood cell volume (abnormal finding).
Lesions	Café au lait spots (light tan or brown macules with well-defined borders, representing areas of increased epidermal melanosis); except for deeper pigmentation, appearance is not different from that of surrounding skin.	More common in normal infants of color. Six or more macules, regardless of spots' size or infant's race, may be pathologically significant, especially if located in the axilla.
	Cutis aplasia (localized or widespread foci of absence of some or all layers of skin); defect may be covered by a thin, translucent membrane or scar tissue, or area may be raw and ulcerated.	Occurs predominantly on the scalp and less frequently on the limbs and trunk.
	Ecchymosis (nonblanching purple or blue-black macule larger than 2 mm in diameter); represents extravasation of blood into subcutaneous tissue.	Results from trauma to underlying blood vessels or fragility of the vessel walls.
	Erythema toxicum (white or yellow papules on red macular base), commonly found on face, trunk, or proximal extremities but not on hands or feet.	Common, benign finding; vesicles are rare, sterile, and composed primarily of eosinophils. When vesicles are pronounced or coalescent, they may mimic postural infectious rash (Furdon & Clark, 2005).
	Harlequin fetus (most severe form of congenital ichthyosis; skin is completely covered with thick, horny scales resembling armor that are divided by deep red fissures).	Most such infants die of dehydration, infection, or respiratory insufficiency within a few hours or days.
	Harlequin sign (vascular phenomenon represented by distinct midline demarcation in side-lying infants; dependent half is deep red, upper half is pale).	Benign finding that lasts a few seconds to 30 minutes, occasionally reverses when position is changed. The physiologic basis is unidentified; without pathologic significance. Occurs most frequently in LBW neonates (Kazin et al, 2005).

Continued

TABLE **39-12**	Abnormalities and Variations Found on Physical Examination of Newborns and Infants—cont'd	
Finding	**Definition/Description**	**Comments**
SKIN—cont'd		
Lesions—cont'd	Strawberry hemangioma (red, raised, circumscribed, soft, compressible, lobulated tumor; may occur anywhere on the body).	Benign tumor of the vascular endothelium that has a proliferative and an involutional phase; most involute spontaneously. Treatment is unnecessary unless vital functions are affected.
	Cavernous hemangioma (similar to strawberry hemangioma; involves dermis and subcutaneous tissue and is soft and compressible on palpation; overlying skin is bluish-red in color).	Cavernous lesions may cause thrombocytopenia (Kasabach-Merritt syndrome) or hypertrophy of bone and soft structures of extremities (Klippel-Trenaunay-Weber syndrome) (Young et al, 2005).
	Mongolian spot (blue-black macule, lacking a sharp border, most frequently seen on sacrum, buttocks, flanks, or shoulders).	Benign lesion, common in dark-skinned neonates, resulting from delayed disappearance of dermal melanocytes; lesion gradually disappears during the first years of life.
	Milia (1 mm, pearly white or yellow papules without erythema; in the mouth these are called Epstein's pearls).	Epidermal inclusion cysts caused by blockage of sebaceous glands; a benign finding that resolves during the first weeks of life.
	Miliaria crystallina (1 to 2 mm, thin-walled vesicles with nonerythematous and nonpigmented base).	Lesions caused by blockage of sweat glands. They are exacerbated by a warm, humid environment and most frequently develop in intertriginous areas and over the face and scalp. They resolve when the environmental factors are eliminated.
	Miliaria rubra (small, erythematous, grouped papules [prickly heat]).	
	Miliaria pustulosis (nonerythematous pustules).	
	Neonatal pustular melanosis (small, superficial vesiculopustules with little or no surrounding erythema; crusted or scaly collarettes appear after vesicles rupture; lesions eventually resolve into hyperpigmented areas).	Transient and benign; frequently confused with infectious lesions. Smears of pustular material reveal predominantly neutrophils and no bacteria.
	Salmon patch (nevus; dull, pink-red, irregularly shaped macules that blanch on pressure; commonly found on nape of neck (stork bite), glabella, forehead, eyelids, and upper lip).	Benign finding; lesions are composed of distended, dilated capillaries, and most lesions (except those on the neck) disappear by 1 year of age.
	Port wine stain (nevus, macular lesion; present at birth but may be pale and hard to discern; initially pink in color with sharply delineated borders; progresses to dark red/purple; some develop small, angiomatous nodules).	Developmental vascular malformation that occurs mostly on the face; does not increase in size but grows with the infant; may occur alone or with structural anomalies (e.g., Sturge-Weber syndrome) (Fletcher, 1998; Young et al, 2005).
	Petechiae (tiny red or purple, nonblanching macules that range from pinpoint to pinhead size).	Caused by minute hemorrhages in the dermal or submucosal layers; may be benign and self-limiting or pathognomonic of serious underlying conditions. They are benign when found on presenting part and when localized areas appear at the same time; progressive, widespread areas require evaluation (Fletcher, 1998).
Redundant skin	More skin than is necessary or normally present in a particular area.	Seen in the neck after resolution of cystic hygroma or in the abdomen in a neonate with prune belly syndrome.
Sclerema neonatorum	Diffuse, stone-hard, nonpitting cutaneous induration; overlying skin appears pale and waxy; face has a mask-like appearance; joints are stiff.	Occurs in debilitated neonates; diffuse systemic process with grave prognosis (Kazin et al, 2005).

TABLE **39-12**	Abnormalities and Variations Found on Physical Examination of Newborns and Infants—cont'd	
Finding	**Definition/Description**	**Comments**
SKIN—cont'd		
Subcutaneous fat necrosis	Firm, nonpitting, poorly circumscribed, reddish violet lesions appearing in the first weeks of life on the face, arms, trunk, thighs, and buttocks. Affected areas may be slightly elevated above adjacent skin (Mangurten, 2006).	Most often seen in areas where a fat pad is present. May occur secondary to cold or trauma and sometimes accompanied by hypercalcemia (Kazin et al, 2005).
HEAD AND NECK		
Acrocephaly	Congenital malformation of the skull caused by premature closure of the coronal and sagittal sutures; accelerated upward growth of the head gives it a long, narrow appearance with a conic shape at the top (also called oxycephaly).	May be associated with premature closure of sutures; found with certain syndromes (e.g., Crouzon's, Apert's) (Cohen, 2006).
Anencephaly	Failed closure of the anterior neural tube without skull formation; the brain is severely malformed, lacking definable structure, although a rudimentary brainstem usually is present.	Most affected neonates (75%) are stillborn; without intervention; the remainder die in the neonatal period (Gressens & Huppi, 2006).
Brachycephaly	Congenital malformation of the skull caused by premature closure of the coronal suture; excessive lateral growth of the head gives it a short, broad appearance.	Condition found with certain syndromes (e.g., trisomy 21, Apert's) (Cohen, 2006).
Bruit	Abnormal murmurlike sound heard on auscultation of an organ or gland that is caused by dilated, tortuous, or constricted vessels. The specific character of the bruit, its location, its association with other clinical findings, and the time of occurrence in a cycle of other sounds is of diagnostic importance.	Bruits heard over the fontanelle or lateral skull associated with signs of congestive heart failure may denote intracranial arteriovenous malformation (Johnson, 2003; Carey, 2003).
Caput succedaneum	Vaguely demarcated pitting edema of the scalp that may extend across suture lines and can shift in response to gravity.	Benign finding that appears at birth (from pressure of the maternal cervix on the fetal skull) and resolves in a few days; incidence of infection with this condition may be higher if internal fetal scalp electrodes are used (Mangurten, 2006; Madan et al, 2005).
Cephalohematoma	Extradural fluid collection caused by bleeding between the skull and periosteum; generally occurs over one or both parietal bones and does not cross the suture lines; has distinct margins and may be fluctuant or tense.	1. May form during labor and enlarges for the first 12 to 24 hours; most resolve spontaneously over several weeks to months (Johnson, 2003). 2. Linear skull fracture is found in 5% of unilateral and 18% of bilateral lesions (Madan et al, 2005). 3. May result in hyperbilirubinemia (Mangurten, 2006).
Craniosynostosis	Premature closure of one or more cranial sutures, causing abnormal skull shape and possibly a palpable ridge along the suture line.	Head growth is restricted in the area perpendicular to the stenotic suture and is excessive in unrestricted areas. Most cases are isolated events, but the condition can occur in some syndromes (Cohen, 2006).
Craniotabes	Congenital thinness of bone at the top and back of the head. Bones may collapse with gentle pressure and recoil (ping-pong).	1. May be a normal variant if present to a mild degree near suture lines. May be caused by the pressure of the skull against the maternal pelvic brim; spontaneous resolution usually occurs in a few weeks (Fletcher, 1998). 2. May be associated with congenital syphilis and other congenital conditions (osteogenesis imperfecta); due to bone resorption or delay in ossification (Sneiderman & Taeusch, 2005).

Continued

TABLE **39-12**	Abnormalities and Variations Found on Physical Examination of Newborns and Infants—cont'd	
Finding	**Definition/Description**	**Comments**
HEAD AND NECK—cont'd		
Dolichocephaly or scaphocephaly	Congenital malformation of the skull in which premature closure of the sagittal suture results in restricted lateral growth. Skull shape often seen in premature babies as a result of prolonged positioning with head turned to the side.	Long narrow head (Cohen, 2006).
Encephalocele	Protrusion of brain tissue through a congenital defect in the cranium; most often occurs in the occipital midline but may also be seen in the frontal, temporal, or parietal areas.	Other cranial defects, congenital anomalies (hydrocephalus, microcephaly, craniosynostosis), and autosomal recessive syndromes Walker-Warburg) are frequently seen (Bach, 2005; Gressens & Huppi, 2006).
Hair whorls	Two or more hair whorls, or abnormally placed whorls (other than parietal area).	May indicate brain anomaly; it has been postulated that the pattern of hair development correlates with underlying brain development (Furdon & Clark, 2003).
Macrocephaly	Excessive head size in relation to weight, length, and gestational age. Occipitofrontal circumference (OFC) is over 90th percentile.	1. Familial; facial features usually are normal. 2. May reflect pathologic condition (e.g., hydrocephaly, hydrancephaly) or chromosomal or neuroendocrine disorder (Bach, 2005).
Microcephaly	Abnormally small head size relative to weight, length, and gestational age. OFC is under 10th percentile.	Associated with either microcephaly (marked reduction in size of brain or cerebral hemispheres) or acquired brain atrophy (Bach, 2005).
Molding	Process by which the head shape is altered as the fetus passes through the birth canal. The biparietal diameter becomes compressed, the head is elongated, and the skull bones may overlap at the suture lines.	Benign finding; condition usually resolves during the first few postnatal days.
Neck masses	May be detected on palpation or inspection. Cystic hygroma (soft, fluctuant mass that is easily transilluminated; usually laterally placed or over clavicles).	Most common neck mass; caused by development of sequestered lymph channels, which dilate into cysts (Johnson, 2003; Berseth & Poenaru, 2005a).
	Goiter (anterior mass caused by hypothyroidism).	Rare in neonates (Johnson, 2003).
	Thyroglossal duct cyst/branchial cleft cyst; a mass may be found high in the neck.	Rare in neonates (Johnson, 2003).
Plagiocephaly	Asymmetry of the skull due to flattening of the occiput. Can be deformational (positional) or due to premature or irregular closure of the coronal or lambdoidal sutures.	1. Posterior plagiocephaly almost always due to mechanical forces (positional; "back to sleep"). 2. Anterior plagiocephaly most commonly due to premature fusion of the sutures (Cohen, 2006).
Subgaleal hemorrhage	Bleeding into the potential space between the epicranial aponeurosis and the periosteum of the skull; manifests as a firm to fluctuant scalp mass with poorly demarcated borders that may extend onto the face, forehead, or neck and may be accompanied by signs of hypovolemia.	May be a life-threatening condition; can be caused by coagulopathy, asphyxia, or vacuum extraction (Ohls, 2001; Madden et al, 2005; Mangurten, 2006).
Webbed neck	Redundant skin at posterolateral region of neck.	Found with Turner's, Noonan's, and Down syndromes (Kirby, 2003).
FACE		
Asymmetry	Unequal appearance or movement of mouth and lips; unequal closure of eyes; uneven appearance of nasolabial folds.	Often caused by in utero positioning but may be due to facial nerve paresis; in mild cases may be evident only only with crying (affected side fails to move or moves less when infant cries).

TABLE 39-12	Abnormalities and Variations Found on Physical Examination of Newborns and Infants—cont'd	
Finding	**Definition/Description**	**Comments**
EARS		
Auricular appendage	Accessory tragi, most commonly in pretragal area; may occur within or behind the ear. These structures contain cartilage and are not truly skin tags.	Primarily of cosmetic significance unless accompanied by other diffuse malformations. Seen in certain congenital syndromes (e.g., Goldenhar's, Treacher Collins); hearing assessment is indicated when other anomalies are present (Fletcher, 1998; Spillman, 2002).
Auricular sinus	Narrow, fistulous tract most often located directly anterior to helix.	May be familial or may be associated with microtia, auricular appendage, facial cleft syndromes, and syndromic anomalies of the outer ear (Fletcher, 1998; Spillman, 2002).
Low-set ears	Superior attachment of pinna lies below imaginary line drawn between both inner canthi and extended posteriorly.	May be associated with chromosomal or renal anomalies (Spillman, 2002).
Microtia	Severely misshapen, dysplastic external ear.	Frequently associated with other malformations that result in conductive hearing loss (i.e., atresia of auditory meatus, abnormalities of middle ear) (Hudgins & Cassidy, 2006; Spillman, 2002).
EYES		
Blepharophimosis	Narrow palpebral fissures in the horizontal measurement; also known as short palpebral fissures.	Usually caused by lateral displacement of the inner canthi; seen in certain dysmorphic or chromosomal syndromes (Gupta et al, 2006; Fletcher, 1998).
Brushfield spots	Pinpoint white or light yellow spots on the iris.	Seen in 75% of neonates with Down syndrome but may also be a normal variant; not always visible at birth (Johnson, 2003).
Coloboma	Cleft-shaped defect in ocular tissue (eyelid, iris, ciliary body, retina, or optic nerve).	Result of incomplete embryologic closure of ocular structures; may be an isolated finding or part of a malformation syndrome (CHARGE, trisomies 13, 18, 22) (Madan & Good, 2005).
Ectropion	Eversion of the margin of the eyelid, which leaves the conjunctiva exposed.	Seen in facial nerve paralysis, in certain syndromes, and in harlequin fetus and collodion baby (Fletcher, 1998; Gupta et al, 2006).
Entropion	Inversion of the eyelid; eyelashes may be in contact with the cornea and conjunctiva.	Congenital condition that usually resolves spontaneously without damage (Fletcher, 1998; Gupta et al, 2006).
Epicanthal folds	Vertical fold of skin at the inner canthus on either side of the nose.	A feature of normal fetal development and may be present in normal infants. Characteristic of trisomy 21 but may occur in malformation syndromes, especially those with a flat nasal bridge; may also be a physical manifestation of in utero compression (Potter facies) (Hudgins & Cassidy, 2006; Cavaliere, 2003).
Exophthalmos	Abnormal displacement of the eye characterized by protrusion of the eyeball.	May be caused by increased volume of the orbit (tumor), swelling secondary to edema or hemorrhage, endocrine disorder (e.g., Graves' disease, hyperthyroidism); known as proptosis when accompanied by shallow orbits (Crouzon's disease) (Gupta et al, 2006; Fletcher, 1998).
Hypertelorism	Increased distance between the orbits, observed clinically as a large interpupillary distance (see Telecanthus) (Hudgins & Cassidy, 2006).	Frequently seen in craniofacial syndromes (Gupta et al, 2006).

Continued

TABLE **39-12**   Abnormalities and Variations Found on Physical Examination of Newborns and Infants—cont'd

Finding	Definition/Description	Comments
EYES—cont'd		
Hypotelorism	Decreased distance between the orbits, observed clinically as smaller than normal interpupillary distance (Hudgins & Cassidy, 2006).	Frequently seen in trisomies 13 and 21 and in other syndromes (Gupta et al, 2006).
Leukocoria	White pupil, denoting an abnormality of the lens, vitreous, or fundus; an indication for further evaluation (Gupta et al, 2006).	May be seen on direct visualization, or as absence of a red reflex (Fletcher, 1998); most commonly seen in cataracts; also found in retinoblastoma, retinal detachment, and vitreous hemorrhage.
Microphthalmia	Small eye; diameter measures less than 2/3 of the normal 16 mm at birth.	Can be hereditary or caused by chromosomal anomalies and environmental influences during development. Associated with multisystem conditions or syndromes (e.g., CHARGE, trisomy 13, fetal rubella effects) (Gupta et al, 2006).
Nystagmus	Involuntary, rhythmic movements of the eye; may be horizontal, vertical, rotary, or mixed. Optokinetic nystagmus reflexive response to a moving target.	Occasional, intermittent nystagmus in an otherwise healthy newborn may be normal in the neonatal period; however, it must be evaluated if frequent or persistent (or both). Pathologic forms may be due to ocular, neurologic, or vestibular defects (Gupta et al, 2006).
Ptosis (blepharoptosis)	Abnormal drooping of one or both upper eyelids; lid does not rise to normal level.	Caused by congenital or acquired weakness in the levator muscle or paralysis of the third cranial nerve; may be difficult to detect in neonates unless unilateral with asymmetry between the eyelids (Gupta et al, 2006).
Strabismus	Misalignment of the visual axes:	Refer for ophthalmologic evaluation if present by third month of age.
	Esotropia—crossed eyes	Results from inheritance, paralysis of the lateral rectus muscle, or refractive errors; may be due to diseases that reduce visual acuity in one eye.
	Exotropia—wall eye	Rare in neonates; usually does not appear until 1 to 2 years of age (Gupta et al, 2006).
Subconjunctival hemorrhage	Bright red area on sclerae.	Caused by rupture of a capillary in the mucous membrane that lines the conjunctiva; commonly seen after vaginal delivery, does not reflect ocular trauma unless massive and associated with other findings; usually resolves in 7 to 10 days (Mangurten, 2006).
Synophrys	Meeting of the eyebrows in the midline.	Seen in multisystem conditions or syndromes (e.g., Cornelia de Lange's, congenital hypertrichosis) (Gupta et al, 2006).
Telecanthus	Lateral displacement of the inner canthi; eyes appear too widely set because of a disproportionate increase between the inner canthi; interorbital distance is appropriate (Hudgins & Cassidy, 2006).	Evident in fetal alcohol syndrome and other syndromes; not synonymous with hypertelorism, although its presence can lead to a false impression of hypertelorism (Gupta et al, 2006).
NOSE		
Choanal atresia	Obstruction of posterior nasal passages.	Patency is assessed in the quiet state. If condition is bilateral, neonate is cyanotic at rest and pink when crying; if unilateral, baby is unable to breathe if mouth is held closed and unaffected naris is occluded with examiner's finger. Atresia/stenosis may be confirmed by passing a catheter.

TABLE **39-12**	Abnormalities and Variations Found on Physical Examination of Newborns and Infants—cont'd	
Finding	**Definition/Description**	**Comments**
NOSE—cont'd		
Nasal deformation	May result from pressure in utero. May be due to dislocation of the septal cartilage.	Benign condition that resolves in a few days. Attempts to restore normal anatomy are unsuccessful; nares remain asymmetric when tip of nose is compressed (Johnson, 2003; Mangurten, 2006).
MOUTH		
Cleft lip/palate	Failure of midline fusion during first trimester.	May occur alone or with other malformations.
Epstein's pearls	Small, white, pearl-like inclusion cysts that appear on the palate and gums.	Benign finding that disappears spontaneously by a few weeks of age (Johnson, 2003).
Macroglossia	Abnormally large tongue; failure of tongue to fit inside a closed mouth (Fletcher, 1998).	Seen in certain congenital syndromes (e.g., Beckwith-Wiedemann) and hypothyroidism; protruding tongue may indicate poor neuromuscular tone or a small mouth rather than a large tongue (Berseth & Poenaru, 2005a).
Micrognathia	Underdevelopment of the jaw, especially the mandible.	Dysmorphic feature seen in certain malformation syndromes (e.g., Pierre Robin sequence) (Kirby, 2003; Johnson, 2003).
THORAX/CHEST		
Auscultation	Adventitious breath sounds	(Askin, 2003)
	Crackles	Discrete, noncontinuous bubbling sounds during inspiration; classified as fine, medium, or coarse. Previously called rales.
	Rhonchi	Continuous, nonmusical, low-pitched sounds occurring on inspiration and expiration; caused by secretions or aspirated matter in large airways.
	Stridor	Rough, harsh sounds caused by narrowing of upper airways; present during both phases of respiratory cycle but worse during inspiration; common with laryngomalacia, subglottic stenosis, and vascular ring.
	Wheezes	Musical, high-pitched sound generated by air passing at high velocity through a narrowed airway; heard most often on expiration but can be noted during both phases of respiratory cycle if airway diameter is restricted and fixed.
	Grunting	Sound produced by forceful expiration against a closed glottis; compensatory mechanism to prevent or reverse alveolar collapse.
	Murmur	Grades I through VI assigned depending on intensity and presence of thrill.
Asymmetry	May be unequal in shape or excursion.	1. Asymmetric shape caused by positioning in utero or presence of air trapping or space-occupying lesions. 2. Unequal excursion caused by diaphragmatic hernia, phrenic nerve damage, or air leakage or trapping (Askin, 2003).
Barrel chest	Increased anteroposterior diameter of the chest.	Result of air trapping in the pleural space (pneumothorax) or distal airways (aspiration or pneumonia), space-occupying lesions, or overdistention from mechanical ventilation (Fletcher, 1998).

Continued

TABLE **39-12**	Abnormalities and Variations Found on Physical Examination of Newborns and Infants—cont'd	

Finding	Definition/Description	Comments
THORAX/CHEST—cont'd		
Heave	Diffuse, gradually rising impulse seen in the anterior chest overlying the ventricular area.	Usually indicates volume overload.
Pectus carinatum	Deformation of chest wall caused by protuberant sternum; also called pigeon chest.	May be associated with Marfan, Noonan's, and other syndromes (Askin, 2003).
Pectus excavatum	Deformation of chest wall caused by depressed sternum; also called funnel chest.	May be associated with Marfan, Noonan's, and other syndromes (Askin, 2003); may develop after birth in neonates with laryngomalacia.
Retractions	Drawing in of the soft tissues of the chest between and around the firmer tissue of the cartilaginous and bony ribs; seen in intercostal, subcostal, substernal, and suprasternal areas.	Mild subcostal retractions may be seen in healthy newborns; intercostal, substernal, and suprasternal retractions reflect increased work of breathing and suggest respiratory distress.
Supernumerary nipples (polythelia)	Extra nipples; may appear as slightly pigmented linear dimples or may be more defined, with palpable breast nodules.	Normal variant; nipples appear along the mammary line. Prospective studies have refuted the association with renal anomalies; no indication for further evaluation based solely on the presence of supernumerary nipples.
ABDOMEN		
Abdominal wall defects	Exstrophy of the bladder (protrusion and eversion of the bladder through an embryologic defect, resulting in absence of muscle and connective tissue on the anterior abdominal wall).	Often associated with other defects of the genitourinary (GU) and musculoskeletal systems and the gastrointestinal (GI) tract (Zderic, 2005).
	Gastroschisis (protrusion of viscera through an abdominal wall defect arising outside the umbilical ring; the cord therefore is not inserted on the defect, and the herniated organs are not covered by peritoneum).	Defect usually is to the right of the umbilicus (Berseth & Poenaru, 2005b; Magnuson et al, 2006).
	Omphalocele (herniation of viscera through an abdominal wall defect within the umbilical ring; defect usually is covered by a translucent, avascular sac at the base of the umbilicus).	Umbilical cord always inserts into the sac; occasionally the sac may rupture. Defect usually is larger than 4 cm and may be associated with other congenital defects and chromosomal anomalies (Berseth & Poenaru, 2005b; Magnuson et al, 2006).
	Umbilical hernia (failure of the umbilical ring to contract, allowing protrusion of bowel or omentum through the abdominal wall).	Characterized by a fascial defect smaller than 4 cm and intact umbilical skin (Fletcher, 1998; Magnuson et al, 2006).
Bruit	See section under Head and Neck	Persistence after a position change may indicate abnormalities of the umbilical vein or hepatic vascular system, hepatic hemangioma, or renal artery stenosis (Goodwin, 2003).
Diastasis rectus	Midline bulge from xiphoid to umbilicus, seen when abdominal muscles are flexed.	Caused by separation of the two rectus muscles along the median line of the abdominal wall; a common benign finding in newborns that has no clinical significance; resolves without intervention (Goodwin, 2003).
Distention	Increase in abdominal girth caused by an increase in the volume of intraperitoneal, thoracic, or pelvic contents.	May be pathologic or benign. Pathologic causes include GI obstruction, ascites, abdominal mass, organomegaly, and depression of the diaphragm (tension pneumothorax). Benign causes include postprandial state, crying, swallowing of air with feedings, air leakage with mechanical ventilation, and administration of continuous positive airway pressure (CPAP).

TABLE **39-12**	Abnormalities and Variations Found on Physical Examination of Newborns and Infants—cont'd	
Finding	**Definition/Description**	**Comments**
ABDOMEN—cont'd		
Patent urachus	Postnatal persistence of communication between the urinary bladder and the umbilicus; may result in passage of urine from the umbilicus, which otherwise appears normal. Other signs are a large, edematous cord that fails to separate after the normal interval and retraction of the umbilical cord during urination.	Lower urinary tract obstruction should be considered (Cavaliere, 2003; Donlon & Furdon, 2002).
Prune belly syndrome	Congenital deficiency of abdominal musculature, characterized by a large, flaccid, wrinkled abdomen, cryptorchidism, and GU malformations.	Almost always seen in males (Vogt et al, 2006).
Scaphoid abdomen	Abdomen with a sunken anterior wall.	May be present with a diaphragmatic hernia or malnutrition.
Single umbilical artery		Seen in fewer than 1% of neonates; approximately 40% of affected newborns have other major congenital malformations. When condition occurs without other abnormalities, it usually is a benign finding (Lissauer, 2006).
GENITALIA/PERINEUM		
Ambiguous	Presence of a phallic structure not discretely male or female, abnormally placed urethral meatus, and inability to palpate one or both gonads in a male.	May be associated with serious endocrine disorders; rapid evaluation and diagnosis are critical (Cavaliere, 2003; Palmert & Dahms, 2006).
Anal atresia	Absence of an external anal opening; imperforate anus.	May be evident by inspection; infant may fail to pass meconium. However, meconium may be passed through a rectovaginal or rectovestibular fistula in a female or a rectoperineal or rectourethral fistula in a male (Goodwin, 2003).
Chordee	Ventral or dorsal curvature of the penis; most evident on erection.	May occur alone but often accompanies hypospadias (Cavaliere, 2003).
Clitoromegaly	The appearance of an enlarged clitoris, with no regard to cause (Palmert & Dahms, 2006); it may be swollen, enlarged, widened, or merely prominent, as in premature females.	May be a normal finding in a premature female or may represent masculinization from exposure to excess androgens during fetal life (Palmert & Dahms, 2006).
Cryptorchidism	Testis or testes in extrascrotal location (undescended testis or testes); characterized by empty, hypoplastic scrotal sac.	In most cases descent occurs spontaneously by 6-9 months of age; descent after 9 months is rare. Bilateral cryptorchidism occurs in up to 30% of patients; consider intersex disorder until proven otherwise (Zderic, 2005).
Epispadias	Abnormal location of urethral meatus on the dorsal surface of the penis; abnormal urine stream may be seen.	Varies in severity from mild (glanular) to complete version seen in exstrophy of the bladder; all forms are associated with dorsal chordee; may require evaluation by a urologist before circumcision (Zaontz & Packer, 1997).
Hydrocele	Nontender scrotal swelling caused by fluid collection; arises from passage of peritoneal fluid through patent processus vaginalis.	May be seen with inguinal hernia but can be distinguished from hernia because hydrocele appears translucent on transillumination; entire circumference of testis may be palpated; and it cannot be reduced (Cavaliere, 2003).

Continued

TABLE **39-12**	Abnormalities and Variations Found on Physical Examination of Newborns and Infants—cont'd	
Finding	**Definition/Description**	**Comments**
GENITALIA/PERINEUM—cont'd		
Hydrocolpos/hydro-metrocolpos	Manifests as suprapubic mass or protruding perineal mass as a result of accumulation of secretions in vagina or vagina and uterus.	Caused by excessive intrauterine stimulation by maternal estrogens, with obstruction of the genital tract by an intact hymen, hymenal bands, vaginal membrane, or vaginal atresia (Cavaliere, 2003; Fletcher, 1998).
Hypospadias	Abnormal location of urethral meatus on the ventral surface of the penis; caused by incomplete development of the anterior urethra; abnormal urine stream may be seen.	Urethral opening may be found on the glans, scrotum, or perineum. Infants with penoscrotal or perineal type or with glanular form and other genital anomalies or dysmorphic features should be evaluated to rule out disorders of sexual differentiation (Palmert & Dahms, 2006; Zderic, 2005). Evaluation by a urologist may be required before circumcision.
Hymenal tag	Redundant tissue manifesting as an annular tag protruding from the vagina.	Benign finding; most disappear during the first year of life.
Inguinal hernia	Scrotal mass caused by the presence of loops of intestines in the scrotal sac; arises from persistence of processus vaginalis, often associated with hydrocele.	On examination, the entire circumference of the testis is not palpable, and the scrotum cannot be transilluminated. Unless incarcerated, hernias are reducible (Benjamin, 2002; Cavaliere, 2003).
Micropenis/microphallus	Abnormally short or thin penis.	Penis more than two standard deviations below the mean of length and width for age according to standard charts; frequently requires evaluation by an endocrinologist and a geneticist (Palmert & Dahms, 2006).
Phimosis	Intractable foreskin.	Must be differentiated from physiologic phimosis, a nonretractable foreskin that is a normal finding in neonates (Cavaliere, 2003).
Priapism	Constantly erect penis.	Abnormal finding in neonate (Rozinski & Bloom, 1997).
Retractile testis	Normally descended testis that recedes into the inguinal canal because of activity of the cremaster muscle.	May not be seen in the newborn period because of lack of cremaster reflex in this age group; however, some newborns do demonstrate this response (Cilento et al, 1994; Fletcher, 1998).
Testicular torsion	Twisting of the testis or testes on the spermatic cord; manifests as a swollen, red or bluish red scrotum; may be painful, but this is not a universal symptom in the neonate.	Urgent evaluation and management are required, because the blood supply to the testis is compromised, which results in irreversible ischemic damage to the testis; condition may occur in utero (Zderic, 2005).
MUSCULOSKELETAL SYSTEM		
Arachnodactyly	Unusually long, spiderlike digits.	Characteristic of, but not universally present in, Marfan syndrome and homocysteinuria (Hudgins & Cassidy, 2006).
Arthrogryposis	Persistent flexure or contracture of one or more joints.	May be associated with oligohydramnios or an underlying neuromuscular disorder (Hudgins & Cassidy, 2006).
Brachydactyly	Shortening of one or more digits as a result of abnormal development of phalanges, metacarpals, or metatarsals.	Benign trait if an isolated finding; may be a component of skeletal dysplasias (achondroplasia) and syndromes (Down syndrome) (Hudgins & Cassidy, 2006).
Calcaneus foot	Abduction of the forefoot with the heel in valgus position (turned outward).	Associated with external tibial torsion; often caused by in utero positioning (Furdon & Donlon, 2002).
Camptodactyly	Congenital flexion deformity of the finger; bent finger.	Usually involves the little finger; can be a minor variant or familial trait, or part of a syndrome (Hudgins & Cassidy, 2006).

TABLE **39-12**	Abnormalities and Variations Found on Physical Examination of Newborns and Infants—cont'd	
Finding	**Definition/Description**	**Comments**

MUSCULOSKELETAL SYSTEM—cont'd

Finding	Definition/Description	Comments
Clinodactyly	Lateral angulation deformity of a finger with either radial or ulnar deviation.	Usually involves the little finger; may be a benign finding if occurring alone but can be associated with congenital syndromes (Hudgins & Cassidy, 2006).
Crepitus	Crackling sensation produced by the presence of air in tissues (subcutaneous emphysema) or the movement of bone fragments (clavicular fracture).	
Genu recurvatum	Abnormal hyperextensibility of the knee allowing the knee to bend backward.	May be due to trauma, prolonged intrauterine pressure, or general joint laxity. May be a feature of other disorders (Ehlers-Danlos, Marfan syndromes) (Sneiderman & Taeusch, 2005).
Kyphosis	Round shoulder deformity; forward bending of the spine. Caused by congenital failure of formation of all or part of the vertebral body, with preservation of the posterior elements and failure of the anterior segmentation of the spine.	Severe deformities may be apparent at birth; less severe abnormalities may not appear until several years later; a progressive deformity can result in paraplegia (Hudgins & Cassidy, 2006).
Lordosis	Exaggeration of the normal curvature in the cervical and lumbar spine.	Caused by a bony abnormality of the spine (Kirby, 2003).
Lymphedema	Puffiness of the dorsum of the hands or feet.	Characteristic of Noonan's or Turner's syndrome (Hudgins & Cassidy, 2006).
Meningocele	Saclike protrusion of the spinal meninges through a congenital defect in the spinal column.	Herniated cyst is filled with cerebrospinal fluid but does not contain neural tissue; affected infants usually do not show neurologic deficits (Cohen & Walsh, 2006).
Metatarsus valgus	Congenital deformity of the foot in which the forepart rotates outward away from the midline and the heel remains straight.	Fixed deformity of the foot, which cannot be brought into neutral position; compare with metatarsus abductus, a functional deformity in which the foot can be brought into neutral position (Grover, 2000b).
Metatarsus varus	Congenital bony abnormality of the foot in which the forepart rotates inward toward the midline and the heel remains straight.	Fixed deformity; the foot cannot be brought into neutral position. Compare with metatarsus adductus, a functional deformity in which the foot can be brought into neutral position (Grover, 2000b).
Myelomeningocele	Defect identical to meningocele but with associated abnormalities in the structure and position of the spinal cord.	Affected infants usually show neurologic deficits below the level of the abnormality (Cohen & Walsh, 2006).
Polydactyly	Presence of more than the normal number of digits; there may be a complete extra digit (preaxial) that is normal in appearance, or a skin tag (postaxial).	May be an isolated finding, inherited as an autosomal dominant trait, or may occur in a variety of syndromes (trisomy 13, Meckel-Gruber syndrome) (Cooperman & Thompson, 2006; Hudgins & Cassidy, 2006).
Rachischisis	Congenital fissure of the spinal cord in which the incompletely folded cord is splayed apart and exposed along the back.	Caused by incomplete neurulation; often accompanied by anencephaly (Fletcher, 1998; Gressens & Huppi, 2006).
Rocker bottom feet	Deformity of the foot in which the arch is disrupted, giving a rounded appearance (rocker bottom) to the sole.	Usually seen in conjunction with congenital syndromes (trisomies 13 and 18) (Hudgins & Cassidy, 2006).
Scoliosis	Failure of formation or segmentation of the vertebrae; manifests as lateral (side to side) curvature of the spine.	May be congenital or acquired; may occur as part of another condition or may be idiopathic (Cooperman & Thompson, 2006; Fletcher, 1998).
Simian crease	Single transverse line in the palm.	May be benign, but when accompanied by other dysmorphic features (e.g., incurving fifth finger, epicanthal folds, low-set thumb), it may be a sign of Down syndrome (Hudgins & Cassidy, 2006).

Continued

TABLE **39-12**	Abnormalities and Variations Found on Physical Examination of Newborns and Infants—cont'd	
Finding	**Definition/Description**	**Comments**
MUSCULOSKELETAL SYSTEM—cont'd		
Spinal dimple, dermal sinus	Pit or depression that occurs along the midline of the back, often at the base of the spinal cord in the lumbosacral area; may be accompanied by tufts of hair.	May be a benign finding, especially if the base of the defect can be visualized; however, defect can extend into the spinal cord, representing a neural tube defect and tethered spinal cord (Carey, 2003).
Syndactyly	Fusion of two or more digits; may involve only soft tissue (simple) or may include bone or cartilage (complex).	May occur as an isolated defect or as part of a syndrome (e.g., Cornelia de Lange's, Smith-Lemli-Opitz) (Cooperman & Thompson, 2006).
Talipes equinovarus	Clubfoot; congenital deformity of the foot and lower leg marked by adduction of the forefoot (turned inward and pointed medially), varus position of the heel (turned inward), and downward pointing of the toes.	May be congenital (isolated deformity), teratologic (associated with underlying neuromuscular disorder), or positional (normal foot held in equinovarus position in utero) (Cooperman & Thompson, 2006).
Tibial torsion	Abnormal rotation of the feet while the knees are pointing forward; may be internal (toes in) or external (toes out).	Often caused by in utero positioning; resolves spontaneously (Cooperman & Thompson, 2006).
Torticollis	Shortening of the sternocleidomastoid muscle, resulting in head tilt toward the affected muscle and chin rotation toward the unaffected muscle; a palpable mass may appear during the first few weeks of life.	May be due to birth trauma, intrauterine malposition, muscle fibrosis, venous abnormalities in the muscle, or congenital cervical vertebral abnormalities (Cooperman & Thompson, 2006).
NEUROLOGIC EXAMINATION		
Brachial plexus injuries	Peripheral damage to the network of spinal nerves supplying the arm, forearm, and hand.	Multifactorial etiology; interaction between characteristics of the brachial plexus, maternal and fetal risk factors, and birth trauma (Benjamin, 2005).
	Erb-Duchenne palsy (upper arm paralysis): Arm is adducted and internally rotated, with elbow extension, flexion of the wrist, and pronation of the forearm. The arm falls to the side of the body when passively abducted, and the Moro reflex is absent on the affected side but the grasp is intact.	Arises from injury to the fifth and sixth cervical roots; most common brachial plexus injury (Mangurten, 2006).
	Klumpke palsy (lower arm paralysis): Hand is paralyzed, and voluntary movement of the wrist and grasp reflex are absent.	Rare; results from injury to the eighth cervical and first thoracic roots; usually Horner's syndrome (ptosis, miosis, and enophthalmos) is present on the affected side; delayed pigmentation of the iris may be seen (Mangurten, 2006).
	Paralysis of the entire arm: Arm is completely motionless, flaccid, and powerless and hangs limply; all reflexes are absent, and sensory deficit may extend to the shoulder.	(Mangurten, 2006)
Facial nerve palsy	Facial weakness or paralysis arising from compression of the seventh cranial nerve, caused by intrauterine position or forceps delivery; characterized by asymmetry of facial movement (most evident on crying), ptosis, and unequal nasolabial folds.	(Mangurten, 2006)
Phrenic nerve injury	Cause of respiratory distress secondary to paralysis of the diaphragm; arises from upper brachial plexus injury.	Rarely occurs as an isolated phenomenon; accompanies signs and symptoms of Erb-Duchenne palsy (Cooperman & Thompson, 2006; Mangurten, 2006).

modified for follow-up of high-risk infants. More frequent visits can be scheduled as needed. Guidelines for health supervision for the first year of life are summarized in Box 39-1.

Immunizations

The AAP has published recommendations for routine childhood immunization through the first 18 years of age. These recommendations are presented in Figure 39-16.

Text continues on p. 712.

BOX **39-1**

Guidelines for Health Supervision of Infants in the First Year of Life

Newborn

Health Assessment
- This visit may take place while the infant is still in the hospital.
- Ask welcoming questions (e.g., "How is the baby?" "How are you doing?" "How is the feeding going?")

Physical Examination
- Examine the baby with the parents present and demonstrate findings, even normal and minor ones.
- Observe parent-infant interactions.
- Take measurements (length, weight, head circumference).
- Perform a full physical examination.

Testing
- Mother's laboratory tests
- Evidence of blood incompatibility
- Metabolic screening

Immunizations
- Hepatitis B (dose 1) may be given.

Anticipatory Guidance
Nutrition
- Discuss the feeding method the parents have chosen (vitamin and fluoride supplementation as indicated).

Sleep Patterns
- Discuss the infant's sleep position and environment.

Skin Care
- Explain the care of the skin, cord, and circumcision.

Signs and Symptoms Needing Follow-up
- Explain when and how to call the health care provider.
- Discuss the reasons for breast engorgement and vaginal discharge.
- Explain the meaning of jaundice if indicated.
- Discuss the postpartum adjustment of the mother, siblings, and family.

Social and Family Relationships
- Discuss the extent to which family members and friends should visit.
- Discuss the individuality of the infant.

Injury Prevention
- Discuss microwave safety (do not use to heat bottles).
- Discuss hot water heater temperature (should be set at 120° F).
- Discuss car safety seat use.
- Discuss crib safety.
- Discuss siblings.
- Discuss pets.
- Discuss smoke detectors.

Closing the Visit
- Ask the parents if they have any questions or concerns.
- Comment on the parents' strength and capability.
- Carry out discharge planning.

2 to 4 Weeks

Health Assessment
- Ask welcoming questions.
- Ask what issues need to be discussed at this visit.
- Inquire about changes in family life and what stressors have arisen.
- Review the status of concerns discussed at the newborn visit.

Examination of the Infant
- Review the birth history.
- Complete a family history: diabetes, tuberculosis, anemia, emotional problems, other significant conditions, household composition, pets, use of cigarettes, alcohol, or other drugs.

Physical Examination
- Take measurements (length, weight, head circumference).
- Perform a general physical examination.
- Check for red reflex, heart murmurs, abdominal masses, and hip dislocation.
- Check developmental progress.
- Perform metabolic screening.
- Review results of newborn metabolic screening (tests and reporting vary by state).

Immunizations
- Give hepatitis B (dose 1 if not given at birth; dose 2 if first dose was given at birth).

Anticipatory Guidance
Nutrition
- Answer questions about breastfeeding.
- Discuss vitamin and fluoride supplementation if indicated.

Sleep Patterns
- Suggest naps for the mother; advise the parents to share feedings when possible.

Social Interaction with Family
- Suggest ways to encourage interaction with the infant.

Injury Prevention
- Discuss car safety seats.
- Discuss smoke detectors.
- Discuss hot water heater temperature.
- Discuss infant's sleeping position.

Closing the Visit
- Review the problems discussed; devise a management plan for each one.
- Ask the parents if they have other questions or concerns.
- Make positive statements about the baby's development.
- Comment encouragingly on the parents' caregiving skills.
- Provide information on where to call if a problem arises.
- Schedule the next visit.

2 Months

Health Assessment
- Ask welcoming questions.
- Ask if the parents have any concerns.
- Ask about siblings and about changes and stress in the family.
- Inquire about the mother's return to work.
- Review the status of issues discussed at the previous visit.
- Ask specific questions about the infant's nutrition, elimination, sleep pattern, behavior, and development.

Physical Examination
- Take measurements (height, weight, head circumference).
- Perform a general physical examination.

Continued

BOX **39-1**

Guidelines for Health Supervision of Infants in the First Year of Life—cont'd

2 Months—cont'd

Observation of Behavior and Development
- Note developmental milestones.
- Note temperament (ability to cuddle and be consoled, excessive crying or irritability).
- Note parent-infant interaction.

Testing
- Draw blood for hematocrit/hemoglobin if infant was premature or low birth weight or had significant hemolysis or excessive blood loss.

Immunizations
- Provide the family with vaccine information sheets.
- Give diphtheria-tetanus-pertussis (DTaP or DPT) (dose 1); polio (dose 1); *Haemophilus influenzae* type b (Hib) (dose 1); hepatitis B (dose 1 or dose 2).
- Recommend acetaminophen for fever and irritability.

Anticipatory Guidance
Nutrition
- Discuss supplementation of vitamin D, iron, and fluoride as indicated.
- Advise the parents not to feed the baby honey or corn syrup.
- Recommend that no solids be fed until the baby is 4 to 6 months old.

Elimination
- Discuss normal elimination patterns.

Sleep Patterns
Social and Family Relationships
- Urge the parents to play with, talk to, and cuddle the baby.
- Inquire about alternative care arrangements when both parents work.
- Advise the parents to spend time alone with the other children.
- Assess for signs of maternal depression.

Injury Prevention
- Discuss the use of car seats.
- Emphasize the hazard of the infant falling from the bed or table if left unattended.
- Stress the importance of a smoke-free environment.
- Discuss gun safety measures.

Closing the Visit
- Review the problems discussed; devise a management plan for each one.
- Ask the parents if they have other questions or concerns.
- Schedule the next visit.

4 Months

Health Assessment
- Ask welcoming questions.
- Ask if parents have any concerns or questions.
- Ask about stress in the family.
- Inquire about work and child care issues.
- Review the status of issues discussed at the previous visit.
- Ask specific questions about the infant's nutrition, elimination, sleep pattern, behavior, and development; also about family relationships.

Physical Examination
- Take measurements (height, weight, head circumference).
- Perform a general physical examination.

Observation of Behavior and Development
- Note developmental milestones.
- Note interactions with caregivers.
- Note temperament (ability to cuddle and to be calmed).

Testing
- Draw blood for hematocrit/hemoglobin if indicated.

Immunizations
- Provide the family with vaccine information sheets.*
- Give DTaP or DPT (dose 2); polio (dose 2); Hib (dose 2); hepatitis B (dose 2 if not given yet).
- Recommend acetaminophen for fever and irritability.

Anticipatory Guidance
Infections
- Advise the parents to expect about six upper respiratory tract infections a year; explain that antibiotics usually are ineffective against these infections and that unnecessary antibiotic use may be harmful.

Nutrition
- Recommend the introduction of solid foods (one at a time).
- Advise the parents not to feed the baby honey or corn syrup until the infant is 1 year old.
- Discuss iron supplementation (in formula or cereal).

Elimination
- Ask family about elimination patterns.

Sleep Patterns
Developmental Progress
- Consider investigation of persistent "colic."

Social and Family Relationships
- Urge the parents to play with, talk to, and cuddle the baby.
- Inquire about sibling rivalry.
- Recommend parents take "free time" for themselves.

Injury Prevention
- Discuss the use of an appropriate car safety seat.
- Explain how to choose safe toys.
- Repeat warning about the danger of the infant falling from a bed or table if left unattended.
- Discuss appropriate use of a microwave oven to heat the baby's food.

Closing the Visit
- Review the problems discussed; devise a management plan for each one.
- Ask the parents if they have other questions or concerns.
- Make positive statements about the baby's development and temperament.
- Schedule the next appointment.

6 Months

Health Assessment
- Ask welcoming questions.
- Ask what issues need to be discussed.
- Ask about stress in the family.
- Inquire about work and child care issues.
- Review the status of issues discussed at the previous visit.
- Ask specific questions about the infant's nutrition, elimination, sleep pattern, behavior, and development; also about family relationships.

Continued

BOX **39-1**

Guidelines for Health Supervision of Infants in the First Year of Life—cont'd

6 Months—cont'd

Physical Examination
- Take measurements (height, weight, head circumference).
- Perform a general physical examination.

Observation of Behavior and Development
- Note developmental milestones.
- Note interactions with caregivers.
- Note temperament.

Testing
- Draw blood for hematocrit/hemoglobin (at 6 to 12 months).
- Test for sickle cell disease (as indicated).

Immunizations
- Provide vaccine information sheets for the family*; review the benefits and risks of vaccines.
- Give DTaP or DPT (dose 3); polio (dose 3); Hib (dose 3); hepatitis B (dose 3 if due).
- Recommend acetaminophen for fever and irritability.

Anticipatory Guidance
Nutrition
- Advise the introduction of solids (if not already done).
- Recommend offering the infant sips from a cup.
Elimination
- Ask family about elimination patterns.
Sleep Patterns
- Ask family about sleep patterns.
Observation of Development and Behavior
- Note stranger anxiety.
- Note language development (advise parents to talk and read to the infant).
Injury Prevention
- Advise the parents on child-proofing the home (e.g., protecting the infant from hot liquids and surfaces).
- Provide the local poison control telephone number.
- Explain the use of syrup of ipecac.
- Discourage the use of infant walkers.
- Reinforce the proper use of microwave ovens to heat the baby's food.
- Encourage the use of sunscreen.
- Explain that swim classes are not recommended at this age.

Closing the Visit
- Review the problems discussed; devise a management plan for each one.
- Ask the parents if they have other questions or concerns.
- Make positive statements about the baby's development and temperament.
- Schedule the next appointment.

9 Months

Health Assessment
- Ask welcoming questions.
- Ask what issues need to be discussed at this visit.
- Inquire about changes and stress in the family.
- Inquire about the parents' approach to discipline.
- Review the status of issues discussed at the previous visit.

- Ask specific questions about the infant's nutrition, elimination, sleep pattern, behavior, and development; also about family relationships and injury prevention measures.

Physical Examination
- Take measurements (height, weight, head circumference).
- Perform a general physical examination.

Observation of Behavior and Development
- Note developmental milestones.
- Note interactions with caregivers.
- Note temperament.

Testing
- Draw blood for hematocrit/hemoglobin (at 6 to 12 months).
- Perform lead toxicity screening.

Immunizations
- Review immunizations to see if the infant is up-to-date.
- Give PPD (this is given now or at 1 year if the infant is at risk of exposure to tuberculosis).
- Give hepatitis B (dose 3 if due).

Anticipatory Guidance
Nutrition
- Encourage the parents to establish regular mealtimes.
- Recommend the introduction of table foods and drinking from a cup.
Elimination
- Recommend that parents delay toilet training until about 2 years of age or until the baby seems ready.
Sleep Patterns
- Recommend that the parents establish a regular bedtime routine.
Observation of Development and Behavior
- Note separation anxiety.
- Note discipline.
- Note language development.
- Note intensified sibling rivalry.
Injury Prevention
- Advise the parents on child-proofing the home.
- Advise the parents to avoid giving the baby foods that can be aspirated; stress safety while eating.
- Provide the local poison control telephone number.
- Explain the use of syrup of ipecac.
- Discourage the use of infant walkers.
- Recommend changing from an infant car seat to a toddler model.

Closing the Visit
- Review the problems discussed; devise a management plan for each one.
- Ask the parents if they have other questions or concerns.
- Make positive statements about the baby's development and temperament.
- Schedule the next appointment.

12 Months

Health Assessment
- Ask welcoming questions.
- Ask what issues need to be discussed at this visit.
- Inquire about changes or stress in the family.
- Ask about the parents' approach to discipline.

Continued

BOX **39-1**

Guidelines for Health Supervision of Infants in the First Year of Life—cont'd

12 Months—cont'd
Health Assessment—cont'd
- Review the status of issues discussed at the previous visit.
- Ask specific questions about the infant's nutrition, elimination, sleep pattern, behavior, and development; also about family relationships and injury prevention measures.

Physical Examination
- Take measurements (height, weight, head circumference).
- Perform a general physical examination.

Observation of Behavior and Development
- Note developmental milestones.
- Note interactions with caregivers.
- Note temperament.

Testing
- Draw blood for hematocrit/hemoglobin (at 6 to 12 months).
- Perform lead toxicity screening.
- Give PPD (if not administered at 9 months, if the infant is at risk of exposure to tuberculosis).

Immunizations
- Provide the family with vaccine information sheets.*
- Review immunizations to see if the infant is up-to-date.
- Give measles-mumps-rubella (MMR) (per local regulations).
- Varicella vaccine may be administered.

Anticipatory Guidance
Infections
- Advise the parents to expect about six upper respiratory tract infections a year; explain that antibiotics usually are ineffective for these infections and that unnecessary antibiotic use may be harmful.

Nutrition
- Explain that the infant may seem to have less of an appetite; advise the parents not to force food on the child.
- Recommend weaning to a cup.
- Recommend changing from baby food to all table foods.
Elimination
- Advise the parents to delay toilet training until about 2 years of age or until the baby seems ready.
Sleep Patterns
- Recommend parents establish a regular bedtime routine.
- Advise the parents not to allow the baby to sleep with them unless it is a cultural practice.
Observation of Development and Behavior
- Note infant's developing autonomy (explain this to the parents).
- Note discipline.
- Note language development.
- Note cognitive and motor skills.
Injury Prevention
- Recommend ways to child-proof the home; stress window, stair, and bathtub safety.
- Advise the parents to avoid giving the baby foods that can be aspirated.
- Provide the local poison control telephone number.
- Explain the use of syrup of ipecac.
- Discourage the use of infant walkers.
- Stress the importance of using the appropriate car safety seat.

Closing the Visit
- Review the problems discussed; devise a management plan for each one.
- Ask the parents if they have other questions or concerns.
- Make positive statements about the baby's development and temperament.
- Schedule the next appointment.

Modified from American Academy of Pediatrics Committee on Psychosocial Aspects of Child and Family Health (2002). *Guidelines for health supervision III*. Elk Grove Village, IL: American Academy of Pediatrics.
*Available from the American Academy of Pediatrics, Publications Department, 141 Northwest Point Boulevard, Elk Grove Village, IL 60001-1098; 847.434.4000 (phone); 847.434.8000 (fax); www.aap.org.

HEALTH MAINTENANCE FOR HIGH-RISK INFANTS IN THE FIRST YEAR OF LIFE

History
It is important for the primary care provider to review the infant's medical history, including a complete family history and the record of the hospital course. Pertinent history to be reviewed is shown in Table 39-13. In addition to providing routine health care maintenance and anticipatory guidance to the parents, the primary care provider must monitor the status of associated medical conditions and developmental sequelae.

Growth and Nutrition
Expected increases in weight, length/height, and head circumference in the first year are summarized in Table 39-14. Weight, length/height, and OFC are measured and plotted on

the appropriate graphs. The parameters for premature infants must be corrected for preterm birth. Adjustments generally are made until 2 to 2½ years of age. Premature infants frequently show accelerated ("catch-up") growth, which first manifests in the head circumference. This may begin as early as 36 weeks postconceptional age or as late as 8 months adjusted age (Sifuentes, 2000). Increases in the OFC of more than 2 cm per week are worrisome and should be investigated, because they may signify a pathologic process (hydrocephalus) rather than catch-up growth (Sifuentes, 2000).

Weight gain is evaluated in grams per day. Many high-risk infants are placed on special diets (24 calories/ounce) or feeding regimens (feedings every 2 hours or continuous feedings). It is important to review the necessity of continuing or modifying the feeding plan according to the adequacy of growth. The need for dietary supplements (vitamins, minerals, human milk fortifier), medications (ranitidine, metoclopramide),

Vaccine ▼ Age ▶	Birth	1 month	2 months	4 months	6 months	12 months	15 months	18 months	24 months	4–6 years	11–12 years	13–14 years	15 years	16–18 years
Hepatitis B¹	HepB	HepB		HepB¹	HepB					HepB Series				
Diphtheria, Tetanus, Pertussis²			DTaP	DTaP	DTaP		DTaP			DTaP	Tdap	Tdap		
Haemophilus influenzae type b³			Hib	Hib	Hib³	Hib								
Inactivated Poliovirus			IPV	IPV	IPV					IPV				
Measles, Mumps, Rubella⁴						MMR				MMR	MMR			
Varicella⁵						Varicella					Varicella			
Meningococcal⁶								Vaccines within broken line are for selected populations		MPSV4	MCV4		MCV4	MCV4
Pneumococcal⁷			PCV	PCV	PCV	PCV				PCV	PPV			
Influenza⁸					Influenza (yearly)					Influenza (yearly)				
Hepatitis A⁹						HepA series				HepA series				

☐ Range of recommended ages   **☐ Catch-up immunization**   **☐ Assessment at age 11–12 years**

This schedule indicates the recommended ages for routine administration of currently licensed childhood vaccines, as of December 1, 2005, for children through age 18 years. Any dose not administered at the recommended age should be administered at any subsequent visit, when indicated and feasible. ☐ Indicates age groups that warrant special effort to administer those vaccines not previously administered. Additional vaccines might be licensed and recommended during the year. Licensed combination vaccines may be used whenever any components of the combination are indicated and other components of the vaccine are not contraindicated and if approved by the Food and Drug Administration for that dose of the series. Providers should consult respective Advisory Committee on Immunization Practices (ACIP) statements for detailed recommendations. Clinically significant adverse events that follow vaccination should be reported through the Vaccine Adverse Event Reporting System (VAERS). Guidance about how to obtain and complete a VAERS form is available at http://www.vaers.hhs.gov or by telephone, 800-822-7967.

1. **Hepatitis B vaccine (HepB). AT BIRTH: All newborns** should receive monovalent HepB soon after birth and before hospital discharge. **Infants born to mothers who are hepatitis B surface antigen (HBsAg)-positive** should receive HepB and 0.5 mL of hepatitis B immune globulin (HBIG) within 12 hours of birth. **Infants born to mothers whose HBsAg status is unknown** should receive HepB within 12 hours of birth. The mother should have blood drawn as soon as possible to determine her HBsAg status; if HBsAg-positive, the infant should receive HBIG as soon as possible (no later than age 1 week). **For infants born to HBsAg-negative mothers,** the birth dose can be delayed in rare circumstances but only if a physician's order to withhold the vaccine and a copy of the mother's original HBsAg-negative laboratory report are documented in the infant's medical record. *FOLLOWING THE BIRTH DOSE:* The HepB series should be completed with either monovalent HepB or a combination vaccine containing HepB. The second dose should be administered at age 1–2 months. The final dose should be administered at age ≥24 weeks. Administering four doses of HepB is permissible (e.g., when combination vaccines are administered after the birth dose); however, if monovalent HepB is used, a dose at age 4 months is not needed. **Infants born to HBsAg-positive mothers** should be tested for HBsAg and antibody to HBsAg after completion of the HepB series at age 9–18 months (generally at the next well-child visit after completion of the vaccine series).
2. **Diphtheria and tetanus toxoids and acellular pertussis vaccine (DTaP).** The fourth dose of DTaP may be administered as early as age 12 months, provided 6 months have elapsed since the third dose and the child is unlikely to return at age 15–18 months. The final dose in the series should be administered at age ≥4 years. **Tetanus toxoid, reduced diphtheria toxoid, and acellular pertussis vaccine (Tdap adolescent preparation)** is recommended at age 11–12 years for those who have completed the recommended childhood DTP/DTaP vaccination series and have not received a tetanus and diphtheria toxoids (Td) booster dose. Adolescents aged 13–18 years who missed the age 11–12-year Td/Tdap booster dose should also receive a single dose of Tdap if they have completed the recommended childhood DTP/DTaP vaccination series. **Subsequent Td** boosters are recommended every 10 years.
3. **Haemophilus influenzae type b conjugate vaccine (Hib).** Three Hib conjugate vaccines are licensed for infant use. If PRP-OMP (PedvaxHIB® or ComVax® [Merck]) is administered at ages 2 and 4 months, a dose at age 6 months is not required. DTaP/Hib combination products should not be used for primary immunization in infants at ages 2, 4, or 6 months but may be used as boosters after any Hib vaccine. The final dose in the series should be administered at age ≥12 months.
4. **Measles, mumps, and rubella vaccine (MMR).** The second dose of MMR is recommended routinely at age 4–6 years but may be administered during any visit, provided at least 4 weeks have elapsed since the first dose and both doses are administered at or after age 12 months. Children who have not previously received the second dose should complete the schedule by age 11–12 years.
5. **Varicella vaccine.** Varicella vaccine is recommended at any visit at or after age 12 months for susceptible children (i.e., those who lack a reliable history of varicella). Susceptible persons aged ≥13 years should receive 2 doses administered at least 4 weeks apart.
6. **Meningococcal vaccine (MCV4).** Meningococcal conjugate vaccine (MCV4) should be administered to all children at age 11–12 years as well as to unvaccinated adolescents at high school entry (age 15 years). Other adolescents who wish to decrease their risk for meningococcal disease may also be vaccinated. All college freshmen living in dormitories should also be vaccinated, preferably with MCV4, although **meningococcal polysaccharide vaccine (MPSV4)** is an acceptable alternative. Vaccination against invasive meningococcal disease is recommended for children and adolescents aged ≥2 years with terminal complement deficiencies or anatomic or functional asplenia and for certain other high risk groups (see *MMWR* 2005;54[No. RR-7]); use MPSV4 for children aged 2–10 years and MCV4 for older children, although MPSV4 is an acceptable alternative.
7. **Pneumococcal vaccine.** The heptavalent **pneumococcal conjugate vaccine (PCV)** is recommended for all children aged 2–23 months and for certain children aged 24–59 months. The final dose in the series should be administered at age ≥12 months. **Pneumococcal polysaccharide vaccine (PPV)** is recommended in addition to PCV for certain high-risk groups. See *MMWR* 2000;49(No. RR-9).
8. **Influenza vaccine.** Influenza vaccine is recommended annually for children aged ≥6 months with certain risk factors (including, but not limited to, asthma, cardiac disease, sickle cell disease, human immunodeficiency virus infection, diabetes, and conditions that can compromise respiratory function or handling of respiratory secretions or that can increase the risk for aspiration), health-care workers, and other persons (including household members) in close contact with persons in groups at high risk (see *MMWR* 2005;54[No. RR-8]). In addition, healthy children aged 6–23 months and close contacts of healthy children aged 0–5 months are recommended to receive influenza vaccine because children in this age group are at substantially increased risk for influenza-related hospitalizations. For healthy, nonpregnant persons aged 5–49 years, the intranasally administered, live, attenuated influenza vaccine (LAIV) is an acceptable alternative to the intramuscular trivalent inactivated influenza vaccine (TIV). See *MMWR* 2005;54(No. RR-8). Children receiving TIV should be administered an age-appropriate dosage (0.25 mL for children aged 6–35 months or 0.5 mL for children aged ≥3 years). Children aged ≤8 years who are receiving influenza vaccine for the first time should receive 2 doses (separated by at least 4 weeks for TIV and at least 6 weeks for LAIV).
9. **Hepatitis A vaccine (HepA).** HepA is recommended for all children at age 1 year (i.e., 12–23 months). The 2 doses in the series should be administered at least 6 months apart. States, counties, and communities with existing HepA vaccination programs for children aged 2–18 years are encouraged to maintain these programs. In these areas, new efforts focused on routine vaccination of children aged 1 year should enhance, not replace, ongoing programs directed at a broader population of children. HepA is also recommended for certain high risk groups (see *MMWR* 1999;48[No. RR-12]).

The Childhood and Adolescent Immunization Schedule is approved by the Advisory Committee on Immunization Practices (http://www.cdc.gov/nip/acip), the American Academy of Pediatrics (http://www.aap.org), and the American Academy of Family Physicians (http://www.aafp.org).

FIGURE **39-16**

Recommended childhood and adolescent immunization schedule, by vaccine and age—United States, 2006. From Centers for Disease Control and Prevention (2005). Recommended childhood and adolescent immunization schedule—United States, 2006. *Morbidity and mortality weekly report* 54(51 and 52):Q1-Q4.

TABLE **39-13**	Recorded Elements of the History, Medical Course, and Current Needs for Neonates
Component	**Elements**
History	Prenatal and perinatal course
	Hospital course:
	Birth weight, gestation
	Illnesses, surgical procedures
	Radiographic studies
	Discharge examination
	Weight, head circumference, length
Nutrition information	Current diet and feeding schedule
	Feeding problems:
	Gastroesophageal (GE) reflux, feeding intolerance
	Dietary supplements:
	Vitamins, minerals, human milk fortifier
	Current deficiencies:
	Osteopenia/rickets, anemia
Medications	Doses
	Serum levels
	Oxygen requirements
Immunizations	Immunizations given in the hospital
	Respiratory syncytial virus (RSV) prophylaxis
Laboratory data	Most recent values:
	Hemoglobin, hematocrit
	Bilirubin
	Pending laboratory studies
	Need for further testing
	Newborn screening results
Current problems and complications	Retinopathy of prematurity (ROP), ophthalmologic problems (e.g., strabismus)
	Hearing deficits
	Bronchopulmonary dysplasia (BPD)/chronic lung problems
	GE reflux
	Intraventricular hemorrhage (IVH)
	Developmental deficits
	Other

Data from Sifuentes M (2000). *Well-child care for preterm infants.* In Berkowitz CD, editor. Pediatrics: a primary care approach, ed 2. Philadelphia: Saunders.

TABLE **39-14**	Expected Increases in Weight, Length/Height, and Head Circumference in the First Year of Life	
Parameter	**Age (months)**	**Expected Increase**
Weight	Birth to 3	25 to 35 g/day
	3 to 6	12 to 21 g/day
	6 to 12	10 to 13 g/day
Length/height	Birth to 12	25 cm/year
Occipitofrontal circumference (OFC)	Birth to 3	2 cm/month
	4 to 6	1 cm/month
	7 to 12	0.5 cm/month

Data from Grover G (2000). *Nutritional needs.* In Berkowitz CD, editor. Pediatrics: a primary care approach, ed 2. Philadelphia: Saunders.

may be necessary for high-risk infants, such as periodic electrolyte determinations for babies receiving diuretics. Consideration should be given to measuring serum levels for such drugs as anticonvulsants, methylxanthines, and digoxin.

Repeat ophthalmologic examinations may be required to evaluate the extent and progression or regression of retinopathy of prematurity (ROP). Further follow-up may be indicated, because some infants are at risk for strabismus, myopia, amblyopia, glaucoma, and other visual deficits. The infant may need serial auditory evaluations (brainstem auditory evoked response [BAER] behavioral audiograms) and other studies, such as electroencephalography, electrocardiography, echocardiography, radiography, pneumography, and neuroradiologic imaging (computed tomography [CT] or magnetic resonance imaging [MRI]). Infants receiving supplemental oxygen often benefit from periodic pulse oximetry (Sifuentes, 2000).

Immunizations

Vaccines are administered according to chronologic (postnatal) age, not gestational age. The standard doses and intervals are followed, as recommended by the AAP (see Box 39-1). Former premature infants have adequate serologic responses to immunizations without increased incidence of untoward effects (Sifuentes, 2000). There is benefit derived from respiratory syncytial virus (RSV) prophylaxis for high-risk infants, especially premature infants with a history of respiratory distress syndrome (RDS) or RDS/BPD (RSD with bronchopulmonary dysplasia).

Psychosocial Needs

Families of high-risk infants require a great deal of support and anticipatory guidance. Health care providers must seek to understand parental expectations and legitimize their fears while providing support and encouragement. Parents should be given consistent, honest information and realistic appraisals of their infant's status and prognosis (Sifuentes, 2000).

NICU graduates may be at risk for vulnerable child syndrome (VCS) (Box 39-2). Because parents continue to perceive their child as vulnerable and fragile, abnormal parent-infant interactions develop. By assessing for early, subtle signs, health care providers may prevent progression of the disorder.

and biochemical monitoring (e.g., for rickets or osteopenia) should also be addressed.

Physical Examination

A complete physical examination should be performed at each visit. Depending on the infant's history and needs, special attention may be required in certain areas, which are listed in Table 39-15.

Laboratory Tests and Monitoring Examinations

All standard screening tests required for healthy infants should be performed according to AAP recommendations. Other tests

TABLE **39-15**	Monitoring for Subsequent Conditions in High-Risk Infants	
System	**Condition**	**Comments**
Ocular	Retinopathy of prematurity (ROP), strabismus, visual abnormalities	
Oropharyngeal	Palatal groove, high arched palate, abnormal tooth formation	May develop secondary to intubation or may be due to congenital abnormalities.
	Discolored teeth	Caused by high bilirubin levels.
Thoracic/respiratory	Retractions, wheezing, stridor	Sequelae of chronic lung disease. Caused by chest tube placement.
	Chest scars	
Cardiovascular	Hypertension	Blood pressure monitoring is especially important for an infant who had umbilical artery catheters in place.
Abdominal	Hypoplastic umbilicus	Use of umbilical catheters and suturing frequently are the cause of this condition.
Genitourinary	Hernias	Increased risk in preterm babies.
	Cryptorchidism	
Extremities	Developmental hip dysplasia	
	Scars on heels or extremities	Sequelae of blood sampling, placement of intravenous (IV) lines, or extravasation of IV fluid.
Neuromuscular	Abnormal tone, asymmetric movements and reflexes, persistence of primitive reflexes and fisting, sustained clonus, scissoring	Abnormalities must be identified as soon as possible and the patient and family referred to appropriate intervention services.
	Poor suck-swallow coordination	

Data from Sifuentes M (2000). Well-child care for preterm infants. In Berkowitz CD, editor. Pediatrics: a primary care approach, ed 2. Philadelphia: Saunders.

BOX **39-2**

Characteristics of Vulnerable Child Syndrome

- Exaggerated separation anxiety (both infant and parent)
- Sleep difficulties
- Overprotectiveness
- Overindulgence
- Lack of appropriate discipline
- Excessive parental preoccupation with infant's health

SUMMARY

The comprehensive history and physical assessment create the framework for identifying problems and planning interventions. Assessment allows the nurse to gather information and to evaluate and integrate that information as care of the newborn proceeds. Although careful attention to the obvious is important, subtle findings detected by an experienced practitioner also may play a crucial role in the continuing care of the infant and family.

Case Study

IDENTIFICATION OF PATIENT PROBLEM

You are assessing a full-term female infant who was born 15 minutes previously via vaginal delivery. You note a firm but fluctuant cranial mass with ill-defined borders swelling across the suture lines to the ear and neck. The pinna appears to be protuberant.

ASSESSMENT: HISTORY AND PHYSICAL EXAMINATION

Obtain detailed history to include:

- Maternal medications used during pregnancy (aspirin, ibuprofen, phenytoin)
- History of placental insufficiency or fetal asphyxia during delivery
- Length of time spent pushing
- If delivery was vacuum assisted, number of attempts and length of application
- Presentation of fetus at delivery
- Infant's Apgar scores
- History of previous child with clotting or bleeding disorder
- Family history of bleeding or clotting disorders
- Detailed examination (to be performed on open warmer):

Observe general appearance of infant including color of skin and mucous membranes, overall perfusion, size and symmetry of head and face, obvious deformities or evidence of birth trauma.

Monitor vital signs (VS).

Assess state of alertness, tone, resting posture/position, and cry.

Note any arching or posturing with movement.

Continued

Case Study—cont'd

Head

Observe general appearance, size, and movement of head and neck.

Observe shape and symmetry of head, neck, pinna bilaterally.

Inspect and palpate sutures and fontanelles.

Measure head circumference.

Observe hair growth patterns and check for signs of birth trauma or other anomalies.

Auscultate fontanelles.

Face

Observe for symmetrical movement of facial features.

Assess eyes, pupillary response to light, red reflex and blink reflex in response to light.

Inspect for facial, head, neck edema, ecchymosis.

Assess gag, suck/rooting reflex, palate, color of mucous membranes, suck/swallow coordination, tongue, midline, moves freely, color, proportional size.

Observe for facial palsy.

Ears

Assess for any drainage or bleeding from the ear canals.

Inspect shape, placement, swelling and position of ears.

Inspect ears for lesions, cysts, nodules.

Inspect nose: appearance, patency of nares.

Neck

Observe appearance, noting any abnormalities such as short, redundant skin, webbing.

Assess clavicles.

Chest

Assess color and perfusion prior to starting examination and note any changes throughout examination.

Palpate quality of pulses and compare upper to lower.

Observe for active precordium.

Assess capillary refill.

Auscultate lung sounds noting any retractions, grunting, flaring, asymmetrical chest movement, or aeration.

Auscultate chest for murmurs, clicks, and rubs, PMI.

Assess for placement of breasts/nipples, presence of breast tissue, symmetry.

Abdomen

Observe color and size, shape, and symmetry of abdomen.

Auscultate abdomen for bowel sounds.

Palpate for loops, noting any tenderness and guarding with examination.

Palpate for hepatosplenomegaly.

Genitourinary

Inspect external genitalia and inguinal area/suprapubic area.

Inspect labia, clitoris, urethral meatus, and any bleeding or discharge.

Inspect for any discoloration/bruising or other signs of birth trauma.

Assess anus for patency and placement.

Musculoskeletal

Observe for spontaneous, symmetrical movement in all four limbs.

Inspect entire body for ecchymosis and petechiae or other signs of bleeding with careful documentation (mark borders if necessary).

Neuro

Assess reflexes: tonic neck reflex, Moro reflex, grasp reflex, Babinski reflex, and trunk incurvation.

DIFFERENTIAL DIAGNOSIS

Caput succedaneum, cephalohematoma, skull fracture, subgaleal hematoma.

DIAGNOSTIC TESTS

Continuous monitoring: heart rate, respiratory rate, blood pressure, and pulse oximetry.

Blood gas to assess for metabolic acidosis.

Hematocrit, platelets, clotting factors, to assess for blood loss and/or coagulopathy.

Liver function studies, blood glucose level.

Skull radiograph to assess for skull fracture.

Depending on the results of the neuro examination, a head CT may be necessary.

WORKING DIAGNOSIS

Subgaleal hemorrhage.

DEVELOPMENT OF MANAGEMENT PLAN

Admit to NICU for close observation.

Monitor vitals signs closely and continuously (HR, RR, BP); pulse oximetry observing closely for signs of hypovolemic shock (tachycardia, hypotension, respiratory distress).

Monitor neurologic vital signs closely for possible deterioration in level of consciousness.

Monitor intake and output strictly.

Blood work to be done:

* Blood gas (for baseline respiratory function)
* Complete blood count (for baseline hematocrit)
* Coagulation factors (for potential indication of massive bleeding and coagulopathy)
* Bilirubin level (for baseline: during resolution the breakdown of the blood may cause hyperbilirubinemia requiring treatment, thus levels of bilirubin need to be followed closely as well)
* Blood urea nitrogen and creatinine (for baseline of kidney function and hydration)

Case Study—cont'd

Keep the patient NPO for now.

Provide maintenance IV solution.

Blood products or NS boluses can be given as required for replacement of blood volume.

Meet with parents: careful preparation of the parents for the acute side effects and sequelae of subgaleal hemorrhage is important. Parents should be warned of the possibility of swelling and discoloration of the face, head, and neck. They should also know that spontaneous resolution usually occur within 2 to 3 weeks and some infants require close long-term follow-up for sequelae.

IMPLEMENTATION AND EVALUATION OF EFFECTIVENESS

Implement above plan with continuous monitoring for deterioration of infant's cardiovascular or neurologic status.

REFERENCES

American Academy of Pediatrics Committee on the Fetus and Newborn and the American College of Obstetricians and Gynecologists Committee on Obstetrics (1996). Use and abuse of the Apgar score. *Pediatrics* 98:141-142.

American Academy of Pediatrics Committee on Psychosocial Aspects of Child and Family Health (2002). *Guidelines for health supervision III*. Elk Grove Village, IL: American Academy of Pediatrics.

Apgar VA (1953). A proposal for a new method of evaluation of the newborn infant. *Current research in anesthesiology analogs* 32:260-267.

Askin D (2003). Chest and lung assessment. In Tappero EP, Honeyfield ME, editors. *Physical assessment of the newborn*, ed 3 (pp 69-79). Petaluma, CA: NICU Ink.

Bach S (2005). Congenital malformations of the central nervous system. In Taeusch HW et al, editors. *Avery's diseases of the newborn*, ed 8 (pp 938-963). Philadelphia: Saunders.

Ballard JL et al (1991). New Ballard score, expanded to include extremely premature infants. *Journal of pediatrics* 119:417-423.

Benjamin K (2002). Scrotal and inguinal masses in the newborn period. *Advances in neonatal care* 2(3):140-148.

Benjamin K (2005). Part I. Injuries to the brachial plexus. *Advances in neonatal care* 5(4):181-189.

Berseth CL, Poenaru D (2005a). Structural anomalies of the gastrointestinal tract. In Taeusch HW et al, editors. *Avery's diseases of the newborn*, ed 8 (pp 1086-1102). Philadelphia: Saunders.

Berseth CL, Poenaru D (2005b). Abdominal wall problems. In Taeusch HW et al, editors. *Avery's diseases of the newborn*, ed 8 (pp 1113-1122). Philadelphia: Saunders.

Blake WW, Murray JJ (2002). Heat balance. In Merenstein GB, Gardner SL, editors:. *Handbook of neonatal intensive care*, ed 5 (pp 102-116). St Louis: Mosby.

Carey B (2003). Neurologic assessment. In Tappero EP, Honeyfield ME, editors. *Physical assessment of the newborn*, ed 3 (pp 149-172). Petaluma, CA: NICU Ink.

Cavaliere TA (2003). Genitourinary assessment. In Tappero EP, Honeyfield ME, editors. *Physical assessment of the newborn*, ed 3 (pp 107-123). Petaluma, CA: NICU Ink.

Cilento BG et al (1994). Cryptorchidism and testicular torsion. *Pediatric clinics of North America* 40:1133-1149.

Cohen AR (2006). Disorders in head shape and size. In Fanaroff AA et al, editors. *Neonatal-perinatal medicine: diseases of the fetus and infant*, ed 8 (pp 989-1014). St Louis: Mosby.

Cohen AR, Walsh MC (2006). Myelomeningocele. In Fanaroff AA et al, editors. *Neonatal-perinatal medicine: diseases of the fetus and infant*, ed 8 (pp 1014-1034). St Louis: Mosby.

Cooperman DR, Thompson GH (2006). Neonatal orthopedics. In Fanaroff AA et al, editors. *Neonatal-perinatal medicine: diseases of the fetus and infant*, ed 8 (pp 1755-1766). St Louis: Mosby.

D'Harlingue AE, Durand DJ (2001). Recognition, stabilization, and transport of the high-risk newborn. In Klaus MH, Fanaroff AA, editors. *Care of the high risk neonate*, ed 5. Philadelphia: Saunders.

Donlon CR, Furdon SA (2002). Part 2. Assessment of the umbilical cord outside of the delivery room. *Advances in neonatal care* 2(1):187-197.

Engel J (2002). *Pocket guide to pediatric assessment*, ed 4. St Louis: Mosby.

Fletcher MA (1998). *Physical diagnosis in neonatology*. Philadelphia: Lippincott-Raven.

Furdon SA, Clark DA (2003). Scalp hair characteristics in the newborn. *Advances in neonatal care* 3(6):286-298.

Furdon SA, Clark DA (2005). Discriminating between skin lesions in the newborn. *Advances in neonatal care* 1(2):84-90.

Furdon SA, Donlon CR (2002). Examination of the newborn foot. *Advances in neonatal care* 2(5):248-258.

Gardner SL et al (2002). Initial nursery care. In Merenstein GB, Gardner SL, editors. *Handbook of neonatal intensive care*, ed 5 (pp 70-101). St Louis: Mosby.

Goodwin M (2003). Abdomen assessment. In Tappero EP, Honeyfield ME, editors. *Physical assessment of the newborn*, ed 3 (pp 97-105). Petaluma, CA: NICU Ink.

Gressens P, Huppi P (2006). Normal and abnormal brain development. In Fanaroff AA et al, editors. *Neonatal-perinatal medicine: diseases of the fetus and infant*, ed 8 (pp 883-908). St Louis: Mosby.

Grover G (2000a). Nutritional needs. In Berkowitz CD, editor. *Pediatrics: a primary care approach*, ed 2. Philadelphia: Saunders.

Grover G (2000b). Rotational problems of the lower extremities: in-toeing and out-toeing. In Berkowitz CD, editor. *Pediatrics: a primary care approach*, ed 2. Philadelphia: Saunders.

Gupta BK et al (2006). The eye: diagnosis and evaluation. In Fanaroff AA et al, editors. *Neonatal-perinatal medicine: diseases of the fetus and infant*, ed 8 (pp 1721-1747). St Louis: Mosby.

Hegyi T et al (1994). Blood pressure ranges in premature infants. I. The first hours of life. *Journal of pediatrics* 124:627-633.

Honeyfield ME (2003). Principles of physical assessment. In Tappero EP, Honeyfield ME, editors. *Physical assessment of the newborn*, ed 3 (pp 1-8). Petaluma, CA: NICU Ink.

Hudgins L, Cassidy SB (2006). Congenital anomalies. In Fanaroff AA et al, editors. *Neonatal-perinatal medicine: diseases of the fetus and infant*, ed 8 (pp 651-582). St Louis: Mosby.

Johnson CB (2003). Head, eyes, ears, nose, mouth, and neck assessment. In Tappero EP, Honeyfield ME, editors. *Physical assessment of the newborn*, ed 3 (pp 55-68). Petaluma, CA: NICU Ink.

Kazin RA et al (2005). Common newborn dermatoses. In Taeusch HW et al, editors. *Avery's diseases of the newborn*, ed 8 (pp 1511-1519). Philadelphia: Saunders.

Kirby E (2003). Assessment of the dysmorphic infant. In Tappero EP, Honeyfield ME, editors. *Physical assessment of the newborn*, ed 3 (pp 185-200). Petaluma, CA: NICU Ink.

Kliegman RM (2006). Intrauterine growth restriction. In Fanaroff AA et al, editors. *Neonatal-perinatal medicine: diseases of the fetus and infant*, ed 8 (pp 271-306). St Louis: Mosby.

Lissauer T (2006). Physical examination of the newborn. In Fanaroff AA et al, editors. *Neonatal-perinatal medicine: diseases of the fetus and infant*, ed 8 (pp 513-528). St Louis: Mosby.

Madan A, Good W (2005). The eye. In Taeusch HW et al, editors. *Avery's diseases of the newborn*, ed 8 (pp 1539-1555). Philadelphia: Saunders.

Madan A et al (2005). Central nervous system injury and neuroprotection. In Taeusch HW et al, editors. *Avery's diseases of the newborn*, ed 8 (pp 965-992). Philadelphia: Saunders.

Magnuson DK et al (2006). Selected abdominal and gastrointestinal anomalies. In Fanaroff AA et al, editors. *Neonatal-perinatal medicine: diseases of the fetus and infant*, ed 8 (pp 1381-1402). St Louis Mosby.

Mangurten HM (2006). Birth injuries. In Fanaroff AA et al, editors. *Neonatal-perinatal medicine: diseases of the fetus and infant*, ed 8 (pp 529-560). St Louis Mosby.

McLean F, Usher R (1970). Measurements of liveborn fetal malnutrition infants compared with similar gestation and with similar birth weight normal controls. *Biology of the neonate* 16:215-221.

Ohls R (2001). Anemia in the newborn. In Polin RA et al, editors. *Workbook in practical neonatology*, ed 3. Philadelphia: Saunders.

Palmert MR, Dahms WT (2006). Abnormalities of sexual differentiation. In Fanaroff AA et al, editors. *Neonatal-perinatal medicine: diseases of the fetus and infant*, ed 8 (pp 1550-1596). St Louis: Mosby.

Rozinski TA, Bloom DA (1997). Male genital tract. In Oldham KT et al, editors. *Surgery of infants and children: scientific principles and practice* (pp 1543-1558). Philadelphia: Lippincott-Raven.

Sansoucie DA, Cavaliere TA (2002). Neonatal assessment. In Kenner C et al, editors. *Comprehensive neonatal nursing: a physiologic perspective*, ed 2 (pp 308-347). Philadelphia: Saunders.

Seidel HM et al (2003). *Mosby's guide to physical examination*, ed 5. St Louis: Mosby.

Sifuentes M (2000). Well-child care for preterm infants. In Berkowitz CD, editor. *Pediatrics: a primary care approach*, ed 2. Philadelphia: Saunders.

Sneiderman S, Taeusch HW (2005). Initial evaluation: history and physical examination of the newborn. In Taeusch HW et al, editors. *Avery's diseases of the newborn*, ed 8 (pp 301-322). Philadelphia: Saunders.

Southgate WM, Pittard WB (2001). Classification and physical examination of the newborn infant. In Klaus MH, Fanaroff AA, editors. *Care of the high risk neonate*, ed 5. Philadelphia: Saunders.

Spillman L (2002). Examination of the external ear. *Advances in neonatal care* 2(2):72-80.

Stanley FJ (1994). Cerebral palsy trends: implications for perinatal care. *Acta obstetricia et gynecologica Scandinavica (Copenhagen)* 73:5-9.

Tappero EP (2003). Musculoskeletal system assessment. In Tappero EP, Honeyfield ME, editors. *Physical assessment of the newborn*, ed 3 (pp 125-148). Petaluma, CA: NICU Ink.

Trotter CW (2003). Gestational age assessment. In Tappero EP, Honeyfield ME, editors. *Physical assessment of the newborn*, ed 3 (pp 21-40). Petaluma, CA: NICU Ink.

Vargo L (2003). Cardiovascular assessment. In Tappero EP, Honeyfield ME, editors. *Physical assessment of the newborn*, ed 3 (pp 81-96). Petaluma, CA: NICU Ink.

Vogt BA et al (2006). The kidney and urinary tract. In Fanaroff AA et al, editors. *Neonatal-perinatal medicine: diseases of the fetus and infant*, ed 8 (pp 1659-1684). St Louis: Mosby.

Waardenburg PJ (1951). A new syndrome combining developmental anomalies of the eyelids, eyebrows, and nose root with pigmentary defects of the iris and head hair and with congenital deafness. *American journal of human genetics* 3:195.

Wright KW (1999). *Pediatric ophthalmology for pediatrician*. Baltimore: Williams & Wilkins.

Young AZ et al (2005). Cutaneous congenital defects. In Taeusch HW et al, editors. *Avery's diseases of the newborn*, ed 8 (pp 1521-1539). Philadelphia: Saunders.

Zaontz MR, Packer MG (1997). Abnormalities of the external genitalia. *Pediatric clinics of North America* 44(5):1267-1297.

Zderic SA (2005). Developmental abnormalities of the genitourinary system. In Taeusch HW et al, editors. *Avery's diseases of the newborn*, ed 8 (pp 1287-1297). Philadelphia: Saunders.

Preconception and Pregnancy Risk Factors and Risk Reduction Strategies Resources

MARCH OF DIMES QUICK STATS FOR THE UNITED STATES*

- Every 8 seconds a baby is born in the United States.
- Every hour three babies die.
- African American infants are more than twice as likely to die before their first birthday as white infants.
- Birth defects are the leading cause of infant mortality, accounting for more than 1 in 5 infant deaths.
- Every $3\frac{1}{2}$ minutes a baby is born with a birth defect.*
- Prematurity/low birth weight is the leading cause of death in the first month of life.
- Prematurity/low birth weight is the second leading cause of all infant deaths and the leading cause of infant deaths among African Americans.
- About 1 in 8 babies is born preterm (less than 37 weeks' gestation).
- Every 2 minutes a low birth weight baby is born (less than $5\frac{1}{2}$ pounds).
- Every year nearly 4400 babies are born weighing less than 1 pound.
- More than 1 in 28 babies are born to mothers who started prenatal care in the third trimester or received no prenatal care at all.
- The U.S. infant mortality rate is higher than those of 26 other nations.[†]

MARCH OF DIMES PREGNANCY AND NEWBORN HEALTH EDUCATION CENTER[‡]

Nine months of a healthy pregnancy is the best gift you can give your future baby. More and more babies are born too early and those who survive may have serious health problems. We often don't know why premature birth happens. We do know there are things you can do, before you get pregnant, to help give your baby a better chance of a healthy and full-term birth. Plan your pregnancy and see a doctor or nurse **before and during pregnancy** to talk about the following topics.

The March of Dimes List: Nine Questions to Ask Your Doctor or Nurse

1. How can diabetes, high blood pressure, infections, or other conditions affect my pregnancy?
2. How can certain medications (prescription, over-the-counter, or home remedies) affect my pregnancy?
3. How does taking a multivitamin with folic acid daily, especially before pregnancy, help me have a healthy baby?
4. What is my ideal weight?
5. How can I stay away from cigarettes, alcohol, and illegal drugs?
6. How can I manage the stress in my life?
7. How long should I wait between my pregnancies?
8. What if premature birth runs in my family?
9. What are the signs of preterm labor and what should I do?

CENTERS FOR DISEASE CONTROL AND PREVENTION RELEASES RECOMMENDATIONS TO IMPROVE PRECONCEPTION HEALTH AND HEALTH CARE—UNITED STATES[§]

This CDC report (Johnson et al, 2006) is aimed at addressing 4 goals to: (1) improve the knowledge and attitudes and behaviors of men and women related to preconception health; (2) ensure that all women of childbearing age in the United States receive preconception care services (i.e., evidence-based risk screening, health promotion, and interventions) that will enable them to enter pregnancy in optimal health; (3) reduce risks indicated by a previous adverse pregnancy outcome through interventions during the interconception period, which can prevent or minimize health problems for a mother and her future children; and (4) reduce the disparities in adverse pregnancy outcomes.

The following are recognized as preconception risk factors for adverse pregnancy outcomes:

1. Isotretinoins.

---

*Based on 2002 final natality and 2002 final linked birth/infant death data from the National Center for Health Statistics and [†]estimates from the CDC. From March of Dimes—Perinatal Data Center, White Plains, NY; peristats@marchofdimes.com or www.marchofdimes.com/peristats.

[‡]From The March of Dimes, White Plains, NY, www.marchofdimes.com.

[§]From CDC. (2006). *MMWR Recommendations to Improve Preconception Health and Health Care—United States.* Atlanta, GA: CDC.

2. Alcohol misuse.
3. Anti-epileptic drugs.
4. Diabetes (preconception).
5. Folic acid deficiency.
6. Hepatitis B.
7. HIV/AIDS.
8. Hypothyroidism.
9. Maternal phenylketonuria (PKU).
10. Rubella seronegativity.
11. Obesity.
12. Oral anticoagulant.
13. STD.
14. Smoking.

Recommendations

1. Individual responsibility across the lifespan.
   a. Develop, evaluate, and disseminate reproductive life planning tools for women and men in their childbearing years, respecting variations in age; literacy, including health literacy; and cultural/linguistic contexts.
   b. Conduct research leading to development, dissemination, and evaluation of individual health education materials for women and men regarding preconception risk factors, including materials related to biomedical, behavioral, and social risks known to affect pregnancy.
2. Consumer Awareness.
   a. Develop, evaluate, and disseminate age-appropriate educational curricula and modules for use in school health education programs.
   b. Integrate reproductive health messages into existing health promotion campaigns (e.g., campaigns to reduce obesity and smoking).
   c. Conduct consumer-focused research to identify terms that the public understands and to develop messages for promoting preconception health and reproductive awareness.
   d. Design and conduct social marketing campaigns necessary to develop messages for promoting preconception health knowledge and attitudes, and behaviors among men and women of childbearing age.
   e. Engage media partners to assist in depicting positive role models for lifestyles that promote reproductive health (e.g., delaying initiation of sexual activity, abstaining from unprotected sexual intercourse, and avoiding use of alcohol and drugs).
3. Preventive Visits.
   a. Increase health provider (including primary and specialty care providers) awareness regarding the importance of addressing preconception health among all women of childbearing age.
   b. Develop and implement curricula on preconception care and continuing education levels.
   c. Consolidate and disseminate existing professional guidelines to develop a recommended screening and health promotion package.
   d. Develop, evaluate, and disseminate practical screening tools for primary care settings, with emphasis on the 10 areas for preconception risk assessment (e.g., reproductive history, genetic and environmental risk factors).
   e. Develop, evaluate, and disseminate evidence-based models for integrating components of preconception care to facilitate delivery of and demand for prevention and intervention services.
   f. Apply quality improvement techniques (e.g., conduct rapid improvement cycles, establish benchmarks and brief provider training, use practice self-audits, and participate in quality improvement collaborative groups) to improve provider knowledge and attitudes, and practices and to reduce missed opportunities for screening and health promotion.
   g. Use the federally funded collaboratives for community health centers and other federally Qualified Health Centers to improve the quality of preconception risk assessment, health promotion, and interventions provided through primary care.
   h. Develop fiscal incentives for screening and health promotion.
4. Interventions for Identified Risks.
   a. Increase health provider (including primary and specialty care providers) awareness concerning the importance of ongoing care for chronic conditions and intervention for identified risk factors.
   b. Develop and implement modules on preconception care for specific clinical conditions for use in clinical education at graduate, postgraduate, and continuing education levels.
   c. Consolidate and disseminate existing guidelines related to evidence-based interventions for conditions and risk factors.
   d. Disseminate existing evidence-based interventions that address risk factors that can be used in primary care settings (i.e., isotretinoins, alcohol misuse, antiepileptic drugs, diabetes [preconception], folic acid deficiency, hepatitis B, HIV/AIDS, hypothyroidism, maternal phenylketonuria [PKU], rubella seronegativity, obesity, oral anticoagulant, STD, and smoking).
   e. Develop fiscal incentives (e.g., pay for performance) for risk management, particularly in managed care settings.
   f. Apply quality improvement techniques and tools (e.g., conduct rapid improvement cycles, establish benchmarks, use practice self-audits, and participate in quality improvement collaborative groups).
5. Interconception Care.
   a. Monitor the percentage of women who complete postpartum visits (e.g., using the Health Employer Data and Information Set measures for managed care plans and Title V Maternal Child Health Block Grant state measures), and use these data to identify communities of women at risk and opportunities to improve provider follow-up.
   b. Develop, evaluate, and replicate intensive evidence-based interconception care and care coordination models for women at high social and medical risk.
   c. Enhance the content of postpartum visits to promote interconception health.
   d. Use existing public health programs serving women in the postpartum period to provide or link to interventions (e.g., family planning, home visiting, and the Special Supplemental Nutrition Program for Women, Infants, and Children).

e. Encourage additional states to develop preconception health improvement projects with funds from the Title V Maternal Child Health Block Grant, Prevention Block Grant, and similar public health programs.

6. Pregnancy Checkup.
   a. Consolidate existing professional guidelines to develop the recommended content and approach for such a visit.
   b. Modify third party payer rules to permit payment for one prepregnancy visit per pregnancy, including development of billing and payment mechanisms.
   c. Educate women and couples regarding the value and availability of pregnancy planning visits.

7. Health Insurance Coverage for Women with Low Incomes.
   a. Improve the design of family planning waivers by permitting states (by federal waiver or by creating a new state option) to offer interconception risk assessment, counseling, and interventions along with family planning services. Such policy developments would create new opportunities to finance interconception care.
   b. Increase health coverage among women who have low incomes and are of childbearing age by using federal options and waivers under public and private health insurance systems and the State Children's Health Insurance Program.
   c. Increase access to health-care services through policies and reimbursement levels for public and private health insurance systems to include a full range of clinicians who care for women.

8. Public Health Programs and Strategies
   a. Use federal and state agency support to encourage more integrated preconception health practices in clinics and programs.
   b. Provide support for CDC programs to develop, evaluate, and disseminate integrated approaches to promote preconception health.
   c. Analyze and evaluate the preconception care activities used under the federal Healthy Start program, and support replication projects.
   d. Convene or use local task forces, coalitions, or committees to discuss opportunities for promotion and prevention in preconception health at the community level.
   e. Develop and support public health practice collaborative groups to promote shared learning and dissemination of approaches for increasing preconception health.
   f. Include content related to preconception care in educational curricula of schools of public health and other training facilities for public health professionals.

9. Research.
   a. Prepare an updated evidence-based systematic review of all published reports on science, programs, and policy (e.g., through the Agency for Healthcare Research and Quality).
   b. Encourage and support evaluation of model programs and projects, including integrated service delivery and community health promotion projects.
   c. Conduct quantitative and qualitative studies to advance knowledge of preconception risk and clinical and public health interventions, including knowledge of more integrated practice strategies and interconception approaches.
   d. Design and conduct analyses of cost-benefit and cost-effectiveness as part of the study of preconception interventions.
   e. Conduct health services research to explore barriers to evidence-based and guidelines-based practice.
   f. Conduct studies to examine the factors that results in variations in individual use of preconception care (i.e., barriers and motivators that affect health-care use).

10. Monitoring Improvements.
    a. Apply public health surveillance strategies to monitor selected preconception health indicators (e.g., folic acid supplementation, smoking cessation, alcohol misuse, diabetes, and obesity).
    b. Expand data systems and surveys (e.g., the Pregnancy Risk Assessment and Monitoring System and the National Survey of Family Growth) to monitor individual experiences related to preconception care.
    c. Use geographic information system techniques to target preconception health programs and interventions to areas where high rates of poor health outcomes exist for women of reproductive age and their infants.
    d. Use analytic tools (e.g., Perinatal Periods of Risk) to measure and monitor the proportion of risk attributable to the health of women before pregnancy.
    e. Include preconception, interconception, and health status measures in population-based performance monitoring systems (e.g., in national and state Title V programs).
    f. Include a measure of the delivery of preconception care services in the *Healthy People 2020* objectives.
    g. Develop and implement indicator quality improvement measures for all aspects of preconception care. For example, use the Health Employer Data and Information Set measures to monitor the percentage of women who complete preconception care and postpartum visits or pay for performance measures.

AREAS IN NEED OF FURTHER STUDY AND RESOURCES REGARDING RISK REDUCTION OF PREGNANCY AND NEONATAL COMPLICATIONS

1. Near term or late premature birth (34 to 37 weeks' gestation).
2. Use of 17HP (human progesterone) on preconceptional risk factors for adverse pregnancy outcomes.
3. Role of human genome epidemiology and preconceptional risk factors for adverse pregnancy outcomes.
4. Use of the Centering Pregnancy Model (March of Dimes, White Plains, NY) on preconceptional risk factors for adverse pregnancy outcomes.

REFERENCE

Johnson K et al (2006). CDC/ATSDR Preconception Care Work Group, Select Panel on Preconception Care. Recommendations to improve preconception health and health care—United States. A report of the CDC/ATSDR Preconception Care Work Group and the Select Panel on Preconception Care. MMWR *recommendations and reports* 55(RR-6):1-23.

RESOURCES

Ioannidis JPA et al (2005). A network of investigator networks in human genome epidemiology. *American journal of epidemiology* 162(4):302-304.

Ioannidis JPA et al, and the Human Genome Epidemiology Network and the Network for Investigator Networks (2006). A road map for efficient and reliable human genome epidemiology. *Nature genetics* 38(1):3-5.

Langhoff-Roos J et al (2006). Spontaneous preterm delivery in primiparous women at low risk in Denmark: population based study. *BMJ* 332:937-939.

McCormick MC et al (2006). Place of birth and variations in management of late preterm ("near-term") infants. *Seminars in perinatology* 30(1):44-47.

Ness A et al (2006). *Impact of NICHD trial on progesterone use among board certified MFM specialists.* Thomas Jefferson University, Philadelphia, PA; Albert Einstein College of Medicine, Bronx, NY; and March of Dimes, White Plains, NY.

INDEX